The Medical Care of Women

Editors:

PHYLLIS L. CARR, M.D.
Instructor
Harvard Medical School
Visiting Physician
Massachusetts General Hospital
Boston, Massachusetts

KAREN M. FREUND, M.D., M.P.H.
Associate Professor of Medicine
Boston University School of Medicine
Chief, Women's Health Unit
Boston University Medical Center Hospital
Boston, Massachusetts

SUJATA SOMANI, M.D.
Instructor
Harvard Medical School
Assistant in Gynecology
Massachusetts General Hospital
Boston, Massachusetts

W.B. SAUNDERS COMPANY
A Division of Harcourt Brace & Company
Philadelphia London Toronto Montreal Sydney Tokyo

W.B. SAUNDERS COMPANY
A Division of
Harcourt Brace & Company

The Curtis Center
Independence Square West
Philadelphia, Pennsylvania 19106

Library of Congress Cataloging-in-Publication Data

The Medical care of women / editors, Phyllis L. Carr,
Karen M. Freund, Sujata Somani.

p.   cm.

ISBN 0–7216–3779–5

1. Women—Diseases.   2. Women's health services.
   3. Women—Health and hygiene.   4. Gynecology.   I. Carr,
   Phyllis L.   II. Freund, Karen M.   III. Somani, Sujata.

RG101.M473 1995

618—dc20   94–34774

THE MEDICAL CARE OF WOMEN   ISBN 0–7216–3779–5

Printed in the United States of America

Last digit is the print number: 9   8   7   6   5   4   3   2   1

Contributors

Lisa Anderson, M.D.
Assistant Professor, Medical College of Pennsylvania, Philadelphia, Pennsylvania
Cervical Intraepithelial Neoplasia and Cervical Cancer

Elisha H. Atkins, M.D., M.S.
Instructor, Harvard Medical School and Harvard School of Public Health;
Medical Director, Employee Health Service, and Assistant Physician,
Massachusetts General Hospital, Boston, Massachusetts
Occupational and Environmental Health for Women

Phyllis August, M.D.
Associate Professor of Medicine and Obstetrics and Gynecology, Cornell
University Medical College, New York, New York
Hypertension in Pregnancy

Emily R. Baker, M.D.
Assistant Professor, Dartmouth Medical School, Hanover; Perinatologist,
Dartmouth-Hitchcock Medical Center, Lebanon, New Hampshire
Physiologic Adaptations to Pregnancy

M. Anita Barry, M.D., M.P.H.
Assistant Professor of Medicine and Public Health, Boston University; Director,
Communicable Disease Control, Boston Department of Health and Hospitals,
Boston, Massachusetts
Immunization; Toxic Shock Syndrome

Patricia P. Barry, M.D., M.P.H.
Associate Professor of Medicine, Chief of Geriatrics Section, and Director of
Gerontology Center, Boston University School of Medicine, Boston,
Massachusetts
Health Care of the Elderly Woman

Joan Bengtson, M.D.
Assistant Professor of Obstetrics, Gynecology, and Reproductive Biology,
Harvard Medical School; Gynecologic Specialist, Harvard Community Health
Plan, Boston, Massachusetts
Hormonal Contraception; Urinary Incontinence

Terry Beresford
Alexandria, Virginia
Counseling the Patient with an Unintended Pregnancy

Susan Biener Bergman, M.D.
Director of Residency Training and Associate Clinical Professor, Department of Physical Medicine and Rehabilitation, Boston University School of Medicine; Lecturer, Department of Physical Medicine and Rehabilitation, Tufts University School of Medicine; Clinical Director, Spinal Cord Injury, Boston University Medical Center, Boston, Massachusetts
The Disabled Patient

John Bernardo, M.D.
Associate Professor of Medicine, Boston University School of Medicine; Medical Director, Tuberculosis Program, Boston Department of Health and Hospitals, and Director, Allergy Unit, Boston City Hospital, Boston, Massachusetts
Lung Disease in Pregnancy

George Blackburn, M.D., Ph.D.
Associate Professor of Surgery, Harvard Medical School; Director, Center of the Study of Nutrition and Medicine, New England Deaconess Hospital, Boston, Massachusetts
Obesity

Sandra E. Brooks, M.D.
Assistant Professor of Obstetrics and Gynecology, Division of Gynecologic Oncology, University of Massachusetts Medical Center, Worcester, Massachusetts
Postmenopausal Bleeding and Uterine Cancer; Uterine Leiomyomas

Melanie J. Brunt, M.D., M.P.H.
Assistant Professor, Boston University School of Medicine; Assistant Director, Diabetes Clinic, Boston City Hospital, Boston, Massachusetts
Amenorrhea and Oligomenorrhea

Risa Beth Burns, M.D., M.P.H.
Assistant Professor, Boston University School of Medicine; Co-Director, Breast Health Center, Boston University Medical Center Hospital, Boston, Massachusetts
Evaluation and Management of a Palpable Breast Mass

Booker Bush, M.D.
Assistant Professor of Medicine, Harvard Medical School; Staff Physician, Beth Israel Hospital, Boston, Massachusetts
Alcohol and Substance Abuse

Phyllis L. Carr, M.D.
Instructor, Harvard Medical School; Visiting Physician, Massachusetts General Hospital, Boston, Massachusetts
Medication and Substance Use in Pregnancy; Nonhormonal Contraception; Vaginitis

Pamela Charney, M.D.
Associate Professor of Internal Medicine and Assistant Professor of Obstetrics and Gynecology, Albert Einstein College of Medicine of Yeshiva University; Director, General Internal Medicine—Women's Health Residency Track, Bronx Municipal Hospital Center, Bronx, New York
Hypertension

Ellen Cohen, M.D.

Associate Professor of Internal Medicine, Albert Einstein College of Medicine of Yeshiva University; Director of Ambulatory Medical Education, and Associate Director of Primary Care, Montefiore Medical Center, Bronx, New York
Hypertension

Michael L. Corbett, M.D.

Assistant Professor of Orthopedics, Boston University School of Medicine, Boston, Massachusetts
Sports Medicine

Donald E. Craven, M.D.

Professor of Medicine and Public Health, Boston University School of Medicine; Director, Clinical AIDS Program, Boston City Hospital, Boston, Massachusetts
Human Immunodeficiency Virus Infection in Pregnancy: Epidemiology, Management, and Vertical Transmission

Gilbert H. Daniels, M.D.

Associate Professor of Medicine, Harvard Medical School; Co-Director, Thyroid Clinic, and Staff Physician, Massachusetts General Hospital, Boston, Massachusetts
Management of Thyroid Nodules; Thyroid Disorders

Mary Lally Delaney, M.D., M.A.

Visiting Attending Physician, Boston University Medical Center Hospital, Boston; Staff Physician, South Shore Hospital, Weymouth, Massachusetts
Hirsutism

Coleman D. Fowble, M.D.

Department of Orthopedics, University of South Alabama College of Medicine, Mobile, Alabama
Sports Medicine

Karen M. Freund, M.D., M.P.H.

Associate Professor of Medicine, Boston University School of Medicine; Chief, Women's Health Unit, Boston University Medical Center Hospital, Boston, Massachusetts
Domestic Violence; Osteoporosis; Preconceptual Care and Management of Early Pregnancy; Screening in Primary Care for Women; Smoking Cessation

Rochelle Rame Friedman, M.D.

Clinical Instructor in Psychiatry, Harvard Medical School; Staff Psychiatrist, Massachusetts Institute of Technology, and Clinical Associate in Psychiatry, Massachusetts General Hospital, Boston, Massachusetts
Emotional Aspects of Pregnancy and the Postpartum Period

Maxine J. Garbo, M.S., C.O.H.N.

Visiting Lecturer in Occupational Health Nursing, Harvard School of Public Health, Boston, Massachusetts
Occupational and Environmental Health for Women

Elizabeth S. Ginsburg, M.D.
Instructor of Obstetrics, Gynecology, and Reproductive Biology, Harvard Medical School; Instructor, Reproductive Endocrinology and Infertility, Brigham and Women's Hospital, Boston, Massachusetts
Evaluation and Treatment of Infertility; Spontaneous and Recurrent Abortion

Linda M. Grant, M.D., M.P.H.
Associate Clinical Professor of Pediatrics, Boston University Medical School; Attending Physician, Boston City Hospital, Boston, Massachusetts
Adolescent Issues

Gail A. Greendale, M.D.
Assistant Professor of Medicine and Obstetrics and Gynecology, UCLA School of Medicine; Staff Physician, UCLA Medical Center, Los Angeles, California
Hormone Therapy in the Menopause; Menopause

Elizabeth Kling Handleman, Ph.D.
Assistant Clinical Professor of Medicine (Psychology), Boston University School of Medicine; Psychologist, Women's Health Unit, Boston University Medical Center Hospital, Boston, Massachusetts
Sexual Assault

James J. Heffernan, M.D., M.P.H.
Associate Professor of Medicine, Boston University School of Medicine; Associate Director of Medicine and Director of General Medicine Consultation Service, Boston City Hospital, Boston, Massachusetts
Thromboembolic Complications of Pregnancy and the Puerperium

Linda J. Heffner, M.D., Ph.D.
Associate Professor of Obstetrics, Gynecology, and Reproductive Biology, Harvard Medical School; Obstetrician/Gynecologist and Chief of Maternal-Fetal Medicine, Brigham and Women's Hospital, Boston, Massachusetts
Delayed Childbearing

Lisa R. Hirschhorn, M.D., M.P.H.
Assistant Professor of Medicine, Boston University School of Medicine; Clinical AIDS Program, Boston City Hospital, Boston, Massachusetts
Human Immunodeficiency Virus Infection: Pathogenesis, Natural History, and Management

B. Jeanne Horner, M.D.
Assistant Clinical Professor of Psychiatry, Boston University School of Medicine; Assistant Director, Psychiatric Consultation and Liaison Service, Boston University Medical Center Hospital, Boston, Massachusetts
Depression in the Primary Care Setting

Cecelia Jarek, P.A.
Physician's Assistant, Department of Obstetrics and Gynecology, Adult Clinical AIDS Program, Boston City Hospital, Boston, Massachusetts
Human Immunodeficiency Virus Infection in Pregnancy: Epidemiology, Management, and Vertical Transmission

Carolyn Johnston, M.D.

Assistant Professor, Department of Obstetrics and Gynecology, University of Michigan School of Medicine, Ann Arbor, Michigan
Vaginal Intraepithelial Neoplasia and In Utero Exposure to Diethylstilbestrol

Lois Jovanovic-Peterson, M.D.

Clinical Professor of Medicine, University of Southern California School of Medicine, Los Angeles; Senior Scientist, Sansum Medical Research Foundation, Santa Barbara, California
Diabetes in Pregnancy

Howard L. Judd, M.D.

Professor of Medicine and Obstetrics and Gynecology, UCLA School of Medicine, Los Angeles; Chair, Department of Obstetrics and Gynecology, Olive View–UCLA Medical Center, Sylmar, California
Hormone Therapy in the Menopause; Menopause

Elaine T. Kaye, M.D.

Instructor, Department of Dermatology, Harvard Medical School; Assistant Physician, Department of Dermatology, Massachusetts General Hospital, Boston, Massachusetts
Diseases of the Vulva

Carolyn V. Kirschner, M.D.

Assistant Professor of Obstetrics and Gynecology, Rush Medical College of Rush University, Chicago, Illinois
Evaluation and Management of Pelvic Masses; Ovarian Cancer

Howard Libman, M.D.

Assistant Professor of Medicine, Harvard Medical School; Associate in Medicine, Division of General Medicine and Primary Care, Beth Israel Hospital, Boston, Massachusetts
Sexually Transmitted Diseases

Clifford Lo, M.D., M.P.H., Sc.D.

Assistant Professor of Pediatrics and Nutrition, Harvard Medical School and Harvard School of Public Health; Director, Nutrition Support Service, Children's Hospital, Boston, Massachusetts
Nutritional Requirements of Women

Elcinda L. McCrone, M.D., M.S.

Assistant Professor of Medicine, Boston University School of Medicine; Director, Outpatient Infectious Diseases Clinic, and Hospital Epidemiologist, Boston University Center Medical Hospital, Boston, Massachusetts
Human Immunodeficiency Virus Infection: Epidemiology, Risk Assessment, and Testing; Human Immunodeficiency Virus Infection: Pathogenesis, Natural History, and Management

Roseanna H. Means, M.D., M.S.

Clinical Instructor in Medicine, Harvard Medical School, and Assistant Clinical Professor of Medicine, Boston University School of Medicine; Staff Physician, Boston Health Care for the Homeless, Boston City Hospital; Associate Physician,

Brigham and Women's Hospital; Clinical Associate, Massachusetts General Hospital, Boston, Massachusetts
Health Care for Homeless Women

Anne Meneghetti, M.D.
Boston University School of Medicine; Fellow, Boston City Hospital and Boston University Medical Center Hospital, Boston, Massachusetts
Lung Disease in Pregnancy

Audrey B. Miklius, M.D.
Assistant Professor of Medicine, Tufts University School of Medicine; Medical Director, Women's Health Services, St. Elizabeth's Medical Center, Boston, Massachusetts
Management of Thyroid Nodules; Thyroid Disorders

Zoe Miner, Ph.D.
Center for the Study of Human Nutrition, New England Deaconess Hospital, Boston, Massachusetts
Obesity

Donnica L. Moore, M.D.
Vice President, American Medical Women's Association; Attending Physician, Planned Parenthood of New Jersey, East Hanover, New Jersey
Elective Termination of Pregnancy: What the Primary Care Physician Should Know

Elise Pechter Morse, M.P.H., C.I.H.
Massachusetts Department of Labor and Industries, Boston, Massachusetts
Occupational and Environmental Health for Women

Joseph F. Mortola, M.D.
Associate Professor of Obstetrics, Gynecology, and Reproductive Biology and Associate Professor of Psychiatry, Harvard Medical School; Director, Division of Reproductive Endocrinology, Beth Israel Hospital, Boston, Massachusetts
Premenstrual Syndrome

Joanne Murabito, M.D., Sc.M.
Assistant Professor of Medicine, Boston University School of Medicine, Boston; Attending Physician, Women's Health Unit, Boston University Medical Center Hospital, Boston; Co-Director of Clinic, Framingham Heart Study, Framingham, Massachusetts
Cholesterol Screening and Management

Angela Palumbo, M.D.
Instructor, Obstetrics and Gynecology, Harvard Medical School, and Fellow, Reproductive Endocrinology and Infertility, Brigham and Women's Hospital, Boston, Massachusetts
Spontaneous and Recurrent Abortion

Charles M. Peterson, M.D.
Clinical Professor, University of Southern California School of Medicine, Los

Angeles; Director of Research, Sansum Medical Research Foundation, Santa Barbara, California
Diabetes in Pregnancy

Richard Polisson, M.D., M.H.S.
Assistant Professor of Medicine, Harvard Medical School; Clinical Director, Arthritis Unit, Massachusetts General Hospital, Boston, Massachusetts
Connective Tissue and Autoimmune Diseases; Fibromyalgia and Regional Pain Syndromes; Inflammatory and Noninflammatory Arthropathies

Donna Poresky, J.D., B.S.
Glastonbury, Connecticut
Legal Issues in Pregnancy and Abortion

Marianne N. Prout, M.D., M.P.H.
Associate Professor of Public Health and Surgery and Associate Director, Program in Research on Women's Health, Boston University School of Medicine; Co-Director, Breast Health Center, Boston University Medical Center Hospital, Boston, Massachusetts
Breast Cancer: Epidemiology, Screening, and Prevention; Management of Patients with Breast Cancer

Ina Ratner, M.D.
Clinical Assistant Professor of Medicine, Boston University School of Medicine, Boston, Massachusetts
Anemia

Peter A. Rice, M.D.
Professor of Medicine, Boston University School of Medicine; Chief, Section of Infectious Diseases, and Director, Maxwell Finland Laboratory, Boston City Hospital, Boston, Massachusetts
Pelvic Inflammatory Disease

James M. Richter, M.D., M.A.
Assistant Professor of Medicine, Harvard Medical School; Staff Physician, Massachusetts General Hospital, Boston, Massachusetts
Gallbladder Disease

Ellen W. Seely, M.D.
Assistant Professor of Medicine, Harvard Medical School; Director of Clinical Research, Endocrine-Hypertension Division, Brigham and Women's Hospital, Boston, Massachusetts
Thyroid Disease and Pregnancy

Margaret Seton, M.D.
Instructor, Harvard Medical School, Boston; Assistant in Medicine, Arthritis Unit, Massachusetts General Hospital, Boston; Chief, Rheumatology, Cambridge Hospital; Medical Director, City of Cambridge Women's Health Initiative Program, Cambridge, Massachusetts
Connective Tissue and Autoimmune Diseases; Fibromyalgia and Regional Pain Syndromes; Inflammatory and Noninflammatory Arthropathies

Ellen E. Sheets, M.D.
Assistant Professor, Department of Obstetrics, Gynecology, and Reproductive Medicine, Harvard Medical School; Director, Pap Smear Evaluation Center, and Director, Gynecologic Oncology Faculty Practice, Brigham and Women's Hospital, Boston, Massachusetts
Gynecologic History, Examination, and Procedures

Alma Dell Smith, Ph.D.
Assistant Clinical Professor of Medicine (Psychology), Boston University School of Medicine; Psychologist, Women's Health Unit, Boston University Medical Center Hospital, Boston, Massachusetts
Management of Anxiety

Caren G. Solomon, M.D., M.P.H.
Instructor in Medicine, Harvard Medical School; Associate Physician, Brigham and Women's Hospital, Boston, Massachusetts
Thyroid Disease and Pregnancy

Sujata Somani, M.D.
Instructor, Harvard Medical School; Assistant in Gynecology, Massachusetts General Hospital, Boston, Massachusetts
Evaluation and Management of Pelvic Pain

Kathleen A. Steger, M.P.H., R.N.
Assistant Professor of Public Health, Boston University School of Public Health; Associate Director, Adult Clinical AIDS Program, Boston City Hospital, Boston, Massachusetts
Human Immunodeficiency Virus Infection in Pregnancy: Epidemiology, Management, and Vertical Transmission

Judith L. Steinberg, M.D.
Assistant Clinical Professor, Boston University School of Medicine; Assistant Visiting Physician, Boston City Hospital, Boston; HIV/AIDS Program Director, East Boston Neighborhood Health Center, East Boston, Massachusetts
Pelvic Inflammatory Disease

Carol Sulis, M.D.
Assistant Professor of Medicine, Boston University School of Medicine; Epidemiologist, Boston City Hospital and Boston Specialty and Rehabilitation Hospital, Boston, Massachusetts
Infectious Disease in Pregnancy

Deborah M. Swiderski, M.D.
Assistant Professor of Internal Medicine, Albert Einstein College of Medicine of Yeshiva University; Program Director, Residency Program in Social Internal Medicine, Montefiore Medical Center, Bronx, New York
Hypertension

Paulette Thabault, M.S.N., R.N.,C.
Adult Nurse Practitioner, Massachusetts General Hospital, Boston, Massachusetts
Nonhormonal Contraception

Nagagopal Venna, M.D., M.R.C.P.(I), M.R.C.P.(UK)
Associate Professor of Neurology, Boston University School of Medicine;
Director of Clinical Neurology, Boston City Hospital, Boston, Massachusetts
Headache; Neurologic Problems in Pregnancy

Sandra Lee Weiner, M.D.
Clinical Instructor of Obstetrics and Gynecology, Washington Hospital Center,
and Clinical Director of Primary Care Programs for Women with Special Needs,
National Rehabilitation Hospital, Washington, D.C.
The Disabled Patient

Debra F. Weinstein, M.D.
Instructor in Medicine, Harvard Medical School; Director of Graduate Medical
Education, Massachusetts General Hospital, Boston, Massachusetts
Irritable Bowel Syndrome

Robert M. Weiss, M.D.
Assistant Professor of Medicine, Boston University School of Medicine; Director,
Reproductive Endocrinology and Infertility, Boston University Medical Center
Hospital, Boston, Massachusetts
Abnormal Uterine Bleeding; Endometriosis

Dale K. Weldon, M.D.
Clinical Instructor, Harvard University Medical School; Attending Physician,
Brigham and Women's Hospital, Boston, Massachusetts
Preconceptual Care and Management of Early Pregnancy

Nanette K. Wenger, M.D.
Professor of Medicine, Emory University School of Medicine; Director, Cardiac
Clinics, Grady Memorial Hospital, Atlanta, Georgia
Coronary Artery Disease

Mary E. Wheat, M.D.
Assistant Clinical Professor of Epidemiology and Social Medicine, Albert
Einstein College of Medicine of Yeshiva University, Bronx; Director, Student
Health Service, Barnard College, Columbia University, New York, New York
Hypertension

Jocelyn White, M.D.
Assistant Professor of Medicine, Oregon Health Services University; Faculty,
Residency Training Program, Legacy Good Samaritan and Emanuel Hospitals,
Portland, Oregon
Medical Care of Lesbian Patients

Nancy R. Williams, J.D., LL.M., R.N.
Assistant Professor, Department of Community Medicine and Health Care,
University of Connecticut School of Medicine; Director of Risk Management,
John Dempsey Hospital, Farmington, Connecticut
Legal Issues in Pregnancy and Abortion

Frances E. Wiltsie, M.S.N., R.N.,C.
Instructor, College of Nursing, Medical University of South Carolina; Nurse

Practitioner, Department of Family Medicine, Medical University of South Carolina, Charleston, South Carolina
The Mentally Retarded Patient

Elizabeth R. Woods, M.D., M.P.H.

Assistant Professor of Pediatrics, Harvard Medical School; Assistant in Medicine and Director of Health Services Research, Children's Hospital, Boston, Massachusetts
Eating Disorders

Foreword

Medical care of women is moving to center stage in American health care. Whether it be the Women's Health Initiative, begun by the National Institutes of Health under the leadership of its first woman director, Bernadine Healy; the increasingly assertive political movements about women's health issues, such as the efforts of many lay groups and congresswomen toward the prevention and early detection of breast cancer; the opening of women's health clinics around the country; the founding of a women's health journal; or the development of professional interest groups, we are surrounded by signs that the health and health care of women have become legitimate concerns.

It is appropriate that this has happened. It is also not surprising. Women's health has always been important, because women constitute more than half of the population and are responsible for much more than half the health care costs in the United States. Women traditionally have taken advantage of health care services more than men, and they outlive men and therefore attain an age when health problems become more frequent. Now women's health care is attracting the attention it has not received before.

The relative lack of attention to women's health care in the past probably had several roots. First, with so few women physicians until recently, few physicians, and therefore few educators, writers, and researchers, had firsthand experience with women's health problems. (If men had menses, would male physicians have ever doubted the existence of physical menstrual pain or premenstrual syndrome, as the authors did in some gynecology textbooks we used as medical students?) Second, many women in the past were willing to tolerate a role that was subservient and unequal to that of men. Changes in society have produced women who want equality—not only in the home and workplace, but also in the realm of health and health care needs. With this new assertiveness by women, it has become obvious that too much of what has been thought to be acceptable health care for women is based on research done on men. Also, the unique health issues of women are beginning to receive their fair share of investigative energy and medical care, work on breast cancer, menopause, and osteoporosis being but three current examples.

When new interests in medicine take hold, a series of predictable steps occurs. Groups of like-minded people congregate, discuss, and write about their interest. Newsletters turn into journals. Informal groups develop into formal organizations. Courses are developed, taught, and accepted as legitimate. Accreditation and certification often evolve. Investigation grows from individually initiated studies that are usually difficult to fund to proposals more acceptable by study sections to specially mandated research programs with separate review committees. Textbooks begin to appear. Several of these steps are already underway in women's health care.

The *Medical Care of Women* is testimony to the need for a textbook in the field. As the first full textbook on women's health, it brings together topics important to women's health and health care but usually not found under one cover. Women's health care is too often fragmented into the separate disciplines of obstetrics-gynecology, family practice, internal medicine, adolescent medicine, geriatrics, and psychiatry. As a result, textbooks that center on these different disciplines leave gaps in the coverage of many health problems facing large numbers of women today, and information needed by interested clinicians has not been easily accessible from a single source. This textbook answers that need.

In textbooks of internal medicine, there is scant coverage of birth control, pregnancy, physical abuse, depression, and even menopause. We therefore found the content of this text very useful. We suspect physicians trained in other disciplines will also find the book particularly helpful in filling in gaps in their clinical knowledge base. All readers, regardless of specialty training, will find useful and timely the chapters on legal issues in pregnancy and abortion, the homeless patient, and the medical problems of gay women.

The editors' effort to cut across disciplinary boundaries, to go wherever the health care needs of women took them, and to work with researchers and practitioners to present conceptual and practical information to readers makes this a particularly effective textbook for the medical care of women. This is a book whose time has come.

SUZANNE W. FLETCHER M.D., M.S.C.
ROBERT H. FLETCHER M.D., M.S.C.
Professors of Ambulatory Care and
Prevention
Harvard Medical School and
Harvard Community Health Plan

Preface

The 1990s have been called the "Decade of the Woman," and many issues regarding women have come to the fore. Is a medical text devoted to women's health care necessary? Or is this extending a political and social issue into a scientific realm that does not require a gender distinction? As more information is gathered about the medical problems of women, it becomes increasingly clear that there are many differences between men and women in their health care needs and in the presentation and outcome of the various disease processes. Extrapolation of data collected in men to women patients is not always valid. We are finding this in more and more illnesses, from coronary artery disease to AIDS, hypertension, and occupational medicine. The complex effects of the menstrual cycle affect the disease process, the metabolism of drugs, and even the predisposition to illness. More gender-specific information is needed to appropriately diagnose and treat many diseases in women.

The splitting of women's health care into multiple specialties has also contributed to the fragmentation of health care delivery for women. Societal problems affect the health of women and result in higher rates of anxiety and depression in women and an alarming incidence of domestic violence against women. We hope that gathering information from many disciplines, interpreting data as they apply to women patients, and making these data conveniently accessible to primary providers will help practitioners achieve a higher standard of comprehensive medical care for women patients. With this goal in mind, we offer this text.

PHYLLIS L. CARR
KAREN M. FREUND
SUJATA SOMANI

NOTICE

Medicine is an ever-changing field. Standard safety precautions must be followed, but as new research and clinical experience broaden our knowledge, changes in treatment and drug therapy become necessary or appropriate. The editors of this work have carefully checked the generic and trade drug names and verified drug dosages to ensure that the dosage information in this work is accurate and in accord with the standards accepted at the time of publication. Readers are advised, however, to check the product information currently provided by the manufacturer of each drug to be administered to be certain that changes have not been made in the recommended dose or in the contraindications for administration. This is of particular importance in regard to new or infrequently used drugs. It is the responsibility of the treating physician, relying on experience and knowledge of the patient, to determine dosages and the best treatment for the patient. The editors cannot be responsible for misuse or misapplication of the material in this work.

THE PUBLISHER

Contents

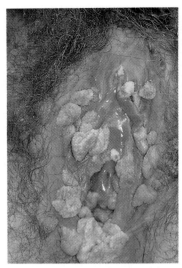

Figure 9–2. Multiple soft, fleshy condylomata acuminata of the vulva. (Courtesy of Richard Reid, M.D.)

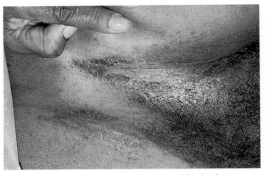

Figure 9–3. Allergic contact dermatitis to fragrance with erythema limited to well-demarcated areas of contact in the pubic area.

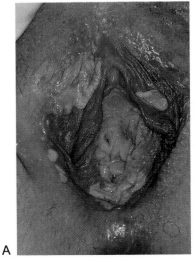

Figure 9–4. Discrete, scaling plaques of psoriasis in the pubic area.

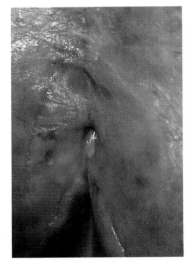

Figure 9–5. Lichen sclerosus with hypopigmented atrophic plaques and erosions. (Courtesy of Richard Reid, M.D.)

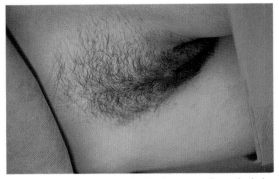

A   B

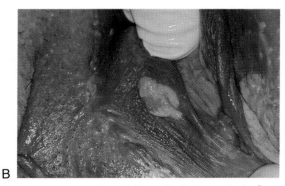

Figure 9–6. *A* and *B*, Pink and whitish macules and plaques of vulvar intraepithelial neoplasia 3 (carcinoma in situ). (Courtesy of Richard Reid, M.D.)

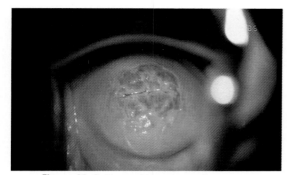

Figure 11–3. Normal transformation zone.

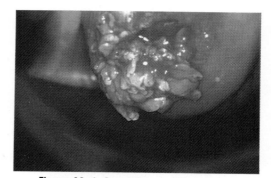

Figure 11–4. Condyloma of the cervix.

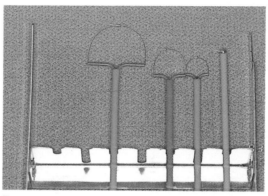

Figure 11–6. Instruments used to perform the loop electroexcision procedure (LEEP).

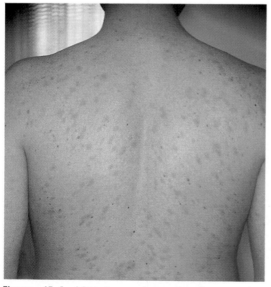

Figure 45–1. Maculopapular rash of secondary syphilis. (From Callen JP, Greer KE, Hood AF, et al. Color Atlas of Dermatology. Philadelphia: WB Saunders, 1993, p 122.)

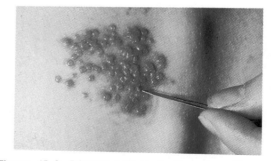

Figure 45–2. Primary herpes simplex virus. (From Lookingbill DP, Marks JG Jr. Principles of clinical diagnosis. In: Moschella SL, Hurley HJ. Dermatology. 3rd ed. Vol. 1. Philadelphia: WB Saunders, 1992, p 219.)

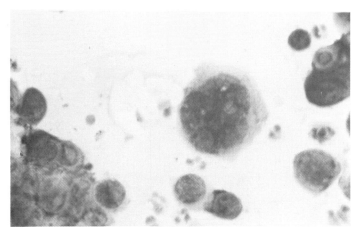

Figure 45–3. A positive Tzanck smear from herpes simplex blister. (From Callen JP, Greer KE, Hood AF, et al. Color Atlas of Dermatology. Philadelphia: WB Saunders, 1993, p 169.)

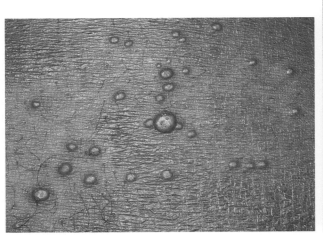

Figure 45–4. Multiple molluscum contagiosum. (From Callen JP, Greer KE, Hood AF, et al. Color Atlas of Dermatology. Philadelphia: WB Saunders, 1993, p 286.)

Figure 45–5. Pruritic papules. (From Callen JP, Greer KE, Hood AF, et al. Color Atlas of Dermatology. Philadelphia: WB Saunders, 1993, p 85.)

PREVENTIVE MEDICINE

1

Screening in Primary Care for Women

Karen M. Freund

The periodic physical examination, which was first popularized in the 1920s, has been refined significantly over the following decades. The role of the primary provider offers major promise in reducing morbidity and mortality for women of all ages not only in the diagnosis and treatment of specific symptoms but also in the prevention and early detection of illness. Screening is the search for disease in the asymptomatic individual and usually implies the administration of specific laboratory or radiologic tests. However, the incorporation of any part of the medical history or physical examination into the evaluation of a patient who has no directly relevant complaints or conditions is, in fact, a screening test. Screening by definition requires the evaluation of a large group of individuals to detect an abnormality in a small proportion of this group. To justify the time, discomfort, and expense of undergoing a screening procedure, the following criteria are useful to evaluate its effectiveness.

1. The screening test should address a common problem in the population being tested. A problem must be sufficiently common to justify investigation of an entire population of patients. If a problem is considered serious but uncommon in the general population, attempts are made to define an "at risk" subgroup of the population toward whom to direct screening efforts. Age is probably the most common factor used to stratify risk; however, family history, socioeconomic status, and lifestyle patterns have also been used to define risk groups.

2. The problem must be of sufficient severity to justify the effort of screening the population. Self-limiting conditions rarely require screening. Most screening is targeted toward conditions with significant morbidity or mortality.

3. The condition must be detectable in a preclinical phase, before the development of any symptoms or signs. For some conditions, such as breast cancer, physical examination has provided a limited means of identifying the disease before it is noticed by the patient. Additional methodologies such as mammography have been developed to detect early stages of disease.

4. Early detection and intervention must lead to a benefit in the identified patients for screening to be useful. Benefit can be broadly defined from prevention of further transmission of a disease to others, as in testing for the human immunodeficiency virus (HIV), to therapy resulting in improved survival, as in mammography for women older than 50.

5. The costs and risks of screening must be acceptable to both patients and providers. Screening that includes the medical history and physical examination adds little additional cost to patient care and therefore requires less justification of its benefits. By contrast, radiologic examinations or invasive procedures require stronger evidence of benefit to justify their costs. Costs of a screening test include not only monetary expense but also discomfort and inconvenience to patients. A stool hemoccult requires no additional visits, the minor discomfort of a rectal examination, and no additional processing of the specimen, whereas sigmoidoscopy requires preparation time and effort, an additional visit, and added discomfort and embarrassment to patients. All of these factors play a role in the less frequent adoption of flexible sig-

moidoscopy, as opposed to occult fecal blood testing, as a screening method.

In deciding on the indications for screening for any particular problem, the previously mentioned criteria are weighed against one another. For example, anemia in premenopausal women may be a common problem that can be verified with an inexpensive and relatively easy test and that can be eliminated by prescribing therapy in the form of iron supplementation. Yet, given the lack of data to indicate that the detection and treatment of mild anemia have any impact on a woman's well-being, routine screening for this disorder is not advocated. In contrast, even though acquired immunodeficiency syndrome (AIDS), which results from HIV, is a much rarer problem than mild anemia, counseling of all women on risks for HIV and screening of women with concerns about their HIV risk is indicated because of its mortality and severe morbidity.

Two major task forces have recently reviewed the indication for screening for a number of conditions. The U.S. Preventive Services Task Force[1] and the Canadian Task Force on the Periodic Health Examination[2] based their recommendations on the strength of available data, requiring at least one randomized controlled trial or several well-controlled nonrandomized trials to consider the evidence for screening to be adequate. Other subspecialty organizations, such as the American Cancer Society, the American College of Physicians, and the American College of Obstetricians and Gynecologists, as well as federal agencies such as the Centers for Disease Control and Prevention, often publish recommendations within their areas of expertise, which usually have not included the rigorous criteria of the two task forces. The result is that the task forces are less likely than the other specialty agencies to recommend a number of screening tests.

SCREENING WITHIN THE MEDICAL HISTORY

The medical history that precedes the physical examination serves multiple purposes. It is the most important means of obtaining information about symptoms and, in most cases, is more useful than the physical laboratory evaluation in narrowing the differential diagnosis on a patient's presenting concerns. The medical history is also used to obtain background information that is frequently useful in the future care of the patient and in establishing the rapport necessary for the collaborative effort in the health care of the patient. In addition, the medical history provides a useful means of screening for a number of common medical problems in a rapid, inexpensive way (Table 1–1). The following are areas for routine inquiry on initial and periodic examinations in women as a method of screening for common and important medical problems and risk factors for future medical problems.

Dietary Habits

Identifying and counseling women with high-fat diets is warranted owing to the risk of developing coronary artery disease, obesity, and possibly breast and colon cancer. All women from adolescence through the postmenopausal period should be counseled on their calcium intake. Fifty-six percent of adult women in the United States do not consume the recommended daily allowance of calcium,[3] and inadequate lifetime dietary calcium may be related to later osteopenia and bone fracture.

Women younger than 30 are at increased risk of developing eating disorders, with prevalence rates of 2 to 10% in many primary care populations.[4, 5] Although patients with anorexia nervosa present with the more obvious signs and symptoms of low weight and amenorrhea, those with bulimia nervosa may present without typical signs or symptoms and are often undetected in primary care practice. One study suggested that the addition of two questions to the medical history, "Do you ever eat in secret?" and "Are you satisfied with your eating patterns?" has sufficient predictive value in detecting bulimia to warrant its addition to the medical history.[6]

Exercise

Exercise has the potential to decrease the risk of multiple common conditions in women, including cardiovascular disease, obesity, hypertension, osteoporosis, diabetes, and depression. The documented benefits of exercise on coronary artery disease in men have not been confirmed in women, although exercise is likely to have the same beneficial effect. Likewise, reducing high blood pressure and reducing diabetes risk have also not been fully evaluated in women. Data support the role of exercise in both prevention and management of obesity.[7] Data on both pre- and postmenopausal women have documented an increase in bone mass with weight-bearing exercise, although a reduction in risk for falls or hip fractures remains to be proved.[8–11] Although exercise is thought to have a

TABLE 1–1. Recommended Screening Tests and Procedures in Women

TESTING	AGES		
	18–35	35–50	50 +
Periodic physical examination	Every 3 yr	1–2 yr	Yearly
History			
Diet			
Fat/fiber	Yes		
Calcium	Yes	Yes	Yes
Eating disorders	Yes	Yes	Yes
Exercise	Yes	Yes	Yes
Smoking	Yes	Yes	Yes
Alcohol use	Yes	Yes	Yes
Drug use	Yes	Yes	Yes
Family planning	Yes	Yes	
STD counseling	Yes	Yes	Yes
Depression or anxiety	Yes	Yes	Yes
Sexual or physical assault	Yes	Yes	Yes
Physical Examination			
Blood pressure	Yes	Yes	Yes
Thyroid examination	Yes	Yes	Yes
Clinical breast examination	Yes	Yes	Yes
Breast self-examination	Yes	Yes	Yes
Skin examination	Yes	Yes	Yes
Pelvic examination	Yes	Yes	Yes
Rectal examination		>40	Yes
Laboratory Tests			
Urinalysis			>60
Fecal occult blood		>40	Yes
Papanicolaou smear	1–3 yr	1–3 yr	1–3 yr
Gonorrhea	1–3 yr	New partner	
Chlamydia	1–3 yr	New partner	
RPR for syphilis	If new STD	If new STD	If new STD
PPD for tuberculosis	High risk	High risk	High risk
Hematocrit			
Rubella titer	Once	Once if unknown	
Glucose	High risk	High risk	High risk
Cholesterol or HDL	Every 5 yr	Every 5 yr	Every 5 yr
HIV	High risk	High risk	High risk
TSH			>60
Other Procedures			
Mammography		Every 2 yr, ages 40–50	Yearly, ages 50–75 2–3 yr, age 75 +
Flexible sigmoidoscopy		High risk	High risk
Chest radiograph			
Electrocardiogram		+ Risk factors	+ Risk factors
CA-125 or ultrasound			
Bone densitometry			Once if questions regarding HT use
Hearing testing		1–3 yr	1–3 yr
Visual acuity and glaucoma testing		1–3 yr	1–3 yr

STD, Sexually transmitted disease; RPR, rapid plasma reagin; PPD, purified protein derivative; HDL, high-density lipoprotein; HIV, human immunodeficiency virus; TSH, thyroid-stimulating hormone; HT, postmenopausal hormone therapy.

beneficial effect on well-being, studies have not determined whether the effect is associational only or is actually causal.[12] The cardiac risks of exercise, mainly from sudden death, are felt to be low, particularly in women who have a lower risk of sudden death than men.

Despite the lack of specific data on the benefits of exercise in women, the benefits studied in men can probably be extrapolated to women. Given the low risk of this intervention, exercise counseling is probably recommended for all patients. Exercise the equivalent of 20 minutes of brisk walking three times weekly has been documented to show a benefit in reducing cardiopulmonary problems.[13, 14] Even less strenuous activities that are of shorter duration may be beneficial, in particular for the elderly and the very sedentary.[15, 16]

Tobacco Use

Given the clearly documented health risks of smoking and the known benefits of brief physician intervention to promote smoking cessation, screening for tobacco use in all patients is indicated (see Chapter 65). Because most smoking begins during adolescence, screening for new smokers can probably be limited to those younger than 25 years of age. All adults should be assessed at initial visits for their smoking habits, and all smokers should be questioned about smoking patterns at each visit for at least 2 years after cessation.

Alcohol Abuse

Alcohol abuse may be present in as many as 10% of women and is clearly underdiagnosed in all age groups. Screening questions about attitudes toward alcohol use have been shown to be more useful than direct inquiry about the amount of alcohol consumed. The CAGE questionnaire (Table 1–2) is the most widely used screening questionnaire for alcoholism.[17] It has been validated mainly in men[17, 18] and may be less valid in women, as many women respond positively to the question on cutting back on alcohol intake for caloric reasons or respond differently from men to the "guilt" question. Cyr and Wartman found that the two questions "Have you ever had a drinking problem?" and "When was your last drink?" had

TABLE 1–2. The Cage Questionnaire for Alcoholism

1. Have you ever CUT back on your drinking?
2. Do you get ANNOYED when people criticize your drinking?
3. Do you ever feel GUILTY about your drinking?
4. Do you ever drink first thing in the morning? (EYE-OPENER?)

From Ewing FA. Diagnosis and treatment of alcoholism: The CAGE questionnaire. JAMA 1984;252:1905–1907. Copyright 1984, American Medical Association.

a high sensitivity for alcohol abuse, although their sample was not stratified by gender.[19] Such a screening tool should be employed for all women patients both at an initial visit and at periodic intervals during their care.

Drug Use

The sensitivity of direct inquiry about drug use, as with that regarding alcohol use, is probably limited because of denial of the problem as well as fear of the associated social stigma and the potential legal implications in acknowledging illicit drug use. However, in the absence of a validated questionnaire to inquire indirectly about drug use, direct inquiry is still useful.

Family Planning

All primary care providers should assess menstruating women on a routine basis regarding family planning. Although unintended pregnancies occur most frequently in adolescent women, the use of termination services is not limited to this group, and unintended pregnancy is a common problem in women beyond their twenties, including those in stable relationships.

Sexually Transmitted Diseases

Separate from the discussion of risk of unintended pregnancy should be a discussion of the risk of sexually transmitted diseases. Regardless of their menstrual status, all women should be asked about the risk factors for sexually transmitted diseases, including multiple sex partners, a partner who has multiple partners or is an intravenous drug user, lack of use of barrier contraceptives, and their history of past sexually transmitted diseases.

Depression and Anxiety Disorders

Extensive evidence documents the fact that primary care physicians underdetect depression as a problem for their patients.[20, 21] This is especially true for patients presenting with somatic complaints and for patients with chronic medical conditions for whom depression is exacerbating their symptoms. Despite a number of lengthy questionnaires for evaluating depression in patients, no short screening instrument has been validated in primary care practice. Given the importance of this problem in medical care, several questions targeted to mood and vegetative symptoms associated with depression, such as sleep disturbance or loss of appetite, libido, or interest in usually pleasurable activities, are probably indicated.

Anxiety disorders are a common problem in women and are often masked as various somatic symptoms, including numbness, chest pain, and difficulty breathing. Inquiring about anxiety or panic episodes in patients with these specific symptoms is indicated.

Trauma History

There is now ample evidence that trauma from intentional violence against women decreases a woman's sense of well-being and increases her health care utilization and her cost of health care.[22, 23] Women are often reluctant to address these problems directly with their providers. Therefore, specific screening questions are useful. One study has found a 12 to 15% increase in the rate of detection of domestic violence owing to the addition of a single screening question.[24] Asking directly whether the patient has been sexually assaulted as an adult, sexually abused as a child, or physically harmed by an intimate partner is the most effective means of identifying earlier trauma.

SCREENING WITHIN THE PHYSICAL EXAMINATION

The notion of a periodic complete physical examination is ingrained in our medical practice for the purposes of establishing a baseline on patients as well as for screening purposes. However, only specific portions of the physical examination have been studied in terms of their sensitivity and usefulness in detecting preclinical disease. The periodic health examination for women should focus on the following aspects, especially because many are often neglected in women's health care.

Blood Pressure

The measurement of blood pressure is an inexpensive method of assessing for high blood pressure, a silent condition with major morbidity associated with it. All groups reviewing blood pressure measurement as a screening test advocate regular blood pressure screening on all patients. For patients with infrequent visits, blood pressure measurements every 3 years before age 40 and yearly thereafter are probably sufficient.

Thyroid Examination

Given the high prevalence of thyroid nodules in women, a screening thyroid examination is probably indicated. The U.S. Preventive Services Task Force limits its recommendation to those who have had upper body irradiation, as this group is at higher risk for thyroid nodules and thyroid cancer.

Breast Examination

Despite the ample evidence that clinical breast examination is useful in the detection of breast cancer, studies indicate that the practice of this examination is declining over time.[25] Although mammography can detect many lesions before their discovery by clinical examination, as many as 10% of all breast cancers are not found on mammography alone.[26, 27] Clinical breast examination may be of increased value in women younger than 50, in whom the sensitivity of mammography is decreased.[28] Most groups advocate a clinical breast screening at least by age 40 and in many cases by age 20.

In elderly patients not considered candidates for mammography screening, clinical breast examination is still a useful screen. Detection of a palpable mass in an elderly patient with multiple medical problems is of value in planning for local therapy to prevent future symptomatology from a fungating mass even if no adjuvant or curative therapy is planned.

Breast self-examination has been advocated as an additional means of breast cancer screening by the American Cancer Society and other groups.[29] Currently, no studies have been able to document its effectiveness; however, these studies may suffer from lack of statistical power in their methods. Breast self-examination may also facilitate the patient's participation in her own health care and, for this reason, is a useful technique to teach all women patients.

Skin Examination

Morbidity decreases with early diagnosis of basal and squamous cell carcinomas, and evidence is ample that improved survival from melanoma is directly related to detection at an early stage of disease. For this reason most groups are currently recommending a complete annual skin examination for all patients. The U.S. Preventive Services Task Force's recommendations limit this screening to persons with a family or personal history of skin cancer or precursor lesions or prolonged sun exposure and educate against sun exposure in all patients. The American Cancer Society has also strongly urged monthly self-examination of the skin for patients.

Pelvic Examination

Pelvic examination has not been demonstrated to reduce mortality from either ovarian or other pelvic cancers or diseases. However, given the severity of late stage ovarian cancer, an annual pelvic examination for all women is prudent. Screening for asymptomatic uterine fibroids is probably not indicated, given that indications for hysterectomy or other therapy usually result from symptoms of pain or bleeding.

Rectal Examination

Digital rectal examination has some value, albeit limited, in the detection of rectal cancers. Current estimates are that less than 10% of colorectal cancers are detectable by digital examination.[30] In women the rectal-vaginal examination has additional efficacy in assessing the posterior fornix for pelvic masses. Given this and the added benefit of fecal occult blood testing with rectal examination, annual rectal examination in women older than 40 is recommended.

LABORATORY AND OTHER TESTS FOR SCREENING

Urinalysis

The urinalysis can potentially screen for bacteriuria and asymptomatic urinary tract infection, glycosuria and diabetes mellitus, and hematuria and proteinuria as first signs of urologic cancers and renal disease. This multitude of findings suggests that urinalysis would be a useful screening test given the relative ease of urine dipstick testing for the detection of abnormalities. However, the low sensitivity and specificity render this test useful only in particular circumstances.

Urine testing for glycosuria as a screen for diabetes is of limited value. Because many diabetics do not spill glucose into the urine at all times, the sensitivity of urine glucose measurements for diabetes may be as low as 30%.[31] However, some individuals have glycosuria at normal blood glucose levels and render false positive results.

Screening for asymptomatic bacteriuria or pyuria has been advocated, as this often detects urinary tract infections before symptoms occur. Such urinary tract infections may be associated with renal insufficiency, hypertension, and low birth weight for pregnant women. The incidence of asymptomatic bacteriuria increases with age and is 10 to 20% in diabetic women.[32] Multipad dipstick reagent strips detect leukocyte esterase as an indirect test for bacteria with a sensitivity of 72 to 97% and a specificity of 64 to 82%.[33] Nitrate reduction testing for bacteria has a sensitivity as low as 35 to 85%; however, its specificity is 92 to 100%.[33] It is felt that in most low-prevalence populations, this dipstick analysis will likely result in more false positive than true positive results. In women younger than 60 years of age, a dipstick testing for bacteria has a positive predictive value of less than 10%.[34] However, the predictive value increases in women who are pregnant, those who are diabetic, and those older than 60. The U.S. Preventive Services Task Force recommends periodic testing for these groups.

Proteinuria and hematuria are often the first detectable signs of end-stage renal disease or urologic cancers. Dipstick testing of urine for protein has a specificity and sensitivity of between 95 and 99%; for hematuria, the sensitivity is between 91 and 100%, with a slightly lower specificity of 65 to 99%.[35] The lower specificity of dipstick testing for hematuria in women is probably due to vaginal contamination during menses in some patients. The positive predictive value of a dipstick test for hematuria and proteinuria in the general population ranges from 6 to 45% for disorders of possible clinical significance, such as mild glomerulonephritis or nonstaghorn calculi, and less than 2% for serious urologic conditions, such as tumors, vasculitis, nephritis, and obstructive lesions.[35] Several studies have indicated that a higher positive predictive value of these tests is achieved in men older than 50 for detection of urologic cancer,[36] and similar results might be anticipated in women older than 50, especially smokers with an increased risk of urologic cancers. The Canadian Task Force recommends screening adults at risk for bladder cancer due to cigarette smoking, and the U.S. Preventive Services Task Force suggests screening of all persons older than 60.

Occult Fecal Blood Testing

Hemoccult screening of stool samples to detect occult fecal blood has been advocated for colon cancer screening. Colon cancer is the third most common cancer in women after breast and lung carcinoma. Although for those with localized disease the estimated 10-year survival rate is 75%, those with regional spread at diagnosis have a 10-year survival rate of less than 30 to 36%.[37] Therefore, early detection is important for this disease. Hemoccult testing involves testing for a positive reaction on a testing card impregnated with guaiac. It has a high false positive rate, which increases with the ingestion of food containing peroxidases and the use of gastric irritants such as salicylates and other anti-inflammatory agents that can produce upper gastrointestinal bleeding. When performed on a group of asymptomatic persons older than 50, the positive predictive value of testing is only 5 to 10% for carcinoma.[38] Screening therefore results in a large number of diagnostic tests on persons who produce false positive results. Nevertheless, at least one randomized control trial has shown that annual testing of three separate stools using hemoccult reagents decreased mortality from colon cancer by 33% after 13 years.[39] Most experts advocate obtaining a Hemoccult test either at the time of the annual rectal examination or with three test cards that the patient sends back to the office. Many also suggest that patients abstain from the use of salicylates or anti-inflammatory agents and from eating large amounts of red meat during testing to prevent false positive reactions.

Cervical Cytology

Cervical cytology, or Papanicolaou (PAP) smears, has clearly been shown to reduce the incidence of as well as to increase the survival rate in cervical cancer by the detection and elimination of premalignant lesions of the cervix. There is no question that cervical cancer screening is indicated and may in fact provide us with the only screening test that prevents cancer on a large scale.

The controversy surrounding PAP smears is not whether to do them but when to begin and when to discontinue and at what interval of testing. Many have argued that annual screening of all women to look for precancerous lesions that may evolve into malignancy only over the course of 5 to 7 years is not cost effective. Data from at least two investigators show that the majority of PAP smears are being performed on women at lower risk and that those women at higher risk are less likely to have access to or obtain primary care services and to receive regular screening.[40] The recommendations of the Canadian Task Force and the U.S. Preventive Services Task Force have been to consider screening every 3 years in women who are considered to be at low risk or who have had several negative smears. In contrast, the American College of Obstetricians and Gynecologists and the American Cancer Society recommend yearly PAP smears for all women.[41]

Annual PAP smear screening of all women beginning at either the age of sexual activity or age 18 and continuing throughout life is probably prudent. The rate of precancerous lesions in young women is increasing, and therefore annual screening in young women who are at higher risk for sexually transmitted diseases is justified. For women who have had normal PAP results in the past and who have one stable sexual partner, screening every 3 years may be adequate. However, obtaining a history of previous abnormal smears is often difficult. It is not unusual to have a woman with several negative smears develop a cervical squamous intraepithelial neoplasia and then recall a similar history in the past.

Screening in elderly women is probably also effective, especially for low-income elderly women whose access to medical care becomes available at age 65 with Medicare. Fahs and colleagues have shown that PAP smears with abnormal results are common in these women, who may not have received screening for a number of years.[42] Currently, nearly 75% of women older than 65 do not receive regular screening.

Periodic screening of women who report no previous sexual activity with men is probably also useful. Despite the very high correlation between exposure to sexually transmitted agents, specifically the condyloma virus, and cervical cancer, not all women who develop cervical cancer have a history of such exposure. Given the high prevalence of rape in our society and of possible patient reluctance to discuss a previous sexual assault, the sexual history may not provide all the necessary information to assess risk. Also, a PAP smear in all women on an annual basis has the added function of ensuring that women receive periodic evaluation and examination of the genitourinary system, including pelvic and rectal examination. When the PAP smear is no longer recommended, some patients and providers interpret this to mean that the whole gynecologic examination can be eliminated. Many other problems are detected in the process of obtaining a PAP smear, including vulvar lesions, symptoms of urinary incontinence, and pelvic and rectal masses.

Screening for Sexually Transmitted Diseases

Both gonorrhea and chlamydia can have an asymptomatic phase of cervical infection. Chlamydial disease, more so than gonorrhea, can lead to asymptomatic pelvic inflammatory disease with subsequent infertility, ectopic pregnancy, and pelvic pain. Data have shown that the cost of screening for chlamydia is less than the cost of subsequent medical treatment when the prevalence of the disease in a population is greater than 7 to 10%, as is found in adolescents, in patients in clinics that treat sexually transmitted diseases, and in patients with multiple sexual partners.[43, 44] However, one can argue that the measure of a screening test should not be its ability to pay for itself, and, given the severe morbidity associated with chlamydia, routine screening of all women of childbearing potential may be indicated, especially those with new sexual partners and those younger than 25.

The data are less compelling for routine screening for gonorrhea, given the lower prevalence and the higher likelihood of symptoms with salpingitis. However, screening in high-risk populations, including adolescents and women presenting to clinics that treat sexually transmitted diseases and family planning clinics, is prudent.

Most data have shown that screening for rapid plasma reagins (RPR) for syphilis results in a much higher rate of false positive than true positive results and that most of those true positive results are titers in patients already treated. However, a rapid plasma reagin test should be obtained whenever another sexually transmitted disease is diagnosed.

Tuberculosis Testing

Skin testing for exposure to tuberculosis has become an important public health issue given the rise of tuberculosis and the increased prevalence of resistant strains. Populations at increased risk include immigrants and refugees exposed in their native countries, American and Alaskan natives, homeless populations, those who provide care within medical settings, and those who volunteer in shelters where they may come in close contact with tuberculosis patients. These populations should obtain periodic screening for exposure to tuberculosis using the Mantoux test. This consists of injecting 5 tuberculin units (5 TU) of purified protein derivative (PPD) intradermally. Induration (not erythema) of 10 ml or more after 48 to 72 hours is considered positive. Multiple puncture tests (e.g., tine) are less expensive and easier to administer, but they have lower sensitivity and specificity compared with those of the Mantoux test. Patients either can be instructed on the signs to look for and told to call with results or can be

asked to return to the testing site for a reading of the test.

For those with a positive PPD result, the current recommendation is a 6-month course of isoniazid for all persons younger than 35. Given that hepatic toxicity increases in those older than 35 years, persons recommended to receive isoniazid prophylaxis in this group are those in high-risk situations, including persons who have a household member or other close contact with active tuberculosis or those who have other illnesses or therapies that may predispose them to active tuberculosis in the future, such as silicosis, diabetes, HIV infection, or steroid therapy.

Screening for Anemia

Routine complete blood counts are often felt by patients to be a standard feature of a complete physical examination. Although the hematocrit and other blood cell indices can be extremely useful diagnostic tools for a large variety of symptoms, the data on routine hemoglobin and hematocrit screening of healthy adult women are less convincing. No adverse effect of asymptomatic anemia has been demonstrated until hemoglobin falls below 10 gm per dl.[45] When anemia is associated with mortality or morbidity, another coexisting illness is usually responsible.

The most common type of anemia in premenopausal women is iron deficiency due to menstrual blood loss. In asymptomatic women, there is no evidence that screening and iron replacement for mild anemia have any specific benefit. An important exception to this is pregnant adult women, in whom low maternal hemoglobin has been linked to a variety of adverse fetal outcomes. It is unclear whether the anemia or the associated conditions, including poor nutrition, are responsible for these poor outcomes. In such a situation, screening and detection of anemia may provide a marker for other obstetric risk factors that might not otherwise be detected.

Rubella Screening

Antibody screening is recommended for all women of childbearing potential for evidence of previous rubella exposure. Rubella antibody, once established, is felt to be lifelong, and further screening is unnecessary. Ideally, this screening should occur before plans are made to conceive, as the live virus vaccine is contraindicated during pregnancy. Alternatively, when a negative rubella titer is noted during early prenatal care, immunization in the immediate postpartum period is recommended.

Diabetes Mellitus

Diabetes affects 11 million persons in the United States, and estimates are that nearly half of these have not been diagnosed. About 90% of all cases are non–insulin-dependent diabetes, which generally occurs in adults after the age of 40. Non–insulin-dependent diabetes can remain undetected in milder forms with ongoing symptoms and morbidity but without the life-threatening ketoacidosis that is characteristic of insulin-dependent diabetes.

Several potential tests are available for screening. Urine dipstick for glycosuria is a poor screen, as there are certain individuals with glycosuria and normal blood sugars and many diabetics without glycosuria. Random or fasting blood glucose measurements are probably the best screening tests. However, basing a diagnosis of diabetes on a single glucose determination is difficult. There is a wide overlap of ranges of glucose within the population. Adopting a threshold of greater than 130 mg per dl results in overdiagnosis of the condition, whereas a more generous threshold of 200 mg per dl that is considered an unequivocal sign of diabetes overlooks many less severe cases. Glucose tolerance testing in nonpregnant women has also been shown to be a poor predictor of diabetes or of the subsequent development of diabetes.

Most expert panels have recommended periodic screening blood glucose determinations for high-risk populations, including the very obese, those with a family history of diabetes, and women with a previous history of gestational diabetes.

Screening for gestational diabetes is advocated for all women, given the high prevalence and the perinatal morbidity and mortality associated with even mild increases in blood sugar (see Chapter 37).

Cholesterol

Cholesterol screening is advocated every 5 years for all adult women. Screening can be done on a nonfasting specimen. Given the large number of young women with high total cholesterol due to a very favorable high-density lipoprotein to low-density lipoprotein ratio, and given the significance of high-density lipoprotein and the ratio of high-density lipoprotein to low-density lipoprotein as independent risk modifiers for coronary artery disease, some investigators argue that the initial cholesterol screening should include a total cholesterol and a high-density lipoprotein cholesterol test. This may be cost effective in populations in which a large number of follow-up studies are obtained for a slightly elevated cholesterol reading. For further management of screening cholesterol, see Chapter 51.

Testing for Human Immunodeficiency Virus

Although counseling on safer sex practices and prevention of HIV infection is recommended in the history for all women, most experts currently recommend HIV screening for patients with risk factors (see Chapter 48). These risk factors have traditionally included women who use intravenous drugs, women whose sexual partners are intravenous drug users or bisexual, prostitutes, and patients with multiple sexual partners. With heterosexual transmission being one of the fastest growing risk factors for HIV transmission in women, counseling of all women on risk factors and screening of all women who express interest or have particular concerns about particular previous sexual partners appears prudent.

Thyroid Function Tests

Routine screening for hyperthyroidism and hypothyroidism in adult women is generally not advocated. However, both the Canadian Task Force and the U.S. Preventive Services Task Force suggest that the screening of elderly women may be prudent, given the increased risk of developing hypothyroidism and the fact that elderly women are much less likely to have the typical signs and symptoms of either hypothyroidism or hyperthyroidism. Given the accuracy of measuring thyroid-stimulating hormone (TSH) levels,[46] this assay may now be used as an initial screen for both hyper- and hypothyroidism in this group.

Mammography

The use of mammography as a screening test for breast cancer has been clearly established in women between the ages of 50 and 75. However, the efficacy of its use in younger and older women is still debated.

There is strong evidence from randomized controlled trials that screening mammography every 1 to 2 years for women between the ages of 50 and

75 not only detects more tumors in earlier stages but also results in a decrease in mortality in this group.[47-53] The data on screening mammography for women aged 40 to 50 are less clear, and none of the recent trials has demonstrated an improvement in mortality.[47-52, 54] Based on this data, some reviewers recommend against screening mammography before the age of 50. Others, however, suggest that given the faster rate of tumor doubling in this population, annual mammography will be found to be effective whereas biennial screening is not. Currently, the Canadian Task Force and U.S. Preventive Services Task Force do not recommend screening mammography before the age of 50. The American Cancer Society recommends screening between the ages of 40 and 50 on a biennial basis.

Screening women older than 75 has not been studied adequately in any of the recent trials. Women who have other comorbid conditions likely to shorten their life span may derive no additional benefit from screening mammography. However, for women who are in otherwise good health, the American Geriatric Society advocates continued screening approximately every 2 years.[55] Although a baseline mammogram at age 35 was initially advocated both by the American College of Radiology and the American Cancer Society, the lack of data on its effectiveness and the concerns regarding high false positive rates and low sensitivity and specificity in this younger age group have resulted in most groups, included the American Cancer Society, no longer recommending it.[29]

Flexible Sigmoidoscopy

The U.S. Preventive Services Task Force found insufficient evidence to recommend for or against sigmoidoscopy as an effective screening for colorectal cancer in asymptomatic persons. Unlike fecal occult blood testing, on which trial data have been reported, the effectiveness of sigmoidoscopy is not yet available from current trials. The American Cancer Society and various gastroenterology groups have recommended sigmoidoscopic screening every 2 to 5 years for women older than 50. The cost, discomfort, and embarrassment of this test limit its use in the general population. Until more definitive information is available, offering screening to women at high risk may be a reasonable approach. This includes women older than 50 with a first-degree relative with colon cancer; women with a personal history of endometrial, ovarian, or breast cancer; and women with a previous history of inflammatory bowel disease or familial polyposis.

Chest Radiograph

Routine chest radiographs have been evaluated for their possible benefit in screening for lung cancer and tuberculosis. A number of well-documented studies have shown that routine chest radiographs with or without sputum cytology are ineffective in reducing mortality from lung cancer in smokers.[56-58] Preventive efforts against lung cancer should focus on smoking cessation counseling and occupational hazards counseling for those who are routinely exposed to asbestos.

Tuberculin PPD is the screening test of choice for tuberculosis, and for those with a positive test result, a chest radiograph is recommended to rule out active infection.

Electrocardiogram

The role of a baseline resting electrocardiogram (ECG) in screening for asymptomatic cardiac disease is controversial. Advocates of this screening include the American College of Cardiology and the American Heart Association, but the Canadian and U.S. task forces recommended against routine screening as secondary prevention for coronary artery disease. The argument for routine screening ECGs includes the fact that certain resting ECG findings are associated with future coronary events, including evidence of previous silent myocardial infarction and ST segment depression. Also, some argue that a baseline cardiogram can be helpful in interpreting subsequent changes. Skeptics of screening ECGs cite the low value of abnormal ECGs as predictors of coronary heart disease (3–15% of asymptomatic persons with between 5 and 30 years of follow-up).[59, 60] These reviewers also cite the negative impact of false positive results, including further testing and difficulties with insurance eligibility and job qualifications in the future. In the past, baseline ECGs were frequently unavailable in acute care settings, when making these comparisons is necessary. However, this problem may be alleviated with the advent of computerized recording and retrieval of ECG results and facsimile transmission, which allows for rapid comparisons with previous studies. Some experts recommend screening ECGs for individuals whose livelihood would endanger public safety if they were to experience a sudden coronary event. There appears to be value in obtaining baseline ECGs for women with other cardiac risk factors, including hypertension, diabetes, a strong family history of heart disease, and hypercholesterolemia.[61]

CA-125 and Ultrasound for Ovarian Cancer

Given the insidious nature of early symptoms of ovarian cancer, the frequency with which this tumor presents in late stages, and the high mortality rates associated with it, a preclinical test would be ideal to reduce morbidity and mortality. Unfortunately, studies to date have not shown that CA-125 or ultrasound alone or both combined have been useful in screening either normal-risk or high-risk women.[62–65] CA-125 is subject to a number of false positive results from other benign ovarian conditions and false negatives for early tumors confined to the ovary. When screening has resulted in increased tumor detection, tumors were still found to be in advanced stages, and survival to date has not been improved. Some investigators have suggested that the usefulness of CA-125 may be greater in postmenopausal women, who may produce fewer false positive results.[66] Women with first-degree family members with ovarian cancer should be enrolled in clinical trials to assess the usefulness of various combinations of CA-125 and ultrasound for screening. However, at this point, routine use of these tests for screening cannot be advocated.

Bone Densitometry

Bone density measurements have been evaluated as a means of determining the risk of osteoporosis and fractures, given that clinical risk factors have a poor predictive value. Many of the initial technologies, including single and dual photon absorptiometry, have sufficiently low reliability and validity to limit their usefulness in screening. Current dual energy x-ray absorptiometry has improved on previous technology, warranting its consideration as a screening tool.[67] Currently, the U.S. and Canadian task forces have not made specific recommendations on bone density studies. Postmenopausal women in whom estrogen therapy is contraindicated should be placed on vitamin D, calcium, and a weight-bearing exercise program. Bone density studies are not indicated until further preventive therapy is available, as their results do not change medical management. For women who for other reasons are planning long-term hormone therapy at menopause, the usefulness of bone densitometry is questionable, as it does not alter therapy. Bone densitometry may be of particular value for women who are unclear on their preference for estrogen therapy or have few demonstrated risk factors for developing osteoporosis. In this group, a finding of low bone density at the time of meno-

pause may help make the patient's decision on whether to commence long-term therapy. The use of follow-up measures is still in question, because in the absence of a noted effect on bone loss, other therapy beyond estrogens is not currently available.

Visual and Hearing Screening

Screening of women older than 65 for hearing impairment and visual acuity, including testing for glaucoma, is recommended. Hearing impairment is reported in nearly one fourth of patients at age 65, one third by age 75, and almost half of those older than 85.[68] The intervention of correction of hearing impairment can have significant benefit on functional status. Screening for intraocular pressure is recommended for those older than 65, given the insidious nature of pressure changes and the fact that irreparable harm can occur in the untreated asymptomatic phase. The U.S. Preventive Services Task Force did not find sufficient evidence to include visual acuity in its recommendations. However, this screening can occur at the time of glaucoma testing, whether done by the primary care provider or an eye specialist.

REFERENCES

1. Report of the U.S. Preventive Services Task Force. Guide to Clinical Preventive Services. Baltimore: Williams & Wilkins, 1989.
2. Canadian Task Force on the Periodic Health Examination. The periodic health examination. Can Med Assoc J 1979;121:1194.
3. Preliminary findings of the first Health and Nutrition Examination Survey, United States, 1971–1972. Anthropometric and clinical findings. DHEW Publication No. (HRA) 75-1229. Rockville, Md: U.S. Department of Health, Education, and Welfare Public Health Service, 1975.
4. Connors ME, Johnson CL. Epidemiology of bulimia and bulimic behaviors. Addict Behav 1987;12:165.
5. Zinkaid H, Cadoret RJ, Widmer RB. Incidence and detection of bulimia in a family practice population. J Fam Pract 1984;18:555.
6. Freund KM, Graham SM, Lesky LM, Moskowitz MA. Detection of bulimia in a primary care setting. J Gen Intern Med 1993;8:236.
7. Epstein LH, Wing RR. Aerobic exercise and weight. Addict Behav 1980;5:371.
8. Cooper C, Barker DJP, Wickham C. Physical activity, muscle strength, and calcium intake in fracture of the proximal femur in Britain. BMJ 1988;297:1443.
9. Aloia JF, Vaswani AN, Yeh JK, Cohn SH. Premenopausal bone mass is related to physical activity. Arch Intern Med 1988;148:121.
10. Dalsky GP, Stocke KS, Ehsame AA, et al. Weight-bearing exercise training and lumbar bone mineral content in postmenopausal women. Ann Intern Med 1988;108:824.
11. Paganini-Hill A, Ross RK, Gerkins JR, et al. Menopausal

estrogen therapy and hip fractures. Ann Intern Med 1981;95:28.

12. Hughes JR. Psychological effects of habitual aerobic exercise: A critical review. Prev Med 1984;13:66.

13. Wenger HA, Bell GJ. The interactions of intensity, frequency and duration of exercise training in altering cardiorespiratory fitness. Sports Med 1986;3:346.

14. American College of Sports Medicine. Position statement on the recommended quantity and quality of exercise for developing and maintaining fitness in healthy adults. Med Sci Sports Exerc 1978;10:7.

15. Badenhop DT, Cleary P, Schaal SF, et al. Physiologic adjustments to higher- or lower-intensity exercise in elders. Med Sci Sports Exerc 1983;15:496.

16. Emes CG. The effects of a regular program of light exercise on seniors. J Sports Med Phys Fitness 1979;19:185.

17. Ewing FA. Detecting alcoholism: The CAGE questionnaire. JAMA 1984;252:1905.

18. Mayfield D, McLeod G, Hall P. The CAGE questionnaire: Validation of a new alcoholism screening instrument. Am J Psychiatry 1974;131:1121.

19. Cyr MG, Wartman S. The effectiveness of routine screening questions in the detection of alcoholism. JAMA 1988;259:51.

20. Perez-Stable EF, Munoz MJ, Ying YW. Depression in medical outpatients: Underrecognition and misdiagnosis. Arch Intern Med 1990;150:1083.

21. Fisch RZ. Masked depression: Its interrelations with somatization, hypochondriasis and conversion. Int J Psychiatry Med 1987;17:367.

22. Koss MP, Woodruff WJ, Koss PG. Relation of criminal victimization to health perceptions among women medical patients. J Consult Clin Psychol 1990;58:147.

23. Koss MP, Koss PG, Woodruff WJ. Deleterious effects of criminal victimization on women's health and medical utilization. Arch Intern Med 1991;151:342.

24. Freund KM, Blackhall LJ. Detection of domestic violence in a primary care setting. Clin Res 1990;38:738A.

25. Coleman EA, Feure EJ, The NCI Breast Cancer Screening Consortium. Breast cancer screening among women from 65 to 74 years of age in 1987–88 and 1991. Ann Intern Med 1992;117:961.

26. Cahill CJ, Boulter PS, Gibb NM, Price JL. Features of mammographically negative breast tumors. Br J Surg 1981;68:882.

27. McClow MV, Williams AC. Mammographic examinations; ten-year clinical experience in a community medical center. Ann Surg 1973;177:616.

28. Tabar L, Dean PB. Mammographic parenchymal patterns: Risk indicator for breast cancer. JAMA 1982;247:185.

29. American Cancer Society. Summary of current guidelines for the cancer-related checkup: Recommendations. New York: American Cancer Society, 1988.

30. Schottenfeld D, Winawer SJ. Large intestine. In: Schottenfeld D, Sherlock R (eds). Colorectal Cancer: Prevention, Epidemiology, and Screening. New York: Raven Press, 1980, p 175.

31. Bitzen PO, Schersten B. Assessment of laboratory methods for detection of unsuspected diabetes in primary health care. Scand J Prim Health Care 1986;4:85.

32. National Diabetes Data Group. Diabetes in America: Diabetes data compiled 1984. Publication No. DHHS (NIH) 85-1468. Washington, DC: U.S. Government Printing Office, 1985.

33. Pels RJ, Bor DH, Woolhandler S, et al. Screening asymptomatic adults for bacteriuria. In: Goldbloom RB, Lawrence RS (eds). Preventing Disease: Beyond the Rhetoric. New York: Springer-Verlag, 1990.

34. Bengtsson C, Bengtsson U, Lincoln K. Bacteriuria in a population sample of women. Acta Med Scand 1980; 208:417.

35. Woolhandler S, Pels RJ, Bor DH, et al. Screening asymptomatic adults for hematuria and proteinuria: Dipstick urinalysis. In: Goldbloom RB, Lawrence RS (eds). Preventing Disease: Beyond the Rhetoric. New York: Springer-Verlag, 1990.

36. Mesing EM, Young TB, Hunt VB, et al. The significance of asymptomatic microhematuria in men 50 or more years old: Findings of a home screening study using urinary dipsticks. J Urol 1987;137:919.

37. National Cancer Institute. Surveillance, epidemiology and end-results: Incidence and mortality data, 1973–77. National Cancer Institute Monograph No. 57. Bethesda, Md: National Cancer Institute, 1981.

38. Knight KK, Fielding JE, Battista RN. Occult blood screening for colorectal cancer. JAMA 1989;261:587.

39. Mandel JS, Bond JH, Church RE, et al. Reducing mortality from colorectal cancer by screening for rectal occult blood. N Engl J Med 1993;328:1365.

40. Woolhandler S, Himmelstein DU. Reverse targeting of preventive care due to lack of health insurance. JAMA 1988;259:2872.

41. Fink DJ. Change in American Cancer Society checkup guidelines for detection of cervical cancer. CA Cancer J Clin 1988;38:127.

42. Fahs MC, Mandelblatt J, Schechter C, Muller C. Cost effectiveness of cervical cancer screening for the elderly. Ann Intern Med 1992;117:520.

43. Phillips RS, Aronson MD, Taylor WL, Safran C. Should tests for *Chlamydia trachomatis* cervical infection be done during routine gynecologic visits? Ann Intern Med 1987;107:188.

44. Nettleman MD, Jones RB, Roberts SD, et al. Cost-effectiveness of culturing for *Chlamydia trachomatis*. Ann Intern Med 1986;105:189.

45. Elwood RC, Waters WE, Greene WJ, et al. Symptoms and circulating hemoglobin level. J Chron Dis 1969;21:615.

46. Ross DS. New sensitive immunoradiometric assays for thyrotropin. Ann Intern Med 1986;104:718.

47. Shapiro S, Venet W, Strax P, et al. Selection, follow-up, and analysis in the health insurance plan study: A randomized trial with breast cancer screening. National Cancer Institute Monograph 1985;67:65.

48. Tabar L, Gad A, Holmberg L, Ljungquist U. Significant reduction in advanced breast cancer: Results of the first seven years of mammography screening in Kopparberg, Sweden. Diagn Imag Clin Med 1985;54:158.

49. Verbeek ALM, Holland R, Sturmans F, Hendriks JHC, Mravunac M, Day NE. Reduction of breast cancer mortality through mass screening with modern mammography: First results of the Nijmegen Project, 1975–1981. Lancet 1984;1:1222.

50. Palli D, Rosselli Del Turco M, et al. A case-control study of the efficacy of a non-randomized breast cancer screening program in Florence (Italy). Int J Cancer 1986;38:501.

51. Seidman H, Gelb SK, Silverberg E, et al. Survival experience in the Breast Cancer Detection Demonstration Project. CA Cancer J Clin 1987;37:258.

52. Andersson I, Aspegren K, Janzon L, et al. Mammographic screening and mortality from breast cancer: The Malmo mammographic screening trial. BMJ 1988;297:943.

53. Miller AB, Baines CJ, To T, Wall C. Canadian national breast screening study: 2. Breast cancer detection and death rates among women aged 50 to 59 years. Can Med Assoc J 1992;147:1477.

54. Miller AB, Baines CJ, To T, Wall C. Canadian national breast screening study: 1. Breast cancer detection and death rates among women aged 40 to 49 years. Can Med Assoc J 1992;147:1459.

55. Screening for breast cancer in elderly women. J Am Geriatr Soc 1989;37:883.
56. Flehinger BJ, Melamed MR, Zaman MB, et al. Early lung cancer detection: Results of the initial (prevalence) radiologic and cytologic screening in the Memorial Sloan-Kettering study. Am Rev Respir Dis 1984;130:555.
57. Frost JK, Ball WC, Levin ML, et al. Early lung cancer detection: Results of the initial (prevalence) radiologic and cytologic screening in the Johns Hopkins study. Am Rev Respir Dis 1984;130:549.
58. Fontana RS, Sanderson DR, Taylor WF, et al. Early lung cancer detection: Results of the initial (prevalence) radiologic and cytologic screening in the Mayo Clinic study. Am Rev Respir Dis 1984;130:561.
59. Kannel WB, Anderson K, McGee DL, et al. Nonspecific electrocardiographic abnormality as a predictor of coronary heart disease: The Framingham Study. Am Heart J 1987;113:370.
60. Knutsen R, Knutsen SF, Curb JD, et al. The predictive value of resting electrocardiograms for 12 year incidence or coronary heart disease in the Honolulu Heart Program. J Clin Epidemiol 1988;41:293.
61. American College of Cardiology. Guidelines for exercise testing a report of the American College of Cardiology/American Heart Association Task Force on Assessment of Cardiovascular Procedures (Subcommittee on Exercise Testing). J Am Coll Cardiol 1986;8:725.
62. Jacobs I. Screening for ovarian cancer by CA-125 measurement. Lancet 1988;1:889.
63. Zurawski VR, Knapp RC, Einhorn N, et al. An initial analysis of preoperative serum CA 125 levels in patients with early stage ovarian carcinoma. Gynecol Oncol 1988;30:7.
64. Campbell S, Goessens L, Goswamy R, et al. Real-time ultrasound for determination of ovarian morphology and volume: A possible early screening test for ovarian cancer? Lancet 1982;1:425.
65. Andolf E, Svalenius E, Astedt B. Ultrasonography for early detection of ovarian carcinoma. Br J Obstet Gynecol 1986;93:1286.
66. Zurawski VR, Broderick SF, Pickens P, et al. Serum CA 125 levels in a group of nonhospitalized women: Relevance for the early detection of ovarian cancer. Obstet Gynecol 1987;69:606.
67. Wahner HW, Dunn WL, Brown ML, et al. Comparison of dual-energy absorptiometry and dual photon absorptiometry for bone mineral measurements of the lumbar spine. Mayo Clin Proc 1988;63:1075.
68. Havlik RJ. Aging in the eighties: Impaired senses for sound and light in persons age 65 years and over. Preliminary data from the supplement on aging to the National Health Interview Survey: United States, January–June 1984. Advance Data from Vital and Health Statistics, No. 125. Publication No. DHHS (PHS) 86-1250. Hyattsville, Md: National Center for Health Statistics, 1986.

2

Immunization

M. Anita Barry

Immunizations reduce morbidity and mortality more effectively than any other preventive health measure. However, the need for routine immunization in adults has received little attention, leaving many adults at risk for vaccine-preventable illnesses.[1] The recent epidemics of diseases such as measles in the United States underscore the importance of appropriate immunization, particularly for women.[2]

Although current data suggest that many health care providers do not routinely assess the need for vaccination in women, immunization status should be routinely assessed as part of primary health care. Consideration should be given to demographics, occupation, lifestyle, and environment in determining the need for immunization in a particular patient. Table 2–1 provides information on immunizations commonly indicated for women by selected risk factors. Women may be candidates for immunization against measles, mumps, rubella, influenza, pneumococcal diseases, hepatitis B, tetanus, and diphtheria, as well as others.

MEASLES

Before the introduction of the measles vaccine in 1963, approximately 500,000 measles cases and 500 measles-related deaths were reported annually in the United States. The number of reported cases declined dramatically following the introduction of the vaccine until the late 1980s, when large measles outbreaks began to be reported. Although inadequately immunized urban preschoolers accounted for many cases, a significant proportion occurred in adults. Of the 9643 cases reported in 1991, 19.6% occurred in adults older than 20 years of age; of these, 27.4% acquired infection in a medical setting.[3]

Measles is associated with significant morbidity in adults. Of adult patients reported in the United States during 1991, 36% required inpatient hospitalization; 20.6% of measles deaths occurred in persons older than age 20.[3] Most reported cases occurred in persons not immunized in accordance with current recommendations of the Advisory Committee on Immunization Practices. Measles can be particularly severe during pregnancy, leading to an increased risk of spontaneous abortion, low infant birth weight, and preterm labor.[4]

Persons born before 1957 are likely to have acquired measles infection, which most believe confers lifelong immunity. Of measles cases reported in the United States from 1985 through 1990, more than 96% occurred in persons born in 1957 or later.[5] Although measles vaccine produces an immune response in 95% of recipients, measles outbreaks in highly vaccinated populations that have resulted from primary vaccine failure or waning immunity have been documented.[6, 7] Factors known to be related to lack of a protective immune response include the administration of vaccine before age 12 months and the administration of killed vaccine (available from 1963 through 1967) either alone or followed by live vaccine.

All adults born after 1956 should be evaluated for measles vaccine unless evidence of immunity to measles is available. Acceptable evidence of immunity to measles includes either (1) serologic evidence of measles antibody at a level believed to be protective or (2) receipt of a measles vaccine given after 1967 when the individual was at least 12 months of age. Women of any age who work in sites where measles may be endemic (e.g., health care facilities) or live in settings where transmission may be facilitated (e.g., college campuses) and who received a single dose of vaccine in childhood should receive a second dose unless a specific contraindication exists. For susceptible persons who are exposed to a case of measles, a single dose of measles vaccine may be effective in preventing or modifying illness if given within 72 hours of exposure.

Serious side effects following measles vaccination are unusual. Approximately 5 to 15% of vaccinees develop a temperature greater than 39.4°C

TABLE 2–1.   Immunization in Women: Indications Based on Demographics, Occupation, and Lifestyle or Environmental Risk Factors

ANTIGEN	DEMOGRAPHIC RISK FACTORS	OCCUPATIONAL RISKS	LIFESTYLE OR ENVIRONMENTAL RISKS
Hepatitis B	Foreign born	Health care workers Laboratory personnel Public safety personnel Staff of institutions for the developmentally disabled	Intravenous drug users Heterosexually active women with multiple partners Correctional facility inmates Residents of institutions for the developmentally disabled Household contacts of hepatitis B carriers Travelers
Influenza	Age >65 yr	Health care workers Public safety personnel Staff of long-term care facilities	Travelers Residents of long-term care facilities
Measles	Birth after 1956* Foreign born	Health care workers	College students Travelers
Meningococcal polysaccharide			Travelers
Mumps	Birth after 1956* Foreign born	Health care workers	College students Travelers
Pneumococcal polysaccharide	Age >65 yr	Staff of long-term care facilities	Residents of long-term care facilities
Rabies		Animal handlers	Travelers
Rubella	18–64 yr	Health care workers	College students Travelers
Tetanus and diphtheria toxoids†	All age groups Foreign born		Travelers

*Persons born before 1956 may be vaccine candidates if in high-risk environments.
†Tetanus and diphtheria toxoids is the preferred product for adults requiring immunization against tetanus.

(103°F) during the fifth to twelfth day following immunization. In addition, approximately 5% of vaccinees develop a rash after immunization. Encephalitis following vaccination has been rarely reported. No data support an increased risk of side effects from vaccine in persons who are already immune by virtue of prior disease or immunization.

Measles vaccine is contraindicated in persons with a history of an immediate type hypersensitivity reaction to eggs or neomycin. Measles is a live virus vaccine and should not be given to women who are immunocompromised or who are pregnant because of a theoretic risk to the fetus. Because the vaccine may suppress reactivity to tuberculin temporarily, tuberculin skin testing should be administered on the same day as measles vaccine or no sooner than 4 to 6 weeks after vaccine administration. Antibody-containing products such as immune globulin preparations and other blood products may interfere with the response to measles vaccine. Immunization should be done at least 14 days before and no sooner than 6 weeks (preferably 3 months) after receipt of these products.

MUMPS

Following the introduction of mumps vaccine in 1967, the incidence of mumps declined sharply in the United States. However, because routine vaccination was not recommended until 1977, young adults may be susceptible to disease.[5] Of the 5712 cases reported in the United States in 1989, 38% occurred in persons older than 15 years of age.[5]

In most persons, mumps is a benign, self-limited illness,[8] with parotitis developing in 60 to 70% of cases. However, meningitis occurs in up to 10% of cases, and oophoritis occurs in approximately 5% of postpubertal women who acquire mumps. In pregnant women, acquisition of mumps during the first trimester has been associated with a significant increase in fetal death.[9]

Women born before 1957 are likely to be immune to mumps as a result of prior disease and subsequent immunity. Women born after 1956 should be considered susceptible to mumps and be offered vaccine unless they meet one of the following criteria: (1) receipt of a mumps vaccine after the age of 12 months or (2) laboratory-documented evidence of immunity to mumps.

A single dose of mumps vaccine produces a protective antibody response in more than 95% of recipients; efficacy in outbreaks has been calculated to be 75 to 91%.[8] Side effects from the mumps vaccine are rare and include parotitis, fever, and allergic reactions. Because of a theoretic risk to the developing fetus, mumps vaccine should be avoided in pregnant women. In general, the vaccine should not be given to persons who are immunocompromised or immunosuppressed. The vaccine is contraindicated in persons with an immediate type hypersensitivity reaction to eggs or neomycin. Mumps vaccine should not be administered for at least 14 days before or no sooner than 6 weeks (preferably 3 months) after administration of immune globulin or other antibody-containing products.

RUBELLA

Following the introduction of rubella vaccine in 1969, the number of reported rubella cases in the United States declined markedly. However, of the 931 cases reported in 1990 for which age was known, 57% occurred in persons older than 15 years of age.[5] In recent outbreaks as many as 40% of cases have occurred in women of childbearing potential.[10] Serologic surveys indicate that 6 to 11% of young women are susceptible to rubella, and sites where these individuals congregate may be conducive to rubella outbreaks.[11] Although postnatal rubella generally is a mild illness, first trimester infection in pregnant women results in congenital rubella syndrome in 20 to 25% of newborns and long-term sequelae in as many as 80%.[12]

A single dose of rubella vaccine produces long-term immunity in approximately 95% of vaccinees.[5] All women should be considered candidates for rubella vaccine unless immunity can be demonstrated through either (1) previous receipt of rubella vaccine on or after the first birthday or (2) laboratory evidence of immunity to rubella.

In large-scale trials, up to 25% of women who receive rubella vaccine develop arthralgias; this occurs more frequently in women who were susceptible to rubella at the time of immunization. In the majority, these complaints usually resolve after a period of 1 to 3 weeks, however, limited evidence suggests that chronic arthritis may follow rubella vaccination. This complication has also been noted following natural infection at a higher rate than that observed following immunization.[13] Transient peripheral neuritis has also been reported

in rare cases following immunization in susceptible women.

Because of a possible risk to the developing fetus, women who are pregnant or who anticipate being pregnant within 3 months should not receive rubella vaccine. Vaccine is contraindicated in persons with a history of an immediate type hypersensitivity reaction to eggs or neomycin. Rubella vaccine should be avoided in immunocompromised or immunosuppressed women. Because rubella is a live vaccine, immunization should be administered at least 14 days before and at least 6 weeks (preferably 3 months) after receipt of immune globulin preparations or other antibody-containing blood products.

Women who are susceptible to measles, mumps, or rubella should be offered immunization with a combined product containing measles, mumps, and rubella antigens (MMR vaccine).

TETANUS

Tetanus cases are rare in the United States, undoubtedly owing to widespread immunization with tetanus toxoid. From 1986 through 1989, only 48 to 64 cases were reported annually. However, of the 513 cases reported between 1982 and 1989 for which age was known, 95% occurred in persons older than 20 years of age.[5] Of women older than 30 years of age who sought care at an urban emergency department, 25% were found to lack antibody to tetanus.[14]

A primary tetanus series for adults consists of three doses of toxoid with at least 4 weeks between the first two doses and 6 to 12 months between the second and third doses. A booster dose is recommended every 10 years; however, following injuries other than clean, minor wounds, a dose of tetanus and diphtheria toxoids (Td) should be given if more than 5 years have elapsed since the last dose. Diphtheria toxoid is usually given with tetanus toxoid to maintain high levels of immunity to diphtheria in the population.

Side effects from Td usually consist of local reactions; fever and other systemic symptoms occur less frequently. More severe local reactions (Arthus-type hypersensitivity) can occur in persons who receive multiple doses of tetanus toxoid. Very severe systemic reactions, including anaphylaxis, occur very rarely after administration of Td; a history of severe reaction (urticaria or anaphylaxis) is a contraindication to the administration of additional doses. For other than clean, minor wounds, tetanus immune globulin should be given to those who cannot be immunized with tetanus toxoid.

INFLUENZA

Influenza continues to cause major morbidity and mortality, particularly among selected populations in the United States. At least 10,000 deaths have been documented in each of 19 epidemics in the United States from 1957 through 1986.[15] The risk of an adverse outcome from the disease is increased in persons older than 65 and in those who have chronic pulmonary conditions, cardiovascular disorders, chronic metabolic diseases, renal dysfunction, hemoglobinopathies, or immunosuppression. Residents and staff of long-term care facilities are also likely to be at increased risk owing to working in an environment that may be conducive to transmission of the virus.

Changes in the predominant circulating influenza viruses as well as waning antibody levels during the 12 months following vaccination mandate that influenza vaccine be offered annually. Although the optimal time to vaccinate is late fall, vaccine should continue to be offered to persons at risk once influenza activity has been documented in a geographic area.

Although most healthy young adults develop an adequately protective antibody response to influenza vaccination, the elderly and those with chronic illnesses have a diminished response. Despite this, vaccinated persons in high-risk groups are less likely to develop severe illness or require hospitalization compared with those who have not been vaccinated.[16] A live attenuated intranasal vaccine used in conjunction with the inactivated vaccine has shown promise in providing additional protection to nursing home residents.[17]

Influenza vaccine is usually associated with few side effects. Fewer than one third of vaccinees develop soreness at the injection site. Infrequently a syndrome of fever, malaise, myalgias, and other systemic symptoms lasting 1 to 2 days may develop, particularly in persons not previously vaccinated. An immediate type hypersensitivity reaction, most likely related to residual egg protein in the vaccine, occurs very rarely. Persons who are unable to eat eggs owing to allergic reactions are not candidates for influenza vaccine. No association between Guillain-Barré syndrome and influenza vaccine has been noted since the use of the 1976 swine influenza product.

PNEUMOCOCCAL POLYSACCHARIDE

Severe pneumococcal disease remains a problem in the United States. Pneumococcal pneumonia is estimated to account for 10 to 25% of all pneumonia and to cause 40,000 deaths annually.[1] The rate of pneumococcal bacteremia is estimated to be 18.7 per 100,000 for all ages and 53 per 100,000 for persons older than 65 years of age.[18] Because pneumococcal disease is associated with mortality in a significant proportion of persons with underlying risk factors despite the availability of appropriate antimicrobial agents, immunization is recommended for those in high-risk groups.[19] These include persons older than 65 and those with chronic cardiovascular diseases, chronic pulmonary disease, diabetes mellitus, alcoholism, cirrhosis, functional or anatomic asplenia, Hodgkin's disease, lymphoma, multiple myeloma, chronic renal failure, nephrotic syndrome, organ transplantation, and human immunodeficiency virus (HIV) infection.[20]

The current pneumococcal polysaccharide vaccine, licensed in 1983, contains capsular polysaccharide antigen from the 23 pneumococcal serotypes associated with 88% of the bacteremic pneumococcal disease in the United States. This product replaced a 14-valent product that was available from 1977 until 1983. Following a single dose of vaccine, most adults develop type-specific antibody responses, which persist for at least 5 years. Persons who are immunocompromised may have an impaired antibody response.

Women at risk for serious pneumococcal disease in the groups listed earlier should be offered vaccine. In addition, persons with cerebrospinal fluid leaks are at increased risk for recurrent pneumococcal disease and should be vaccinated. Crowded living environments (e.g., homeless shelters) may facilitate transmission of the pneumococcus, and persons living in these situations should be considered vaccine candidates.[21] Populations known to be at particularly high risk of pneumococcal disease or its complications (e.g., some Native Americans) are also vaccine candidates.

Based on available data, a single dose of vaccine is recommended for adults. However, revaccination should be considered for persons at highest risk of severe disease (1) if the individual previously received the 14-valent vaccine, (2) if the individual received the 23-valent vaccine more than 6 years previously, or (3) if the individual is from a group in which antibody levels may decline rapidly (e.g., persons with nephrotic syndrome or renal failure or transplant recipients).

Approximately 50% of vaccinees develop mild local side effects; fever, myalgias, and severe local reactions occur in fewer than 1%. Anaphylactic-type reactions have been reported very rarely. Because no data are available on the safety of this vaccine in pregnant women, immunization is optimally provided either before or after pregnancy to women who are vaccine candidates.

HEPATITIS B

More than 18,000 cases of hepatitis B were reported in the United States in 1991.[22] This number undoubtedly represents an underestimate of the problem due to incomplete reporting. Groups at particular risk of infection include immigrants and refugees from endemic areas, Alaskan natives or Pacific Islanders, residents and staff of institutions for the developmentally disabled, intravenous drug users, household contacts of hepatitis B carriers, sexual contacts of hepatitis B patients, hemodialysis patients, inmates of correctional facilities, heterosexually active persons with multiple sexual contacts, and health care workers who have blood contact. Serious sequelae of hepatitis B infection include long-term carriage of the virus, which occurs in approximately 6 to 10% of acutely infected adults.[23, 24] Long-term carriage is associated with a more than 300-fold increased risk of hepatocellular carcinoma.[25] Active hepatitis B infection in pregnant women who test positive for both hepatitis B surface antigen and hepatitis B e antigen results in transmission of the virus to 70 to 90% of newborns unless appropriate prophylaxis is provided.[23]

Vaccine should be offered to persons with risk factors for hepatitis B virus unless laboratory testing indicates prior infection. Recombinant hepatitis B vaccine, the currently available product, consists of hepatitis B surface antigen produced by a plasmid inserted into yeast. A primary vaccine series consists of three doses, with the second and third doses given 1 and 6 months, respectively, after the initial dose. Vaccine should be administered in the deltoid in adults; administration in the buttocks is associated with a lower response rate.[26] More than 90% of healthy adults develop protective levels of hepatitis B surface antibody following a primary series. However, persons who are undergoing hemodialysis or who are immunosuppressed may require either a higher vaccine dose or additional vaccine doses to develop an adequate response. Although booster doses are not recommended for normal, healthy adults based on current data, hemodialysis patients should have hepatitis B surface antibody levels assessed annually with a booster dose of vaccine given when levels decline to less than what is believed to be protective.

Soreness at the injection site is the most com-

monly reported side effect following immunization; other side effects are rare. Data are not available on the safety of hepatitis B vaccine in the fetus, but because the vaccine contains only inactivated particles, the risk is likely to be low. Pregnant women who are at high risk of exposure to hepatitis B and who are susceptible should be offered vaccine.

POLIO

The risk of poliomyelitis in the United States is very small, and most adults are already immune.[27] Therefore, a primary vaccine series is not recommended for the general adult population even if no documentation of receipt of a primary series of immunization as a child can be obtained. However, individuals who are traveling to areas in which the disease is endemic or epidemic and those who work in a specific medical occupation that may result in exposure to the virus may be at increased risk. For individuals in high-risk situations who are previously unvaccinated, enhanced inactivated polio vaccine (eIPV) is the vaccine of choice. A primary series consists of two doses given 4 to 8 weeks apart with a third dose given 6 to 12 months after the second dose. Persons at high risk who have completed a partial series of either eIPV or oral polio vaccine (OPV) should be given the remaining doses of vaccine to complete the series. A primary OPV series consists of two doses given 6 to 8 weeks apart with a third dose given 6 to 12 months after the second. Travelers to areas of risk who have previously completed a primary series of OPV should be given a booster dose of OPV. Those who have completed a primary series of inactivated polio vaccine should receive a dose of either OPV or eIPV.

Oral polio vaccine should not be given to immunosuppressed or immunocompromised persons. Furthermore, OPV should not be used to vaccinate household contacts of immunosuppressed or immunocompromised persons because of an association between OPV and paralysis among healthy recipients and their contacts. Unlike other live virus vaccine products such as MMR, antibody-containing blood products do not interfere with the immune response to OPV.

No serious side effects of eIPV have been documented. Because eIPV contains trace amounts of streptomycin and neomycin, persons with an immediate type hypersensitivity response to these agents should not be given eIPV. In general, vaccination of pregnant women should be avoided. However, pregnant women who require immediate protection against polio should be offered OPV rather than IPV.

RABIES

Rabies continues to be rare in the United States, but persons at risk include travelers to countries in which rabies is endemic, animal handlers, and laboratory personnel who work with the rabies virus. These individuals should be offered preexposure immunization with rabies human diploid cell vaccine (HDCV). This vaccine is available for intramuscular injection (injection volume 1.0 ml) and for intradermal injection (injection volume 0.1 ml); a complete series consists of three injections on days 0, 7, and 28. Persons at continuing risk of exposure should have rabies antibody titer periodically assessed and receive a booster dose of vaccine when levels fall below those believed to be protective.[28]

Rabies vaccine is also used for postexposure prophylaxis. In assessing the need for postexposure prophylaxis, consideration should be given to the type of exposure, the species of biting animal, and the circumstances of the biting incident. Unless the person has been immunized previously or has a prior documented adequate rabies titer, both human rabies immune globulin and a five-dose series of HDCV should be given. Those who were previously vaccinated or who have a previously documented adequate antibody titer require only two doses of HDCV. Only the intramuscular preparation is approved for postexposure situations.

Side effects following receipt of HDCV include swelling, itching, and pain in 74% of recipients, and mild systemic symptoms (headache, myalgias, abdominal pain, dizziness) in 5 to 40%. Following booster doses, up to 6% of recipients may develop an immune complex–mediated reaction with hives, itching, and angioedema. Corticosteroids may interfere with response to HDCV and should be avoided during preexposure prophylaxis. Chloroquine phosphate may also interfere with response to the vaccine.

MENINGOCOCCAL POLYSACCHARIDE

Meningococcal disease occurs sporadically in the United States, with serogroups B and C reported most frequently. Those at risk for meningococcal disease include persons with terminal complement component deficiencies, persons with asplenia, and travelers to areas in which meningococcal disease is endemic.

A single quadrivalent vaccine is licensed for use in the United States and may be indicated for persons in specific risk groups. Side effects of the vaccine consist mainly of local reactions.[5] Safety of the vaccine in pregnant women has not been established.

VACCINATION IN TRAVELERS

Travelers to certain geographic areas, particularly those who will be outside urban areas with tourist accommodations, may be candidates for additional vaccines, including plague, cholera, yellow fever, and typhoid. Some immunizations may be required for entry into specific countries. Requirements for immunization and information on disease risk in different geographic areas is generally available through state or local health departments.

CONSIDERATIONS IN PREGNANCY

Women of childbearing potential should be questioned about pregnancy before the administration of vaccines (Table 2–2). However, routine pregnancy testing before immunization is not recommended. Although immunization in general should be avoided during pregnancy, it is important to evaluate risks and benefits for each situation. When a vaccine is indicated in a pregnant woman, waiting until after the first trimester if possible is a reasonable step to minimize the risk of teratogenicity. Live viral vaccines are of particular concern because of a theoretic risk to the fetus; women who are pregnant or anticipate being pregnant within 3 months should not receive these products except in unusual circumstances. Risk to the fetus when a pregnant woman is inadvertently vaccinated is likely to vary according to the particular product that was administered, but data on the specific risk for some vaccines used during pregnancy are sparse. With rubella vaccine, risk to the fetus appears to be very small.[29] Inactivated products such as hepatitis B vaccine and tetanus diphtheria toxoids are unlikely to be a problem when given during pregnancy.

REFERENCES

1. Williams WW, Hickson MA, Kane MA, et al. Immunization policies and vaccine coverage among adults: The risk for missed opportunities. Ann Intern Med 1988;108:616.
2. Centers for Disease Control. Measles prevention: Recommendations of the Immunization Practices Advisory Committee (ACIP). MMWR 1989;38(No.S-9):1.
3. Centers for Disease Control. Measles surveillance—United States, 1991. MMWR 1992;41(No.SS-6):1.

TABLE 2–2. Use of Selected Immunobiologics in Pregnancy

IMMUNIZING AGENT	RISK FROM DISEASE TO PREGNANT WOMAN	RISK FROM DISEASE TO FETUS OR NEONATE	RISK FROM IMMUNIZING AGENT TO FETUS	INDICATIONS FOR IMMUNIZATION DURING PREGNANCY	DOSE SCHEDULE	COMMENTS
Hepatitis B (HB)	Possible increased severity during third trimester	Possible increase in abortion rate and prematurity; perinatal transmission may occur if mother is a chronic carrier or is acutely infected	None reported	Indications for prophylaxis not altered by pregnancy	1.0 ml intramuscularly at 0, 1, and 6 mo	Infants born to HB_sAg-positive mothers should receive 0.5 ml HB immune globulin as soon as possible after birth, plus 0.5 ml HB vaccine within 1 wk of birth; vaccine should be repeated at 1 and 6 mo
Influenza	Possible increase in mortality during epidemic of new antigenic strain	Possible increased abortion rate; no malformation confirmed	None confirmed	Usually recommended only for patients with serious underlying diseases; public health authorities to be consulted for current recommendation	Consult with public health authorities because recommendations change each year	Criteria for vaccination of pregnant women same as for all adults
Measles	Significant morbidity; low mortality (not altered by pregnancy)	Significant increase in abortion rate; may cause malformation	None confirmed	Contraindicated	One or two doses, depending on school or work status (see text)	Vaccination of susceptible women should be part of postpartum care
Meningococcus	No increased risk during pregnancy; no increase in severity of disease	Unknown	No data available on use during pregnancy	Indications not altered by pregnancy; vaccination recommended only in unusual outbreak situations	Public health authorities to be consulted	
Mumps	Low morbidity and mortality (not altered by pregnancy)	Probable increased rate of abortion in first trimester; questionable association of fibroelastosis in neonates	None confirmed	Contraindicated	Single dose	

Disease	Risk from disease to pregnant woman	Risk from disease to fetus or neonate	Risk from immunizing agent to fetus	Indications for immunization during pregnancy	Dose schedule	Comments
Pneumococcus	No increased risk during pregnancy; no increase in severity of disease	Unknown	No data available on use during pregnancy	Indications not altered by pregnancy; vaccine used only for persons at high risk	In adults one dose only, unless they are at highest risk of fatal infection or antibody loss; such persons may be revaccinated >6 yr after the first dose	
Poliomyelitis	No increased incidence in pregnancy but may be more severe if it does occur	Anoxic fetal damage reported; 50% mortality in neonatal disease	None confirmed	Not routinely recommended for adults in United States, except persons at increased risk of exposure	Primary: two doses of eIPV 4–8 wk apart and a third dose 6–12 mo after the second dose; two doses of OPV with a 6- to 8-wk interval and a third dose at least 6 wk later, customarily 8–12 mo later	OPV indicated for susceptible pregnant women traveling in endemic areas or in other high-risk situations; no data on safety of eIPV in pregnancy
Rabies	Near 100% fatality (not altered by pregnancy)	Determined by maternal disease	Unknown	Indications for prophylaxis not altered by pregnancy; each case considered individually	Public health authorities to be consulted for indications and dosage	
Rubella	Low morbidity and mortality (not altered by pregnancy)	High rate of abortion and congenital rubella syndrome	None confirmed	Contraindicated	Single dose	Teratogenicity of vaccine is theoretic, not confirmed to date; vaccination of susceptible women should be part of postpartum care
Tetanus and diphtheria toxoids	Severe morbidity; tetanus mortality, 60%; diphtheria mortality, 10% (both of which are not altered by pregnancy)	Neonatal tetanus mortality, 60%	None confirmed	Lack of primary series or no booster within past 10 yr	Primary: two doses at 1- to 2-mo interval with a third dose 6–12 mo after the second; booster: single dose every 10 yr after completion of the primary series	Updating of immune status should be part of antepartum care; unvaccinated women should be vaccinated, preferably after first trimester

eIPV, Enhanced inactivated polio vaccine; OPV, oral polio vaccine.
Adapted from Update on Adult Immunization: Recommendations of the Immunization Practices Advisory Committee (ACIP). MMWR 1991;40 (RR-12):82.

4. Atmar RL, Englund JA, Hammill H. Complications of measles during pregnancy. Clin Infect Dis 1992;14:217.

5. Centers for Disease Control. Update on adult immunization. MMWR 1991;40(No.RR-12):1.

6. Gustafson TL, Lievens AW, Brunell PA, et al. Measles outbreak in a fully immunized secondary-school population. N Engl J Med 1987;316:771.

7. Mathias RG, Meekison WG, Arcand TA, Schechter MT. The role of secondary vaccine failures in measles outbreaks. Am J Public Health 1989;79:475.

8. Wharton M, Cochi SL, Hutcheson RH, et al. A large outbreak of mumps in the post vaccine era. J Infect Dis 1988;158:1253.

9. Siegel M, Fuerst HT. Comparative fetal mortality in maternal virus diseases: A prospective study on rubella, measles, mumps, chickenpox, and hepatitis. N Engl J Med 1966;274:768.

10. Goodman AK, Friedman SM, Beatrice ST, Bart SW. Rubella in the workplace: The need for employee immunization. Am J Public Health 1987;77:725.

11. Stehr-Green PA, Cochi SL, Preblud SR, Orenstein WH. Evidence of increasing rubella seronegativity among adolescent girls. Am J Public Health 1990;80:88.

12. Centers for Disease Control. Rubella prevention: Recommendations of the Immunization Practices Advisory Committee (ACIP). MMWR 1990;39(No.RR-15):1.

13. Howson CP, Katz M, Johnston RB, Fineberg HV. Chronic arthritis after rubella vaccination. Clin Infect Dis 1992;15:307.

14. Koblin BA, Townsend TR. Immunity to diphtheria and tetanus in inner-city women of childbearing age. Am J Public Health 1989;79:1297.

15. Centers for Disease Control. Prevention and control of influenza: Recommendations of the Immunization Practices Advisory Committee (ACIP). MMWR 1992;41(No. RR-9):1.

16. Patriarca PA, Weber JA, Parker RA, et al. Efficacy of influenza vaccine in nursing homes: Reduction in illness and complications during an influenza A (H3N2) epidemic. JAMA 1985;253:1136.

17. Treanor JJ, Mattison R, Dumyati G, et al. Protective efficacy of combined live intranasal and inactivated influenza A virus vaccines in the elderly. Ann Intern Med 1992; 117:625.

18. Breiman RF, Spika JS, Navarro VJ, et al. Pneumococcal bacteremia in Charleston County, South Carolina: A decade later. Arch Intern Med 1990;150:1401.

19. Austrian R, Gold J. Pneumococcal bacteremia with especial reference to bacteremic pneumococcal pneumonia. Ann Intern Med 1964;60:759.

20. Centers for Disease Control. Pneumococcal polysaccharide vaccine. MMWR 1989;38:64.

21. DeMaria A, Browne K, Berk SL, et al. An outbreak of type 1 pneumococcal pneumonia in a men's shelter. JAMA 1980;244:1446.

22. Centers for Disease Control. Summary of notifiable diseases, United States, 1991. MMWR 1992;40:6.

23. Centers for Disease Control. Protection against viral hepatitis: Recommendations of the Immunization Practices Advisory Committee (ACIP). MMWR 1990;39:(No.RR-2):1.

24. Ganem D. Persistent infection of humans with hepatitis B virus: Mechanisms and consequences. Rev Infect Dis 1982;4:1026.

25. Beasley RP, Lin CC, Hwang LY, et al. Hepatocellular carcinoma and hepatitis B virus: A prospective study of 22,707 men in Taiwan. Lancet 1981;2:1129.

26. Centers for Disease Control. Suboptimal response to hepatitis B vaccine given by injection into the buttock. MMWR 1985;34:105.

27. Strebel PM, Sutter RW, Cochi SL, et al. Epidemiology of poliomyelitis in the United States one decade after the last reported case of indigenous wild virus-associated disease. Clin Infect Dis 1992;14:568.

28. Centers for Disease Control. Rabies prevention—United States, 1991: Recommendations of the Immunization Practices Advisory Committee (ACIP). MMWR 1991; 40(No.RR-3):1.

29. Centers for Disease Control. Rubella prevention: Recommendations of the Immunization Practices Advisory Committee (ACIP). MMWR 1990;39(No.RR-15):4.

Nutritional Requirements of Women

Clifford Lo

Women have particular nutritional concerns and nutritional needs. During childhood and adolescence, young women have distinct growth patterns and susceptibilities to nutritional problems such as obesity and anorexia nervosa. During pregnancy and lactation, women must provide for the growing fetus or child as well as for their own nutrition. Premenopausal and postmenopausal women are also at special risk for nutritional problems such as osteoporosis. Dietary factors have been related to breast cancer and other malignancies, and it has been estimated that approximately 35% of cancer deaths can be attributed to diet.[1, 2] Nutrition is also a major factor in the development of other chronic diseases such as coronary heart disease, diabetes, and dental caries that afflict many women. Excessive or inadequate intake of energy sources and many specific nutrients probably affects the majority of American women today despite increased consciousness and concern about nutrition.

Historically, nutritionists have been particularly concerned with malnutrition and nutritional deficiencies in the world. Although specific vitamin deficiency syndromes still occur in many parts of the world, classic deficiency diseases such as pellagra (niacin), beriberi (thiamin), scurvy (vitamin C), and rickets (vitamin D) are now quite uncommon in the United States. Although iron deficiency is still very common among certain groups of women, the typical American diet contains most nutrients in abundance, so that the majority of nutritional problems come from excessive intake rather than inadequate intake. Except in the case of special dietary restrictions or circumstances such as pregnancy, routine vitamin supplements are probably not necessary for most American women. Inadequate dietary intake of minerals such as calcium, iron, or fluoride is more likely to be a problem.

The typical American diet provides too much total fat, saturated fat, cholesterol, sugar, and sodium for optimal health. Approximately 20 million women, or 26% of all adult American women, and as many as 61% of African American women aged 45 to 54 are overweight,[3] leading to excess morbidity and mortality from coronary heart disease, hypertension, and diabetes. By contrast, 46% of American women[3, 4] try to lose weight by dieting or exercise, but many risk endangering their health with fad or crash diets while being unsuccessful in maintaining long-term weight loss. The social stigma of obesity contributes to body image problems, which in some young women leads to bulimia or anorexia.

The Food and Nutrition Board of the National Research Council of the National Academy of Science has periodically issued revisions of its recommended dietary allowances (RDA), which lists "levels of intake of essential nutrients . . . to be adequate to meet the known nutritional needs of practically all healthy persons."[5] These age- and sex-specific guidelines are listed in Table 3–1 and in general are lower for women than men, except during pregnancy and lactation. These levels have been set by expert panels that meet periodically and review published research by a variety of techniques such as absorption and balance studies.[6] They were first issued in 1941, and the emphasis was on avoiding deficiencies of specific nutrients by intentionally exceeding the nutrient requirements for most people; they generally do not address levels of overnutrition.

National nutrition surveys such as the Ten-State Nutrition Survey[7] and the Health and Nutrition Examination Surveys[8, 9] have identified specific nutritional problems in the American population by analyzing dietary, anthropometric, biochemical, and clinical variables of a large statistical sample (more than 10,000), concentrating on low-income groups at greater nutritional risk. Although few

TABLE 3–1. Food and Nutrition Board, National Academy of Sciences–National Research Council Recommended Dietary Allowances* Revised 1989

Designed for the maintenance of good nutrition of practically all healthy people in the United States

CATEGORY	AGE (years) OR CONDITION	WEIGHT† (kg)	(lb)	HEIGHT† (cm)	(in)	PROTEIN (gm)	FAT-SOLUBLE VITAMINS Vitamin A (μg RE)‡	Vitamin D (μg)§	Vitamin E (mg α-TE)∥	Vitamin K (μg)	WATER-SOLUBLE VITAMINS Vitamin C (mg)	Thiamin (mg)	Riboflavin (mg)	Niacin (mg NE)¶	Vitamin B₆ (mg)	Folate (μg)	Vitamin B₁₂ (μg)	MINERALS Calcium (mg)	Phosphorus (mg)	Magnesium (mg)	Iron (mg)	Zinc (mg)	Iodine (μg)	Selenium (μg)
Females	11–14	46	101	157	62	46	800	10	8	45	50	1.1	1.3	15	1.4	150	2.0	1200	1200	280	15	12	150	45
	15–18	55	120	163	64	44	800	10	8	55	60	1.1	1.3	15	1.5	180	2.0	1200	1200	300	15	12	150	50
	19–24	58	128	164	65	46	800	10	8	60	60	1.1	1.3	15	1.6	180	2.0	1200	1200	280	15	12	150	55
	25–50	63	138	163	64	50	800	5	8	65	60	1.1	1.3	15	1.6	180	2.0	800	800	280	15	12	150	55
	51+	65	143	160	63	50	800	5	8	65	60	1.0	1.2	13	1.6	180	2.0	800	800	280	10	12	150	55
Pregnant						60	800	10	10	65	70	1.5	1.6	17	2.2	400	2.2	1200	1200	320	30	15	175	65
Lactating	1st 6 mo					65	1300	10	12	65	95	1.6	1.8	20	2.1	280	2.6	1200	1200	355	15	19	200	75
	2nd 6 mo					62	1200	10	11	65	90	1.6	1.7	20	2.1	260	2.6	1200	1200	340	15	16	200	75

*The allowances, expressed as average daily intakes over time, are intended to provide for individual variations among most normal persons as they live in the United States under usual environmental stresses. Diets should be based on a variety of common foods in order to provide other nutrients for which human requirements have been less well defined.

†Weights and heights of Reference Adults are actual medians for the U.S. population of the designated age, as reported by NHANES II.

‡Retinol equivalents. 1 retinol equivalent = 1 μg retinol or 6 μg β-carotene.

§As cholecalciferol. 10 μg cholecalciferol = 400 IU of vitamin D.

∥α-Tocopherol equivalents. 1 mg d-α tocopherol = 1 α-TE.

¶NE (niacin equivalent) is equal to 1 mg of niacin or 60 mg of dietary tryptophan.

Reprinted with permission from National Academy of Sciences–National Research Council. Recommended Dietary Allowances. 10th ed. Copyright 1989 by the National Academy of Sciences. Courtesy of the National Academy Press, Washington, DC.

24

TABLE 3–2. Median Heights and Weights and Recommended Energy Intake

CATEGORY	AGE (years) OR CONDITION	WEIGHT (kg)	WEIGHT (lb)	HEIGHT (cm)	HEIGHT (in)	REE* (kcal/day)	MULTIPLES OF REE	AVERAGE ENERGY ALLOWANCE (kcal)† Per kg	AVERAGE ENERGY ALLOWANCE (kcal)† Per day‡
Females	11–14	46	101	157	62	1310	1.67	47	2200
	15–18	55	120	163	64	1370	1.60	40	2200
	19–24	58	128	164	65	1350	1.60	38	2200
	25–50	63	138	163	64	1380	1.55	36	2200
	51 +	65	143	160	63	1280	1.50	30	1900

*Calculation based on FAO equations, then rounded.
†In the range of light to moderate activity, the coefficient of variation is ±20%.
‡Figure is rounded.
REE, Recommended energy expenditure.
Reprinted with permission from National Academy of Sciences–National Research Council. Recommended Dietary Allowances. 10th ed. Copyright 1989 by the National Academy of Sciences. Courtesy of the National Academy Press, Washington, DC.

overt clinical signs of specific nutritional deficiency were found, the following problems in dietary intake and nutrition were highlighted:

- Of all women older than 45 years, 24.7% of all women and 32.4% of African American women were considered to be obese[8]
- Of females of all ages, 95% consumed less than recommended dietary intake of iron, and biochemical evidence of iron deficiency was found especially in young children and adolescents, with as many as 22% of African American children younger than 5 years having abnormal transferrin saturation[9]
- Of women older than 18, 56% received less than the recommended dietary intake of calcium[9]
- Up to 73% of women received less than the recommended intakes of vitamins A and C

In 1980, the Surgeon General of the U.S. Public Health Service issued a report that listed several goals and guidelines for the diet of Americans. In addition to recommending a varied diet and maintenance of a desirable weight, the report suggested avoiding excessive total fat, saturated fat, cholesterol, sodium, sugar, and ethanol. In women and children, increased dietary intake of calcium, iron, and fluoride was recommended.

ENERGY REQUIREMENTS

Because such a large percentage of American women are obese, knowing ideal body weight and approximate energy requirements of individuals patients is often of importance to primary care providers. Basal energy requirements can be measured by using a whole-body room direct calorim-

eter, expired gas indirect calorimetry ("metabolic cart"), or the doubly labeled water method. However, these methods are not available in most clinical settings, and standard equations have been devised that usually estimate basal metabolic rate within about 10 to 20%. The Harris-Benedict equation for women is

$$655 + 9.56 \times \text{weight(kg)} + 1.85 \times \text{height(cm)} - 4.68 \times \text{age(yr)}$$

The U.S. RDAs use the World Health Organization (1985) standards based on weight and age (Table 3–2). This basal metabolic rate must be adjusted for activity levels, which can range from a factor of 1.3 for a sedentary person to 2.0 for a very active person. A factor of 1.5 is usually used for bedridden hospitalized patients, and the RDAs use a factor of 1.5 to 1.7 depending on age.

If a patient is obese, ideal body weight is usually used for calculations of energy needs rather than actual weight. Ideal body weight for women can be estimated as

$$100 \text{ lb} + 5 \text{ lb per inch over 5 ft}$$

The most recent RDAs use reference data based on the NHANES II survey with the fifteenth, fiftieth, and eighty-fifth percentiles shown in Table 3–3.[4] This gives an RDA for females aged 11 to 50 of 2200 kcal per day and for females older than 51 of 1900 kcal per day. An extra 300 kcal per day are recommended for women in the second or third trimester of pregnancy for safe weight gain and an extra 500 kcal per day for lactating women.

It is interesting to note that an extra 200 kcal per day in dietary intake (equivalent of a doughnut) without a corresponding increase in activity

TABLE 3–3. Weights for Height of Adult Women in the United States*

HEIGHT cm (in)	WEIGHT, kg (lb) by PERCENTILE		
	15th	50th	85th
147 (58)	45 (99)	55 (122)	72 (159)
152 (60)	49 (107)	60 (132)	75 (164)
157 (62)	51 (112)	60 (132)	77 (170)
163 (64)	54 (118)	63 (139)	79 (175)
168 (66)	55 (122)	64 (141)	81 (179)
173 (68)	59 (130)	67 (148)	83 (184)
178 (70)	61 (133)	69 (152)	78 (171)
183 (72)			
188 (74)			
193 (76)			

*Unpublished data from NHANES II (1976–1980) provided by the National Center for Health Statistics. Values rounded to nearest whole number. Subjects were 18–74 years old. Height determined without shoes. Weight includes clothing weight, ranging from an estimated 0.09 to 0.28 kg (0.20 to 0.62 lb).

Reprinted with permission from National Academy of Sciences–National Research Council. Recommended Dietary Allowances. 10th ed. Copyright 1989 by the National Academy of Sciences. Courtesy of the National Academy Press, Washington, DC.

would theoretically lead to an increased weight of 18 lb of fat within a year. The typical American woman gains an average of a pound of weight per year after the age of 20.

PROTEINS AND AMINO ACIDS

Contrary to what some believe, the typical American diet contains more than adequate protein for nutritional needs, and the excess protein is usually excreted as nitrogen in the urine. Lean body mass is increased by exercise, not by excess protein intake. The typical American diet contains 11 to 14% of total calories as protein, with 48% from meat, fish, and poultry; 16 to 20% from cereal grains; 17% from dairy products; and 4% from eggs. Adult women typically consume 65 to 70 gm of protein per day.

Proteins are made up of amino acids containing nitrogen. About 16% of protein is nitrogen, so that 6.25 gm of protein contains 1 gm of nitrogen. Although amino groups are readily exchanged by transamination, certain essential amino acids cannot be synthesized by humans, including leucine, isoleucine, lysine, methionine, cystine, phenylalanine, tyrosine, tryptophan, threonine, valine, and possibly histidine, arginine, and taurine for infants.

Traditionally, protein requirements have been determined by nitrogen balance techniques, measuring urinary and fecal nitrogen excretion on a set protein intake over a period of time (usually 10–15 days) in a controlled situation. For a young male adult to stay in nitrogen balance, the mean protein intake is about 0.6 gm per kg per day, an amount that must be extrapolated to reach a figure for women because few studies have measured the protein needs of young women. The RDA for protein intake has been set generously at 0.8 gm per kg per day for adults older than 15 years, or about 44 to 50 gm per day for most adult women. An additional 10 gm per day are recommended during pregnancy and 12 to 15 gm per day during lactation.

Vegetarians, especially vegetarians who consume eggs and dairy products, can get enough protein in their diet by ingesting a wide variety of vegetables, cereals, and legumes. A wide variety usually ensures a favorable amino acid balance that may not be achieved with a more limited selection, which may lack one or more of the essential amino acids.

CARBOHYDRATES AND FIBER

Carbohydrates make up a major portion of caloric intake in most diets, with an average of 177 gm per day providing 46% of the energy in the diet of adult American women. There is no absolute requirement for carbohydrates in the diet, because glucose can be formed from glycerol or amino acids, but a carbohydrate-free diet often leads to ketosis and muscle protein breakdown. Of the total dietary carbohydrates, 41% comes from grain products, mostly complex starches; 28% from fruits and vegetables; and almost 25% from added sweeteners, mostly sucrose and corn syrup.[10] These added simple sugars are probably responsible for much of the dental caries found and especially those found in children. Dietary fibers are undigestible complex carbohydrates from plant cell walls such as cellulose, hemicellulose, and pectin. They hold water in the colon and promote softer, bulky stools, which may reduce constipation and other diseases such as diverticulosis, colon cancer, and cardiovascular disease. Therefore, one dietary goal is to reduce simple sugars in favor of complex carbohydrates and fiber.

LIPIDS

Dietary lipids consist mainly of triglycerides and cholesterol and make up about 37% of the caloric intake of Americans. They provide a concentrated form of energy, 9 kcal per gm, versus 4 kcal per gm for carbohydrates and protein. The saturated fats contain no double bonds and come mainly from animal sources (meats, milk, butter, and eggs), whereas the polyunsaturated fats come mainly from vegetable sources (e.g., corn oil, margarine). Linoleic acid, linolenic acid, and arachidonic acid are essential fatty acids for the formation of prostaglandins and cell membranes. Unlike other fatty acids, they cannot be synthesized by humans and must be supplied in the diet, although only 2 to 3% of total calories, or 3 to 6 gm per day, is probably sufficient.

Recent epidemiologic evidence suggests that diets lower in total fats, especially saturated fats and cholesterol, may reduce the risk of coronary heart disease and certain cancers, and the American Heart Association and American Cancer Society recommend a reduction of total fat to under 30% of dietary calories. Although these recommendations have had a considerable effect on modifying Americans' dietary choices, some warnings have also been raised concerning excessive amounts of unsaturated trans fatty acids, as found in margarine and some other vegetable oils, which may predispose to oxidant stress and free radical formation. Therefore, the wisest strategy is to select a variety of foods to avoid excess or deficiency of any particular category.

VITAMINS

Vitamins are a heterogeneous group of organic substances that are required in the diet in trace quantities because humans generally cannot synthesize them. They are present in most foods, especially in fresh fruits and vegetables, and, with a few possible exceptions, in sufficient quantities in typical American diets to prevent any widespread deficiency syndromes. The classic vitamin deficiency diseases such as pellagra (niacin deficiency), beriberi (thiamin), rickets (vitamin D), and scurvy (vitamin C) are rarely seen in the United States today but are still prevalent in some developing countries, where there may be an insufficient variety of grains or availability of fresh vegetables. In many American foods, vitamins are added as supplements, so that RDAs are usually exceeded; in most persons, excess vitamin intake is merely excreted in the urine. Therefore, it is usually not necessary to advise the use of vitamin supplements for healthy adults with unrestricted American diets, except for pregnant and lactating women, who should receive multivitamin supplements with special attention to folate (RDA 400 μg/day) and pyridoxine (vitamin B_6, RDA 2.2 mg/day). Certain vegetarian diets may be lacking in adequate vitamin B_{12}, which, like iron, is found mainly in foods of animal origin.

Considerable controversy has accompanied claims for preventive and therapeutic efficacy of megavitamin supplements. Certain vitamins, especially vitamins A, E, and C, have a role in epithelial differentiation or as antioxidants in reducing free radical formation and therefore may help prevent cancer. Most authorities dispute claims of therapeutic efficacy of megadoses of vitamin C in cancer.[11] There is more evidence for the preventive relationship of vitamin A to cancer because of its role in epithelial differentiation, but studies are not clear whether vitamin A or its precursor carotene is more important.

Most multivitamin supplements are probably harmless. One notable exception is vitamin A, which is stored in the liver and may lead to toxicity if ingested in excessive quantities, usually in the form of megavitamin supplements. Excessive dietary carotene may cause yellowing of the skin but does not lead to vitamin A toxicity. Likewise, very large excessive oral doses of vitamin D may lead to hypercalcemia, although skin production of vitamin D by exposure to sunlight does not. Megadoses of vitamin C may predispose to oxalate kidney stones. Toxicity is probably very rare with vitamin E and most of the water-soluble vitamins.

MINERALS

Minerals perform a wide variety of functions in the human body, from providing structural strength in the skeleton to serving as essential cofactors of metabolic reactions to conducting electrical signaling between muscle and nerve cells. Some, such as selenium and manganese, are trace elements that are present only in milligram quantities in the body; others make up a large proportion of the bone mass. Most are consumed in quantities far above the necessary minimum, so that dietary deficiencies are extremely rare; others, such as calcium, are underconsumed so that the RDAs are met only by a minority of the population.

Sodium is an example of a mineral that is ingested in quantities far above the necessary minimum, with American dietary intakes averaging 2 to 6 gm per day (5–15 gm of salt, including discretionary salt sprinkling) and some Asian diets ranging up to 25 gm (60 gm salt) per day. Almost all of this sodium is excreted in the renal glomeruli, with only a small percentage reabsorbed in the tubules according to hormonal control and fluid needs. Without excessive sweating and with adequate renal conservation, only about 115 mg per day of sodium (300 mg salt) is absolutely necessary under most conditions; the minimum RDA is 500 mg sodium (1.2 gm salt). Any excess can usually be excreted by the kidneys, but compensatory mechanisms may be impaired in patients with hypertension or congestive heart failure, so dietary goals suggest a reduction in daily intake to 2.4 gm (5 gm salt).

Potassium balance is also regulated closely by the kidneys, but deficiencies may occur with diuretic use, diabetes, diarrhea, vomiting, or laxative abuse. Potassium is widely distributed in foods, especially in fruits and vegetables. Dietary intakes range from as little as 1 gm per day in some urban blacks to 8 to 11 gm per day, with the minimum requirement for adults estimated at 1.6 to 2.0 gm per day.

Calcium forms the bulk of bone mineral where it is stored (about 1200 gm) but is also required for many cellular processes such as muscle contraction, nerve conduction, clotting, and enzyme function. Serum levels are regulated to a narrow range by several hormones, especially 1,25 dihydroxycholecalciferol and parathyroid hormone, so that dietary calcium deficiency results not in hypocalcemia but in osteopenia. Postmenopausal women experience rapid loss of bone mineral because of estrogen withdrawal and are particularly prone to osteoporosis and debilitating hip or spine fractures (see Chapter 62). Adequate calcium intake in childhood and adolescence is probably important in ensuring maximal peak bone mass to prevent premature osteoporosis. However, the average dietary intake of calcium, about 530 mg in adult American women, is far below the U.S. RDA of 800 mg (1200 mg for adolescence, pregnancy, and lactation). Supplemental calcium may also be helpful in adult women to avoid excessive bone loss.

Phosphorus is also a major component of bone mineral and participates in many metabolic processes, as in adenosine triphosphate (ATP). However, in contrast to calcium, it is widely distributed in most foods and is well absorbed in the intestinal tract, so dietary deficiency of phosphorus is rare in healthy adults. The average dietary intake of phosphorus is at least 1000 to 1500 mg per day and is often higher because of food additives in processed and convenience foods. The RDA is similarly 800 mg (1200 mg for adolescence, pregnancy, and lactation).

Magnesium is another mineral that plays a crucial role as an enzyme cofactor or activator, often in conjunction with ATP, although the bulk of magnesium is stored in bone or soft tissue (20–28 gm). Like phosphorus deficiency, dietary magnesium deficiency is rare in healthy adults and is usually only associated with diarrhea, renal dysfunction, malnutrition, alcohol abuse, or iatrogenic causes. The RDA is 4.5 mg per kg, or 280 mg for

adult women and 320 to 355 mg in pregnancy and lactation.

Iron deficiency is one of the most common nutrient deficiencies in women because of regular menstrual blood loss, with estimates of up to 14% of adult females having impaired iron status.[12] Iron stores are much lower in women than in men, averaging about 300 mg, and anemia may ensue when stores are depleted. Only 4% of women in national surveys actually had iron deficiency anemia with low hemoglobin levels, on an average intake of 10 to 11 mg per day of elemental iron. Heme iron from animal sources is absorbed better than nonheme iron, so those on vegetarian diets may be at more risk. The RDA has been set at 10 mg in children and 15 mg in adults, but increased needs in pregnancy, estimated at 30 mg, cannot be achieved easily in the diet, so daily iron supplements are recommended. Daily iron supplements up to 25 to 75 mg are probably safe in premenopausal women, but a certain percentage of the population is prone to iron overload or hemochromatosis so that extra iron may be deleterious after menopause.

Zinc and copper are essential components of many metalloenzymes. Although a zinc deficiency syndrome of hypogonadism and growth retardation has been described in Iran,[13] the most recognized form of zinc deficiency in the United States is the rare inherited syndrome of acrodermatitis enteropathica. Likewise, copper deficiency is rarely seen, mostly in patients on parenteral nutrition or in those with the rare inherited Menkes' kinky hair syndrome. Other essential trace elements include selenium, manganese, molybdenum, chromium, fluoride, iodine, and their RDAs are listed in Table 3–4.

SPECIAL REQUIREMENTS

Special mention should be made of certain nutrients that are often critical during certain stages of life in women.[14, 15] Ideally, infants should be fed breast milk, which provides the many nutrients and especially the high density of fat calories (55%) to sustain their rapid rate of growth. Even so, their iron and vitamin D status may be marginal. Cow's milk–based formulas are usually supplemented with vitamin D, but whole cow's milk should probably not be introduced before the age of 1 year because of the possibility of occult blood loss from the gastrointestinal tract.[16, 17] Gastrointestinal uptake of cow's milk proteins may provoke a wide range of allergic reactions in some infants,[18] but claims of delayed effects on subsequent devel-

TABLE 3–4.   Estimated Salt and Adequate Daily Dietary Intakes of Selected Vitamins and Minerals*

CATEGORY	VITAMINS	
	Biotin (μg)	Pantothenic Acid (mg)
Adults	30–100	4–7

CATEGORY	TRACE ELEMENTS†				
	Copper (mg)	Manganese (mg)	Fluoride (mg)	Chromium (μg)	Molybdenum (μg)
Adults	1.5–3.0	2.0–5.0	1.5–4.0	50–200	75–250

*Because there is less information on which to base allowances, these figures are not given in the main table of RDA and are provided here in the form of ranges of recommended intakes.

†Since the toxic levels for many trace elements may be only several times usual intakes, the upper levels for the trace elements given in this table should not be habitually exceeded.

Reprinted with permission from National Academy of Sciences–National Research Council. Recommended Dietary Allowances. 10th ed. Copyright 1989 by the National Academy of Sciences. Courtesy of the National Academy Press, Washington, DC.

opment of eczema and food allergies are controversial.[19]

In childhood, frequent growth monitoring (every 6–12 months) is the best way to prevent obesity or failure to thrive, as children's dietary habits and activity vary widely. The avoidance of excess simple sugars and the addition of fluoride (in the water supply or as a supplement) do much to prevent dental caries. It may be necessary to determine whether a local water supply has fluoride supplementation, as excess fluoride may promote teeth staining (fluorosis).

As adolescents undergo the pubertal growth spurt and menarche, they are all too frequently prone to cycles of binge eating (bulimia) and anorexia nervosa. They often prefer high-energy "junk" food, which should be balanced by exercise to prevent bad dietary habits from leading to obesity. Although not every obese adolescent becomes an obese adult, obesity in adolescence may be more predictive of later morbidity than obesity in adulthood.[20] There is some evidence that adequate calcium intake in adolescence may be beneficial in establishing maximal peak bone mass to prevent future osteoporosis.[21]

Pregnancy and lactation impose additional requirements on the nutrition of the mother, especially during the third trimester. A moderate weight gain of 15 to 25 lb during pregnancy is suggested, with daily supplements of vitamins and minerals, including iron (30 mg/day), calcium (total 1200 mg/day), folate (400 μg/day), and pyridoxine, as well as avoidance of smoking, alcohol, and drugs.

Adult women are now more conscious of their risk for coronary heart disease and various cancers, which probably can be substantially reduced by reducing the total fat in the diet to 30% or less of calories and especially in reducing saturated fats and cholesterol. Women should also be particularly aware of the need to meet requirements for iron and calcium in their diets. The high percentage of women who are obese, especially in lower socioeconomic groups, is of continued frustration both to the women and to the health care professionals. This group needs to be managed with both caloric restriction and exercise.

Postmenopausal women are particularly prone

TABLE 3–5.   Proportions of Cancer Deaths Attributed to Various Factors*

FACTOR OR CLASS OF FACTORS	PERCENT OF ALL CANCER DEATHS	
	Best Estimate	Range of Acceptable Estimates
Tobacco	30	25–40
Alcohol	3	2–4
Diet	35	10–70
Food additives	1	(−5†)−2
Reproductive and sexual behavior	7	1–13
Occupation	4	2–8
Pollution	2	1–5
Industrial products	1	1–2
Medicines and medical procedures	1	0.5–3.0
Geophysical factors	3	2–4
Infection	10?	1–7
Unknown	7	?

*It should be understood that these figures are speculative, and there is considerable uncertainty associated with them.

†Some factors (e.g., food fortification) may be protective.

From Surgeon General's Report on Nutrition and Health. Publication No. 88-50211. Washington, DC: Department of Health and Human Services, 1988.

TABLE 3–6. Reported Relationship Between Selected Dietary Components and Cancer

SELECTED CANCER SITES IN DESCENDING ORDER OF INCIDENCE	FAT	BODY WEIGHT AND CALORIES	FIBER	FRUITS AND VEGETABLES	ALCOHOL	SMOKED, SALTED, AND PICKLED FOODS
Lung				−	+ *	
Breast	+	+		−	+	
Colon	+	+	−	−		
Bladder				−		
Rectum	+				+	
Endometrium	+	+				
Oral Cavity				−	+	
Stomach				−		+
Kidney		+				
Cervix		+		−		
Thyroid		+				
Esophagus					+	+

*Synergistic with smoking.

+, Positive association; increased intake with increased cancer. −, Negative association; increased intake with decreased cancer.

From Surgeon General's Report on Nutrition and Health. Publication No. 88-50211. Washington, DC: Department of Health and Human Services, 1988.

to rapid bone loss that leads to osteoporosis, and although adequate calcium intake[22] and exercise may help prevent this, many authorities are also suggesting estrogen supplements (see Chapter 61). In addition, elderly women are at risk for many illnesses and nutritional deficiencies and may need to restrict sodium because of hypertension or heart disease.

It has been estimated that as much as 35% of cancer mortality can be attributed to diet[1] (Table 3–5). Many international epidemiologic comparisons show an association of breast and colon cancer with increased dietary fat, but it is not clear whether certain types of fat (saturated fats, trans-fatty acids, or cholesterol) or kinds of food (e.g., meat, butter) are more important or what mechanisms are involved[23–27] (Table 3–6). Indeed, excess caloric intake and obesity may also be partly responsible for these cancers and those of the kidney, cervix, and thyroid. Excessive alcohol intake may also increase the risk of developing breast or colon cancer as well as head and neck cancers. However, increasing dietary fiber, especially by eating fruits and vegetables, may reduce the incidence of colon and other cancers.

Although vitamins A, C, and E and selenium probably play a protective role against oxidant stress and some cancers, it is too early to recommend widespread dietary supplementation, because it is not clear that benefits outweigh risks.

Much is still to be learned about the nutritional requirements of women and the relationship of diet to disease, but tremendous progress has been made in the last few years, both in identifying specific

goals that women can reliably follow and in actually modifying the diets of American women. These goals are to eat a variety of foods; maintain desirable weight; avoid too much fat, saturated fat, and cholesterol; eat foods with adequate starch and fiber; and avoid excess sugar, sodium, and alcohol.[2]

REFERENCES

1. Doll R, Peto R. The causes of cancer: Quantitative estimates of avoidable risks of cancer in the United States today. J Natl Cancer Inst 1981;66:1191.
2. The Surgeon General's Report on Nutrition and Health. DHHS (PHS) Publication No. 88-50210. Washington, DC: US Department of Health and Human Services Public Health Service, 1988, p 180.
3. The Surgeon General's Report on Nutrition and Health. DHHS (PHS) Publication No. 88-50210. Washington, DC: US Department of Health and Human Services Public Health Service, 1988, p 278.
4. Stephenson MG, Levy AS, Saas NL, McGavvey WE. 1985 NIHS findings: Nutrition knowledge and baseline data for the weight-loss objectives. Health Rep 1987;102:61.
5. National Research Council Subcommittee on the Tenth Edition of the RDAs: Recommended Dietary Allowances. 10th ed. Washington, DC: National Academy of Sciences, 1989.
6. Irwin MI. Nutritional Requirements of Man: A conspectus of Research. New York: The Nutrition Foundation, 1980.
7. Ten State Nutrition Survey: 1968–1970. DHEW Publication No. (HSM). Washington, DC: US Department of Health, Education and Welfare, 1972, p 72.
8. Preliminary Findings of the First Health and Nutrition Examination Survey, United States, 1971–1972: Dietary Intake and Biochemical Findings. DHEW Publication No. (HRA) 75-1229. Rockville, Md: US Department of Health, Education and Welfare, Public Health Service, 1975.
9. Preliminary Finding of the First Health and Nutrition Ex-

amination Survey, United States, 1971–1972: Anthropometric and Clinical Findings. DHEW Publication No. (HRA) 75-1229. Rockville, Md: US Department of Health, Education, and Welfare, Public Health Service, 1975.

10. National Research Council Subcommittee on the Tenth Edition of the RDAs: Recommended Dietary Allowances. 10th ed. Washington, DC: National Academy of Sciences, 1989, p 40.

11. Moertel CG, Fleming TR, Creagan ET, et al. High-dose vitamin C versus placebo in the treatment of patients with advanced cancer who have had no prior chemotherapy. N Engl J Med 1985;312:137.

12. Expert scientific working group. Summary of a report on assessment of the iron nutritional status of the United States population. Am J Clin Nutr 1985;42:1318.

13. Prasad AS. Clinical manifestations of zinc deficiency. Ann Rev Nutr 1985;5:341.

14. Winick M, ed. Nutritional Disorders of American Women. New York: John Wiley & Sons, 1977.

15. Moghissi KS, Evans TN (eds). Nutritional Impacts on Women. Hagerstown, Md: Harper & Row, 1977.

16. Fomon SJ, Ziegler EE, Nelson SE, Edwards BB. Cow milk feeding in infancy: Gastrointestinal blood loss and iron nutritional status. J Pediatr 1981;98:540.

17. Ziegler EE, Fomon SJ, Nelson SE, et al. Cow milk feeding in infancy: Further observations on blood loss from gastrointestinal tract. J Pediatr 1990;116:11.

18. Bahna S, Heiner D. Allergies to Milk. New York: Grune & Stratton, 1980.

19. Kramer MS, Moroz B. Do breast-feeding and delayed introduction of solid foods protect against subsequent atopic eczema? J Pediatr 1981;98:546.

20. Must A, Jacques PF, Dallal GE, et al. Long-term morbidity and mortality of overweight adolescents: A follow-up of the Harvard growth study of 1922 to 1935. N Engl J Med 1992;327:1350.

21. Johnston CC, Miller JZ, Slemenda CW, et al. Calcium supplementation and increases in bone mineral density in children. N Engl J Med 1992;327:82.

22. Reid IR, Ames RW, Evans MC, et al. Effect of calcium supplementation on bone loss in postmenopausal women. N Engl J Med 1993;328:460.

23. Committee on Diet, Nutrition, and Cancer. Diet Nutrition and Cancer. Washington, DC: National Academy Press, 1982, p 55.

24. Winick M (ed). Nutrition and Cancer. New York: John Wiley & Sons, 1977.

25. London S, Willett W. Diet and the risk of breast cancer. Hematol Oncol Clin North Am 1989;3:559.

26. Willet WC, Stampfer MJ, Culditz GA, et al. Relation of meat, fat, and fiber intake to the risk of colon cancer in a prospective study among women. N Engl J Med 1990;323:1664.

27. Willett WC, MacMahon B. Diet and cancer—An overview. N Engl J Med 1984;310:633.

4

Adolescent Issues

Linda M. Grant

Adolescence is a period of unique growth in an individual's life. Biologically, the adolescent experiences major changes in her body, different from any growth she has experienced before. Emotionally and psychologically, she gradually develops the capacity to think critically, to develop relationships, and to make independent decisions that will have an impact on her future health. This growth can span a decade and challenge the medical practitioner to keep pace with the development.

Medical practitioners who care for adolescents must be aware of this uniqueness. Adolescents are neither big children nor little adults. Pediatricians accustomed to problem solving with parents must learn to interact with the adolescent and deal with a new repertoire of medical conditions, traditionally more familiar to the internist. The internist, comfortable with the medical problems of adolescents, must deal with the psychosocial and cognitive limitations of the age group and accept the adolescent as different from the adult patient. Effective work with adolescents requires interest, sensitivity, flexibility, and patience, as well as a strong knowledge of the developmental process.

Adolescence is, in general, a period relatively free of system pathology. Adolescents have survived the risks of infectious disease and congenital defects of childhood and have not yet developed the chronic medical conditions of adulthood. This makes each medical encounter an opportunity to prevent the development of detrimental habits and morbid conditions of adulthood.

At the same time that adolescents enjoy a period of relative physical health, they are burdened with a relatively high mortality rate. The reason for this is rooted in adolescent behavior. Adolescent pregnancy, violence between or among adolescents, sexually transmitted diseases, accidents, and suicide are all the results of behavioral actions. Even when an adolescent has a chronic illness such as diabetes or asthma, the psychosocial and behavioral issues predominate and interfere with management of the disease.

Although adolescent males have higher mortality rates from homicide, suicide, and motor vehicle accidents, adolescent females bear a disproportionate morbidity from other behaviors. More than 50% of adolescent girls are sexually experienced by their eighteenth birthday. This has led to an increase in the nonmarital birth rate among adolescents younger than 20 years of 300% for whites and 16% for blacks over the last 40 years. In that same period, cases of reported gonorrhea among 15- to 19-year-old females have increased almost 40%, and 4% of 15 to 19 year olds terminate pregnancies each year.

Although the rates of physical and emotional abuse are very similar for males and females, rates of sexual abuse are four times greater for females. Adolescent females consistently report higher rates of sad feelings than males. And although males are four times more likely to complete a suicide, adolescent girls are four to five times more likely to attempt it. Boys and girls have equal rates of trying alcohol and drugs, but adolescent females have a higher daily smoking rate—up to 20% of female high school seniors in 1987.

Therefore, to prevent adolescent females from becoming statistics, the practitioner must take an active role in screening for the antecedents of high-risk behavior and in guiding adolescents toward more health-enhancing behaviors.

There is some debate as to the optimal frequency of health care visits during adolescence. The guidelines of the American Academy of Pediatrics recommend screening at ages 10, 12, 14, 16, 18, and 20. Other practitioners recommend annual assessment for non–sexually active adolescents to update the ever-changing risk-profile. For the sexually active adolescent, it is prudent, especially in areas of high rates of sexually transmitted diseases (STDs), to examine the adolescent female every 6 months to monitor for asymptomatic STDs and discuss sexual risk taking. Most practitioners agree that waiting for the adolescent to seek services is rarely as effective as scheduling routine visits.

THE SETTING

Because adolescents are not, in general, active health consumers, every effort should be made to market appropriate health services to them. For adolescents, an office crowded with mothers and infants is not as appealing as one filled with peers or even adult patients. This issue can be solved by having separate adolescent appointment hours after school or in the evening. The availability of brochures geared to sensitive teen issues in the waiting area helps to create an atmosphere friendly to adolescents. They set a tone of a safe environment where these topics may be discussed.

In the last decade, schools have gained prominence as a setting for adolescent health services. Many school systems across the country have developed school-based and school-linked services with the intent of making health care more accessible. Services in the schools range from extended diagnostic support for the school nurse to comprehensive health services, including mental health. Although this system works only for students, it is still an improvement over waiting for adolescents or parents or guardians to recognize and utilize services.

THE INITIAL VISIT

The key to engaging adolescents is to provide a nonjudgmental atmosphere of trust, confidentiality, openmindedness, and sincerity. For adolescents to share the intimate details of their lives, they must be assured that this will not put their relationships with their family, friends, or the community at risk. Adolescents often resist medical visits with their childhood providers because they fear that the information will be shared with their parents.

Whenever possible, an initial interview and physical examination should be scheduled for 40 to 60 minutes. If this is not possible within the constraints of the practice, consider dividing the visit into two sessions.

CONFIDENTIALITY

It is important to establish ground rules for the adolescent and her family before any personal discussions ensue. This is most easily accomplished by addressing the patient and family together at the first appointment. If the adolescent and the family are new to the practitioner, this interview serves as an introduction to the philosophy of the clinic. If the parent is a patient of the practitioner and is requesting services for a child, the practitioner must explicitly clarify that the relationship with the daughter will be confidential and separate and information will not necessarily be shared.

Confidentiality, however, is not absolute. There are four areas in which confidentiality must be waived (1) if the patient is suicidal and is in immediate danger of hurting herself, (2) if the patient is making threats against another and is felt to be homicidal, (3) if there is sexual or physical abuse that the law mandates reporting, or (4) if there is a life-threatening illness (Table 4–1). These guidelines are the least restrictive recommendations for the practitioner. The practitioner should be aware of the laws in his or her own state regarding adolescent confidentiality and parental notification.

RIGHTS OF MINORS

Legally, the care of minors generally requires consent of the parents or guardian. When parents agree with the provider to accept the previously mentioned guidelines, they are consenting to this approach. However, when an adolescent presents for care without a parent, issues may arise. The categories of mature and emancipated minor are meant to address the circumstances of treating a child without parental consent.

In most states, an adolescent is considered to be emancipated if she is married, pregnant, in the armed services, or living independently from the family unit. Many states have waivers for specific issues such as pregnancy-related care, diagnosis and treatment of STDs, contraception, substance abuse, and mental health. In these circumstances, an adolescent can consent to treatment without parental notification. Care for life-threatening events may also be performed without any consent (Table 4–2).

The concept of mature minor is less clearly defined. The profile of a mature minor is that of an adolescent who, although supported by a parental

---

TABLE 4–1.   Limits of Confidentiality in Adolescence

Confidentiality may be waived
1. If the patient is suicidal and is in immediate danger of hurting herself.
2. If the patient is making threats against another and is felt to be homicidal.
3. If there is sexual or physical abuse that the law mandates reporting.
4. If there is a life-threatening illness.

TABLE 4–2 Legal Guidelines for Minors by State

STATE	AGE OF MAJORITY (yr)	MAY CONSENT FOR MEDICAL CARE			MAY CONSENT FOR			
		In General Conditions (E = emancipated) (M = married)	Emergency (X = yes) (O = not required in emergencies)	Contraception (X = yes)	Pregnancy-Related	VD Care	Substance Abuse	Other
Alabama	18	Age 14, or M or E; parent; divorced	O		X	X	X	
Alaska	18	M or E	X		X	X		Rape—age 12
Arizona	18	M or E	X, if parents unavailable			X	Age 12	
Arkansas	18	M or E	O	X	X	X		
California	18	M or E (age 15)	X	X	X	Age 12	X	Rape—age 12
Colorado	18	M or E (age 15)	O	X		X	X	Mental health—age 15
Connecticut	18	M				Age 12	X	
Delaware	18	M	X, if parents unavailable		Age 12	Age 12		
District of Columbia	18					X (notify parents)	X	
Florida	18		O	X, if likely to face health hazards if services not rendered	X	X	X	Mental health—age 12
Georgia	18	M	O	X	X	X	X	
Hawaii	18	M		X	Age 14	Age 14	X	
Idaho	18		O	X		Age 14	Age 16	
Illinois	18	M or pregnant	O	X, if limit to access would have an adverse effect on health	X	Age 12	Age 12	Mental health—age 14
Indiana	18	M or E	O			X	X	
Iowa	18	M	O			X	X	
Kansas	18 or M (age 16)	M or E	O		X	X	X	
Kentucky	18	M or E	O	X	X	X	X	
Louisiana	18	M	O		X	X	X	
Maine	18					X	X	Mental health—age 16
Maryland	18	M, parent	X	X	X	X	X	
Massachusetts	18	M or E	O		X	X	X, if 2 doctors agree	Mental health—age 16

State	Age of majority	Exceptions						
Michigan	18	M; parent; court action; armed services				Age 12	X	
Minnesota	18	M or E	O			X	X	
Mississippi	18	M or E; sufficient intelligence	O	X, if referred by physician, clergy, school, governmental agency, or family-planning clinic		X	Age 15	Urgent psychiatric treatment
Missouri	21	18 or M; parent	O			X	X	
Montana	18	M or E; parent; high school graduate	O	X	X	X	X	
Nebraska	19 or M	M	O		X	X	X	
Nevada	18	M or E; parent	X		X	X	X	
New Hampshire	18	M	O		Age 14	Age 14	Age 12	
New Jersey	18	M or E	O		X	X	X	Mental health
New Mexico	18	M or parent	O	X	X	X	X	Mental health
New York	18	E	O	X	X	X	Alcohol	
North Carolina	18		X	X	X	X	X	
North Dakota	18		X		Age 14	Age 14	Age 14	
Ohio	18				X	X	X	
Oklahoma	18	M or E; parent; armed services	X	X		X	X	
Oregon	18	15 or M		X	Age 12	Age 12	X	
Pennsylvania	18	M; pregnant; high school graduate	O	X	X	X	X	
Rhode Island	18	M or 16 (except surgery)	16 or M		X	X		
South Carolina	18		O		X			
South Dakota	18		O		X	X	Alcohol	
Tennessee	18		O	X	X	X	X	
Texas	18, M or E	E (age 16); armed services		X	X	X	Age 13	
Utah	18, M	M		X	X	X	Age 12	
Vermont	18				X	Age 12	X	
Virginia	18	M	X	X	X	X	Age 14	Mental health
Washington	18	M	O		Age 14	Age 14	X	
West Virginia	18				X	X	X	
Wisconsin	18				X	X	X	
Wyoming	19	M	X		X	X	X	

From Neinstein L: Legal issues. In: Adolescent Health Care. 2nd ed. Baltimore, Urban & Schwarzenberg, 1991, p 123. Copyright Williams & Wilkins, 1991.

figure, functions independently of the family on most decisions, contributes significantly to her own financial stability, and is able to initiate and follow through on health care interventions. Circumstances may reveal that she cannot communicate either meaningfully or safely with her parents. Likewise, an adolescent can refuse consent to treatment under the same constructs. Even in states without a specific consent law for minors, physicians have never been sued for providing an adolescent with contraceptives without parental consent.

Consent issues are more likely to arise when the adolescent expects to be rebuked by an angry parent. When an adolescent is seen for routine care or an acute nonconfidential complaint, it is optimal to include the parent in the treatment plan. Whatever the consent situation, adolescents should always be encouraged to discuss their issues with their parents.

The practitioner can facilitate better communication between adolescent and parent through the following approaches. Once the parent is aware of and agrees to the guidelines of confidentiality, the interview can begin with a joint discussion of the reasons for the visit. This affords an excellent opportunity to observe the interactions between parent and child, providing an insight into family dynamics and the reasons for risk-taking behaviors. Then the parent, having been prepared that the child will need some private time alone with the practitioner, can be asked to leave the room before sensitive questioning. The parent may also want some time to talk to the physician privately, and the practitioner needs to offer this opportunity to the parent.

DEVELOPING RAPPORT

The first 5 minutes alone with the adolescent patient are absolutely crucial to the bonding process. In those first few moments, the adolescent judges whether the practitioner is sympathetic to and understanding of her needs. Body language, eye contact, and a conversational tone are very important to an adolescent. Emphasis should be on maximal listening and minimal writing so that the adolescent feels as though she has the practitioner's undivided attention.

It is helpful to preface the interview with an acknowledgment that some of the questions may appear to be intrusive or may seem not to have a bearing on the presenting complaint. An explanation that the questions help the practitioner understand and get to know the adolescent is useful. Questions need to be open ended, such as ''Tell me about your family'' instead of ''Is everything all right at home?'' Open-ended questions allow for discussion, whereas yes-no questions or leading questions may limit information. Above all, the tone of the questioning must be nonjudgmental. The adolescent must be separated from her behavior. However, this does not mean that practitioners cannot express their concerns about an adolescent's behavior. It simply means that the practitioner needs to be sensitive to the antecedents of the behavior and honest in the presentation of the risks associated with the behavior. Adolescents are looking for guidance and support rather than paternalistic dictates.

ADOLESCENT DEVELOPMENT

To provide guidance effectively, the practitioner needs to be aware of adolescent development (Table 4–3). Adolescence is a period of high-risk behavior, much of which has direct impact on an adolescent's health. Substance abuse, pregnancy, violence, and acquired immunodeficiency syndrome (AIDS), all have a behavioral common pathway, which varies depending on the developmental level of the adolescent.

Adolescence is generally defined by the individual's ability to master several tasks: individuation and emancipation, acceptance of a new physical and emotional identity, and emergence of a cognitive thought process involving abstract reasoning and complex decision making. These tasks are accomplished in stages that reflect three relatively distinct periods: early, middle, and late adolescence. The underpinning of each of these stages is risk taking. At no other time in life is risk as prominent as in adolescence when the relative lack of experience in judgment further amplifies the risk. Each of these periods has different hallmarks, with progress toward achievement, building on the previous stage's experience. Because of this, health promotion strategies that may work with older adolescents are usually ineffective with adolescents just experiencing puberty. The practitioner should, therefore, be aware of these different stages.

Early Adolescence

The hallmark of early adolescence is adjustment to a new physical identity. With the development of secondary sex characteristics of puberty comes a preoccupation with a new body and a coming to terms with the disruption of one's former body image. In addition, cognitive thinking is concrete,

TABLE 4–3. Anticipatory Guidance

ADOLESCENCE	MEDICAL	DEVELOPMENTAL
		HEADS should be done at least once a year and specific areas reviewed more frequently as needed.
Early Early Puberty 10–12 yr	• Height, weight, and vital signs • Breast asymmetry is normal; teach BSE • Menarche preparation • Scoliosis screening prior to growth spurt peak • Vision screening • Auditory screening • MMR #2, PPD (if not recently) • Dental review • Height, weight, and vital signs • Acne	• Masturbation is a normal behavior that relieves sexual tension • Body disproportions distort self-image; early maturers at risk for early sex activity • Dietary-nutrition reviewed • Discussion of tampons and pads • Physical activity encouraged • Independence needs acknowledged • Safety issues; bicycle helmet • Parental discussions on decision making, respect for privacy, communication; sexuality dialogues
Late Puberty 12–14 yr	• Menstrual irregularity—usually anovulatory • Weight control—screen for bulimia and anorexia • Sports fitness	• Discussions of risk-taking behaviors and suggestion of alternative behaviors • Assessment of sexuality knowledge • Social skill assessment; dating concerns • Parental discussions on negotiating rules, periods of estrangement, allowing decision making, supervision, role modeling
Middle 14–17 yr	• Height, weight, and vital signs • Contraception • Sexually transmitted diseases (STDs) • Routine pelvic examination (if sexually active) every 6 mo (in high STD area) • GC, chlamydia every 6 mo • PAP, VDRL annual • Pubertal completion • Cholesterol and triglyceride check if parent died of heart disease	• Discussions of drinking and driving • Development of decision-making skills • Relationship issues: intimacy • Safety issues repeated • Parental discussions on accepting teen's independence, encouraging self-responsibility
Late 18–21 yr	• Check for completeness of immunization status • Height, weight, and vital signs	• Discussing future plans (e.g., work, marriage, college) • Planning health care (e.g., termination if seeing a pediatrician) • Dealing with being away from home • Dealing with college or work group peer pressure • Relationship involves mutual reciprocity; couple discussions with feelings

HEADS, Home, education, activities, affect, ambition, anger, drugs, sex; BSE, breast self-examination; MMR, measles-mumps-rubella; PPD, purified protein derivative; STD, sexually transmitted disease; GC, gonorrhea; PAP, Papanicolaou smear; VDRL, Veneral Diseases Research Laboratory titer.

with limited ability to discern complicated cause and effect scenarios. Although their academic decision making may be of a higher order, in social situations, young adolescents are inexperienced and their decisions are emotionally driven. Therefore, young adolescents, although striving for independence, still require strong guidance and limits.

Nowhere in adolescence is there such physical variability as in this period of early middle school. Although early puberty and physical maturation may carry distinct advantages for males in a society that highly values sports achievements, early

maturation in females is associated with problems in adaptation and self-esteem. Girls who mature early are not only set apart from their peers and subject to ostracism but also are more at risk for early sexual initiation as they become differentially attractive to older adolescent boys.

Middle Adolescence

By middle adolescence, the new physical identity has become well established, the repertoire of social experiences has expanded, and the ability to understand cause and effect has begun to develop. Peer influences, although not replacing parental influences, begin to have increasing prominence in the adolescent's decision making. This often coincides with a greater degree of autonomy both in the home as well as in society. Adolescents at this age begin to experience that others are affected by their actions and may appreciate this power of being acknowledged and becoming "significant."

In young adolescents, same sex peer groups are the norm, while the adolescent consolidates gender identity issues. As the adolescent matures, the same sex peer group may become less influential than a single partner. Males and females use their peer groups differently. In sexual decision making, for example, boys seek support for their decisions from their peers. Girls, however, look to their partners for their sexual decision making, using their peer group's perceived sexuality as a roadmap for guiding their own sexual experiences.

Late Adolescence

By late adolescence, cognitive thinking has attained adult levels, and the adolescent is able to think abstractly and make sophisticated decisions based on complicated constructs. This culminates in a strong sense of identity and individuality in both males and females. However, there is also evidence that since early childhood, males and females have been forging separate, distinct identities and perspectives that follow them through adult life. Young adult women define themselves in a context of human relationships and judge themselves in their ability to care. Young adult men judge themselves on the basis of their competitive success and define themselves in relation to their positional social orientation. Therefore, understanding the psyche of an adolescent female requires not only an appreciation of growth over time, but also of differential growth by gender and an appreciation of the importance of relationships in this framework.

With these developmental stages in mind, the practitioner should (1) develop a risk profile, based on information gathered, (2) try to determine what need the risk behavior is fulfilling, (3) provide concrete guidance and suggestions for an alternative response that more safely meets those needs, and (4) focus on the benefits of the alternative behavior in the present rather than focusing on long-range benefits.

THE INTERVIEW

The interview should contain the usual information on past medical history, family history, and history of present illness; however, the psychosocial history is the most important part of the adolescent interview. It is this information that describes the adolescent's lifestyle and provides clues to her compliance with medical regimens, her ability to comprehend her problem, and the extent to which she engages in risk-taking behavior. The problems facing adolescents are largely psychosocial and behavior based, and every encounter needs to include a screening update on these behaviors. An annual psychosocial examination is at least as important as a yearly physical examination.

The HEADS system, which was originated in 1972 by D. Harvey Berman, has been utilized and augmented by many adolescent providers as a screening tool for psychosocial issues (Table 4–4). Each letter stands for a psychosocial area that has a significant impact in an adolescent's life: *H*ome, *E*ducation, *A*ctivities, *A*ffect, *A*mbition, *A*nger, *D*rugs, *S*ex. Each area has a set of questions designed to help the provider assess the adolescent's functioning and risk-taking behavior. Often, the adolescent is unaware that she has any risk behaviors or that help may exist for problems that she thought were hopeless. Based on the responses, the practitioner develops a risk profile of the patient and can then offer appropriate interventions.

Home

These questions assess the stability of the home situation. The home is where the adolescent develops her value system and her sense of support. Questions should be directed toward screening for abusive situations, intrafamilial conflicts, familial patterns of behavior (such as alcoholism or depression), and family cohesiveness. Absence of a parent should be gently probed. The absence may be related to parental alcohol or substance abuse, and this in turn presents a risk factor for the child. Questions such as "How does your family deal with discipline?" or "What does home mean to you?" provide more information than directed questions such as "Are there problems at home?"

Education

The second most important place of socialization and support is the school. Screening should focus on school absenteeism, school performance, and the presence of possible learning disabilities or attention deficit disorder. In the larger cities, school absenteeism and dropout rates are almost

Table 4–4. Psychosocial Assessment of Adolescents

HEADS	OBJECTIVE	QUESTIONS
Home	To assess stability, interpersonal violence in the home, support systems	What is home to you? Who lives there? How do your family members get along? What number child are you? What are your home responsibilities? Does anyone at home fight physically with anyone else? How do people in your family deal with problems? If you could change one thing about home, what would it be? Do you know if there are any money worries at home? Can you tell me about any recent problems in your home?
Education	To assess school performance and attendance, the role of school in the child's life	Are you in school? Where? If not, what are you doing with your time? How much school did you miss last semester? Why? What are your favorite subjects? What are your least favorite subjects? Are you having any difficulties? What kind of grades do you get in school?
Activities	To assess developmental milestones, such as separation from family, identification with peers; signs of depression	(If in school) What do you do after school? Do you have an after school job? Do you have friends you mostly group with? Do you have a best friend? What's his or her name? What activities do you do together? Do your parents (guardian, etc.) approve of your friends? Do you wear seatbelts in cars? Do you wear a helmet when you ride a bike? Have you had a problem with the law?
Affect	To assess current affect (chances are, if they seem depressed, they are), body language	Does the patient make eye contact with interviewer?* Does the patient fidget throughout interview? Does the patient appear: • hostile • depressed • disoriented • silly • physically uncomfortable? Does the patient initiate questions? Does the patient respond with yes or no only? Have you ever felt so sad you felt like hurting yourself?
Ambition	To assess future orientation	What do you want to do in 5 years (or after high school/college)
Anger	To assess risks of violence in patient's life	How do you deal with your anger? (fight, hit, yell, cry, withdraw) How do people in your family deal with anger? Have you ever been physically hurt by someone out of anger? Have you ever hurt someone yourself out of anger? Do you carry a weapon?
Drugs	To assess history of family and patient substance use	Does anyone in your family smoke cigarettes? If so how much? Does anyone in your family drink alcohol? Do you think anyone in your family drinks too much? Does anyone in your family do drugs? When you are with your friends, do they ever drink or do drugs? How many cigarettes have you had in the last week; month; year; ever tried? How much alcohol have you had to drink in the last week; month; year; ever tried? How much marijuana have you had in the last week; month; year; ever tried? How much cocaine have you had in the last week; month; year; ever tried? How much of other substances of potential abuse have you had in the past week; month; year; ever tried? Have you ever tried intravenous drugs? Do you use substances and drive? Have you ever felt bad about your drinking or drug use? Have you ever done something stupid while on drugs? What was it? Do you ever drink or do drugs alone? Do you ever drink to calm down or relax?
Sex	To assess sexual activity and high-risk behaviors	Are you currently in a relationship? Does this relationship include intercourse? Do you use any protection? (Do you know what it means?) Have you ever had any sexually transmitted disease? How many partners have you had? How old were you when you first had intercourse? Has anyone ever forced you to have sex? Have you ever been pregnant? Tell me what you know about AIDS? Have you ever had sex with someone of the same sex? Have you ever had rectal or oral sex? Is sex an enjoyable experience for you?

*Need to be aware of cultural differences within the serviced population. Eye contact may not be within a cultural repertoire.
AIDS, Acquired immunodeficiency syndrome.

epidemic. An adolescent's boredom in school can manifest in poor grades, as can an undiagnosed learning disability. Problems in school can be the first warning signs of depression or substance abuse. With permission from the adolescent and the parent, the practitioner can initiate further educational evaluation as necessary.

Activity

With these questions, the practitioner is evaluating the cognitive level of functioning, peer relationships, vegetative signs of depression, and history of suicidal ideation. An adolescent without friends, one who has sleeping problems, or one who works 20 hours a week while in school may be of concern.

Much can be gained by asking about the adolescent's peer group. A strong association with a peer group is part of the process of achieving a new identity separate from the family. Peer influence varies with gender, race, age, and behavior. The activities engaged in by the peer group often reflect the activities of the individual and should be noted.

Affect

Adolescents express a great deal through body language. Depression, hostility, agitation, and confidence can all be observed in the way an adolescent responds to questioning while seated directly across from the examiner. In general, if a practitioner senses that an adolescent is displaying an affect, it is helpful to acknowledge the emotion. ''I notice that you seem a little sad or down (or angry or nervous) . . . Is there something you'd like to talk about?'' This serves the dual purpose of not only increasing data collection but also reinforcing to the adolescent that you are paying attention and care about what she is telling you. It is always wise to routinely ask if an adolescent has ever thought of hurting herself. This is especially portentous with the adolescent who appears to be depressed.

Ambition

An adolescent's sense of the future barely reaches to tomorrow. Future orientedness is a learned, nurtured, and mature behavior. Establishing an adolescent's sense of where she would like to be in 5 years tells the practitioner the extent of the nurturing and the cognitive functioning of the

adolescent. A 16 year old who wants to be a surgeon but has dropped out of school is not being realistic and could benefit from guidance and support in both returning to school and working toward appropriate goals. Well-adjusted, supported adolescents have dreams for their futures. Giving up on these dreams raises other issues for the child.

Anger

Adolescents today deal with more interpersonal violence than ever before. Whether it be in the home or in the streets, homicide and assault are becoming increasingly more common in young women. Adolescents should be asked how they deal with their anger: by crying or screaming, hitting, or silence. How does the family, in general, deal with anger? As many patterns of violence have their roots in the family's behavior, the family's style in dealing with anger should be assessed. In studies done on pregnant adolescents, there is evidence that drug use is more strongly associated with assault by a mate, whereas alcohol use is more often associated with the victim's family of origin. The abused child may evolve into the battered woman. It is necessary to ask the heterosexual adolescent if she has ever been hurt by her boyfriend and whether she knows how to avoid getting into dangerous situations. The practitioner should be able to help her think of nonviolent, acceptable ways to diffuse a violent situation. It is also helpful for the provider to acknowledge concern about violence and elicit the adolescent's thoughts on why it occurs and what would help to prevent it. When questioning unearths abuse by a family member or battering by a boyfriend, mandated reporting to the appropriate authorities may be required.

Drugs

Many adolescents who have been willing to answer questions about family, friends, and school are unwilling to answer questions about alcohol or drugs. It is helpful to preface this questioning with a reiteration of confidentiality and a qualifying statement such as ''Up until now we have been talking mostly about your family, friends, and school. Now I'd like to ask you a few questions about your own behavior. Once again, everything is confidential and won't automatically be shared with your parents.'' If prior questions revealed familial or peer substance abuse, this may help introduce the topic and reveal information on the adolescent's own habits. If not, a statement such as "It's not unusual for people your age to take some risks and experiment with things they've never tried before, such as alcohol. When was the last time you tried some alcohol?" Asking yes or no questions about whether someone uses drugs or alcohol should be avoided. If the adolescent indicates she is familiar with alcohol, an indication of frequency needs to be obtained. Unlike an adult, an adolescent who drinks heavily at one point in time may not be drinking 6 months later as she progresses through developmental stages. The effects of alcohol on other risk behaviors need to be acknowledged by asking questions about driving or engaging in sexual activity while intoxicated. Surveys have repeatedly shown that adolescent girls who are intoxicated are more likely to be sexually victimized and are less likely to use appropriate protection in sexual behaviors.

Sex

The intent of this question is to determine whether there is sexual activity and if so, whether it is protected activity. Questioning needs to be direct and comprehensive, making no assumptions. Practitioners need to be sensitive to sexual identity issues and include questions asked about same sex sexual relationships. Sexual practices should be discussed, given that an increasing number of heterosexual couples are turning to rectal sex as an alternative method to avoid pregnancy. Knowledge of AIDS, number of partners, STDs, and condoms should be discussed.

Throughout adolescence, cognitive and emotional developmental progression influences sexual practices. A 13 year old understands the concept of contraception in a different way from that of a 19 year old. Male-oriented methods of contraception, such as withdrawal and condoms, tend to be more prevalent with the younger age group, whereas middle adolescents opt for oral contraceptives. As adolescents mature and develop comfort with their own bodies, they may express interest in barrier methods. At this point they may choose diaphragms, condoms, or other methods. As educational efforts about safer sexual practices grow, it is hoped that abstinence, monogamy, and condoms will, for those who are sexually active, become a more acceptable means of protection.

Adolescents also need an opportunity to discuss their feelings as part of a relationship. Involvement of the partner in the visit can help to facilitate joint sexual decision making and may improve compliance with safer sexual practices.

An adolescent needs to hear that abstaining from sexual activity is normal and is becoming increasingly more common. She also needs to hear that sexuality is a part of being human. Too often, sexuality is linked with AIDS and implies death. Instead, the message should be that the adolescent has control of her body, and responsible sexuality in a mutually caring relationship is part of that control. Responsible choices are part of this control. No one has to get AIDS or an STD.

Using the HEADS interviewing technique with adolescents helps the provider establish a trusting relationship with the patient at the same time that it offers a comprehensive screening tool. In many ways, the interview may become an intervention.

Some clinics have adolescents complete a health assessment survey in the waiting room. This technique, although time efficient, does not replace the interaction of the practitioner with the adolescent.

PHYSICAL EXAMINATION

Screening

Every effort should be made to provide privacy to the adolescent. All interviewing should be done with the adolescent fully clothed, followed by private disrobing and provision of an adequate cover-up garment. The physical examination of adolescents should include several elements not in the adult examination. Vision and hearing screening examinations should be done at least once between the ages of 12 and 17 years. Vision screening can be done on the initial visit and then every 3 years thereafter, assuming there are no visual complaints. Auditory screening, if available, is advisable at least once during the adolescent years. The examination also provides an opportune time to demonstrate breast self-examination. Postural screening for scoliosis and kyphosis is particularly important in the early pubertal phase before the growth spurt. The hallmark of the adolescent examination, however, is Tanner staging.

An adolescent's progression through puberty is measured by standard milestones in breast and pubic hair development. Determining the Tanner staging can alert the practitioner to delays or precocity. It is important to be aware of any self-esteem issues that may arise secondary to perceptions of body distortions. Concern over breast asymmetry is a major physical concern of the young adolescent. Although breasts differ slightly in size in almost all women, occasionally there may be a significant size difference in adolescence. The difference may be an illusion, as in an adolescent with scoliosis, or it may be actual and due to a different rate of maturation of the two breasts. In any case reassurance is appropriate. In extreme cases, when discrepancy in breast size is significant, no intervention should be initiated until development is complete, usually when both nipples measure greater than 9 mm.

Eating disorders may also appear at any time during adolescence and may or may not be indicated by weight patterns that deviate from the growth chart tracking. Careful observation of weight gains or losses should be coupled with questions of body image and dietary habits in all female adolescents.

The Pelvic Examination

A pelvic examination is appropriate in any adolescent who is voluntarily sexually active, no matter what the age. There is some debate, however, as to when to initiate a pelvic examination in an adolescent who is not sexually active. The variables include (1) the patient's request, (2) the nature of the gynecologic complaint, and (3) the gynecologic versus the chronologic age.

Many adolescents request a pelvic examination as a right of passage or in anticipation of sexual activity and initiation of contraception. Some practitioners use this opportunity to discuss the first sexual encounter and assess the adolescent's expectations of the event. In some cases, practitioners may opt to forego the first pelvic examination until after the first intercourse, with appropriate anticipatory contraceptive guidance.

In the young, virginal adolescent with a gynecologic complaint, it is rarely necessary to do a pelvic examination. For example, dysfunctional uterine bleeding in an adolescent is more often due to immaturity of the hypothalamic-pituitary-ovarian axis and anovulation than to any structural lesion that could be appreciated on speculum visualization. When a gynecologic evaluation is necessary, external visualization and bimanual rectal palpation or pelvic ultrasound or both are usually sufficient. Use of a vaginal speculum and bimanual palpation is difficult at best when the hymen is intact and the patient is virginal. The development of a lifelong habit of regular pelvic examinations begins with the positive experience of the first pelvic examination. The more mature the adolescent, the more likely she will be to experience the examination positively and painlessly.

Some young adults do not become sexually experienced until they are into their twenties. The same is true for young women with significant cognitive impairment. It is difficult to specify the appropriate time to initiate a pelvic examination in a young adult who is not yet, and may never become, sexually active. Assuming no pelvic pathology is suspected, many practitioners start at 18 years. By this age, the hymen may be broken or the opening enlarged enough to facilitate easy examination.

It is helpful to have the adolescent be as involved in her pelvic examination as possible. The patient can be asked if she wants to look at her cervix and external genitalia in a hand-held mirror. She should also be told that the examination will be stopped if she feels discomfort. Each step should be anticipated so that there are no surprises for the patient.

WORKING WITH THE PARENT

Although it is important to understand adolescent psychological and physical development when working with teenagers, it is also important to understand how their parents are coping. Parenting an adolescent is a daunting task. Parents must deal not only with the child's sense of frustration and emotional lability but also with their own feelings of being rejected and challenged as well. Adolescents need to make decisions, but these need to be bounded by consistent parental guidelines. Adolescents need to take risks, but these need to be directed by an adult who is experienced in the magnitude and consequences of the risk involved. There needs to be communication and a parental willingness to listen.

By anticipating the issues and bringing them up separately with the parents, practitioners can assist parents through this often difficult time. The practitioner should be knowledgeable about written resources for parents and provide waiting room literature.

SUMMARY

Caring for the adolescent patient is a challenge. Although system pathology in the adolescent is usually limited, the psychosocial issues are paramount and require sensitive nonjudgmental evaluation. By involving the adolescent in her own health care and promoting positive health habits, the practitioner optimizes the chances for a healthier adult lifestyle.

Bibliography

Committee on Psychosocial Aspects of Child and Family Health. Guidelines for Health Supervision. Elk Grove Village, Ill, American Academy of Pediatrics, 1988.

Berenson A, San Miguel VV, Wilkin GS. Violence and its relationship to substance use in adolescent pregnancy. J Adolesc Health Care 1992;13(5), 470–474.

Gans J, Blythe DA, Eisler A, Gavenas L. America's Adolescents: How Healthy Are They? Chicago, American Medical Association, 1991.

Gilligan C. In a Different Voice. Cambridge, Mass, Harvard University Press, 1982.

Glantz L, Annas G. The Rights of Doctors, Nurses, and Allied Health Professionals. Cambridge, Mass, Ballinger Publishing Co, 1981.

Goldenberg J, Cohen E. Getting into adolescent heads. Contemp Pediatr 1988; 75.

Greydanus D. Caring for Your Adolescent. New York, Bantam Books, 1991.

Neinstein LS. Adolescent Health Care, A Practical Guide. Baltimore, Urban and Schwarzenberg, 1984.

DISEASES OF THE GYNECOLOGIC ORGANS

5

Gynecologic History, Examination, and Procedures

Ellen E. Sheets

Although gynecologic care has often been separated from other medical care, the gynecologic examination is an integral part of a complete history and a thorough physical examination. Women who present to a gynecologist for a yearly Papanicolaou (PAP) smear and pelvic examination benefit greatly from a complete examination as they frequently do not see another health care provider unless specific problems arise. An opportunity exists during this yearly examination to fully evaluate and subsequently treat any underlying disorder that is not apparent to the patient. Likewise, patients seeking routine care from a nongynecologist also benefit from integrating the entire physical examination. This chapter provides a summary on how the gynecologic history, examination, and appropriate diagnostic procedures are approached in the patient presenting for routine care.

GYNECOLOGIC HISTORY

The tendency to focus only on topics related to the reproductive history of the woman presenting for examination can lead to serious problems if that patient's complete medical history is not known. Time should be spent obtaining general health information such as allergies to medication, current medications, previous surgical procedures, and medical problems as would be done at any initial patient contact. Once this general information has been obtained, focus is then turned to the presenting complaint, which is best discussed in the patient's own words. This information usually provides a sound basis for diagnosis and helps focus the rest of the history and examination.

MENSTRUAL HISTORY

The menstrual history should include questions regarding the onset of menses (menarche) and the frequency, duration, and character of menstrual bleeding, which can provide important clues regarding the function of the hypothalamic-pituitary-gonadal axis. The range of normal values are present in Table 5–1. One should also note the date of onset of the last menstrual period and of the previous menstrual period. Any associated menstrual discomfort such as cramps (dysmenorrhea), diarrhea, or nausea should be noted along with the age at onset and the degree of discomfort. Mid-

TABLE 5–1. Characteristics of Normal Menstrual Cycle

Menarche	Average age 13 y.o. (range 8–16 yr)
Frequency	Every 28 days (range 25–34 days)
Duration	Average range 3–7 days
Menopause	Average age 50 y.o. (range 45–55 yr)

cycle pain (mittelschmerz) may indicate ovulatory cycles. For older patients, the age at cessation of menses (menopause) and any subsequent bleeding should be noted.

PAST GYNECOLOGIC HISTORY

Although past obstetric history is more pertinent in the pregnant patient, an understanding of previous pregnancies is also helpful in the gynecologic patient. Each pregnancy (gravidity), delivery before 20 weeks (miscarriage or abortion), pregnancy termination (abortion), delivery after 20 weeks (parity), or ectopic pregnancy should be noted. Depending on the patient's age and presenting symptoms, questions regarding secondary sexual development can be important (Table 5–2). Previous PAP smear results and findings on previous pelvic examinations are useful for the subsequent evaluation. In patients who have undergone vaginal delivery, the possibility of problems with urinary incontinence or difficult defecation should be explored. Any surgical procedure such as tubal ligation, exploratory surgery, or treatment for an abnormal PAP smear or abnormal-appearing cervix should be noted. Results of previous mammography, if the patient is 40 years of age or older, should be noted along with a discussion of appropriate follow-up.

SEXUAL HISTORY

Although the sexual history is often viewed as a difficult topic of discussion, important information can be acquired from a thorough history. It is helpful for the practitioner to keep focused and to view this segment of history taking as an integral part of the interview. Age of onset of sexual activity, number of past and current sexual partners, and history of venereal diseases are often the most difficult questions to be asked. Inquiry concerning the health of previous sexual partners is also important. History of past and current contraceptive use should be noted. Advising patients about safe sex practices should be routine. Often patients do not initiate such discussions, and a tactful comment by the practitioner may put the patient at ease so that she can raise her own questions. Inquiry regarding difficulty with intercourse should also be addressed. Pain with intercourse (dyspareunia), postcoital bleeding, or difficulty with sexual enjoyment should be noted and evaluated. Patients complaining of difficulty with sexual enjoyment or orgasm or with dyspareunia when no physical cause is found need further evaluation and can be referred to a therapist knowledgeable in the management of sexual dysfunction.

PHYSICAL EXAMINATION

Pelvic Examination

Practitioners outside the arena of obstetrics and gynecology are sometimes anxious about performing a pelvic examination and PAP smear. This anxiety often stems from a lack of frequency of performing the examination and a sense of violating the patient's privacy. The patient's gynecologic examination is an important part of her overall assessment. It is important to put the patient at

TABLE 5–2. Characteristics of Secondary Sexual Development

STAGE	BREAST DEVELOPMENT (MEDIAN AGE)	PUBIC HAIR (MEDIAN AGE)
Stage 1 (prepubertal)	Elevation of papilla	Absent
Stage 2	Elevation of breast and papilla, areola enlarged (9.8 yr)	Occasional hair along labia majora (10.5 yr)
Stage 3	Breast continues to enlarge, breast and areola still continuous (11.2 yr)	Sparse dark hair, tends to be coarse and curled (11.4 yr)
Stage 4	Areola and papilla become separate from breast as secondary mound (12.1 yr)	Adult-type hair over mons only (12.0 yr)
Stage 5	Areola recedes into contour of breast (14.6 yr)	Adult-type hair in normal distribution (13.7 yr)

Modified from Tanner JM. Growth at Adolescence. 2nd ed. Oxford, Blackwell Scientific Publications, 1962.

ease and never appear to be in a hurry during the examination. Time should be taken to explain each procedure and to answer questions as they arise. Approaching the examination in a consistent, systematic fashion as one would other parts of the physical examination helps the practitioner develop a routine despite possible infrequency of performing a gynecologic examination.

Visual inspection and subsequent palpation of the inguinal region bilaterally should be done as part of the pelvic examination because this region drains the lymphatics from the vulva and lower one third of the vagina and may be abnormal when vulva abnormalities, such as cancer or infection, are present. The overall appearance of the vulva should be assessed before placement of the speculum. Abrasion of the epithelium can occur in patients who have never been sexually active or in postmenopausal patients suffering from vulvar atrophy. Care should be taken to note the character and distribution of hair, the prominence or atrophy of the labia, the status of the hymen (imperforate or open) and the degree of laxity of the introitus. Any lesions of the labia or perineum should be noted and inquiry made whether they had been previously noted. Undiagnosed vulvar lesions require biopsy, and, if necessary, appropriate referral should be made. The Bartholin's gland area should be inspected and any inflammation, exudate, or cyst noted. Evaluation of the urethra and Skene's glands for purulent exudate should also be completed. If the patient is multiparous, the perineum should be inspected for signs of perineal relaxation, scarring, or both.

The introitus should always be inspected before the speculum examination because the status of the hymen and laxity of the introitus may dictate the speculum type and size that should be used. Care should be taken to warm and lubricate the speculum with warm water for patient comfort. Only water can be used when a PAP smear or cultures are to be done as gels can interfere with both evaluations. The patient should be told when the practitioner is about to insert the speculum and the labia should be spread to expose the introitus. The speculum should be inserted in the transverse position with pressure posteriorly toward the perineum and rectum to avoid the urethra, which is very sensitive to pressure. Once the top of the vagina has been reached, careful opening of the blades of the speculum to avoid pressure on the urethra is done allowing the practitioner to visualize the cervix. If locating the cervix is difficult, the speculum can be repositioned downward into the vagina, which solves the problem in most cases. If the cervix still cannot be located, the speculum should be moved upward toward the bladder be-

cause the cervix can be anterior in patients with a retroverted and retroflexed uterus. If these maneuvers fail, the next step is to insert a gloved, wet finger into the vagina to locate the cervix, thus allowing for repositioning of the speculum as necessary. Once visualized, the cervix should be evaluated for its size, shape, and color. The characteristics of the cervix should be noted, such as the location of the squamocolumnar junction, the presence or absence of childbirth trauma, and the presence or absence of discharge. Any lesion on the cervix that appears abnormal requires biopsy even if the PAP smear is normal.

The speculum should be rotated 90 degrees as it is removed from the vagina to allow for visualization of all the vaginal mucosa. Relaxation of the anterior wall (cystocele) can be assessed by using only the bottom blade of the speculum to open the posterior aspect of the vagina while the patient performs a Valsalva maneuver. With the speculum removed entirely, a Valsalva maneuver is performed again, and relaxation of the posterior vaginal wall (rectocele) is assessed.

Once the cervix is visualized, a PAP smear should be obtained. Obtaining a specimen for cervical cytology is one of the most important parts of the pelvic examination. It is also one of the easiest examinations to perform incorrectly. Studies estimate that up to 62% of false negative smears are the result of sampling errors.[1, 2] These errors can result from not obtaining an adequate number of cells owing to technical errors on the part of the clinician, to lack of exfoliation of abnormal cells, or to air-drying artifact.[1] The endocervical brush obtains a better sample and is superior to the cotton swab for sampling the endocervical canal.[2, 3] The presence of endocervical cells in the PAP smear is important to ensure that the transformation zone has been sampled and the PAP smear is adequate for the cytologist to read.[4] To minimize error in sampling, the endocervix should be sampled first. The endocervical brush should be inserted as deep into the canal as possible and turned clockwise three to five times. This specimen should be plated onto the glass slide first as the sample contains more moisture than the cervical scrape obtained with the Ayre's spatula. The Ayre's spatula is then used to sample the exocervix. One edge of the spatula should be placed into the os and with firm pressure the spatula should be rotated three to five times. Once both the endocervical and ectocervical specimens have been plated on the slide, fixation should occur immediately. This approach, coupled with minimizing the time to fixation, decreases air-drying artifact. This can be done by using one of the commercially available fixatives or by dropping the slide into a 10% alcohol solution. When removing the speculum, it is again important to avoid the urethral meatus due to its sensitivity.

Before doing the bimanual examination, it is important that the patient empty her urinary bladder. A full bladder not only can be a source of discomfort during the examination but also can inhibit palpation of the uterus and adnexa (consisting of the fallopian tubes and ovaries), which is the primary goal of a bimanual examination. In general, the nondominant hand is the one used inside the vagina. To initiate the examination, the hand opposite from the internal hand should be used to separate the labia and facilitate entry of the lubricated index finger of the examining hand. Next, pressure is exerted on the posterior vaginal wall, allowing entry of a lubricated middle finger. Both fingers course the entire length of the vagina to the cervix. Compromise of the examination can occur in patients who are obese owing to the thickness of the anterior abdominal wall or who experience significant discomfort, which makes relaxation of the anterior abdominal wall difficult. Patients who are not able to relax, who have pain, or who have increased abdominal girth may be candidates for a pelvic ultrasound or an examination under anesthesia in the operating room.

The sequence of the bimanual examination may vary from one examiner to the next, but some type of systematic approach should be utilized. Initially, the vagina itself is palpated to rule out any subepithelial lesions that were not seen on speculum examination. Palpation of the cervix can be of use in identifying cervical leiomyomata and sometimes invasive cervical cancer. Then attention is directed to evaluation of the uterus. Its position within the pelvis (e.g., tilted anterior, posterior) is noted along with its shape, consistency, and size. Often the size of the uterus is equated to the size of a pregnant uterus at different stages of gestation. Tenderness on movement of the cervix can sometimes indicate problems with the adnexal structures as they are put on slight traction on the opposite side from the cervical movement. Once the uterus has been assessed, attention is turned to the adnexal region by moving the vaginal hand to the lateral fornix on the side to be examined. The external hand starts at the anterior iliac crest and with slow firm pressure is moved downward toward the mons. This brings the tube and ovary downward toward the internal hand, and the adnexa is felt between the two hands. The rectovaginal examination is performed by placing the middle finger through the anal sphincter into the rectum. The index finger remains in the vagina. With this position, the rectal-vaginal septum can be evaluated and the cul-de-sac checked for masses that may have fallen behind the uterus and cervix.

Technique for Wet Preparation and Vaginal Culture

The initial history may indicate concern regarding abnormal vaginal discharge, odor, or symptoms such as itching or vulvovaginal discomfort. The presence of vaginal discharge in asymptomatic women need not be pursued unless there is suspicion of chlamydia or gonorrhea. The sequence of obtaining vaginal specimens depends on the patient's presenting symptoms. Cultures and samples for microscopic evaluation are generally obtained before the PAP smear. Chlamydia and gonorrhea testing should be done before any other samples are obtained.

Some practitioners advocate prescribing treatment based solely on the characteristics of the discharge. However, relying only on the characteristics of the discharge misclassifies many patients, who receive treatment when no infection is present.[5, 6] An inexpensive and more specific approach is to evaluate for infection by a wet preparation. Generally, a saline-moistened swab is used to obtain a sample of discharge or to sample the surface of the vaginal fornices and cervix. The swab is then rolled in a drop of saline and subsequently in a drop of 10% potassium hydroxide. It is important to do the saline preparation first because the purpose of the 10% potassium hydroxide is to lyse normal cellular elements, allowing for the buds and hyphae of yeast to be detected.

Typical microscopic findings on the saline preparation are bacteria, white blood cells, "clue" cells, or trichomonads. In the potassium hydroxide portion, ghosts of cells that represent the shell of cell membranes that were lysed can be seen. This sample typically contains branched hyphae and rounded buds if a yeast infection is present. Culture of material from the vagina increases diagnostic accuracy and in fact doubles the number of trichomonal infections detected.[5] Bacteria and white blood cells can indicate bacterial vaginosis, but the diagnosis is classically made by the presence of clue cells. These cells are epithelial cells covered with bacteria and are identified by a typical stippled birefringence that obscures the normal cell boundaries. See Chapter 44.

Cultures can be obtained for bacterial, yeast, and viral infections. Genital herpes infections can be diagnosed in a variety of ways but the most specific is by tissue culture. Typical herpetic vesicles can be ruptured and their fluid used for culture. In the vagina and cervix, samples are taken from the endocervical os. *Chlamydia trachomatis,* found as an obligate intracellular parasite in the epithelium of the reproductive tract, can be identified by cell culture technique. Enzyme-linked immunosorbent assay (ELISA) and direct fluorescent antibody slide-staining techniques and DNA probes have been developed. These tests are not as sensitive as culture when used to screen the general population; however, their specificity is excellent.[7, 8] General culture tubes detect bacteria and yeast. Specific culture media tubes are required for herpes samples. For *Chlamydia,* the sample is obtained from the endocervical canal with the second swab. The first swab is used to cleanse the cervix and is discarded. Special specimen collection tubes are used for transport to the appropriate laboratory.

OFFICE PROCEDURES

Depending on the patient's presenting complaint, her gynecologic history, or her gynecologic examination, she may require an office procedure. Some of the most common procedures are colposcopy with cervical biopsies and endometrial biopsies. Other procedures that are done in the office include diagnostic hysteroscopy and treatment of cervical intraepithelial neoplasia with cryocautery, laser, or loop excision by electrocautery. Another procedure is evaluation of abnormal vulvar lesions with vulvar biopsies.

Colposcopy

Evaluation of the abnormal PAP smear is the most common reason that colposcopy and cervical biopsies are done. Colposcopy, using a binocular microscope to visualize the cervical epithelium under magnification, is performed to identify areas of abnormal epithelium. The cervix is painted with a dilute 3 to 5% acetic acid solution and abnormal areas are identified by colposcopy. These areas appear white following acetic acid application owing to their high nuclear content. There are also abnormal vessels with mosaicism and punctation present in areas with intraepithelial neoplasia. These abnormal areas are sampled by biopsy and provide a histologic diagnosis for the abnormality seen on cytologic examination. An endocervical curettage or scraping of the endocervical canal is also done to look for any abnormalities that are not seen by colposcopy. The procedure takes 5 to 10 minutes, and patient discomfort from the procedure is generally minimal with mild cramping and discomfort. Vaginal intraepithelial neoplasia is

evaluated in a manner similar to that for cervical colposcopy with vaginal biopsies from abnormal areas.

Endometrial Biopsy

The indications for endometrial biopsy include excessive, prolonged, or frequent bleeding episodes or evaluation of postmenopausal bleeding. The endometrial biopsy is generally done without any local anesthesia; however, a paracervical block may be used in patients who have marked discomfort or in patients with cervical stenosis when cervical dilation may be needed. The most commonly used method of endometrial biopsy is by the Pipelle. The Pipelle endometrial suction curette (Unimar, Wilton, Conn.), compares favorably with previous office devices and with surgical dilation and curettage. Its diagnostic accuracy is excellent compared with that of the other endometrial sampling techniques.[9] The Pipelle is a 3.1 mm hollow plastic tube that has an internal plunger and an opening opposite the plunger handle. After cleansing the cervix with povidone-iodine (Betadine), the tube is easily inserted through the cervical os into the endometrial cavity. A gentle suction is created by drawing back on the plunger, and endometrial tissue is aspirated into the catheter. Rotation of the catheter back and forth into the endometrial cavity ensures that an adequate sample is obtained. The major complaint from patients is uterine cramping during the procedure. Other sampling devices for office endometrial sampling include the Novak's curet, which is a metal catheter that is connected to a syringe to create a vacuum and aspirate endometrial contents. This is generally associated with more patient discomfort. In patients with a large amount of blood or tissue in the cavity, a Karman cannula can be used. It is a plastic catheter similar to the Pipelle but one that can be attached to a large suction syringe.

Vulvar Biopsy

A vulvar biopsy is done to evaluate abnormal areas on the vulva. A vulvar colposcopy can precede vulvar biopsies. The procedure is similar to that for cervical colposcopy. Administration of a local anesthetic is necessary before a vulvar biopsy owing to its sensitivity. Following injection of local anesthesia, a biopsy of 3 to 6 mm of tissue is obtained, and the area is cauterized with silver nitrate for hemostasis. Sutures are sometimes necessary for larger areas of biopsy.

Treatment Methods for Cervical Intraepithelial Neoplasia

Treatment of preinvasive disease of the cervix is another common gynecologic office procedure. Cryocautery is done by freezing the cervix with liquid nitrogen. The procedure takes 12 to 15 minutes, is done without local anesthesia, and is associated with mild cramping. Laser ablation with the carbon dioxide laser is also usually done without local anesthesia or sometimes with a local anesthetic infiltrated into the cervix. The procedure takes 15 to 20 minutes and is also associated with mild uterine cramping. The loop excision of the transformation zone is a newer method to treat cervical intraepithelial neoplasia. A thin wire loop is used to remove the transformation zone after local anesthetic is injected into the cervix. The advantage of loop excision over the other two methods is that it provides a specimen for pathologic evaluation including the margins of excision, which is of prognostic value in determining recurrence rates. Loop excision takes 5 to 10 minutes and is also associated with mild uterine cramping. The success of treatment and cure rates are similar for all three methods.

Hysteroscopy

Diagnostic hysteroscopy is done in patients with persistent abnormal bleeding, in patients in whom an endometrial polyp or submucous fibroid is suspected, in patients with infertility, and in patients with persistent postmenopausal bleeding with normal endometrial biopsies. Flexible 3- to 5-mm hysteroscopes can be inserted into the uterine cavity without dilation or anesthesia. Normal saline, lactated Ringer's solution, or carbon dioxide is used to expand the endometrial cavity for adequate visualization. The procedure takes 5 to 10 minutes and can be associated with moderate cramping. Use of prostaglandin inhibitors before the procedure can relieve some discomfort.

REFERENCES

1. Gay JD, Donaldson LD, Goeliner JR. False-negative results in cervical cytologic studies. Acta Cytol 1985;29:1043.
2. Kristensen GB, Holund B, Grinsted P. Efficacy of the Cytobrush versus the cotton swab in the collection of endocervical cells. Acta Cytol 1989;33:849.
3. Selvaggi SM. Spatula/cytobrush vs. spatula/cotton swab detection of cervical condylomatous lesions. J Reprod Med 1989;34:629.
4. National Cancer Institute Workshop. The 1988 Bethesda System for reporting cervical/vaginal cytological diagnoses. JAMA 1989;262:931.
5. Fouts AC, Kraus SJ. *Trichomonas vaginalis:* Reevaluation of its clinical presentation and laboratory diagnosis. J Infect Dis 1980;141:137.
6. McLellan R, Spence MR, Brockman M, et al. The clinical diagnosis of trichomoniasis. Obstet Gynecol 1982;60:30.
7. Livengood CH 3rd, Schmitt JW, Addison WA, et al. Direct fluorescent antibody testing for endocervical *Chlamydia trachomatis:* Factors affecting accuracy. Obstet Gynecol 1988;72:803.
8. Kellogg JA, Seiple JW, Levisky JS. Efficacy of duplicate genital specimens and repeated testing for confirming positive results for chlamydiazyme detection of *Chlamydia trachomatis* antigen. J Clin Microbiol 1989;27:1218.
9. Koonings PP, Moyer DL, Grimes DA. A randomized clinical trial comparing pipelle and tis-u-trap for endometrial biopsy. Obstet Gynecol 1990;75:293.

Evaluation and Management of Pelvic Masses

Carolyn V. Kirschner

A pelvic mass may be detected incidentally on routine pelvic examination, during physical examination of a patient with specific symptoms, or during radiologic evaluation of a patient with specific symptoms. The evaluation and management of a pelvic mass varies depending on the differential diagnosis, which is based on the patient's age; the size of the mass; the characteristics on ultrasound, such as simple cyst, complex cyst, and solid mass; and associated symptoms such as acute pain.

DIFFERENTIAL DIAGNOSIS OF A PELVIC MASS

A mass in the pelvis may arise from any structure that lies in the pelvic area. It is important to consider all possible structures that may be involved with the abnormal process and to recognize those organs that are more commonly associated with pelvic masses.

A palpable pelvic mass on examination may be due to an enlarged uterus. In patients in the reproductive age, pregnancy must be excluded. Other common etiologies of benign uterine enlargement include uterine leiomyoma and adenomyosis. Malignant conditions of the uterus, more common in women older than 40, may result in uterine enlargement from sarcoma and carcinoma.

The most common causes of ovarian enlargement in a woman of reproductive age are functional cysts, endometriomas, or benign neoplastic cysts. Functional cysts are follicular or corpus luteum cysts that can sometimes be as large as 7 to 8 cm in diameter. They are usually simple on ultrasound without septations or solid areas. Hemorrhages can develop within functional cysts,

and these are difficult to distinguish from endometriomas on ultrasound. Endometriomas develop from ectopic endometrial tissue that attaches to the ovary and forms a cyst that is due to repetitive bleeding from hormonal stimulation during the menstrual cycle. Both endometriomas and functional cysts can appear asymptomatically on routine examination or can manifest with acute pain from rupture or torsion. Benign ovarian tumors such as a mature cystic teratoma or dermoids are common in young women, but a woman of any age can develop neoplastic cysts or solid tumors.

The fallopian tube may be involved with a tubo-ovarian complex or a paratubal cyst. Paratubal cysts can occur in women of any age group. They arise from the peritoneum surrounding the tube and are filled with clear fluid. Paratubal cysts can be multiple and can be as large as 12 to 15 cm. They are of no clinical significance except in their differentiation from ovarian masses on examination and ultrasound. Tubo-ovarian masses can develop during an acute episode of pelvic inflammatory disease or from a remote history of pelvic infection, in patients with current or past use of an intrauterine device, and in patients with appendicitis or diverticulitis. Ectopic pregnancy can be a cause of a pelvic mass but usually has other clinical findings that point toward that diagnosis. Fallopian tube malignancy is rare but must be considered in an older woman with an adnexal mass.

Bowel complaints are frequent and may be referred to the pelvis. Feces or gas in the colon may appear to be a pelvic mass. Inflammatory conditions such as diverticular disease or appendiceal inflammation may be detected as a pelvic mass. Either cecal or rectosigmoid carcinoma, in addition, may appear as a pelvic mass. Metastatic tumors to the ovary, which are most commonly from the gastrointestinal tract and breast, could also occur in a similar manner.

Other conditions that are less common include a pelvic kidney, a distended bladder, a urachal cyst, an abdominal wall hematoma or abscess, a retroperitoneal neoplasm such as lymphoma, or a hernia—all of which could appear as a pelvic mass.

Table 6–1 lists the most common diagnoses for women with a pelvic mass.

DIAGNOSTIC EVALUATION

Both the history and the physical examination are important in the diagnostic work-up of a patient with a pelvic mass. In a young woman, attention to the last menstrual period is necessary. Any abnormal uterine bleeding or irregular menses should be noted. Uterine bleeding in the postmenopausal patient should be investigated promptly. Urinary complaints including pain or dysuria should be evaluated.

Symptoms from pelvic masses are generally related to tumor size or manifestations of associated ascites. An expanding ovarian lesion in the pelvis may cause pressure on the bladder or rectum. In addition, ovarian tumors may undergo torsion, which results in acute pelvic pain from infarction or rupture. In any woman, bowel complaints, including blood in the stool, diarrhea, constipation, or gastrointestinal upset, must be evaluated.

Examination

Pelvic examination may indicate a midline mass, more suggestive of uterine disease, rather than a mass in either the right or the left pelvis. It may be possible to ascertain whether the mass moves with the uterus or appears to be separate from it. Pelvic examination may be helpful in distinguishing a benign from a malignant neoplasm. In general, a benign neoplasm is mobile, more likely to be unilateral, and more likely to be cystic. A solid, fixed, or bilateral tumor, associated with nodularity in the cul-de-sac on rectovaginal examination or associated with ascites, is more likely to be malignant. Women with bilateral masses have a 2.6-fold increased risk of malignancy compared with women with unilateral masses.[1]

Although ascites is classically associated with ovarian cancer, other malignant or nonmalignant conditions such as cirrhosis or congestive heart failure may also appear with ascites. Physical examination can identify the presence or absence of a fluid wave. Examination of a patient with a pelvic mass must include a careful node survey for metastatic disease, particularly in the cervical, inguinal, and axillary areas. Careful breast examination, abdominal examination, and pelvic examination are also important. The extremities should be evaluated for the presence of edema and varicosities. Finally, a general assessment of the patient's overall health is important, in the event that the patient needs surgical exploration.

ULTRASOUND IN THE EVALUATION OF A PELVIC MASS

The role of ultrasound in the evaluation of the pelvis has greatly expanded with higher resolution scanners. The resolution afforded by vaginal

---

TABLE 6–1. Differential Diagnosis of Adnexal Mass

ORGAN	CYSTIC	SOLID

Ovary	Functional cyst
	Neoplastic cyst
	  Benign
	  Malignant
	Endometriosis
		Neoplasm
		  Benign
		  Malignant

Fallopian tube	Tubo-ovarian abscess Hydrosalpinx Parovarian cyst	Tubo-ovarian abscess Ectopic pregnancy Neoplasm
Uterus	Intrauterine pregnancy in a bicornate uterus	Pedunculated or interligamentous myoma
Bowel	Sigmoid or cecum distended with gas and/or feces	Diverticulitis Ileitis Appendicitis Colonic cancer
Miscellaneous	Distended bladder Pelvic kidney Urachal cyst	Abdominal wall hematoma or abscess Retroperitoneal neoplasm

From DiSaia PJ, Creasman WT (eds). Clinical Gynecologic Oncology. 4th ed. St. Louis: Mosby-Year Book, 1992, p 293.

probes, which operate at a higher frequency than standard transducers, has allowed for detection of much smaller structures. In addition, a cystic unilocular adnexal mass on abdominal ultrasonography may, in fact, display septation on vaginal ultrasonography.

Ultrasound may be particularly useful in the evaluation of a patient who is obese or unable to cooperate with a physical examination. Ultrasound is the best imaging method available for the uterus, fallopian tubes, and ovaries and is, in addition, less expensive than computed tomography and magnetic resonance imaging studies. An ultrasound may distinguish a uterine from a tubal or an ovarian mass, which may be helpful before surgery so that a gynecologic oncologist is available if malignancy is suspected.

Rulin and Preston assessed the utility of pelvic examination in detecting ovarian masses.[2] In their study, pelvic examination missed 10% of tumors less than 10 cm in diameter. It is apparent, therefore, that pelvic examination alone is not optimal for assessing patients, and ultrasound evaluation should be considered in patients with suspected ovarian enlargement or with pelvic pain or tenderness on examination.

Many investigators have attempted to predict malignancy based on the appearance of the mass on ultrasound. Andolf and Jorgensen compared ultrasound with clinical examination and found ultrasound superior to examination in terms of sensitivity (83% and 67%, respectively), whereas specificity was high for both methods (96% versus 94%, respectively).[3] Sassone and colleagues attempted to develop a scoring system using transvaginal sonographic characterization of pelvic lesions.[4] The variables studied on ultrasound included inner wall structure (smooth, irregular, or papillary), wall thickness (thin, thick, or solid), septa (none, thin, or thick), and echogenicity (sonolucent low echogenicity, mixed echogenicity, and high echogenicity). They were able to distinguish benign from malignant masses with a specificity of 83% and a sensitivity of 100%. Although tumor size has frequently been identified as a risk factor for malignancy, these researchers did not find that inclusion of this characteristic in their score improved the sensitivity. In general, benign ovarian tumors tend to be unilateral, cystic, mobile, and smooth. Malignant lesions tend to be bilateral, solid, fixed, irregular, and associated with ascites, nodules in the cul-de-sac, and a rapid increase in size.

OTHER RADIOLOGIC STUDIES

Intravenous pyelogram is useful in patients who are scheduled for surgical exploration to assess the location and anatomy of the ureters to avoid ureteral injury during surgery. Intravenous pyelogram also detects the rare pelvic kidney.

Barium enema has been utilized extensively in the preparation of a patient for surgical exploration of a pelvic mass. In addition to evaluation of the colonic mucosa for lesions suggesting malignancy, diverticular disease in the pelvis can be suggestive of an inflammatory process. It should be noted, however, that diverticular disease may coexist with another gynecologic disorder.

Computed tomography may be helpful in evaluation of the retroperitoneum, specifically the pancreas and para-aortic node area. The liver may also be assessed for metastatic disease. The presence of ascites may also be noted on a computed tomography scan. Computed tomography is not particularly accurate in distinguishing uterine from adnexal disease, and ultrasound is superior in this area.

Serum CA-125

The utility of the CA-125 tumor marker in the preoperative evaluation with a pelvic mass is limited. CA-125 is elevated in approximately 80% of nonmucinous epithelial ovarian malignancies. The marker is also elevated, however, in a variety of other conditions, including endometriosis, other pelvic and abdominal malignancies, congestive heart failure, and other chronic diseases.[5] A mildly elevated CA-125 is particularly nonspecific in the premenopausal woman, in whom pelvic inflammatory disease, endometriosis, and uterine leiomyomata may cause an increase in CA-125 levels.[6] The marker is, therefore, best reserved for patients in whom a malignancy has already been diagnosed and in whom serial CA-125 levels may be drawn to follow the patient's clinical course during and after treatment.

MANAGEMENT OF THE PREMENOPAUSAL WOMAN WITH A PELVIC MASS

A mass that is larger than 8 cm in diameter should be explored promptly because of the risk of malignancy, torsion, rupture, or hemorrhage. A mass smaller in size that appears cystic on examination or ultrasound may be followed conservatively. Many of these lesions prove to be functional cysts and will resolve during the course of one or two menstrual cycles. Reexamination in 4 to 6 weeks with resolution of the mass confirms this diagnosis. Many physicians prescribe oral contraceptives to accelerate involution of a functional cyst. If the mass persists, surgical exploration is indicated. Spanos studied 286 patients who had cystic pelvic masses, were prescribed oral contraceptives, and then reexamined in 6 weeks.[7] In 72% of these women the masses disappeared. Of the 81 patients in whom cystic enlargement remained, all were neoplastic and five were malignant. Solid ovarian masses are not functional and do not resolve with time and therefore should be explored promptly. In addition, tender or painful masses require consideration of at least a laparoscopy to rule out ovarian torsion or rupture.

In a woman younger than 30 with an ovarian mass with solid components, serum alpha-fetoprotein and human chorionic gonadotropin levels should be obtained in the event that a germ cell tumor of the ovary exists. A CA-125 level is less helpful in this age group, as this may be indicative of endometriosis, salpingo-oophoritis, or other fairly common pelvic disorders. If findings on ultrasound are most compatible with a benign lesion, that is, a unilocular unilateral cystic and smooth-bordered lesion, laparoscopy can be considered. The presence or absence of peritoneal fluid may also be assessed at the time of ultrasound.

MANAGEMENT OF THE POSTMENOPAUSAL WOMAN WITH A PELVIC MASS

In the premenopausal woman, an ovarian cyst may be physiologic, but in the postmenopausal woman any enlargement of the ovary is considered abnormal. The ovaries are no longer functioning in the production of follicles and corpora lutea, and therefore ''functional'' cysts should not occur.

In the postmenopausal patient with an adnexal mass, ultrasound and serum CA-125 tests should be performed. If both these tests are suggestive of benign disease, that is, normal CA-125 and lesions with ultrasound findings showing unilocular unilateral smooth-bordered lesion without fluid in the cul-de-sac, and if family history is negative for carcinoma, the decision should then be made whether to proceed with surgical removal or with observation. Although there are no long-term follow-up studies, some data suggest that with informed consent, conservative follow-up without intervention may be appropriate.[8, 9] Conservative follow-up has been advocated for unilateral, unilocular, simple adnexal masses of sizes ranging from 2 to less than 5 cm. The mass may be followed every 1 to 3 months with ultrasound and serum CA-125 level tests. This may be particularly

appropriate for a patient who is a poor surgical risk, in whom the morbidity of surgery may outweigh any potential benefit.

Any pelvic mass thought to be malignant in a postmenopausal woman should be explored promptly. Preoperative studies should include intravenous pyelogram, barium enema, chest radiograph, and CA-125. The patient should be prepared for surgery with a thorough cleansing of the bowel, preferably with an isotonic solution that provides catharsis without dehydration. Other important preoperative considerations include evaluation of the patient's medical status. Blood should be available for transfusion if required, and consideration should be given to perioperative prophylactic antibiotics and to thromboembolic prophylaxis.

OPERATIVE PROCEDURES

Laparoscopy is indicated in patients who are at low risk for malignancy, for example, a young patient with signs and symptoms suggestive of a benign cyst or an endometrioma. A small cystic mass of less than 5 cm in a postmenopausal woman could be managed laparoscopically if ultrasound and normal CA-125 levels suggest that it is benign.

Maiman and Seltzer reported on 42 patients who had undergone laparoscopic management of ovarian neoplasms that were subsequently found to be malignant.[10] At least 50% of these patients had stage II, III, or IV ovarian cancer. Thirty-one percent of these patients had prelaparoscopic ultrasound, which had shown unilateral unilocular cystic lesions less than 8 cm in diameter, all suggestive of a benign lesion.

Laparotomy is reserved for patients in whom pelvic malignancy cannot be excluded or in whom the danger of subsequent complications (e.g., rupture, torsion, or hemorrhage of an ovarian mass) mandates definite treatment. It should be emphasized that patients who are medically unable to tolerate laparotomy will very likely be even less able to tolerate laparoscopy, owing to the steep Trendelenburg position required for a laparoscopic procedure as well as the instillation of many liters of carbon dioxide into the abdomen.

EXPLORATORY LAPAROTOMY

In the operating room, an examination under anesthesia is performed to confirm the presence of the mass. The patient should be explored through a low midline (subumbilical, vertical) incision.

Washings for cytology should be taken from the right hemidiaphragm, the right and left gutters, and the pelvis. The abdomen and pelvis should then be explored thoroughly.

Every attempt should be made to remove the mass intact. In the past, the standard treatment included a bilateral salpingo-oophorectomy as well as total abdominal hysterectomy. Patients often question the necessity for hysterectomy if the mass proves to be benign. The addition of the hysterectomy adds little to the morbidity and avoids the potential of another procedure if final pathology reveals the mass to be malignant. The risk of a subsequent malignancy in this organ is also avoided, and postoperative estrogen replacement therapy is simplified.

POSTMENOPAUSAL PALPABLE OVARY SYNDROME

Barber and Graber's classic paper on the postmenopausal patient with a palpable ovary, written in 1971,[11] emphasized the need for any postmenopausal woman in whom the adnexa is palpable to undergo surgical exploration with excision of the mass because of the risk of malignancy. The most common diagnosis, however, is ovarian fibroma or other benign solid tumor, and ultrasound evaluation of the ovaries is helpful in evaluating the need for surgical exploration. Barber has recently modified his recommendations and appended that surgical exploration need not be performed on the asymptomatic patient with a nonpalpable ovarian mass detected on ultrasound.[9]

ROLE OF PROPHYLACTIC OOPHORECTOMY

The role of prophylactic oophorectomy for women undergoing pelvic surgery for benign disease after childbearing has been completed is debated. In retrospective studies of patients with ovarian carcinoma, up to 12% of patients have undergone previous pelvic surgery with retention of ovarian function.[12] Further, up to 4% of patients

undergoing pelvic surgery require reoperation because of a benign ovarian disorder.[13] However, the risk of future coronary artery disease and osteoporosis are increased with oophorectomy, and these risks must be carefully weighed against potential benefits.

Although no prospective studies have been reported, prophylactic oophorectomy should be discussed with all perimenopausal patients (ages 40–50 years) who are undergoing pelvic surgery for benign disease. The patients must be informed of all potential risks as well as benefits. The patient should also be aware of the risk of ovarian cancer from germinal tissue remnants and of primary peritoneal carcinoma after bilateral oophorectomy.

REFERENCES

1. Koonings PP, Grimes DA, Campbell K, Sommerville M. Bilateral ovarian neoplasms and the risk of malignancy. Am J Obstet Gynecol 1990;162:167.
2. Rulin MC, Preston AL. Adnexal masses in postmenopausal women. Obstet Gynecol 1987;70:578.
3. Andolf E, Jorgensen C. A prospective comparison of clinical ultrasound and operative examination of the female pelvis. J Ultrasound Med 1988;7:617.
4. Sassone AM, Timor-Tritsch IE, Artner A, et al. Transvaginal sonographic characterization of ovarian disease: Evaluation of a new scoring system to predict ovarian malignancy. Obstet Gynecol 1991;78:70.
5. Bast RC, Klug TL, St. John E, et al. A radioimmunoassay using a monoclonal antibody to monitor the course of epithelial ovarian cancer. N Engl J Med 1983;309:883.
6. Malkasian GD, Podratz KC, Stanhope CR, et al. CA-125 in gynecologic practice. Am J Obstet Gynecol 1986;155:515.
7. Spanos W. Preoperative hormonal therapy of cystic adnexal masses. Am J Obstet Gynecol 1973;116:551.
8. Seltzer VL, Maiman M, Boyce J, et al. Laparoscopic surgery in the management of ovarian cysts. Female Patient 1992;17:16.
9. Barber H. A second look at the postmenopausal palpable ovary. Female Patient 1988;13:13.
10. Maiman M, Seltzer V, Boyce J. Laparoscopic excision of ovarian neoplasms subsequently found to be malignant. Obstet Gynecol 1991;77:563.
11. Barber HRK, Graber EA. The PMPO syndrome (postmenopausal palpable ovary syndrome). Obstet Gynecol 1971;38:921.
12. Gibbs EK. Suggested prophylaxis for ovarian cancer. Am J Obstet Gynecol 1971;111:756.
13. McKenzie LL. On discussion of the frequency of oophorectomy at the time of hysterectomy. Am J Obstet Gynecol 1968;100:724.

Evaluation and Management of Pelvic Pain

Sujata Somani

Pelvic pain is a common complaint among women presenting to emergency departments and primary care offices. More than half of all women are affected by pelvic pain at some time in their lives, and approximately 10% have persistent pelvic pain of greater than 6 months' duration. There are numerous causes of both acute and chronic pelvic pain. These may involve gynecologic as well as gastrointestinal, urologic, and musculoskeletal causes. The diagnosis and management of pelvic pain depends on whether it is acute, chronic, or an acute exacerbation of recurrent or chronic pain. Acute pelvic pain is generally an emergency and indicates potentially serious and at times life-threatening problems, which require prompt evaluation and appropriate management. Chronic pelvic pain and recurrent pelvic pain associated with the menstrual cycle are usually not life threatening but can lead to long-term suffering and disability. This chapter is intended to help the primary care provider distinguish and manage the various causes of acute and chronic pelvic pain.

ANATOMY OF THE FEMALE PELVIS

The female pelvis is bounded anteriorly by the pubis, laterally by the ilium and ischium, and posteriorly by the sacrum and coccyx. It is in direct communication with the abdominal cavity. The upper limit of the pelvis is at the level of the iliac crest. The anterior wall of the pelvis is formed by the rectus muscles, and the lateral walls are formed by the iliopsoas and obturator muscles. Inferiorly, the pelvic outlet is bounded by the levator ani and pubococcygeus muscles, which form the pelvic diaphragm. The visceral contents of the pelvis include the bladder and urethra anteriorly; the geni-

tal organs, including the upper vagina, uterus, fallopian tubes, broad ligaments, and ovaries medially; and the rectum posteriorly. Also contained within the pelvis are loops of ileum, the sigmoid colon, the ureter, and the appendix.

Innervation of the Pelvis

The pelvic viscera is innervated by autonomic and somatic nerves. The sympathetic plexus is derived from T11–L2 and the parasympathetic from S2–4. The bladder and urethra derive their autonomic innervation from the hypogastric plexus, the uterus and the proximal fallopian tubes from the uterovaginal plexus, and the rectum from the rectal plexus. All of these combine to form the inferior hypogastric nerves, which arise from the presacral nerve of the hypogastric plexus. The ovaries and the lateral portion of the fallopian tubes are supplied from the ovarian plexus, and the rectal autonomic nerve supply originates from the rectal plexus.

The visceral pelvic peritoneum covers the upper one third of the bladder, the uterus, and the upper third of the rectum. It is also innervated by the autonomic nerves supplying these viscera. The peritoneum is insensitive to touch but responds with pain to traction, distention, spasm, or ischemia.

There is common sympathetic and parasympathetic innervation of the bladder, genital organs, and rectum. This common innervation makes it difficult for the patient to pinpoint the exact location of the origin of pelvic pain.

ACUTE PELVIC PAIN

Acute pelvic pain can result from gynecologic and nongynecologic causes. Acute pain from gynecologic causes may originate from the vulva, vagina, uterus, fallopian tubes, or ovaries (Table 7–1). Vulvar pain and dyspareunia are usually due to infections such as candidal vulvitis, herpes, and infections of the Skene's or paraurethral glands and the Bartholin's glands. Vaginal pain is also usually due to infections such as candidal infections and herpetic ulcerations. Uterine pain may be due to complications from pregnancy, such as threatened or incomplete abortion; dysmenorrhea; uterine fibroids; and adenomyosis. Tubal pain may be due to ectopic pregnancy; complications following abortion, such as pelvic infections or hemorrhage; and pelvic infections leading to pelvic inflammatory disease (PID) or tubo-ovarian abscesses. Ovarian-related causes of pelvic pain can be ruptured ovarian cysts, endometriomas, or ovarian torsion. Acute exacerbation of chronic pain originating in the genital tract can be caused by endometriosis, adenomyosis, or pelvic adhesions or can be related to dysmenorrhea, premenstrual syndrome, and uterine fibroids with degeneration.

Nongynecologic causes of acute pelvic pain may be from the urinary, gastrointestinal, or musculoskeletal systems (Tables 7–2, 7–3). Urinary causes of pelvic pain include cystitis, urethritis, or urinary calculi. Gastrointestinal causes of pelvic pain may be appendicitis, diverticulitis, bowel obstruction, inflammatory bowel disease, strangulated hernias, and Meckel's diverticulum with bowel obstruction or adhesions. Musculoskeletal causes of pelvic pain may be psoas muscle abscess or hemorrage, lumbosacral disk disease, or musculoskeletal tumors.

Approach to the Patient with Acute Pelvic Pain

Acute pelvic pain can represent a life-threatening emergency. Patients with acute pelvic pain usually require an immediate evaluation to determine the need for hospitalization and referral to a gynecologist or general surgeon. The history should include the patient's age, menstrual and sexual history, contraceptive use, and past gynecologic, surgical, and medical problems. The duration and location of the pain should be noted as well as its relation to posture and movement. Patients should be questioned for symptoms such as fever, nausea, vomiting, constipation, dysuria, unusual vaginal discharge, or bleeding. A menstrual and sexual history should be obtained to rule out first trimester complications related to pregnancy. In a patient complaining of an acute exacerbation of chronic pelvic pain, one needs to consider the duration of the pain, its timing in association with

TABLE 7–1. Common Gynecologic Causes of Acute Pelvic Pain

Vulva	Infections
	Candida
	Herpes
	Skene's glands
	Bartholin's glands
Vagina	Infections
	Candida
	Herpetic ulcerations
Uterine	Pregnancy complications
	Incomplete abortion
	Threatened abortion
	Dysmenorrhea
	Uterine fibroids with degeneration
	Adenomyosis
Tubal	Ectopic pregnancy
	Infections—PID, tubo-ovarian abscess
	Torsion
Ovarian	Ruptured ovarian cyst
	Endometrioma
	Torsion

PID, Pelvic inflammatory disease.

TABLE 7–2. Nongynecologic Causes of Pelvic Pain

Skin	Herpes zoster, scabies, granuloma inguinale, actinomycosis, pilonidal cysts
Fat	Infection and inflammation, tumor (lipoma, sarcoma), necrobiosis lipoidica diabeticorum
Muscle	(Especially the rectus, psoas, obturator, and obliques) Strain, bruise, hematoma, tumor
Fascia (Hernias)	Inguinal femoral, obturator, spinelian, umbilical, epigastric, incisional
Nerve	(Especially the intercostal, iliohypogastric, ilioinguinal, genitofemoral, obturator, sciatic) Compression, ischemia, traction, friction, injection, irradiation, laceration, neuroma, neuritis
Artery	Aneurysm, ischemia (e.g., abdominal angina)
Vein	Thrombophlebitis
Nodes	Inflammation, tumor
Bone	Osteomyelitis, osteitis, arthritis, tumor, fracture, disk, posture (lordosis, scoliosis), coccydynia, ligamentous injuries
Peritoneum	Peritonitis, tuberculosis
Mesentery	Cysts
Kidney	Stones, infection, tumor
Ureter	Stones, external obstruction from inflammation, tumor, fibrosis, infection
Bladder	Infection, tumor, dysfunctional
GI tract	See Table 7–3

GI, Gastrointestinal.
Courtesy of Dr. Patricia Numann.

TABLE 7–3. Gastrointestinal Sources of Pelvic Pain

Inflammation	Gastroenteritis, diverticular disease, regional enteritis, Meckel's diverticulum, appendicitis, proctitis, hemorrhoids, mesenteric venous occlusion, cholecystitis (usually secondary to gallstones), pancreatitis
Tumor	Polyps, carcinoma of colon, carcinoma of small bowel
Perforation	Ulcer
Obstruction	Adhesions, hernias, tumors, volvulus, irradiation
Infarction	Bowel, appendices epiploicae
Metabolic	Lactose intolerance, sprue and steatorrhea, constipation
Psychogenic	Functional bowel disorders, anxiety

Courtesy of Dr. Patricia Numann.

the menstrual cycle, and any other factors, such as a history of pelvic infections, pregnancy complications, or surgeries. One also needs to ask whether there is a history of previous episodes of similar pain, its diagnosis or management, and the duration of similar symptoms in the past.

The physical examination of the patient presenting with acute pain is directed toward evaluation of the various organ systems within the pelvic cavity. Inspection of the vulva and vagina is important. Mucopurulent discharge from the cervix may be a sign of PID. A bimanual examination should be performed with special attention to cervical motion tenderness, midline or adnexal tenderness, and the presence of uterine enlargement or adnexal masses. Cervical motion tenderness is generally a sign of intraperitoneal inflammation, which may result from PID, ruptured ovarian cyst, or ruptured ectopic pregnancy with hematoperitoneum. A rectal examination with tenderness on the right side suggests appendicitis, and a stool sample for guaiac testing is helpful in the diagnosis for diverticulitis.

Common Causes of Acute Pelvic Pain

The most common gynecologic causes of acute pelvic pain are PID, ectopic pregnancy, rupture of an ovarian cyst, and adnexal torsion. The most common nongynecologic causes include acute appendicitis and ureteral stones (Fig. 7–1).

Gynecologic Causes

PELVIC INFLAMMATORY DISEASE. Pelvic inflammatory disease is one of the most common causes of acute pelvic pain. The incidence of PID is 10 to 13 per 1000 women in the reproductive age; it is highest in women between 15 and 24 years, with an incidence of 18 to 20 per 1000 women.[1-4] One in 10 American women develop PID during their lifetime,[5] and PID accounts for 5 to 20% of all gynecologic admissions. One fourth of patients with PID are younger than 25 years old, and early diagnosis and adequate treatment is especially important in this age group because up to 15% of women become infertile after one episode of PID, and 17 to 20% develop chronic pelvic pain.[6]

Risk factors for PID include multiple sexual partners, low socioeconomic status, and a previous episode of PID and concurrent use of an intrauterine device.[7-9] The infection is usually caused by ascending organisms from the cervix. Multiple organisms may be involved, but PID is most often caused by gonococcus, *Chlamydia,* and other vaginal organisms such as alpha streptococcus, *Escherichia coli, Staphylococcus aureus,* and *Bacteroides.*

Patients with PID may not develop symptoms until weeks to months after contact with an infected partner. They usually present with acute onset of moderate to severe lower abdominal and pelvic pain approximately 1 week after menses. The pain secondary to PID is often worse with defecation and urination. The patient usually has an elevated temperature, often as high as 40°C (104°F). The patient may also have other complaints such as abnormal vaginal bleeding or nausea and vomiting. Unlike appendicitis, nausea and vomiting are present in less than half of patients with PID, and the pain and tenderness is usually bilateral in PID compared with the right lower quadrant pain with appendicitis.

The abdominal examination in patients with PID usually reveals lower abdominal tenderness. Pelvic examination shows a mucopurulent vaginal discharge and marked cervical motion tenderness with pelvic and bilateral adnexal tenderness. One may also palpate a pelvic mass on examination, and these patients should be evaluated by ultrasound to rule out pelvic abscesses.

Unlike patients with PID with bacterial infection, patients with PID due to *Chlamydia* may present with subtle signs and a normal temperature or a low-grade fever. They may have only mild lower abdominal pain and minimal adnexal or cervical motion tenderness. Subclinical infections may be entirely asymptomatic; however, they can lead to pelvic adhesions and infertility. Therefore, it is important to obtain culture samples from patients with mild symptoms of pelvic pain to test for *Chlamydia* and to treat patients with suspected

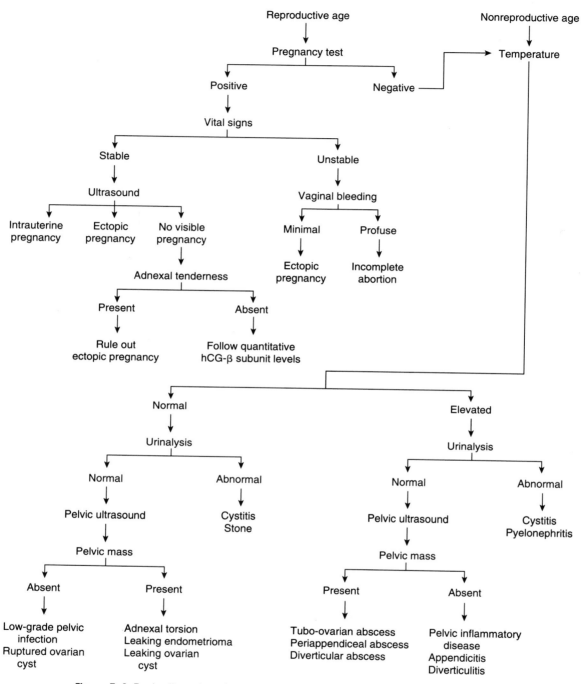

Figure 7–1. Evaluation of acute pelvic pain. hCG, Human chorionic gonadotropin.

low-grade pelvic infection with doxycycline. Pelvic inflammatory disease can also occur after therapeutic or spontaneous abortion, endometrial biopsy, dilation and curettage, hysterosalpingogram, hysteroscopy, and any other pelvic surgery such as

hysterectomy during which the vaginal flora come in contact with the peritoneal cavity.

Definitive diagnosis of PID is sometimes difficult, and up to one third of the patients admitted with a diagnosis of PID have no evidence of pelvic infection at laparoscopy.[10] Patients are often treated empirically with antibiotics if signs and symptoms suggest pelvic infection. Definitive diagnosis of PID can be made by laparoscopy; however, the cost and risks of surgery prohibit diagnostic laparoscopy in most patients. Laparoscopy is indicated in patients who do not respond to antibiotic therapy or in whom the diagnosis of PID is uncertain or in patients who have suspected pelvic abscesses who do not respond to antibiotic therapy.

PREGNANCY COMPLICATIONS. Pregnancy complications require urgent diagnosis and management and should always be considered in the evaluation of any woman with acute pelvic pain. Ectopic pregnancy occurs in approximately one in 100 pregnancies. Risk factors for ectopic pregnancy include a previous history of PID, a history of intrauterine device use, pelvic adhesions, tubal disease or surgery, and in utero diethylstilbestrol exposure. The most common presenting symptoms are abnormal uterine bleeding and lower abdominal pain. The pain is usually more severe on one side but may be diffuse in a patient with a ruptured ectopic pregnancy and hemoperitoneum.

All women of childbearing age who present with acute abdominal pain should have a pregnancy test to rule out an ectopic pregnancy. If the pregnancy test is positive and vital signs are stable, a quantitative level of hCG-β subunit and an ultrasound should be done. Any patient with a positive pregnancy test and hypotension, elevated heart rate, or signs of peritoneal inflammation should be checked for a ruptured ectopic pregnancy, and prompt referral to a gynecologist for surgical management is warranted. Any suspicion of an ectopic pregnancy should also be promptly referred to a gynecologist for further evaluation.

RUPTURED OVARIAN CYST. Rupture of an ovarian cyst can lead to spillage of fluid contents or blood into the peritoneal cavity, which can cause peritoneal inflammation and acute pelvic pain. This can occur during any time of the menstrual cycle but is most common in midcycle during ovulation or in the luteal phase of the cycle with a corpus luteum cyst. The patient usually presents with acute onset of diffuse lower abdominal and pelvic pain, which is usually more severe on one side. Examination reveals lower abdominal and pelvic tenderness and mild to moderate cervical motion tenderness. Absence of fever or leukocytosis is helpful in distinguishing patients with PID from those with a ruptured ovarian cyst. Diagnosis can be made by ultrasound or culdocentesis or by a laparoscopy in some patients. Culdocentesis is done by insertion of a spinal needle through the posterior fornix into the peritoneal cavity. Aspiration of clear fluid on culdocentesis confirms a diagnosis of a ruptured ovarian cyst, whereas bloody fluid can be a sign of both cyst rupture and ectopic pregnancy. The presence of blood on culdocentesis requires close monitoring of the patient for hemodynamic instability. Surgical intervention by laparoscopy or laparotomy may be required in patients with a ruptured ovarian cyst and hemoperitoneum.

ADNEXAL TORSION. Adnexal torsion is an uncommon but important cause of acute pelvic pain that requires urgent diagnosis and treatment. Patients usually present with acute onset of unilateral lower abdominal pain, which is the result of vascular occlusion of the twisted organ. Arterial perfusion into the torsed adnexa continues, and venous return is decreased or absent, causing organ edema, distention, and eventual necrosis. The pain is usually quite severe and is generally described as sharp and colicky in nature, with localization to the side with the torsion, although there are occasional instances of bilateral adnexal torsion. Often the patients have a mild fever, nausea, vomiting, and a mild leukocytosis. In contrast to patients with appendicitis, patients with adnexal torsion generally have pain before the initiation of nausea and vomiting.

Physical examination usually reveals a low-grade fever, lower abdominal tenderness, and an adnexal mass. Unlike patients with acute PID or ruptured ovarian cyst, patients with adnexal torsion do not have tenderness in the cul-de-sac. The adnexal mass is usually 5 to 10 cm in size, because masses larger than 10 to 12 cm are too large to undergo torsion owing to their limited mobility. Many patients with adnexal torsion report previous episodes of similar pain that resolved spontaneously, suggesting previous episodes of torsion and spontaneous detorsion.[11, 12]

Torsion can occur in a normal ovary or fallopian tube but generally occurs in an enlarged ovary or a dilated fallopian tube. Patients with endometriomas or PID rarely develop torsion because these masses cause adhesions and are generally fixed to other pelvic structures.

Early diagnosis and management is important because the torsed adnexa undergoes necrosis with time. A suspicion of adnexal torsion requires prompt consultation with a gynecologist and surgical management by either laparoscopy or laparotomy. If the adnexal torsion is detected before the onset of necrosis, it can simply be untorsed at surgery. Patients with one episode of adnexal torsion are at risk for future torsion on the same or the opposite side and should be warned to seek medical consultation early if recurrent symptoms develop.

Gastrointestinal Causes

APPENDICITIS. Appendicitis is the most common nongynecologic cause of acute abdominal and pelvic pain. It usually appears with fever, anorexia, nausea, and periumbilical to right lower quadrant abdominal pain. Classically, the pain begins in the periumbilical region and evolves to the right lower quadrant within 24 hours. Examination frequently reveals an elevated temperature, right lower quadrant tenderness on abdominal and pelvic examination, and tenderness on the right side on rectal examination. Patients may have psoas inflammation with appendicitis that is manifested by increased pain with extension of the hip. Most patients have an elevated white blood cell count and sedimentation rate. Patients suspected to have acute appendicitis should have prompt evaluation by a general surgeon.

DIVERTICULITIS. Diverticulitis occurs most commonly in older women and appears with left lower abdominal and pelvic pain associated with fever and an elevated white blood cell count. Patients may also present with a pelvic mass on physical examination. Diagnosis is usually made by the exclusion of other causes of pelvic pain and the findings of diverticuli on barium enema or computed tomography scan. Patients with suspected diverticulitis are usually treated with antibiotics unless a large mass is present, in which case surgical intervention may be required.

Urologic Causes

CYSTITIS. Cystitis is a very common infection in women. Presenting symptoms include lower abdominal or midline pelvic pain associated with dysuria, urinary frequency, and occasional hematuria or pyuria. The diagnosis is made by examination of the urine for white blood cells and bacteria and is confirmed by culture samples. Treatment with antibiotics relieves symptoms rapidly.

RENAL STONES. Renal stones can appear with acute colicky abdominal or pelvic pain. Patients with renal stones usually have costovertebral angle tenderness and back pain. Urinalysis frequently reveals hematuria. Definitive diagnosis is based on an intravenous pyelogram and should be done in patients with a suspicion of renal stones. Treatment is generally conservative with intravenous hydration and analgesia. Surgery may be required in patients who fail conservative therapy.

Causes of Recurrent Pelvic Pain

Causes of recurrent pelvic pain include ovulatory pain, dysmenorrhea, and dyspareunia. Ovulatory pain (mittelschmerz) occurs during midcycle and is related to ovulation. It is usually felt as mild unilateral pelvic discomfort for 24 to 36 hours and can be associated with vaginal spotting.

Dysmenorrhea

Dysmenorrhea can be primary or secondary. Primary dysmenorrhea is pain during menses without any identifiable pelvic pathologic condition, whereas secondary dysmenorrhea is menstrual pain associated with pelvic disease such as adhesions, endometriosis, adenomyosis, leiomyomas, intrauterine devices, or obstructed outflow of menstrual blood secondary to anatomic causes.

Dysmenorrhea is a common complaint among women. More than half of all menstruating women complain of some degree of discomfort for 48 to 72 hours, and 10% of women are incapacitated for 1 to 3 days each month. In one study, three fourths of women reported experiencing some degree of dysmenorrhea, and 15% suffered from enough pain to limit physical activity.[13] Dysmenorrhea usually begins with the onset of menses and lasts from 8 to 72 hours. The pain can be felt as an aching heaviness in the pelvis, lower back, and upper thighs. Some women have associated symptoms of nausea, vomiting, diarrhea, headaches, and fatigue.

It is believed that dysmenorrhea is caused by increased concentrations of prostaglandins in the endometrium, which increase uterine contractility.[14, 15] Increased prostaglandin $F_{2\alpha}$ has been shown in patients with endometriosis, uterine myomas, and intrauterine devices.[16, 17] Hormonal factors are also important in the etiology of dysmenorrhea. Dysmenorrhea is known to occur only in ovulatory cycles and is therefore uncommon in women for 6 to 12 months after menarche until ovulatory cycles are established.

In the evaluation of the patient presenting with dysmenorrhea, it is important to assess whether any pelvic pathologic condition is present. Endometriosis should be suspected in patients who have associated dyspareunia, infertility, or premenstrual spotting. Pelvic adhesions are suspected in patients with a history of pelvic infections, previous pelvic surgeries, or use of an intrauterine device. Pelvic examination may reveal cervical stenosis or an enlarged uterus that is suggestive of uterine fibroids or adenomyosis. Ultrasound may be needed in some women to evaluate for congenital abnormalities or fibroids. Hysterosalpingography can identify uterine anomalies, and hysteroscopy can be helpful in diagnosing endometrial polyps. Diagnostic laparoscopy may be needed in some patients who do not respond to conservative management for diagnosis and treatment of pelvic adhesions or endometriosis.

TREATMENT OF DYSMENORRHEA. The treatment of dysmenorrhea depends on the etiology. Patients with primary dysmenorrhea can be treated with oral contraceptives if they also require contraception and have no contraindication to their use. Anovulatory cycles due to oral contraceptives decrease the prostaglandin content of the uterine cavity and result in decreased contractions of the uterine muscle, resulting in relief of dysmenorrhea. Eighty percent of patients achieve complete relief of dysmenorrhea with oral contraceptives.[18, 19]

In women who do not require contraception, prostaglandin synthetase inhibitors can be used. Studies have shown that prostaglandins and their metabolites are reduced with the use of prostaglandin inhibitors, resulting in decreased uterine contractility and menstrual pain. These medications also decrease the amount of menstrual blood loss. The various types of prostaglandin inhibitors are equally efficacious in the relief of dysmenorrhea.[19–22] They are most effective if given as soon as menses begin before the onset of cramping and pain. Their side effects include headaches, gastrointestinal upset, and occasional feelings of disorientation or ''spaciness.'' A more serious complication from these drugs is renal disease, including nephrotic syndrome, acute interstitial cystitis, and acute papillary and tubular necrosis.[23, 24] Most of these complications occur in older women who take these medications for a long period of time.

In patients who remain symptomatic after using oral contraceptives or prostaglandin inhibitors, a diagnostic laparoscopy may be indicated to rule out pelvic pathology. Patients with a normal pelvis at laparoscopy are candidates for either laparoscopic uterosacral nerve ablation or presacral neurectomy to control their symptoms. Laparoscopic uterosacral nerve ablation is accomplished by laser or electrocautery and separation of the nerves along the uterosacral ligaments, which carry the pain fibers from the uterus. Presacral neurectomy is done via laparotomy and removal of the nerve fibers along the presacral region.

Endometriosis

Endometriosis is defined as the presence of endometrial glands and stroma outside of the uterine cavity. The presence of endometrial tissue within the uterine muscle is called adenomyosis.

The incidence of endometriosis in the general population is believed to be 1 to 2% but is much higher in infertile women and women presenting with pelvic pain and dysmenorrhea. Endometriosis is found in 25% of all laparoscopies performed.[25] Patients with endometriosis usually present with infertility or pelvic pain. The presenting complaints include worsening dysmenorrhea; dyspareunia; noncyclic pelvic, abdominal, and lower back pain; and pain and cramping before the menstrual cycle. Premenstrual spotting for 4 to 7 days before the onset of menses is another sign of endometriosis. Physical findings with endometriosis are rarely specific. Patients may have thickened, nodular uterosacral ligaments on examination or may have adnexal masses or tenderness. A retroverted and fixed uterus may also be present in advanced cases. The severity of pain does not correlate with the extent of disease, however, and many patients with advanced endometriosis have no symptoms.

The definitive diagnosis of endometriosis can be made only by surgery and direct visualization or biopsy because there are no symptoms or signs that are pathognomonic for the disease. Endometriosis can be suspected in patients presenting with worsening dysmenorrhea, especially if it is not relieved by nonsteroidal agents or oral contraceptives. Patients with dyspareunia or infertility have a high likelihood of endometriosis. The definitive diagnosis is made by laparoscopy by direct visualization of the endometriotic implants in the pelvis or by biopsy and microscopic evaluation of suspected areas.

The treatment of endometriosis can be surgical, medical, or a combination of both. The initial treatment can be done at the time of diagnostic laparoscopy with lysis of adhesions and ablation of all visible lesions by electrocautery or laser. Medical treatment can be done for patients with extensive disease who cannot be treated by laparoscopy or for patients who are thought to have recurrent disease. Agents used to treat endometriosis include danazol, gonadotropin-releasing hormone agonists, or, less commonly, oral contraceptives. This is discussed in greater detail in Chapter 8.

Dyspareunia

Dyspareunia, or painful intercourse, is another complaint causing recurrent pelvic pain. There are numerous causes for dyspareunia (Table 7–4). It is important to ask the patient whether the pain occurs during each act of intercourse or intermittently. Intermittent pain may be related to infections or cyclic causes such as ovarian cysts or

TABLE 7–4. Causes of Dyspareunia

Vulva	Infections
	Herpes vulvitis
	Candida vulvitis
	Folliculitis
	Bartholin's gland infection
	Anatomic
	Episiotomy scar
	Perineorrhaphy scar
	Other
	Vestibulitis
Vagina	Infections
	Candida vaginitis
	Gardnerella vaginitis
	Congenital
	Imperforate hymen
	Vaginal septum
	Anatomic
	Postsurgical shortening of vagina
	Tender vaginal cuff after hysterectomy
	Other
	Atrophic vaginitis
	Insufficient lubrication
	Urethritis
	Urethral diverticulum
Pelvic	Infection
	Pelvic inflammatory disease
	Other
	Pelvic masses
	Endometriosis
	Adhesions
	Cystitis

endometriosis. Physical examination should include inspection for signs of vulvar, vaginal, or cervical infections, and cultures should be obtained in all patients. Scarring secondary to previous surgeries, including episiotomies or perineorrhaphy, can be a cause of dyspareunia. Pain in the vagina can also be due to tenderness of the levator muscles, and injection of local anesthetics at the trigger points may be helpful for both diagnosis and therapy. Congenital abnormalities such as a vaginal septum or imperforate hymen should also be considered at the time of vaginal examination. Pelvic examination to evaluate for any masses, such as fibroids or ovarian cysts; tenderness from PID; adhesions; or endometriosis is indicated. Patients should be asked to pinpoint the location of the pain, whether it is more external or deep in the vagina or is related to the vaginal apex, cervix, uterus, or other pelvic organs.

Patients may also complain of burning in the vulvar region, which is exacerbated with intercourse (vulvodynia). Colposcopy of the vulva may reveal characteristic aceto-white changes consistent with human papilloma virus infection. Numerous treatment methods, including xylocaine ointment, 5-fluorouracil cream, interferon or alcohol injections, tricyclic antidepressants, and surgical therapy, have been used but with limited success (see Chapter 9).

CHRONIC PELVIC PAIN

Chronic pelvic pain is generally defined as pain localized to the pelvic area of longer than 6 months' duration. Chronic pelvic pain accounts for 2 to 10% of all outpatient gynecologic referrals and is the reason for 10 to 35% of laparoscopies[26] and 12% of hysterectomies per year.[27, 28] The differential diagnosis, evaluation, and management of chronic pelvic pain are much less straightforward than those of acute pain. The patient usually presents after months or years of chronic pain and numerous visits to many health care providers. One needs a careful, unhurried approach in the history and diagnostic evaluation of patients with chronic pelvic pain.

A thorough evaluation may be required by several different specialty providers including primary care providers, gynecologists, psychologists, urologists, gastroenterologists, and anesthesiologists. It is important to have appropriate communication among the various specialists to avoid inconsistencies in the diagnosis and delivery of information. A large percentage of patients have a concomitant history of psychiatric illnesses. The psychological component of chronic pelvic pain should be recognized, and a psychological evaluation should be considered as a routine part of the evaluation of chronic pelvic pain.

Differential Diagnosis

The causes of chronic pelvic pain can be divided into gynecologic, nongynecologic, and chronic pelvic pain without obvious cause.

The most common gynecologic causes for chronic pelvic pain are endometriosis and pelvic adhesions. Other less common findings on laparoscopy include ovarian cysts, a retroverted uterus, small uterine fibroids, and other uterine anomalies; however, their role in the etiology of chronic pelvic pain is controversial. Many nongynecologic causes of pelvic pain should be considered before performing a diagnostic laparoscopy (Table 7–5). The most common are gastrointestinal, including constipation, irritable bowel syndrome, inflammatory bowel disease, hernia, and diverticulitis. Urologic causes of chronic pelvic pain include interstitial cystitis and urethral syndrome that manifests with urinary frequency, urgency, and dysuria without bacteriuria. Orthopedic and musculoskeletal

TABLE 7–5. Causes of Chronic Pelvic Pain in Patients with Negative Results on Laparoscopy

Gastrointestinal tract
Constipation
Irritable bowel syndrome
Inflammatory bowel disease
Diverticulitis
Urinary tract
Urethral syndrome
Interstitial cystitis
Musculoskeletal/neurologic
Pelvic floor tension myalgia
Piriformis syndrome
Nerve entrapment
Ventral hernia
Rectus tendon strain
Myofascial pain
Back or pelvic postural changes
Gynecologic
Pelvic vascular congestion
Cervical stenosis

causes include degenerative hip or spine disease, pelvic floor tension myalgia, contraction of the levator plate, pain arising from the lumbar musculature, or spasm of the piriformis muscle. Myofascial pain arising from the abdominal wall can result from entrapment of the genitofemoral or ilioinguinal nerves, which can occur after a Pfannenstiel's or transverse incision. It may also be due to fibrosis and retraction of previous incisions or occasional wound endometriosis or suture granulomas. Myofascial pain has been reported in up to 30% of patients with normal findings at diagnostic laparoscopy.[29, 30]

Evaluation

A thorough history and physical examination can help guide the evaluation of women with chronic pelvic pain. The history should include the duration of the pain and its relationship to the menstrual cycle, because this is important in differentiating among functional causes of long-term pain such as ovulatory pain (mittelschmerz) and dysmenorrhea. Patients should be asked to describe the location and severity of the pain and variation over time. It is important to ask whether there is any dyspareunia and whether this has affected the frequency of intercourse. It is also important to take a thorough developmental history because a large percentage of patients with chronic pelvic pain have a history of childhood sexual abuse. The degree of functional impairment and interference with sleep and work should also be assessed. Any associated urologic symptoms such

as exacerbation before or with voiding would suggest urethral syndrome, and tenderness of the urethra and bladder should be assessed. Gastroenterologic symptoms such as intermittent diarrhea or constipation or episodes of painful gaseous distention suggest a diagnosis of irritable bowel syndrome. A history of previous surgery or pelvic infections may lead to the suspicion of pelvic adhesions or myofascial pain.

The physical examination is important but is often nondiagnostic in the evaluation of chronic pelvic pain. In one study, up to 50% of patients with normal results on examination had abnormal pelvic findings at laparoscopy; thus, laparoscopy should not be reserved only for patients with abnormalities on examination.[31] It is important, however, to evaluate for urethral or bladder tenderness and for myofascial or musculoskeletal tenderness. Because there are multiple tissues between the abdominal wall and the vagina, it may be difficult to locate the exact area of tenderness during the bimanual examination. Myofascial pain is suspected when pain is localized to the anterior abdominal wall and is reproduced by direct palpation or contraction of the rectus muscle. It is helpful to identify the source of the pain by palpation of small areas of tissue with a cotton tip or a single finger or by placement of a needle and local anesthetic into the tissue either by the vaginal or the abdominal route. The exact location of the pain can be confirmed if it is completely blocked by the local anesthetic. Discomfort in the cul-de-sac or uterosacral ligaments or a fixed retroverted uterus may suggest endometriosis.

Psychological and Behavioral Assessment

Psychosocial and behavioral assessment should be an integral part of the evaluation of women presenting with complaints of chronic pelvic pain. Numerous reports have been published regarding the psychological profile of women with chronic pelvic pain. Women with chronic pelvic pain are at increased risk for major depression, substance abuse, and sexual dysfunction.[32] Many studies have shown that the prevalence of childhood or adult sexual abuse is high in women with chronic pelvic pain.[33–37] Patients with chronic pelvic pain also report a high incidence of marital and sexual dysfunction.[38] The initial psychological assessment is most commonly done by the Minnesota Multiphasic Personality Inventory (MMPI), which is helpful in identifying patients who may require more intensive evaluation.[39, 40] The psychological factors that are important to assess are the affective state, the response of family members to the pain, any relationship or sexual problems, and the impact of the pain on the patient's life.[41]

All patients should undergo an evaluation by a psychologist interested and knowledgeable in the management of patients with chronic pain. In dealing with patients who present with chronic pelvic pain, it is important to avoid implying that the pain is imagined or "in their minds." It should be explained to the patient that the psychological evaluation is part of the overall evaluation of all patients with chronic pain and should be done before any operative intervention.

Laboratory evaluation should include a complete blood count, a sedimentation rate to screen for chronic PID, a stool sample for guaiac testing, a urinalysis and culture, and cervical cultures and cytology. Pelvic ultrasound is helpful in patients with a pelvic mass or tenderness on examination or in patients who are obese or unable to relax so that an adequate pelvic examination can be performed. If urinary symptoms are present, an intravenous pyelogram or a cystoscopy is indicated. Patients with gastrointestinal symptoms such as intermittent diarrhea, constipation, or rectal bleeding should undergo sigmoidoscopy or barium enema. Hysteroscopy or hysterosalpingogram should be done in patients with abnormal bleeding to look for intrauterine disease. Diagnostic laparoscopy is the most helpful in the evaluation of patients with chronic pelvic pain. Patients with chronic pelvic pain are often anxious that the pain is indicative of a more serious underlying disorder, and a negative laparoscopy provides reassurance to the patient that no serious abnormalities are present. Up to 30% of patients can have improvement of symptoms even after a negative laparoscopy.[42]

Treatment

Medical Therapy

The treatment of patients with chronic pelvic pain should consist of an integrated approach with equal attention to somatic and psychological causes. A randomized study has shown that patients who are managed using an integrated approach have greater symptom control over time than those managed by the traditional approach with routine laparoscopy and subsequent referral to psychotherapy if no pathologic condition is found.[43] Psychotherapy in patients with chronic pelvic pain can be helpful in stress reduction, muscle relaxation, self-hypnosis, and specific behavioral and sexual therapy.

Treatment of specific causes is based on the diagnosis. Endometriosis can be treated by surgical or medical therapy. Chronic pelvic adhesions require surgical therapy, preferably by laparoscopy because a majority of adhesions recur after a laparotomy. Chronic pelvic infection may respond to antibiotic therapy. Patients with gastrointestinal diseases may respond to increased dietary fiber and medical therapy, based on the specific diagnosis. Patients with urethral syndrome may respond to urethral dilation and antibiotic therapy. Interstitial cystitis is difficult to eradicate, but symptoms may be controlled by hydrodilation and by dietary modification. Long-term therapy of myofascial pain can be accomplished by long-acting anesthetics or steroid injections. Some patients may require revision of incisional scars. Success has also been reported in some patients with portable transcutaneous nerve stimulation therapy.

Pharmacotherapy has been widely studied in chronic pain syndromes, and advocates for its use recommend that analgesics be taken continually to avoid medication-reinforced pain behavior.[44, 45] This approach, however, can result in long-term serious side effects with both nonsteroidal agents and narcotics because of their addiction potential. Antidepressants are also commonly used for chronic pain because there is a strong association between chronic pain and depression; however, studies using antidepressants with pelvic pain patients have not been done. Biofeedback and relaxation training has been used extensively in patients with chronic pain.

Operative Management

The initial operative management in most patients with chronic pelvic pain is diagnostic laparoscopy. Abnormal findings range from 14 to 92% in different studies.[46, 47] It is generally believed that 50 to 60% of patients with chronic pelvic pain have some abnormal findings at diagnostic laparoscopy.[48] The most common findings are endometriosis and pelvic and abdominal adhesions; however, the area of pathology does not always correlate with the location of the pain. Endometriosis is found in up to 40% of adolescents and 28% of adults at laparoscopy in patients with chronic pelvic pain.[48] Pelvic adhesions are found in 15 to 20% of patients with pelvic pain, and several studies have shown that lysis of adhesions improves pain in up to 65% of patients.[49, 50] Other laparoscopic findings include pelvic congestion and laceration of the broad ligament (Allen-Masters syndrome), but their role in the causation of pelvic pain is debated.[51, 52]

Presacral neurectomy has been used in the past

mostly in patients with dysmenorrhea and endometriosis and less commonly in patients with chronic pelvic pain. Initial success with presacral neurectomy in patients with dysmenorrhea and endometriosis was 60 to 80%; however, this procedure has lost popularity because a large percentage of patients have recurrence of pain in 18 to 30 months, presumably due to reinnervation of the pelvic nerves.[53] Patients with chronic pelvic pain, the origin of which is in the abdominal wall or the dorsal sacrum, which is outside the area of the presacral innervation, would not benefit from a presacral neurectomy.

Laparoscopic uterosacral nerve ablation is a newer alternative to presacral neurectomy in the surgical management of dysmenorrhea, endometriosis, and chronic pelvic pain. Sympathetic and parasympathetic fibers traveling along the uterosacral ligaments are cauterized and transected through the laparoscopic approach. In one double-blind randomized trial with a small number of patients, 80% had relief of pain at 3 months and 45% had continued relief at 1 year.[54]

REFERENCES

1. Centers for Disease Control. Pelvic inflammatory disease: United States. MMWR 1980;28:605.
2. World Health Organization. Non-gonococcal urethritis and other sexual diseases of public health importance. WHO Tech Rep Ser 1981;660:98.
3. Westrom L. Incidence, prevalence, and trends of acute pelvic inflammatory disease and its consequences in industrialized countries. Am J Obstet Gynecol 1980;138:880.
4. Eschenbach DA, Harnisch JP, Holmes KK. Pathogenesis of acute pelvic inflammatory disease: Role of contraception and other risk factors. Am J Obstet Gynecol 1977;128:838.
5. Aral SO, Mosha WD, Cates W Jr. Self reported pelvic inflammatory disease in the United States, 1988. JAMA 1991;266:2570.
6. Brunham RC. Therapy for acute pelvic inflammatory disease: A critique of recent treatment trials. Am J Obstet Gynecol 1984;148:235.
7. Sweet RL. Diagnosis and treatment of acute salpingitis. J Reprod Med 1977;19:21.
8. Holmes KK, Eschenbach DA, Knapp JS. Salpingitis: Overview of etiology and epidemiology. Am J Obstet Gynecol 1980;138:893.
9. Flesh G, Weiner JM, Corlett RC Jr, et al. The intrauterine contraceptive device and acute salpingitis: A multifactor analysis. Am J Obstet Gynecol 1979;135:402.
10. Jacobsen L, Westrom L. Objectivized diagnosis of acute pelvic inflammatory disease. Am J Obstet Gynecol 1969;105:1088.
11. Lee RA, Welsh JS. Torsion of the uterine adnexa. Am J Obstet Gynecol 1967;97:974.
12. McGowan L. Torsion of cystic or diseased adnexal tissue. Am J Obstet Gynecol 1964;88:135.
13. Andersch B, Milson I. An epidemiologic study of young women with dysmenorrhea. Am J Obstet Gynecol 1982;144:655.
14. Downie J, Poyser NL, Wunderlich M. Levels of prosta-

glandins in human endometrium during the normal menstrual cycle. J Physiol 1974;236:465.
15. Chan WY, Hill JC. Menstrual prostaglandin levels in nondysmenorrheic and dysmenorrheic subjects. Prostaglandins 1978;15:365.
16. Williams EA, Collins WP, Clayton SG. Studies in the involvement of prostaglandins in uterus symptomatology and pathology. Br J Obstet Gynaecol 1976;83:337.
17. Roy S, Shaw ST Jr. Role of prostaglandins in the IUD associated uterine bleeding—effect of a prostaglandin synthetase inhibitor (ibuprofen). Obstet Gynecol 1981;58:101.
18. Chan WY, Dawood MY. Prostaglandin levels in menstrual fluid of nondysmenorrheic and dysmenorrheic subjects with and without oral contraceptive or ibuprofen therapy. Adv Prostaglandin Thromboxane Leukot Res 1980;8:1445.
19. Chan WY, Dawood MR, Fuchs F. Prostaglandins in primary dysmenorrhea: Comparison of prophylactic and nonprophylactic treatment with ibuprofen and the use of oral contraceptives. Am J Med 1981;70:535.
20. Anderson ABM, Haynes PJ, Fraser IS, Turnbull AC. Trial of prostaglandin-synthetase inhibitors in primary dysmenorrhea. Lancet 1978;1:345.
21. Dingfelder JR. Primary dysmenorrhea treatment with prostaglandin inhibitors: A review. Am J Obstet Gynecol 1981;140:874.
22. Owen PR. Prostaglandin synthetase inhibitors in the treatment of primary dysmenorrhea. Outcome trials reviewed. Am J Obstet Gynecol 1984;148:96.
23. Carmichael J, Shankel SW. Effects of nonsteroidal anti-inflammatory drugs on prostaglandins and renal function. Am J Med 1985;78:992.
24. Reeves WB, Foley RJ, Weinman EF. Nephrotoxicity from nonsteroidal anti-inflammatory drugs. South Med J 1985;78:318.
25. Williams TJ, Pratt JH. Endometriosis in 1000 consecutive celiotomies: Incidence and management. Am J Obstet Gynecol 1977;129:255.
26. Levitan S, Eibschitz I, DeVries K, et al. The value of laparoscopy in women with chronic pelvic pain and a "normal pelvis." Int J Gynecol Obstet 1985;23:71.
27. Dicker RC, Greenspan JR, Strauss LT, et al. Complications of abdominal and vaginal hysterectomy among women of reproductive age in the United States. Am J Obstet Gynecol 1982;144:841.
28. Lee N, Dicker RC, Rubin GL, Ory HW. Confirmation of the preoperative diagnosis for hysterectomy. Am J Obstet Gynecol 1984;150:283.
29. Slocumb J. Neurological factors in chronic pelvic pain: Trigger points and the abdominal pelvic pain syndrome. Am J Obstet Gynecol 1984;149:536.
30. Reiter RC, Gambone JC. Demographic and historic variables in women with idiopathic chronic pelvic pain. Obstet Gynecol 1990;75:428.
31. Lundberg WI, Wall JE, Mathers JE. Laparoscopy in the evaluation of pelvic pain. Obstet Gynecol 1973;42:872.
32. Walder EW, Katon W, Harrop-Griffiths J, et al. Relationship of chronic pelvic pain to psychiatric diagnosis and childhood sexual abuse. Am J Psychiatry 1988;145:75.
33. Castelnuovo-Tedesco P, Krout BM. Psychosomatic aspects of chronic pelvic pain. Int J Psychiat Med 1970;1:109.
34. Beard RW, Belsey EM, Lieberman BA, et al. Pelvic pain in women. Am J Obstet Gynecol 1977;128:566.
35. Gross R, Doerr H, Caldirola D. Borderline syndrome and incest in chronic pelvic pain patients. Int J Psychiatry Med 1980–81;10:79.
36. Raskin DE. Diagnosis in patients with chronic pelvic pain (letter). Am J Psychiatry 1984;141:824.
37. Haber J, Roos C. Effects of spouse abuse and/or sexual abuse in the development and maintenance of chronic pain in women. Adv Pain Res Ther 1985;9:889.

38. Stout AL, Steege JF. Psychosocial and behavioral self-reports of chronic pelvic pain patients. Paper presented at the meeting of the American Society for Psychosomatic Obstetrics and Gynecology. Houston, TX, March 1991.

39. Blazer D. Chronic pain: A multiaxial approach to psychosocial assessment and intervention. South Med J 1981;74:203.

40. Aronoff GM, Evans WO. Evaluation and treatment of chronic pain at the Boston Pain Center. J Clin Psychiatry 1982;43(8):3.

41. Steege JF, Stout AL, Somduti SG. Chronic pelvic pain in women: Towards an integrative model. Obstet Gynecol Surv 1993;48(2):95.

42. Beard RW, Belsey EM, Leiberman BA, et al. Pelvic pain in women. Am J Obstet Gynecol 1977;128:566.

43. Peters AAW, Dorst E, Jellis B, et al. A randomized clinical trial to compare two different approaches in women with chronic pelvic pain. Obstet Gynecol 1991;77(5):740.

44. Sternbach RA. The Psychology of Pain. New York: Raven Press, 1986.

45. Fordyce WE. Behavioral Methods of Control of Chronic Pain and Illness. St. Louis: CV Mosby, 1976.

46. Goldstein DP, deCholnoky C, Emans SJ, Leventhal JM. Laparoscopy in the diagnosis and management of pelvic pain in adolescents. J Reprod Med 1980;24:251.

47. Levitan S, Eibschitz I, deVries K, et al. The value of laparoscopy in women with chronic pelvic pain and a normal pelvis. Int J Obstet Gynecol 1985;23:71.

48. Howard FM. The role of laparoscopy in chronic pelvic pain: Promise and pitfall. Obstet Gynecol Surv 1993;48:357.

49. Chan CLK, Wood C. Pelvic adhesiolysis: The assessment of symptom relief by 100 patients. Aust N Z J Obstet Gynaecol 1985;25:295.

50. Daniell JF. Laparoscopic enterolysis for chronic abdominal pain. J Gynecol Surg 1989;5:61.

51. Chatman DI. Pelvic peritoneal defects and endometriosis: Allen-Masters syndrome revisited. Fertil Steril 1981;36:751.

52. Glezerman M. The Allen-Masters syndrome revisited: Successful treatment by laparoscopy. Int J Gynaecol Obstet 1984;22:325.

53. Lee RB, Stone K, Magelssen D, et al. Presacral neurectomy for chronic pelvic pain. Obstet Gynecol 1986;68:517.

54. Lichten EM, Bombard J. Surgical treatment of primary dysmenorrhea with laparoscopic uterine nerve ablation. J Reprod Med 1987;32:37.

Endometriosis

Robert M. Weiss

Endometriosis is one of the most common benign conditions found in women of reproductive age. It is a major cause of infertility, chronic pelvic pain, and dysmenorrhea. Endometriosis is defined as the presence of tissue outside the uterus that both structurally and functionally resembles normal endometrium. Adenomyosis is a type of endometriosis in which the endometrial glands are found in the myometrium of the uterus (endometriosis interna). This is a common cause of dysmenorrhea in a woman in her thirties and forties.

PATHOGENESIS

Despite years of investigation and hundreds of articles written since its first description in 1921, the pathogenesis of endometriosis is still not fully understood. Retrograde menstruation of endometrial tissue through the fallopian tubes during menses is the most frequently noted theory of pathogenesis and explains most cases of endometriosis. However, as endometriosis has been found in such distant sites from the uterus as the lung, pleura, and breast and has been found in the urinary bladder, retrograde menstruation does not explain all cases of endometriosis. The growth of endometriosis at a site distant from the uterus points to the ability of endometriosis to spread via vascular and lymphatic channels. In addition, some endometriosis may be the result of coelomic epithelial metaplasia. Although retrograde menstruation probably occurs in all women, it is not known why certain women show a propensity to have the endometrial glands implant in the abdominal cavity. Factors that may be involved in the development of endometriosis are an increased amount of endometrium entering the peritoneal cavity and an altered immunologic status in certain women.[1]

LOCATION

Endometriosis is most commonly found on the ovaries. In 60 to 75% of women with endometriosis, ovarian involvement is found. Both ovaries are involved in approximately 50% of patients. Other common sites of endometriosis are the posterior peritoneum, posterior cul-de-sac, uterosacral ligaments, broad ligaments, fallopian tubes, peritoneum of the uterus, vesicouterine fold, and rectosigmoid. Less common sites of involvement are the cecum, appendix, bladder, cervix, vagina, small bowel, lymph nodes, and omentum. Sites distal to the abdominal cavity have also been noted to have endometriosis. These occurrences are extremely rare.[2]

EPIDEMIOLOGY

Establishing the exact incidence of endometriosis has remained elusive to date, although best estimates place the incidence at 1 to 7% of all women of reproductive age.[3] In one study of hospital discharges, 7 to 8% of women admitted for gynecologic reasons were found to have endometriosis. Approximately 10 to 15% of women undergoing pelvic surgery and 30 to 50% of women having laparoscopies as part of an infertility work-up were found to have endometriosis. Endometriosis has been found in girls as young as 10 to 15 years old. Although endometriosis is very rare after menopause, it has been found in women in their fifties and sixties, particularly those on hormone replacement therapy. The average age of diagnosis is 27 years old.[4]

Studies by Cramer and colleagues[5] have noted that women with menstrual cycle lengths of 27 days or less have a twofold increased risk of endometriosis and women who have blood flow durations of 8 days or more have a 2.5-fold increased risk of having endometriosis compared with women who have less frequent and less lengthy menstrual periods (Table 8–1). As part of this study, it was noted that women with mild, moderate, and severe menstrual pain have a 1.7-, 3.4-, and 6.7-fold increased risk, respectively, of having endometriosis compared with women who have no

TABLE 8–1. Menstrual Characteristics in Relation to Relative Risk for Endometriosis

CYCLE LENGTH (days)	RELATIVE RISK OF ENDOMETRIOSIS
≤ 27	2.1
28–34	1.0
≥ 35	0.6
DURATION OF FLOW	
≤ 7	1.0
≥ 8	2.4

menstrual pain (Table 8–2). A woman whose sibling has endometriosis has a sixfold increase in risk and the daughter of a woman with endometriosis has a tenfold increased risk of endometriosis over the general population.[6]

SYMPTOMS AND SIGNS

Classic symptoms of endometriosis include secondary dysmenorrhea, dyspareunia, and infertility (Table 8–3). The dysmenorrhea generally occurs months or even years after the onset of menarche and is progressive in nature. Women with primary dysmenorrhea generally do not have endometriosis. In the unusual circumstance of a müllerian abnormality, in which the uterus is malformed and the menstrual flow through the cervix is blocked, endometriosis can be associated with severe primary dysmenorrhea in the very young patient. Endometriosis is often associated with dyspareunia, particularly when pain occurs during deep penetration of the penis. Some patients may present with premenstrual staining or painful defecation. The degree or number of symptoms of endometriosis is often unrelated to the amount of endometriosis found during laparoscopy.

Classic signs of endometriosis on physical examination include induration of the cul-de-sac and thickened, nodular, and occasionally painful uterosacral ligaments, which are located posterior to the

TABLE 8–2. Menstrual Characteristics in Relation to Relative Risk for Endometriosis

MENSTRUAL PAIN	RELATIVE RISK OF ENDOMETRIOSIS
None	1.0
Mild	1.7
Moderate	3.4
Severe	6.7

TABLE 8–3. Symptoms and Signs of Endometriosis

SYMPTOMS	SIGNS
• Progressive dysmenorrhea	• Cul-de-sac tenderness
• Chronic pelvic pain	• Uterosacral ligament nodularity
• Dyspareunia	• Ovarian mass
• Infertility	

uterus (see Table 8–3). Endometriosis can also appear as an adnexal mass. Although pain is the most common symptom in women with endometriosis, often due to uterosacral or ovarian involvement, many patients initially present with otherwise asymptomatic infertility.

Endometriosis causes infertility in a number of ways. The most obvious is tubal scarring and adhesions that prevent the sperm from fertilizing the egg or prevent the early embryo from migrating into the uterus. Numerous studies have shown that minimal endometriosis may be associated with infertility as well. Endometriosis may be associated with increased anovulation, luteinized unruptured follicle, and luteal phase defect.[7] Increased peritoneal prostaglandin levels in patients with endometriosis may also affect tubal mobility and prevent ovum pickup by the fallopian tubes.[8]

In addition, many studies point to altered immunologic factors as a cause of infertility in patients with endometriosis. Increased numbers of total leukocytes and activated macrophages as well as other immunologic abnormalities have been found in the peritoneal fluid in patients with endometriosis.[9] However, the exact cause of infertility in patients with mild disease is not fully understood.

DIAGNOSIS

A careful history and physical examination and a high index of suspicion in the woman of reproductive age are crucial to early diagnosis and treatment of endometriosis. Unfortunately, radiologic studies are rarely helpful in diagnosing endometriosis. Although the transvaginal ultrasound is helpful in picking up endometriomas, it is not able to pick up small implants. Magnetic resonance imaging (MRI) can reveal the presence of smaller implants. However, a high percentage of patients with endometriosis have normal results on an MRI scan.

Much has been written about the clinical use of CA-125 in helping to diagnose endometriosis. CA-125 is a complex glycoprotein that is expressed in some derivatives of coelomic epithelium. The level of CA-125 is frequently elevated with endometriosis, but it is also frequently expressed in other benign and malignant tumors of the ovaries and uterus. CA-125 has not been found to be helpful as a screening test and has shown limited ability in diagnosing endometriosis in patients with pelvic pain and infertility. CA-125 may be useful in monitoring patients with endometriosis, but even in this role it has shown limited capabilities to date.

Studies of the use of CA-125 in patients with pelvic pain and infertility have revealed that 58% of patients with stage I and stage II endometriosis and nearly 100% of patients with stage III and stage IV endometriosis have CA-125 levels 16 μ per ml or higher. However, approximately 19% of patients without endometriosis had levels above this cutoff.[10] Other studies have confirmed these findings, revealing low levels of CA-125 in patients with early stage endometriosis and high levels in women with stages III and IV endometriosis. These studies also confirmed a high false positive rate, up to 70% in certain populations.[1] Unfortunately, the use of CA-125 is only minimally helpful in the diagnosis of endometriosis.

Laparoscopy or laparotomy with biopsy of endometrial implants remains the only definitive method of diagnosing endometriosis. The woman of reproductive age with pelvic pain or severe dysmenorrhea should be referred to a physician who is able to perform a laparoscopy to make a diagnosis of endometriosis.

Endometriosis classically appears as powder-burned brown or purple lesions on the peritoneum. However, endometriosis can manifest in many other ways including atypical blood vessels, peritoneal defects, and small red lesions. The physician performing the laparoscopy must be aware of these atypical appearances of endometriosis and must have a low threshold for biopsies of any abnormal areas on the peritoneum.

STAGES OF ENDOMETRIOSIS

The staging of endometriosis is controversial. Although not perfect and without carefully controlled studies to prove its true prognostic value, the American Fertility Society's 1985 revision of its staging system has become a standard staging system throughout the United States. This staging system is presented in Figure 8–1.

TREATMENT OF ENDOMETRIOSIS

The treatment of endometriosis varies according to the individual's present and future desire for pregnancy. Additional modifications of treatment should be made for the patient who presents with infertility as opposed to the patient who presents with chronic pelvic pain or dyspareunia. More aggressive and prolonged medical management is often needed in cases of pelvic pain. More radical surgical treatment can be offered to the patient who has completed her family.

Initial treatment of endometriosis should occur during the initial laparoscopy if possible. The use of the laser or cautery to ablate endometrial implants and remove endometriosis should be part of the initial laparoscopy. In addition, resection of peritoneal tissue around endometrial implants may be helpful in decreasing the chance of recurrence and increasing the chance of proper diagnosis.

After this initial therapeutic laparoscopy, medical treatment is nearly always indicated unless immediate fertility is desired. Medical treatment of endometriosis is based on the fact that the tissue of endometriosis, like the endometrium of the uterine cavity, responds to hormonal manipulation. Endometrial tissue proliferates during estrogen stimulation, becomes secretory under progesterone stimulation, and becomes atrophic in the face of a high dose of progestin or androgen. Also, in the absence of all hormonal stimulation, such as that which happens during menopause, the endometrium becomes atrophic. Medical treatment of endometriosis is based on numerous studies that show that endometriosis responds to hormonal manipulation as does uterine endometrial tissue.

MEDICAL TREATMENT OF ENDOMETRIOSIS

Although numerous medications have been used in the past to treat endometriosis, four basic types are utilized today. These include progestins, danazol sulfate, gonadotropin-releasing hormone (Gn-RH) agonists, and occasionally the combination estrogen-progestin oral contraceptive pill. The use of high-dose estrogens and androgens, although effective, leads to many side effects that limit their use. They are included here only for historical interest.

Some of the earlier treatments of endometriosis were the use of diethylstilbestrol (DES) and methyltestosterone. The effectiveness of DES and other high-dose estrogen compounds has been mixed. Methyltestosterone has been shown to be very effective in treating endometriosis, but its use is associated with many androgenic side effects. Robert Kistner at the Boston Hospital for Women popularized the use of high-dose progestins as well as continuous oral contraceptive pills in his "pseudo-

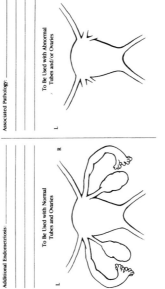

Figure 8–1. American Fertility Society endometriosis classification system. (From American Fertility Society. Revised American Fertility Society classification of endometriosis: 1985. Fertil Steril 1985;43:351. Reproduced with permission of the publisher, The American Fertility Society, Birmingham, Alabama.)

pregnancy'' regimen. These medications, as well as danazol sulfate and Gn-RH agonists, have become the mainstays of modern medical treatment of endometriosis.

Medroxyprogesterone Acetate

Progestins have been used for the treatment of endometriosis for many years. However, very few randomized clinical trials exist using medroxyprogesterone acetate or other progestogens. Most of the early studies with this medication dealt with infertility problems and were very difficult to control, as there are many factors involved with fertility. Medroxyprogesterone acetate, 30 mg daily, has been used for 3 to 6 months with good results in patients with infertility problems. The most common side effect when using continuous progestins is breakthrough bleeding. Other side effects include nausea, breast tenderness, fluid retention, and depression.[11] The use of oral contraceptive pills in either a cyclic or a continuous fashion is fairly common. However, to date few well-controlled studies have shown it to be efficacious.

Depot medroxyprogesterone acetate, which was approved by the U.S. Food and Drug Administration for use as a contraceptive, has had very few clinical trials as a treatment for endometriosis. This medication may become important in the treatment of the patient with pelvic pain related to endometriosis. However, the time to return of ovulation is highly variable with the use of depot medroxyprogesterone acetate, and it should not be prescribed for the infertile woman.

Danazol Sulfate

Until recently, danazol sulfate was the most commonly used medication for treatment of severe endometriosis. Danazol is a derivative of ethisterone and is a potent inhibitor of gonadotropin release. This medication blocks ovulation, suppresses follicular development, and leads to a hypoestrogenic state. In high doses, danazol is also mildly androgenic and may act directly on the endometrium. All of these effects cause a markedly atrophic endometrium and lead to amenorrhea. The dose of danazol required for treating patients with endometriosis varies from 400 to 800 mg daily. Most experts feel that danazol sufficient to prevent menses is necessary for the drug to be effective. Studies have shown that 98% of patients on 800 mg daily and 80% of patients on 600 mg daily become amenorrheic.[12] In general 200 mg of

danazol given orally three times per day is an appropriate initial dose that can be titrated higher if menses continue. Treatment with this medication should last 3 to 6 months.

Although danazol is highly effective in treating patients with endometriosis, it has many side effects. Common side effects of danazol therapy are weight gain (85%), muscle cramps (52%), decreased breast size (48%), flushing (42%), mood changes (38%), oily skin (37%), and depression (32%). In addition, 27% of patients complain of increased acne, and 7% of patients complain of deepening of the voice. Unfortunately, this last side effect is irreversible. Danazol sulfate is metabolized in the liver, and therefore the patient who is on this medication for longer than 6 months should have liver function tests biannually.

Gonadotropin-releasing Hormone Agonists

Gonadotropin-releasing hormone agonists have become the treatment of choice for many cases of endometriosis. These agonists cause an initial increase in follicle-stimulating hormone (FSH) and luteinizing hormone (LH) release from the pituitary and cause increased estrogen production for approximately 7 to 10 days. Following this initial flare response, rapid down regulation of the pituitary causes a sustained decrease in production of FSH and LH from the pituitary. This decrease in pituitary production of FSH and LH leads to a hypoestrogenic state that continues throughout treatment with Gn-RH agonists. All available Gn-RH agonists, including leuprolide acetate, nafarelin acetate, and goserelin acetate, cause this rapid and prolonged suppression of gonadal steroid production.

These medications are very effective in causing atrophy of endometrial tissue and in treating endometriosis. Unfortunately, the severely hypoestrogenic state, caused by the Gn-RH agonists, leads to many short-term and long-term hypoestrogenic side effects, which limit their use. Patients on Gn-RH agonists frequently experience hot flashes, vaginal dryness, and decreased libido. In addition, loss of bone mass and bone mineral density is noted to occur after 6 months of treatment. Spinal bone mineral density loss is 3 to 15%,[13] and femoral neck bone mineral density loss up to 3% has been noted in numerous studies. This bone loss is nearly completely reversible if the medication is discontinued after 6 months. Thus, nafarelin acetate, goserelin acetate, leuprolide acetate, and depot leuprolide acetate are approved by the Food and Drug Administration for the treatment of en-

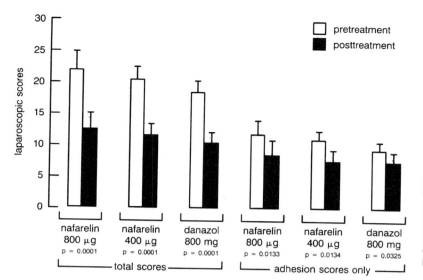

Figure 8–2. Treatment effects reflected by mean scores of laparoscopic findings. The American Fertility Society classification system was used to assign scores to laparoscopic findings. All P values are based on the t-test and confirmed by the signed-rank test. Bars indicate ±1 SEM. (From Henzl MR, Corson SL, Moghissi K, et al. Administration of nasal nafarelin as compared with oral danazol for endometriosis: A multi-centered double blind comparative clinical trial. N Engl J Med 1988;318:485. Reprinted by permission of the New England Journal of Medicine. Copyright 1988, Massachusetts Medical Society.)

dometriosis for only up to 6 months owing to this effect on bone loss.

Patients treated with Gn-RH agonists must have had laparoscopically proven endometriosis. The patient must be monitored closely, and treatment must not begin until the clinician is sure that the patient is not pregnant. To ensure this, treatment is best begun with the onset of menses.

Numerous studies comparing treatment with Gn-RH agonists with that with high-dose danazol have shown equal efficacy in decreasing pain and severity of disease. In one study comparing treatment with nafarelin acetate with that with danazol sulfate,[14] more than 80% of patients treated with nafarelin acetate and danazol showed a reduction in the extent of disease, which was assessed by laparoscopy (endometriosis scores decreased by nearly 50% in each category) (Fig. 8–2). The percentage of women with ''severely painful'' symptoms of endometriosis decreased from 40% to 5% after 6 months of treatment, whereas the percentage of patients with ''none to mild pain'' increased from 25% to approximately 80% after 6 months of treatment (Fig. 8–3). Approximately 39% of patients who attempted pregnancy after treatment were able to get pregnant. Although danazol and the Gn-RH agonists showed equal effectiveness in the treatment of endometriosis, patients on danazol had a higher percentage of serious side effects. Danazol was shown to cause a decrease in high-density lipoproteins (HDL) and an increase in low-density lipoproteins (LDL).

Studies utilizing leuprolide acetate have shown this medication to be as effective as nafarelin ace-

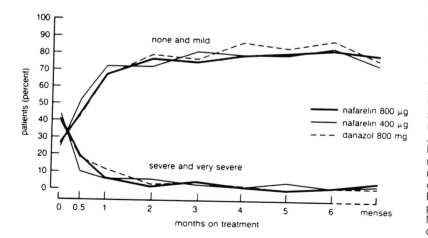

Figure 8–3. Percentage of patients with none and mild symptoms or severe and very severe symptoms of endometriosis. Mild corresponds to a symptom-profile score of 0 to 2, severe to a symptom-profile score of 6 to 10, and very severe to a symptom-profile score of 11 to 15. (From Henzl MR, Corson SL, Moghissi K, et al. Administration of nasal nafarelin as compared with oral danazol for endometriosis: A multi-centered double blind comparative clinical trial. N Engl J Med 1988;318:485. Reprinted by permission of the New England Journal of Medicine. Copyright 1988, Massachusetts Medical Society.)

tate in treating endometriosis.[15] Unfortunately, all available Gn-RH agonists need to be given parenterally. The effective daily dose of nafarelin acetate is 0.4 to 0.8 mg administered intranasally, and that of leuprolide acetate is 0.5 to 1.0 mg administered subcutaneously daily. A monthly depot form of leuprolide acetate (3.75 mg intramuscularly) has been shown to be equally effective. The Food and Drug Administration has approved this depot form of leuprolide acetate, and many patients and their physicians prefer this simpler form of treatment.

Although Gn-RH agonists alone should be utilized only for up to 6 months, studies utilizing Gn-RH agonists along with the addition of progestin and estrogen or bone-sparing agents such as etidronate have shown promising effects in controlling the endometriosis while preventing further bone loss. Ongoing studies are attempting to define the dosage of medication that will continue suppressing the endometriosis while protecting against bone mineral loss.[16, 17] It is hoped that these studies will yield useful protocols to be utilized by the clinician for long-term treatment of endometriosis. However, at present, utilization of Gn-RH agonists for longer than 6 months must be considered experimental.

SURGICAL MANAGEMENT

Surgical management of endometriosis can often be accomplished via the laparoscope. With the more common use of the intra-abdominal laser, this surgery has become not only more effective but safer as well. The carbon dioxide, potassium titanyl phosphate, argon, or YAG laser and unipolar and bipolar cautery are all equally effective in the treatment of endometriosis. However, unlike what is possible with unipolar or bipolar cautery, the depth of destruction can be controlled well using the laser. Although numerous studies have compared the various lasers and cautery, none has shown that one specific agent is clearly more effective than another. In the proper hands, any one of these instruments should be able to treat the disease via the laparoscope safely and effectively. Certainly, in some patients the extent of the disease requires a laparotomy to treat the endometriosis. Studies have shown that in patients with known advanced disease, preoperative medical treatment of endometriosis with Gn-RH agents can improve success rates.[18]

The definitive treatment of the woman with advanced and symptomatic endometriosis is total abdominal hysterectomy and bilateral salpingo-oophorectomy. The bilateral salpingo-oophorec-

tomy is crucial in causing a permanent hypoestrogenic state in which the endometriosis does not recur. Some physicians advocate leaving one ovary. However, more than 50% of women treated with hysterectomy and unilateral salpingo-oophorectomy require reoperation because of persistent endometriosis.[1] However, in the patient with mild to moderate endometriosis, a hysterectomy and unilateral salpingo-oophorectomy may be indicated.

SPECIAL CONSIDERATIONS IN THE MANAGEMENT OF PATIENTS WITH ENDOMETRIOSIS

Infertility

Treatment of the patient with infertility varies according to the patient's stage of endometriosis. Numerous studies have shown that medical treatment of the patient with minimal or mild endometriosis is no more effective than expectant management. In the older infertile patient, the 3 to 6 months of treatment for endometriosis seems to be an unnecessary delay without improving fecundity rates. Even the initial laparoscopic ablation of the endometriosis is felt by some to be unnecessary. However, most gynecologists feel that decreasing the amount of endometriosis during laparoscopy is helpful with only a minimal amount of risk. Although this issue remains controversial, there is consensus that postoperative medical treatment for the infertile patient with minimal endometriosis is unnecessary.

The patient with stage III or IV endometriosis should undergo conservative surgical management. Following conservative surgical debulking of the endometriosis, a 4- to 6-month course of medical treatment with a high-dose progestin, danazol, or a Gn-RH agonist is usually indicated.[1] Overall pregnancy rates following danazol therapy may be as high as 40 to 70%.[19] However, with the increased accessibility to in vitro fertilization, many infertile patients with stage III to IV endometriosis should be referred directly for in vitro fertilization. For the patient with severely damaged fallopian tubes, ovaries, or both, in vitro fertilization is often more effective than conservative laparotomy followed by medical treatment. Of course, this decision needs to be addressed following a careful staging by laparoscopy. Even in the patient who is to be referred for in vitro fertilization, postoperative medical treatment of stage III to IV endometriosis is often beneficial. In vitro fertilization can often be performed directly following long-term treatment with a Gn-RH agonist.

Pelvic Pain

Unlike asymptomatic infertility patients with early stage endometriosis who receive no benefit from medical management, all patients with pelvic pain caused by endometriosis should undergo a course of medical treatment. In most circumstances a 4- to 6-month course of aggressive medical treatment should be undertaken following operative treatment. In addition, the patient requiring repeat surgery should undergo preoperative medical treatment.

Treatment of patients with pelvic pain related to endometriosis can be difficult. Quite often, patients respond to a 4- to 6-month course of medical treatment only to have symptoms recur shortly after discontinuing the medication. For the patient treated with a Gn-RH agonist, a 3- to 6-month wait for recovery of bone density may be indicated before having the patient undergo another course of medical treatment. It is hoped that new protocols that allow use of Gn-RH agonists for longer than 6 months will be available soon. For the woman no longer interested in bearing children, a total abdominal hysterectomy and bilateral salpingo-oophorectomy are often indicated.

The Young Patient

Management of the teenager or woman in her early twenties who is diagnosed with endometriosis and is not interested in getting pregnant in the near future must be handled carefully. For the patient who had been symptomatic before her laparoscopy or is diagnosed with advanced disease, a 4- to 6-month course of postoperative medical treatment with either a Gn-RH agonist or danazol is indicated. Following this, the young woman should be placed on an oral contraceptive pill to decrease the recurrence of endometriosis. Oral contraceptive pills with potent progestins (e.g., norgestrel [Lo/Ovral]) or a high progestin to estrogen ratio (e.g., Loestrin 1/20) are theoretically the oral contraceptives of choice in these situations. One might also consider continuous use of these oral contraceptive pills.

Some physicians manage women with minimal to mild endometriosis with close observation and oral contraceptives only. In young women diagnosed with endometriosis, the clinician must follow the patient closely for recurrence or spread of the disease with annual or biannual examinations.

Hormone Therapy

Whether hormone therapy should be offered the patient with a history of endometriosis is another difficult question. In the patient with active endometriosis who undergoes a total abdominal hysterectomy and bilateral salpingo-oophorectomy, hormone replacement therapy should be delayed for 4 to 6 months postoperatively. In the woman who has had endometriosis in the past but did not have a hysterectomy and has had no symptoms for a few years, hormone therapy is justifiable. In all of these situations, recurrence of endometriosis while the patient is on hormone replacement therapy is possible. Cases of endometrial cancer arising from endometriosis are rare, but even so, women with a history of endometriosis should not be given unopposed estrogen for the first 6 to 12 months but should be on a hormone replacement regimen that includes a progestin (see Chapter 61).

Adenomyosis (Endometriosis Interna)

Adenomyosis is defined as the presence of endometrial tissue within the myometrium of the uterus. Women in their thirties or forties with adenomyosis often present with menorrhagia, dysmenorrhea, or pelvic pain. Physical findings consistent with adenomyosis are an enlarged, regular globular uterus, one that is usually smaller than 12 weeks' gestational size.

Although this disease is fairly common and is found in up to 20% of all specimens from hysterectomies, definitive diagnosis in the past was only possible by the pathologist with such a specimen. Preoperative attempts at diagnosis with a hysterogram, ultrasound, or MRI scan have shown mixed results in the last decade. The ability to obtain biopsy samples of the myometrium via operative hysteroscopy or laparoscopy has made it possible to make a diagnosis without a hysterectomy specimen.

The definitive treatment for symptomatic adenomyosis remains removal of the uterus. Although there have been a few case reports of medical management of adenomyosis with danazol or Gn-RH agonists, the feasibility and cost effectiveness of a nonsurgical approach remains to be seen.

REFERENCES

1. Barbieri RL. Endometriosis. Curr Probl Obstet Gynecol Fertil 1989;12(1):1.
2. Mishell DR, Davajan V. Reproductive Endocrinology, Infertility and Contraception. Philadelphia: FA Davis, 1979.
3. Barbieri RL. Etiology and epidemiology of endometriosis. Am J Obstet Gynecol 1990;162(2):565.
4. Cramer DW. Epidemiology of endometriosis. In: Wilson EA (ed). Endometriosis. New York: Alan R Liss 1987;5.
5. Cramer DW, Wilson E, Stillman RJ, et al. The relation of endometriosis to menstrual characteristics, smoking and exercise. JAMA 1985;255:1904.

6. Simpson JL, Elias S, Malinack LR, Buttram VC Jr. Heritable aspects of endometriosis I. Genetic Studies. Am J Obstet Gynecol 1980;137:327.

7. Schenken RS, Asch RD, Williams RF, Hodgen GD. Etiology of infertility in monkeys with endometriosis: Luteinized unruptured follicles, luteal phase defects, pelvic adhesions, and spontaneous abortions. Fertil Steril 1984;41:122.

8. Suginami H, Yano K, Watanabe K, Matsaura S. A factor inhibiting ovum capture by the oviductal fimbriae present in endometriosis peritoneal fluid. Fertil Steril 1986;46:1140.

9. Hill JA, Faris HMP, Schiff I, Anderson DJ. Characterization of leukocyte subpopulations in the peritoneal fluid parameters of infertile patients and the subsequent occurrence of pregnancy. Fertil Steril 1988;50:216.

10. Pittaway DE, Douglas JW. Serum Ca-125 in women with endometriosis and chronic pelvic pain. Fertil Steril 1989;51:68.

11. Moghissi KS, Boyce CR. Management of endometriosis with oral medroxyprogesterone acetate. Obstet Gynecol 1976;47:265.

12. Young MD, Blackmore WP. The use of danazol in the management of endometriosis. J Int Med Res 1977; 5(3):86.

13. Dawood MY, Lewis V, Ramos J. Cortical and trabecular bone mineral content in women with endometriosis: Effect of GnRH agonist and danazol. Fertil Steril 1989;52:21.

14. Henzl MR, Corson SL, Moghissi K, et al. Administration of nasal nararelin as compared with oral danazol for endometriosis: A multi-centered double blind comparative clinical trial. N Engl J Med 1981;318:485.

15. Dlugi AM, Miller JD, Knittle J. Lupron depot (leuprolide acetate for depot suspension) in the treatment of endometriosis: A randomized, placebo-controlled, double-blind study. Fertil Steril 1990;54(3):419.

16. Surrey ES, Fournet N, Voight B, Judd HL. Effects of sodium etidronate in combination with low dose norethindrone in patients administered a long acting GnRH agonist. A preliminary report Obstet Gynecol 1993;81:581.

17. Cedars MI, Lu JK, Meldrum D. Treatment of endometriosis with a long acting GnRH agonist plus medroxyprogesterone acetate. Obstet Gynecol 1990;75:641.

18. Buttram VC Jr. Conservative surgery for endometriosis in the infertile female: A study of 206 patients with implications for both medical and surgical therapy. Fertil Steril 1979;31:117.

19. Buttram VC Jr, Reiter RC, Ward SM. Treatment of endometriosis with danazol. Report of a 6 year prospective study. Fertil Steril 1985;43:353.

Diseases of the Vulva, Vagina, and Cervix

9

Diseases of the Vulva

Elaine T. Kaye

ANATOMY OF THE VULVA

The vulva encompasses the labia majora, labia minora, clitoris, and vaginal vestibule (Fig. 9–1). Its lateral boundaries are the labiocrural folds medial to the thighs and its central boundary is the hymenal ring. Its anterior boundary is the mons pubis, a fatty prominence overlying the symphysis pubis, which is covered with pubic hair. Its posterior border is the anus.

The labia majora are made up of adipose and connective tissue and are covered by keratinizing epithelium. They are prominent in the neonate and then again in puberty and later become less prominent after menopause as fatty tissue is lost. They develop sexual hairs and contain sebaceous, apocrine, and sweat glands.

The labia minora represent a transition to mucosal epithelium. Laterally, they contain sebaceous glands, and medially they are smooth and blend with mucosa of the vestibule. The line that separates these two portions is referred to as Hart's

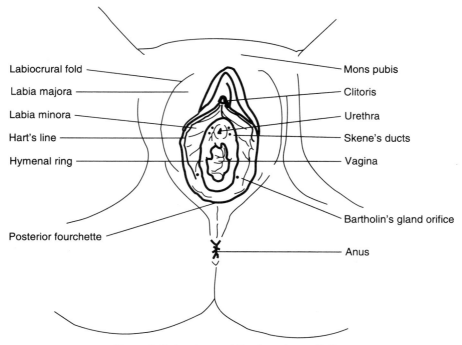

Figure 9–1. Anatomy of the female genitalia.

line. The labia minora also may atrophy after menopause.

The clitoris is composed of erectile tissue with two corpora cavernosa within fibrous tissue. It corresponds embryologically to the dorsal aspect of the penis.

The vestibule is bound anteriorly and posteriorly by the clitoris and posterior fourchette, laterally by the labia minora, and medially by the hymenal ring. It is covered by a very thinly keratinizing epithelium. It includes the vaginal introitus, the duct openings for Bartholin's glands, the urethral meatus, and Skene's (periurethral) duct openings.

The hymen separates the vulvar vestibule from the vagina. The vagina contains stratified squamous epithelium and does not have any glands. It also can become atrophic and dry in response to the hormonal changes of menopause.

EVALUATION OF THE VULVA

Evaluating a patient with a vulvar complaint necessitates an accurate description of the onset, duration, periodicity, and quality of the patient's discomfort. A history of preexisting dermatologic conditions such as eczema, contact dermatitis, psoriasis, or lichen planus may be relevant and should be recorded. A sexual, obstetric, and medical history should also be obtained.

After a thorough history, attention can then be given to the physical examination. It is often helpful to begin with examination of the cutaneous surface of the entire body and of the oral mucosa. When that is completed, careful inspection of the vulva should be performed with the patient's legs in stirrups. The urethra, Skene's glands, and Bartholin's glands should be palpated; sensitivity of small lesions and glandular elements can be tested by probing gently with a cotton-tipped swab.

When indicated, a speculum examination is performed next. The vaginal walls should be inspected with regard to their color, evidence of atrophy, or specific lesions such as papillomas that indicate human papillomavirus (HPV) infection. The cervix should be examined for signs of inflammation or discharge.

VULVOVAGINAL INFECTIONS

Infections Associated with Vaginal Discharge

Women who present with a complaint of an abnormal discharge or vulvar discomfort should be evaluated for a vaginitis. The vulva is rarely the source of discharge. Rather, vaginal discharge by acting as an irritant may cause vulvar erythema with an accompanying burning or itching sensation.

Bacterial Vaginosis

Bacterial vaginoses account for one third of vaginal infections in women of childbearing age. It is a frequent complaint of women visiting their primary care physicians. In addition, studies demonstrate its prevalence to be 10 to 25% in women presenting in obstetric clinics.

Although it has been called nonspecific vaginitis, bacterial vaginosis can most often be attributed to *Gardnerella vaginalis.* Increased numbers of *Bacteroides* species (Prevotella), *Mobiluncus* species, and *Mycoplasma hominis* as well as a reduction in the number of *Lactobacillus* have also been implicated.

Four diagnostic criteria, of which three must be present, confirm a diagnosis of bacterial vaginosis.

1. A thin, frothy gray, odorous discharge
2. Vaginal pH greater than 4.5 with nitrazine pH paper
3. A wet mount of the vaginal smear with normal saline revealing "clue cells," clusters of coccobacilli on the surface of desquamated epithelial cells
4. A positive "whiff" test for amines, with a fishy odor detected when 10% potassium hydroxide is added to the discharge

Traditionally, oral metronidazole or clindamycin has been the mainstay of therapy. Effective topical preparations of both these antibiotics have been developed. It is still unclear whether bacterial vaginosis is sexually transmitted. Therefore, indications for the treatment of the asymptomatic male sexual partner remain controversial.

Trichomonal Vaginitis

Trichomonal vaginitis is a protozoan infection that manifests with a copious, frothy yellow-green discharge that is highly irritating to the vulva. The pH of the vagina is elevated from the normal pH of 3.8 to 4.2; it is generally in the range of 5.0 to 7.0. A normal saline wet mount of the vaginal smear demonstrates the diagnostic motile, pear-shaped trichomanads. Treatment is similar to that for bacterial vaginosis. Sexual partners should be treated as well.

Candida *Vulvovaginitis*

Candida is responsible for more than 90% of vulvovaginal infections. More than 75% of women are affected during their lifetimes. The reservoir for *Candida* is the gastrointestinal tract, which by local transmission may then colonize the genital tract; 10% of women harbor *Candida* as part of their genital flora.

Several factors increase the incidence of *Candida* infection. One predisposing factor is systemic antibiotics, which alter the bowel and vaginal flora. Normally, the *Lactobacillus* and *Corynebacterium* metabolize glycogen to lactic and acetic acid, thus creating an acidic environment that inhibits *Candida* growth. A second factor is high estrogen levels in women who are pregnant, are in midmenstrual cycle, or are taking exogenous estrogen. A third factor is immunosuppression, which can be local, as seen with the use of a topical steroid, or systemic. Candidal vaginitis is an increasingly recognized problem in women who are infected with the human immunodeficiency virus (HIV). Women who demonstrate recurrent or refractory infections should be considered candidates for HIV testing. Women with diabetes are also susceptible to candidal infections.

The vulva may be directly infected by *Candida,* or it may demonstrate an irritant dermatitis to the discharge of the candidal vaginitis. On examination, the vulva shows a range of mild to prominent erythema. This may be accompanied by a curd-like white exudate that will demonstrate pseudohyphae and spores with a 10% potassium hydroxide stain. The potassium hydroxide preparation has a sensitivity of 22 to 65% in symptomatic women with positive cultures.

The labiocrural folds can become infected as opposing skin folds set up a warm, moist environment that is conducive to the growth of *Candida.* This appears as a beefy red dermatitis with delicate ''cigarette-paper'' scale and frequently with satellite pustules.

Topical therapy is the treatment of choice for all initial vulvar and vaginal infections. It is advisable to treat both the vulva and the vagina. Imidazoles, such as clotrimazole and miconazole, are now available over the counter as tablet and cream preparations. Systemic antifungal therapy with imidazoles or the newer triazoles is best reserved for persistent or recurrent candidiasis.

Other Considerations

When patients present with a complaint of vulvar itching or discharge, the physician's time and effort are well spent establishing the correct diagnosis. Although it is essential to evaluate for evidence of infection, the cause may be noninfectious. Women can have a copious discharge from a normal physiologic state such as mucorrhea, a profuse cervical discharge that may occur around the time of ovulation; generally, it is asymptomatic and not malodorous. Physiologic vaginal secretions may also be due to the increased rate of epithelial turnover associated with high progesterone states such as during pregnancy and oral contraceptive use.

In addition, women with atrophic vaginitis associated with menopause may present with a complaint of dyspareunia and a scant discharge; an elevated pH of 6.0 to 7.0 of the vaginal secretions in the absence of infection is a helpful diagnostic clue.

Other Infections

Folliculitis and furuncles caused by *Staphylococcus aureus* commonly affect the pubic area. Treatment is the same as in other locations; for persistent cases, consideration should be given to treatment for nasal carriage of *S. aureus* with topical mupirocin. Tinea cruris caused by dermatophyte infection and erythrasma caused by *Corynebacterium minutissimum* are other causes of vulvar dermatitis, especially in the labiocrural folds.

Infestations

Scabies is an infestation of the human mite, *Sarcoptes scabiei*. The fertile female mite lays eggs and deposits feces (scybala), antigens to which the body develops a pruritic hypersensitivity reaction. Transmission can occur from skin-to-skin contact, as in children's play, or from sexual contact. Examination of the patient demonstrates linear burrows especially in interdigital spaces, axillae, groin, and labia majora.

Pediculosis pubis represents an infestation of the pubic louse, *Phthirus pubis*. Patients present with itching, and examination of the pubic area reveals the ''freckle-like'' lice and the ''dandruff-like'' nits.

Both infestations are treated successfully with a permethrin lotion and the accompanying treatment of human contacts and clothing. Special consideration of treatment options is appropriate in pregnant and lactating women.

Viral Infections of the Female Genitalia

Human Papillomavirus

Human papillomavirus has become the most common viral cause of sexually transmitted disease in the United States. It is estimated that in 1989 220,000 initial visits were made to physicians' offices for treatment of genital HPV.

Human papillomavirus is often asymptomatic. It has been identified by the presence of koilocytes in cervical smears in 1 to 2% of all women screened and in 10% of young women screened. In a clinic treating sexually transmitted diseases, 10% of randomly selected women with normal Papanicolaou smears and colposcopic examinations had HPV as identified by DNA sequencing.

Human papillomavirus is most commonly transmitted through sexual contact. It can also be transmitted nonsexually through direct entry through small abrasions in the skin. In addition, there have been some reports of patient-to-patient transmission through the use of unsterilized specula or biopsy equipment. The incubation period of HPV is long, ranging from 6 weeks up to 6 to 8 months. The infectivity rate of the virus in a woman who has sexual contact with an infected male is high; she will become infected 65% of the time.

Condylomata acuminata, the genital warts caused by HPV, typically appear as hyperplastic or papillomatous warty growths (Fig. 9–2). Initially they appear acuminate, meaning sharp, or

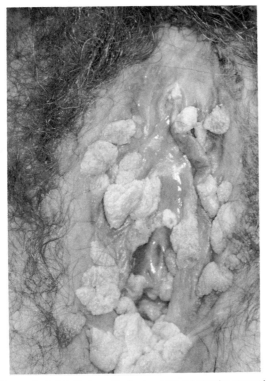

Figure 9–2. Multiple soft, fleshy condylomata acuminata of the vulva (see also color section). (Courtesy of Richard Reid, M.D.)

filiform, but eventually they can grow polypoid and pedunculated. A solution of 5% acetic acid applied for 5 minutes may help to identify early lesions. In about 10% of patients with vulvar condylomata, lesions may be found internally on the vagina or cervix. Papanicolaou smears and colposcopically directed biopsies can be useful in the detection of infection.

Studies have shown that HPV is a factor in the development of cancer in the female genital tract. Approximately 95% of cervical cancers and 15% of vulvar cancers have been associated with HPV. Most condylomata are caused by HPV type 6 or 11, both of which have a low malignancy potential. However, viral types 16, 18, 31, and 33 have been implicated as the HPV types with high malignancy potential.

The treatment options for condylomata include cryotherapy, podophyllin, and trichloroacetic acid. These methods require a series of treatments either weekly or biweekly. Several studies have shown that cryotherapy with liquid nitrogen appears to be marginally more effective than podophyllin. Podophyllin in a 25% concentration in a tincture of benzoin or alcohol is painted onto lesions and washed off in 4 to 6 hours. It is often useful in patients who cannot tolerate the discomfort of cryotherapy or as supplemental therapy in patients with bulky or refractory condylomata immediately following cryotherapy. Trichloroacetic acid, 50 to 85% concentration in aqueous solution, is a long-used treatment that is helpful in limited disease. Laser therapy and interferon are used as well, whereas surgery is seldom used any longer because of high recurrence rates. Also, examination of the sexual partner is necessary to identify condylomata that might provide a source of reinfection.

Herpes Simplex Virus

Patients with vulvar herpes simplex virus (HSV) can be categorized into three groups. In the first group are patients who are having their first episode of the disease with primary infection; they have no circulating HSV antibodies. In the second are patients who have recurrences of previously recognized episodes of genital herpes. In the third are patients who experience their initial clinical episode of genital herpes who already have circulating HSV 1 or HSV 2 antibodies; their episodes generally parallel the course of the second group of patients with recurrences.

The groups are distinguished by their clinical syndromes. The first group without previous exposure generally has systemic symptoms such as fever, adenopathy, and malaise 2 to 7 days after exposure. The vulva may be edematous, and lesions are often severe and bilateral; they usually resolve over a 2-week period. Members of the second and third group with existing immunity generally present with more mild local symptoms lasting about 1 week. These patients usually do not have systemic symptoms but may experience a prodrome 1 to 2 days before the appearance of local lesions.

Vulvar herpes lesions generally progress through several clinical stages. Initially, they are vesicular with a characteristic erythematous halo; they then become pustular, eroded, and finally crusted. Herpes infection in the immunocompromised host, especially the HIV-infected patient, may have unusual manifestations, such as verrucous plaques or extensive chronic ulcers that persist for months despite therapy.

In establishing the diagnosis of a herpes infection, the physician should consider a broad differential diagnosis, including infectious etiologies such as chancroid and the syphilitic chancre and vesicobullous diseases such as pemphigus vulgaris, ulcerating neoplastic lesions, aphthous ulcers, and Behçet's syndrome.

The diagnosis of herpes can be confirmed by a Tzanck smear, in which a scraping of the base of the lesion demonstrates multinucleated giant cells. Additional laboratory confirmation can be provided by tissue culture, which identifies virus in 94% of patients with vesicular lesions, or the rapid antigen assay, which is less sensitive.

Treatment of HSV includes local therapy with application of cool compresses of tap water or Domeboro (aluminum sulfate; calcium acetate) solution (see instructions for use in contact dermatitis section). Acyclovir, 200 mg five times daily, should be considered in primary infection or in recurrences that are detected early, especially in the prodromal stage. A daily prophylactic dose of acyclovir may be beneficial for HSV suppression in individuals who experience frequent recurrences.

Poxvirus (Molluscum Contagiosum)

Molluscum contagiosum is caused by a poxvirus that is sexually transmitted in adults. It manifests as multiple, asymptomatic, shiny, dome-shaped papules, often with a central umbilication. It is commonly located on the inner thighs and the pubic and anogenital areas. Diagnosis can be made by the distinctive clinical appearance. However, if the lesions do not have the classic appearance, the diagnosis can be confirmed by expressing the cheesy core in the center of the lesions and placing it on a slide. Staining with Wright's stain reveals

large molluscum bodies that are cytoplasmic inclusion bodies that fill the keratinocytes. Lesions respond well to cryotherapy, curettage, or other physically destructive modalities.

VULVAR DERMATOSES

Contact Dermatitis

Contact dermatitis, a form of eczematous dermatitis, is manifested by erythema, edema, and a burning or an itching sensation (Fig. 9–3). It usually affects the vulva and sometimes the vagina. Contact dermatitis is caused by an irritant or an allergen.

Irritant dermatitis is common and generally causes discomfort almost immediately after contact. Irritants may be found in clothing, laundry detergents, soaps, vaginal creams, and contraceptive jellies as well as in antiviral treatments such as podophyllin, 5-fluorouracil (5-FU), and trichloracetic acid. Major culprits include alcohol contained in some soaps and shampoos and propylene glycol, a vehicle common in many creams. Other factors implicated are excessive douching, which may change the vaginal pH, and chronic urinary incontinence.

Allergic contact dermatitis is uncommon, requires a prior sensitization to the allergen, and appears 2 to 3 days after exposure. Allergens include topical benadryl, benzocaine, neomycin, fragrance, nickel, and formaldehyde found in nail polish and fabric softeners.

Diagnosis requires a careful history that should include identification of all products that come in contact with the genital area as well as products used by sexual partners.

The most important element in treatment is the

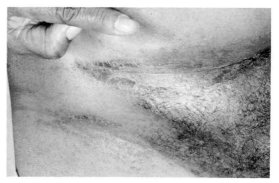

Figure 9–3. Allergic contact dermatitis to fragrance with erythema limited to well-demarcated areas of contact in the pubic area (see also color section).

removal of the offending contact agent. An allergic dermatitis may still take up to 3 weeks to resolve once the allergen is removed. Symptomatic relief can be accomplished with sitz baths or Domeboro soaks. Domeboro or aluminum acetate solution prepared by combining a tablet or packet with cool water in a 1:40 dilution can be directly applied as a compress for 20 to 30 minutes three or four times daily. If necessary, topical steroids of low and intermediate potency, preferably in a cream formulation, may be used for a short course. Emollients are poorly tolerated in this area.

Atopic Dermatitis

Patients who have a history of atopic dermatitis or eczema may complain of burning, itching, or dryness of the vulva. Examination often reveals only mild erythema and occasional scaling. This vulvar condition can be treated effectively with low-potency topical steroids.

Lichen Simplex Chronicus

Lichen simplex chronicus is a common eczematous condition that has also been termed hyperplastic vulvar dystrophy in the past. It manifests as a well-demarcated plaque most often on the labia majora with hyperpigmentation and lichenification (increased skin markings), which give it a leathery appearance. It may also cause hyperkeratosis appearing as white patches; if persistent, biopsy samples should be taken to rule out dysplasia.

Pruritus is the primary symptom. Long after the inciting factor (e.g., *Candida,* irritant) has gone, the skin remains intensely pruritic, thus creating an "itch-scratch-itch" cycle. The chronic rubbing and scratching of this neurodermatitis may even result in nodules, termed prurigo nodularis ("picker's nodule").

Treatment includes topical steroids and antihistamines to help diminish scratching, especially at night. Intralesional steroids are sometimes useful for refractory cases, but scarring and sloughing are occasional adverse effects. Patient awareness of the role of scratching in perpetuating lichen simplex chronicus and even behavior modification techniques are helpful.

Psoriasis

Psoriasis is common in the anogenital area. It appears on the mons and the labia majora as well-defined, erythematous plaques (Fig. 9–4); these are

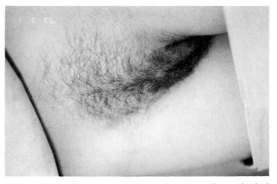

Figure 9–4. Discrete, scaling plaques of psoriasis in the pubic area (see also color section).

sometimes covered by a characteristic silver-white micaceous scale. They are variably pruritic. When involving the labiocrural or interlabial folds, the appearance is smooth and red, often with accompanying painful fissures. Lesions do not extend into the vagina. Diagnosis is aided by general skin examination, which often reveals typical psoriatic plaques commonly present on the elbows, knees, and scalp.

The primary treatment is soaks and topical low-potency steroids or occasionally the short-term use of higher-potency steroid preparations. Tar or anthralin preparations for vulvar psoriasis are generally too irritating for most patients.

Hidradenitis Suppurativa

Hidradenitis suppurativa is a chronic disease affecting the axillary, vulvar, perineal, and gluteal skin. Pathogenesis begins with follicular occlusion in sites where apocrine glands are present. Follicular retention products can cause rupture of the follicle, and inflammation can ensue. Although not a primary bacterial infection, superinfection is common, and careful hygiene by cleansing with an antibacterial soap or a solution such as chlorhexidine gluconate (Hibiclens) is essential. Staphylococcal and streptococcal infection are most common, although gram-negative organisms such as *Escherichia coli* and *Proteus* as well as anaerobic organisms have been isolated. Purulent drainage not controlled by local measures may require systemic antibiotics directed at the predominating flora. The condition begins after puberty, generally in the second and third decades. It can be progressive, with abscess-like nodules, hypertrophy, and scarring with sinus tracts. Oral retinoids such as isotretinoin (Accutane) and corticosteroids have been found to be useful in limited trials. Surgical excision is reserved for aggressive cases that are refractory to medical treatment.

Vesicobullous Diseases

PEMPHIGUS VULGARIS. Pemphigus vulgaris is a chronic intraepidermal blistering disorder that affects predominantly individuals of Jewish or Mediterranean origin. It often appears with oral erosions, followed by generalized involvement that can include the vulva. Occasionally, superficial vulvar erosions may be the sole presenting finding; intact flaccid bullae are only rarely found owing to their fragility. Bullous pemphigoid, a subepidermal blistering disease most common in the elderly, can also occur, rarely, with localized vulvar involvement.

The diagnosis of pemphigus is accomplished through a skin biopsy, which demonstrates intraepidermal blister formation, and immunofluorescent staining of skin and serum to identify intercellular antibodies. Treatment usually requires the use of a systemic agent, often prednisone in combination with azathioprine or methotrexate.

HAILEY-HAILEY DISEASE. Hailey-Hailey disease, a rare dominantly inherited bullous disease that affects intertriginous areas, appears as moist, vegetative, eroded plaques in the labiocrural folds. Treatment is directed at débridement of crusts with soaking and control of the frequent bacterial and *Candida* superinfection.

ERYTHEMA MULTIFORME. Erythema multiforme predominantly causes cutaneous lesions that are most prominent on distal extremities. However, in severe erythema multiforme ''major,'' Stevens-Johnson syndrome, as well as in toxic epidermal necrolysis, vulvovaginal mucosa may be focally erosive or diffusely desquamative. Careful attention to local care is important to prevent late scarring. Of course, removal of the offending medication or treatment of underlying infection as well as aggressive supportive care is required.

Lichen Planus

Lichen planus of the vulva often manifests as an erosive or a desquamative vulvitis accompanying a desquamative vaginitis. Patients are often women older than 40 years who generally present with complaints of chronic burning and pruritus and occasionally a serosanguinous discharge.

Examination of the vulva may reveal either white, reticulated papules or erosions. The more keratinized areas of the perineum may demonstrate the characteristic violaceous, flat-topped, polygonal plaques that are characteristic for lichen planus on nonmucosal surfaces. Later in the disease, the labia minora may be lost, the clitoral hood may become fused, and hypopigmentation of the vulva may occur secondarily to scarring. Examination of the vagina usually reveals erosions; later, the vagina may be foreshortened, making insertion of the speculum difficult.

Examination of the oral mucosa is essential for diagnosis. Many patients have oral erosions or papules with a white, lacy, reticulated pattern (Wickham's striae) that are diagnostic. The glabrous skin should also be examined, but it seldom reveals lesions in patients with erosive vulvar lichen planus.

A skin biopsy of a noneroded but clinically involved area should be performed to establish the diagnosis. Pathology can be helpful in ruling out lichen sclerosus, an entity often in the differential diagnosis for lichen planus. White, hypertrophic plaques should also be biopsied to rule out dysplasia.

Treatment usually requires the use of medium- and even high-potency topical steroids. Intralesional injection or systemic corticosteroids are sometimes necessary. Hydrocortisone suppositories that can be inserted vaginally may be helpful both symptomatically and in preventing adhesions later.

An expensive but effective treatment is the application of topical cyclosporine. In addition, oral dapsone, retinoids, and griseofulvin have all been used but are not especially promising in patients with vulvovaginal lichen planus.

Lichen Sclerosus

Lichen sclerosus is a chronic disorder that most often affects the anogenital area of postmenopausal women and, less commonly, prepubertal girls. This disease was managed by dermatologists and gynecologists, and gradually different terminology for the disease evolved. To clarify terminology, the International Society for the Study of Vulvar Disease (ISSVD) in 1989 reclassified non-neoplastic diseases into three categories: lichen sclerosus (et atrophicus has been dropped), squamous cell hyperplasias, and other vulvar dermatoses. The terms leukoplakia and kraurois are currently out of favor.

The appearance of lichen sclerosus is distinctive, with polygonal ivory-colored papules that show central delling that may coalesce into plaques. In the anogenital area, lesions appear as pink or hypopigmented plaques with fine crinkling secondary to atrophy. As the disease becomes more chronic, purpura and abrasions may be present (Fig. 9–5). Eventually, resorption of the labia minora, scarring of the clitoral hood, and contraction of the introitus may occur. The classic area of involvement creates an hourglass pattern around the clitoris, down the inner aspect of the labia majora and labia minora (with relative sparing of the vestibule), and extending posteriorly around the anus. In contrast to the pattern with lichen planus, the vaginal mucosa is generally spared.

The first symptom of lichen sclerosus is pruritus, which can become debilitating as the disease progresses. In addition, scratching and rubbing can extend the disease (Koebner's phenomenon) and can create additional thickening of the skin.

The clinical appearance may be so characteristic that biopsy is unnecessary. However, evaluation is helpful in distinguishing it from other entities such as lichen planus, morphea, and vitiligo. In prepubertal girls who present with inflammation and bleeding, biopsy may be particularly useful in evaluating the suspicion of sexual abuse.

Evidence of the pathogenesis of lichen sclerosus is sparse. Human leukocyte antigen associations have been found, including B21, B40, B44, and AW31. Minor associations have been made with achlorhydria, vitiligo, autoimmune thyroiditis, and pernicious anemia. Some cases have been identified as having an absence of collagenase and an increased elastase activity. Also, changes of levels of testosterone and dihydrotestosterone with testosterone therapy suggest that 5-alpha reductase might be playing a role. *Borrelia* infection has been weakly linked to some cases of lichen sclerosus.

The course of the disease in older women is usually chronic and progressive. There is an increased risk of vulvar malignancy, perhaps as high as 6%; therefore, patients should be seen regularly, and biopsies should be performed on suspicious lesions. In prepubertal girls, early reports indicated a clearing of lichen sclerosus at puberty, although more recent studies suggest that the disease may reappear later in life.

Bland emollients and topical steroids are the mainstay of treatment. Sedating antihistamines may be necessary as well. Two percent testosterone ointment is of benefit to some patients but should not be used in children. Its potential side effects may include deepening of the voice, change in libido, and clitoral hypertrophy. Progesterone ointment has been used as well. Surgical excision or laser ablation is generally contraindicated because of recurrences following the procedures.

VULVODYNIA

Vulvodynia is defined as a condition of chronic vulvar discomfort often described by the patient as burning, stinging, or rawness. Physical findings are often minimal. It is distinctive from the condition pruritus vulvae, in which the prominent complaint is itching.

Vulvodynia is not a specific entity and probably has multiple causes. McKay has subdivided vulvodynia into five groups. In the first group are the vulvar dermatoses, which include lichen sclerosus, lichen planus, and contact dermatitis, as discussed earlier. In the second group is cyclic candidiasis, in which recurrent *Candida* infection may be approached by aggressive anticandidal treatment. In the third group is squamous papillomatosis. Small papillae around the vulvar vestibule and posterior introitus were previously felt to be a normal variant but may represent subclinical or latent HPV infection. The significance of data demonstrating HPV infection is unclear as most women with subclinical infection are asymptomatic.

In the fourth category is vulvar vestibulitis, which is characterized by pain to vestibular touch

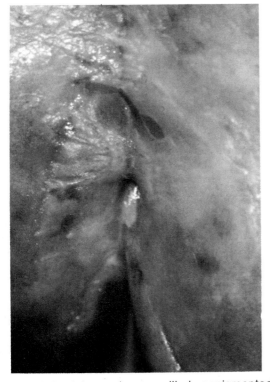

Figure 9–5. Lichen sclerosus with hypopigmented atrophic plaques and erosions (see also color section). (Courtesy of Richard Reid, M.D.)

or vaginal entry, vulvar erythema, or both. Tenderness can be elicited by palpation with a cotton-tipped swab, especially at the site of Bartholin's gland orifices. Xylocaine preparations applied directly to painful areas provide important temporary relief. Intralesional injections with interferon three times weekly for 4 weeks have been associated with significant (partial to total) relief in one study; transient flu-like symptoms are a tolerable but uncomfortable side effect of this therapy. Surgical excision of the affected vestibule has a good success rate in a well-selected population of patients who have had unremitting vestibulitis for 1 to 2 years without response to medical therapy. Carbon dioxide laser ablation has been disappointing when attempted in severe cases.

The last category is "essential" or dysesthetic vulvodynia, in which no cause can be identified. This diagnosis should be made only after an evaluation reveals no evidence of infection or inflammatory dermatoses. The diagnosis can be elusive, as often the physical findings such as erythema may be minimal or even absent. However, the patient's description of an often debilitating burning sensation or a soreness and extreme discomfort to palpation are the key factors in establishing the diagnosis. Occasionally, one can identify hyperesthesia or hypoesthesia objectively in the area extending from the mons pubis to the posterior fourchette and laterally by the inner thighs. Essential vulvodynia may be considered a dysesthesia or a pudendal neuralgia similar to postherpetic neuralgia or glossodynia (burning tongue). The success of tricyclic antidepressants in these other chronic pain syndromes suggested the use of amitriptyline in essential vulvodynia. Dosing should start at 10 mg at bedtime and can be increased from there up to the minimal dose effective to control symptoms (often less than 75 mg).

VULVAR MANIFESTATIONS OF SYSTEMIC DISEASES

In much the same way as the glabrous skin or oral mucosa may reveal clues of underlying disease, the vulva, with its combination of keratinizing and mucosal type of epithelium, demonstrates important manifestations of systemic pathology.

Necrotizing Fasciitis

Necrotizing fasciitis is an acute, potentially fatal infection of the superficial fascia and subcutaneous tissue. It may appear in the vulvar area following an episiotomy or minor trauma. Diabetic women appear to be more susceptible to this infection. Although the overlying skin may initially appear unremarkable, blunt probing reveals a loss of integrity of the underlying tissue. Débridement and antibiotics are required.

Other Infections

Chronic infections that may affect the vulva include tuberculosis, filariasis, schistosomiasis, amebiasis, and deep mycotic infections. These may manifest in the vulva as ulcerations or fungating masses. In addition, recurrent candidiasis is an infection often found in individuals with diabetes or HIV infection.

Aphthosis

Aphthae are small, tender, recurrent punched-out ulcers that can appear in the mouth or on the vulva. Aphthae are common and usually are not a reflection of underlying disease. However, in some individuals with frequent aphthae, an association with Behçet's disease or inflammatory bowel disease is established.

Behçet's Disease

The classic characterization of Behçet's disease is the triad of recurrent oral ulcers, recurrent genital ulcers, and uveitis. Oral and genital ulcers may not appear concurrently. Other systemic findings include arthritis, central nervous system involvement, and thrombophlebitis.

In the vulvar area, lesions appear initially as shallow ulcers, usually on the labia minora, and rarely extend into the vagina. Later in the disease, ulcerations become larger and deeper and may cause scarring. Destruction of vulvar tissue can be marked and can even penetrate through the labia minora to form a "keyhole ulcer."

Diagnosis is established by the fulfillment of criteria set by the International Study Group for Behçet's Disease. These criteria include recurrent oral ulceration and two of the following: genital ulceration, specific eye lesions, typical defined skin lesions (folliculitis, papulopustular lesions, acneiform nodules, or erythema nodosum), or a positive pathergy test. Pathergy is defined as the development of a sterile pustule at the site of a needle prick over a 24- to 48-hour period.

Patients with severe disease, especially that involving the eye and the central nervous system, require prompt treatment with systemic steroids, sometimes in combination with cyclophosphamide or cyclosporine. Individuals who primarily are symptomatic with orogenital lesions may respond to local care and to less toxic medications such as colchicine.

Crohn's Disease

A small number of women with Crohn's disease develop primary lesions on the vulva consisting of noncaseating granulomas. These may appear as painful, indurated swellings with draining sinuses or fistulas; when discontiguous with gastrointestinal lesions, they are termed metastatic Crohn's disease. Recalcitrant disease often indicates active gastrointestinal disease, and surgery is sometimes required when conservative treatment is not successful. Secondary manifestations include aphthae, erythema nodosum, and pyoderma gangrenosum.

Pyoderma Gangrenosum

Pyoderma gangrenosum is an inflammatory, noninfectious condition that begins as a pustule that expands into an ulceration with a suppurative base and an undermined, erythematous border. It is frequently associated with inflammatory bowel disease, immunoglobulin A (IgA) gammopathy, rheumatoid arthritis, and myeloproliferative disorders. Lesions involving the vulva appear either as broad, "dirty" ulcers or as deep, narrow, "knife-cut" ulcers in skin folds. Corticosteroids are the mainstay of treatment.

Lupus Erythematosus

Lupus erythematosus is a disease with protean manifestations. Women with systemic lupus erythematosus or chronic cutaneous disease may rarely present with vulvar ulcers or an erosive vulvovaginitis.

Endocrine and Metabolic Conditions

ESTROGEN DEFICIENCY. Estrogen deficiency may be physiologic and most commonly occurs with naturally occurring menopause. Absence of hormonal stimulation on the vulva may result in atrophy, dryness, and increased fragility, which cause fissures, erosions, and sometimes dyspareunia. The labia majora become atrophic and hypopigmented and develop a sparsity of pubic

hair. In some cases, the labia minora are reabsorbed into the labia majora and the vaginal introitus becomes stenotic. In addition, changes in the vaginal mucosa, pH, and flora may lead to an atrophic vulvovaginitis (see discussion of vulvovaginitis earlier).

Acrodermatitis enteropathica is a syndrome of acquired or genetic zinc deficiency causing a triad of dermatitis, diarrhea, and alopecia. Necrolytic migratory erythema is a dermatitis associated with the glucagonoma syndrome along with diabetes mellitus and high fasting blood glucagon levels. Both entities may begin as an erosive, crusted, psoriasiform eruption. Involvement around the vulva and perineum may precede involvement around other periorificial areas.

Acanthosis nigricans is a velvety, brown thickening of the skin in intertriginous areas, classically involving the axillae and sometimes involving the pubic area, inner thighs, and vulva. Obesity, diabetes, and other endocrine disturbances, malignancy, and drugs have been associated with it.

PIGMENTED LESIONS OF THE VULVA

Studies suggest that pigmented vulvar lesions are present in 10 to 12% of the population. Benign pigmented lesions include seborrheic keratoses, postinflammatory hyperpigmentation, warts, lentigines, and melanosis. In addition, diffuse hyperpigmentation can be caused by hormonal changes of pregnancy, excess melanocyte-stimulating hormone in Cushing's disease and Addison's disease, or increased testosterone production. Some chemotherapeutic agents, antimalarial drugs, metals, and even radiation can result in hyperpigmentation.

Vulvar melanosis is distinguished from lentigines by its larger size and border irregularity. Although it is not believed to be a precursor of melanoma, it can mimic melanoma, and biopsy may be required to distinguish it histologically.

Approximately 2% of women have true moles or nevocellular nevi on the vulva. It is controversial whether nevi on the genitalia are more likely to undergo malignant transformation than nevi elsewhere. Although the great majority of vulvar nevi are unremarkable and indistinguishable from nevi elsewhere on the body, dysplastic nevi are not uncommon. A thorough examination of the female genitalia is warranted; lesions that are larger than 5 mm or have irregular borders or pigment variegation should be considered for excision for definitive histologic diagnosis.

Vulvar melanoma accounts for 8 to 10% of all vulvar malignancies. Two to five percent of melanomas are found on the vulva. Most patients with vulvar melanoma are postmenopausal; the peak incidence occurs in the sixth through the eighth decades. The presenting symptoms of patients with vulvar melanoma include a new mass, a changing mole, bleeding, pruritus, or a burning sensation. The morphology of a vulvar melanoma is the same as melanoma located elsewhere. Thin melanomas diagnosed early have an excellent prognosis. Unfortunately, vulvar melanomas tend to be diagnosed at more advanced stages, which emphasizes the importance of vigilant surveillance of the vulva by patient and physician for suspicious pigmented lesions.

BENIGN VULVAR TUMORS

The following is a brief summary of the more commonly encountered benign vulvar lesions. Although these lesions often have a distinctive clinical appearance, they are at times sufficiently nondescript to require biopsy.

Seborrheic keratoses are common benign lesions in middle-aged and older individuals. They appear as well-demarcated, flesh-colored to brown plaques with a verrucous nature that resembles warts. Because they can be deeply pigmented, they often require differentiation from nevi.

Acrochordons or skin tags are fibroepithelial polyps frequently found in the labiocrural folds bordering the vulva. They are generally flesh colored or brown, soft, and pedunculated. If symptoms develop owing to external irritation, they can be removed easily.

Adnexal tumors include syringomas, which are common, benign tumors derived from eccrine ducts. They appear as multiple, small, flesh-colored asymptomatic papules on the eyelids and sometimes the labia majora. Hidradenoma papilliferum is a rarer sweat gland tumor that appears as a solitary nodule on the vulva, particularly the labia majora. Fox-Fordyce disease (apocrine miliaria) can occur in the pubic area as well as in the axilla.

Vascular tumors include hemangiomas, which may be congenital but are commonly acquired, as in the case of the small, sharply demarcated "cherry" angiomas. Other vascular anomalies include angiokeratomas (analogous to the male scrotal angiokeratoma), varices, and lymphangiomas.

Epidermal inclusion cysts are not uncommon in the pubic and hair-bearing areas of the vulva. Generally, they require excision only if they become recurrently inflamed or infected. Mucous cysts most frequently occur on the vestibule. Excision is preferred over incision and drainage because of concern for secondary infection.

The Bartholin's duct cyst is common. Treatment is either excision or marsupialization. Incision and drainage alone may result in secondary infection. In older women, biopsy samples should be taken from suspicious lesions to rule out Bartholin's gland carcinoma. Cysts of Skene's ducts occur only rarely.

Cysts of the canal of Nuck are the female equivalent of the male hydrocele. They occur from incomplete embryologic closure as the peritoneovaginal canal separates from the peritoneal cavity. Cysts may be found in the mons, groin, or labia majora. The treatment is surgical.

Lipomas of the vulva as elsewhere appear as soft, compressible, asymptomatic subcutaneous masses. Endometriosis has been identified in the vulva as well as in the accessory nipples because the milk line extends down to the vulva.

MALIGNANT VULVAR TUMORS

Classification

To introduce common terminology that can be used across the medical community, the ISSVD established the following system to classify vulvar intraepithelial neoplasia (VIN) (Table 9–1). This terminology is designed to replace the more confusing terms that include Bowen's disease, carcinoma in situ, Queyrat's erythroplasia, bowenoid papulosis, bowenoid dysplasia, and hyperplastic dystrophy with atypia.

Vulvar Intraepithelial Neoplasia of Squamous Origin

Presenting symptoms of VIN include pruritus, pain, or bleeding if ulceration has occurred; alternatively, it may be asymptomatic. On examination, VIN can have variable clinical manifestations (Fig. 9–6A and B). On the nonkeratinized epithelium of

---

TABLE 9–1.   ISSVD Classification of Vulvar Intraepithelial Neoplasia

Squamous
  VIN1—mild dysplasia
  VIN2—moderate dysplasia
  VIN3—severe dysplasia or carcinoma in situ
Nonsquamous
  Paget's disease
  Melanoma in situ

From Wilkinson EJ, Kneale B, Lynch PJ. Report of the ISSVD Terminology Committee. J Reprod Med 1986;31:973.

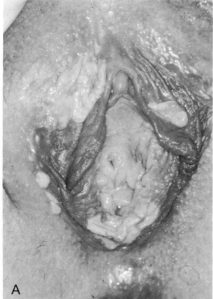

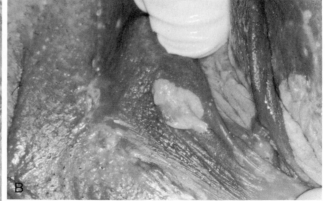

Figure 9–6. *A* and *B,* Pink and whitish macules and plaques of vulvar intraepithelial neoplasia 3 (carcinoma in situ) (see also color section). (Courtesy of Richard Reid, M.D.)

the vestibule, it may appear as an erythematous macule or patch. On the keratinized epithelium, such as that of the labia majora where it is most common, it may appear as a white, hyperkeratotic or papillomatous lesion with irregular borders. Aceto-whitening with 5% acetic acid is sometimes helpful in identifying lesions.

Vulvar intraepithelial neoplasia is generally found in sexually active women. The number of young women with VIN has increased dramatically, with more than half the patients now younger than 40 years of age. Vulvar intraepithelial neoplasia of squamous origin is graded by degree of dysplasia. Presumably this reflects the increase in HPV infection, particularly HPV 16 and rarely HPV 18 and HPV 31. One study demonstrated the presence of HPV 16 in more than 80% of patients with VIN 3 (carcinoma in situ). Unlike younger women who often have multifocal disease, postmenopausal women generally have solitary lesions, sometimes arising in a region of lichen sclerosus. Invasive disease is more likely to occur in the older population.

There is a striking association of VIN with other concurrent or subsequent carcinomas. This link is strongest with cervical cancer but also is seen with vaginal carcinomas, ovarian and endometrial carcinomas, and even more distant carcinomas of the colon and pancreas. A thorough examination of the anogenital area as well as a complete gynecologic evaluation is critical in these patients.

The management of VIN is in evolution. Partial or total vulvectomy is still advocated in older or immunosuppressed patients. Local excision, laser therapy, or other locally destructive therapy is usually reserved for younger women in whom risk of invasion is lower. Clear margins are important in trying to achieve a cure in this disease. Because of the multicentric nature and 20% recurrence rate of VIN, regular surveillance and biopsy of suspicious lesions are critical.

Invasive Squamous Cell Carcinoma

Invasive squamous cell carcinoma represents 5% of all female genital tract cancers and accounts for the great majority of vulvar malignancies. Vulvar squamous cell carcinoma may appear as a hyperkeratotic plaque, a polypoid mass, or an ulceration. The association with VIN is strong. Seventeen percent of patients presenting with clinical signs of VIN have evidence of invasion; 20 to 80% of patients with invasive squamous cell carcinoma have adjacent VIN.

Squamous cell carcinoma is generally a disease of women older than 60 years of age. However, reports are increasing of disease in younger women who are immunocompromised, such as renal transplant patients or HIV-infected individuals. Staging of disease is done using a TNM system, with stage I (T1 N0 M0) representing disease less than 2 cm confined to the vulva without palpable lymph nodes. The 5-year survival rate for stage I disease is 85%, but it is as low as 10% for advanced stage IV disease.

Verrucous Carcinoma

One distinct variant of vulvar squamous cell carcinoma is verrucous carcinoma. In the past, it has also been termed giant condyloma of Buschke-Löwenstein, and HPV association is likely. The carcinoma is locally aggressive but rarely metastatic. Treatment is surgical; radiotherapy may cause further aggressive transformation.

Vulvar Intraepithelial Neoplasia of Nonsquamous Origin

Vulvar Paget's disease is an intraepithelial neoplasm of mucin-containing cells. Unlike Paget's disease of the breast with certain underlying carcinoma, extramammary Paget's disease is associated with other carcinomas in less than half the cases. In about 25% of cases, there is adenocarcinoma of contiguous skin appendages or Bartholin's glands. In 10 to 20% of cases, there is more distant carcinoma from sites such as the uterus, rectum, or breast.

Extramammary Paget's disease is rare, accounting for only 2% of vulvar neoplasms. Its clinical appearance may be deceptive, manifesting as an ill-defined eczematous plaque unresponsive to the topical steroids; biopsy of these persistent plaques reveals the diagnostic intraepithelial Paget cells. Treatment is surgical excision, although recurrences are common.

Other Neoplasms

Basal cell carcinomas account for 2% of vulvar carcinomas. Complaints of a new growth, ulceration, or bleeding are often presenting symptoms. The labia majora are the most common location. On examination, the classic appearance of a basal cell carcinoma is a firm papule or nodule with a rolled, translucent border and frequent central ulceration. If left untreated, basal cell carcinomas become locally invasive although only very rarely metastatic.

Metastasis from genital tract neoplasms and infrequently from more distant neoplasms may appear on the vulva. Histologic differentiation from a primary adenocarcinoma is sometimes difficult.

Bibliography

Baker DA, Mead PB. Viral STDs in the female patient: A therapeutic update. Proceedings of a Symposium at the annual meeting of the American College of Obstetricians and Gynecologists. IntraMed Communications/Burroughs Wellcome Co, 1991.

Blickstein I, Feldberg E, DGani R, et al. Dysplastic vulvar nevi. Obstet Gynecol 1991;78:968.

Crum CP. Carcinoma of the vulva: Epidemiology and pathogenesis. Obstet Gynecol 1992;79:448.

Edwards L. Vulvar lichen planus. Arch Dermatol 1989; 125:1677.

Edwards L. Desquamative vulvitis. In: Turner MLC, Marinoff SC (eds). Vulvar Diseases. Dermatol Clin 1992;10:325.

Friedrich EG Jr, Kalra PS. Serum levels of sex hormones in vulvar lichen sclerosus and the effect of topical testosterone. N Engl J Med 1984;310:488.

Friedrich EG Jr, Wilkinson EJ, Fu YS. Carcinoma in situ of the vulva: A continuing challenge. Am J Obstet Gynecol 1980;136:830.

Hood AF, Lumadue J. Benign vulvar tumors. In: Turner MLC, Marinoff SC (eds). Vulvar Diseases. Dermatol Clin 1992;10:371.

International Study Group for Behçet's Disease. Criteria for diagnosis of Behçet's Disease. Lancet 1990;335:1078.

Mann MS, Kaufman RH. Erosive lichen planus of the vulva. Clin Obstet Gynecol 1991;34:605.

Marinoff SC, Turner MLC. Vulvar vestibulitis syndrome: An overview. Am J Obstet Gynecol 1991;165:1228.

Marinoff SC, Turner MLC, Hirsch RP, Richard G. Intralesional alpha interferon: Cost-effective therapy for vulvar vestibulitis syndrome. J Reprod Med 1993;38:19.

McCance DJ, Campion MJ, Baram A, Singer A. Risk of transmission of human papillomavirus by vaginal specula. Lancet 1986;2:816.

McCue JD. Evaluation and management of vaginitis. Arch Intern Med 1989;149:565.

McKay M. Vulvodynia. Arch Dermatol 1989;125:256.

McKay M. Vulvar dermatoses. Clin Obstet Gynecol 1991; 34:614.

McKay M. Vulvitis and vulvovaginitis: Cutaneous considerations. Am J Obstet Gynecol 1991;165:1176.

McKay M. Dysesthetic ("essential") vulvodynia: Treatment with amitriptyline. J Reprod Med 1993;38:9.

Pincus SH. Vulvar dermatoses and pruritus vulvae. In: Turner MLC, Marinoff SC (eds). Vulvar Diseases. Dermatol Clin 1992;10:297.

Reid R, Greenberg MD. Human papillomavirus–related diseases of the vulva. Clin Obstet Gynecol 1991;34:630.

Ridley CM. Lichen sclerosus. In: Turner MLC, Marinoff SC (eds). Vulvar Diseases. Dermatol Clin 1992;10:309.

Rock B. Pigmented lesions of the vulva. In: Turner MLC, Marinoff SC (eds). Vulvar Diseases. Dermatol Clin 1992;10:361.

Schulman D, Beck LS, Roberts IM, Schwartz AM. Crohn's disease of the vulva. Am J Gastroenterol 1987;82:1328.

Sobel JD. Vulvovaginitis. In: Turner MLC, Marinoff SC (eds). Vulvar Diseases. Dermatol Clin 1992;10:339.

Tovell HMM, Young AW. Diseases of the Vulva in Clinical Practice. New York: Elsevier Science Publishing Co, 1991.

Turner MLC. Vulvar manifestations of systemic diseases. In: Turner MLC, Marinoff SC (eds). Vulvar Diseases. Dermatol Clin 1992;10:445.

Turner MLC, Marinoff SC. Pudendal neuralgia. Am J Obstet Gynecol 1991;165:1233.

Wilkinson EJ. Normal histology and nomenclature of the vulva and malignant neoplasms, including VIN. In: Turner MLC, Marinoff SC (eds). Vulvar Diseases. Dermatol Clin 1992;10:283.

Wilkinson EJ, Kneale B, Lynch PJ. Report of the ISSVD Terminology Committee. J Reprod Med 1986;31:973.

Vaginal Intraepithelial Neoplasia and In Utero Exposure to Diethylstilbestrol

Carolyn Johnston

Although uncommon, premalignant diseases of the vagina are to some degree predictable as a consequence of previous lower genital tract dysplasia, viral infection (e.g., human papillomavirus [HPV]), or exposure to diethylstilbestrol (DES). Vaginal intraepithelial neoplasia occurs most frequently in the older woman who has a history of cervical dysplasia or carcinoma. Human papillomavirus infection is a multifocal disease of the lower genital tract and is often on the vaginal mucosa as well as the vulva. Cervical and vaginal adenosis is increased in women with a history of in utero exposure to DES. Furthermore this group of women who were exposed to DES have a higher subsequent incidence of squamous dysplasia and clear cell carcinoma. This chapter focuses on these diseases, their interrelationships, and an approach to their evaluation, follow-up, and treatment.

VAGINAL INTRAEPITHELIAL NEOPLASIA

Vaginal intraepithelial neoplasia (VAIN) is markedly less common than cervical intraepithelial neoplasia (CIN) and occurs at an older age. The frequency, however, appears to be increasing as Papanicolaou (PAP) smears and colposcopy are performed more routinely and as HPV infections become more prevalent. The rate and time interval of progression from VAIN to squamous cell carcinoma of the vagina is unknown. In the largest reported series of persons with VAIN, the average age of patients was 50 years with a range of 23 to 75 years.[1] The majority (75%) of women have had a prior hysterectomy for a variety of indications,

including both benign and malignant conditions, but most often for CIN or cervical carcinoma.[1–3] Vaginal intraepithelial neoplasia occurs at varying intervals after hysterectomy but appears more quickly following hysterectomy performed for CIN than for benign disease; 53.7 months versus 153.5 months, respectively.[1] Similarly, vaginal carcinoma appears more quickly after hysterectomy for premalignant disease (68.4 months vs. 156 months) and with a comparable time course to VAIN.[4] Originally, the occurrence of VAIN after hysterectomy for cervical dysplasia was attributed to an inadequate vaginal cuff margin, which led several investigators to recommend a margin of at least 1.5 to 2.0 cm below the cervix.[5, 6] Creasman and Rutledge, however, found no relationship between cuff length and recurrent dysplasia in a large review of 861 females who underwent hysterectomy for carcinoma in situ.[7] Others found a higher frequency of VAIN if the vaginal margin was positive for dysplasia.[8] Thus, although absolute cuff length may not be relevant, involved margins probably are significant. Therefore, careful colposcopic examination of the vaginal fornices, as well as the cervix, is warranted in the preoperative evaluation of the female with cervical dysplasia.

The vagina and cervix arise from the same urogenital sinus epithelium, so it is not surprising that lower genital tract dysplasia is often a multifocal process. One would also expect risk factors for dysplasia to be similar at the different sites. Brinton and colleagues attempted to define risk factors for VAIN.[9] Although several common risk factors with CIN were noted, including low socioeconomic status, a history of HPV infection, vaginal discharge, and a prior abnormal PAP smear result, there was one glaring exception: the use of tobacco. Cervical intraepithelial neoplasia has been associated with tobacco use but not VAIN. This is curious given its detrimental effect on cervical and vulvar dysplasias. It is possible that their series of patients was too small to make this distinction. Human papillomavirus infection is associated with VAIN, and as the incidence of HPV infection continues to increase, so probably will the incidence of VAIN as well as its persistence and recalcitrance to treatment.[10, 11]

Diagnosis

Vaginal dysplasia is usually asymptomatic[1, 12] and is detected incidentally by PAP smear[13]; therefore, it is important to perform routine PAP smears in women after hysterectomy. Cytologic follow-up should be long term because of the relatively long latency period to development of VAIN even after hysterectomy for dysplasia: Yearly PAP smears for at least 6 years, and preferably for a lifetime, are warranted in light of longitudinal data from Audet-Lapointe and associates[1] and Stuart and coworkers.[4] Whenever an abnormal result on a cytologic study is detected, colposcopy should be performed. Colposcopic technique is similar to that advocated for the evaluation of the cervix, with a few modifications to facilitate the examination. The disease usually occurs in the upper one third of the vagina and may be difficult to evaluate colposcopically owing to involvement of the vaginal angles and rugae. Various tricks to improve the accuracy of the examination include the use of the largest speculum feasible to distend the vaginal angles and rugae, 2 to 4 weeks of estrogen cream vaginally in postmenopausal females before the colposcopy, 5% acetic acid, and a dilator in women who have had prior radiation therapy, especially intracavitary brachytherapy.[1, 12] Lugol's solution may be used at the discretion of the examiner. This strong iodine solution is preferentially absorbed by the normally glycogenated epithelium of the vagina and may aid in defining the borders of the dysplastic epithelium, which does not absorb it. Use of this dark brown solution makes the acetic acid examination difficult and may mislead the examiner in the absence of adequately glycogenated epithelium such as in the atrophic mucosa of a postmenopausal woman. After the application of acetic acid, the dysplastic epithelium appears as white, slightly raised punctate areas. Mosaicism is rarely present, but abnormal blood vessels are present in the more severe lesions. It is important to examine the entire vagina and take biopsy samples of at least the most abnormal looking area. If carcinoma in situ is of concern, then biopsy samples should be taken from multiple areas within the lesion to rule out invasion, particularly if ablative therapy is planned. Alternatively, a wide local excision or partial vaginectomy provides both the evidence to rule out invasion and, potentially, a cure. Partial vaginectomy may also be necessary if the PAP smear results remain significantly abnormal despite negative colposcopic biopsy results by an experienced colposcopist.

Therapy

Several treatment options exist, and the one chosen depends on the severity and focality of the dysplasia, concern for the possibility of underlying carcinoma, distensibility of the vaginal area to be treated, a history of prior radiation therapy, and the general medical condition of the patient.

Historically, radiation therapy, via a vaginal cylinder or tandem designed to give 6000 cGy to the vaginal surface, was used.[14, 15] However, recurrences (12%) and persistence led to concern regarding its use.[1, 12] Presumably rugae and limited distensibility of the vaginal angles cause incomplete contact of the entire vaginal epithelium with the radiation source. Radiation therapy also causes vaginal stenosis, foreshortening, and dyspareunia, which is of concern to the sexually active woman.[15] These issues, in turn, led others to advocate the use of surgical excision.[12] However, this procedure also carries a similar risk of recurrence (18%), presumably because approximately one third of patients have multifocal disease on thorough evaluation.[12, 16, 17] Partial vaginectomy is most useful (1) to rule out invasion, (2) to obtain a diagnosis when colposcopic biopsies are nondiagnostic and the PAP smear results suggest VAIN, (3) to treat disease in the apical vaginal angles, and (4) to treat recurrent disease after topical or ablative therapy fails.

Other therapeutic methods include the carbon dioxide laser, which has replaced cryosurgery and electrocautery, which have poor depth control, and 5% 5-fluorouracil (5-FU) cream (Efudex). Large comparative studies on these newer modalities do not exist; however, several small series in patients with VAIN using the carbon dioxide laser have reported a success rate of approximately 70%.[1, 7-19] Vaginal intraepithelial neoplasia is a disease of the epithelium only; thus, laser vaporization should be performed to a depth of 1.0 to 2.0 mm. Careful attention should be given to adequate distention of the vaginal walls and angles to avoid missing areas of epithelium obscured by the skin folds. The liberal use of skin hooks[18] and retractors is encouraged, as is careful patient selection. The major risks of laser ablation are treatment failure, vaginal vault agglutination, and inadvertent damage to subepithelial structures such as bowel and bladder. Postoperative healing can be enhanced by the immediate use of intravaginal silver sulfadiazine cream and, after 1 to 2 weeks, the use of acidifying agents such as vinegar douches or boric acid suppositories.[20]

If the VAIN is associated with HPV infection, then the adjunctive use of 5-FU cream after laser ablation may help reduce recurrences.[12, 16] Some patients, especially those who are immunosuppressed, may require long-term suppression to avoid recurrent dysplasia.[16] Several different regimens exist, but the use of 2 gm per vagina per week for 1 month is well tolerated and efficacious.[20] Alternatively, a subcutaneous injection of 1 million units of interferon-α into the introital skin can be used weekly for 1 month or longer.[20] Patients are often reluctant to self-administer a vaginal injection, whereas 5-fluorouracil cream is easily inserted using an applicator and thus may be more practical.

5-Fluorouracil cream alone provides an effective treatment for VAIN, especially if the lesions are multifocal or, as previously discussed, associated with HPV infection.[12, 16] The 85% initial success rate is comparable to that of radiation therapy and laser ablation.[16] It is unlikely to be well absorbed by hyperkeratotic lesions, so other methods should be used to treat these lesions. Topical 5-FU is generally well tolerated, although complaints of vulvar irritation and dysuria are common. Patients can apply zinc oxide or petroleum jelly as protection to the vulva before inserting the cream intravaginally. They should also be instructed to treat themselves at bedtime to improve the initial retention of the 5-FU cream in the vagina. Vaginal ulceration and agglutination can occur; thus, the patient should be evaluated shortly after, or during, longer courses of therapy. These lesions will resolve after a short respite off 5-FU. Therapy using 5-FU can then be reinstituted at either a lower dose or a longer cream-free interval, or both. As with use on the skin, no systemic toxicity has been reported.[17] Despite this, use in pregnancy is not recommended because of the concern of fetal cytotoxicity. Many treatment regimens exist that are characterized by different patient tolerances but comparable efficacies.[1, 17, 20–23] (Table 10–1). Reevaluation of the vaginal epithelium immediately after the completion of 5-FU therapy is complicated by the excoriating effect of 5-FU that can yield false positive PAP smear results. A repeat PAP smear should be performed 8 to 12 weeks

TABLE 10–1. Various 5% 5-FU Cream Treatment Regimens for Vaginal Intraepithelial Neoplasia

5 gm/night	5 nights (1,17)*
¼ applicator BID†	1 mo; if tolerated after 3–4 days (21)
2 gm/night	5 nights and repeat if persists (20)
2 gm/night	2 wk (22)
1.5 gm/week	8–10 wk (23)

*Reference numbers in parentheses.
†5-FU concentration only 1–2% and appeared to be well tolerated over the long term.

after completion of therapy, when the vault epithelium has healed. If this result shows resolution of disease, then evaluation with PAP smears every 3 to 4 months the first year and every 6 months thereafter is adequate.[1] Another course of 5-FU may be pursued or alternative therapies sought if disease persists.[1, 20]

HUMAN PAPILLOMAVIRUS INFECTION OF THE VAGINA

The incidence of genital HPV infection is increasing, especially in the young and sexually active population. The significance and epidemiology have been reviewed extensively elsewhere.[24–27] The increase is clearly associated with an increase in both occurrence and progression of CIN.[28–30] In contrast, high spontaneous regression rates (approximately 30–40%) have also been reported.[29, 31]

Less certain is the role of HPV infection in vaginal dysplasias and carcinomas. Vaginal intraepithelial neoplasia and vaginal squamous cell carcinoma have been associated with HPV infection,[9, 11, 32] but because these lesions are much less common than comparable disease in the cervix, less information has been gathered. However, the presence of concomitant HPV infection and VAIN appears to increase the recurrence rates of VAIN.[1]

Diagnosis

Vaginal HPV infection has three manifestations: *overt*, with grossly apparent warts; *subclinical*, or detectable by cytology or histology; and *latent*, requiring HPV DNA analysis for diagnosis. As for the cervix, the clinical relevance of a latent infection is unknown. A significant proportion of patients are asymptomatic; however, others complain of a vaginal discharge and dyspareunia referred to as HPV colpitis.[20] Itching and burning are more likely if the patient also has vulvar condyloma.

Once detected, either grossly or on PAP smear, colposcopy with biopsy is mandatory to assess the extent of disease and to rule out associated dysplasia. Typically when viewed with a colposcope after the application of 5% acetic acid, acetowhite, slightly raised, spiculated areas are seen.[20] Although the patient may complain of a vaginal discharge and other irritating symptoms, colposcopic findings are hyperplastic, not inflammatory.

The importance of a biopsy, both to rule out dysplasia and to rule in HPV infection, cannot be overemphasized. A diagnosis of HPV infection can have a significant emotional and psychological impact. There are overt and histologic findings that are suggestive of HPV infection that on closer analysis using either HPV DNA technology or more stringent histologic criteria do not represent HPV infection.[33] These include grossly papillary vaginal surfaces and histologic papillomatosis and perinuclear clearing without nuclear atypia.[33] Gynecologists and pathologists are encouraged to have good evidence of HPV infection before making the diagnosis.

Therapy

Treatment of vaginal HPV infection is controversial, as is therapy elsewhere in the lower genital tract. Clearly, if it is associated with VAIN, then the dysplasia should be treated. Contributing to the uncertainty is the variety of equally mediocre treatment options available and the high rates of reinfection and spontaneous regression.[29, 31] As expressed in the Centers for Disease Control and Prevention guidelines on sexually transmitted diseases (1989): "The effect of genital treatment on HPV transmission and the natural history of HPV is unknown. Therefore the goal of therapy is removal of exophytic warts and the amelioration of signs and symptoms, not the eradication of HPV."[34] The basic indications for treatment are given in Table 10–2. Although approximately three fourths of the partners also have HPV infec-

TABLE 10–2. Indications for Treatment of Vaginal Human Papillomavirus Infection

Concomitant vaginal dysplasia
Presence of an irritating vaginal discharge or dyspareunia
Obvious exophytic lesions
Psychologic or emotional distress created by an untreated sexually transmitted disease

tions,[35] treatment or evaluation of the partner cannot be recommended at this time unless he is symptomatic. In the largest evaluation of the effect of treatment of male HPV infections on recurrence rates in concurrently treated females, no difference in recurrence rates was noted whether or not the males were treated.[36] Condoms may be protective but do not cover the scrotum, which is affected in approximately 22% of men.[35]

Treatment options include carbon dioxide laser, topical 85% trichloroacetic acid, 5-FU cream, and interferon. These are tailored to the disease characteristics. Hyperkeratotic lesions require either trichloroacetic acid or laser ablation, the latter being preferable and more useful.

Trichloroacetic acid is useful for introital lesions, although solitary vault lesions may also be amenable to such treatment. It can be used during pregnancy. If trichloroacetic acid is used intravaginally, then the speculum should be left in place for 1 to 2 minutes to prevent diffuse burning. Applications are usually repeated weekly. Topical podophyllum preparations cannot be used intravaginally or during pregnancy because of the risk of systemic toxicity.

Laser ablation is useful for multifocal disease. (See the section on VAIN for details of therapy.) The laser can be used in pregnancy, but bleeding can be quite troublesome.

Five percent 5-FU cream is useful for extensive disease with minimal hyperkeratosis and may be more cost effective than the laser.[37] See Table 10–1 for the possible treatment regimens; all of them appear to be equally efficacious but variably tolerated by the patient. Two grams of 5-FU cream intravaginally once a week for 8 to 10 weeks is probably the best tolerated regimen. Vaginal examination every 2 weeks is recommended to assess for response, vault wall agglutination, disruption of synechiae, and epithelial ulceration.[20] This therapy can be continued indefinitely. Intravaginal 5-FU is contraindicated in pregnancy because of the potential for absorption and fetal cytotoxicity.

Minimal data are available on the use of interferon-α alone for vaginal condyloma, but extrapolating from data on the vulva, one would expect some benefits from its use. Interferon-α (1 million units, subcutaneously three times per week) has been shown to improve the success rate when given adjunctively after laser ablation of vulvar condyloma and may potentially be useful for distal vaginal disease.[38] For treatment of vaginal condyloma, Hatch recommends initially using 1 million units subcutaneously at the introitus for 1 month and then continuing it weekly for 8 weeks in responders.[20] Fifty percent of patients experience flulike symptoms, which, albeit short-lived (2–6 hours), can be debilitating. A nonsteroidal anti-inflammatory drug or acetaminophen is often beneficial.

Vaginal condyloma can be particularly troublesome during pregnancy when they can enlarge and increase in number, possibly secondary to the stimulus of progesterone or to an altered immune state during pregnancy.[39] Many regress after delivery but in the interim may cause bleeding and dystocia at the time of delivery. For this reason, intrapartum removal may be necessary. A biopsy should be performed before ablation to rule out malignancy or dysplasia. If treatment is necessary, laser ablation and cryotherapy are most useful. Cryotherapy avoids the risk of anesthesia and is probably associated with less bleeding.[40] More than one treatment is usually required.[40]

The other major concern is the risk of viral transmission to the upper respiratory tract of the fetus and the development of juvenile laryngeal papillomatosis. The viral types most commonly associated with this condition are identical to those found in simple genital warts: types 6 and 11. Juvenile laryngeal papillomatosis is rare, with 150 to 300 cases per year.[41] Because of the apparently low rate of transmission and the possibility that HPV may be transmitted in utero, the routine performance of cesarean section cannot be recommended for cervical and vaginal HPV infection.[42]

EXPOSURE TO DIETHYLSTILBESTROL

Diethylstilbestrol, a nonsteroidal estrogen, was promoted in the United States in the 1940s for the treatment of habitual abortion and other pregnancy complications.[43] However, these benefits were not confirmed in a randomized, double-blind study, conducted at the University of Chicago in the 1950s, which included 840 women treated with DES and 806 women who received a placebo.[44] Following this report, its use declined but continued until 1971 when a retrospective, controlled study by Herbst and colleagues suggested that maternal ingestion of DES during pregnancy increased the risk of vaginal clear cell carcinoma in female offspring.[45] By this time, an estimated 2 to 3 million females in the United States had received DES.[46] In response to the increased frequency of clear cell carcinoma in these offspring who were exposed to DES, the Registry for Research on Hormonal Transplacental Carcinogenesis was established at the University of Chicago in 1971 to characterize the clinical, pathologic, and epidemiologic aspects of all cases of clear cell carcinoma that occurred after 1940.[47] The findings of the Registry are updated periodically.[48–50] The incidence of cervical and vaginal clear cell carcinoma has steadily declined since a peak of 31 cases in 1975. In utero exposure to DES has been consistently documented in 60% of the patients, and another 12% were exposed to another hormone or unknown medication.[48] The median age at diagnosis was 19 years (range 15–34 years). Ninety percent of cases have developed in females 15 to 27 years old.[48] Although apparently increased, the risk of clear cell carcinoma developing after prenatal DES exposure is still low at 0.14 to 1.4 cases per 1000 women.[48, 50] This relatively low risk and the long latency period led Herbst and colleagues to suggest that DES is an incomplete carcinogen and that an as yet unidentified factor or factors are also important.[50]

Although DES is not clearly a carcinogen, its role as a teratogen is better substantiated, with approximately 35% and 20% of DES daughters demonstrating vaginal adenosis and structural anomalies of the genital tract, respectively.[51] A dose-response effect is suggested for structural anomalies but not for clear cell carcinoma.[52] Most apparent is that maternal exposure before 18 weeks of gestation is associated with development of both nonmalignant and malignant conditions in the offspring.[50, 52]

Vaginal and Cervical Clear Cell Carcinoma

Clear cell carcinoma is best treated with surgery, radiation therapy, or a combination of both. As with most gynecologic malignancies, recurrences most often develop in the first 3 years after diagnosis and are located in the pelvis (60%), lungs (36%), and supraclavicular lymph nodes (20%).[53] Particular attention should be directed to these sites at follow-up visits.

Most patients present initially with abnormal vaginal bleeding; however 16% are reportedly asymptomatic and diagnosed at the time of routine pelvic examination.[49] Papanicolaou smears are useful for detection, but false negative rates of up to 21% have been reported.[49] Thus, prompt evaluation of any abnormal bleeding, vaginal discharge, or cytologic finding in this cohort is important.

Adenosis

Adenosis refers to the persistence of müllerian-type glandular epithelium in the vagina after vaginal development is completed. Three types of glandular epithelium can be represented and are, in order of decreasing frequency, mucinous endocervical, tuboendometrial, and embryonic colum-nar types.[54] Adenosis can involve the surface epi-thelium or manifest as glands in the superficial stroma. Although adenosis is the most common genital tract abnormality reported after in utero DES exposure, it has also been reported with an identical appearance in females with no history of DES exposure.[54] Presumably it occurs because DES or another agent, or both, interferes with the normal growth of the urogenital sinus epithelium as it advances to cover the müllerian epithelium of the vagina and cervix.[55]

In DES patients, adenosis is most commonly found on the anterior vaginal wall in the upper third of the vagina, where it appears as red velvety lesions, palpable nodules, or both. Varying degrees of squamous metaplasia are often present. This sequential involution has been documented with serial histology and cytology.[56, 57] The rate of squa-mous metaplasia is more rapid in sexually active women.[56] Also the use of oral contraceptive pills appears to be associated with less adenosis[51] and is not contraindicated in DES daughters.

Adenosis and its subsequent squamous metapla-sia can potentially be altered by any process that alters the normal transitional zone on the cervix, to which it is analogous. Glandular[58] dysplasias and microglandular hyperplasia as well as squa-mous dysplasias[59] have been documented by bi-opsy in association with vaginal adenosis. Transi-tions between normal and dysplastic glandular cells have been identified, whereas a transition from dysplastic glandular epithelium to frank ade-nocarcinoma has been difficult to document de-spite the observation of adenosis in clear cell car-cinomas of patients who were exposed to DES.[58] Robboy and Welch presented five cases of micro-glandular hyperplasia in association with oral con-traceptive use and prenatal DES exposure and re-viewed the distinctive microscopic features, noting that many of these lesions were initially mistaken for adenocarcinoma.[60] In the three patients who discontinued oral contraceptive pill use, the lesions spontaneously resolved in 3 to 13 months.

Squamous Dysplasia

The risk of squamous dysplasia in patients with in utero exposure to DES continues to be debated. The difficulty stems from both referral bias and confusion between the histologic appearance of immature squamous metaplasia and squamous dysplasia.[61] In the 1970s, one group reported squa-mous dysplasia in 17% of females exposed to DES,[62] whereas several others reported frequencies of only 0 to 5%.[51, 59, 61, 63–66] Generally the dysplasia

was mild and appeared to be more common in the cervix than in the vagina.[61, 63] Subsequently in 1984, a follow-up report of the same women en-rolled in the diethylstilbestrol adenosis (DESAD) project demonstrated a markedly increased inci-dence of cervical and vaginal dysplasia and carci-noma in situ in DES daughters compared with that in controls.[67] In 1981, the rate of dysplasia in this same group was similar to that of controls (1.8%), whereas 3 years later it was more than twice that of controls. With the exception of more extensive squamous metaplasia in the exposed group, the two groups were identical.[67] These investigators postulated that there was more dysplasia because there was essentially a larger "transformation zone" in these patients who had been exposed to DES. They recommended at least annual cytologic examinations of the cervices and of any abnormal vaginal epithelium of DES daughters.[67] Despite the increased incidence of preinvasive disease, the in-cidence of cervical and vaginal squamous cell car-cinoma does not appear to be increased in patients who were exposed to DES prenatally.

Little attention has been paid to the role of HPV infection in DES-associated vaginal dysplasias since Robboy first postulated the possible interac-tion of herpes simplex virus or HPV infection with immature squamous metaplasia.[67] Vaginal lesions from five of 959 patients with a history of prenatal DES exposure and subsequent development of moderate vaginal dysplasia were examined by in situ hybridization for HPV 6 or 16 DNA.[68] Four of the five had lesions positive for HPV 6, and one of five had an HPV 16–positive lesion. They pos-tulated that the higher incidence of VAIN in DES patients was due to a greater susceptibility of their vaginal mucosa to HPV infection.[68]

Genital Tract Abnormalities

Although less common than adenosis, a number of upper genital tract abnormalities have been re-ported in the female offspring of mothers who took DES while pregnant.

Female

Structural abnormalities apparently associated with prenatal exposure to DES include transverse cervical ridges (cockscomb or cervical collars), cervical pseudopolyps, hypoplastic cervices, T-shaped uterine cavities, uterotubal constrictions, cervical widening, and hypoplastic uteri.[52, 69, 70] The postulated mechanism for cervical abnormalities comes from mouse and human data suggesting that DES at 9 to 20 weeks gestation preferentially af-

TABLE 10–3.   Management of the Female with Prenatal Exposure to Diethylstilbestrol (DES)

1. Careful examination of the cervix and vagina.
2. Palpation of vault for adenosis: felt as raised or indurated lesions.
3. Papanicolaou (PAP) smear from cervix and upper ⅓ of vagina and any other abnormal vaginal area. Provide the cytologist with information regarding oral contraceptive pill and hormone use.
4. Colposcopy with acetic acid ± Lugol's solution at the initial visit and as indicated thereafter.
5. Biopsy: for initial diagnosis of adenosis, new indurated or raised areas detected on subsequent examinations and sites found to be dysplastic on PAP smear, colposcopy, or both. If in doubt, perform a biopsy.
6. Treat dysplasia as indicated. Laser ablation is preferable to cryotherapy on the cervix because of less potential stenosis.
7. Perform bimanual rectovaginal examination.
8. Perform breast examination and mammographic follow-up as recommended for all patients of a similar age.
9. Consider screening for autoimmune disorders.
10. Oral contraceptive pills and postmenopausal hormone replacement therapy are not contraindicated for a past history of exposure to DES.
11. Have a higher index of suspicion and a lower threshold for evaluation of abnormal bleeding and new vaginal discharge in the female with prenatal exposure to DES.

From Herbst AL, Scully RE, Robboy SJ. Problems in the examination of the DES-exposed female. Obstet Gynecol 1975;46:353. Reprinted with permission from The American College of Obstetricians and Gynecologists.

fects the developing cervical stroma, thereby preventing normal development.[52] An unusual-appearing cervix should prompt one to seek a history of DES exposure. When followed serially, some of these cervical abnormalities appear to regress, especially after a pregnancy.[52, 56]

Pregnancy outcome in females prenatally exposed to DES is worse than in controls, with an increased frequency of ectopic pregnancies, first and second trimester losses, and preterm deliveries.[71–73] This seems to be associated with upper genital tract abnormalities.[74]

Effects on fertility have been more difficult to elucidate. Reports exist on both sides of the issue and are confounded by different definitions of infertility and referral bias.[72, 75, 76] Kaufman and associates addressed the issue of whether any upper genital tract anomaly was associated with increased infertility in DES daughters.[69] Within a defined subgroup of females who had failed to conceive after 1 year of unprotected intercourse, 73% had abnormal hysterosalpingograms, which was similar to the prevalence (74%) in the group that had successfully conceived within 1 year's time. However, when specific hysterosalpingogram abnormalities were compared with infertility rates, the researchers observed that the presence of a constriction of the upper uterus was associated with a 2.3 times greater likelihood of infertility. When both a constricted upper uterus and a T-shaped cavity were present, the risk for infertility was 2.6 times higher than the general population.[69] Thus, specific uterine abnormalities are associated with infertility. This should not translate into a recommendation to perform hysterosalpingograms on all females who were exposed to DES but rather be used for counseling as part of an infertil-

ity work-up performed for the indication of infertility and not for a history of prenatal DES exposure.

Despite the heightened risk of pregnancy losses, in vitro fertilization has been used in patients exposed to DES with success rates equivalent to those for nonexposed patients.[77] The number of DES-exposed patients who have gone through in vitro fertilization is very small, however. Still, in vitro fertilization offers hope to women who may have cervical or tubal abnormalities secondary to prenatal DES exposure and ectopic pregnancies.

Autoimmune Defects

Concern over the possibility of autoimmune defects in females with in utero exposure to DES arose because of detrimental immunologic effects noted in mice following DES administration after birth. These included transient decreases in the size of the spleen and thymus and persistent impairment of lymphocytes and cell-mediated immune responses.[78] Altered T cell and natural killer cell function in DES-exposed females has been reported.[79, 80] Extrapolating from this information, others have examined the occurrence of specific autoimmune diseases in DES-exposed offspring and found it to be significantly increased, although the patient numbers are small and the confidence intervals large.[81, 82] These findings have led Ways and colleagues[80] to suggest that all DES-exposed females be screened for autoimmune disorders and, conversely, that young women with newly diagnosed autoimmune disorders be queried regarding a history of in utero DES exposure.[82]

Other Malignancies in Women Exposed to Diethylstilbestrol during Pregnancy

Breast cancer is the only malignancy to date that might be increased in mothers who were treated with DES while gravid. Although two small studies failed to show an increased risk,[83, 84] a larger study with 85,000 woman-years of follow-up demonstrated a slightly increased relative risk of 1.4 (confidence interval 1.1–1.9) in DES-exposed mothers.[85] It is prudent to warn women of this potentially increased risk and to encourage regular monthly breast self-examinations and mammographic follow-up. No recommendation can be made at this time to begin screening mammograms earlier or to perform mammograms more frequently than that already recommended (see Chapter 17).

Management of Patients with in Utero Exposure to Diethylstilbestrol

Because DES is no longer being used for pregnancy preservation, fewer females will be presenting for a first time evaluation of in utero exposure to DES. The incidence of clear cell carcinoma has decreased, but pregnancy outcome, fertility effects, and squamous dysplasia remain pertinent issues as the last females exposed are now in their midtwenties. Diethylstilbestrol still exists, however, and is used as a ''morning after'' pill to prevent implantation, a treatment for breast and prostatic carcinomas, and a growth enhancer in livestock; thus, it cannot be forgotten.

At this time, unless other specific indications for more frequent follow-up exist, patients should have annual gynecologic examinations commencing at age 14 or age of first coitus or menstruation, whichever comes first.[86] More frequent examinations should be performed when indicated. The recommended examination procedure is given in Table 10–3.

REFERENCES

1. Audet-Lapointe P, Body G, Vauclair R, et al. Vaginal intraepithelial neoplasia. Gynecol Oncol 1990;36:232.
2. Lenechan PM, Meffe F, Lickrish GM. Vaginal intraepithelial neoplasia: Aspects and management. Obstet Gynecol 1986;68:333.
3. Ireland D, Monaghan JM. The management of the patient with abnormal vaginal cytology following hysterectomy. Br J Obstet Gynecol 1988;95:973.
4. Stuart GC, Allen HH, Anderson RJ. Squamous cell carcinoma of the vagina following hysterectomy. Am J Obstet Gynecol 1981;139:311.
5. Funnell JP, Merrill JA. Recommendations following treatment of carcinoma in situ of the cervix. Surg Gynecol Obstet 1963;117:15.
6. Copenhaver EH, Salzman FA, Wright KA. Carcinoma in situ of the vagina. Am J Obstet Gynecol 1964;89:962.
7. Creasman WT, Rutledge F. Carcinoma in situ of the cervix. Obstet Gynecol 1972;39:373.
8. Rasmussen J, Diernaes E. Neoplasia in the vagina following hysterectomy for dysplasia or carcinoma in situ of the uterine cervix. Acta Obstet Gynecol Scand 1983;62:437.
9. Brinton LA, Nasca PC, Mallin K, et al. Case-control study of in situ and invasive carcinoma of the vagina. Gynecol Oncol 1990;38:49.
10. Schneider A, deVilliers EM, Schneider V. Multifocal squamous neoplasia of the female genital tract: Significance of human papillomavirus infection of the vagina after hysterectomy. Obstet Gynecol 1987;70:294.
12. Gallup DG, Morley GW. Carcinoma in situ of the vagina. Obstet Gynecol 1975;46:334.
13. Hernandez-Linares W, Puthawala TA, Nolan JF, et al. Carcinoma in situ of the vagina. Past and present management. Obstet Gynecol 1980;56:356.
14. Perez CA, Arneson AN, Galakatos A, et al. Malignant tumors of the vagina. Cancer 1973;31:36.
15. Brown GR, Fletcher GH, Rutledge FN. Irradiation of in situ and invasive squamous cell carcinoma of the vagina. Cancer 1971;28:1278.
16. Sillman FH, Sedlis A, Boyce J. A review of lower genital intraepithelial neoplasia and the use of topical 5-fluorouracil. Obstet Gynecol Surv 1985;40:190.
17. Petrilli ES, Townsend DE, Morrow CP, Nakao CY. Vaginal intraepithelial neoplasia: Biologic aspects and treatment with topical 5 FU and CO_2 laser. Am J Obstet Gynecol 1980;138:321.
18. Curtin JP, Twiggs LE, Julian TM. Treatment of vaginal intraepithelial neoplasia with the CO_2 laser. J Reprod Med 1985;30:942.
19. Townsend DE, Levine RO, Crum CP, Richart RM. Treatment of vaginal CIS with the CO_2 laser. Am J Obstet Gynecol 1982;143:565.
20. Hatch KD. Handbook of Colposcopy. Diagnosis and Treatment of Lower Genital Tract Neoplasia and HPV. Boston: Little Brown & Co, 1989, p 56.
21. Woodruff JD, Parmely TH, Julian CG. Topical 5 FU in the treatment of vaginal carcinoma in situ. Gynecol Oncol 1975;3:124.
22. Ballon SC, Roberts JA, Lagasse LD. Topical 5-fluorouracil in the treatment of intraepithelial neoplasia of the vagina. Obstet Gynecol 1979;54:163.
23. Krebs HB. Treatment of vaginal condyloma by weekly application of topical application of 5-FU. Obstet Gynecol 1987;70:68.
24. Krebs HB (ed). Genital HPV infections in men. Clin Obstet Gynecol 1989;32(1):180.
25. Wright TC, Richart RM. Role of human papillomavirus in the pathogenesis of genital tract warts and cancer (review). Gynecol Oncol 1990;37:151.
26. Villa LL, Bretani RR. Human papillomavirus update. Int J Cancer 1991;48:163.
27. Gall SA. Update on HPV infection and how to manage it. Contemp Obstet Gynecol Oct 1991;37.
28. Rome RM, Chanen W, Pagano R. The natural history of human papillomavirus atypia of the cervix. Aust N Z J Obstet Gynecol 1987;27:287.
29. Nash JD, Burke TW, Hoskins WJ. Biologic course of cervical human papillomavirus infection. Obstet Gynecol 1987;69:160.
30. Koutsky LA, Holmes KK, Critchlow CW, et al. A cohort study of the risk of cervical intraepithelial neoplasia grade

2 or 3 in relation to papillomavirus infection. N Engl J Med 1992;327:1272.

31. Carmichael JA, Maskens PD. Cervical dysplasia and human papillomavirus. Am J Obstet Gynecol 1989;160:916.

32. Ikenberg H, Runge M, Goppinger A, Pfleiderer A. Human papillomavirus DNA in invasive carcinoma of the vagina. Obstet Gynecol 1990;76:432.

33. Nuovo GJ, Blanco JS, Silverstein SJ, Crum CP. Histologic correlates of papillomavirus infection of the vagina. Obstet Gynecol 1988;72:770.

34. Centers for Disease Control. Sexually transmitted disease treatment guidelines. MMWR 1989;38:19.

35. Rosenberg SK. Sexually transmitted papillomaviral infection in men. Dermatol Clin 1991;9:317.

36. Krebs HB, Helmkamp BF. Treatment failures of genital condylomata acuminata in women: Role of the male sexual partner. Am J Obstet Gynecol 1991;165:337.

37. Ferenczy A. Comparison of 5-fluorouracil and CO_2 laser for treatment of vaginal condylomata. Obstet Gynecol 1984;64:773.

38. Reid R, Greenberg MD, Pizzuti DJ, et al. Superficial laser vulvectomy. V. Surgical debulking is enhanced by adjuvant systemic interferon. Am J Obstet Gynecol 1992;166:815.

39. Schneider A, Hotz M, Gissman L. Increased prevalence of human papillomaviruses in the lower genital tract of pregnant women. Int J Cancer 1987;40:198.

40. Bergman A, Matsunaga J, Bhatia NN. Cervical cryotherapy for condylomata acuminata during pregnancy. Obstet Gynecol 1987;69:47.

41. Smotkin D. Human papillomavirus infection of the vagina. Clin Obstet Gynecol 1993;36:188.

42. Sedlacek TV, Lindheim S, Eder C, Hasty L. Mechanism for HPV transmission at birth. Am J Obstet Gynecol 1989;161:55.

43. Smith OW, Smith LG. The influence of DES on the progress and outcome of pregnancy as based on a comparison of treated and untreated primigravidas. Am J Obstet Gynecol 1949;58:994.

44. Dieckmann WJ, Davis ME, Rynkiewicz SM, et al. Does the administration of DES during pregnancy have therapeutic value? Am J Obstet Gynecol 1953;66:1062.

45. Herbst AL, Ulfelder H, Poskanzer DC. Adenocarcinoma of the vagina: Association of maternal stilbestrol therapy with tumor appearance in young women. N Engl J Med 1971;284:878.

46. Stillman RJ. In utero exposure to DES: Adverse effects on the reproductive tract and reproductive performance in male and female offspring. Am J Obstet Gynecol 1982;142:905.

47. Adenocarcinoma registry (abstract). Am J Obstet Gynecol 1972;113:718.

48. Melnick S, Cole P, Anderson D, Herbst AL. Rates and risks of diethylstilbestrol-related clear cell adenocarcinoma of the vagina and cervix. An update. N Engl J Med 1987;316:514.

49. Herbst AL, Robboy SJ, Scully RE, Poskanzer DC. Clear cell adenocarcinoma of the vagina and cervix in girls: Analysis of 170 registry cases. Am J Obstet Gynecol 1974;119:713.

50. Herbst AL, Cole P, Colton T, et al. Age incidence and risk of diethylstilbestrol related clear cell adenocarcinoma of the vagina and cervix. Am J Obstet Gynecol 1977;128:43.

51. Herbst AL, Poskanzer DC, Robboy SJ, et al. Prenatal exposure to stilbestrol: A prospective comparison of exposed female offspring with unexposed controls. N Engl J Med 1975;292:334.

52. Jeffries JA, Robboy SJ, O'Brien PC, et al. Structural anomalies of the cervix and vagina in women enrolled in

the diethylstilbestrol adenosis (DESAD) project. Am J Obstet Gynecol 1984;148:59.

53. Herbst AL, Norusis MJ, Rosenow PJ, et al. An analysis of 346 cases of clear cell adenocarcinoma of the vagina and cervix with emphasis on recurrence and survival. Gynecol Oncol 1979;7:111.

54. Robboy SJ, Hill EC, Sandberg EC, Czernobilsky B. Vaginal adenosis in women born prior to the diethylstilbestrol era. Hum Pathol 1986;17:488.

55. Ulfelder H, Robboy SJ. The embryologic development of the human vagina. Am J Obstet Gynecol 1976;126:769.

56. Frank AR, Krumholz BA, Deutsch S. Regression of cervicovaginal abnormalities in DES-exposed women. A comparison of changes in sexually inactive women and the effects of the onset of sexual activity. J Reprod Med 1985;30:400.

57. Noller KL, Townsend DE, Kaufman RH, et al. Maturation of vaginal and cervical epithelium in women exposed in utero to diethylstilbestrol (DESAD) project. Am J Obstet Gynecol 1983;146:279.

58. Antonioli DA, Rosen S, Burke L, Donahue V. Glandular dysplasia in diethylstilbestrol-associated vaginal adenosis. A case report and review of the literature. Am J Clin Pathol 1979;71:715.

59. Robboy SJ, Kaufman RH, Prat J, et al. Pathologic findings in young women enrolled in the National Cooperative Diethylstilbestrol Adenosis (DESAD) Project. Obstet Gynecol 1979;53:309.

60. Robboy SJ, Welch WR. Microglandular hyperplasia in vaginal adenosis associated with oral contraceptives and prenatal diethylstilbestrol exposure. Obstet Gynecol 1977;49:430.

61. Robboy SJ, Keh PC, Nickerson RJ, et al. Squamous cell dysplasia and carcinoma in situ of the cervix and vagina after prenatal exposure to diethylstilbestrol. Obstet Gynecol 1978;51:528.

62. Mattingly RF, Stafl A. Cancer risks in diethylstilbestrol exposed offspring. Am J Obstet Gynecol 1976;126:543.

63. Robboy SJ, Szyfelbein WM, Goellner JR, et al. Dysplasia and cytologic findings in 4589 young women enrolled in diethylstilbestrol adenosis (DESAD) project. Am J Obstet Gynecol 1981;140:579.

64. Bibbo M, Gill WB, Azizi F, et al. Follow-up study of male and female offspring of DES exposed mothers. Obstet Gynecol 1977;49:1.

65. Ng AB, Regan JW, Nadji M, et al. Natural history of vaginal adenosis in women exposed to diethylstilbestrol in utero. J Reprod Med 1977;18:1.

66. Hart WR, Townsend DE, Aldrich JO, et al. Histopathologic spectrum of vaginal adenosis and related changes in stilbestrol-exposed females. Cancer 1976;37:763.

67. Robboy SJ, Noller KL, O'Brien P, et al. Increased incidence of cervical and vaginal dysplasia in 3980 diethylstilbestrol-exposed young women. Experience of the national collaborative diethylstilbestrol adenosis project. JAMA 1984;252:2979.

68. Bornstein J, Kaufman RH, Adam E, Adler-Storthz K. Human papillomavirus associated with vaginal intraepithelial neoplasia in women exposed to diethylstilbestrol in utero. Obstet Gynecol 1987;70:75.

69. Kaufman RH, Adam E, Noller K, et al. Upper genital tract changes and infertility in diethylstilbestrol-exposed women. Am J Obstet Gynecol 1986;154:1312.

70. Kaufman RH, Binder GL, Gray PM Jr, et al. Upper genital tract changes associated with exposure in utero to DES. Am J Obstet Gynecol 1977;128:51.

71. Herbst AL. Clear cell adenocarcinoma and the current status of DES-exposed females. Cancer 1981;48:484.

72. Herbst AL, Hubby MM, Blough RR, Azizi F. A compari-

son of pregnancy experience in DES-exposed and DES-unexposed daughters. J Reprod Med 1980;24:62.

73. Cousins L, Karp W, Lacey C, Lucas WE. Reproductive outcome of women exposed to diethylstilbestrol in utero. Obstet Gynecol 1980;56:70.

74. Kaufman RH, Noller K, Adam E, et al. Upper genital tract abnormalities and pregnancy outcome in diethylstilbestrol-exposed progeny. Am J Obstet Gynecol 1984;148:973.

75. Barnes AB, Colton T, Gundersen J, et al. Fertility and outcome of pregnancy in women exposed in utero to diethylstilbestrol. N Engl J Med 1980;302:609.

76. Menczer J, Dulitzky M, Ben-Baruch G, Modan M. Primary infertility in women exposed to diethylstilbestrol in utero. Br J Obstet Gynecol 1986;93:503.

77. Muasher SJ, Garcia JE, Jones HW. Experience with diethylstilbestrol-exposed infertile women in a program of in vitro fertilization. Fertil Steril 1984;42:20.

78. Blair PB. Immunologic consequences of early exposure of experimental rodents to diethylstilbestrol and steroid hormones. In: Herbst AL, Bevin HA (eds). Developmental Effects of DES in Pregnancy. New York: Thieme-Stratton, 1981, p 193.

79. Ford CD, Johnson GH, Smith WG. NK cells in in utero DES-exposed patients. Gynecol Oncol 1983;16:400.

80. Ways SC, Mortola JF, Zvaifler NJ, et al. Alterations in immune responsiveness in women exposed to DES in utero. Fertil Steril 1987;48:193.

81. Noller KL, Blair PB, O'Brien PC, et al. Increased occurrence of autoimmune disease among women exposed in utero to diethylstilbestrol. Fertil Steril 1988;49:1080.

82. Turiel J, Wingard DL. Immune response in DES-exposed women (letter). Fertil Steril 1988;49:928.

83. Vessey MP, Fairweather DVI, Norman-Smith B, Buckley J. A randomized double-blind controlled trial of the value of stilbestrol therapy in pregnancy: Long-term follow up of mothers and their offspring. Br J Obstet Gynecol 1983;90:1007.

84. Brian DD, Tilley BC, Labarthe DR, et al. Breast cancer in DES-exposed mothers: Absence of association. Mayo Clin Proc 1980;55:89.

85. Greenberg ER, Barnes AB, Resseguie L, et al. Breast cancer in mothers given diethylstilbestrol in pregnancy. N Engl J Med 1984;311:1393.

86. Herbst AL, Scully RE, Robboy SJ. Problems in the examination of the DES-exposed female. Obstet Gynecol 1975;46:353.

Cervical Intraepithelial Neoplasia and Cervical Cancer

Lisa Anderson

Squamous cell carcinoma of the cervix is the second most common cancer in women worldwide and is a leading cause of death among young women in Third World countries.[1] Cervical cancer is a preventable disease. Its preinvasive phase progresses slowly, and the treatment for early stage disease is extremely effective. The Papanicolaou (PAP) test for cervical cancer screening is simple and easily performed. The effectiveness of cervical cancer screening is evident in the dramatic decline in the incidence and mortality from cervical cancer in the United States over the past 35 years. Although surveys for cervical cancer in Great Britain[2–4] and New Zealand[5] have shown recent increases in the incidence and mortality among young women, data from the Surveillance, Epidemiology and End Results Program reveal no increase of cervical cancer in the United States.[6] These trends have remained fairly stable except for the impressive increase in preinvasive disease. This reflects, in part, the increased detection of precursor lesions and significant increases in the prevalence of known and putative risk factors.

EPIDEMIOLOGY OF CERVICAL CANCER

Sexual Behavior

Sexual behavior has the strongest association with the subsequent development of cervical intraepithelial neoplasia (CIN) and invasive cervical carcinoma. This includes earlier age at first intercourse, multiple sexual partners, and a male partner who has had multiple sexual partners (Table 11–1). The significance of a woman's early age of first intercourse relates to the adolescent cervix, which undergoes a process of squamous metaplasia involving the transformation of endocervical columnar epithelium to squamous epithelium. It is hypothesized that this active metaplasia renders the adolescent cervix more susceptible to the incorporation of potential carcinogens.[7, 8] Early age of first intercourse also implies a longer lifetime exposure to carcinogens and infectious agents.[9]

The risk of cervical cancer is strongly influenced by the number of male sexual partners and by a promiscuous male partner. Women who have had more than one sexual partner have a two- to threefold increased risk of developing cervical cancer compared with monogamous women.[10] This finding has been interpreted as evidence for the important role of a sexually transmitted agent. However, sexually monogamous women may be at risk for cervical cancer depending on the sexual history of their male partner. The most direct evidence for a male factor derives from several studies in which the sexual histories of husbands of cervical cancer patients were compared with the sexual histories of control husbands.[11–13] In all these studies, case husbands reported significantly more female sexual partners and a higher incidence of venereal disease than the control husbands. The incidence of cervical cancer in the

TABLE 11–1. Risk Factors for Cervical Cancer

1. Early age coitus
2. Multiple sex partners
3. High-risk male partner
4. Cigarette smoking
5. Immunosuppression
6. History of genital human papillomavirus infection
7. History of cervical intraepithelial neoplasia

second wives of husbands whose first wives had cervical cancer is also 3.5 times higher than that in a control population.[14] In addition, there is an association between cervical cancer and penile cancer in the male sexual partner, with a significantly higher incidence of cervical cancer in the wives of men with penile cancer.[14, 15]

Human Papillomavirus

Human papillomavirus infection (HPV) may represent the most common sexually transmitted disease in the United States. It is a highly infectious disease, transmitted by genital contact, with approximately 60% of sexual partners of persons with condylomata acuminata developing the infection.[16]

The incubation period can be from 3 weeks to 9 months before a lesion becomes clinically apparent.[17] Distribution of the virus is fairly ubiquitous, often involving the entire lower genital tract. Characteristically, some of these lesions regress spontaneously; others persist or may progress to invasive cervical cancer. Prolonged latency phases of up to 20 years before the onset of clinical disease have been recorded. This may be a function of immune status changes related to age.

Current epidemiologic and molecular-biologic data support the belief that genital HPV infection plays an important, if not causal, role in the etiology of CIN and cervical cancer. There is compelling evidence in support of this hypothesis. The epidemiology of HPV infection in women closely parallels that of CIN and cervical cancer, each sharing similar risk factors such as early age of first intercourse and increased number of sexual partners, cigarette smoking, and immunosuppression. Evidence linking HPV infection with cervical cancer was based on the recognition that certain cytologic features on PAP smears suggesting dysplasia were actually manifestations of HPV infection.[18] These infected cells were called koilocytes because of their perinuclear cytoplasmic clearing or ''halos'' and nuclear atypia.[19] The term koilocytosis is now considered pathognomonic of HPV's cytopathic effect on superficial cervical squamous epithelium. The direct relationship between HPV and cervical neoplasia is further substantiated by the detection of HPV in 80 to 90% of cervical intraepithelial neoplasias and cervical cancers.[20] At the molecular level, HPV has been shown to be capable of in vitro malignant human cell transformation.[21, 22] Clinical evidence from one prospective study showed that women with normal cytologic findings who are HPV positive have a significantly higher rate of development of CIN than HPV-negative women with normal cytologic findings.[23]

The actual prevalence of genital HPV is unknown because only clinically evident disease is reported and the majority of HPV infection remains subclinical or latent. More important, population studies using the newly applied polymerase chain reaction estimate that as many as 40 to 70% of sexually active, ''disease-free'' women with normal PAP smear, normal colposcopy, and normal cervical biopsy results are infected with HPV.[24, 25] Infection with HPV alone does not translate into cervical cancer because only about 5% of sexually active women develop HPV-associated lesions. Because of this discrepancy, progression from latent HPV infection to CIN appears to depend on the cumulative effect of other cofactors, such as smoking, immune status, or the presence of other sexually transmitted diseases that may be involved in the initiation and promotion of cervical cancer.

Currently more than 60 different subtypes of HPV have been identified. Much research has been directed toward analyzing the prevalence and distribution of genital HPV subtypes and their relationship to the natural history of CIN. Human papillomaviruses 6 and 11 have been associated with benign condylomata and low-grade cervical intraepithelial lesions (CIN 1). These viruses have been considered low risk because they are rarely associated with invasive carcinomas. Human papillomaviruses 16, 18, and 33 appear to be the most oncogenic and have been associated with high-grade lesions and invasive cervical cancer.

For HPV typing to be clinically useful it must serve a defined role in clinical management. Proponents of HPV typing see it as a useful adjunct to the standard approach of PAP screening and colposcopy. Women with latent HPV infection or low-grade lesions associated with high-risk HPV types could be identified. However, the natural history of low-risk and high-risk HPV types remains unknown and unpredictable. The data regarding the appropriate evaluation, treatment, and follow-up of women infected with latent genital HPV are insufficient. Currently, there is no effective therapy to eliminate the virus. Symptomatic lesions are treated by local therapy, and HPV-related CINs are managed according to the grade of dysplasia. The standard treatment of women with CIN and cervical cancer is based on histopathologic diagnosis regardless of HPV subtype.

Immunosuppression and the Human Immunodeficiency Virus

Immunologic status plays an important role in the clinical expression of genital HPV infection and CIN. Increased prevalences of HPV and CIN have been associated with the mild immunodeficiency state of pregnancy[26] and with medically immunosuppressed renal transplant patients.[27] Human papillomavirus and human immunodeficiency virus (HIV) have been clearly associated with cervical cancer. They are sexually transmitted diseases and share common behavioral risk factors. Studies have shown that HIV-seropositive women have increased rates of genital HPV infection and CIN.[28–30] In one study, 70% of symptomatic HIV-positive women had genital HPV infection, and more than 50% of these had abnormal results on PAP tests.[30] Cervical intraepithelial neoplasia and cervical cancer appear to have a more aggressive course in HIV-positive women than in uninfected women.

In women who are HIV positive, recurrence rates for CIN after standard therapy are significantly higher than those in controls and are related to the degree of immunosuppression.[31] Compared with uninfected women, HIV-positive women with cervical cancer had an overall poorer prognosis, with higher recurrence and death rates.[32] The increased deaths were caused by the cervical cancer and not by the opportunistic infection due to acquired immunodeficiency syndrome (AIDS). Infection with HIV appears to impair local cervical immunity, increasing the likelihood of oncogenic progression of HPV-related lesions.[33] Human papillomavirus may assume an important role in the sexual transmission of HIV infection either by disruption of normal mucosal integrity or by diminution of local immune surveillance.[30] As of January 1, 1993, the Centers for Disease Control and Prevention included invasive cervical cancer as one of four neoplastic and 23 AIDS-defining illnesses: A woman with cervical cancer who is HIV positive has AIDS.

Cigarette Smoking

Winkelstein in 1977 was the first to observe the association between cervical cancer and cigarette smoking.[34] Numerous reports have confirmed the increased risk of invasive cervical cancer and CIN in women who smoke. Exposure to passive smoke seems to have the same impact as active smoking.[35] Women who smoke are about twice as likely to develop cervical cancer even after controlling for the number of sexual partners. The risk correlates with the number of cigarettes smoked daily, the number of pack years, the age of onset of smoking, and the use of nonfiltered cigarettes.[35–37] Nicotine is known to be secreted in the cervical mucus,[38] and although it is not itself a carcinogen, its metabolic intermediates, the nitrosamines, are proven carcinogens. Women who smoke shed higher levels of mutagens in their cervical mucus, suggesting a direct carcinogenic effect.[39] Cigarette smoking has been shown to depress local immune defenses in the cervical epithelium, with an observed reversal of the T4 to T8 ratio and a diminution of Langerhans' cells, which are responsible for cell-mediated immunity.[40] Also, cervical HPV infection and CIN have been associated with a local reduction in the number of Langerhans' cells and decreased T-cell counts.[41] Cigarette smoking and cervical HPV infection appear to be cofactors in the etiology of cervical neoplasia.[42]

SCREENING

Since Papanicolaou's introduction of cervical cytology in 1945, there has been a 70% reduction in deaths due to cervical cancer in the United States. In 1992 approximately 55,000 cases of carcinoma in situ (CIS) of the cervix and 13,500 new cases of cervical cancer were diagnosed and 4400 deaths occurred due to cervical cancer.[43] It has been estimated that approximately 50% of women diagnosed with cervical cancer have never had a PAP smear.[44] However, one third of invasive cancers occurred in women who had recent negative smears.[45]

Cervical cytology screening in theory should eliminate cervical cancer, but technical limitations and nonmedical or social variables affect access to and acceptance of preventive health care. The eradication of cervical cancer has many confounding factors related to failures inherent in PAP smear screening (Table 11–2).

There have been numerous debates regarding the optimal guidelines for effective cervical screening. In 1988, the American College of Obstetricians and Gynecologists, the American Can-

---

TABLE 11–2. Failures in Papanicolaou Smear Screening

1. Access to health care
2. High false negative rate (20–30%)
3. Lack of appropriate action regarding abnormal smears
4. Inability to detect aggressive precursor lesions
5. Laboratory and sampling errors

cer Society, and the National Cancer Institutes endorsed the following recommendations regarding the frequency of cervical screening: "All females who are or who have been sexually active or who have reached age 18 should undergo an annual PAP test and pelvic examination. After she has had three or more consecutive, satisfactory annual examinations with normal findings, the PAP test may be performed less frequently at the discretion of the physician."

The risk factors for cervical cancer are well established. An early age at first intercourse, a history of multiple sexual partners, and a prior history of abnormal cervical cytologic findings should influence the frequency of subsequent screening. It has been shown that after evaluating factors involved in classifying a woman as high risk, most sexually active women fall into that category.[46] For this reason (in most clinical settings) yearly screening is recommended for all women and should be lifelong. The rationale for indefinite lifelong screening is based on the documentation of preinvasive disease and cancer from vaginal vault cytologic findings in women who have had hysterectomies. There is a pervasive belief that older women or women who have had a hysterectomy no longer require PAP screening. Surveys have shown that the utilization of PAP screening decreases with increasing age. However, approximately 20% of cervical cancer patients are elderly, and these women often present with advanced disease. Two separate long-term studies evaluating vaginal cytologic findings in women following hysterectomy for cervical dysplasia reported a 2.5% and a 4% incidence of abnormal vaginal cytology.[47, 48] Both investigators concluded that continued screening is important to identify abnormal cytologic findings particularly in the first 2 years following a hysterectomy. Further support for lifelong screening comes from a report that demonstrated a 4.1% incidence of HPV DNA detected on routine cervical smears in women older than 65.[49]

Cervical Cytology: The Bethesda System

Until recently, there has been much variation and lack of standardization in the reporting of cervical cytologic findings. Cytologic descriptions of "squamous atypia with koilocytosis" or "HPV effect" have presented a management dilemma for the clinician. The Bethesda System resulted from a 1988 workshop of pathologists and clinicians that was sponsored by the National Cancer Institute (Table 11–3). The system was further revised

in 1991. It reflects currently held views of the biologic behavior of preinvasive lesions and HPV infection and links cytologic findings with current guidelines for clinical management.[50] The Bethesda System offers a new terminology for reporting cervicovaginal cytology and replaces the original Papanicolaou and the more recent CIN classification (Fig. 11–1).

The Bethesda System consists of three elements: a statement of specimen adequacy, a general categorization (normal or abnormal), and a descriptive diagnosis regarding abnormal cytologic results. In the category of epithelial cell abnormalities, the term squamous atypia is now reserved for smears with abnormal cytologic features for which the cytopathologist is unable to render a definitive judgment. Squamous atypia excludes the diagnosis of low-grade squamous intraepithelial lesions, reactive, inflammatory, and HPV changes. The diagnosis of squamous cell atypia is further qualified as to whether a reactive or a premalignant or malignant process is favored.

The approach to patients with atypical cytologic findings is not a matter of general agreement. However, the practice of simply repeating the PAP smear is discouraged. The rate of having an underlying dysplasia is substantial (20–30%) in some studies, and there is a 20% false negative rate in PAP smear screening.[51–53] Further evaluation and therapy for patients in this category should be based on the colposcopic findings.

The term squamous intraepithelial lesion (SIL) now replaces CIN, although the latter term still exists in the histopathologic terminology. Squamous cell intraepithelial abnormalities are currently subclassified into two categories: low-grade and high-grade intraepithelial lesions. This subclassification is based on the different morphologic and molecular features and HPV type distribution that distinguish moderate (CIN 2) and severe dysplasias (CIN 3) from mild dysplasia (CIN 1). Low-grade SILs include cytologic features consistent with koilocytosis or HPV changes and mild dysplasia (CIN 1). The rationale for including HPV changes in the same category as low-grade SILs is supported by the following: (1) the cytologic differences between the two are very subjective, (2) their natural history and behavior are unpredictable, and (3) the majority of these lesions tend to regress or persist but usually do not progress to high-grade lesions.

High-grade SILs include lesions that correspond to moderate (CIN 2) and severe dysplasia (CIN 3) or CIS. The elimination of an intermediate grade is based on the similar biologic behavior, greater oncogenic potential, and lack of reproducible consistency in distinguishing between moderate (CIN

TABLE 11–3. The 1991 Bethesda System

ADEQUACY OF THE SPECIMEN
Satisfactory for evaluation
Satisfactory for evaluation but limited by (specify
  reason)
Unsatisfactory for evaluation (specify reason)
GENERAL CATEGORIZATION (OPTIONAL)
Within normal limits
Benign cellular changes: See descriptive diagnosis
Epithelial cell abnormality: See descriptive diagnosis
DESCRIPTIVE DIAGNOSES
Benign Cellular Changes
Infection
Trichomonas vaginalis
Fungal organisms morphologically consistent with
  Candida spp
Predominance of coccobacilli consistent with shift in
  vaginal flora
Bacteria morphologically consistent with *Actinomyces*
  spp
Cellular changes associated with herpes simplex virus
Other
Reactive Changes
Reactive cellular changes associated with:
  Inflammation (includes typical repair)
  Atrophy with inflammation (''atrophic vaginitis'')
  Radiation
  Contraceptive intrauterine device (IUD)
  Other

EPITHELIAL CELL ABNORMALITIES
Squamous Cell
Atypical squamous cells of undetermined significance
  (qualify)*
Low-grade squamous intraepithelial lesion
  encompassing: HPV†, mild dysplasia/CIN 1
High-grade squamous intraepithelial lesion
  encompassing: Moderate and severe dysplasia, CIS/
  CIN 2, and CIN 3
Squamous cell carcinoma
Glandular Cell
Endometrial cells, cytologically benign, in a
  postmenopausal woman
Atypical glandular cells of undetermined significance
  (qualify)*
Endocervical adenocarcinoma
Endometrial adenocarcinoma
Extrauterine adenocarcinoma
Adenocarcinoma, NOS
Other Malignant Neoplasms (specify)
**Hormonal Evaluation (applies to vaginal smears
  only)**
Hormonal pattern compatible with age and history
Hormonal pattern incompatible with age and history
  (specify)
Hormonal evaluation not possible due to (specify)

CIN, Cervical intraepithelial neoplasia; CIS, carcinoma in situ; NOS, not otherwise specified.
  *Atypical squamous or glandular cells of undetermined significance should be further qualified as to whether *a reactive or a premalignant-malignant
process is favored.*
  †Cellular changes of human papillomavirus (HPV)—previously termed koilocytosis, koilocytotic atypia, or condylomatous atypia—are included in
the category of low-grade squamous intraepithelial lesion.

Descriptive Convention							
Class System	Class I (Normal)	Class II Inflammation	Class III Mild Dysplasia or Moderate Dysplasia		Class IV Severe Dysplasia CIS	Class V Suggestive of Cancer	
CIN System	Normal	Inflammatory	CIN I *or*	CIN II	CIN III	Suggestive of Cancer	
Bethesda System	Within Normal Limits	Inflammatory a) Without atypia / b) With atypia	Low Grade SIL		High Grade SIL	Squamous Cell Cancer	

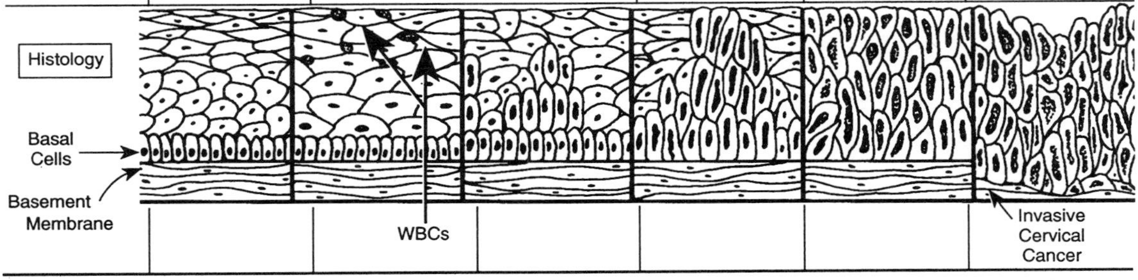

Histology
Basal Cells
Basement Membrane
WBCs
Invasive Cervical Cancer

Figure 11–1. Comparisons of Papanicolaou smear descriptive conventions. CIN, Cervical intraepithelial neoplasia; SIL, squamous intraepithelial lesion. (From Beckmann CRB, Ling FW, Barzansky BM, et al. Cervical neoplasia and carcinoma. In: Beckmann CRB, Ling FW (eds). Obstetrics and Gynecology for Medical Students. Baltimore: Williams & Wilkins, 1992, p 386.)

2) and severe dysplasia (CIN 3). Prognostically, the majority of these lesions tend to persist or to progress and require treatment, whereas low-grade lesions may be treated or followed conservatively. All women with the cytologic diagnosis of SIL require colposcopy and appropriate colposcopically directed biopsies for a histopathologic diagnosis (Fig. 11–2).

THE CLINICAL MANAGEMENT OF CERVICAL DYSPLASIA

Natural History

It is generally accepted that cervical dysplasia progresses from mild to severe dysplasia to invasive cancer. Reports differ regarding the time frame for a preinvasive lesion to become invasive. Peterson followed 127 women with untreated CIS for 9 years and found that one third of these cases progressed to invasive cancer.[54] Masterson found that 28% of 25 untreated cases of CIS progressed to invasive cancer in 5 years.[55]

Nasiell and co-workers followed 410 women with cytologic evidence of moderate dysplasia (CIN 2) and reported a regression rate of 50% over an average of a 50-month follow-up period.[56] These same researchers in a more recent study observed a 62% regression and a 16% progression to CIS or invasive cancer in women with mild dysplasia.[57] However, Campion and associates present different results.[58] In 100 women with mild dysplasia, they found a regression rate of only 11% with progression to CIS in 26% and persistence in 64%. Mitchell and associates followed 846 women with cytologic evidence of HPV infection alone. Carcinoma in situ developed in 30 women

(3.5%) over a 6-year period.[59] Koutsky and colleagues studied the temporal relationship between HPV infection and the development of CIN in women with negative cervical cytologic findings.[23] Twenty-eight percent of the women followed developed CIN 2 and CIN 3 lesions within 24 months after the first positive test result for HPV.

Problems in these studies include the varying length of follow-up, the individual criteria used in determining the grade of lesions, and the actual effect of cervical biopsies on the natural history of the lesion. In most clinical settings, the management of moderate to severe dyplasias (CIN 2–3) is straightforward, and these women are treated by an excisional or a destructive method. The management of women with mild dyplasia (CIN 1) is more variable. If a patient is reliable, she may be followed conservatively with cytology and colposcopy until the lesion either disappears or progresses and thus requires definitive treatment. Because there is no method of predicting which lesions will regress or progress to become a more serious lesion, treatment of mild dysplasia can also be done by an excisional or a destructive method. Treatment of HPV alone is not recommended because it is impossible to eradicate the virus.

Anatomy

The anatomic junction where the mucus-secreting columnar cells of the endocervical canal meet the squamous cells of the ectocervix is called the squamocolumnar junction. The site of this junction is influenced by several factors. Beginning at menarche, a change in the hormonal milieu and a shift to an acidic vaginal pH cause the junction to shift toward the endocervix. The endocervical columnar

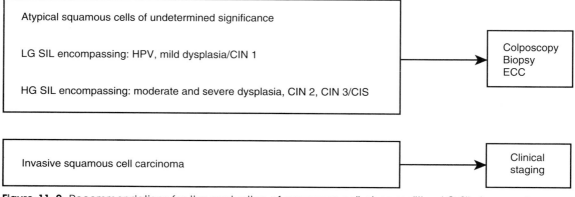

Figure 11–2. Recommendations for the evaluation of squamous cell abnormalities. LG SIL, Low-grade squamous intraepithelial lesion; HPV, human papillomavirus; CIN, cervical intraepithelial neoplasia; HG SIL, high-grade squamous intraepithelial lesion; CIS, carcinoma in situ; ECC, endocervical curettage.

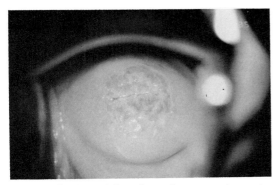

Figure 11–3. Normal transformation zone (see also color section).

cells undergo a process of metaplasia with their transformation into squamous cells. This area appears as a circular zone around the external os and is called the transformation zone (Fig. 11–3). The location of the transformation zone is influenced by age, parity, estrogen support, and a history of previous cervical procedures. Because of the ongoing process of squamous metaplasia, the majority of preinvasive lesions and cervical cancers originate in the transformation zone.

Colposcopy

Most cervical dysplasias and early invasive cervical cancers are subclinical and asymptomatic. The PAP smear detects asymptomatic disease and identifies the woman who needs colposcopic evaluation and possible treatment. Colposcopy and directed biopsies provide a histopathologic diagnosis on which definitive treatment is based.

The colposcope is a binocular microscope capable of magnifying the surface contour of the cervix. The fundamental principle of colposcopy is based on satisfactory visualization of the transformation zone. A 3% acetic acid solution is applied to the cervix. Metaplastic and dysplastic epithelia become opacified, thus enabling the colposcopist to evaluate any abnormal lesions. Suspicious aceto-white lesions include abnormal vascular patterns (mosaicism, punctation), atypical vessels, and condylomata (Fig. 11–4). A skilled colposcopist can identify the most abnormal-appearing lesion on which to perform a biopsy. Colposcopy eliminates the previous practice of performing multiple random cervical biopsies and the historical use of diagnostic cone biopsies in the evaluation of abnormal cervical cytologic findings.

An algorithm representing the appropriate triage of an abnormal PAP smear is shown in Figure 11–

5. Colposcopy is considered either satisfactory or unsatisfactory depending on whether the transformation zone is fully visualized. This zone usually can be visualized in women throughout their reproductive years but may be located higher in the endocervical canal in postmenopausal women or in women who have undergone prior treatment for CIN. If the entire lesion cannot be visualized fully or if colposcopy is unsatisfactory, a diagnostic cone biopsy is required. At the time of colposcopically directed biopsies, it is also recommended that all women undergo an endocervical curettage. This step decreases the chance of missing an occult lesion in the nonvisualized endocervical canal. Before definitive treatment, other sources of abnormal cervical cytologic findings must be excluded. Lesions in the adjacent vaginal fornices can inadvertently contaminate cervical cytologic results.

Evaluation of the pregnant woman with abnormal cervical cytologic findings follows the previously mentioned algorithm except that routine sampling of the endocervical canal is contraindicated and colposcopically directed biopsies are performed only on lesions that are highly suggestive of malignancy. The pregnant woman is followed antenatally approximately every 2 to 3 months with repeat PAP smears and colposcopy to assess for progression. Definitive therapy is delayed until 2 to 3 months after childbirth. If cancer is suspected during pregnancy, a colposcopically directed biopsy should be done, and if necessary a diagnostic conization or colposcopically guided wedge biopsy may be required. This is done to avoid any delay in treatment should an invasive cancer be present. Because colposcopy is technically more difficult in the pregnant patient and management relies on the colposcopic assessment, this procedure should be performed by an experienced colposcopist.

It is usually unnecessary to perform a sampling of the endometrial cavity at the time of colposcopy

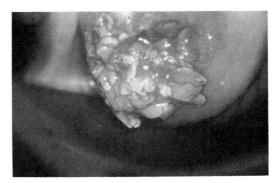

Figure 11–4. Condyloma of the cervix (see also color section).

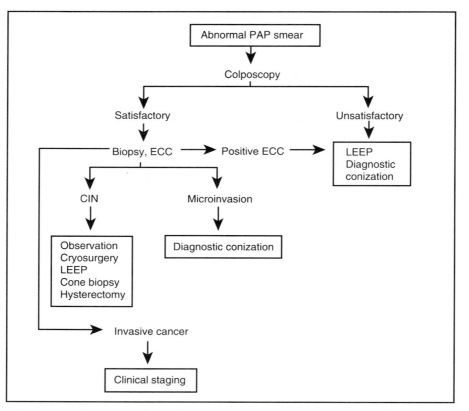

Figure 11–5. Management of the patient with an abnormal Papanicolaou smear. ECC, Endocervical curettage; CIN, cervical intraepithelial neoplasia; LEEP, loop electroexcision procedure.

because CIN is not a precursor lesion or a risk factor for endometrial carcinoma. However, the presence on a PAP smear of either cytologically abnormal or, in the latter half of the cycle, normal endometrial cells or endometrial cells in the postmenopausal woman should alert the clinician to the possibility of endometrial pathology. Approximately 25 to 40% of women who have cytologically abnormal endometrial cells on routine cytologic findings have endometrial carcinoma.[60] Further diagnostic evaluation should be performed by an endometrial biopsy or a fractional dilation and curettage.

Concepts in the Treatment of Cervical Intraepithelial Neoplasia

The choice of treatment for CIN is influenced by several factors, including the patient's desire for future fertility, preference for and likelihood of following a treatment regimen, pregnancy, and co-existing gynecologic and medical conditions. Various methods are available for the treatment of CIN. The pretreatment evaluation should include cytologic and histopathologic correlation and colposcopic documentation of the extent and location of the lesion.

Standard treatments for CIN include cryosurgery, laser surgery, loop electroexcision procedure (LEEP), conization, and, in limited cases, hysterectomy. Regardless of the method selected, the aim of therapy is the complete destruction or excision of the transformation zone. Treatment is directed at the lesion topography, which is more significant than the histologic grade. The reported success rates for all these methods are in the range of 85 to 95%.

Specific Treatments

Destructive Methods

Cryosurgery and laser vaporization physically destroy the transformation zone without providing a surgical specimen for histopathologic confirmation. For this reason strict pretreatment criteria, as shown in Table 11–4, must be fulfilled before choosing a destructive method.

TABLE 11–4. Criteria for Choosing Destructive Therapy (Cryosurgery, Laser Therapy)

1. The entire transformation zone must be fully visualized.
2. The lesion must be seen in its entirety without extension into the endocervical canal.
3. The endocervical curettings must be negative for dysplasia or cancer.
4. There must be agreement among the results of cytology, colposcopy, and colposcopically directed biopsies.
5. There is no microinvasion on biopsy samples.

CRYOSURGERY. Cryosurgery is the most cost-effective method available for the treatment of CIN. It is ideal for the outpatient setting as it is easily performed and requires no anesthesia. The technique employs application of a cryoprobe to the entire transformation zone, which freezes the tissue to approximately −60°C. This results in the formation of intracellular ice crystals, thermal shock, and local cryonecrosis with a subsequent sloughing of the necrotic tissue. Standard therapy is done by two 3-minute freezes with an interim partial thaw of 5 minutes.

Cryosurgery when coupled with colposcopy is extremely effective in treating CIN. In a long-term follow-up study of 96 women with CIN 2 or 3 lesions treated by cryosurgery, the overall cure rate was 92%.[61] Cumulative series by various researchers show equivalent results,[61–63] but some series reveal lower success rates.[64–65] Most treatment failures involve inappropriate technique and patient selection. The disadvantage of cryosurgery is its lack of precision compared with that of laser vaporization, which controls for the depth and width of tissue destruction. Failure with cryosurgery seems to be related to lesion size rather than to its histologic grade; patients with large lesions have a higher failure rate.[66–68]

Complications from cryotherapy are rare. Women can expect to have a watery foul-smelling vaginal discharge that lasts approximately 1 month. Healing occurs in 4 to 8 weeks. Infection occurs in less than 5% of cases.[67, 69] There seems to be little effect on subsequent fertility or labor. A disadvantage of cryotherapy is the more frequent retraction of the new squamocolumnar junction into the endocervical canal. Jobson and Homesley reported that the transformation zone was completely visualized in 86% of patients treated by laser vaporization compared with 52% treated by cryotherapy.[70] The advantage of a fully visualized new transformation zone is that it allows for adequate colposcopic evaluation should abnormal cytologic findings recur.

CARBON DIOXIDE LASER VAPORIZATION. Laser is an acronym for "light amplification by stimulated emission of radiation." The most efficient of the lasers used in gynecology is the carbon dioxide laser. When used for the treatment of CIN, the laser is coupled with a colposcope, and the laser beam is directed onto the cervix by the use of a hand-held micromanipulator.

Because laser vaporization is considered a destructive method, patient selection criteria are the same as for cryotherapy. Successful employment of the laser involves vaporization of the entire transformation zone to a depth of 7 mm. The light energy of the laser beam is converted to heat, which instantly vaporizes intra- and extracellular water. Because the tissue is destroyed by vaporization, the base of the crater is clean. Minimal necrotic tissue remains, and rapid epithelial regeneration occurs within 4 weeks.

Laser therapy offers several advantages over cryotherapy. It provides greater surgical precision in destroying the lesion to a desired depth. Adequate visualization of the transformation zone is more common following laser vaporization. The laser beam can also be used to perform an excisional cone biopsy when criteria for a destructive method are not met. Disadvantages of laser vaporization include the initial high investment cost, the need for greater surgical expertise, the longer operative time, and the greater patient pain, requiring either local or general anesthesia.

Diagnostic and Excisional Procedures

In specific clinical circumstances (Table 11–5), invasive cervical cancer cannot be ruled out by either colposcopy or directed biopsies. In these cases a combined diagnostic and, it is hoped, therapeutic procedure must be performed to provide a surgical specimen for definitive histopathologic diagnosis.

LOOP ELECTROEXCISION PROCEDURE. The LEEP has gained wide popularity in the treatment of CIN. The LEEP (Fig. 11–6) is

TABLE 11–5. Indications for an Excisional Biopsy

1. Inability to visualize the transformation zone
2. Inability to visualize the full extent of a lesion
3. Positive endocervical curettings
4. Microinvasion on colposcopically directed biopsy
5. Cytologic suspicion of adenocarcinoma in situ
6. Discrepancy between the results of cytology (2 grades) and histology tests
7. Colposcopic suspicion of an invasive lesion

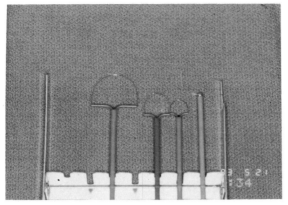

Figure 11–6. Instruments used to perform the loop electroexcision procedure (LEEP) (see also color section).

performed using a hand-held electrical surgical device that employs a fine wire loop (electrode) that delivers a high-frequency, low-voltage current that excises and coagulates tissue as it passes through it. This greatly diminishes the bleeding encountered during the excision and protects the specimen from unnecessary thermocoagulative damage. The wire loops are available in various sizes and provide the desired width and depth of excision.

The LEEP provides several advantages over other methods employed in the treatment of CIN. Like cryotherapy, the LEEP is an easily learned, relatively inexpensive and cost-effective outpatient technique. Effects on cervical healing are similar to those of laser vaporization. In a randomized study comparing the effects on women of the LEEP and laser vaporization, women who had a LEEP experienced less discomfort, a shorter operative time, and decreased postoperative hemorrhage.[71]

Unlike laser vaporization or cryotherapy, which are destructive techniques, the LEEP method provides a surgical specimen. This allows significant lesions not suspected on colposcopy or cervical biopsy to be detected. Two separate reports have documented an unsuspected 3% incidence of either microinvasive or invasive cancer found in LEEP specimens that would have been missed if a destructive method had been used.[72, 73] Cumulative large series on women undergoing LEEP therapy for CIN report excellent cure rates in the range of 95%. Some providers advocate performing colposcopy and LEEP at the same time, citing increased patient convenience and compliance; however, performing a LEEP before histopathologic diagnosis by biopsy would overtreat a significant proportion of patients and is therefore not recommended.

CONE BIOPSY. Cone biopsy describes the procedure of excising the transformation zone and producing a specimen suitable for histologic examination.[74] Technically, the excision may be performed using the scalpel as in the traditional cone biopsy, by a laser excisional cone biopsy, or more recently by the LEEP. The advantage of a cone biopsy is that it provides a specimen for definitive histopathologic diagnosis and in most cases is also therapeutic. Indications for performing a cone biopsy (excisional method) are listed in Table 11–5.

The traditional cold knife cone biopsy has several disadvantages. It is a surgical procedure requiring general or regional anesthesia and is not suitable for the office or clinic setting. Complications include hemorrhage, sepsis, cervical stenosis, infertility, and cervical incompetence, which occur in about 2 to 12% of patients depending on the depth and geometry of the excised specimen.[75–77] The traditional cone biopsy has been largely replaced by the LEEP. The latter method is quick to perform, is suitable for the office setting, and offers equivalent cure rates.

In certain clinical situations, the traditional cone biopsy remains a useful tool. In a postmenopausal woman or in a patient who has already undergone several cervical procedures, the cervix may be flush with the vaginal fornices. The scalpel provides greater technical control in preventing inadvertent entry into the bladder or bowel. The traditional cone biopsy is an extremely effective therapeutic method for the treatment of CIN, with cure rates in the range of 95%. Cumulative series report an overall recurrence rate of 30% if the margins of resection on the cone specimen are involved with dysplasia.[78–80]

HYSTERECTOMY. Hysterectomy, whether abdominal or vaginal, is the most radical method of treatment for CIN. The comparatively higher cost, the related surgical morbidity, the loss of reproductive function, and the potential for disease recurrence involving the vaginal cuff limit its indications for the treatment of CIN.

Hysterectomy is acceptable in the following instances, presuming the standard pretreatment evaluation, which includes adequate colposcopy and directed biopsies to rule out an invasive process, has been performed: (1) coexisting benign gynecologic conditions that require a hysterectomy or (2) involvement of the upper margins of a cone biopsy specimen with CIN in the postmenopausal woman or in a younger woman who does not desire future fertility.

At the time of hysterectomy, it is unnecessary to remove the upper vagina unless the vaginal mucosa is also involved with vaginal intraepithelial neoplasia as documented by colposcopically directed biopsies. Cumulative data indicate that the

TABLE 11–6. Clinical Stages in Carcinoma of the Cervix Uteri (FIGO System)

Stage 0	Carcinoma in situ, intraepithelial carcinoma.
Stage I	The carcinoma is confined strictly to the cervix (extension to the corpus should be disregarded).
Stage IA	Preclinical carcinomas of the cervix, i.e., those diagnosed only by microscopy.
Stage IA1	Minimal microscopically evident stromal invasion.
Stage IA2	Lesions detected microscopically that can be measured. The upper limit of the measurement should not show a depth of invasion of more than 5 mm taken from the base of the epithelium, either surface or glandular, from which it originates, and a second dimension, the horizontal spread, must not exceed 7 mm. Larger lesions should be staged as IB.
Stage IB	Lesions of greater dimension than stage IA2, whether seen clinically or not; preformed space involvement should not alter the staging but should be specifically recorded to determine whether it should affect future treatment decisions.
Stage II	The carcinoma extends beyond the cervix but has not extended to the pelvic wall. The carcinoma involves the vagina but not as far as the lower third.
Stage IIA	No obvious parametrial involvement.
Stage IIB	Obvious parametrial involvement.
Stage III	The carcinoma has extended to the pelvic wall. On rectal examination, there is no cancer-free space between the tumor and the pelvic wall. The tumor involves the lower third of the vagina. All patients with hydronephrosis or a nonfunctioning kidney are included.
Stage IIIA	No extension to the pelvic wall.
Stage IIIB	Extension to the pelvic wall and/or hydronephrosis or a nonfunctioning kidney.
Stage IV	The carcinoma has extended beyond the true pelvis or has clinically involved the mucosa of the bladder or rectum. A bullous edema as such does not permit a case to be allotted to stage IV.
Stage IVA	Spread to adjacent organs.
Stage IVB	Spread to distant organs.

incidence of persistent disease or recurrent cancer involving the vagina following hysterectomy is less than 1%. However, follow-up screening in these patients is essentially the same as that in patients undergoing more conservative methods of therapy for CIN and should be for the lifetime of the patient.

Follow-up Management

There is no standard protocol regarding the appropriate follow-up of women who have been treated for cervical dysplasia. However, in most clinical settings, these women are initially reevaluated at approximately 3 to 4 months following therapy. By this time, the destroyed or excised transformation zone has regenerated and can be evaluated cytologically and colposcopically. Providing this initial assessment is satisfactory, further cervical screening is recommended every 3 months for the first year and biannually during the second year following therapy. Thereafter, the patient should receive annual PAP smears. If an abnormality is reported on follow-up screening, then the patient should undergo the appropriate triage of an abnormal PAP smear as outlined in Figure 11–5.

INVASIVE CERVICAL CANCER

Cervical intraepithelial neoplasia, including CIS, is a preinvasive condition. This is important to remember because prognosis of CIN is excellent and survival is 100%. Approximately 85% of invasive cervical cancers are squamous cell carcinomas, which arise from the transformation zone of the cervix. Another 15% of cervical cancers originate from the glandular component of the endocervix and are called adenocarcinomas. These two histologic types are treated identically and are considered to have similar survival outcomes when matched for stage and grade.

Histopathologically, the earliest evidence of invasion is recognized as a disruption of the basement membrane by malignant cells penetrating into the underlying stroma. At the clinical level, early invasive lesions tend to be asymptomatic and are detected by abnormal cells on routine cervical screening. Occasionally women complain of postcoital spotting or a foul-smelling vaginal discharge. Symptoms associated with more locally advanced disease include lower back pain, sciatic pain, and lower extremity edema, which relates to the lateral spread of tumor within the pelvis with subsequent entrapment of the pelvic ureters or sciatic nerve or obstruction to lymphatic return. Hematogenous metastasis to the liver or lung is a late manifestation of advanced or recurrent disease.

Cervical cancer is staged by clinical examination and radiologic procedures (Tables 11–6, 11–7). Therapy is planned according to whether the patient has disease localized to the cervix, advanced disease confined locally to the pelvis, or systemic metastases. The two methods for primary treatment are surgery and radiotherapy. Radiation therapy may be employed in all stages of cervical cancer, whereas surgery alone is limited to women with stage I and IIA disease. Microinvasive cervical cancer that is invasive disease up to 3 mm beneath the basement membrane without lymphatic or vascular spread identifies a subset of patients who are not at risk for pelvic lymph node metastases and may be treated with less radical surgery such as conization or simple hysterectomy. Patients with stages IB to IIA cervical cancer are treated by radical hysterectomy with pelvic lymph node dissection or external beam radiation to the pelvis followed by one or two intracavitary implants. The 5-year survival rate for stage I disease in patients with negative results on pelvic lymph node tests is approximately 90%.[81] For patients with stages IIB to IVA cervical cancer, whole pelvic radiation therapy is the treatment of choice. Extended field radiation is added to pelvic radiation when there is surgical documentation of periaortic lymph node metastases without evidence of distant spread. The 5-year survival rate for stage III and IV disease treated by radiation alone is 30% and 10%, respectively.[82] Treatment is individualized in patients who present with systemic disease. Cisplatin is considered the single most effective chemotherapeutic agent for squamous cell carcinoma of the cervix, with an overall response rate of 30%.

Treatment for recurrent cervical cancer depends on the primary treatment method and the site of the recurrence. In patients with recurrent cancer in the pelvis who were initially treated with surgery, pelvic radiation is advised. A 25% survival rate is reported in patients treated with radiation for a postsurgical recurrence.[83] If the initial therapy consisted of pelvic radiation and the recurrence is within the pelvis without involvement of the pelvic sidewall, a pelvic exenteration with removal of the bladder, vagina, cervix, uterus, and rectum has a 5-year survival of 20 to 46%.[84–86] Chemotherapy for cervical cancer is palliative and should be lim-

ited to patients who are considered incurable by surgery or radiation therapy.

REFERENCES

1. Parkin DM, Laara E, Muir CS. Estimates of the worldwide frequency of sixteen major cancers in 1980. Int J Cancer 1988;41:184.
2. MacGregor JE, Teper S. Mortality from carcinoma of cervix uteri in Britain. Lancet 1978;2:774.
3. Cook GA, Draper GJ. Trends in cervical cancer and carcinoma in situ in Great Britain. Br J Cancer 1984;50:367.
4. Doll R. Invasive cervical and combined oral contraceptives (letter). BMJ 1985;290:1210.
5. Green GH. Rising cervical cancer mortality in young New Zealand women. N Z Med J 1979;89:89.
6. Devesa SS, Silverman DT, Young JL Jr, et al. Cancer incidence and mortality trends among whites in the United States, 1947–1984. J Natl Cancer Inst 1987;79:701.
7. Rotkin ID, Cameron JR. Clusters of variables influencing risk of cervical cancer. Cancer 1986;21:663.
8. Rotkin ID. Relation of adolescent coitus to cervical cancer risk. JAMA 1962;179:486.
9. La Vecchia C. The epidemiology of cervical neoplasia. Biomed Pharmacother 1985;39:426.
10. Herrero R, Brinton LA, Reeves WC, et al. Sexual behavior, venereal disease, hygiene practices and invasive cervical cancer in a high-risk population. Cancer 1989;65:380.
11. Pridan H, Lilienfeld AM. Carcinoma of the cervix in Jewish women in Israel, 1960–67. An epidemiological study. Israel J Med Sci 1971;7:1465.
12. Buckley JD, Harris RWC, Doll R, et al. Case-control study of the husbands of women with dysplasia or carcinoma of the cervix uteri. Lancet 1981;2:1010.
13. Zunzunegui MV, King MC, Coria CF, Charlet J. Male influence on cervical cancer risk. Am J Epidemiol 1986;123:302.
14. Graham S, Priore R, Graham M, et al. Genital cancer in wives of penile cancer patients. Cancer 1979;44:1870.
15. Martinez I. Relationship of squamous cell carcinoma of the cervix uteri to squamous cell carcinoma of the penis. Cancer 1969;24:777.
16. Barrasso R, DeBrux J, Croissant O, Orth G. High prevalence of papillomavirus-associated penile intraepithelial neoplasia in sexual partners of women with cervical intraepithelial neoplasia. N Engl J Med 1987;317:916.
17. Oriel JD. Natural history of genital warts. Br J Vener Dis 1971;47:1.
18. Meisels A, Fortin R. Condylomatous lesions of the cervix and vagina. I. Cytologic patterns. Acta Cytol (Baltimore) 1976;20:505.
19. Koss LG, Durfee GR. Unusual patterns of squamous epithelium of the uterine cervix: Cytologic and pathologic study of koilocytotic atypia. Ann N Y Acad Sci 1956;63:1245.
20. Lorincz AT, Temple GF, Kurman RJ, et al. Oncogenic association of specific human papillomavirus types with cervical neoplasia. J Natl Cancer Inst 1990;7:158.
21. Kreider JW, Howert MK, Wolfe SA, et al. Morphological transformation in vivo of human uterine cervix with papillomavirus from condylomata acuminata. Nature 1985;317:639.
22. Pirisi L, Yasumoto S, Feller M, et al. Transformation of human fibroblasts and keratinocytes with human papillomavirus type 16 DNA. J Virol 1987;61:1061.
23. Koutsky L, Holmes K, Critchlow C, et al. A cohort study of the risk of cervical intraepithelial neoplasia grade 2 or 3

in relation to papillomavirus infection. N Engl J Med 1992;327:1272.

24. Melchers W, van den Brule A, Walboomers J, et al. Increased detection rate of human papillomavirus in cervical scrapes by the polymerase chain reaction as compared to modified FISH and Southern blot analysis. J Med Virol 1989;27:329.

25. Young LS, Bevan IS, Johnson MA, et al. The polymerase chain reaction: A new epidemiological tool for investigating cervical human papillomavirus infection. BMJ 1989;298:14.

26. Noffsinger A, White D, Fenoglio-Preiser CM. The relationship of human papillomaviruses to anorectal neoplasia. Cancer 1992;70:1276.

27. Halpert R, Ruchter RG, Sedlis A, et al. Human papillomavirus and lower genital neoplasia in renal transplant patients. Obstet Gynecol 1986;68:251.

28. Feingold AR, Vermund SH, Burk RD, et al. Cervical cytologic abnormalities and papillomavirus in women infected with human immunodeficiency virus. J Acquir Immune Defic Syndr 1990;3:896.

29. Maiman M, Tarricone N, Vieira J, et al. Colposcopic evaluation of human immunodeficiency virus seropositive women. Obstet Gynecol 1991;78:84.

30. Vermund SH, Kelley KF, Klein RS, et al. High risk of human papillomavirus infection and cervical squamous intraepithelial lesions among women with symptomatic human immunodeficiency virus infection. Am J Obstet Gynecol 1991;165:392.

31. Maiman M. Recurrent cervical intraepithelial neoplasia (CIN) in human immunodeficiency virus (HIV) seropositive women. Presented at the 24th Annual Meeting of the Society of Gynecologic Oncologists, February 10, 1993, Palm Desert, CA.

32. Maiman M, Fruchter RG, Guy L, et al. Human immunodeficiency virus infection and invasive cervical carcinoma. Cancer 1993;71:402.

33. Spinillo A, Tenti P, Zappatore R, et al. Langerhans' cell counts and cervical intraepithelial neoplasia in women with human immunodeficiency virus infection. Gynecol Oncol 1993;48:210.

34. Winkelstein W. Smoking and cancer of the uterine cervix: Hypothesis. Am J Epidemiol 1977;106:257.

35. Brinton LA, Schairer C, Haenszel W, et al. Smoking and invasive cervical cancer. JAMA 1986;255:3265.

36. Trevathan E, Layde P, Webster LA, et al. Cigarette smoking and dysplasia and carcinoma in-situ of the cervix. JAMA 1983;250:449.

37. La Vecchia C, Franceschi S, Decarli A, et al. Cigarette smoking and the risk of cervical neoplasia. Am J Epidemiol 1986;123:22.

38. Hellberg D, Nilsson S, Haley NJ, et al. Smoking and cervical intraepithelial neoplasia: Nicotine and continine in serum and cervical mucus in smokers and non-smokers. Am J Obstet Gynecol 1988;158:910.

39. Holly EA, Petrakis NL, Friend NF, et al. Mutagenic mucus in the cervix of smokers. J Natl Cancer Inst 1986;76(6):983.

40. Barton SE, Maddox PH, Jenkins D, et al. Effect of cigarette smoking on cervical epithelial immunity: A mechanism for neoplastic change? Lancet 1988;17:652.

41. Tay SK, Jenkins D, Maddox P, et al. Subpopulations of Langerhans cells in cervical intraepithelial neoplasia and human papillomavirus infection. Br J Obstet Gynaecol 1987;94:16.

42. Barton SE, Hollingworth A, Maddox PH, et al. Possible co-factors in the etiology of cervical intraepithelial neoplasia. An immunopathologic study. J Reprod Med 1989; 34(9):613.

43. Cancer Facts and Figures—1992. Atlanta, GA: American Cancer Society, 1992.

44. Fruchter RG, Boyce J, Hunt M. Missed opportunities for early diagnosis of cancer of the cervix. Am J Public Health 1980;70:418.

45. Reid R. What does an abnormal Papanicolaou smear really mean? Colpo Gynecol Laser Surg 1984;1:199.

46. Ginsberg C. Exfoliative cytologic screening: The Papanicolaou test. J Obstet Gynecol Neonatal Nurs 1991;20:39.

47. Wiener JJ, Sweetnam PM, Jones JM. Long term follow-up of women after hysterectomy with a history of pre-invasive cancer of the cervix. Br J Obstet Gynaecol 1992;99:907.

48. Gemmell J, Holmes DM, Duncan ID. How frequently need vaginal smears be taken after hysterectomy for cervical intraepithelial neoplasia? Br J Obstet Gynaecol 1990;97:58.

49. Schneider A, deVilliers E-M, Schneider V. Multifocal squamous neoplasia of the female genital tract: Significance of human papillomavirus infection of the vagina after hysterectomy. Obstet Gynecol 1987;70:294.

50. Ambros RA, Kurman RJ. Current concepts in the relationship of human papillomavirus infection to the pathogenesis and classification of precancerous squamous lesions of the uterine cervix. Semin Diagn Pathol 1990;7:158.

51. Davis GL, Hernandez E, Davis JL, et al. Atypical squamous cells in Papanicolaou smears. Obstet Gynecol 1987;69:43.

52. Jones DED, Creasman WT, Dombroski RA, et al. Evaluation of the atypical Pap smear. Am J Obstet Gynecol 1987;157:544.

53. Noumoff JS. Atypia in cervical cytology as a risk factor for intraepithelial neoplasia. Am J Obstet Gynecol 1987;156:628.

54. Peterson O. Spontaneous course of cervical precancerous conditions. Am J Obstet Gynecol 1956;72:1063.

55. Masterson JG. Analysis of untreated intraepithelial carcinoma of the cervix. Proceedings of the Third National Cancer Conference. Philadelphia: JB Lippincott, 1957.

56. Nasiell K, Nasiell M, Vaclavinkova V. Behavior of moderate cervical dysplasia during long-term follow-up. Obstet Gynecol 1983;61:609.

57. Nasiell K, Roger V, Nasiell M. Behavior of mild cervical dysplasia during long-term follow-up. Obstet Gynecol 1986;67:665.

58. Campion MJ, McCance DJ, Cuzick J, Singer A. Progressive potential of mild cervical atypia: Prospective cytological colposcopic and virological study. Lancet 1986;2:237.

59. Mitchell H, Drake M, Medley G. Prospective evaluation of risk of cervical cancer after cytological evidence of human papillomavirus infection. Lancet 1986:2:573.

60. Zucker PK, Kasdon EJ, Feldstein ML. The validity of Pap smear parameters as predictors of endometrial pathology in menopausal women. Cancer 1985;56:2256.

61. Walton LA, Edleman DA, Fowler WC Jr, et al. Cryosurgery for the treatment of cervical intraepithelial neoplasia during the reproductive years. Obstet Gynecol 1980;55:353.

62. Benedet JL, Miller DM, Nickerson KG. The results of cryosurgical treatment of cervical intraepithelial neoplasia at one, five, and ten years. Am J Obstet Gynecol 1987;157:268.

63. Andersen ES, Thorup K, Larsen G. The results of cryosurgery for cervical intraepithelial neoplasia. Gynecol Oncol 1988;30:21.

64. Creasman WT, Hinshaw WM, Clarke-Pearson DL. Cryosurgery in the management of cervical intraepithelial neoplasia. Obstet Gynecol 1984;63:145.

65. Hatch KD, Shingleton HM, Austin JM Jr, et al. Cryosurgery of cervical intraepithelial neoplasia. Obstet Gynecol 1981;57:692.

66. Chanen W, Hollyock VE. Colposcopy and the conservative management of cervical dysplasia and carcinoma in situ. Obstet Gynecol 1971;43:527.

67. Popkin DR, Scali V, Ahmed MN. Cryosurgery for the treatment of cervical intra-epithelial neoplasia. Am J Obstet Gynecol 1978;130:551.

68. Tredway DR, Townsend DE, Hovland DN, Upton RT. Colposcopy and cryosurgery in cervical intraepithelial neoplasia. Am J Obstet Gynecol 1972;114:1020.

69. Hemmingsson E, Stendahl U, Stension S. Cryosurgical treatment of cervical intraepithelial neoplasia with follow-up of five to eight years. Am J Obstet Gynecol 1981;139:144.

70. Jobson VW, Homesley HD. Comparison cryotherapy and CO_2 laser for cervical intraepithelial neoplasia. Colpo Gynecol Laser Surg 1984;1:176.

71. Gunasekera PC, Phipps JH, Lewis BV. Large loop excision of the transformation zone (LLETZ) compared to carbon dioxide laser in the treatment of CIN: A superior mode of treatment. Br J Obstet Gynaecol 1990;97:995.

72. Chappatte QA. Histological difference between colposcopic-directed biopsy and loop excision of the transformation zone (LETZ): A cause for concern. Gynecol Oncol 1991;43:46.

73. Turner MJ, Rasmussen MJ, Flannelly GM, et al. Outpatient loop diathermy conization as an alternative to inpatient knife conization of the cervix. J Reprod Med 1992;37:314.

74. Anderson M, Jordan J, Morse A, Sharp F. A Text and Atlas of Integrated Colposcopy. St. Louis: Mosby Year Book, 1991, p 92.

75. Luesley D, McCrum A, Terry PB, Wade-Evans T. Complications of cone biopsy related to the dimensions of the cone and the influence of prior colposcopic assessment. Br J Obstet Gynaecol 1985;92:158.

76. Larson G, Gullberg B, Grundsell H. A comparison of laser and cold knife conization. Obstet Gynecol 1983;62:213.

77. Jordan JA. Symposium on cervical neoplasia. I. Excisional methods. Colpo Gynecol Laser Surg 1984;1:271.

78. Bjerre B, Eliasson G, Linell F, et al. Conization as only treatment of carcinoma in situ of the uterine cervix. Am J Obstet Gynecol 1979;125:143.

79. Kolstad P, Klem V. Long-term follow-up of 1121 cases of carcinoma in situ. Obstet Gynecol 1979;125:143.

80. Larsson G, Alm P, Grundsell H. Laser conization versus cold knife conization. Surg Gynecol Obstet 1982;154:59.

81. Martinbeau P, Kjorstad K, Iversen T. Stage IB carcinoma of the cervix. The Norwegian Radium Hospital. II. Results when pelvic nodes are involved. Obstet Gynecol 1982;60:215.

82. Campodonico I, Escudero P, Suarez E: Carcinoma of the cervix uteri. In: Pettersson F, Kolstad P, Ludwig H, Ulfelder H (eds). Annual Report on the Results of Treatment in Gynecological Cancer. Stockholm: Tryckeri Balder AB, 1985.

83. Krebs HB, Helmkamp BF, Sevin B-U, et al. Recurrent cancer of the cervix following radical hysterectomy and pelvic node dissection. Obstet Gynecol 1982;59:422.

84. Morley GW, Lindenauer SM. Pelvic exenteration therapy for gynecologic malignancy: An analysis of 70 cases. Cancer 1976;38:581.

85. Rutledge FN, Smith JP, Wharton JT, O'Quinn AG. Pelvic exenteration: An analysis of 296 patients. Am J Obstet Gynecol 1977;129:991.

86. Averette HE, Lichtinger M, Sevin BU, Girtanner RE. Pelvic exenteration: A 150-year experience in a general hospital. Am J Obstet Gynecol 1984;150:179.

Diseases of the Uterus

12

Abnormal Uterine Bleeding

Robert M. Weiss

Abnormal uterine bleeding can be defined as vaginal bleeding that occurs at an abnormal frequency or for an abnormal length of time or that is unusually heavy in a woman of reproductive age. Dysfunctional uterine bleeding is the most common cause of abnormal bleeding and results from ovarian dysfunction and chronic anovulation. Vaginal bleeding that occurs in a postmenopausal woman has different implications and is discussed in Chapter 14. Abnormal vaginal bleeding is one of the most common clinical problems faced by the clinician who treats women of reproductive age. Despite this, the proper diagnosis, treatment, and long-term management of this disorder remains among the most confusing issues faced by the clinician.

The proper diagnosis of abnormal vaginal bleeding is difficult because of the broad differential diagnosis, which includes hundreds of causes. These diagnoses are assignable to groups as varied as pregnancy complications, anatomic lesions, drug-induced bleeding, systemic disorders, coagulopathies, and chronic anovulation. Recent advances in diagnostic modalities have increased the likelihood of appropriate diagnosis but have also made the proper choice of laboratory and diagnostic tests more complex. Endometrial biopsy, office hysteroscopy, and transvaginal ultrasound have all increased the ability to diagnose both malignant and benign causes of abnormal bleeding in the outpatient setting.

The treatment of abnormal bleeding can also be confusing. The choice of a progestational agent, estrogenic agent, or combination estrogen and progestational agent can be difficult. In addition, gonadotropin-releasing hormone (Gn-RH) agonists are now available and can be an effective medication for patients resistant to all other methods of management.

THE NORMAL MENSTRUAL CYCLE

Any discussion of abnormal vaginal bleeding should begin with a brief review of the normal parameters of uterine bleeding as well as an understanding of the basic physiology of normal menses. Menarche occurs between the ages of 9 and 13, and the average age of menopause in the United States is 51.7 years. During these 40 years, most women have cyclic menstrual bleeding every 24 to 35 days. Bleeding that occurs more or less frequently is associated with either anovulatory cycles or an anatomic cause of abnormal bleeding. Normal menses lasts between 2 and 9 days. However, most patients with more than 7 days of bleeding complain of prolonged or heavy menses. During normal menses, 30 to 60 ml of blood, with an average hemoglobin content of 30 to 50%, is lost daily.[1]

In an idealized 28-day menstrual cycle, estrogen production is significant during the first 14 days of the cycle. During this "proliferative" phase, estrogen stimulates rapid and dramatic changes in the endometrium. Estrogen acts as a mitogen on the endometrial cells, causing rapid replication and growth of endometrial glands; mitoses are prominent during this phase. At ovulation, which occurs midcycle, formation of the corpus luteum leads to the secretion of progesterone and estrogen. Progesterone changes the endometrium to a secretory pattern. The endometrium grows from 0.5 mm up to 5.0 mm during the proliferative phase and differentiates during the secretory phase. During this time, the endometrial glands become tortuous, the stroma edematous, and the endometrium prepared for implantation of an early embryo. With lack of implantation and an ongoing pregnancy, estrogen and progesterone levels drop rapidly in the late luteal phase, leading to a rapid rise in local production of prostaglandin F2-α. These events lead to intense vasospasm and rhythmic contractions of arterioles in the endometrium, which lead to necrosis and sloughing of the upper layers of the endometrium. The top layers of the endometrium are lost; however, the bottom 0.5 mm (the basalis) is retained. As the sloughing begins, small amounts of estrogen are being produced, and reparation of the endometrium begins. Thrombin platelet plug formation is also essential to limit bleeding during this period.[2]

CAUSES OF ABNORMAL UTERINE BLEEDING

The causes of abnormal bleeding fall into six basic categories: (1) pregnancy complications, (2) anatomic lesions, (3) drug-induced bleeding, (4) systemic disorders, (5) coagulopathies, and (6) anovulation, that is, dysfunctional uterine bleeding (Table 12–1).[3]

PREGNANCY COMPLICATIONS. Bleeding in pregnancy is common and potentially life threatening. Threatened and incomplete spontaneous abortions, ectopic pregnancies, and gestational trophoblastic disease can manifest as very irregular, abnormal bleeding. The nonsurgical clinician might consider referring all patients with a positive pregnancy test who are experiencing vaginal bleeding to a trained gynecologist.

ANATOMIC LESIONS. Both benign and malignant lesions of the vulva, vagina, cervix, and uterus can appear as abnormal bleeding. Vulvar and vaginal atrophy and cancer, cervical polyps, and cervical ectropion caused by oral contraceptives or early pregnancy can all lead to abnormal bleeding. Cervical cancer often manifests as postcoital bleeding or highly irregular bleeding.

Lesions of the uterus that cause abnormal bleeding are often not as readily identifiable as vulvar, vaginal, or cervical causes of bleeding. Endometrial polyps often appear as asymptomatic intermenstrual bleeding. Submucous myomas are often associated with heavy menstrual periods. The presence of adenomyosis, which is growth of the endometrial glands into the myometrium of the uterus, can be signaled by heavy menstrual periods in women in their forties. Patients with endometrial hyperplasia, or cancer, often present with inter-

TABLE 12–1. Causes of Abnormal Uterine Bleeding

I. Pregnancy complications
  A. Threatened spontaneous abortion
  B. Incomplete spontaneous abortion
  C. Ectopic pregnancy
  D. Gestational trophoblastic disease
II. Anatomic lesions
  A. Vulva and vagina
    1. Atrophy
    2. Cancer
  B. Cervix
    1. Polyps
    2. Ectropian
    3. Preinvasive and invasive carcinoma
  C. Uterus
    1. Endometrial polyps
    2. Submucous myomas
    3. Adenomyosis
    4. Endometrial hyperplasia
    5. Endometrial cancer
    6. Sarcoma
III. Drug-induced bleeding
  A. Contraceptive pills
  B. Oral progestational agents
  C. Progestin injections or implants
IV. Systemic disorders
  A. Hypothyroidism
  B. Renal failure
  C. Liver failure
  D. Adrenal disease
V. Coagulopathies
  A. Thrombocytopenia
  B. Thrombasthenia
  C. Von Willebrand's disease
  D. Leukemia
VI. Chronic anovulation (i.e., dysfunctional uterine bleeding)
  A. Immature hypothalamic-pituitary-ovarian axis
  B. Perimenopausal state
  C. Obesity
  D. Polycystic ovarian syndrome (many causes)

menstrual bleeding. These lesions are not uncommon causes of abnormal bleeding in the perimenopausal woman.

DRUG-INDUCED BLEEDING. Women on oral contraceptive pills can have breakthrough bleeding. Women who are on the ''mini'' pill or who are on long-acting progestin injections (e.g., Depo-Provera) or progestin implants (e.g., Norplant) can also experience breakthrough bleeding. In addition, although Gn-RH agonists are an important treatment for abnormal uterine bleeding, women can experience acute heavy bleeding using these agents as well.

SYSTEMIC DISORDERS. These illnesses are often listed as causes of abnormal uterine bleeding, but they are uncommon. Hypothyroidism, renal failure, liver failure, and adrenal disease can all manifest as abnormal bleeding. Hypothyroidism, renal failure, and liver failure can all lead to altered metabolism and excretion of sex steroids. In many cases a decrease in sex hormone–binding globulin leads to elevated levels of free estradiol, resulting in abnormal bleeding. Hypothyroidism is one of the more common systemic causes of irregular bleeding. It often appears as menorrhagia although it can appear as amenorrhea as well.[4] Also, many adrenal diseases, including Cushing's syndrome, Addison's disease, and congenital adrenal hyperplasia, can lead to abnormal bleeding secondary to altered hormonal production and metabolism.

COAGULOPATHIES. These are fairly uncommon causes of abnormal bleeding in the woman of reproductive age. However, in the adolescent, it can be a more common cause of abnormal bleeding. Thrombocytopenia and thrombasthenia can lead to menorrhagia. Von Willebrand's disease can lead to an increase in bleeding time and often manifests as severe menorrhagia. It is uncommon for this disease to be initially diagnosed in a woman in her thirties or forties. In addition, leukemia and other blood dyscrasias can lead to abnormal bleeding.

CHRONIC ANOVULATION (DYSFUNCTIONAL UTERINE BLEEDING). Dysfunctional uterine bleeding is by definition abnormal bleeding caused by unopposed estrogenic stimulation of the endometrium brought about by chronic anovulation. Chronic anovulation has a number of causes: (1) an immature hypothalamic-pituitary-ovarian axis as seen in the adolescent, (2) ovarian failure as seen in the perimenopausal patient, and (3) polycystic ovarian syndrome. In all of these cases, estrogen is secreted by the ovaries, but progesterone is not produced. This state of unopposed estrogen production leads to estrogen breakthrough bleeding, which can appear as irregular and heavy menses.

Polycystic ovarian syndrome has many causes, including elevated ovarian or adrenal androgen levels, hyperprolactinemia, and obesity. Insulin resistance, as a primary cause of polycystic ovarian syndrome, has been described. In these cases, elevated levels of insulin and insulin-like growth factor 1 stimulate the ovaries to produce elevated androgen levels, which can lead to polycystic ovarian syndrome.[5] An abnormal hypothalamic pituitary secretion of Gn-RH and gonadotropins may also be a cause of polycystic ovarian syndrome in certain patients. Polycystic ovarian syndrome can be the end product of any cause of chronic anovulation. Whatever the cause, chronic anovulation that leads to dysfunctional uterine bleeding is certainly one of the most common causes of abnormal bleeding.

EVALUATION OF ABNORMAL BLEEDING

Clues from the History

A careful history can lead the clinician toward a proper diagnosis of abnormal bleeding. The following parameters in the history can help pinpoint the cause:

1. The pattern of the bleeding
2. The age (or phase of reproductive life) of the patient
3. Associated medical illnesses and medications that the patient is taking

Ascertaining the exact pattern of bleeding is very important when initially evaluating the patient. A history of regular cycles in length and duration is important in determining whether the patient is having normal ovulatory menstrual periods. Ovulatory cycles are generally accompanied by premenstrual symptoms (molimina) that include breast tenderness, bloating, and menstrual cramps with the onset of bleeding. In a patient with cycle lengths of 24 to 35 days and premenstrual molimina, the patient is most certainly having ovulatory cycles. In the patient with suspected ovulatory cycles, irregular or intermenstrual bleeding should suggest an organic cause for the bleeding. In a woman who appears to be having regular, ovulatory menses but has very heavy bleeding, one must consider the diagnoses of submucous fibroids, polyps, coagulopathies, and systemic illnesses. However, for patients who appear to be having breakthrough bleeding and are not experiencing premenstrual molimina, the diagnosis of chronic anovulation or dysfunctioinal uterine bleeding must be strongly considered.

The age of the patient is the second most important factor to consider when taking a history. In an adolescent, the most common diagnosis is that of chronic anovulation due to an immature hypothalamic-pituitary-ovarian axis. In adolescents, 75% of abnormal bleeding is caused by chronic anovulation, 20% is caused by coagulopathies, and 5 to 10% is caused by other factors. However, in this age group, one must be aggressive in ruling out a coagulopathy. Approximately 20% of adolescents admitted to the hospital for abnormal bleeding have coagulopathies, and up to 33% of patients who require transfusion are diagnosed with a coagulopathy.[6, 7]

At the other end of the age spectrum, chronic anovulation is again a very common cause of abnormal bleeding. In perimenopausal patients, anovulation is related to a decrease in functioning ovarian follicles. In women older than 40 with abnormal uterine bleeding, endometrial hyperplasia and endometrial cancer must always be ruled out by an endometrial biopsy or a dilation and curettage of the uterus.

The third part of the history must focus on daily medications and major medical illnesses that the patient may have. Questions related to undiscovered medical problems include the presence of easy bruisability, increased hair growth or breast discharge, and rapid changes in weight. All are important in helping to rule out coagulopathies, hirsutism, prolactinomas, obesity, Cushing's syndrome, or anorexia nervosa as causes of abnormal bleeding. Among medications, any hormonal drug, including those given for contraception or treatment of hypertension or thyroid or adrenal disease, can effect menstrual bleeding. Drugs that decrease the coagulability of the blood or increase the hepatic metabolism of enzymes may also alter the menstrual pattern.

The Importance of the Physical Examination

The physical examination is also important in diagnosing the cause of abnormal bleeding. Important points in this examination should include a careful thyroid examination and a search for evidence of hirsutism, that is, excessive midline hair above the lip, on the chin, between the breasts, below the umbilicus, and on the upper inner thighs. Looking for evidence of bruises or bleeding is important. Noting the general body habitus of the patient is important as obesity alone can be a cause of chronic anovulation. Evidence of striae and a buffalo hump may lead the clinician to rule out hypercortisolism. The clinician must do a careful abdominal examination, looking for evidence of liver disease or abdominal masses.

Finally, a careful pelvic examination is crucial. Inspection of the vulva, vagina, and cervix is important to diagnose a benign or malignant pelvic cause of abnormal bleeding. Bimanual examination to determine uterine enlargement resulting from uterine fibroids or adenomyosis is also important. Patients with polycystic ovaries often have bilaterally enlarged ovaries. Estrogen-producing or androgen-producing ovarian tumors might manifest as a unilaterally enlarged ovary.

Laboratory Tests

After completing the history and physical examination, the following laboratory tests should be performed on all patients: a serum or urine β-hCG

(pregnancy test), a complete blood count with differential, and a Papanicolaou smear (Table 12–2). The β-hCG is always an initial step to rule out a normal or abnormal pregnancy. A complete blood count can determine whether anemia is present as well as serve as a preliminary screen for blood dyscrasias or thrombocytopenia. The Papanicolaou smear is a routine evaluation for undiagnosed cervical dysplasia or cancer.

A luteal phase serum progesterone, drawn approximately 1 week before the expected next menses, can be very helpful in confirming ovulation and in narrowing the cause of abnormal bleeding. A serum progesterone level of 5 ng per ml or greater is indicative of the formation of a corpus luteum and ovulation. Abnormal bleeding associated with ovulatory cycles must lead the clinician to look more aggressively for either a systemic or an anatomic cause. If the serum progesterone level is below 5 ng per ml, it is doubtful that the patient ovulated, and determining the cause of chronic anovulation and dysfunctional uterine bleeding is indicated.[8] In this situation, hormonal manipulation of the menses before more invasive tests is indicated. Another important but more invasive method for diagnosing ovulation is analysis of endometrial tissue obtained by a luteal phase endometrial biopsy.

In addition to these four initial tests, numerous other tests may be indicated depending on the findings of the history and physical examination. Results of a prothrombin time, partial thromboplastin

---

TABLE 12–2. Evaluation of Abnormal Uterine Bleeding

INITIAL STUDIES
1. Pregnancy test
2. Complete blood count with differential and platelet count
3. Papanicolaou smear

ADDITIONAL STUDIES (AS NEEDED)
1. Prothrombin time, partial thromboplastin time, bleeding time (to rule out coagulopathy)
2. Thyroid-stimulating hormone, total thyroxin (T4) (to rule out hypothyroidism)
3. Luteal phase serum progesterone or endometrial biopsy (to rule out anovulation)

If Symptoms Indicate Further Testing
4. Follicle-stimulating hormone for menopause symptoms
5. Prolactin level for galactorrhea or oligomenorrhea
6. Testosterone, dehydroepiandrosterone sulfate, 17-hydroxyprogesterone (follicular phase) for hirsutism
7. Dexamethasone suppression test for symptoms of Cushing's syndrome

For Ovulatory Abnormal Bleeding or Refractory Anovulatory Bleeding (If Diagnosis is Obscure)
7. Transvaginal ultrasound
8. Dilation and curettage, hysteroscopy
9. Hysterosalpingogram

time, and bleeding time may point to an abnormality in clotting as a cause of abnormal bleeding. Although a bleeding time is not part of the initial work-up on all patients, it is certainly an important test if initial evaluation has not uncovered a cause of heavy, irregular menstrual periods.

A thyroid-stimulating hormone and total thyroxin (T4) level may be indicated to rule out thyroid disease. In the perimenopausal patient with hot flashes, an elevated follicle-stimulating hormone level may reveal menopause. A serum prolactin level is indicated in the woman with galactorrhea or oligomenorrhea. In the patient with evidence of hirsutism, a testosterone, dehydroepiandrosterone sulfate level, and follicular phase 17-hydroxyprogesterone are important in ruling out ovarian or adrenal hypersecretion of androgens. Finally, in the patient with symptoms suggestive of Cushing's syndrome, a low-dose dexamethasone suppression test or 24-hour urinary free cortisol is indicated.

Invasive Tests

More advanced and invasive tests are sometimes indicated when evaluating the cause of abnormal bleeding. A common and important test to perform is the in-office endometrial biopsy. In the woman 35 years of age or older who is experiencing either heavy menstrual bleeding (menorrhagia) or intermenstrual bleeding (metrorrhagia), an endometrial biopsy is indicated to rule out endometrial hyperplasia or cancer. In the woman younger than 35 an endometrial biopsy is rarely indicated. However, as stated earlier, a late luteal endometrial biopsy can be helpful in any woman to confirm ovulation. However, one must keep in mind that in-office endometrial biopsies are very poor at diagnosing endometrial polyps or submucous fibroids. A dilation and curettage of the uterus performed in the operating room may be more helpful in diagnosing uterine polyps or submucous myomas, but this procedure may also fail to diagnose up to 35% of anatomic lesions of the uterus.[9] A dilation and curettage may be indicated in patients who had negative results on office endometrial biopsies but who are at high risk for endometrial hyperplasia or cancer.

New methods that have greatly increased the ability to diagnose anatomic causes of abnormal bleeding have become available over the last few years. Transvaginal ultrasonography has improved the ability to diagnose pathologic conditions within the endometrial cavity, the uterine myometrium, and the ovaries. Ultrasonographic measurement of the endometrial thickness may reveal important clues as to the diagnosis of abnormal uterine bleeding. An endometrial thickness of less than 5 mm all but rules out hyperplasia or cancer and may be associated with atrophy of the endometrium (which can be a cause of breakthrough bleeding). Nonetheless, an endometrial thickness of greater than 15 mm can be abnormal, and, in this situation, an endometrial biopsy is indicated to rule out hyperplasia or endometrial cancer. In addition, abnormalities noted in the endometrial stripe can help the clinician diagnose uterine polyps and submucous myomas as the cause of abnormal bleeding.[10] This new technology is greatly dependent on the ability of the ultrasonographer and of the radiologist or gynecologist who interprets these studies.

Office hysteroscopy is another method that is becoming more common in practice. Hysteroscopy can be performed in the office without analgesia or with oral or local injectable anesthesia. The diameter of office hysteroscopes ranges from 3.6 to 5.0 mm. Using carbon dioxide or normal saline as a distending medium, the inside of the uterine cavity can be well visualized and suspicious areas biopsied. Hysteroscopy has become a very effective tool in the diagnosis of uterine polyps and submucous myomas, which are often missed on endometrial biopsy and dilation and curettage.[9, 10]

Hysterosalpingography, which utilizes fluorescence to outline the uterine cavity, is another method that can be utilized to diagnose an organic cause of abnormal bleeding. This test has been used for decades, and many practicing radiologists and gynecologists have experience with it.

In general, all of the previously mentioned invasive tests and radiologic dye studies are not indicated in the majority of patients. However, when the diagnosis is not clear or when the patient does not respond to medical management, these methods may be helpful in further evaluating the patient.

TREATMENT AND LONG-TERM MANAGEMENT OF ABNORMAL UTERINE BLEEDING

Any anatomic lesion, medical illness, or medication that is causing abnormal bleeding must first be addressed. If a submucous myoma or polyp is causing the abnormal bleeding, surgical management is indicated. A nonovarian endocrine cause of the bleeding must be controlled. In addition, medication that may be causing the abnormal bleeding may need to be changed.

In treating abnormal uterine bleeding that is related to a hormonal imbalance, three factors are very important. These factors are (1) the degree of anemia and symptomatology, (2) the degree of bleeding, and (3) the age of the patient (Table 12–3).

In the patient with very heavy uterine bleeding who may have severe anemia, the goal of management must be to stop the bleeding quickly. There are two common regimens to stop menorrhagia. In an outpatient setting, a 50 μg ethinyl estradiol/0.5 mg norgestrel–containing oral contraceptive pill can be utilized. The patient takes two pills twice a day for 3 to 5 days until the bleeding stops and then finishes the remaining pills in the contraceptive pack. With this regimen, the estradiol causes stabilization of the endometrium, and the norgestrel, an androgenic progestin, leads to vasospasm of uterine vessels and atrophy of the endometrium, significantly decreasing the bleeding. Another common regimen entails the administration of intravenous conjugated estrogen. Premarin, 25 mg, can be given every 2 to 4 hours for up to six doses until the bleeding stops.[11] This regimen is based solely on the estrogenic effects of stabilizing the endometrium, which leads to a rapid decrease in bleeding. If these two regimens do not decrease or stop the bleeding, emergency surgical management may be indicated (see subsequent discussion).

For patients who have experienced continuous, prolonged, and chronic uterine bleeding that has not compromised their hemodynamic status, other regimens are useful. In this case, the oral contraceptive regimen described earlier may be indicated. Alternatively, 12 days of an oral progestin may be helpful. Common progestins that may be utilized are medroxyprogesterone, 20 mg daily, or norethindrone, 0.7 mg daily. Norethindrone is available in a 0.35-mg dose in two of the "mini" pills, Nor-QD or Micronor. Two of these 0.35-mg tablets can be given to decrease the bleeding. In any of these regimens, the patient should expect additional but light bleeding following discontinuation of the medication.

Long-term management of patients with chronic anovulation and dysfunctional uterine bleeding is fairly straightforward. Patients with no contraindications can be managed easily on a standard low-dose oral contraceptive pill, either a triphasic or a low-dose pill, containing 30 to 35 μg of ethinyl estradiol. If the patient has a contraindication against taking a pill that contains estrogen or would prefer not to be on the oral contraceptive pill, the patient can be cycled monthly with a progestin. Either 10 mg of medroxyprogesterone acetate or 0.35 mg of norethindrone should be taken the first 12 days of each month. This dose should be sufficient to control any abnormal uterine bleeding associated with anovulation or altered sex steroid metabolism. In most situations of heavy menses, nonsteroidal, anti-inflammatory drugs utilized throughout the period of bleeding have been shown to decrease menstrual flow. Mefenamic acid (Ponstel), 500 mg initially followed by 250 mg every 6 hours, has been shown to decrease menstrual flow significantly.[12]

TABLE 12–3. Treatment of Uterine Bleeding

ACUTE DYSFUNCTIONAL BLEEDING*
Medical
1. Conjugated equine estrogen 25 mg intravenously every 4 h for a maximum of 6 doses
2. 35 μg ethinyl estradiol/norgestrol-containing oral contraceptive pill. Two pills orally twice a day for 3–5 days
Surgical
1. Curettage of uterus
2. Radiologic embolization
3. Hysterectomy

CHRONIC DYSFUNCTIONAL BLEEDING
Medical
1. Cyclic oral contraceptive pills
2. Medroxyprogesterone, 10 mg, or norethindrone, 0.35 mg orally, for the first 12–14 days of each month
Surgical
1. Endometrial ablation
2. Hysterectomy

ADDITIONAL THERAPY
Nonsteroidal anti-inflammatory drugs:
1. Mefenamic acid 500 mg orally, then two 250-mg tablets every 6 h
Gn-RH agonists:
1. Leuprolide acetate, 3.75 mg intramuscular monthly
2. Nafarelin acetate, 200 mg intranasally twice a day

---

*Hospitalize if patient has hemoglobin <8 gm/dl or hematocrit <24% or orthostatic hypotension.

Reproduced with permission from Weiss R. The management of abnormal uterine bleeding. Hosp Pract 1992;27(10A):68.

MANAGEMENT OF REFRACTORY ABNORMAL UTERINE BLEEDING

In the patient who is not responsive to one of these acute or long-term management plans, the administration of a second tier of laboratory tests is necessary. Repeating the initial laboratory tests and ordering a full coagulation profile, including a bleeding time, liver function and renal function tests, and complete endocrine testing, are indicated. If the results of these laboratory tests are normal, transvaginal ultrasonography, hysteroscopy, or a hysterosalpingogram must be performed to rule out an anatomic lesion as a cause of abnormal bleeding. Also, even if the endometrial biopsy revealed a normal endometrial pattern, a full dilation and curettage of the uterus at the time of hysteroscopy may be indicated. Endometrial polyps, submucous myomas, and malignancies are often missed by office biopsy.

Medical Management

If the results of all repeat laboratory tests are normal and the patient continues to experience menorrhagia, medical management may still help control the bleeding. High-dose progestins including medroxyprogesterone, 40 mg daily; megestrol acetate (Megace), 80 to 160 mg daily; or norethindrone, 1.05 mg daily, may be given. Danazol (Danocrine), a testosterone derivative utilized for endometriosis, can be very effective in causing atrophy of the endometrial glands and a decrease in uterine bleeding. Generally, 600 to 800 mg of danazol daily are required to cause amenorrhea. However, numerous androgenic side effects from the danazol often cause patients to discontinue the medication. These side effects include deepening of the voice, hirsutism, acne, weight gain, and possibly clitorimegaly.[13]

Gn-RH agonists have been utilized in some patients to cause amenorrhea. Leuprolide acetate is available as a monthly or daily injection. Nafarelin acetate is available as a nasal inhaler for daily use. Both of these medications are approved by the U.S. Food and Drug Administration for the treatment of endometriosis. When used properly, both are highly effective in causing amenorrhea. Approximately 90% of patients treated with Gn-RH agonists become amenorrheic within 3 months of using these medications. They are highly effective agents to be utilized when other therapy fails.[14]

Gn-RH agonists cause a down regulation and desensitization of follicle-stimulating hormone and luteinizing hormone production from the pituitary gland, thereby causing a rapid decrease in estrogen and progesterone production. However, these agents do lead to a pseudomenopausal state in which patients experience hypoestrogenic side effects. These side effects include hot flashes, vaginal dryness, insomnia, headaches, and possible decrease in breast size. It is important to note that Gn-RH agonists cause an initial flare in estrogen production that may cause an acute exacerbation of symptoms and may lead to an increase in bleeding during the first 2 weeks of therapy. Following this period, even the most refractory patients with abnormal bleeding become amenorrheic.

The antifibrolytic agent aminocaproic acid has been utilized to control menorrhagia. A 5-gm dose can be infused into the uterine cavity via a pediatric feeding tube.[15] In patients with certain types of von Willebrand's disease, desmopressin acetate given before menses has been shown to decrease menstrual flow significantly.

Surgical Management

In the patient with acute bleeding that is refractory to medical management, an office suction curettage or full dilation and curettage may be required to stop the bleeding. Radiologic embolization of pelvic vessels is another method that can be employed to control acute bleeding. Finally, ligation of pelvic vessels or a hysterectomy may be indicated.

In nonacute situations, the patient diagnosed with a uterine polyp or submucous fibroid can be treated via hysteroscopic removal of the lesion. Patients recover from these short procedures within 1 to 2 days. Occasionally, an exploratory laparotomy and myomectomy may be indicated to control abnormal bleeding. In the perimenopausal patient, hysterectomy may be the procedure of choice.

Hysteroscopic ablation of the endometrium via the cervical os, either with electrocautery or laser, is becoming a more common procedure to control menorrhagia in patients resistant to medical management. This short outpatient procedure allows the patient to return to full activities within 1 to 2 days following surgery. When performed by an experienced surgeon, this procedure leads to complete amenorrhea in 80% of patients. The majority of the remaining patients continue to have only minimal cyclic bleeding. Endometrial ablation is somewhat experimental, as the long-term side effects, including its effect on endometrial cancer, are not well known. However, it shows promise as a very safe and effective treatment for persistent abnormal uterine bleeding.[16]

REFERENCES

1. Higham JM, O'Brien PMS, Shaw RW. Assessment of menstrual blood loss using a pictorial chart. J Obstet Gynecol 1990;97:734.
2. Speroff L, Glass R, Kase N. Clinical gynecologic endocrinology and infertility. Baltimore: 4th ed. Williams and Wilkins, 1989, p 265.
3. Weiss RM. The management of abnormal uterine bleeding. Hosp Pract 1992;27(10A):55.
4. Wilansky D, Greisman B. Early hypothyroidism in patients with menorrhagia. Am J Obstet Gynecol 1989;160:673.
5. Giudice L. Insulin-like growth factors and ovarian follicular development. Endocrine Rev 1992;13(4):641.
6. Claessens EA, Cowell CA. Acute adolescent menorrhagia. Am J Obstet Gynecol 1981;139:277.
7. Cowan B, Morrison J. Management of abnormal genital bleeding in girls and women. N Engl J Med 324;24:1710.

8. Wathen NC, Perry L, Lilford RJ, et al. Interpretation of single progesterone measurement in diagnosis of anovulation and defective luteal phase. BMJ 1984;288:7.

9. Loffer FD. Hysteroscopy with selective endometrial sampling compared with D&C for abnormal uterine bleeding: The value of a negative hysteroscopic view. Obstet Gynecol 1989;73:16.

10. Fedele L, Bianchi S, Dorta M, et al. Transvaginal ultrasonography vs. hysteroscopy in the diagnosis of uterine submucous myomas. Obstet Gynecol 1991;77:745.

11. Devore GR, Owens O, Kase N. Use of intravenous Premarin in treatment of dysfunctional uterine bleeding—A double blind randomized control study. Obstet Gynecol 1982;59:285.

12. Hall P, Maclachlan N, Thorn N, et al. Control of menorrhagia by the cyclo-oxygenase inhibitors, naproxen sodium and mefenamic acid. Br J Obstet Gynaecol 1987;94:544.

13. Barbieri RL, Evans S, Kistner RW. Danazol in the treatment of endometriosis: Analysis of 100 cases with a 4 year follow-up. Fertil Steril 1982;37:737.

14. Shaw RW, Marshall JC (eds). LHRH and its Analogues and the Control of Menstrual Bleeding: Their Use in Gynecologic Practice. London: Butterworth, 1989.

15. Cedars MI. Acute management of DUB. Infertil Reprod Med Clin North Am 1992;3(4):811.

16. Derman S, Rehnstrom J, Neuwirth R. The long-term effectiveness of hysteroscopic treatment of menorrhagia and leiomyomas. Obstet Gynecol 1991;77(4):591.

Uterine Leiomyomas

Sandra E. Brooks

Uterine leiomyomas, commonly called fibroids, are smooth muscle tumors of the uterus that occur in approximately 20 to 30% of women older than 30. The true incidence of leiomyomas is unknown. The reported finding of myomas in 50% of postmortem examinations suggests a higher incidence than is clinically evident. Multiple leiyomyomas have been found to be equally present in uteri of women with and without a clinical diagnosis of myomas.[1]

PATHOLOGY

Leiomyomas are nonencapsulated, spherical tumors composed primarily of smooth muscle admixed with connective tissue. On cut surface, the smooth muscle bundles can be identified in a whorl-like arrangement. Leiyomyomas are thought to arise from smooth muscle cells of the uterus and blood vessels. The size of myomas varies widely. They are described in terms of their relative anatomic location and position in relation to the layers of the uterus. Leiomyomas may be confined to the myometrium (intramural); may project into the uterine cavity, distorting the endometrium and contour of the cavity (submucous); or may project out of the peritoneal surface of the uterus (subserous) (Fig. 13–1).

Leiomyomas contain a pseudocapsule of loose areolar tissue that separates them from the surrounding uterine smooth muscle. Myomas are generally firm, except when degenerative changes have occurred. Their color is light gray to pinkish white, depending on the blood supply. Microscopically, the cells form uniform bundles of spindle-shaped muscle cells. Mitotic figures are rare, with fewer than 3 mitoses per 10 high-power fields (HPF) in the majority of leiomyomas. The cells within leiomyomas differ from those of normal myometrium in terms of increased nuclear size, greater number of mitochondria, and increased numbers of free ribosomes.

Smooth muscle tumors with increased mitotic

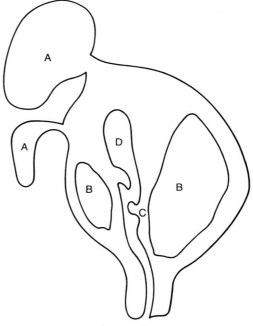

Figure 13–1. Schematic diagram of a uterus with multiple myomas. A, Subserous myomas; B, intramural myomas; C, submucous myomas; D, endometrial cavity.

activity and cellular atypia must be distinguished from both leiomyomas and leiomyosarcomas. Tumors with 5 to 9 mitoses per 10 HPF that lack cytologic atypia are termed smooth muscle tumors of uncertain malignant potential. The natural history of these tumors is unknown; however, benign clinical behavior demonstrated in one report suggests that these tumors should be designated mitotically active leiomyomas rather than smooth muscle tumors of uncertain malignant potential.[2] Tumors with more than 10 mitoses per 10 HPF or those with 5 to 9 mitoses per 10 HPF with cytologic atypia are considered leiomyosarcomas.

Leiomyomas are hormonally responsive tumors that grow under increased estrogenic conditions.

Such conditions during the reproductive years include pregnancy and, less commonly, oral contraceptive use. A growth spurt is frequently seen in the perimenopausal period and is likely due to anovulatory cycles with a relative estrogen excess that is commonly experienced during this period. Pregnancy is a condition of both elevated estrogen and progesterone, and although progesterone exerts an antiestrogenic effect and is associated with a decrease in the size of myomas, the enhanced blood supply during pregnancy leads to an overall trophic effect on the uterine leiomyomas.[3] With continued growth, degeneration can occur from outgrowth of the blood supply.

A more common type of degenerative change is hyaline degeneration, which refers to a loss of cellular detail as a result of a decrease in vascularity. Liquefaction necrosis results in cystic degeneration, an entity that is uncommon but important, as it lends a softer consistency to the myomas and may be confused with an ovarian mass. Calcification can occur over a period of time and is usually seen in postmenopausal women.

Myomas regress under conditions of estrogen deficiency. Although malignant degeneration is rare, occurring in 0.3 to 0.7% of myomas, the appearance of a new uterine growth or an increase in the size of the uterus after the menopause should increase one's suspicion of a malignancy. The true incidence of malignant degeneration is difficult to estimate owing to the very common occurrence of leiomyomas and the rarity of sarcomas.

SYMPTOMS

Uterine leiomyomas may be completely asymptomatic or may cause life-threatening hemorrhage and anemia. Symptoms relate to the location and size of the myomas. Menorrhagia and hypermenorrhea are believed to result from enlargement of the uterine vasculature with resultant congestion of the endometrium and myometrium. Ulceration and distortion of the endometrium surrounding submucous myomas may also be responsible for abnormal bleeding.

Approximately one third of women with myomas experience pelvic pain. Dysmenorrhea has been linked to an increase in myometrial activity.[4] Milder pelvic discomfort or pelvic "heaviness" is also described. Pain may also be experienced as a result of torsion of a pedunculated myoma or cervical dilation caused by a myoma protruding through the cervical os.

Pressure symptoms can occur when myomas are located near the bladder or rectum. Some patients experience urinary retention or incontinence. Ureteral obstruction as a result of lateral growth of myomas is an indication for early intervention. Hydronephrosis is reversible once the pressure is relieved.

Although a pregnant patient with uterine myomas can be completely asymptomatic, rapid growth of myomas during pregnancy can lead to degeneration of the myomas with resultant acute or chronic pain. This condition is best managed conservatively, as operative intervention is associated with excessive blood loss and the risk of premature labor. Implantation of the placenta over a submucous myoma may result in abnormal bleeding during pregnancy. Unusual complications associated with leiomyomas include premature rupture of membranes, placenta previa, placenta accreta, dystocia, uterine inversion, and postpartum hemorrhage. Disseminated intravascular coagulation and infection are rare complications that may occur. Rarely, myomas have been associated with the autonomous production of erythropoietin with resulting polycythemia.[6]

DIAGNOSIS

The diagnosis of uterine myomas is usually made by palpation of an enlarged, firm, and irregular uterus on pelvic examination. Myomas that have undergone cystic degeneration may be confused with an adnexal mass, as they may have a softer consistency. Movement of the mass independently from the uterus may be helpful in distinguishing uterine from adnexal masses. Direct observation of submucous myomas is possible with hysteroscopy or indirect observation via hysterosalpingogram. Office hysteroscopy can be performed easily with flexible 3- and 5-mm hysteroscopes, which can be inserted into the uterine cavity and which usually require no cervical dilation or anesthesia. Hysterosalpingogram is done by instillation of radiopaque dye into the uterine cavity using a catheter inserted into the cervix. The endometrial cavity as well as the fallopian tubes can be viewed under fluoroscopy.

Ultrasound is the most commonly used method of confirming the diagnosis of uterine leiomyomas. In particular, ultrasound can specify the number, size, location, and homogeneity of the leiomyomas as well as any calcific changes. Transvaginal ultrasound can provide information about the adnexa in the presence of uterine myomas.[6] Of note, ultrasound cannot differentiate between benign and malignant uterine masses. The role of other imaging modalities such as computed tomography or magnetic resonance imaging is limited in defining the extent of tumors not adequately visualized by ultrasound. Magnetic resonance imaging provides excellent contrast of soft tissue and is useful in the evaluation of the adnexa and endometrial stripe and in the differentiation of uterine fibroids from an adnexal mass.[7]

THERAPY

The treatment of patients with leiomyomas is guided by the patient's age, severity of symptoms, and desire for future fertility. The management of a patient with small asymptomatic myomas requires observation. Mild pelvic discomfort and anemia can be managed with nonsteroidal anti-inflammatory agents and iron supplements. It is appropriate to perform ultrasound and pelvic examinations at intervals of 3 to 4 months initially to document size and growth. The interval can be lengthened once growth has been found to be stable.

Symptoms that warrant consideration of intervention include (1) excessive bleeding that results in symptomatic anemia, requires blood transfusion, or forces the patient to curtail usual activity secondary to heavy bleeding on a regular basis during menses; (2) pelvic pain unresponsive to nonsteroidal anti-inflammatory agents; (3) extreme pressure and abdominal bloating; or (4) urinary frequency secondary to compression of the bladder from the fibroids. Patients may seek treatment before the development of these extreme symptoms and should be managed according to the extent to which the leiomyomas interfere with their daily activities. The patient's age and desire to maintain fertility should be taken into consideration.

Surgery is sometimes indicated based on the size of the leiomyomas alone; however, there are no absolute criteria for surgical intervention. Intervention is considered if the uterus rises above the pelvic brim (12–14 week size), because at this size, the ovaries are generally not palpable on pelvic examination. Another option is to follow asymptomatic patients who have large fibroids by yearly pelvic ultrasound to look for ovarian abnormalities.

Women with abnormal bleeding should be investigated for concurrent problems such as endometrial hyperplasia. An endometrial biopsy is warranted in patients with frequent menses; prolonged, heavy menses; or intermenstrual bleeding. If symptoms do not improve, either medical or operative intervention should be considered.

MEDICAL MANAGEMENT

Uterine leiomyomas have estrogen and progesterone receptors and are responsive to hormonal manipulation.[8] Progestational agents such as norethindrone and medroxyprogesterone acetate have been used successfully to reduce the size of leiomyomas. These agents inhibit the secretion of pituitary gonadotropins and produce a hypoestrogenic milieu, which results in a decrease in the size of the uterine myomas.

Gonadotropin-releasing hormone (Gn-RH) agonists also induce a state of hypoestrogenism. Histologic evaluation of myomas after treatment with Gn-RH agonists reveals hyaline degeneration with retention of estrogen receptors.[9] Gonadotropin-releasing hormone analogs have been used to reduce the size of leiomyomas by 40 to 50%. Patients can be followed with ultrasound and pelvic examinations to determine the success of treatment. After discontinuation of treatment, uterine size increases, and a return to pretreatment menstrual patterns often occurs. For this reason, short-term use of Gn-RH agonists is not definitive therapy for fibroids in younger women. However, Gn-RH agonists can be used before surgery or as an alternative to surgery in perimenopausal patients with symptomatic fibroids.

After 3 to 4 months of Gn-RH treatment, myomectomy or hysterectomy is accomplished with reduced blood loss and less difficulty owing to reduction in the size of the myomas.[10] A hysteroscopic submucous resection is also easier to accomplish with decreased blood loss after treatment with Gn-RH agonists for 2 to 3 months. Reduction in the size of myomas preoperatively has also allowed vaginal rather than abdominal hysterectomy in selected patients. During Gn-RH agonist therapy, most women become amenorrheic, and this allows for correction of anemia, which further minimizes operative morbidity.

The natural history of fibroids is such that their size usually stabilizes or declines after menopause. For this reason, some perimenopausal women can be treated with Gn-RH agonists to avoid surgery. Gonadotropin-releasing hormone analogs have been used in perimenopausal patients for a 3- to 6-month period in an effort to decrease myomatous growth, which then stabilizes when the patient enters menopause.

Gonadotropin-releasing hormone agonists may also be considered for use in patients with submucous myomas, which are thought to be implicated in infertility or recurrent abortion. Shrinkage of fibroids can be followed by assisted reproduction.[11] Submucous resection is also indicated in patients with infertility or recurrent abortion.

Long-term treatment of young patients with Gn-RH agonists has not been practical because of concerns about the safety of long-term hypoestrogenism. Currently, therapy for young patients with symptomatic leiomyomas consists of 3 to 6 months of Gn-RH agonists followed by surgical management. Studies are currently ongoing to evaluate the addition of estrogen and progesterone in combination with Gn-RH agonists. Preliminary reports suggest that reduced uterine volume can be maintained and menopausal symptoms controlled without loss of bone mass or alteration in high-density lipoprotein cholesterol.

CA-125, a marker for ovarian cancer, has been found to be elevated in approximately one third of patients with uterine myomas. When elevated, this marker may be used to follow the results of therapy.[12] As new technology and drugs become available, the treatment of uterine myomas is evolving, with fewer patients requiring hysterectomy for relief of symptoms.

SURGICAL MANAGEMENT

The surgical therapeutic options for the treatment of leiomyomas include myomectomy or hysterectomy. This determination is made based on the basis of the patient's age, parity, and desire for preservation of fertility. The presence of myomas is seldom a cause of infertility; however, when a relationship is seen, it is generally the location of the myoma that interferes with the establishment or maintenance of a successful pregnancy. The mechanism by which myomas are thought to cause infertility is by alteration in sperm transport, disruption of implantation, or compression of the uterotubal junction.[13] Myomectomy is indicated in patients with long-standing infertility and in cases of recurrent abortion after all other potential factors have been investigated.[14]

Removal of myomas can be accomplished via laparotomy or laparoscopy.[15] Patients with abnormal bleeding or infertility due to submucous myomas may also undergo hysteroscopic resection of the leiomyomas.[16, 17] Pregnancy rates after myomectomy have been reported to be about 30 to 50% and are dependent on coexisting factors impeding fertility.[15, 18–20] Myomas recur in 10% of patients after myomectomy, and therefore patients are advised to attempt to conceive within a short interval following surgery.

The mode of delivery in patients with uterine myomas who have undergone myomectomy is controversial. In the past it was felt that a prior uterine scar mandated cesarean section to decrease the risk of uterine rupture. Uterine rupture has been reported to occur in approximately one in 1500 deliveries. Uterine rupture after myomectomy is even rarer, accounting for approximately one in 50 to 60 cases of uterine rupture.[21, 22] Pa-

tients in whom the operation has been uncomplicated by infection or bleeding should be expected to heal satisfactorily and may undergo vaginal delivery under proper monitoring conditions. It is not currently known whether the rate of uterine rupture after laparoscopic myomectomy is equivalent to that after abdominal myomectomy.[23] Myomectomy may also be indicated for the removal of a pedunculated subserous myoma or one that is causing hypermenorrhea. Myomas that enlarge rapidly in a nonpregnant patient or those that cause pressure symptoms may also be removed.

Some symptomatic women may desire myomectomy rather than hysterectomy for preservation of the uterus even when childbearing is not of primary concern. This can be performed after careful evaluation for the presence of any coexisting pathologic condition in the uterus. Patients should be counseled, however, that multiple myomectomies may be associated with significant blood loss, infection, or extreme distortion of the uterus and that such complications may necessitate hysterectomy.

Hydronephrosis should be investigated promptly. Rapid enlargement of the uterus, especially in a postmenopausal women, should prompt an evaluation. In some cases, the patient will have an unrecognized ovarian neoplasm. The incidence of malignant degeneration of a uterine fibroid is very low, however, less than 1%.[24]

REFERENCES

1. Cramer SF, Patel A. The frequency of uterine leiomyomas. Am J Clin Pathol 1990;94(4):435.
2. Prayson RA, Hart WR. Mitotically active leiomyomas of the uterus. Am J Clin Pathol 1992;97(1):14.
3. Cramer SF, Robertson AL, Ziats NP, et al. Growth potential of human uterine leiomyomata: Some in vitro observations and their implications. Obstet Gynecol 1985; 66:36.
4. Iosif CS, Akerlund M. Fibromyomas and uterine activity. Acta Obstet Gynecol Scand 1983;62:165.
5. Weiss DB, Aldor A, Aboulafia Y. Erythrocytosis due to erythropoietin-producing uterine fibromyoma. Am J Obstet Gynecol 1975;12:358.
6. Coleman BL, Arger PH, Grumbach K, et al. Transvaginal and transabdominal sonography: Prospective comparison. Radiology 1988;168:639.
7. Weinreb JC, Barkoff ND, Megibow A, Demopoulos R. The value of MR imaging in distinguishing leiomyomas from other solid pelvic masses when sonography is indeterminate. AJR 1990;154:295.
8. Rein MS, Friedman AJ, Stuart JM, et al. Fibroid and myometrial steroid receptors in women treated with gonadotropin-releasing hormone agonist leuprolide acetate. Fertil Steril 1990;53:1018.
9. Uamura T, Mori J, Yushimura Y, Minaguchi H. Histologic effects of GnRH agonists of leiomyomas. Asia Oceania J Obstet Gynaecol 1991;17:315.
10. Stovall TG, Ling FW, Henry LX, Woodruff MR. A ran-

domized trial evaluating leuprolide acetate before hysterectomy as treatment of leiomyomas. Am J Obstet Gynecol 1991;164:1420.

11. Volpe A, Adamo R, Coukos G, et al. Pregnancy following regression of uterine submucosal leiomyoma with Gn RH therapy; a case report. Eur J Obstet Gynecol Reprod Biol 1991;39:223.

12. Bischof P, Galfetti MA, Seydoux J, et al. Peripheral CA 125 levels in patients with uterine fibroids. Hum Reprod 1992;7:35.

13. Markha S. Cervico-utero-tubal factors in infertility. Curr Opin Obstet Gynecol 1991;3:191.

14. Berkely AS, DeCherney AH, Polan ML. Abdominal myomectomy and subsequent fertility. Surg Gynecol Obstet 1983;156:3190.

15. Starks GC. CO_2 laser myomectomy in an infertile population. J Reprod Med 1988;33:184.

16. Brooks PG, Loffer FD, Serden SP. Resectoscopic removal of symptomatic intrauterine lesions. J Reprod Med 1989;34:435.

17. Corson SL, Brooks PG. Resectoscopic myomectomy. Fertil Steril 1991;55:1041.

18. Prien-Larsen JC. Myomectomy as treatment of infertility in women with uterine fibromyoma. Ugesknif fur Laeger 1989;151:2584.

19. Egwatu VE. Fertility and fetal salvage among women with uterine leiomyomas in a Nigerian teaching hospital. Int J Fertil 1989;34:341.

20. Garcia CR, Tureck RW. Submucosal leiomyomas and infertility. Fertil Steril 1984;142:16.

21. Golan D, Aharoni A, Gonen R, et al. Early spontaneous rupture of the post myomectomy gravid uterus. Int J Gynaecol Obstet 1990;31:167.

22. Garnet JD. Uterine rupture during pregnancy. Obstet Gynecol 1980;56:549.

23. Harris WJ. Uterine dehiscence following laparoscopic myomectomy. Obstet Gynecol 1992;80:595.

24. Montaue AC, Swartz DP, Woodruff JD. Sarcoma arising in a leiomyoma of the uterus. Am J Obstet Gynecol 1965;92:421.

Postmenopausal Bleeding and Uterine Cancer

Sandra E. Brooks

POSTMENOPAUSAL BLEEDING

Postmenopausal bleeding may arise from any organ of the reproductive tract, although most commonly it is uterine in origin. The appearance of bleeding in a woman more than 6 months beyond her last menstrual period requires evaluation. The patient may experience a brownish discharge or a frank hemorrhage with the passage of clots. Prompt evaluation should be undertaken irrespective of the amount of bleeding. Care must be taken not to call all bleeding in perimenopausal women dysfunctional, because 20% of patients with endometrial carcinoma are between the ages of 40 and 50 (see Chapter 12). A history and physical examination, cervical cytology, and endometrial tissue sampling are part of the evaluation of a patient with postmenopausal bleeding. A summary of possible causes of postmenopausal bleeding is listed in Table 14–1.

Differential Diagnosis

Nongynecologic

Bleeding from either the urinary tract or the rectum may be reported by the patient as vaginal bleeding. A careful history and, if necessary, a catheterized urine specimen or a cystoscopic or proctoscopic examination can aid in the determination of the source of the bleeding.

Gynecologic

VULVA. Patients with vulvar carcinoma may present with postmenopausal bleeding. Vulvar cancer is uncommon, comprising approximately 3 to 5% of all female genital tract malignancies. The mean age of diagnosis is approximately 65 years. Nonmalignant conditions of the vulva such as vul-

var dystrophy and psoriasis may cause irritation and lead to bleeding. A biopsy should be performed on any abnormal areas on the vulva to rule out vulvar cancer.

VAGINA. Patients with atrophic vaginitis may present with postmenopausal bleeding that may be difficult to distinguish from bleeding of uterine origin based on the history alone. The patient may experience staining or pinkish discharge and may only notice a scant amount of blood on a piece of tissue after urination. On examination, the estrogen-deficient tissues are friable and thin. Once bleeding of uterine origin has been excluded, estrogen therapy via vaginal, oral, or transdermal routes can be administered.

Patients with invasive carcinoma of the vagina may also present with painless bleeding, which may be accompanied by a discharge. Metastasis from the cervix, endometrium, and ovary should be excluded before classifying the tumor as being primarily vaginal in origin. According to the International Federation of Gynecology and Obstetrics

---

TABLE 14–1.   Causes of Postmenopausal Bleeding

NONGYNECOLOGIC CAUSES OF BLEEDING
Gastrointestinal tract
Urinary tract
GYNECOLOGIC CAUSES OF BLEEDING
Benign tumors
   Cervical polyps
   Endometrial polyps
Preneoplastic diseases
   Endometrial hyperplasia
Malignant tumors
   Cervical cancer
   Endometrial cancer
   Vaginal cancer
   Fallopian tube cancer
Exogenous estrogens
Atrophic endometrium or vagina

(FIGO), a primary vaginal cancer can involve neither the portio of the cervix nor the vulva. The mean age of patients with squamous cell carcinoma of the vagina is approximately 60 years. Definitive diagnosis is made by performing a biopsy. Coloposcopy can aid in determining the area from which to take the sample for biopsy and allow for a complete evaluation of the vagina and lower genital tract.

CERVIX. Premalignant diseases of the cervix rarely cause bleeding. Cervical polyps may cause postcoital spotting and should be removed. Invasive carcinoma of the cervix or the vagina may also cause postcoital bleeding. The average age of a patient with invasive carcinoma of the cervix is 48 years. Bleeding is often ascribed to perimenopausal hormonal disturbances. The appropriate diagnostic work-up includes a biopsy of any suspicious lesions. A patient with a normal-appearing cervix should have a Papanicolaou (PAP) smear and a colposcopic examination if the PAP smear results are abnormal.

UTERINE BLEEDING. In addition to a history and physical examination, a PAP smear and an endometrial biopsy or dilation and curettage (D&C) should be performed on all patients with suspected postmenopausal uterine bleeding. Specific attention should be paid to risk factors for endometrial cancer (Table 14–2). The presence of atypical glandular cells or endometrial cells on a PAP smear in a postmenopausal patient is abnormal and mandates evaluation. Patients in whom the endometrial biopsy results are negative should undergo a D&C. Fifty percent of women with endometrial cancer have abnormal PAP smear results.

The presence of normal endometrial cells on a PAP smear in a postmenopausal woman is an abnormal finding unless she is on hormonal therapy. This finding is associated with malignancy in approximately 6% of patients.[1, 2] Patients on continuous estrogen and progesterone hormonal therapy may experience irregular bleeding, which may continue for 1 year. An endometrial biopsy should

TABLE 14–2.   Risk Factors for Endometrial Cancer

Obesity
Hypertension
Diabetes
Chronic anovulation
Late onset of menopause
Exogenous estrogens
Family history of breast, ovary, colon, or endometrial cancer

be performed if bleeding is prolonged or heavy or if it persists for longer than 12 months.

FALLOPIAN TUBE. Fallopian tube cancer is a rare malignancy that comprises 0.3% of female genital tract malignancies. The majority of patients are postmenopausal. The triad of watery vaginal discharge, pelvic pain, and a pelvic mass is present in 15 to 20% of patients with tubal cancer.

Diagnostic Methods

Formerly, fractional D&C was the standard method used to assess uterine bleeding. This is done by performing an endocervical curetting before dilation of the cervix and sharp curettage of the uterine cavity. An endometrial biopsy is now a commonly used alternative to the fractional D&C. The overall results with endometrial biopsy are comparable to those with D&C.[3] In 1982, a review of the role of the diagnostic D&C was published after analysis of 33 reports comparing 13,598 D&Cs with 5851 Vabra aspirations, an endometrial biopsy technique.[4] The D&C was associated with a higher rate of bleeding complications, infection, and perforation than the Vabra aspirator. When D&C or hysterectomy results are used as the standard, then the diagnostic accuracy of the Vabra aspirator is approximately 96% for detecting endometrial carcinoma and 86% for detecting endometrial polyps. Several other instruments that vary in cannula size and material, suction technique, and cost are now available for endometrial sampling.[5] These include the Karman and the Pipelle. The Pipelle is currently used most widely and has been compared favorably with the Vabra aspirator when evaluated for ease of use, tissue obtained, pain, and cost.

Dilation and curettage is mandated in the following circumstances:

1. Patients in whom an endometrial biopsy is not technically feasible
2. Patients with an unclear result on endometrial biopsy
3. Atypical endometrial hyperplasia detected on endometrial biopsy in a patient undergoing treatment with progestins
4. Persistent bleeding after a negative endometrial biopsy
5. Patients in whom an examination under anesthesia is necessary

Hysteroscopy can be a valuable adjunct in the evaluation of the patient with postmenopausal bleeding as it allows for direct examination of the endometrial cavity. It can aid in the detection of small lesions missed by either curettage or biopsy.

Endometrial polyps can also be removed. In addition, hysteroscopy can add valuable information in the patient with bleeding due to atrophic changes as the biopsy or curettage may yield insufficient tissue for evaluation. Because of the frequent difficulty in cannulating the cervical os owing to cervical stenosis, it is sometimes necessary to perform this technique under anesthesia.[6, 7]

Ultrasonography can also be useful in the evaluation of the postmenopausal patient with bleeding. Commonly, patients at high risk for the development of endometrial cancer are obese, and the pelvic examination is limited. Ultrasonography can serve to assess the adnexa and the endometrial thickness. Although it has not replaced endometrial sampling, the presence of an endometrial stripe of less than 4 mm provides reassurance and can eliminate the need for fractional D&C in selected patients with a nondiagnostic endometrial biopsy. An approximately 80% correlation has been found between histology and ultrasound in determining atrophic conditions and endometrial carcinoma. A thickened endometrial stripe of greater than 9 mm correlates with the presence of uterine pathology, and patients should undergo a D&C if endometrial sampling is not technically feasible.[8–10]

Benign Causes of Uterine Bleeding

Atrophy

The diagnosis of bleeding secondary to atrophic changes of the estrogen-dependent tissues is made after a thorough evaluation of the lower genital tract and endometrial cavity. Atrophic vaginal epithelium along with a predominance of parabasal cells on PAP smear may suggest estrogen deficiency. Careful examination and sampling of the endometrial cavity should be performed. Hysteroscopy can be valuable in the evaluation of these patients, as negative results on hysteroscopic examination provide assurance to both the patient and the physician in the event that insufficient tissue is obtained for histologic review.

Endometrial Polyps

Endometrial polyps may be solitary or multiple and are commonly composed of hyperplastic endometrium. They are generally found in women between the ages of 40 and 55. Cystic hyperplasia may be present on microscopic evaluation. The tip of the polyp can become necrotic and inflamed, and this may represent the site of abnormal bleeding.

Patients receiving tamoxifen as adjuvant therapy for breast carcinoma may also develop endometrial polyps. Such polyps are associated with coexisting carcinoma of the endometrium in about 10% of patients. Removal of the polyp may be accomplished under direct vision through the hysteroscope or with polyp forceps at the time of D&C.

Endometrial Hyperplasia

The peak incidence of endometrial hyperplasia is between 40 and 50 years of age. A classification of endometrial hyperplasia based on the presence or absence of nuclear atypia is recommended based on the finding that lesions with nuclear abnormalities are clearly associated with the development of endometrial cancer. This information allows the physician to direct patients to medical therapy or to more aggressive evaluation and possible hysterectomy. Kurman and colleagues devised a classification system based on observations made from 170 women with untreated endometrial hyperplasia.[11] The following trends have been observed:

- *Simple hyperplasia* is associated with a 1% risk of progression to endometrial cancer. The endometrium is thicker than normal with cystic dilation of glands and crowding.
- *Complex hyperplasia* describes crowding of the glands and epithelial pseudostratification. The absence of nuclear atypia places these patients in a low-risk category, roughly 3%, for the development of endometrial cancer.
- *Atypical hyperplasia* describes the presence of cytologic atypia of the glands. The simple type, without back-to-back glands, is associated with an 8% risk of progression to invasive cancer, whereas complex atypical hyperplasia is associated with a 29% risk of progression to endometrial cancer.[11] In addition, 15 to 25% of these patients may have a coexisting endometrial carcinoma at the time of initial diagnosis. Patients with atypical hyperplasia who are treated medically should undergo a D&C to rule out the possibility of an occult malignancy.[12]

MANAGEMENT. Postmenopausal patients with atypical endometrial hyperplasia should undergo hysterectomy. Patients who are not considered to be surgical candidates can be treated with high-dose progestin therapy with periodic endometrial sampling.

Patients with simple hyperplasia can be treated with progestin therapy, that is, megestrol acetate (Megace), 40 to 160 mg daily, until regression of the hyperplasia is documented. A repeat endometrial biopsy should be performed after 3 months of treatment to assess results. Patients with persistent hyperplasia should undergo hysterectomy. Postmenopausal patients who are obese may require progestin therapy indefinitely.

ENDOMETRIAL CANCER

Carcinoma of the endometrium is the most common malignancy of the female reproductive tract. The American Cancer Society estimates that 31,000 women will be affected by endometrial cancer in 1994. In 75% of cases, the tumor is confined to the uterine corpus at the time of surgery. The primary mode of therapy is surgical. A minority of patients are not surgical candidates owing to unrelated underlying medical conditions.

Etiology

Carcinoma of the endometrium may arise in normal, atrophic, or hyperplastic endometrium. Estrogen serves as a promoter of endometrial carcinoma, and carcinoma of the endometrium is more common in patients with long-term exposure to unopposed endogenous or exogenous estrogen.

Obese women have a higher rate of conversion of androstenedione to estrone in peripheral adipose tissue and therefore have higher levels of endogenous estrogen.[13] Obese patients who are more than 50 pounds over their ideal weight are at a tenfold increased risk for the development of endometrial cancer. The relative risk directly correlates with the degree of obesity. Diabetes and hypertension, diseases that occur coincident with obesity, are associated with a 2.8-fold and 1.5-fold increased risk of developing endometrial cancer.[14, 15] A history of infertility and chronic anovulation is also associated with an increased risk for endometrial cancer.[16]

Several studies have shown the association of unopposed estrogen use with a four- to fifteen-fold increased risk of endometrial cancer. The addition of progesterone for 10 to 14 days of each month neutralizes the increased risk of endometrial cancer associated with estrogen use.[17, 18] In addition, atypical hyperplasia if left untreated has a 29% risk of development of invasive cancer.[19]

Tamoxifen, an antiestrogen, exerts a local estrogenic effect on the endometrium. Patients receiving tamoxifen should be monitored carefully, as endometrial cancer has been reported to occur in 1 to 5% of patients on tamoxifen; however, the optimal frequency of monitoring is undetermined at this time.[20, 21] Bleeding while on tamoxifen needs to be evaluated promptly by endometrial biopsy.

Some advocate yearly endometrial biopsies for patients receiving tamoxifen therapy.

Coexistent endometrial cancer is found in 15% of patients with estrogen-secreting tumors, such as ovarian granulosa cell tumors. The endometrial cancer tends to be well differentiated and localized to the uterus in these patients.

A smaller percentage of patients with endometrial cancer may not have any of the classic risk factors. In these individuals, the tumors do not seem to be under any hormonal influence. The surrounding endometrium in these patients may be normal or atrophic. Genetic events have been implicated in the development of endometrial carcinoma. Lynch and colleagues have reported on the Lynch syndrome II. This syndrome describes an inherited predisposition to colon cancer at an early age along with an excess incidence of adenocarcinomas from other sites such as the endometrium and the ovary.[22]

On a molecular level, point mutations in the K-*ras* gene, 17p and 18q, have been reported. K-*ras* proto-oncogene activation may play a role in the aggressiveness of endometrial cancer.[23] Mutations of p53 have also been reported to be overexpressed in women with endometrial cancer.[24] Although these reports are preliminary, they provide potential molecular models for disease progression and behavior. It is not known whether these mutations confer a more virulent phenotype or whether genetic lesions are accumulated during disease progression. The numbers of allelic loci have been shown to correlate with the stage of disease.

Symptoms

The majority of patients with endometrial cancer are postmenopausal with an average age at diagnosis of 60 years. Only 5% of patients are younger than 40 years old. Symptoms include abnormal vaginal discharge (90%), bleeding (80%), or leukorrhea (10%). Pain is not generally reported until the disease has advanced beyond the uterus. Because virtually all women have symptoms of bleeding or discharge even with early disease, screening is not routinely recommended.

Screening

Screening with endometrial biopsy may be justified for some postmenopausal patients, including morbidly obese patients, patients with hypertension or diabetes, and those with a family history of endometrial cancer. Patients receiving tamoxifen therapy or hormonal therapy should be observed carefully and should undergo endometrial biopsy with the onset of any abnormal uterine bleeding. Any postmenopausal patient who experiences bleeding should undergo endometrial biopsy. Abnormal bleeding in patients older than 40, especially patients with risk factors for the development of endometrial cancer, should be investigated by endometrial sampling.

The PAP smear is not a screening test for endometrial cancer, but results may be abnormal in up to 50% of patients with endometrial cancer. In one study, the presence of atypical or suspicious cells on PAP smear was associated with endometrial pathology in 56% of patients and adenocarcinoma of the endometrium in 45% of patients.[25]

Vaginal probe ultrasonography can be a useful tool in the evaluation of the patient with postmenopausal bleeding. The presence of an endometrial stripe of greater than 5 mm has been associated with endometrial pathology, whereas an endometrial thickness of less than 4 mm is usually associated with negative findings or minimal tissue at the time of endometrial sampling.[26]

Diagnosis

The diagnosis of endometrial cancer is made either by endometrial biopsy or fractional D&C. In a fractional curettage, the endocervical canal is curetted before the endometrial canal and the specimens are sent separately. Although endocervical curettage has been performed routinely, it has been reported to produce false positive results in up to 50% of patients owing to contamination from the endometrial canal. Preoperative endocervical sampling may become less important now that the information is no longer used for staging, because staging for endometrial cancer is now done at the time of exploratory laparotomy.[27]

Patients with a history of atypical endometrial hyperplasia should be followed aggressively, as 15 to 25% of these patients may have a coexistent endometrial cancer.[28] Postmenopausal patients with this condition should undergo hysterectomy, as up to 30% of patients may develop endometrial cancer.[19]

The preoperative history and the physical examination of the majority of patients reveal evidence of endogenous estrogen production. The liver and upper abdomen should be palpated carefully to discern the presence of hepatomegaly or an abdominal or omental mass. A complete blood count, blood urea nitrogen (BUN), creatinine, and liver function tests as well as a baseline CA-125

test should be performed. An elevation of the serum CA-125 level may suggest the presence of extrauterine disease and may be helpful in monitoring the results of therapy.[29] A chest radiograph should also be performed.

Additional tests such as cytoscopy and sigmoidoscopy are performed if advanced disease is suspected. Pelvic ultrasound, although not routinely performed, may aid in the assessment of the adnexa if a mass is suspected on clinical examination. Similarly, abdominal-pelvic computed tomography is not performed routinely; however, it may be useful in the evaluation of the liver, upper abdomen, and pelvis in a symptomatic patient with abnormal liver function test results, a palpable mass, or ascites. Although findings on magnetic resonance imaging have been found to correlate with the depth of myometrial invasion, the role of this newer imaging method in patients with endometrial cancer is yet to be determined.[30]

Pathology

Endometrial carcinomas are classified by a grading system of well-differentiated, moderately differentiated, and poorly differentiated adenocarcinomas. Classification affects therapy and prognosis. Distinguishing well-differentiated adenocarcinoma of the endometrium from atypical hyperplasia can sometimes be difficult. The presence of stromal invasion with a desmoplastic response, confluent ''back-to-back'' glands, papillary epithelium-lined processes, and squamous epithelium that replaces glandular epithelium (i.e., squamous metaplasia) are characteristic findings of adenocarcinoma. The histologic subtypes of endometrial cancer are listed in Table 14–3. Our discussion is divided into endometrioid carcinoma and histologic subtypes such as papillary serous, clear cell, and squamous carcinoma of the endometrium.

TABLE 14–3.   Histologic Subtypes of Endometrial Cancer

Endometrioid
   Adenosquamous
     Adenoacanthoma
Mucinous
Papillary
Squamous
Papillary serous
Clear cell
Mixed
Undifferentiated

Endometrioid Carcinoma

Endometrioid carcinoma is the most common type of endometrial cancer, comprising approximately 75% of cases.[31] The grade of tumor correlates with its prognosis and propensity for myometrial invasion. Well-differentiated tumors form distinct glands in at least 90% of the tumor. Poorly differentiated tumors form glands in less than one half of the tumor and are associated with a higher rate of deep myometrial invasion and lymph node metastasis.

Adenosquamous and papillary adenocarcinomas are variants of endometrioid adenocarcinoma, and although previous reports have suggested distinctive behavior of these tumors, their biologic potential has been shown to correlate more with their architecture and nuclear grade.[32, 33]

Papillary Serous Carcinoma

Papillary serous carcinomas comprise less than 10% of endometrial carcinomas and must be distinguished from papillary cancer, which is a variant of endometrioid adenocarcinoma. They are important because they display a marked propensity for myometrial and lymphatic invasion. Nuclear atypia and prominent papillary growth are common, and psammoma bodies are seen frequently.

Papillary serous carcinoma of the endometrium is histologically and biologically similar to serous carcinoma of the ovary and frequently involves peritoneal surfaces in the pelvis and abdomen. The recurrence rate is high even with tumors confined to the uterus at the time of surgery. Its aggressive behavior leads to a poor prognosis.[34]

Clear Cell Carcinoma

Clear cell carcinoma occurs in approximately 4% of women with endometrial cancer and is histologically similar to that seen in the cervix, vagina, and ovary. It occurs in a slightly older population than that with endometrioid cancer. Solid, cystic, tubular, and papillary patterns can be found; however, the solid pattern is most common. The characteristic cell found in these tumors is the "hobnail" cell. These cells have extruded their cytoplasm, leaving the bare nuclei protruding into the glandular lumen. Psammoma bodies can be found in the papillary areas of the tumor. Nuclear atypia is prominent, and mitotic figures are frequently found. These tumors are generally high-grade lesions and behave more aggressively than endometrioid adenocarcinomas.

Squamous Carcinoma

The diagnosis of squamous cell carcinoma of the endometrium is made only when squamous cell carcinoma of the cervix has been excluded. It is a very rare tumor and is also associated with a poor prognosis.[35]

Management

Historically, a variety of treatment approaches have been used in patients with endometrial carcinoma. Traditionally, patients who are not surgical candidates owing to medical illness have been offered primary radiation therapy. This is done less frequently today owing to advances in preoperative and postoperative care and anesthesia. In support of a surgical approach, valuable prognostic information can be obtained, and postoperative radiation can subsequently be tailored to the individual.[36, 37]

Endometrial cancers rarely occur in young women, but preservation of fertility is of importance in this population. The majority of the tumors that occur in young women are well differentiated. Selected patients may be offered a trial of a progestational agent such as megestrol acetate (Megace). Once disease regression has been documented, regular withdrawal bleeding with cyclic progesterone treatment must be continued, as many of these young women are anovulatory. Persistence of the lesion mandates hysterectomy. Grade 2 and 3 tumors are unlikely to respond to progestational therapy and should be treated with hysterectomy.[38]

Surgical Staging

Multiple prognostic factors are important in endometrial cancer (Table 14–4). The importance of these prognostic factors was documented by two Gynecologic Oncology Group surgical staging

TABLE 14–4. Poor Prognostic Factors in Endometrial Cancer

Histologic subtype
  Clear cell
  Papillary serous
High tumor grade
Deep myometrial invasion
Involvement of the uterine cervix
Vascular space invasion
Positive peritoneal cytology
Lymph node metastases

trials.[39] Patients were surgically staged using total abdominal hysterectomy, bilateral salpingo-oophorectomy, peritoneal cytologic examination, and selective pelvic and para-aortic lymph node sampling. Based on these trials, the importance of a primary surgical approach for determining prognosis was recognized and resulted in the development of a new staging system in 1988[40] (Table 14–5).

It is recognized that the presence of clear cell or papillary serous histology, deep myometrial invasion, and high tumor grade are important in the determination of prognosis for patients with endometrial cancer. The extension of tumor to the uterine cervix and the presence of vascular space invasion are also poor prognostic factors. The recognition of these factors allows identification of patients at high risk for recurrence in whom postoperative radiation therapy is indicated.

Surgical staging includes careful examination of the abdominal and pelvic cavities for evidence of extrauterine spread and peritoneal washings for cytology. A total abdominal hysterectomy and bilateral salpingo-oophorectomy are then performed. The uterus is evaluated intraoperatively by the pathologist, and a frozen section is performed to determine the depth of myometrial invasion.[41] Suspicious pelvic and para-aortic lymph nodes are removed. In the absence of suspicious nodes, a selective pelvic and para-aortic lymph node sampling is performed in patients with high-grade tumors, clear cell or papillary serous histology, and invasion of the outer one half of the myometrium or involvement of the cervix or adnexa.[42]

Patients with stage IA, grade 1 disease have a less than 1% risk of lymph node metastases and do not require lymph node sampling. Controversy exists over the necessity of sampling lymph nodes in patients with grade 2 and 3 tumors limited to the inner one half of the myometrial cavity, as the risk of lymph node metastases is approximately 5%.[43] The presence of positive para-aortic lymph nodes correlates with metastases in the pelvic lymph nodes, adnexa, or upper abdomen or involvement of the outer one third of the myometrium.

Disadvantages of Surgical Staging

Surgical staging adds additional operative time and blood loss. Patients who subsequently receive radiotherapy may be at higher risk for bowel complications as a result of adhesion formation. The overall surgical complication rate has been reported to be as high as 20% with a major complication rate of 6%, although several reports do not show clinically significant increases in morbidity or mortality.[44, 45] Some surgeons may choose not to sample pelvic lymph nodes in patients with high-grade tumors and deep myometrial invasion, because in some centers, patients receive radiation therapy irrespective of nodal status. The positive finding on para-aortic lymph node testing, however, results in extension of the radiation field to a para-aortic "chimney," and therefore patients at high risk for pelvic lymph node metastasis should undergo para-aortic lymph node sampling when possible.

Treatment

A schematic diagram for use as a guide to treatment can be found in Figure 14–1.

Stage I

A primary surgical approach is recommended for the treatment of endometrial cancer clinically confined to the uterus. Selected patients found to be at higher risk based on surgical findings may then receive radiation therapy tailored to their clin-

---

TABLE 14–5.   Corpus Cancer Surgical Staging, FIGO 1988

STAGE	DESCRIPTION
IA grade 123	Tumor limited to the endometrium
IB grade 123	Invasion to $< \frac{1}{2}$ myometrium
IC grade 123	Invasion to $> \frac{1}{2}$ myometrium
IIA grade 123	Endocervical glandular involvement only
IIB grade 123	Cervical stromal invasion
IIIA grade 123	Tumor invades serosa or adnexa or positive peritoneal cytologic results
IIIB grade 123	Vaginal metastases
IIIC grade 123	Metastases to pelvic or para-aortic lymph nodes
IVA grade 123	Tumor invasion of bladder or bowel mucosa or both
IVB	Distant metastases, including intra-abdominal, inguinal lymph node, or both

From International Federation of Gynecology and Obstetrics (FIGO). Corpus cancer staging. Int J Gynaecol Obstet 1989;28:190.

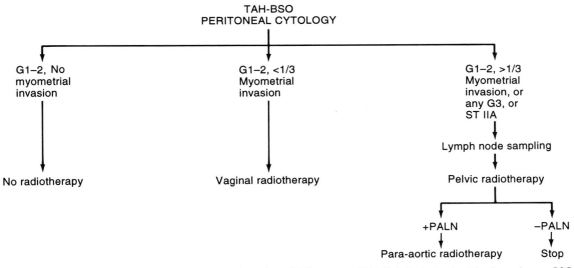

Figure 14–1. Guidelines for the treatment of endometrial cancer. TAH, Total abdominal hysterectomy; BSO, bilateral salpingo-oophorectomy; G, grade; ST, stage; PALN, para-aortic lymph nodes.

ical situation. The 5-year survival rate for patients with disease confined to the uterus is 72%.

Treatment consisting of preoperative radiation to the whole pelvis and Heyman's intrauterine capsules plus vaginal ovoids has been recommended for patients with grades 2 and 3 disease. Total abdominal hysterectomy and bilateral salpingo-oophorectomy are performed 6 weeks later. This order of therapy seems to result in overtreatment of patients with tumor limited to the superficial myometrium and delays treatment of patients in whom para-aortic lymph node metastases are discovered after the patient has undergone radiation. Radiation therapy alone for treatment of endometrial cancer is reserved for patients with medical contraindications to surgery. Adequate control can be achieved in patients with low-grade lesions without significant myometrial invasion; however, the outcome is poor in patients with enlarged uteri, advanced disease, or high-grade lesions.[46]

Stage II

Patients with gross involvement of the cervix may be treated with primary surgery followed by radiation or external beam irradiation followed by an intracavitary radioactive implant and surgery. Survival rates of 70 to 85% have been reported with this approach.[47] Grade has been shown to be an important predictor of survival. In one report 63% of patients with grade 3 tumors developed distant metastases.[48] Combination therapy does incur a higher risk of bowel obstruction and fistula formation in up to 9% of patients.[49] Because of the

high rate of false positive findings on endocervical curettage, patients with possible occult cervical involvement are best managed with primary surgery followed by radiation after evaluation of the surgicopathologic findings.[50]

Stages III and IV

Patients who present with disease outside of the uterus at the time of initial diagnosis are generally treated with a combination of radiation and surgery. Hormonal or cytotoxic chemotherapy may also be offered. Although the role of chemotherapy remains undefined, the need for effective regimens is clear, as the risk for distant recurrence is quite high in these patients. When the extrauterine disease is confined to the pelvic or para-aortic lymph nodes, radiation therapy can be given with reported survival rates of approximately 50%. One of the goals of surgery in these patients is the relief of symptoms such as bleeding or pain. The 5-year survival rates for patients with stages III and IV endometrial cancer are 31.5% and 10%, respectively.[51]

Vaginal Hysterectomy

Although the optimal approach to patients with endometrial cancer is hysterectomy using an abdominal approach, morbid obesity and coexistent medical problems may place some patients at high risk for abdominal surgery. A vaginal hysterectomy may be performed in these patients. A vaginal approach precludes nodal sampling. Survival rates of more than 90% have been reported in patients with disease clinically confined to the uterus who have been treated in this manner.[52]

Postoperative Treatment

Patients with grade 1 or 2 tumors confined to the endometrium do not require any further therapy. The 5-year survival rate in these patients approaches 100%.

Whole Pelvic Radiation Therapy

Radiation therapy is indicated in patients with poorly differentiated tumors with deep myometrial invasion. Patients with a positive finding on lymph node sampling and extrauterine pelvic spread should also receive radiation therapy. The survival benefit of whole pelvic radiotherapy has not been shown clearly in patients with superficial and intermediate myometrial invasion in the absence of other risk factors, although regional and local control appear to be improved.

Nine percent of patients with endometrial carcinoma have pelvic lymph node metastases. Para-aortic lymph node metastases are present in about 60% of patients with positive results on pelvic lymph node tests. The risk of lymph node metastases is increased in the presence of deep myometrial invasion or extrauterine spread. Doses of 5000 cGy are needed to eradicate microscopic disease. Five-year survival rates of up to 72% and 47% have been reported with postoperative radiation therapy to the pelvic and para-aortic region, respectively.[53] Tolerance to the para-aortic region is limited by the spinal cord and small bowel because they are within the para-aortic radiation port, and consideration of this must be made when radiating this area, owing to an associated 12% complication rate.[54]

Brachytherapy (Vaginal Cylinder or Ovoids)

The application of a vaginal cylinder has been recommended for patients with superficial and intermediate myometrial invasion with grade 1 or 2 tumors who are at low risk for nodal metastases. The risk of vaginal recurrence has been reported to be reduced from 12 to 14% to 0 to 1.7% in patients treated postoperatively with vaginal vault radium or cesium.[55]

Treatment of Positive Peritoneal Cytology

Positive peritoneal cytologic findings have also been reported to be a poor prognostic factor. Pa-

tients commonly have extrauterine disease. Approximately 5% of patients with endometrial cancer have positive peritoneal cytologic findings without other high-risk factors. The optimal approach to treatment in these patients has not been clearly defined. Some experts have advocated the use of intraperitoneal ^{32}P, and others have used progestins or whole abdominal radiotherapy.[56–58]

Estrogen Therapy

Historically, estrogen therapy has been contraindicated in all patients with surgically treated carcinoma of the endometrium. No clear evidence indicates that this therapy significantly increases the risk of recurrence. As data are limited, estrogen therapy is usually offered only to symptomatic patients with well-differentiated, superficially invasive tumors. Proper counseling should precede the institution of such therapy.[59, 60]

Survival and Surveillance

The 5-year survival rates of patients with stages I and II disease are 75% and 52%, respectively. Patients with advanced disease have 30% and 11% 5-year survival rates for stages III and IV disease, respectively. As 80% of recurrences are detected within 2 years, patients should be examined frequently and pelvic examinations and PAP smears performed regularly. Serum CA-125 levels have been reported to be elevated in up to 80 to 87% of patients with extrauterine disease, and thus may be a useful marker in patients with advanced endometrial cancer.[61, 62] Serial chest radiography should also be performed.

Recurrent Disease

As postoperative treatment with radiation therapy becomes more defined, it is apparent that many recurrences of endometrial cancer occur outside of the pelvis and therefore are not amenable to treatment with radiation or surgery. Isolated recurrences in the vaginal vault may be cured with radiation therapy. Exenterative surgery can be offered in the minority of patients who display a central vaginal recurrence who have received previous radiation therapy.[63] Hormonal therapy and cytotoxic chemotherapy are recommended in patients who require systemic therapy for recurrent disease.

Hormone Therapy and Receptor Status

Although progestin therapy has not been found useful as an adjuvant treatment for endometrial

TABLE 14–6. Classification of Uterine Sarcomas

PURE SARCOMAS	MIXED SARCOMAS (HOMOLOGOUS OR HETEROLOGOUS) MIXED MÜLLERIAN TUMORS
Pure homologous	Müllerian adenosarcoma
Leiomyosarcoma	(homologous or heterologous)
Low-grade endometrial stromal sarcoma	Malignant mixed müllerian tumors
High-grade endometrial stromal sarcoma	(homologous or heterologous)
Angiosarcoma	**SARCOMA, UNCLASSIFIED**
Pure heterologous	**MALIGNANT LYMPHOMA**
Rhabdomyosarcoma (including sarcoma botryoides)	
Chondrosarcoma	
Osteosarcoma	

From Kurman RJ (ed). Blaustein's Pathology of the Female Genital Tract, 3rd ed. New York: Springer-Verlag, 1993. Copyright Springer-Verlag.

carcinoma, approximately one third of patients with recurrent disease respond.[64–66] Well-differentiated tumors have a greater number of estrogen and progesterone receptors and respond more readily to hormonal treatment. Responses of up to 70% have been reported. Between 13 and 16% of patients with poorly differentiated tumors respond to hormonal therapy.[67, 68] The presence of both estrogen and progesterone receptors correlates well with response even without regard to differentiation of tumor. Megestrol acetate (Megace), 40 mg four times per day, is commonly used.

Tamoxifen, a nonsteroidal antiestrogen, has also been used in doses of 20 to 40 mg daily to treat patients with recurrent endometrial cancer. Response rates have varied; however, some responses may be seen in patients otherwise refractory to progestational agents.[69]

Patients who do not have receptors may be offered cytotoxic chemotherapy for treatment of recurrent disease.

Chemotherapy

Chemotherapy plays a limited role in the treatment of metastatic carcinoma of the endometrium. The most active agents are doxorubicin and cisplatin, with response rates of 38 to 40%. Unfortunately, the duration of response is limited. The median survival time is less than 12 months in most studies. Future directions include the use of novel chemotherapeutic agents and combination regimens in an effort to improve survival rates in patients with metastatic disease.

UTERINE SARCOMAS

Uterine sarcomas are rare tumors that comprise approximately 3% of cancers of the uterine corpus. They contrast greatly with endometrial carcinoma in that they behave aggressively and carry a poor

prognosis. A classification of uterine sarcomas can be found in Table 14–6. The most common uterine sarcomas are carcinosarcomas, leiomyosarcomas, and endometrial stromal sarcomas.

Previous radiation to the pelvis is the only known risk factor for the development of uterine sarcomas, although a history of intrauterine device use and therapeutic abortions has been reported. Sarcomatous degeneration of a benign leiomyoma is an uncommon occurrence (0.21%).[70] Leiomyosarcomas and carcinosarcomas are more common in women of African American descent; however, specific etiologic factors have not been delineated.

The age-specific incidence of uterine sarcomas varies by histologic subtype. The average age of patients with carcinosarcoma and leiomyosarcoma is 65 and 52, respectively. Early lymphatic and hematogenous metastases are common characteristics of the majority of uterine sarcomas. Patients frequently have more advanced disease than is clinically suspected. Tumors that are not as biologically aggressive are the low-grade stromal sarcomas, leiomyosarcomas of uncertain malignant potential, and adenosarcomas.

Clinical Presentation

Patients generally present with perimenopausal or postmenopausal bleeding. Pelvic or abdominal pain is reported in about one third of patients. On examination, a malodorous discharge may accompany a polypoid mass protruding through the cervical os. The uterus may be enlarged.

Diagnosis

The diagnosis of uterine sarcoma is not commonly made before surgery. Patients with abnormal uterine bleeding should undergo an endometrial biopsy or a fractional D&C. The epithelial component of a carcinosarcoma may be detected on an endometrial biopsy. Leiomyosarcomas are rarely diagnosed preoperatively. Suspicion for malignancy should be increased in patients older than 60 years of age with a history of uterine fibroids and a rapidly enlarging abdominal mass.[71] Endometrial stromal sarcomas may be completely intramural and therefore inaccessible to curettage.

Uterine sarcomas are a heterogeneous group of tumors with unique pathologic characteristics. Our discussion here is limited to the most common uterine sarcomas: carcinosarcomas, leiomyosarcomas, and endometrial stromal sarcomas.

Carcinosarcoma

Carcinosarcomas, or malignant mixed müllerian tumors of the uterus, contain both malignant mesenchymal and epithelial elements. They are classified as homologous or heterologous according to the mesenchymal elements present in the tumor. The epithelial component is usually an endometrioid adenocarcinoma. The presence of a high-grade tumor and clear cell or serous histology is associated with a higher frequency of metastases. The mesenchymal components do not determine clinical behavior.[72] Depth of myometrial invasion, lymphatic or vascular space invasion, and extent of disease are important predictors of survival.

Leiomyosarcoma

Leiomyosarcomas comprise approximately 25% of uterine sarcomas. In contrast to benign leiomyomas, they commonly occur as solitary masses. The diagnosis of leiomyosarcoma is made on the basis of number of mitotic figures per 10 high-power fields (HPF) and the extent of cellular atypia. A leiomyosarcoma is characterized by the presence of at least 10 mitoses per 10 HPF.[73] Neoplasms with 5 to 9 mitoses per 10 HPF with moderate cellular atypia are also considered leiomyosarcomas. The category of smooth muscle tumors of uncertain malignant potential applies to tumors with 5 to 9 mitotic figures per 10 HPF with minimal atypia.

Endometrial Stromal Sarcoma

Endometrial stromal sarcomas are divided into two types: a high-grade tumor with at least 10 mitoses per 10 HPF and a low-grade tumor with minimal atypia and fewer than 10 mitoses per 10 HPF. Grossly, the tumors are commonly smooth surfaced and polypoidal. In some cases, low-grade stromal sarcomas diffusely infiltrate the myometrium. The cells resemble stromal cells of the endometrium. Invasion into lymphatic and vascular channels is common.[74]

Smooth Muscle Tumors of Uncertain Malignant Potential

The diagnosis of smooth muscle tumor of uncertain malignant potential is generally not made until after myomectomy or hysterectomy. The recurrence risk for postmyomectomy patients is uncertain; however, these patients are encouraged to undergo hysterectomy at the completion of childbearing. The presence of cytologic atypia appears to be an important indicator of biologic behavior. A small study from the Cleveland Clinic followed six women with smooth muscle tumors with 5 to 15 mitoses per HPF and found no evidence of recurrence or metastasis.[75]

Staging

Because there is no separate staging system for uterine sarcomas, the endometrial cancer staging system is used.

Treatment

A surgical approach should be undertaken in a patient with a suspected uterine sarcoma. Total abdominal hysterectomy and bilateral salpingo-oophorectomy and pelvic washings are performed. Additional treatment is dependent on the histologic subtype of the tumor.

Carcinosarcoma

After performance of hysterectomy and bilateral salpingo-oophorectomy, lymph node sampling for carcinosarcomas may be performed. Although sampling may add additional prognostic information, it has not proved to alter survival rates. Similarly, aggressive cytoreduction in patients with stage III or IV carcinosarcoma has not been shown to improve outcome. These tumors are very aggressive. Five-year survival rates of 20 to 40% have been reported for patients with clinically localized disease.[76]

The value of adjuvant treatment has been difficult to assess owing to the rarity of the tumors. Local and distant recurrence rates of 20 to 56% have been reported.[77, 78] Adjuvant whole pelvic radiotherapy has been reported to reduce the risk of local recurrence to 16 to 17%; however, data supporting its efficacy in prolonging survival time are lacking.[79] Chemotherapy has not been found to be of absolute benefit in decreasing the risk of distant metastases in patients with stages I and II disease, although clinical trials are currently in progress.

Positive peritoneal cytologic findings carry a poor prognosis, and patients should be considered for whole abdominal radiotherapy or chemotherapy.

Low-Grade Endometrial Stromal Sarcoma

Low-grade endometrial stromal sarcoma can be treated readily with a radical surgical approach, as the tumor is infiltrative but slow growing. It is important that the ovaries be removed in these patients as these tumors are responsive to hormone stimulation. Recurrences occur in up to 50% of patients; however this is often a late occurrence, and the tumor is responsive to progestational agents.[80]

High-Grade Endometrial Stromal Sarcoma

Patients with endometrial stromal sarcoma are best treated with a combination of surgery and radiation therapy.[81, 82] Progestational agents are not usually effective in the treatment of high-grade stromal sarcomas; however, estrogen and progesterone receptors may identify patients that may respond to hormonal treatment. Five-year survival rates are approximately 50 to 62% for patients with early stage disease.

Leiomyosarcoma

Leiomyosarcomas are treated using a surgical approach. Enlarged lymph nodes should be removed at the time of surgery; however, the routine sampling of nonenlarged lymph nodes has not proved to be useful. Radiation therapy has not been shown to be beneficial. Survival rates of 29 to 50% have been noted for patients with early stage disease.[83] Virtually all patients who present with extrauterine disease succumb to their disease within 2 years.[84] Recurrent disease is difficult to treat, as neither radiation nor chemotherapy is very effective. Isolated recurrences may be amenable to surgical treatment.

Chemotherapy

Clinical studies have been limited owing to the rarity of these tumors. Some information has been gained from multi-institutional, prospectively ran-

domized trials. Cisplatin and ifosfamide have shown individual activity in the treatment of carcinosarcomas.[85, 86] Ifosfamide is currently under study either singly or in combination with cisplatin as adjuvant therapy. Although doxorubicin has demonstrated little activity in patients with carcinosarcoma, it has been found to be active as a single agent in the treatment of patients with leiomyosarcomas.[87]

In the treatment of uterine sarcomas, there has not been a successful trial of combination chemotherapy or adjuvant chemotherapy to routinely support its use. To date, the use of chemotherapy is restricted to experimental protocols or the use of single-agent chemotherapy for advanced or recurrent disease.

REFERENCES

1. Ng ABP, Reagan JW, Hawliczek CT, Wentz BW. Significance of endometrial cells in the detection of endometrial carcinoma and its precursors. Acta Cytol 1974;18:356.
2. Bibbo M, Rice AM, Wied GL, Zuspan FP. Comparative specificity and sensitivity of routine cytologic examination and the Gravlee jet wash technique for diagnosis of endometrial changes. Obstet Gynecol 1974;43:253.
3. Kaunitz AM, Masciello A, Ostrowski M, et al. Comparison of endometrial biopsy with endometrial Pipelle and Vabra aspirator. J Reprod Med 1988;33:427.
4. Grimes DA. Diagnostic dilatation and curettage: A reappraisal. Am J Obstet Gynecol 1992;142:1.
5. Kaunitz AM. Endometrial sampling in menopausal women. The tools and techniques. Menopause Management 1990;3(3):7.
6. Loffer FD. Hysteroscopy with selective endometrial sampling compared with dilatation and curettage for abnormal uterine bleeding: The value of a negative hysteroscopic view. Obstet Gynecol 1989;73:16.
7. Chao YC, Mak KC, Hsu C, et al. Postmenopausal uterine bleeding of nonorganic cause. Obstet Gynecol 1985;55:225.
8. Smith P, Bacos O, Heimer G. Transvaginal ultrasound for identifying endometrial abnormalities. Acta Obstet Gynecol Scand 1991;70:591.
9. Nasri MN, Shephard JH, Setchell ME, et al. The role of vaginal scan in measurement of endometrial thickness in a post menopausal woman. Br J Obstet Gynecol 1991;98:480.
10. Granberg S, Wikland M, Karlsson B, et al. Endometrial thickness as measured by endovaginal ultrasonography for identifying endometrial abnormality. Am J Obstet Gynecol 1991;164:47.
11. Kurman RJ, Kaminski PF, Norris HJ. The behavior of endometrial hyperplasia. A long-term study of "untreated" hyperplasia in 170 patients. Cancer 1985;56:403.
12. Tavassoli F, Kraus FT. Endometrial lesions in uteri resected for atypical endometrial hyperplasia. Am J Clin Pathol 1978;70:770.
13. Jasonni VM, Lodi S, Preti S, et al. Extraglandular estrogen production in postmenopausal women with and without endometrial cancer. Comparison between in vitro and in vivo results. Cancer Detect Prev 1981;4:469.
14. MacMahon B. Risk factors for endometrial cancer. Gynecol Oncol 1974;2:122.
15. Folson AR, Kay SA, Potter JD, et al. Association of inci-

dent carcinoma of the endometrium with body weight and fat distribution in older women: Early findings of the Iowa Women's Health Study. Cancer Res 1989;49:6828.

16. Dahlgren E, Friberg LG, Johanson S, Lindstrom B. Endometrial carcinoma: Ovarian dysfunction—A risk factor in young women. Eur J Obstet Gynaecol Reprod Biol 1991;41(2):142.

17. Robboy SJ, Miller AW III, Kurman FJ. The pathologic features and behaviour of endometrial carcinoma associated with exogenous estrogen administration. Pathol Res Pract 1982;174:237.

18. Dahlgren E, Johanson S, Oden A. A model for prediction of endometrial cancer. Acta Obstet Gynecol Scand 1989;68:507.

19. Kurman RJ, Kaminski PF, Norris HJ. The behavior of endometrial hyperplasia. A long-term study of ''untreated'' hyperplasia in 170 patients. CA Cancer J Clin 1985;56:403.

20. DeMuylder X, Neven P, DeSomer M, et al. Endometrial lesions in patients undergoing tamoxifen therapy. Int J Gynaecol Obstet 1991;36:127.

21. Andersson M, Storm HH, Mouridsen HT. Carcinogenic effects of adjuvant tamoxifen treatment and radiotherapy for early breast cancer. Acta Oncol 1992;31:259.

22. Lynch HT, Kimberling WJ, Albano WA. Hereditary nonpolyposis colorectal cancer (Lynch syndromes I and II) Parts I and II. Cancer 1985;56:934.

23. Mizuchi H, Nasim S, Kudo R, Silverberg SG. Clinical implications of K-*ras* mutations in malignant epithelial tumors of the endometrium. Cancer Res 1992;52(10):2777.

24. Kohler MF, Berchuck A, Davidoff AM, et al. Overexpression and mutation of p53 in endometrial cancer. Cancer Res 1992;52:1622.

25. Yancey M, Magelssen D, Demaurez A, Lee R. Classification of endometrial cells on cervical cytology. Obstet Gynecol 1990;76:1000.

26. Goldstein S, Nachtigall M, Snyder J, et al. Endometrial assessment by vaginal ultrasonography before endometrial sampling in patients with postmenopausal bleeding. Am J Obstet Gynecol 1990;163:119.

27. Wallin TE, Malkasian GD, Gaffey TA, et al. Stage II cancer of the endometrium: A pathologic and clinical study. Gynecol Oncol 1984;18:1.

28. Tavassoli F, Kraus FT. Endometrial lesions in uteri resected for atypical endometrial hyperplasia. Am J Clin Pathol 1978;70:770.

29. Berchuck A, Soisson AP, Clarke-Pearson DL, et al. Immunohistochemical expression of CA-125 in endometrial adenocarcinoma: Correlation of antigen expression with metastatic potential. Cancer Res 1989;49:2091.

30. Sironi S, Taccagni G, Garancini P, et al. Myometrial invasion by endometrial carcinoma: Assessment by MR imaging. AJR 1992;158:656.

31. Fanning J, Evans MC, Peters AJ, et al. Endometrial adenocarcinoma histologic subtypes: Clinical and pathologic profile. Gynecol Oncol 1989;32:288.

32. Sutton GP, Brill L, Michael H, et al. Malignant papillary lesions of the endometrium. Gynecol Oncol 1987;27:294.

33. Zaino RJ, Kurman RJ, Herbold D, et al. The significance of squamous differentiation in endometrial carcinoma. Cancer 1991;68:2293.

34. Hendrickson MR, Ross J, Eifel P, et al. Uterine papillary serous carcinoma. A highly malignant form of endometrial adenocarcinoma. Am J Surg Pathol 1982;6:93.

35. Abeler V, Kjorstad KE. Endometrial squamous cell carcinoma: Report of three cases and review of the literature. Gynecol Oncol 1990;36:321.

36. Patterson E, Spratt D, Tenkiewicz Z, et al. Management of stage I carcinoma of the uterus. Obstet Gynecol 1982;59:755.

37. Boronow RC, Morrow CP, Creasman WT, et al. Surgical staging in endometrial cancer: Clinical-pathologic findings of a prospective study. Obstet Gynecol 1984;63:825.

38. Farhi DC, Nosanchuk J, Silberberg SG. Endometrial adenocarcinoma in women under 25 years of age. Obstet Gynecol 1986;68:741.

39. Creasman WT, Morrow CP, Bundy L, et al. Surgical pathological spread patterns of endometrial cancer. Cancer 1987;60:2035.

40. International Federation of Gynecology and Obstetrics. Corpus cancer staging. Int J Gynaecol Obstet 1989;28:190.

41. Malviya VK, Deppe G, Malone JM Jr, et al. Reliability of frozen section examination in identifying poor prognostic indicators in stage I endometrial adenocarcinoma. Gynecol Oncol 1989;34:299.

42. Creasman WT, Morrow CP, Bundy L, et al. Surgical pathological spread patterns of endometrial cancer. Cancer 1987;60:2035.

43. Morrow CP, Bundy BN, Kumar RJ, et al. Relationship between surgical-pathological risk factors and outcome in clinical stages I and II carcinoma of the endometrium. A Gynecologic Oncology Group study. Gynecol Oncol 1991;40:55.

44. Orr JW Jr, Holloway RW, Orr PF, Holimon JL. Surgical staging of uterine cancer: An analysis of perioperative morbidity. Gynecol Oncol 1991;42:209.

45. Larson DM, Johnson K, Olson KA. Pelvic and par-aortic lymphadenectomy for surgical staging of endometrial cancer: Morbidity and mortality. Obstet Gynecol 1992;79:998.

46. Lehoczky O, Bosze P, Ungar L, Tottossy B. Stage I endometrial cancer: Treatment of nonoperable patients with intracavitary radiation therapy alone. Gynecol Oncol 1991; 43:211.

47. Greven K, Olds W. Radiotherapy in the management of endometrial carcinoma with cervical involvement. Cancer 1987;60:1737.

48. Resinger SA, Staros EB, Mohiuddin M. Survival and failure analysis in stage II endometrial cancer using the revised 1988 FIGO staging system. Int J Radiat Oncol Biol Phys 1991;21:1027.

49. Kinsella TJ, Bloomer WD, Lavin PT, Knapp RC. Stage II endometrial carcinoma: 10 year follow-up of combined radiation and surgical treatment. Gynecol Oncol 1980;10:290.

50. Mannell RS, Berman ML, Walker JL, et al. Management of endometrial cancer with suspected cervical involvement. Obstet Gynecol 1990;75:1016.

51. Pettersson F (ed). Annual Report on the Results of Treatment in Gynecologic Cancer, Vol 20. Stockholm: International Federation of Gynecology and Obstetrics, 1988.

52. Peters WA III, Andersen WA, Thornton N Jr, Morley GW. The selective use of vaginal hysterectomy in the management of adenocarcinoma of the endometrium. Am J Obstet Gynecol 1983;146:285.

53. Potish RA, Twiggs LB, Adcock LL, et al. Para-aortic lymph node radiotherapy in cancer of the uterine corpus. Obstet Gynecol 1985;654:251.

54. Rose PG, Cha SD, Tak WK, et al. Radiation therapy for surgically proven para-aortic node metastases in endometrial carcinoma. Int J Radiat Oncol Biol Phys 1992;24:229.

55. Graham J. The value of preoperative or postoperative treatment by radium for carcinoma of the uterine body. Surg Gynecol Obstet 1971;132:855.

56. Heath R, Rosenman J, Varia M, Walton L. Peritoneal fluid cytology in endometrial cancer; its significance and the role of chromic phosphate (^{32}P) therapy. Int J Radiat Oncol Biol Phys 1988;15:815.

57. Piver MS, Lele SB, Gamarra M. Malignant peritoneal cytology in stage I endometrial adenocarcinoma: The effect

of progesterone therapy (a preliminary report). Eur J Gynaecol Oncol 1988;9:187.

58. Potish RA, Twiggs LB, Adcock LL, Prem KA. Role of whole abdominal radiation therapy in the management of endometrial cancer; prognostic importance of factors indicating peritoneal metastases. Gynecol Oncol 1985;21:80.

59. Creasman WT. Recommendations regarding estrogen replacement therapy after treatment of endometrial cancer. Oncology 1992;6:23.

60. Lee RB, Burke TW, Park RC. Estrogen replacement therapy following treatment for stage I endometrial carcinoma. Gynecol Oncol 1990;36:189.

61. Patsner B, Mann WJ, Cohen H, et al. Predictive value of preoperative serum CA 125 in clinically localized and advanced endometrial carcinoma. Am J Obstet Gynecol 1988;158:399.

62. Niloff JM, Klug TL, Schaetzl E, et al. Elevation of serum CA 125 in carcinomas of the fallopian tube, endometrium, and endocervix. Am J Obstet Gynecol 1984;148:1057.

63. Phillips GL, Prem KA, Adcock LL, Twiggs LB. Vaginal recurrence of adenocarcinoma of the endometrium. Gynecol Oncol 1982;13:323.

64. Kauppila A, Gornroos N, Nieminen U. Clinical outcome in endometrial cancer. Obstet Gynecol 1982;60:473.

65. Kohorn EI. Gestagens and endometrial carcinoma. Gynecol Oncol 1976;4:398.

66. Bonte J. Medroxyprogesterone in the management of primary and recurrent or metastatic uterine adenocarcinoma. Acta Obstet Gynecol Scand (Suppl) 1972;19:21.

67. Thigpen JT, Homesley HD. A randomized study of medroxyprogeterone acetate (MPA) 200 mg versus 1000 mg in the treatment of advanced, persistent or recurrent carcinoma of the endometrium. In: Gynecologic Oncology Group Statistical Report. Buffalo: Gynecologic Oncology Group, 1990, p 177.

68. Ehrlich CE, Young PC, Stehman FB, et al. Steroid receptors and clinical outcome in patients with adenocarcinoma of the endometrium. Am J Obstet Gynecol 1988;158:796.

69. Slavik M, Petty WM, Blessing JA, et al. Phase II clinical study of tamoxifen in advanced endometrial adenocarcinoma: A Gynecologic Oncology Group study. Cancer Treat Rep 1984;68:809.

70. Montaue AC, Swartz DP, Woodruff JD. Sarcoma arising in a leiomyoma of the uterus. Am J Obstet Gynecol 1965;92:421.

71. Leibsohn S, d'Ablaing G, Mishell DR, et al. Leiomyosarcoma in a series of hysterectomeies performed for presumed uterine leiomyoma of the uterus. Am J Obstet Gynecol 1990;162(4):968.

72. Silverberg SG, Major FG, Blessing JA, et al. Carcinosarcoma (malignant mixed mesodermal tumor) of the uterus. A Gynecologic Oncology Group pathologic study of 203 cases. Int J Gynecol Pathol 1990;9:1.

73. Taylor HB, Norris HJ. Mesenchymal tumors of the uterus. IV. Diagnosis and prognosis of leiomyosarcomas. Arch Pathol 1966;82:40.

74. Hart WR, Yoonessi M. Endometrial stromatosis of the uterus. Obstet Gynecol 1977;49:393.

75. Prayson RA, Hart WR. Mitotically active leiomyomas of the uterus. Am J Clin Pathol 1992;97:14.

76. Macasaet MA, Waxman M, Fruchter RG, et al. Prognostic factors in malignant mesodermal (Müllerian) mixed tumors of the uterus. Gynecol Oncol 1985;20:32.

77. Hornback NB, Omura G, Major FJ. Observations on the use of adjuvant radiation therapy in patients with stage I and II uterine sarcoma. Int J Radiat Oncol Biol Phys 1986;12:2127.

78. Salazar OM, Bonfiglio TA, Patten SF, et al. Uterine sarcomas—analysis of failures with special emphasis on the use of adjuvant radiation therapy. Cancer 1978;42:1161.

79. Olah KS, Gee H, Blunt S, et al. Retrospective analysis of 318 cases of uterine sarcoma. Eur J Cancer 1991;27:1095.

80. Berchuck A, Rubin SC, Hoskins WJ, et al. Treatment of endometrial stromal tumors. Gynecol Oncol 1990;36:60.

81. Salazar OM, Bonfiglio TA, Patten SF, et al. Uterine sarcomas: Natural history, treatment, and prognosis. Cancer 1978;42:1152.

82. Wheelock JB, Krebs H-B, Schneider V, Goplerud DR. Uterine sarcoma: Analysis of prognostic variables in 71 cases. Am J Obstet Gynecol 1985;151:1016.

83. Marchese MJ, Liskow AS, Crum CP, et al. Uterine sarcomas: A clinicopathologic study, 1965–1981. Gynecol Oncol 1984;18:299.

84. Berchuck A, Rubin SC, Hoskins WJ, et al. Treatment of uterine leiomyosarcoma. Obstet Gynecol 1988;71 (6 pt 1):845.

85. Sutton GP, Blessing JA, Rosenshein N, et al. Phase II trial of ifosamide and mesna in mixed mesodermal tumors of the uterus (A Gynecologic Oncology Group study). Am J Obstet Gynecol 1989;161:309.

86. Thigpen JT, Blessing JA, Orr JW Jr, DiSaia PJ: Phase II trial of cisplatin in the treatment of patients with advanced or recurrent mixed mesodermal sarcomas of the uterus. J Clin Oncol 1987;5:618.

87. Omura GA, Major FJ, Blessing JA, et al. A randomized study of Adriamycin with or without dimethy triazinoimidazole carboxamide in advanced sarcomas. Cancer 1983;52:626.

Ovarian Diseases

15

Ovarian Cancer

Carolyn V. Kirschner

Ovarian cancer is the leading cause of death from gynecologic malignancies in the United States. In 1994 it was estimated that ovarian cancer would have an incidence of 24,000 and a mortality rate of 13,600.[1] The primary reason for the high mortality rate in ovarian cancer remains its insidious onset and lack of symptoms until dissemination into the peritoneal cavity results in ascites. Because ovarian cancer remains asymptomatic until it has reached an advanced stage, it is much less likely to be diagnosed at an early stage.

EPIDEMIOLOGY

Epithelial ovarian cancer may in some way be related to repeated stimulation of the ovarian epithelium by ovulation.[2] Factors that suppress ovulation, such as pregnancy and use of oral contraceptives, are associated with a decreased incidence of ovarian cancer.[3] Asymptomatic mumps appears to be associated with an increased risk[4] and so is the use of talc-containing dusting powders.[5] The Collaborative Ovarian Cancer Group published its analysis of risk factors for developing invasive epithelial ovarian cancer.[6] The group reported a decreasing risk with increasing number of pregnancies, increasing duration of breast-feeding, and use of oral contraceptives. Increasing risk was reported with the use of fertility drugs in patients who did not subsequently become pregnant. No risk relationships were observed regarding age at menarche, age at menopause, or use of postmenopausal estrogen therapy. These data remain to be reproduced, however.

FAMILIAL OVARIAN CANCER

The term "familial ovarian cancer" is not well defined currently in the medical literature. It may be used to describe ovarian cancer in a woman with a hereditary ovarian cancer syndrome as well as ovarian cancer in a woman who has one or more relatives with ovarian cancer. The term "hereditary ovarian cancer syndrome" includes three separate cancer syndromes: breast-ovarian cancer syndrome, site-specific ovarian cancer syndrome, and hereditary nonpolyposis colorectal cancer or Lynch syndrome II.[7, 8] Women with hereditary ovarian cancer syndrome tend to be younger at diagnosis of ovarian cancer than the population mean and are most likely to have serous cystadenocarcinoma.[9] Hereditary ovarian cancer syndromes may have an autosomal dominant inheritance. Both maternal and paternal lines of inheritance have been demonstrated. The first-degree relatives of a woman with ovarian cancer syndrome may have a lifetime risk as high as 50% of developing ovarian cancer.[10]

The proportion of all cases of ovarian cancer that are hereditary is unknown. Several studies suggest that these represent less than 1% of ovarian cancer cases.[11, 12]

SCREENING FOR OVARIAN CANCER

Because ovarian cancer is usually detected at advanced stages, when it is less likely to be curable, the therapeutic goal in this disease is prevention and early detection. The use of CA-125, a serum ovarian cancer antigen, has been investigated extensively.[13] Serum CA-125 levels are elevated in approximately 80% of advanced-stage epithelial ovarian cancer. A retrospective Norwegian study analyzed specimens collected from more than 100,000 patients.[14] Only 3% of patients identified with stage I ovarian cancer had an elevated CA-125 level. In addition, CA-125 levels have been found to be elevated in various other conditions, both benign and malignant, including cancers of the uterus, lung, breast, pancreas, and colon, as well as in endometriosis, liver disease, congestive heart failure, pregnancy, menses, pelvic inflammatory disease, and uterine leiomyomas. Currently, the specificity and sensitivity of serum CA-125 in early stage disease are considered too low to be of value as a screening test for ovarian cancer.

Transvaginal ultrasound as a screening method for ovarian masses and early ovarian cancer has been proposed since the mid 1980s. If epithelial ovarian carcinoma arises by malignant transformation of benign tumors, then theoretically the detection and removal of benign or borderline epithelial ovarian tumors could prevent the subsequent development of ovarian cancer. Van Nagell and colleagues screened 1300 asymptomatic postmenopausal women with vaginal ultrasound.[15] Twenty-seven (2%) were found to have a persistent ovarian abnormality. Fourteen patients (1%) had ovarian serous cystadenomas, and two had ovarian carcinomas. The two women with ovarian cancers had normal results on pelvic examination and normal serum CA-125 values.

Concerns about the use of ultrasound in screening for ovarian cancer include the performance of unnecessary surgery and the cost of repeat ultrasound when necessary. It is estimated that each diagnosis of stage I ovarian cancer would cost approximately $1 million.[16] The role of ultrasound in the screening of high-risk women, if such a definition can be determined, may be more cost effective.

Patients at increased risk for ovarian cancer who may benefit from the screening procedures include patients with a family history of ovarian cancer. In women who have two or more first-degree relatives with a diagnosis of ovarian cancer, physical surveillance in the form of pelvic and abdominal examinations and CA-125 assay every 6 months with pelvic ultrasound every year is advocated by some practitioners.[17] Prophylactic oophorectomy is sometimes performed in these women when childbearing has been completed. The patient should be warned, however, that peritoneal carcinomatosis after prophylactic oophorectomy has been reported.[18]

Another area of controversy includes the role of prophylactic oophorectomy at the time of hysterectomy for benign disease. An average of 7% of ovarian cancer occurs in women who have had a hysterectomy but who have ovarian conservation after age 40.[19] Routine prophylactic oophorectomy for women age 40 or older who are undergoing hysterectomy would therefore prevent 6 to 8% of all ovarian cancer in the United States, or an additional 1242 to 1656 cases each year. Opponents to prophylactic oophorectomy fear the consequences of surgically induced menopause, such as osteoporosis, cardiovascular disease, and increased medical costs in the form of estrogen therapy. Oophorectomy may also be more difficult when a vaginal approach for hysterectomy is utilized, as opposed to an abdominal approach.

CLINICAL PRESENTATION

Early ovarian cancer is usually asymptomatic. Symptoms of ovarian cancer that prompt the patient to seek the attention of a physician are often those associated with advanced disease, such as abdominal pain, distention, and a mass.

The earliest symptoms are usually insidious and include vague abdominal discomfort, dyspepsia, indigestion, slight anorexia, distention, and urinary frequency. These often prompt the physician, if consulted at this point, to pursue gastrointestinal and urologic work-ups, often with negative results. Patients, therefore, who present with vague abdominal complaints should undergo a pelvic examination. Ultrasound, CA-125 testing, or both should be considered, as discussed later.

PHYSICAL FINDINGS

Pelvic examination most suggestive of ovarian malignancy includes a mass in the ovary, fixation with subsequent immobility of the mass, irregularity and nodularity in the cul-de-sac, a mass that is relatively nontender, and bilaterality of the mass.

EVALUATION

A careful history and physical examination should be performed for diagnosis and to alert the physician to any preoperative or perioperative complications that may occur as a result of intercurrent medical problems. The physician should undertake a number of laboratory and radiographic studies, including Papanicolaou smear, complete blood count, blood chemistry, CA-125, chest radiograph, intravenous pyelogram, and barium enema. Upper gastrointestinal radiographs may be of benefit in a patient whose symptoms suggest obstruction. A computed tomography scan may be of benefit in the patient in whom a definite mass is not palpable.

MANAGEMENT

Surgical staging is recommended for all cases of ovarian cancer and is outlined in Table 15–1.

TABLE 15–1. Surgical Staging of Ovarian Cancer

1. A midline incision is made.
2. Ascitic fluid is aspirated and sent for cytologic analysis. If no ascites is present, washings for cytology are taken from the right diaphragm, right and left abdominal gutters, and pelvis.
3. The upper abdomen and pelvis are explored.
4. Total abdominal hysterectomy and bilateral salpingo-oophorectomy are performed. Exceptions to this may include ovarian neoplasms that have low potential for malignancy and germ cell malignancies.
5. Infracolic omentectomy is performed.
6. If no metastatic tumor is present grossly in the upper abdomen, peritoneal biopsies and a selective pelvic and para-aortic node sampling are performed. If gross tumor is noted, an attempt is made to remove as much tumor as possible (cytoreduction or debulking).

The goal in the surgical management of ovarian cancer is to remove as much of the cancer as possible without causing high morbidity or mortality. The incision must be vertical, so that it can be extended to gain access to the upper abdomen. A small incision also increases the risk of rupture of the mass, with potential spread of the malignancy. Washings of the peritoneal cavity for cytology testing are taken, followed by a full abdominal exploration. A total abdominal hysterectomy and bilateral salpingo-oophorectomy are then performed, with care taken to avoid tumor rupture, if at all possible. Exceptions to the recommendation for a hysterectomy would be a young patient with a germ cell tumor in which bilaterality is unlikely and a young woman with stage IA epithelial ovarian carcinoma in whom future fertility is desired. Complete surgical staging also includes multiple random peritoneal biopsies, omentectomy, and a sampling of the pelvic and para-aortic lymph nodes.

TREATMENT OF EARLY OVARIAN CANCER

The optimal treatment for stages I and II ovarian cancer is unknown. Stage IA, low-grade tumors may be followed after surgical removal without further therapy. Other early lesions, however, may benefit from adjunctive treatment in the form of radioactive chromic phosphate or a short course of chemotherapy.

TREATMENT OF ADVANCED OVARIAN CANCER

An attempt should be made to remove as much cancer as possible, as well as to perform a total abdominal hysterectomy, a bilateral salpingo-oophorectomy, and an omentectomy. After cytoreductive surgery, the patient is a candidate for chemotherapy.

Chemotherapy

Since the early 1980s, platinum-based chemotherapy has been the mainstay of treatment for advanced epithelial ovarian carcinoma in the United States. Cisplatin and cyclophosphamide are considered first-line treatment. With this regimen approximately 60 to 80% of patients experience a clinical response, with 40 to 50% of patients experiencing complete clinical remission.[20, 21]

Cisplatin and other chemotherapeutic agents have also been investigated via the intraperitoneal route. There is appeal to this regimen, with active agents being applied directly to the peritoneal cavity, which is the most common site of spread of ovarian cancer. Toxic side effects include adhesions with subsequent bowel obstruction, peritonitis, and catheter dysfunction. The exact role of intraperitoneal therapy also remains to be seen.

Other agents, including carboplatin, paclitaxel (Taxol), altretamine (Hexalen), ifosfamide, and biologic response modifiers have been investigated. The role of these regimens in frontline treatment or salvage treatment remains to be delineated.

Second-Look Exploratory Laparotomy

Standard therapy in the past has included a reassessment laparotomy to determine the extent, if any, of residual tumor.[22] Traditionally, this has been done because of the insensitivity of various tumor markers, scans, and radiographic studies in determining the effectiveness of chemotherapy. Recently, however, the utility of second-look laparotomy has been questioned. Up to 50% of patients with negative results on second-look laparoscopy eventually relapse. This issue continues to be addressed in the literature and remains a source of controversy.[23, 24]

OVARIAN CARCINOMA OF LOW MALIGNANT POTENTIAL

Ovarian carcinoma of low malignant potential (''borderline'' ovarian tumors) is classified pathologically as intermediate between cystadenomas and cystadenocarcinomas.[25] Full surgical staging for these tumors is recommended, if possible. The long-term prognosis is excellent.[26] Chemotherapy appears to offer no advantage over surgery alone.[27]

REFERENCES

1. Boring CC, Squires TS, Tong T, Montgomerry S. Cancer statistics, 1994. CA Cancer J Clin 1994;44:7.
2. Casagrande JT, Lowe EW, Pike MC, et al. "Incessant ovulation" and ovarian cancer. Lancet 1979;2:170.
3. Oral contraceptive use and the risk of ovarian cancer: The Centers for Disease Control cancer and steroid hormone study. JAMA 1983;249:1596.
4. Cramer DW, Welch WR, Cassells S, Scully RE. Mumps, menarche, menopause and ovarian cancer. Am J Obstet Gynecol 1983;147:1.
5. Cramer DW, Welch WR, Scully RE, Wojciechowski CA. Ovarian cancer and talc: A case-control study. Cancer 1982;50:372.
6. Whittemore AS, Harris R, Itnyre J, et al. Characteristics relating to ovarian cancer risk: Collaborative analysis of 12 U.S. case-control studies. Am J Epidemiol 1992; 136:1175.
7. Kerlikowske K, Brown JS, Grady DG. Should women with familial ovarian cancer undergo prophylactic oophorectomy? Obstet Gynecol 1992;80:700.
8. Lynch HT, Conway T, Lynch J. Hereditary ovarian cancer: Pedigree studies, part II. Cancer Genet Gytogenet 1991;51:161.
9. Lynch HT, Watson P, Bewtra C, et al. Hereditary ovarian cancer: Heterogeneity in age at diagnosis. Cancer 1991; 67:1460.
10. Lynch HT, Fitzsimmons M, Conway TA, et al. Hereditary carcinoma of the ovary and associated cancers: A study of two families. Gynecol Oncol 1990;36:48.
11. Greggi S, Genuardi M, Benedetti Panici P, et al. Analysis of 138 consecutive ovarian cancer patients: Incidence and characteristics of familial cases. Gynecol Oncol 1990;39:300.
12. Schildkraut JM, Thompson WD. Familial ovarian cancer: A population-based case-control study. Am J Epidemiol 1988;128:456.
13. Bast RC, Klug TL, St. John E, et al. A radioimmunoassay using a monoclonal antibody to monitor the course of epithelial ovarian cancer. N Engl J Med 1983;309:883.
14. Zurawski VR, Orjaseter H, Andersen A, et al. Elevated serum CA-125 levels prior to diagnosis of ovarian neoplasm: Relevance of early detection of ovarian cancer. Int J Cancer 1988;42:677.
15. Van Nagell JR Jr, DePriest P, Puls L, et al. Ovarian cancer screening in asymptomatic postmenopausal women by transvaginal sonography. Cancer 1991;68:458.
16. Piver MS, Recio FO. Issues in ovarian cancer screening. Contemp Oncol 1992;10:26.
17. Piver MS, Mettlin CG, Tsukada Y, et al. Familial ovarian cancer registry. Obstet Gynecol 1984;64:195.
18. Chen KT, Schooley JL, Flam MS. Peritoneal carcinomatosis after prophylactic oophorectomy in familial ovarian cancer syndrome. Obstet Gynecol 1985;66:93S.
19. Boike G. Surgical prevention of ovarian cancer. Contemp Obstet Gynecol 1992;8:66.
20. Cohen CJ, Goldberg J, Holland JF, et al. Improved therapy with cisplatin regimens for patients with ovarian carcinoma (FIGO stages III and IV) as measured by surgical end-staging (second-look operation). Am J Obstet Gynecol 1983;145:955.
21. Ozols RF. The case for combination chemotherapy in the treatment of advanced ovarian cancer. J Clin Oncol 1985;3:1445.
22. Smith JP, Delgado G, Rutledge F. Second-look operation in ovarian carcinoma. Cancer 1976;38:1438.
23. Potter ME, Hatch KD, Soong S-J, et al. Second-look laparotomy and salvage therapy: A research modality only? Gynecol Oncol 1992;44:3.
24. Young RC. A second look at second-look laparotomy. J Clin Oncol 1987;5:1311.
25. Serov SF, Scully FE, Sobin LH. International Classification of Tumors. No. 9: Histological typing of ovarian tumors. Geneva: World Health Organization, 1973.
26. Leake JF, Currie JL, Rosenshein NB, Woodruff JD. Long-term follow-up of serous ovarian tumors of low malignant potential. Gynecol Oncol 1992;47:150.
27. Sutton GP, Bundy BN, Omura GA, et al. Stage III ovarian tumors of low malignant potential treated with cisplatin combination therapy (A Gynecologic Oncology Group study). Gynecol Oncol 1991;41:230.

DISEASES OF THE BREAST

16

Evaluation and Management of a Palpable Breast Mass

Risa Beth Burns

A major concern of primary care physicians is the evaluation of a patient with a palpable breast mass. This concern is driven by the incidence of breast cancer that has increased dramatically since 1980, from 84.8 per 100,000 to 111.9 per 100,000 in 1987.[1] In addition, current estimates from the American Cancer Society suggest that one of every two women will consult a physician in her lifetime to evaluate a breast disorder, that one in three women will have a biopsy, and that one in nine will have cancer diagnosed.[2] This chapter is designed to provide primary care physicians with a comprehensive framework for evaluating and managing a patient who presents with a palpable breast mass. The chapter includes a discussion of benign breast disease; a discussion of diagnostic tools, including breast examination, radiologic studies, and needle aspiration; and an algorithm for evaluating and managing a patient with a breast mass. A section is included at the end of the chapter on how to evaluate and manage a palpable mass in the pregnant patient. The reader is referred to Chapters 17 and 18 for a discussion of breast cancer.

BENIGN BREAST DISEASE

Palpable breast masses fall into two broad categories: benign and malignant. Benign disease is a broad and heterogenous group of clinical and pathologic entities, including nonproliferative disease, proliferative disease without atypia, and atypical hyperplasia. Nonproliferative disease is the most common and encompasses normal breast tissue, fibroadenoma, cysts, and ductal ectasia.[3]

Traditionally, women who have diffuse changes with prominent glandular breast tissue have been diagnosed as having fibrocystic breast disease. This term has now been discarded in favor of "physiologic nodularity." The reason for this change in terminology is the understanding that some variation in breast lumpiness is normal and is not indicative of "disease."[4] In addition, fibrocystic disease is a pathologic and not a clinical diagnosis. Fibrocystic disease, as a pathologic diagnosis, encompasses all categories of benign breast disease (nonproliferative, proliferative without atypia, and atypical hyperplasia) and has wide-ranging clinical significance. Women with biopsy-proven atypical hyperplasia have been shown in both retrospective and prospective studies to be at significantly increased risk for development of breast cancer, whereas women with nonproliferative disease and proliferative disease without atypia are not at any increased risk.[3,5] Women who clinically are thought to have physiologic nodularity are not at increased risk of developing breast cancer.

The two most common benign breast conditions

that manifest as dominant masses are cysts and fibroadenomas. Haagensen estimates that approximately 7% of adult women in the United States have gross cystic disease.[6] Peak incidence is in the fifth decade, dropping dramatically in the menopause. On pathologic inspection cysts are brown to blue and contain semitranslucent or turbid fluid.[7] There are two basic types of cysts: simple and complex. Simple cysts are fluid filled, whereas complex cysts contain debris, either cellular material or blood. Women who have gross cysts are not at increased risk of developing breast cancer.[3, 5]

Fibroadenomas are the most frequent benign tumor in young women. In Haagensen's series, the mean age at diagnosis was 33.9 years.[6] Fibroadenomas are painless, slowly growing masses, which may appear as single or multiple lesions. Grossly, they are firm, freely movable nodules with sharp boundaries. They can vary in size from a few millimeters up to giant forms that occupy nearly the entire breast, although they are generally several centimeters in size when removed.[7] Fibroadenomas are generally considered to be benign[3, 5]; however, there have been reports of carcinoma occurring within fibroadenomas. One series found the mean age of this occurrence was 42.4 years for all patients and 47.0 years for patients with infiltrating carcinoma.[8] This mean is considerably higher than the average age of patients with simple fibroadenomas (33.9 years). A possible explanation for the differences in the peak age is that the two lesions, the benign and the malignant, occur independently. Furthermore, the cancer is thought to represent an incidental finding that is found at an earlier, in situ stage, because of the easily palpable fibroadenoma.

A review of benign disorders of the breast in older women found that older women do indeed experience benign problems of the breast and that even though the age-specific incidence of benign disorders drops dramatically after the menopause, benign disorders are more frequently encountered than carcinoma up to age 75. The most common problem after age 55 remains breast nodularity with or without pain. Discrete benign lumps (cysts and fibroadenomas) are proportionally much less common in women over age 55, but they do occur. The possibility of cystic carcinoma remains in any postmenopausal woman who develops a new breast cyst.[9]

DIAGNOSTIC METHODS

The initial evaluation of a patient with a breast mass is the performance of a careful history and breast examination. Historical information that helps to establish the patient's baseline risk for breast cancer includes age, menstrual status, parity, family history, alcohol use, exogenous hormone use (birth control pills and hormone therapy), and previous biopsy results showing atypical hyperplasia. Information that needs to be obtained specifically about the palpable mass is whether the patient has been performing breast self-examination for a significant period of time, whether the mass has changed over time or changes during a given cycle, and whether there is any pain or tenderness.

A complete breast examination should be performed. Findings suggestive of a cancer are masses that are hard, have irregular, indistinct borders, or are fixed to underlying or overlying structures. A lack of tenderness is a characteristic but not dependable sign. Dimpling of the skin and retraction of the nipple are suggestive of malignancy. Bloody nipple discharge also requires evaluation, as it is associated with malignancy in up to 5% of cases. Benign breast masses are soft to firm in consistency; have discrete, regular margins; and are freely mobile. Physiologic nodularity is soft and irregular, with areas of thickened bands or firm bead-like lumps or cysts, and has been said to feel like "lumpy oatmeal." The tissue is generally uniform in consistency, although it may be denser with prominent ridges in both upper outer quadrants.

Radiologic studies that can help in the evaluation of a dominant mass are mammography and ultrasound. Computed tomography and magnetic resonance imaging do not currently provide useful clinical information. Mammography is an important part of the evaluation of a palpable mass for women aged 35 and older. Women younger than this typically have very dense breast tissue that decreases the accuracy of mammography. The ability to detect cancers of the breast by mammography is increased in breasts that contain predominantly fat.[10–12] Older women generally have large amounts of fat in their breasts, and therefore the ability to detect early breast cancers is enhanced.[13] Mammography should be performed on women younger than 35 only if suspicion for malignancy is high. In this instance, mammography can help to characterize the mass and evaluate the breasts for clinically occult lesions. Women 35 years of age and older should have mammography performed in conjunction with a careful clinical breast examination. Even if a woman has had a mammogram performed in the past year, a repeat mammogram should be performed if a new palpable mass is appreciated.

Studies have found that clinical examination and mammography are complementary in screening for breast cancer and that neither one should be used in isolation. In one study, 16% of all breast cancers were found based on clinical examination alone and would have been missed if only mammography had been performed, whereas 45% of cancers were found on mammography alone and would have been missed if only a clinical breast examination were performed.[14] A second study found that 9.3% of clinically palpable tumors were not detected by mammography. On retrospective review, 9% (9/30) of these clinically palpable tumors could still not be seen on mammography. There was no statistically significant difference in tumor type, size, or lymph node involvement between the radiologically positive and negative groups.[15] These studies illustrate two points. First, neither clinical breast examination nor mammography should be performed in isolation, and second, a clinically palpable mass requires a thorough evaluation independent of whether the mass is visualized on mammography.

Breast ultrasound can be used alone or in conjunction with mammography. The rationale for using breast ultrasound is twofold. First, it portrays the breast tissue in a different format from that of mammography. Mammography displays a summation image in which three dimensions of tissue are shown in one plane, which may result in the superimposition of structures. Ultrasound acquires data in a slice-type format and therefore does not have this problem. Second, ultrasound is able to determine with essentially 100% accuracy whether a mass is a cyst or not. This distinction cannot be made by mammography.[16]

The principal indications for the use of breast ultrasound are (1) distinguishing a cystic from a solid mass, (2) evaluating a palpable mass with negative results on mammogram, (3) evaluating a palpable mass in a young patient (30 years of age or younger), and (4) providing guidance for interventional procedures.[17] The exact role ultrasound should play in the evaluation of a palpable breast mass is controversial. Although one investigator recommends its use,[18] another does not.[19] In his article, Feig suggests that ultrasound be the primary imaging study performed to evaluate a breast mass for women younger than 35 unless they have a family history of breast cancer.[18] The reasons for this recommendation are the lower breast cancer incidence among women younger than 35, the lower sensitivity of mammography in women of this age group, and the theoretic radiation risk from mammography. He suggests that women older than 35 should have a mammogram first. Ultrasound is then used as a second method, whether the mass is visualized by mammography or not, to determine whether the mass is cystic.[14]

Donegan states that ultrasound has no role in the evaluation of a palpable breast mass.[19] He suggests using needle aspiration as a routine part of evaluating a palpable mass, reasoning that it is a safe, a simple, and an inexpensive means of immediately distinguishing cystic from solid masses.[15] The difficulties with this position are that some women may prefer not to have the mass aspirated; others may have multiple masses, making aspiration less practical; and aspiration may result in a hematoma, making subsequent management more difficult.

Needle aspiration fluid should be sent for cytologic testing only if it is blood stained. This recommendation is based on a study that found routine cytologic examination of breast fluid was not cost effective, as only blood-stained breast fluids were associated with significant pathology, intracystic papilloma, and occult in situ lobular carcinoma.[20]

Solid masses can be further evaluated with the use of fine-needle aspiration (FNA). Fine-needle aspiration has been shown to be a safe, inexpensive, rapid method of establishing the diagnosis of breast cancer.[21–24] The role of FNA in the diagnosis of palpable breast masses remains uncertain because of the false positive and false negative cytologic diagnoses. In a review of the literature, Hammond and colleagues found that the specificity of FNA ranged from 98 to 100%, and the sensitivity ranged from 65 to 99%.[23] False positive results may occur with atypical epithelial proliferations, fibroadenomas, or inflammatory lesions. False negative aspirates may occur because of technical errors, cystic lesions, and underdiagnosis of low-grade neoplasms.[25] Given the significant false negative rate for FNA, it should not be used alone when formulating management decisions. It is ideally used as an adjunct to other diagnostic methods such as clinical breast examination and mammography (see subsequent discussion). The techniques for needle aspiration and FNA are described in two recent articles.[26, 27] Because sampling error can greatly affect the reliability of FNA, it is important that any person using the technique gain personal experience first by sampling lumps that will be excised and submitted for histologic evaluation.[28]

Each method—physical examination, mammography, and FNA—has a fixed false negative rate. The "triplet" management of breast lesions—palpation, mammography, and FNA—has been proposed to overcome the limitations of each individual method.[25, 29] Butler and co-workers found that all 86 patients who underwent these three studies with negative results had benign conditions. The incidence of cancer in patients who had a single suspicious or malignant test result was 6%; it was 64% in those who had two suspicious or malignant test results and 97% in those who had three suspicious or malignant test results.[29] Layfield and associates found cancer in 3 out of 457 (0.7%) cases in which all three test results were negative.[25] These findings do suggest that when this triplet management approach is applied prospectively, false negative results can occur. Close follow-up is therefore mandatory, and the ultimate decision on which masses to perform biopsies depends on clinical judgment.

EVALUATION

The first step in evaluating a patient with a dominant mass is to determine whether the finding represents a true dominant mass or merely prominent glandular tissue. The second step is to determine whether the dominant mass represents a cyst, a benign solid mass, or a cancer. These steps are discussed in what follows.

Clinical parameters that are helpful in distinguishing a dominant mass from physiologic nodularity are (1) presence of distinct borders on all sides, (2) difference in texture from background breast tissue (harder, firmer, or more rubbery), (3) persistence in both a sitting and a lying position, and (4) persistence over time. The patient's age must be considered when a decision cannot be made as to whether the patient has a breast mass based on these parameters alone. Women younger than 35 should have a repeat examination after one or two menstrual cycles, on day 7 to 14 of their menstrual cycle. If a question still remains, a breast surgeon can be consulted to repeat the examination. Women older than 35 should have a mammogram performed, and if the mass cannot be visualized an ultrasound should be obtained. If neither of these methods can visualize the mass, a breast surgeon should repeat the examination.

The evaluation of a dominant mass is based on the woman's age because both the differential diagnosis and the diagnostic studies used vary depending on age (Figs. 16–1, 16–2). Women in their twenties and thirties are most likely to have benign breast conditions, such as cysts and fibroadenomas, and breast cancer is fairly rare. Older women (especially those older than 50) have a higher incidence of breast cancer, although they continue to have benign breast conditions.

Women younger than 35 should be evaluated using ultrasound initially. An ultrasound examination can determine whether the mass is a cyst. If the mass is not a cyst, it could represent normal glandular tissue, a solid benign tumor, or a cancer. Ultrasound cannot distinguish among these possibilities. The distinction must be made based on

clinical examination. The previous section suggests maneuvers to help determine, on clinical examination, whether the woman has physiologic nodularity or a dominant mass. Mammograms are generally of less help in making this distinction because the glandular breast tissue is too dense for the study to be meaningful. This study should be reserved for situations in which the suspicion of breast cancer is high. Women who are thought to have a solid dominant mass can be watched carefully if the mass is less than 1 cm, is old, and is unchanging. An FNA biopsy can be performed for additional assurance that the mass is benign. Biopsies should be performed on solid masses that do not meet these criteria or masses in which the FNA is positive.

An alternative management plan suggested by Donegan is to start the evaluation using needle aspiration. The fluid from a simple cyst is not bloody, and the mass will disappear leaving only a temporary defect in the breast tissue. Failure to aspirate cyst fluid suggests a solid mass.[9]

Women older than 35 should have a mammogram first, as the incidence of breast cancer in these women is higher and the study can also be helpful in finding other abnormalities. An ultrasound should be performed if the mass appears to be benign (to determine if it is a cyst) or if the mass cannot be visualized on mammogram. A mass that cannot be visualized on mammography or ultrasound should be referred to a surgeon for repeat examination and consideration for biopsy. All suspicious lesions (on clinical examination or mammography) should be referred directly to a surgeon for evaluation.

MANAGEMENT

All patients regardless of their diagnosis should be encouraged to perform monthly breast self-examinations and to report any change immediately. Patients who are thought to have physiologic nodularity should receive routine follow-up, yearly clinical breast examinations. More frequent follow-up is recommended, every 3 to 6 months, if the examination is particularly difficult, allowing the examiner to maintain familiarity. Patients who were evaluated initially for a dominant mass, whether detected by the patient or a health care provider, and subsequently determined to have physiologic nodularity, need to be followed very closely. A repeat examination should be done at least every 3 months for 1 year to ensure that the patient does not have a dominant mass. A surgical referral should be made if there is any change or uncertainty. Patients who are at high risk for breast

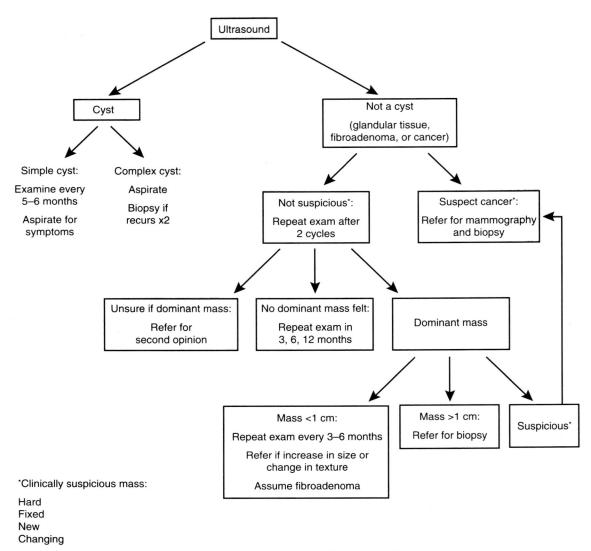

Figure 16–1. Work-up of a patient who is younger than 35 years and has a dominant breast mass.

cancer (who have first-degree relatives with breast cancer) but who do not have a dominant mass should receive a clinical breast examination every 6 months. If these women are found to have a dominant mass, they should be managed as discussed subsequently and always with careful and close follow-up.

Premenopausal women who have a simple cyst or cysts should receive clinical breast examinations every 6 months. There is no medical necessity to aspirate the cyst. The decision to aspirate is based on the patient's preference or the symptoms. A complex cyst needs to be aspirated and the fluid sent for cytologic testing. A biopsy should be performed on a complex cyst that recurs twice. A

postmenopausal woman who develops a new simple or complex cyst or cysts should have a biopsy performed on the cyst to exclude an intracystic carcinoma or a partially cystic cancer. A postmenopausal woman with an existing simple cyst that is unchanging should be examined every 6 months. A biopsy should be performed if there is any change in the cyst.

Patients who have a solid, benign-appearing mass are presumed to have a fibroadenoma. If this mass is under 1 cm, is old, and is unchanged, it can be observed with repeat examinations every 6 months. An FNA biopsy can be performed to provide additional evidence that this solid mass is benign. Evaluation by a surgeon for possible bi-

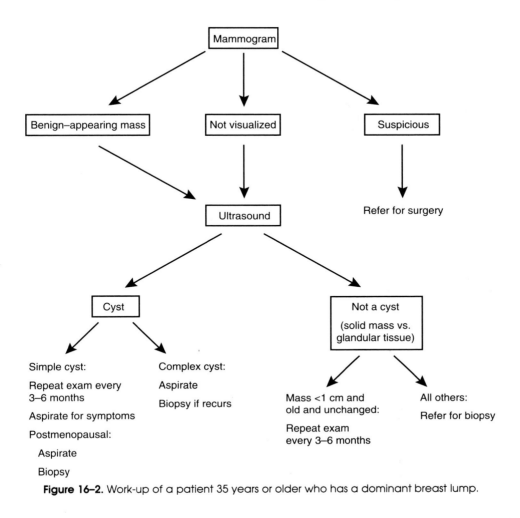

Figure 16–2. Work-up of a patient 35 years or older who has a dominant breast lump.

opsy is recommended when a woman has a solid mass that does not meet these criteria or when the results of the needle aspiration are positive.

Patients with suspicious masses either on clinical examination (hard, fixed, new, changing) or on mammography should be referred for surgical evaluation. These masses include ones that are appreciated on clinical examination that cannot be visualized radiographically. An FNA biopsy can be performed preoperatively. A positive result on biopsy allows the surgeon to plan the most appropriate procedure or to provide preoperative chemotherapy.

EVALUATION AND MANAGEMENT OF A PALPABLE BREAST MASS IN PREGNANT AND LACTATING WOMEN

Benign breast lesions frequently appearing as palpable masses in pregnant or lactating women include fibroadenomas, lipomas, papillomas, cystic disease, galactoceles, and inflammatory processes (mastitis and abscesses). A new breast lesion found during pregnancy can also represent a breast cancer. Nearly 3% of breast cancers in women younger than 41 appear during pregnancy. Historically, breast cancer occurring during pregnancy has been thought to offer a poor prognosis. Improved results suggest that the earlier findings may have been due to delays in diagnosis and treatment (delayed diagnosis averages 2 to 7 months longer for pregnant than for nonpregnant patients) rather than to differences in tumor characteristics. The histologic types of tumors found in pregnant and lactating women are the same as those found in nonpregnant women; inflammatory carcinoma is not more common.[30]

The emphasis is therefore placed on prompt diagnosis and treatment. Prompt diagnosis depends on the performance of careful clinical breast examination and the appropriate use of radiologic and other diagnostic studies. Clinical breast examination during pregnancy is difficult owing to breast engorgement, and it can be difficult to define the usually palpable tumor. Radiologic studies that can be used to evaluate a clinically palpable abnormality include mammography and ultrasound. Mammography is an indicated diagnostic tool even in pregnancy, particularly for the high-risk patient or for those with a suspicious palpable lesion, although it is limited by the density of breast tissue.[26, 31] Ultrasound is a useful technique to distinguish cystic from solid masses and is not limited by the density of breast tissue. Alternatively, needle aspiration can be performed to distinguish cystic from solid masses. Fine-needle aspiration has been shown to be a useful diagnostic tool for evaluating a solid breast mass. It can distinguish benign breast masses associated with pregnancy from those with marked atypia that require biopsy. Fine-needle aspiration in pregnancy has two major limitations. First, pregnancy-related changes in the breast can result in false positive results. Second, a negative FNA result does not exonerate the clinically or mammographically suspicious lesion. Patients with such lesions require further evaluation, including, if appropriate, an excisional biopsy.[32, 33]

Inflammatory processes should be considered in the pregnant or lactating woman presenting with a palpable breast mass. Mastitis typically appears as unilateral localized tenderness, redness, and heat along with systemic symptoms of fever, malaise, and sometimes nausea and vomiting. It is important to distinguish mastitis from breast engorgement or a plugged duct. Engorgement occurs early in the postpartum period and is bilateral and generalized over both breasts; it is not associated with fever or systemic illness. A plugged duct is usually unilateral and is noticed after feeding when there is a small discrete mass remaining. There is no fever or systemic illness. The management of mastitis includes continued breast-feeding to drain the affected lobules, local hot compresses, and treatment with a penicillinase-resistant penicillin or a cephalosporin for at least 10 days.[34, 35]

Breast abscess develops in 5 to 11% of women with infectious mastitis. The chance of abscess formation is increased with unnecessary weaning and subsequent milk stasis or with delay in antibiotic treatment of the mastitis. Treatment consists of incision and drainage along with antibiotics.[36]

Inflammatory processes, infectious mastitis, and breast abscesses also occur in the nonpuerperal period. Generally, in this period are premenopausal women with an average age of 40 years. Common presenting signs and symptoms are tenderness, pain and swelling, warmth and erythema, mass, chills and fever, and nipple discharge. There is no association between the development of mastitis and antecedent trauma or puerperal infections. Treatment of mastitis and breast abscesses is identical to that during the puerperal period.[37]

Confusion can occur between inflammatory breast carcinoma and benign inflammatory processes. On mammography the two processes can be identical; however, several days of antibiotics should dramatically improve a benign process. Ultrasound is more sensitive than mammography in detecting an abscess cavity, and FNA can confirm the presence of pus. A suggested management plan is to make a distinction on the basis of history and physical examination as to whether carcinoma or infection is the more likely. If carcinoma is a strong consideration, the patient should receive a mammogram and potentially a biopsy. If infection is a likely possibility, an ultrasound can be performed to look for an abscess cavity. Treatment is then directed as discussed earlier. If all signs and symptoms do not resolve completely within 7 to 14 days, or if there is still any clinical suspicion of a malignancy, a mammogram should be obtained.[33]

MASTALGIA

Mastalgia, or breast tenderness, also referred to as mastodynia, is a common symptom, occurring in more than half the women who present for routine breast screening. Because it rarely indicates a significant pathologic condition, there is relatively little study of its cause or of effective management. Many women present with mastalgia with a concern that the tenderness is an indicator of other pathologic processes, and once this possibility has been excluded, they do not require treatment for their symptoms. Other women seek relief of symptoms and require management for symptomatic improvement.

Mastalgia can be cyclic or noncyclic in nature. Cyclic symptoms usually begin during the luteal phase of the menstrual cycle and remit with onset of menses, similar to the process with other premenstrual symptoms (see Chapter 21). Mastalgia is not necessarily associated with nodularity on clinical breast examination; however, in one study an association was noted between cyclic mastalgia and glandular as opposed to fatty tissue on mammography.[38] The etiology of cyclic mastalgia is presumed to be related to hormonal changes of the menstrual cycle, given its relation to the menses, the increased prevalence through the third and fourth decades, and the decrease in symptoms after the menopause.

Noncyclic breast pain is infrequently associated with a palpable mass, benign or malignant. One study has suggested a link between previous breast pain and breast cancer, although the use of retrospective data collection from patients with breast cancer and controls may have resulted in significant recall bias.[39] No other data to suggest such a link have been demonstrated. Breast cysts that enlarge rapidly or that hemorrhage can be painful. Fibroadenomas are rarely painful. Mastitis also needs to be considered in a patient presenting with breast pain.

Evaluation of the patient presenting with mastalgia begins with a thorough breast examination and ancillary studies as indicated based on findings from the physical examination. Evaluation of suspected dominant masses proceeds as discussed previously. Mammography is reserved for evaluation of abnormal findings on clinical examination or for screening as appropriate based on the patient's age. Biopsy is not indicated for evaluation of mastalgia alone without other findings on physical examination or radiographic studies to suggest a dominant mass.

A number of therapies have been suggested, especially for cyclic mastalgia; however, only a few have been tested on large groups of subjects in a randomized, double-blind fashion. Bromocriptine and danazol have been the most thoroughly investigated agents. However, despite the fact that studies reported significant improvement in symptoms with both of these medications, large numbers of women in both sets of trials withdrew owing to severe side effects from the medications. Bromocriptine, in doses of 5 mg daily, improved scores of breast pain in 20 to 47% of women, but as many as one third of them dropped out of the treatment group owing to side effects of nausea, dizziness, vomiting, and postural hypotension.[40, 41] Danazol, in initial doses of 200 mg daily tapering to 100 mg on alternate days during the second half of the menstrual cycles over 4 to 6 months, also relieved symptoms, but side effects including irregular menses and hirsutism occurred in more than half of all patients.[40]

Other therapies studied in small series without controls include luteinizing hormone releasing hormone analogues,[42] diuretics, hypnosis, beta-carotene,[43] and vitamin B_6. Tamoxifen has been shown to reduce mastalgia in doses of 10 to 20 mg daily, but given the unknown effects of this medication on premenopausal women, its use is not recommended for this purpose. Evening primrose oil, in doses of 3 gm daily, has been shown to benefit some women, with results similar to those for bromocriptine. Randomized trials of progestins have not shown them to be effective.[44] Vi-

tamin E is often advocated, but studies have shown little effect. Its use in doses of 200 to 400 mg daily is probably not harmful and has no side effects.

Caffeine and other methylxanthines have been suggested as etiologic agents of mastalgia, although in at least one study, there was no difference in mean levels of consumption between women with and without symptoms.[45] One study found a statistically significant, although small, improvement in a group of women who discontinued caffeine for 4 months compared with the results in a control group.[46] Another study found that a diet with fewer fats and more complex carbohydrates decreased symptoms.[47]

Given the current data, it is prudent to attempt those therapies that produce minimal or no side effects, which may provide some relief for the majority of women. A trial of discontinuing all caffeine products for several months should be attempted, with a warning to heavy consumers of caffeine that sudden discontinuation will lead to withdrawal headaches. Local measures including cool compresses can be effective. The use of athletic support brassieres when symptoms are present, including use at night if nocturnal symptoms are reported, can be effective. A trial of diet modification to lower fat and increase carbohydrates may be of help and is clearly of benefit for other preventive indications. Use of bromocriptine or danazol should be reserved for patients with the most severe symptoms and no response to other measures.

REFERENCES

1. Ries LG, Hankey BF, Edwards BK. Cancer Statistics Review 1973–1987. Bethesda, Md: Department of Health and Human Services, Public Health Service, No. 90-2789, 1990.
2. Bland KI, Love N. Evaluation of common breast masses. Postgrad Med 1992;92:95.
3. London SJ, Connolly JL, Schnitt SJ, Colditz GA. A prospective study of benign breast disease and the risk of breast cancer. JAMA 1992;267:941.
4. Love SM, Gelman RS, Silen W. Fibrocystic ''disease'' of the breast—A nondisease? N Engl J Med 1982;307:1010.
5. Dupont WD, Page DL. Risk factors for breast cancer in women with proliferative breast disease. N Engl J Med 1985;312:146.
6. Haagensen CD. Diseases of the Breast. 3rd ed. Philadelphia: WB Saunders, 1986.
7. Tobon H, Doshi N. Breast pathology synopsis. Semin Ultrasound CT MR 1989;10:139.
8. Pick PW, Iossifides IA. Occurrence of breast carcinoma within a fibroadenoma. A review. Arch Pathol Lab Med 1984;108(7):590.
9. Devitt JE. Benign disorders of the breast in older women. Surg Gynecol Obstet 1986;162:340.
10. Clark RL, Copeland MM, Egan RL, et al. Reproducibility of the technic of mammography (Egan) for cancer of the breast. Am J Surg 1965;109:127.
11. Strax P, Venet L, Shapiro S, Gross S. Mammography and

clinical examination in mass screening for cancer of the breast. Cancer 1967;12:2184.

12. McClow MV, Williams AC. Mammographic examinations (4030): Ten-year clinical experience in a community medical center. Ann Surg 1973;177:616.

13. Tabar L, Dean PB. Mammographic parenchymal patterns. Risk indicator for breast cancer. JAMA 1982;247:185.

14. Moskowitz M. The predictive value of certain mammographic signs in screening for breast cancer. Cancer 1983;51:1007.

15. Cahill CJ, Boulter PS, Gibbs NM, Price JL. Features of mammographically negative breast tumors. Br J Surg 1981;68:882.

16. Dempsey PJ. The importance of resolution in the clinical application of breast sonography. Ultrasound Med Biol 1988;14:43.

17. Reynolds HE, Jackson VP. The role of ultrasound in breast imaging. Appl Radiol 1991; p 55.

18. Feig SA. The role of ultrasound in a breast imaging center. Semin Ultrasound CT MR 1989;10:90.

19. Donegan WL. Evaluation of a palpable breast mass. N Engl J Med 1992;327:937.

20. Ciatto S, Cariaggi P, Bulgaresi P. The value of routine cytologic examination of breast cyst fluids. Acta Cytol 1987;31:301.

21. Adye B, Jolly PC, Bauermeister DE. The role of fine-needle aspiration in the management of solid breast masses. Arch Surg 1988;124:37.

22. Goodson WH, Mallman R, Miller TR. Three year follow-up of benign fine-needle aspiration biopsies of the breast. Am J Surg 1987;154:58.

23. Hammond S, Keyhani-Rofagha S, O'Toole RV. Statistical analysis of fine needle aspiration cytology of the breast. Acta Cytol 1987;31:276.

24. Wilkinson EJ, Schuettke CM, Ferrier CM, et al. Fine needle aspiration of breast masses. Acta Cytol 1989;33:613.

25. Layfield LJ, Glasgow BJ, Cramer H. Fine-needle aspiration in the management of breast masses. Pathol Annu 1989;24:23.

26. Herbst AL. Breast biopsy techniques. Clin Obstet Gynecol 1989;32:800.

27. Wilkinson EJ, Bland KI. Techniques and results of aspiration cytology for diagnosis of benign and malignant diseases of the breast. Surg Clin North Am 1990;70:801.

28. Abele JS, Miller TR, Goodson WH, et al. Fine-needle aspiration of palpable breast masses. A program for staged implementation. Arch Surg 1983;118:859.

29. Butler JA, Vargas HI, Worthen N, Wilson SE. Accuracy of combined clinical-mammographic-cytologic diagnosis of dominant breast mass. Arch Surg 1990;125:893.

30. Donegan WL. Cancer and pregnancy. CA Cancer J Clin 1983;33:194.

31. Parente JT, Amsel M, Lerner R, Chinea F. Breast cancer associated with pregnancy. Obstet Gynecol 1988;71:861.

32. Novotny DB, Maygarden SJ, Shermer RW, Frable WJ. Fine needle aspiration of benign and malignant breast masses associated with pregnancy. Acta Cytol 1991; 35:676.

33. Finley JL, Silverman JF, Lannin DR. Fine-needle aspiration cytology of breast masses in pregnant and lactating women. Diagn Cytopathol 1989;5:255.

34. Lawrence RA. The puerperium, breastfeeding, and breast milk. Curr Opin Obstet Gynecol 1990;2:23.

35. Marshall BR, Hepper JK, Zirbel CC. Sporadic puerperal mastitis. JAMA 1975;233:1377.

36. Olsen CG, Gordon RE. Breast disorders in nursing mothers. AFP 1990;41:1509.

37. Leveque J, Lorino CO, Ferrara JJ. Inflammatory disease of the breast. Cancer Res 1990;119:18.

38. Leinster SJ, Whitehouse GH, Walsh PV. Cyclical mastalgia: Clinical and mammographic observations in a screened population. Br J Surg 1987;74:220.

39. Plu-Bureau G, Thalabard JC, Sitruk-Ware R, et al. Cyclical mastalgia as a marker of breast cancer susceptibility: Results of a case-control study among French women. Br J Cancer 1992;65:946.

40. Gateley CA, Mansel RE. Management of the painful and nodular breast. Br Med Bull 1991;47:284.

41. Mansel RE, Dogliotti L. European multicentre trial of bromocriptine in cyclical mastalgia. Lancet 1990;335:190.

42. Hamed H, Caleffi M, Chaudary MA, Fentiman IS. LHRH analogue for treatment of recurrent and refractory mastalgia. Ann R Coll Surg Engl 1990;72:221.

43. Santamaria DL, Santamaria AB. Cancer chemoprevention by supplemental carotenoids and synergism with retinol in mastodynia treatment. Med Oncol Tumor Pharmocother 1990;7:153.

44. Maddox PR, Harrison BJ, Horobin, JM, et al. A randomised controlled trial of medroxyprogesterone acetate in mastalgia. Ann R Coll Surg Engl 1990;72:71.

45. Campbell BG, Tachtenbarg DE, Barclay A. Cyclic breast pain. J Fam Pract 1984;19:549.

46. Ernster VL, Mason L, Goodson WH, et al. Effect of caffeine-free diet on benign breast disease: A randomized trial. Surgery 1982;91:263.

47. Boyd NF, Shannon P, Kriukov V, et al. Effect of a low-fat high-carbohydrate diet on symptoms of clinical mastopathy. Lancet 1988;2:128.

Breast Cancer: Epidemiology, Screening, and Prevention

Marianne N. Prout

EPIDEMIOLOGY OF BREAST CANCER

The magnitude of breast cancer as a health problem for women in the United States and around the world is not easily summarized by a single statistical measure. Familiarity with the cumulative incidence, incidence rates, mortality rates, case-survival rates, secular trends in the United States, and international data is helpful in understanding current strategies for breast cancer screening and prevention.

The lifetime cumulative incidence is often cited in promotional literature by advocacy groups to highlight the impact of this disease and to emphasize its increasing frequency in aging populations. The recent revision of lifetime risk of breast cancer for U.S. women from one in 10 to one in nine and now one in eight reflects the increasing incidence of breast cancer noted from 1980 to 1987 and the inclusion of data on women older than 85.[1-10]

Incidence rates of breast cancer in women vary by age, increasing sharply until about age 45 in the United States, plateauing (Clemmesen's hook) for women aged 45 to 50, and then increasing through age 75.[2] Secular trends in the age-standardized incidence rates for women in the United States include a steady slow increase since the 1960s with a rapid increase of approximately 4% per year from 1982 to 1987; incidence rates are level in the 1988 and 1989 data. Many reasons have been proposed for the rapid increase in incidence during most of the 1980s, including that increased screening has diagnosed cases that would otherwise remain undetected for 2 to 7 years and that delayed childbirth has led to an increased number of women in the high-risk category.[3-5] Internationally, the high U.S. incidence rate is shared by most Western countries but is five times the rate in Japan, where there is almost no increase in incidence rate with increasing age.

Breast cancer was projected to be the cause of 46,000 deaths in women in the United States in 1994. Breast cancer mortality rates have changed little over the past 50 years. Increasing case-survival rates account for the stable overall mortality rate, with the 5-year survival rate from breast cancer in U.S. women increasing from 60% in the 1950s to 75% in the 1980s. This stable mortality rate unfortunately represents a conglomerate of increasing and decreasing mortality rates. Breast cancer mortality rates have increased in women older than 55, and they have decreased in younger women. In addition, differences in case-survival rates for breast cancer in black and white women are striking. In the United States, 63% of black women live for 5 years after diagnosis of breast cancer compared with 78% of white women. Additional analyses have attributed most of the decreased survival in groups of women who are elderly, minority, and of low socioeconomic status to more advanced stage at diagnosis, implicating delayed diagnosis or inadequate screening as a risk for mortality in these groups.[6-10]

Factors associated with a statistically increased risk of breast cancer have been identified in abundance in case-control and cohort studies. Any discussion of such risk factors must be read with caution, however, as *all* U.S. women must be regarded and screened as high risk for breast cancer. In spite of the dramatic international variations in breast cancer rates and the plethora of epidemiologic studies in the United States, few breast cancers can be attributed to these identified risks because most factors are prevalent and accompanied by small relative risks.[11, 12] In addition, whether the risk factors are causal or independent of each other is unclear.

FAMILY HISTORY

After age, the strongest risk factor for breast cancer is a family history of breast cancer. Both the number of family members with breast cancer and the age at diagnosis of breast cancer strongly affect the relative risk.[13, 14] For example, a maternal history of breast cancer after age 60 increases the relative risk to 1.5. A family history of breast cancer in multiple first-degree relatives (mother, sisters, daughters) or of premenopausal breast cancer is associated with relative risks of 2.0 to 6.0. Studies have explored the association of prostate and breast cancer in male relatives with breast cancer in women and identified the need to obtain paternal family cancer histories.[15]

HORMONAL FACTORS

A number of hormonal factors, both endogenous and exogenous, have been associated with increased risk for breast cancer.[11, 12] The timing of hormonal events, the dose and duration of exogenous hormones, and the underlying genetic risk may all eventually prove important, but currently the interactions are poorly understood. Early menarche is a weak risk factor, with a relative risk of 1.2 associated with menarche before age 12 versus after age 14. Nulliparity or late age at first childbirth (note risk decreases with early childbirth, not with pregnancy) increases the relative risk to approximately 2 compared with first childbirth before age 20. Late menopause, after age 55, is also associated with a doubling of relative risk compared with menopause before age 45.

The effects of exogenous hormones on breast cancer risk have been intensely studied, and the data defy simple interpretations or translation into clinical guidelines.[16–21] Oral contraceptive use has repeatedly been associated with a lower risk for benign breast disease, even considering the problems of definition of benign breast disease. The most consistent association of oral contraceptive use and increased risk of breast cancer is an increase in risk for breast cancer for women younger than 45. This subset analysis, however, is based on small numbers. Other subset analyses have looked at family history, type of oral contraceptive used, duration of use, parity, and other known risk factors and have not produced consistent results.[16, 17] Equally controversial is the association of postmenopausal estrogen therapy with increased breast cancer risk.[18–21] Most studies have shown a positive association, although not a statistically significant increase, in breast cancer risk with estrogen use. Thus, the conclusion of many epide-

miologists is that a weak but positive association is indicated by current data. Further work is concentrating on identifying subgroups of women at significantly increased risk and on types or patterns of hormone therapy associated with increased risk, but conclusions are premature. Data are insufficient on the effects of adding progesterone to estrogen on breast cancer risk in postmenopausal women. Increased risk for breast cancer has been noted among women who used diethylstilbestrol during pregnancy; further studies of their daughters are ongoing to assess their breast cancer risks.

DIET

The role of diet in the etiology and growth of breast cancers has generated many studies and even more controversies.[22–29] Ecologic analyses correlate international variations in breast cancer mortality rates with dietary fat intake. Case-control and cohort analyses in the United States and elsewhere provide mixed estimates of the association between total dietary fat intake or polyunsaturated fat intake and breast cancer risk. Other investigations have concentrated on the roles of obesity, body mass, and body fat distribution as indicators of breast cancer risk. The most frequently proposed mechanism of dietary fat influence on breast cancer evolution is an increase in the production of estrogenic compounds from androgenic precursors in postmenopausal women. If this is the primary mechanism, dietary factors must be integrated into other endogenous and exogenous hormonal events, and the potential confounders in studies of dietary factors are indeed complex. Alcohol consumption has been associated with an increased risk for breast cancer in the majority of studies that have included it as a dietary factor; consumption of five to seven drinks per week is associated with relative risks of approximately 1.5.[30–34] Pathophysiologic mechanisms are being investigated, and alcohol-induced increases in estrogen levels have been reported.[35]

Exposure to ionizing radiation, especially in early adolescence, is associated with increased risk for breast cancer. The potential risk of very low levels of exposure to radon, electromagnetic fields, and low-energy fields is undefined but has created consumer concerns about such exposure from electric blankets and from living near an electrical substation.[11]

Early reports that benign breast disease was associated with an increased risk of breast cancer have been clarified for pathologic distinctions within this category. Women with nonproliferative disease or proliferative disease without atypia have no increased risk, whereas hyperplasia is associated with increased risk (see Chapter 16).

THE BIOLOGIC BASIS FOR SCREENING RECOMMENDATIONS

An understanding of the natural history of breast cancer serves as a basis for appreciating the dilemmas in breast cancer screening and early detection. Breast cancers exhibit a wide range from indolent to aggressive biologic behaviors.[36, 37] Bloom and colleagues reported the median survival period of untreated patients with breast cancer (those who declined treatment) as 2.7 years, with several patients living decades.[38] The median tumor doubling time for breast lesions observed on mammograms is about 200 days; a 1-cm tumor containing 10^9 cells would represent 30 doublings or about 10 years of growth. Estimated doubling times have ranged from 25 to 1800 days; therefore, the calculated duration of the preclinical phase of breast cancer, of the time from a single cancer cell to a 1-cm tumor, ranges from under 2 years to well over 15 years. Of particular importance for early detection is the duration of the *detectable* preclinical phase of cancer. If mammography detects 1 mm of cancer and clinical examination detects 1 cm, the lead time for mammography would be nine doubling times. Cancers with doubling times as short as 30 days would progress from undetected to clinically apparent in 9 months, whereas cancers with doubling times of 100 days would not be apparent on mammograms for almost 3 years.

Early Detection and Screening for Breast Cancer

Three methods are commonly advocated for the early detection of breast cancer in individuals and have been applied for the mass screening of populations: mammography, clinical breast examination, and breast self-examination (BSE). The utility of these and other potential screening examinations is evaluated and compared for specific populations or subgroups by measures of sensitivity (the percentage of women with cancer who have a positive result on examination), specificity (the percentage of women without breast cancer who have a negative result on examination), and predictive value of a positive result (the percentage of women with a positive result who have cancer). Many other measures have been used to compare potential screening approaches, including changes in mortality and costs per year of life saved.

Breast Self-Examination

The value of BSE is debated.[39–41] Its evaluation by standard screening parameters such as sensitivity, specificity, and predictive value has been limited by unreliable methods to measure and to validate the actual practice by individual women, both in terms of frequency and quality of their examinations. Studies using breast models have estimated the mean sensitivity for detection of lumps in the models in a testing situation as 55%; for untrained volunteer women the detection rate was estimated as 25% for a broad range of sizes of lumps. Several retrospective studies have shown an association between smaller tumor size at diagnosis and self-reported regular practice of BSE; however, the issues of recall bias and the variation in examination quality limit the assessment of the impact of BSE. The independent role of BSE is even harder to assess because clinical breast examinations and mammograms are additional healthy habits selected by adherents to BSE. In the Breast Cancer Detection Demonstration Project, the sensitivity of BSE was 26% in women who were also being screened by clinical examination and mammography.[42] Theoretically, the impact of BSE in women participating in regular mammography and clinical breast examinations should be confined to the early detection of interval cancers; these cancers are also more aggressive biologically, and thus their size and stage at diagnosis are subject to length bias when compared with cancers diagnosed at annual screening.

The efficacy of clinical breast examination is also difficult to evaluate because the skill of the examiner and the characteristics of the individual breast can each affect the sensitivity and specificity of the examination. Estimated sensitivity of physician breast examination is 85 to 90% for lumps of 1.0 cm in diameter. Specificity generally decreases as sensitivity increases for physical examination. Preliminary data comparing mammography and clinical breast examination from the Canadian breast cancer screening trial are available but controversial.[41]

Mammography remains the gold standard for breast cancer screening, with evaluation in randomized controlled studies estimating mortality reductions from breast cancer of 30% for screened versus unscreened populations.[43, 44] An ongoing Canadian trial has challenged the role of mammography versus clinical breast examination in reduction of breast cancer mortality, but the results are still preliminary.[45, 46] Questions remain about the age at which mammographic screening should begin, the optimal interval between examinations to achieve best sensitivity and control costs, and

TABLE 17–1. American Cancer Society Recommendations: Breast Cancer Screening in Asymptomatic Women

TEST	AGE	FREQUENCY
Breast self-examination	20 and older	Every mo
Breast clinical examination	20–40	Every 3 yr
	Older than 40	Every yr
Mammography	40–49	Every 1–2 yr*
	50 and older	Every yr

*The National Cancer Institute does not recommend the routine use of mammography for breast cancer screening in this age group.
From Cancer Manual. 8th ed. Boston: American Cancer Society, Massachusetts Division, 1990.

the sensitivity and specificity of the test in various age groups.[43–53] Randomized controlled studies of mammography have not demonstrated a statistically significant effect on breast cancer mortality for women in the 40 to 49 age group; however, a 30% decrease in mortality at 10 years has been reported for women in the 50 to 60 age group, as emphasized in a highly publicized review.[54] Criticisms of this review focus on problems of pooling data from studies conducted in several countries over a 25-year time span. In addition, some studies used single-view mammography, several studies used screening intervals of 24 or more months, and technical quality was poorly controlled in many studies.[55] Quality control of mammography has become a major concern of women's groups and has resulted in passage of regulations nationally.[56]

The sensitivity of mammography varies by age, with improved sensitivity accompanying the glandular atrophy that occurs after menopause. Estimated sensitivities are generally reported as about 80% for women older than 50 and 60% for women younger than 50. The issues on the effectiveness of screening women younger than 50 include not only the lower incidence of breast cancer in this age group, which lowers the predictive value of an abnormal mammogram, but also the lower sensitivity of the test in this age group.[50, 53] The specificity of mammography is high, an estimated 95%. The predictive value of a positive finding on mammography remains low, and controversies abound about what percentage of mammographically indicated biopsies should reveal cancer. Currently biopsies are recommended when the probability of cancer is 10 to 20%.

The costs of breast cancer screening have created many controversies. Eddy has modeled the costs per year of life saved when women older than 50 are screened annually for 10 years: clinical breast examinations cost approximately $15,000 per year of life saved; adding mammography raises this cost to $20,000 to $90,000 per year of

life saved.[51] Note that screening studies to date have not addressed the issue of screening women older than 65 and that cost models have looked at a relatively short time period of screening.[52]

GUIDELINES FOR BREAST CANCER SCREENING

Guidelines for breast cancer screening have been issued for populations and for individuals by several groups who have placed different emphases on costs, sensitivity, specificity, and predictive value.[49, 53] Guidelines issued by the American Cancer Society are summarized in Table 17–1, which also notes how these guidelines vary from recent recommendations by the National Cancer Institute. Unresolved issues in breast cancer screening include both the effectiveness and the cost-effectiveness of screening women younger than 50 and older than 65, the optimal periodicity of screening mammograms for various ages, the utility of baseline mammograms, and the role of BSE.[54, 55] The National Cancer Institute no longer recommends breast cancer screening by mammography for all women aged 40 to 49 but advises such women to discuss the use of mammography individually with their physicians.

Special groups fall outside the screening guidelines and require individualized special management. Women with family histories of premenopausal breast cancer generally begin regular mammography when they are 5 years younger than the age at diagnosis of their relatives. Thus, a woman whose mother had breast cancer at age 40 would begin mammographic screening at age 35. For women whose relatives had breast cancer at very young ages, the management strategy should incorporate consideration of pregnancies, the total number of mammograms that would be performed, the clarity of physical examination and mammograms, and the patient's adherence to BSE. Patients should be managed during pregnancy with clinical breast examination at 3- to 4-month intervals and should have new baseline postpartum mammograms after the clinical examination stabilizes. Patients with multiple relatives with cancers at young ages should be considered for genetic testing to further refine their risk.

Quality control of mammographic screening has received both medical and political attention. The American College of Radiology, in conjunction with the American Cancer Society, has defined standards for quality control of facilities and staff performing mammograms and physicians reading mammograms. These have been incorporated into regulations in the Mammography Quality Standards Act of 1992 enacted by the U.S. Congress but with no allocation of funds to establish a review and accrediting program. Concerns of regulators include the machines used, the maintenance and monitoring of machines for image quality and radiation doses, the procedures used in performing studies and in notifying patients and their physicians, and the training and experience of personnel performing mammography and physicians interpreting the results.[56]

Additional techniques for detecting breast cancer have no established role in screening asymptomatic women for cancer, although they may be under investigation or have diagnostic value. Thermography was evaluated early in the Breast Cancer Demonstration and Detection Project and classified as ineffective. Ultrasonography is a useful procedure to complement mammography by quickly distinguishing masses as cystic or solid, as a first diagnostic procedure in young women with palpable abnormalities, and in localizing nonpalpable lesions for biopsy. Current studies include combining ultrasonography with Doppler studies to define whether enhanced blood flow can differentiate benign from malignant tumors. Ultrasonography is not, however, useful as an initial cancer screening technique. Magnetic resonance imaging is also being studied for its role in evaluating small lesions seen mammographically, especially in women with dense breasts on mammograms. It is unlikely to be useful in initial screening in the near future because of its high cost and time considerations.

The underutilization of breast cancer screening by U.S. women remains a persistent problem.[57–64] In repeated national surveys, the percentage of women who report having a mammogram in the previous 12 months has been steadily increasing: in 1990, 40% of women aged 40 to 49 but only 28% of women aged 60–69 had mammograms in the prior year. Other factors associated with lower rates of mammograms included lower income, lower education, and minority status. The most frequently cited reasons for not having mammography were that women did not know they needed a mammogram or their doctor had not advised them to have a mammogram. Approaches to improve breast cancer screening utilization have stressed public education and physician practice. The impact of such approaches requires evaluation using population-based data from cancer registries and vital statistics bureaus to identify trends in incidence and mortality rates for targeted geographic areas and groups.

FOLLOW-UP OF ABNORMAL RESULTS ON MAMMOGRAPHY

Clinicians must incorporate the information from mammograms as one more test result, appreciating the limitations of the examinations. A normal result on mammography in the setting of an abnormal finding on clinical breast examination does not rule out cancer[65] or preclude further evaluation. Only 80 to 85% of breast cancers present mammographically as a mass, a cluster of calcifications, or both. Clinicians must integrate clinical information and mammographic reports with an appreciation of the probability of cancer based on a given mammographic finding and review of all earlier mammograms. Current mammograms should always be compared with prior mammograms to enhance the detection of subtle changes and to evaluate the stability of any abnormalities. Comparisons should include not just the earlier study but the earliest good quality films, so that indolent cancers can be appreciated.

Nonpalpable mammographic findings result in biopsies for 0.5 to 2% of women undergoing screening mammography; lower rates apply to women receiving repeated mammograms. Many reports address the cancer yield on biopsies for various types of mammographic abnormalities; generally the rate is 15 to 30%.[66] High yields of cancer (over 25%) are associated with changes from a prior mammogram, architectural distortion, irregularly defined or stellate masses, densities with microcalcifications, and clusters of more than 10 microcalcifications.[67] Careful follow-up of a large series of "abnormal, probably benign" mammograms reported subsequent cancer diagnosis in 0.5%; noncalcified, well-defined solid nodules constituted the initial mammographic picture for most of these cancers.[68] Small calcifications account for more than half of abnormal mammograms and classifications as suspicious or benign calcifications can be subjective.

Mammographic patterns have also been evaluated as independent predictors of breast cancer risk. Mammograms with dense tissue are problematic as such patterns not only reduce the sensitivity of mammography for detecting early breast cancers but densities on mammograms in women over age 45 are associated with increased risk for breast cancer, with relative risks of 1.5 to 2.[69, 70]

Women with suspicious mammographic findings, clinical breast examinations, or both must have tissue evaluation; localization techniques are used for nonpalpable abnormalities. The types of biopsies range from excisional to incisional to fine-needle aspiration, and surgical controversies remain about the sensitivity, specificity, morbidity and costs of these approaches.[71] Breast biopsy should be routinely done as an outpatient procedure. A patient should be followed up in 3 to 4 months following a biopsy to establish a new ''baseline'' mammogram and to ensure that a small cancer was not missed by the biopsy.

PREVENTION OF BREAST CANCER

The prevention of breast cancer is a goal with very high appeal to clinicians, researchers, and the general public, at least in theory. The many controversies that have surrounded the initiation of the Breast Cancer Prevention Trial of the National Surgical Adjuvant Breast and Bowel Project, however, provide lessons on the complexities and uncertainties that surround cancer prevention.[72–74] Individual patients at high risk for breast cancer have few preventive options; current choices include prophylactic mastectomies, low-fat diets, and participation in clinical trials of tamoxifen and 4-HPR, the synthetic retinoid *N*-(4-hydroxyphenyl)retinamide. These approaches employ very different strategies to control breast cancer evolution and progression, but all inherently involve risk versus benefit determinations. Accurately estimating a woman's risk for breast cancer remains difficult despite a computer model now widely utilized.[12] Balancing the risk of breast cancer and other chronic diseases with the risks of each prevention strategy is even more tenative.

The various approaches to breast cancer prevention attempt to control different steps of carcinogenesis. Prophylactic mastectomy attempts to remove the tissue at risk for development of breast cancer; in actuality, such surgeries often just reduce the amount of tissue at risk, leaving a small amount of breast tissue attached to the nipple and areolar complex. Dietary modifications to reduce the risk of breast and other cancers have been recommended by several groups.

Many recommendations, based on animal studies and international variations, include reduction of dietary fat intake to prevent breast cancer; increased intake of fruits and vegetables is also suggested. Disagreements abound concerning the level of dietary fat intake needed to test whether reduction in dietary fat reduces breast cancer risk and what biologic markers can be used to verify dietary adherence and to correlate with breast cancer risks. Dietary fat intakes of 20% or less and monitoring of serum cholesterol and estradiol levels have been proposed. Some large-scale clinical trials of low-fat diets have been postponed pending further development of biomarkers for effective dietary intervention and better understanding of the age-specific effects on breast cancer risk.[75–78]

Chemoprevention utilizes specific pharmacologic agents aimed at interrupting or inhibiting events in carcinogenesis such as the mutation, proliferation, or dedifferentiation of cells.[79, 80] Tamoxifen, an antiestrogen with weak estrogenic activity, is being evaluated in a randomized, double-blind, placebo-controlled clinical trial of healthy women who have a risk for breast cancer equivalent to that of a 60-year-old woman. The trial is designed to test whether tamoxifen decreases the incidence of invasive breast cancer, the mortality from breast cancer or heart disease, or the incidence of bone fractures.[81] 4-HPR, a synthetic retinoid that concentrates in breast tissue, is being evaluated in Italy in women who have had unilateral breast cancer to see if contralateral breast cancer is prevented.[82]

All approaches for breast cancer prevention require years of systematic evaluation in thousands of women to establish efficacy. These studies depend on the support of primary care clinicians in the recruitment and follow-up of their patients in breast cancer prevention trials.[83, 84]

REFERENCES

1. Boring C, Squires T, Tong T. Cancer statistics, 1993. CA Cancer J Clin 1993;43:7.
2. Kessler L. The relationship between age and incidence of breast cancer. Cancer 1992;69:1896.
3. Miller B, Feuer E, Hankey B. Recent incidence trends for breast cancer in women and the relevance of early detection: An update. CA Cancer J Clin 1993;43:27.
4. Tarone R, Chu K. Implications of birth cohort patterns in interpreting trends in breast cancer rates. J Natl Cancer Inst 1992;84:1402.
5. White E, Lee C, Kristal A. Evaluation of the increase in breast cancer incidence in relation to mammography use. J Natl Cancer Inst 1990;82:1546.
6. Bassett M, Krieger N. Social class and black-white differences in breast cancer survival. Am J Public Health 1986;76:1400.
7. Dayal H, Power R, Chiu C. Race and socio-economic status in survival from breast cancer. J Chronic Dis 1982;35:675.
8. Freeman H, Wasfie T. Cancer of the breast in poor black women. Cancer 1989;63:2562.

9. Mandelblatt J, Andrews H, Kerner J, et al. Determinants of late stage diagnosis of breast and cervical cancer: The impact of age, race, social class, and hospital type. Am J Public Health 1991;81:646.

10. Silliman R, Balducci L, Goodwin J, et al. Breast cancer care in old age: What we know, don't know, and do. J Natl Cancer Inst 1993;85:190.

11. Harris J, Lippman M, Veronesi U, Willett W. Breast cancer. N Engl J Med 1992;327:319, 390, 473.

12. Gail M, Brinton L, Byar D. Projecting individualized probabilities of developing breast cancer for white females who are being examined annually. J Natl Cancer Inst 1989;81:1879.

13. Lynch H, Guirgis H, Brodkey F. Early age of onset in familial breast cancer: Genetic and cancer control implications. Arch Surg 1976;111:126.

14. Roseman D, Straus A, Shorey W. A positive family history of breast cancer: Does its effect diminish with age? Arch Intern Med 1990;150:191.

15. Anderson D, Badzioch M. Breast cancer risks in relatives of male breast cancer patients. J Natl Cancer Inst 1992;84:1114.

16. Bernstein L, Ross R, Henderson B. Relationship of hormone use to cancer risk. J Natl Cancer Inst Monographs 1992;12:137.

17. McGonigle K, Huggins G. Oral contraceptives and breast disease. Fertil Steril 1991;56:799.

18. Bergkvist L, Adami H, Persson I, et al. The risk of breast cancer after estrogen and estrogen-progestin replacement. N Engl J Med 1989;321:293.

19. Ernster V, Bush T, Huggins G, et al. Risks and benefits of menopausal hormone use. Prev Med 1988;17:201.

20. Harris R, Namboodiri K, Wynder E. Breast cancer risk: Effects of estrogen replacement therapy and body mass. J Natl Cancer Inst 1992;84:1575.

21. Wingo P, Layde P, Lee N, et al. The risk of breast cancer in postmenopausal women who have used estrogen replacement therapy. JAMA 1987;257:209.

22. Chu S, Lee N, Wingo P, et al. The relationship between body mass and breast cancer among women enrolled in the cancer and steroid hormone study. J Clin Epidemiol 1991;44:1197.

23. Graham S, Marshall J, Mettlin C, et al. Diet in the epidemiology of breast cancer. Am J Epidemiol 1982;116:68.

24. Howe G, Friedenreich C, Jain M, Miller A. A cohort study of fat intake and risk of breast cancer. J Natl Cancer Inst 1991;83:336.

25. Hulka B. Dietary fat and breast cancer: Case-control and cohort studies. Prev Med 1989;18:180.

26. Hursting S, Thornquist M, Henderson M. Types of dietary fat and the incidence of breast cancer at five sites. Prev Med 1990;19:242.

27. Jones D, Schatzkin A, Green S, et al. Dietary fat and breast cancer in the National Health and Nutrition Examination Survey I epidemiologic follow-up study. J Natl Cancer Inst 1987;79:465.

28. Kushi L, Sellers T, Potter J, et al. Dietary fat and postmenopausal breast cancer. J Natl Cancer Inst 1992;84:1092.

29. La Vecchia C, Decarli A, Franceschi S, et al. Dietary factors and the risk of breast cancer. Nutr Cancer 1987;10:205.

30. Hiatt R, Bawol R. Alcoholic beverage consumption and breast cancer incidence. Am J Epidemiol 1984;120:676.

31. Longnecker M, Berlin J, Orza M, Chalmers T. A meta-analysis of alcohol consumption in relation to risk of breast cancer. JAMA 1988;260:652.

32. Schatzkin A, Jones D, Hoover R, et al. Alcohol consumption and breast cancer in the epidemiologic follow-up study of the First National Health and Nutrition Examination Survey. N Engl J Med 1987;316:1169.

33. Simon M, Carman W, Wolfe R, Schottenfeld D. Alcohol consumption and the risk of breast cancer: A report from the Tecumseh Community Health Study. J Clin Epidemiol 1991;44:755.

34. Willett W, Stampfer M, Colditz G, et al. Moderate alcohol consumption and the risk of breast cancer. N Engl J Med 1987;316:1174.

35. Reichman M, Judd J, Longcope C, et al. Effects of alcohol consumption on plasma and urinary hormone concentrations in premenopausal women. J Natl Cancer Inst 1993;85:722.

36. Henderson I. Biologic variations of tumors. Cancer 1992;69:1888.

37. Wolman S, Dawson P. Genetic events in breast cancer and their clinical correlates. Crit Rev Oncog 1991;2:277.

38. Bloom H, Richardson W, Harries E. Natural history of untreated breast cancer (1805–1933). BMJ 1962;2:213.

39. Atkins E, Solomon L, Worden J, Foster R. Relative effectiveness of methods of breast self-examination. J Behav Med 1991;14:357.

40. Baines C. Breast self-examination. Cancer 1992;69:1942.

41. Janz N, Becker M, Haefner D, et al. Determinants of breast self-examination following a benign biopsy. Am J Prev Med 1990;6:84.

42. Seidman J, Gelb S, Silverberg E, et al. Survival experience in the Breast Cancer Detection Demonstration Project. CA Cancer J Clin 1987;37:258.

43. Chu K, Smart C, Tarone R. Analysis of breast cancer mortality and stage distribution by age for the Health Insurance Plan Clinical Trial. J Natl Cancer Inst 1988;80:1125.

44. Tabar L, Fagerberg C, Gad A. Reduction in mortality from breast cancer after mass screening with mammography. Lancet 1985;1:829.

45. Miller A, Baines C, To T, Wall C. Canadian National Breast Screening Study: 2. Breast cancer detection and death rates among women aged 50 to 59 years. Can Med Assoc J 1992;147:1477.

46. Miller A, Baines C, To T, Wall C. Canadian National Breast Screening Study: 1. Breast cancer detection and death rates among women aged 40 to 49 years. Can Med Assoc J 1992;147:1459.

47. Moskowitz M. Breast cancer: Age-specific growth rates and screening strategies. Radiology 1986;161:37.

48. Tabar L, Fagerberg G, Day N. What is the optimum interval between mammographic screening examinations? An analysis based on the latest results of the Swedish two-county breast cancer screening trial. Br J Cancer 1987;55:547.

49. United States Preventive Services Task Force. Guide to Clinical Preventive Services: An Assessment of the Effectiveness of 169 Interventions. Report of the US Preventive Services Task Force. Baltimore: Williams & Wilkins, 1989.

50. Vanchieri C. Europeans say screen only women age 50 and older. J Natl Cancer Inst 1993;85:350.

51. Eddy D. Screening for Cancer: Theory, Analysis, and Design. Englewood Cliffs, NJ: Prentice-Hall, 1980.

52. Mushlin A, Fintor L. Is screening for breast cancer cost-effective? Cancer 1992;69:1957.

53. Dodd G. American Cancer Society guidelines on screening for breast cancer: An overview. CA Cancer J Clin 1992;42:177.

54. Fletcher S, Black W, Harris R, et al. Report of the International Workshop on Screening for Breast Cancer. J Natl Cancer Inst 1993;85:1644.

55. Sickles E, Kopans D. Deficiencies in the analysis of breast cancer screening data. J Natl Cancer Inst 1993;85:1621.

56. Evans P, Gaskill S. Quality control of mammography in the '90s. Contemp Oncol 1992;2:37.

57. Smith R, Haynes S. Barriers to screening for breast cancer. Cancer 1992;69:1968.

58. Bastani R, Marcus A, Hollatz A. Screening mammography rates and barriers to use: A Los Angeles county survey. Prev Med 1991;20:350.

59. Cohen S, Jackson V, Booher P, Loehrer P. Failure to comply with a mammography appointment: an analysis of indigent patients' reasons. Breast Dis 1991;4:107.

60. Fox S, Stein J. The effect of physician-patient communication on mammography utilization by different ethnic groups. Med Care 1991;29:1065.

61. Harris R, Fletcher S, Gonzalez J, et al. Mammography and age: Are we targeting the wrong women? A community survey of women and physicians. Cancer 1991;67:2010.

62. Hayward R, Shapiro M, Freeman H, Corey C. Who gets screened for cervical and breast cancer? Arch Intern Med 1988;148:1177.

63. Lerman C, Rimer B. Psychosocial impact of cancer screening. Onocology 1993;7:67.

64. Lerman C, Rimer B, Trock B, Engstrom P. Factors associated with repeat adherence to breast cancer screening. Prev Med 1990;19:279.

65. Donegan W. Evaluation of palpable breast mass. N Engl J Med 1992;327:937.

66. Hall F, Storella J, Silverstone D, Wyshak G. Nonpalpable breast lesions: Recommendations for biopsy based on suspicion of carcinoma at mammography. Radiology 1988;167:353.

67. Skinner M, Swain M, Simmons R, et al. Nonpalpable breast lesions at biopsy. Ann Surg 1988;208:203.

68. Sickles E. Periodic mammographic follow-up of probably benign lesions: Results in 3,184 consecutive cases. Radiology 1991;179:463.

69. Boyd N, Jensen H, Cooke G, Han H. Relationship between mammographic and histologic risk factors for breast cancer. J Natl Cancer Inst 1992;84:1170.

70. Saftlas A, Hoover R, Brinton L, et al. Mammographic densities and risk of breast cancer. Cancer 1991;67:2833.

71. Arishita G, Cruz B, Harding C, Arbutina D. Mammogram-directed fine-needle aspiration of nonpalpable breast lesions. J Surg Oncol 1991;48:153.

72. Fisher B, Redmond C. Should healthy women take tamoxifen? (letter). N Engl J Med 1992;327:1596.

73. Fugh-Berman A, Epstein S. Should healthy women take tamoxifen? (letter). N Engl J Med 1992;327:1596.

74. Kiang D. Chemoprevention for breast cancer: Are we ready? J Natl Cancer Inst 1991;83:462.

75. Freedman L, Prentice R, Clifford C, et al. Dietary fat and breast cancer: Where are we? J Natl Cancer Inst 1993;85:764.

76. Henderson M, Kushi L, Thompson D, et al. Feasibility of a randomized trial of a low-fat diet for the prevention of breast cancer: Dietary compliance in the Women's Health Trial Vanguard Study. Prev Med 1990;19:115.

77. Whittemore A, Henderson B. Dietary fat and breast cancer: Where are we? J Natl Cancer Inst 1993;85:762.

78. Wynder E. Cancer prevention: Optimizing life-styles with special reference to nutritional carcinogenesis. J Natl Cancer Inst Monographs 1992;12:87.

79. Bernstein L, Ross R, Henderson B. Prospects for the primary prevention of breast cancer. Am J Epidemiol 1992;135:142.

80. Will M, Fontana J. Chemoprevention of breast cancer. Dev Oncol 1991; 62:169.

81. Nayfield S, Karp J, Ford L, et al. Potential role of tamoxifen in prevention of breast cancer. J Natl Cancer Inst 1991;83:1450.

82. Veronesi U, De Palo G, Costa A, et al. Chemoprevention of breast cancer with retinoids. J Natl Cancer Inst Monographs 1992;12:93.

83. Kuller LH. Recruitment strategies for a possible tamoxifen trial. Prev Med 1991;20:119.

84. Engstrom P. Specific compliance issues in an antiestrogen trial of women at risk for breast cancer. Prev Med 1991;20:125.

Management of Patients with Breast Cancer

Marianne N. Prout

Management of the newly diagnosed patient with breast cancer requires knowledge of the many diagnostic and prognostic tests. Following a brief but targeted staging of her cancer, the patient should be presented with an array of therapeutic options appropriate for her prognosis and her individual characteristics. This chapter focuses on the principles of initial staging and triage to therapy and the rehabilitation and follow-up of women treated for breast cancer.

PROGNOSTIC FACTORS

Prognostic uncertainty results from the biologic variability among patients with breast cancer. The success of early detection depends not just on timely screening but also on the course of metastatic events. Prognostic factors that have been correlated with disease-free survival in previous patients are used to predict the probability of relapse-free survival and to select appropriate therapy. The most useful prognostic information continues to be precise clinical and pathologic staging, with additional precision provided by histologic classification and steroid hormone receptor status.[1-7]

The stage of cancer at diagnosis remains the most available and useful prognostic indicator. Table 18-1 summarizes the tumor-node-metastasis (TNM) categories and staging system.[1] Primary tumor size is both an important predictor of regional spread to the axillary lymph nodes and of survival, but approximately 20% of patients with tumors smaller than 1.0 cm have involvement of axillary lymph nodes at diagnosis and 12% of women with these small tumors have a recurrence of disease within 20 years. Clinical studies suggest that disease will recur within 10 years in 20% of patients with negative findings on axillary lymph node testing.[2]

Histologic classification must accurately define both in situ and invasive breast cancers and the subtype of breast cancer. Careful review of all in situ lesions is required to rule out areas of invasive disease; specimen orientation and identification of all margins is likewise critical to ensure the microscopic review of biopsy specimen margins. For in situ breast cancers, important issues to consider prognostically are the probability of multicentric disease and the subsequent risk for invasive disease. One study noted that ipsilateral breast cancer developed in more than 16% of patients with ductal carcinoma in situ within 5 years after excision only.[8] Lobular carcinoma in situ is considered a risk factor for invasive breast cancer, with a relative risk for invasive cancer seven to 10 times that of women without lobular carcinoma in situ at 15 years of follow-up.

Infiltrating ductal cancers comprise approximately 75% of breast cancers; infiltrating lobular cancers account for 5 to 10%. Special types of invasive breast cancer with prognoses more favorable than those of ductal cancers account for up to 15%: 2% are tubular, 5 to 7% are medullary, and 3% are colloid. The disease-free survival rates for these other histologic types is reported as 10 to 15% better than those for ductal cancers at more than 10 years of follow-up in small numbers of patients.[4]

The impact of estrogen and progesterone receptor status on the prognosis for patients with stage I breast cancers has been debated. Fisher and colleagues report small but significant survival advantages for patients with estrogen receptor–positive tumors, but other studies have not confirmed this finding.[6] For patients with stage II and higher stages of breast cancer, positive estrogen and progesterone receptor status is more clearly associated with a better prognosis. For the smallest tumor sizes, the quality of estrogen receptor assay results may be a confounder in the conflicting data be-

TABLE 18–1.   Breast Cancer Staging

T0	No evidence of primary tumor		
T1	≤2 cm: T1a ≤0.5 cm		
	T1b >0.5–1 cm		
	T1c >1–2 cm		
T2	>2–5 cm		
T3	>5 cm		
T4	Includes any inflammatory carcinoma, any cancer with direct extension to skin or chest wall		
N0	No regional lymph node metastasis		
N1	Ipsilateral axillary lymph node metastasis(es)		
N2	Fixed ipsilateral lymph node metastasis(es)		
N3	Metastasis to internal mammary or other lymph nodes		
M0	No distant metastasis		
M1	Distant metastasis(es)		

STAGE GROUPING			
Stage 0	Tis	N0	M0
Stage I	T1	N0	M0
Stage II	T0	N1	M0
	T1	N1	M0
	T2	N0	M0
	T2	N1	M0
	T3	N0	M0
Stage III	T3	N1,N2	M0
	T4	any N	M0
	any T	N2,N3	M0
Stage IV	any T	any N	M1

Adapted from American Cancer Society. Cancer Manual. 8th ed. Boston: American Cancer Society, Massachusetts Division, 1990.

cause simultaneous histologic control of tissue used for the assay is difficult with low tumor volumes. Immunocytochemical methods combined with image analysis to perform tumor-specific analyses are being assessed for accuracy in determining estrogen and progesterone receptor status on in situ cancers, but these assays provide qualitative and not quantitative results.

Tumor kinetics are replacing pathologic morphology such as histologic and nuclear grade for evaluating the biologic characteristics of early breast cancers. Flow cytometry and image analysis are used to evaluate ploidy status and S-phase fraction, which have been correlated with disease-free survival in patients with both stage I and higher stages of breast cancer.[9–11] Other markers such as HER-2/neu, epidermal growth factor receptors, cathepsin D, and p53 are still considered investigational until their association with disease-free survival is elucidated.[12–15] Further work on the integration of multiple factors into models to predict prognosis is under way.[16] Table 18–2 outlines traditional indicators of prognosis for breast cancer patients with negative axillary nodes; these indicators should be obtained for all patients. Table 18–2 also cites examples of indicators that have undergone preliminary evaluations and are under scrutiny for use in the 50% of breast cancer pa-

tients with negative axillary nodes, tumor sizes of 1 to 5 cm, and intermediate or unknown receptor status. The expanding research on the biology of breast cancer is adding potential prognostic markers, but the clinical utility of any single marker or combination of markers requires further study. Such studies are appropriately incorporated into clinical trials to unravel the role of each marker in predicting response to therapy versus indicating prognosis independent of therapy.

INITIAL THERAPY FOR NEWLY DIAGNOSED BREAST CANCERS

The number of women in the United States diagnosed with early stage breast cancer, which is defined as tumor size under 2 cm and negative axillary lymph nodes, has risen rapidly from approximately 12,000 cases in 1982 to 32,000 in 1986.[17] These women require information on the choice between mastectomy and breast conservation and the role of adjuvant therapy in general and in their particular case.

Breast conservation treatment involves excision of the primary tumor with adjacent breast tissue plus radiation therapy. It has been compared with total mastectomy in many studies with long-term

TABLE 18–2. Prognostic Indicators for Node-Negative Breast Cancer

TRADITIONAL INDICATORS	FAVORABLE CATEGORY
Tumor size	<1 cm
Differentiation	Well-differentiated
	Moderately well-differentiated
Histologic type	Pure tubular, colloid, cribriform
Receptor status	ER +, PR + (for tumors of 1–5 cm)

TYPES OF INDICATORS UNDER ACTIVE INVESTIGATION Examples	Favorable Category
Histologic	
Tumor angiogenesis	Low microvessel density
Tumor proliferation rate markers	
S-phase fraction	<10%
Growth suppressor genes	
p53	No mutation, no accumulation in tissue
Growth factors	
(Epidermal growth factor receptors)	—

ER, Estrogen receptor; PR, progesterone receptor.

follow-up and has shown comparable results over-all. Most patients with stage I or II breast cancers should be offered a choice between mastectomy or breast conservation. Keeping in mind that the goals of such therapy are good local control of cancer with good cosmesis, specific circumstances contraindicate breast conservation: multicentric breast cancers, large tumor size with respect to breast size, prior radiation to the breast area, and pregnancy in the first or second trimester. Conservation approaches should be considered with caution in women who have extensive intraductal carcinoma around the primary tumor as radiation toxicity of tissues may be increased in this group (in women with collagen vascular diseases).[18–24]

The presentation of options for breast conservation or mastectomy is now considered a professional responsibility for providers of care to patients with breast cancer, based on equivalent cancer outcomes for carefully evaluated and appropriately treated patients. Unfortunately, many surgeons in the United States do not accept the therapies as equally effective in spite of these results. Psychosocial outcomes in women treated with mastectomy and those treated with breast conservation have also been evaluated and have shown few differences in overall adaptation or fear of recurrence. Body image, however, is generally better in women treated with breast conservation, and autonomy in choosing one's therapy was rated highly by some but not all women.[19, 20]

Breast conservation therapy requires teamwork among experienced surgeons, radiation therapists, medical oncologists, and mammographers to ensure good cosmesis, good cancer control, and early detection of any recurrence. Surgical concerns include use of arcuate incisions, good hemostasis, and careful marking of all margins to ensure that they are microscopically free of tumor. In addition, patients should generally have a separate incision for axillary dissection.[23] Radiation principles include treatment with megavoltage to the whole breast to 4500 or 5000 cGy; boost irradiation is added if the tumor was close to or microscopically involved the surgical margins.[24] Mammographic follow-up is advised after surgery but before radiation, at 6-month intervals in the first year and then at least annually. The role of early mammograms after radiation requires further clarification; however, the importance of clinical examinations for detecting recurrence in the treated breast must be emphasized because palpable abnormalities account for up to half of all recurrences.[25, 26]

ADJUVANT THERAPY FOR BREAST CANCER

Systemic therapy after initial treatment of breast cancer has been studied extensively during the last 20 years. Meta-analyses and overviews of the results of clinical trials have been conducted by the National Institutes of Health Consensus Development Conferences and the Early Breast Cancer Trialists' Collaborative Group; they concluded that chemotherapy and hormonal therapy are effective for both node-positive and node-negative breast cancer patients.[27] Questions abound about which therapies should be used for which subgroups of patients and for what duration. In addition, the criteria to identify a "good risk" subgroup who need no systemic therapy are debated.[28-34]

For node-positive premenopausal patients, combination chemotherapy is the standard in the United States. The role of additional hormonal therapy in patients with positive estrogen receptors and the duration of chemotherapy are under investigation, with early data suggesting that short but intensive chemotherapy regimens are most effective. For postmenopausal patients with positive nodes, tamoxifen is standard therapy when estrogen receptors are positive, and its role in estrogen receptor–negative patients is being defined; longer duration of tamoxifen treatment is associated with decreasing mortality. Appropriate adjuvant therapy reduces recurrences by 20 to 30% and reduces mortality by 10 to 20% in node-positive and node-negative patients; the absolute number of node-negative patients who benefit is much lower because of the lower risk of recurrence than that in node-positive patients.[27, 32-34]

Patients with tumors 1 cm or smaller are generally considered at minimal risk for recurrence and are not candidates for standard adjuvant therapy.[30] Such patients may appropriately be enrolled in clinical trials; indeed, because of the range of unanswered questions, all patients could appropriately be enrolled in clinical trials of adjuvant therapy. Currently fewer than 5% of new breast cancer patients in the United States enroll in clinical adjuvant trials, resulting in a slow evolution of therapeutic regimens appropriate to various subgroups.

Table 18–3 outlines some of the therapeutic options that should be discussed with patients who have stage I and II breast cancer. Consideration should be given to enrolling all such patients in clinical trials when they are available. Disease-free survival is a critical endpoint in clinical trials to evaluate and compare initial treatment regimens for breast cancer. Patterns of recurrence and implications of types of recurrence should guide therapeutic choices.

About one third of recurrences after initial therapy are local or regional, involving the breast, chest wall, or regional lymph nodes. In patients who had initial breast-conserving therapy, 75% of breast recurrences occur at or near the initial tumor location, and more than half of these patients are again disease-free following mastectomy.[27, 30] After mastectomy, local and regional relapses are generally followed by distant relapse. Common sites of distant relapse are bone, soft tissue, liver, lung, and brain.

REHABILITATION AND SUPPORT

Rehabilitation and support needs must be assessed for each woman both at the time of initial diagnosis and therapy and during the follow-up period. These needs may include physical, psychological, social, sexual, and economic issues. Most patients should be asked if they would like to be contacted by volunteers who have had breast cancer, as the trained volunteers provided by the American Cancer Society can assist with frank discussions of how to handle myriad details in addition to providing role models of recovery and peer support. Some patients may benefit from physician-initiated or facilitated discussions with their

TABLE 18–3. **Adjuvant Therapy Strategies for Categories for Breast Cancer Patients**

TUMOR SIZE	NODES	MENOPAUSAL STATUS	ER/PR	CLINICAL OPTIONS
<1 cm	N0	post-	+	Tamoxifen, clinical trial
<1 cm	N0	post-	−	No therapy, clinical trial
<1 cm	N0	pre-	+	No therapy, clinical trial
<1 cm	N0	pre-	−	No therapy, clinical trial*
2–5 cm	N0	post-	+	Tamoxifen, clinical trial
2–5 cm	N0	post-	−	Consider chemotherapy, clinical trial
2–5 cm	N0	pre-	+	Chemotherapy ± tamoxifen, clinical trial
2–5 cm	N0	pre-	−	Chemotherapy, clinical trial
2–5 cm	N1	post-	+	Tamoxifen, clinical trial
2–5 cm	N1	post-	−	Chemotherapy, clinical trial
2–5 cm	N1	pre-	+	Chemotherapy, clinical trial
2–5 cm	N1	pre-	−	Chemotherapy, clinical trial

*For poorly differentiated cancers, consider chemotherapy.

partners or family members. Additional support by clergy or referral to cancer support groups can also be offered. Some patients may benefit from individual or family counseling. Primary care physicians should be sensitive and attentive to patients who are having serious problems coping with the diagnosis, therapies, or both and should initiate referrals to specialized counselors; such patients are often more willing to accept their need for assistance in coping when it is mentioned by their long-term provider of care. The potential economic consequences of cancer should be assessed, and resources for management of economic sequelae should be identified if possible. The effects of the diagnosis of cancer on medical insurance for the patient and her family and on employment and the indirect costs of cancer care are a source of ongoing stress for many.

Breast reconstruction or appropriate prostheses can mitigate the psychosocial morbidity associated with mastectomy. Ideally, appropriate consultations should be incorporated as part of the initial therapeutic planning. Most patients are candidates for reconstruction, and the timing of the procedure, the type of reconstruction, and the procedures planned for the contralateral breast should be thoroughly explored. Many patients prefer immediate reconstruction, but delayed reconstruction may be advised for those who are at high risk for local recurrence. Adequate skin flaps must be provided at the time of initial mastectomy to facilitate later reconstruction. Myocutaneous flaps and implants are the two general categories of reconstruction. In spite of the current controversies surrounding implants, they allow immediate reconstruction with a simple surgical technique. Myocutaneous flaps require special surgical expertise, a longer surgical procedure, and a higher risk of blood transfusion. Symmetry is a major issue and goal for reconstruction and often requires a procedure on the contralateral breast. Reconstruction of the nipple or areolar area may also be accomplished for those women who prefer such a cosmetic result.[18, 35]

LONG-TERM FOLLOW-UP OF BREAST CANCER PATIENTS

Several areas require special concern by the primary care physician who is following a patient with a history of breast cancer: timing and patterns of recurrence, risk for second primary cancers, late sequelae of therapies, and management of reproductive and menopausal options.

Recurrences of breast cancer can occur many years after diagnosis: in a large cohort of women with axillary node-negative breast cancers, sur-

vival was 88% at 5 years but 78% at 8 years. Estimates for recurrence for women with negative axillary nodes are from 25 to 40% by 10 years after diagnosis.[7, 22] Patterns of recurrence include local, either in the preserved breast or on the chest wall postmastectomy; regional; and distant; common metastatic sites include bone, lung, liver, and brain. Local recurrence rates vary by primary tumor size, other prognostic factors, and the quality of local therapy; rates of 5 to 20% at 10 years are often reported. Local recurrences are common as the first site of recurrence but generally also predict risk for distant recurrence.[18, 25, 26] Follow-up visits are recommended at 3- to 6-month intervals for the first 3 years after diagnosis, at 6-month intervals through 5 years, and then at least annually. Follow-up evaluations should include careful history and physical examinations, mammograms of both the preserved and the contralateral breast, and other tests as justified by signs or symptoms. The value of bone scans or other testing in asymptomatic patients is uncertain.[18]

The risk of second malignancies from several long-term follow-up studies is estimated at 10% for new cancers in the contralateral breast and approximately 10% for a nonbreast malignancy, with lower rates in younger women. The overall non–breast cancer rate is considered equivalent to the age-matched population rate. The risk for contralateral breast cancer is higher with an initial histology of lobular carcinoma.[7]

Late sequelae of therapies for breast cancer are changing; lymphedema of the upper extremity associated with mastectomy plus radiation is now an infrequent complication, although mild lymphedema remains a problem, especially in older women and women with advanced stages of cancer. The risk of contralateral breast cancer has been reported as increased in patients who receive radiotherapy for breast cancer; however, whether techniques to reduce the dose to the contralateral breast can reduce this risk is unclear.[36] The risk of leukemia in patients receiving adjuvant chemotherapy containing alkylating agents such as cyclophosphamide (Cytoxan) or melphalan has been calculated as 5 per 10,000 patients.[37] The risks of premature menopause in women receiving adjuvant therapy for breast cancer have not been well assessed but potentially include accelerated osteoporosis and atherogenesis.[38]

The management of two major hormonal events remain controversial for women with a personal history of breast cancer: pregnancy and menopause. Studies have shown that pregnant women are at increased risk of advanced disease at diagnosis, but the paucity of data does not provide a good assessment of the risk of subsequent pregnancy on the prognosis of breast cancer. Although most oncologists counsel that the high hormone levels associated with pregnancy are contraindicated in patients with prior breast cancer, recommendations on future risk with pregnancy are considered theoretic or extrapolations from other situations. Similarly, menopausal hormone therapy has been considered contraindicated; indeed, controversies continue on the role of ovarian ablation as adjuvant therapy in premenopausal women. Some investigators propose that the effectiveness of adjuvant chemotherapy is explained by its effects on the ovaries. At this time, careful consideration of options for the management of menopausal symptoms and the risks of chronic disease must include nonhormonal approaches and tamoxifen and careful explanation of the potential risks of estrogen.[39, 40]

REFERENCES

1. American Cancer Society. Cancer Manual. 8th ed. Boston: American Cancer Society, Massachusetts Division, 1990.
2. Clayton F. Pathologic correlates of survival in 378 lymph node-negative infiltrating ductal breast carcinomas. Cancer 1991;68:1309.
3. Elledge R, McGuire W, Osborne C. Prognostic factors in breast cancer. Semin Oncol 1992;19:244.
4. Gilchrist K. Routine histoprognostic factors in early-stage breast carcinoma. Cancer Invest 1992;10:565.
5. Sigurdsson H, Baldetorp B, Borg A, et al. Indicators of prognosis in node-negative breast cancer. N Engl J Med 1990;322:1045.
6. Fisher E, Redmond C, Fisher B. Prognostic factors in NSABP studies of women with node-negative breast cancer. J Natl Cancer Inst Monographs 1992;11:151.
7. Rosen P, Groshen S, Kinne D. Survival and prognostic factors in node-negative breast cancer: Results of long-term followup studies. J Natl Cancer Inst Monographs 1992;11:159.
8. Fisher B, Costantino J, Redmond C, et al. Lumpectomy compared with lumpectomy and radiation therapy for the treatment of intraductal breast cancer. N Engl J Med 1993;328:1581.
9. Kornstein M. DNA flow cytometry in the prognosis of node-negative breast cancer. N Engl J Med 1989;321:473.
10. Merkel D, McGuire W. Ploidy, proliferative activity and prognosis. Cancer 1990;65:1194.
11. Stal O, Dufmats M, Hatschek T, et al. S-phase fraction is a prognostic factor in Stage I breast carcinoma. J Clin Oncol 1993;11:1717.
12. Allred D, Clark G, Elledge R, et al. Association of p53 expression with tumor cell proliferation rate and clinical outcome in node-negative breast cancer. J Natl Cancer Inst 1993;85:200.
13. Isola J, Visakorpi T, Holli K, Kallioniemi O. Association of overexpression of tumor suppressor protein p53 with rapid cell proliferation and poor prognosis in node-negative breast cancer patients. J Natl Cancer Inst 1992;84:1109.
14. Paik S. Clinical significance of erbB-2 (HER-2/neu) protein. Cancer Invest 1992;10:575.
15. Gasparini G, Pozzo F, Harris A. Evaluating the potential usefulness of new prognostic and predictive indicators in node-negative breast cancer patients. J Natl Cancer Inst 1993;85:1206.
16. Spyratos F, Martin P, Hacene K, et al. Multiparametric prognostic evaluation of biological factors in primary breast cancer. J Natl Cancer Inst 1992;84:1266.
17. Consensus Development Panel. Consensus statement: Treatment of early-stage breast cancer. J Natl Cancer Inst Monographs. 1992;11:1.
18. American College of Radiology, American College of Surgeons, College of American Pathologists, Society of Surgical Oncology, Winchester D, Cox J. Standards for breast-conservation treatment. CA Cancer J Clin 1992;42:134–162.
19. Lasry J, Margolese R. Fear of recurrence, breast-conserving surgery, and the trade-off hypothesis. Cancer 1992;69:2111.
20. Schain W, Fetting J. Modified radical mastectomy versus breast conservation: Psychosocial considerations. Semin Oncol 1992;19:239.
21. Weil M, Borel C, Auclerc G, et al. Nonsurgical approach in stage I and stage II breast cancer. Cancer Invest 1992;10:581.
22. Fisher B, Redmond C, and Others for the NSABP Project. Lumpectomy for breast cancer: An update of the NSABP experience. J Natl Cancer Inst Monographs 1992;11:7.
23. Margolese R. Surgical considerations in selecting local therapy. J Natl Cancer Inst Monographs 1992;11:41.
24. Fowble B. Radiotherapeutic considerations in the treatment of primary breast cancer. J Natl Cancer Inst Monographs 1992;11:49.
25. Orel S, Troupin R, Patterson E, Fowble B. Breast cancer recurrence after lumpectomy and irradiation: Role of mammography in detection. Radiology 1992;183:201.
26. Vicini F, Recht A, Abner A, et al. Recurrence in the breast following conservative surgery and radiation therapy for early-stage breast cancer. J Natl Cancer Inst Monographs 1992;11:33.
27. Straus K, Lichter A, Lippman M, et al. Results of the National Cancer Institute Early Breast Cancer Trial. J Natl Cancer Inst Monographs. 1992;11:27.
28. Love R. Tamoxifen in axillary node-negative breast cancer: Multisystem benefits and risks. Cancer Invest 1992;10:587.
29. McWhorter W, Mayer W. Black/white differences in type of initial breast cancer treatment and implications for survival. Am J Public Health 1987;77:1515.
30. Rosner D, Lane W. Should all patients with node-negative breast cancer receive adjuvant therapy? Identifying additional subsets of low-risk patients who are highly curable by surgery alone. Cancer 1991;68:1482.
31. Silliman R, Balducci L, Goodwin J, et al. Breast cancer care in old age: What we know, don't know, and do. J Natl Cancer Inst 1993;85:190.
32. Sledge G, McCaskill-Stevens W. Adjuvant therapy for node-negative breast cancer. Cancer Invest 1992;10:595.
33. Gelber R, Goldhirsch A. Reporting and interpreting adjuvant therapy clinical trials. J Natl Cancer Inst Monographs 1992;11:59.
34. McGuire W, Tandon A, Allred D, et al. Treatment decisions in axillary node-negative breast cancer patients. J Natl Cancer Inst Monographs 1992;11:173.
35. Baker R, Robinson R. The management of breast cancer with immediate or delayed reconstruction. Adv Surg 1992;25:51.
36. Boice J, Harvey E, Blettner M, et al. Cancer in the contralateral breast after radiotherapy for breast cancer. N Engl J Med 1992;326:781.

37. Harris J, Lippman M, Veronesi U, Willett W. Breast Cancer. N Engl J Med 1992;327:319, 390, 473.
38. American College of Physicians. Guidelines for counseling postmenopausal women about preventive hormone therapy. Ann Intern Med 1992;117:1038.
39. Creasman W. Estrogen replacement therapy: Is previously treated cancer a contraindication? Obstet Gynecol 1991;77:308.
40. Zemlickis D, Lishner M, Degendorfer P, et al. Maternal and fetal outcome after breast cancer in pregnancy. Am J Obstet Gynecol 1992;166:781.

ENDOCRINE DISORDERS IN WOMEN

19

Amenorrhea and Oligomenorrhea

Melanie J. Brunt

Primary amenorrhea is defined as the failure to menstruate by age 16 years in girls who have breast or pubic hair development, or both, or the failure to menstruate by age 14 in girls who have not developed secondary sex characteristics. Secondary amenorrhea is defined as cessation of menstrual periods for at least three menstrual cycles in a previously normally menstruating woman. Oligomenorrhea is scant or infrequent menses with intermenstrual intervals of at least 35 days. With the exception of anatomic or genetic disorders resulting in primary amenorrhea, the etiologies of amenorrhea and oligomenorrhea are similar and are discussed in this chapter as a single entity.

ETIOLOGY AND DIFFERENTIAL DIAGNOSIS

Primary Amenorrhea

The disorders discussed in this section are those in which a normal menarche is prohibited by the nature of the disorder and for which a presentation as secondary amenorrhea is therefore not possible. The causes of primary amenorrhea are summarized in Table 19–1. All other disorders are discussed under secondary amenorrhea.

Girls who present at the expected time of puberty without menstrual periods can be divided into two groups: those with no evidence of pubertal development and those who have complete or partial development of normal secondary sex characteristics.

Absence of Secondary Sex Characteristics

When primary amenorrhea occurs in association with the absence of breast or pubic hair development, the usual diagnosis is Turner's syndrome, or gonadal dysgenesis. This occurs in females who

---

TABLE 19–1.   Differential Diagnosis of Primary Amenorrhea

ABSENCE OR INCOMPLETE DEVELOPMENT OF SECONDARY SEX CHARACTERISTICS
Turner's syndrome
Constitutional delayed adolescence
Kallmann's syndrome
Severe chronic illness (anorexia nervosa, Crohn's disease, sickle cell anemia)
Strenuous exercise
Panhypopituitarism
Hypothalamic tumor or infiltrative disorder
Pituitary tumor or infiltrative disorder
Hyperprolactinemia
Primary hypothyroidism
Primary ovarian failure (autoimmune, viral, postchemotherapy, or irradiation)

PRESENCE OF SECONDARY SEX CHARACTERISTICS
Anatomic defects
    Müllerian agenesis
    Vaginal atresia
    Asherman's syndrome
    Congenital cervical stenosis
Testicular feminization

---

have only one normal X chromosome; it has a frequency of one in 10,000 female births. The usual chromosome abnormality is 45,X, occurring in approximately 50% of Turner's syndrome patients, with the remaining cases due to other X chromosome abnormalities, such as an abnormal long arm of the X chromosome or mixed 45,X/46X,X or 45,X/46X,Y chromosomal patterns. Turner's syndrome is sometimes diagnosed at birth, manifesting as low birth weight with lymphedema of the hands and feet. However, it is often not diagnosed until later in childhood in girls who experience growth delay, which affects 95 to 100% of all Turner's syndrome patients. The occasional patient with no obvious Turner's stigmata and minimal growth delay may not present to a physician until mid or late adolescence when primary amenorrhea becomes apparent.

In addition to short stature, the stigmata of Turner's can include epicanthal folds (25%), high arched palate (36%), short broad neck (74%), webbed neck (pterygium coli)(46%), shield-like rectangular contour chest (53%), coarctation of the aorta or ventricular septal defect (10–16%), renal abnormalities (38%), pigmented nevi (63%), nail hypoplasia (66%), and skeletal deformities such as cubitus valgus (54%) or short fourth metacarpals (48%). The ovaries consist of streaks of connective tissue with minimal or absent follicles, and gonadotropins are elevated. Treatment with estrogen is essential to increase growth and promote development of secondary sex characteristics; it must be maintained indefinitely to avoid complications of estrogen deficiency such as osteoporosis. Growth hormone may also be used to achieve a more normal adult height.

Constitutional delayed adolescence refers to a physiologic delay in puberty, which is more common in boys than in girls but can be seen in girls. The family history often reveals delayed menarche. Birth weight is normal, but growth velocity is slow. The growth curve may remain less than the fifth percentile, but the slope of the curve is normal. Skeletal age is delayed, and pubertal development begins at the appropriate skeletal age and progresses normally.

Kallmann's syndrome is rare and occurs more commonly in men, but it can occur in women. It is a genetic defect that results in agenesis of the olfactory apparatus in association with hypothalamic hypogonadism. Both gonadotropin-releasing hormone (Gn-RH) neurons and olfactory nerves fail to migrate into the hypothalamus during embryologic development. The resultant clinical syndrome consists of anosmia or hyposmia, primary amenorrhea, and variable degrees of development of secondary sex characteristics, ranging from no development to moderate breast development. Long-term continuous pulsatile administration of Gn-RH via an infusion pump device induces normal pubertal development and fertility.

Presence of Secondary Sex Characteristics

Primary amenorrhea occurring in association with normal breast or pubic hair development is most often due to müllerian agenesis or testicular feminization syndrome. Disorders of müllerian agenesis are congenital anatomic abnormalities due to incomplete development of the structures arising embryologically from the müllerian ducts, which consist of the fallopian tubes, uterus, and upper vagina. Affected individuals are otherwise genetically and phenotypically normal females with normally functioning ovaries. These abnormalities occur in 0.02% of the female population. Specific abnormalities can include a bicornuate or septate uterus, a transverse vaginal septum, or an imperforate hymen. Patients with the last two disorders can present with monthly pelvic pain, a vaginal mass due to retained menstrual blood, or both. Patients with müllerian agenesis have a high frequency of associated renal abnormalities (15–40%), usually a pelvic or missing kidney.

Intrauterine exposure to diethylstilbestrol is associated with müllerian agenesis and, most commonly, abnormalities of the uterus. It is estimated that 1.0 to 1.5 million women were exposed to diethylstilbestrol in utero from the late 1940s until the 1970s. Depending on the adequacy of the endometrial lining and outflow tract, these women can present with primary amenorrhea, or they may have normal menstrual periods. In the latter case, diagnosis of the disorder is delayed until infertility or repeated early pregnancy loss occurs due to uterine structural abnormalities.

The lower third of the vagina has a different embryologic origin, arising from the urogenital sinus. Vaginal atresia is a condition in which this lower third does not develop, but structures derived from the müllerian duct are normal. Similarly to an imperforate hymen or a transverse vaginal septum, it can manifest as monthly pelvic pain, but the vagina is absent on physical examination.

Testicular feminization, or complete androgen resistance, is an X-linked recessive disorder with a prevalence of one in 64,000. The individual is genetically male with a 46 X,Y karyotype. Serum testosterone levels are in the normal adult male range, but there is end-organ insensitivity to androgen effects, presumably due to a receptor defect. In the absence of androgen stimulation, phenotypically female features develop. Breast development occurs, often only to Tanner stage 3 or 4 (Fig. 19–1), but little or no pubic or axillary hair is present. Stature is usually normal. Female reproductive organs are absent, and the vagina is small, as only the distal third, of urogenital sinus origin, is present. Testes are present and may be intra-abdominal, inguinal, or labial and are at increased risk for neoplasia. Inguinal hernias are common and should raise suspicion of this disorder when they occur in prepubertal girls. Incomplete testicular feminization is a variant in which there is some response to androgen, such that clitoral enlargement and labioscrotal fusion occur at puberty, resulting in earlier detection.

Secondary Amenorrhea

The types of disorders that cause secondary amenorrhea are best thought of in terms of whether they occur in association with sufficient or insufficient estrogen production. Table 19–2 summarizes the causes of secondary amenorrhea.

Adequate Estrogen Production

To establish adequate estrogen levels, progesterone can be administered to note whether withdrawal bleeding occurs. Adequate stimulation of the endometrium by estrogen is essential for a bleeding response to progesterone. Gonadotropin levels should also be normal in this setting. If there is no withdrawal bleeding and gonadotropin levels are normal, acquired anatomic problems causing outflow tract obstruction should be ruled out before assuming that estrogen production is inadequate. Asherman's syndrome is the most common anatomic cause of secondary amenorrhea due to outflow tract obstruction. It is characterized by scarring or adhesions of the intrauterine cavity. This syndrome may appear as amenorrhea, hypomenorrhea, infertility, or recurrent pregnancy loss. Surgical procures such as dilation and curettage, myomectomy, or cesarean section can all result in this syndrome. Acute bacterial pelvic inflammatory disease that results in scarring can be another cause, as can chronic pelvic infections such as tuberculosis or schistosomiasis. The last two disorders should be considered in women from countries in which these diseases are endemic. Chronic

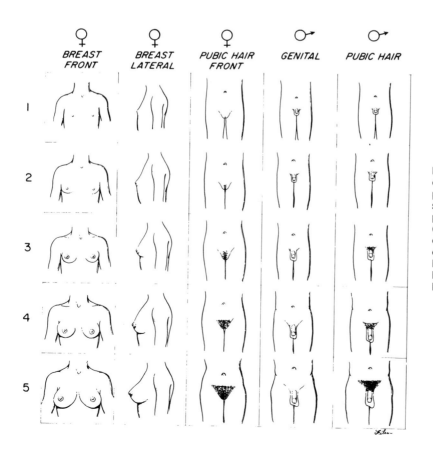

Figure 19–1. Tanner stages of development. Five stages of puberty for females with two staging criteria. Stage 1 is pre-puberty and stage 5 is adult. (Modified from Lee PA. Physiology of puberty. In: Becker KL, et al. (eds). Principles and Practice of Endocrinology and Metabolism. Philadelphia: JB Lippincott, 1990, p 744.)

TABLE 19–2.   Differential Diagnosis of Secondary Amenorrhea

ADEQUATE ESTROGEN PRODUCTION
Anatomic Defects
Asherman's syndrome
Acquired cervical stenosis
Chronic Anovulation
Polycystic ovary syndrome
Late-onset congenital adrenal hyperplasia
Adrenal or ovarian tumors
Cushing's disease
Hypothyroidism
Hyperthyroidism

INADEQUATE ESTROGEN PRODUCTION
Low or Normal Gonadotropins
Hypothalamic amenorrhea
    Midline cerebral tumors (craniopharyngioma, germinoma)
    Infiltrative disorders (tuberculosis, sarcoidosis)
    Functional hypothalamic amenorrhea (stress-related)
    Strenuous exercise
    Malnutrition
    Anorexia nervosa
    Weight loss
    Head trauma

Pituitary disorders
Hyperprolactinemia
    Prolactinoma
    Medications
    Primary hypothyroidism
    Renal failure
    Cerebral tumor or infiltrative disorder
Panhypopituitarism
Head trauma (pituitary infarct or necrosis)
Sheehan's syndrome
Autoimmune hypophysitis
Elevated Gonadotropins
Primary ovarian failure
Genetic defect (47,XXX or galactosemia)
Chemotherapy
Irradiation
Viral infection
Autoimmune
Idiopathic

pelvic infections are also seen in women with HIV disease. The diagnosis of Asherman's syndrome requires a hysterosalpingogram or hysteroscopy, which usually shows multiple filling defects or adhesions. If chronic infection is suspected, an endometrial biopsy can be performed for culture and histology to look for plasma cells.

Cervical stenosis is another anatomic lesion that can result in amenorrhea. Rarely, it is due to a congenital defect, but more commonly it follows a surgical procedure such as conization of the cervix.

If the anatomy is normal, chronic anovulation due to inappropriate hypothalamic pituitary axis feedback is the usual cause of estrogen-sufficient secondary amenorrhea. Polycystic ovary syndrome (PCOS), previously known as Stein-Leventhal syndrome, is the most common cause. Clinical findings may include late menarche, irregular menses or amenorrhea, hirsutism, and obesity. A history of an irregular menstrual pattern commencing within a few years of menarche is typical. Multiple ovarian cysts may be present due to chronic stimulation of ovarian follicles without ovulation, but cystic ovaries are not essential to make the diagnosis. Free testosterone, androstenedione, and luteinizing hormone (LH) are elevated, with an LH to follicle-stimulating hormone (FSH) ratio greater than two. Obesity associated with androgen overproduction may be present. In those who are obese, hyperinsulinemia is seen, which appears to be a consequence of the android, or central, fat distribution pattern. All of the features of PCOS

can be ameliorated with weight loss; thus, obesity is a key component of the pathogenic process.

Most likely, the excess androgen levels are the primary defect in PCOS, causing both the obesity and the hirsutism. The primary source of androgen overproduction is controversial; both the ovaries and the adrenals have been implicated. However, in some individuals with PCOS there clearly is an ovarian defect consisting of a deficiency in the ovarian enzyme 17-ketosteroid reductase, which converts androstenedione to testosterone and estrone to estradiol. The elevated androgen levels, principally androstenedione, in combination with the excess adiposity, result in increased conversion of androstenedione to estrone by peripheral fat tissue, such that estrone levels are elevated. The elevated estrone has in turn been implicated as the cause of the abnormal hypothalamic pituitary function that results in anovulation. The estrone appears to exaggerate hypothalamic Gn-RH release, resulting in higher pituitary LH secretion with loss of the LH surge. The absence of an LH surge means that ovulation cannot occur (Fig. 19–2). Thus, individuals with PCOS are hyperandrogenemic, hyperestrogenemic, hyperinsulinemic, and anovulatory.

The hormonal abnormalities seen in PCOS are similar to those that occur in certain other disorders that cause chronic anovulation, such as late-onset adrenal hyperplasia, hyperthecosis, Cushing's disease, and androgen-secreting adrenal tumors, suggesting that androgen excess of any

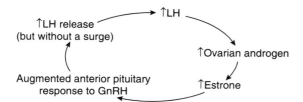

Figure 19–2. The pathophysiology of the polycystic ovary syndrome can be viewed as a self-reinforcing cycle. The event initiating the cycle is unknown and may be different in different patients. The elements of the cycle include an acyclic, surgeless increase in the release of luteinizing hormone (LH), increased ovarian androgen production, and increased production of estrone. GnRH, Gonadotropin-releasing hormone. (From Federman DD. Ovary. In: Rubenstein E, Federman DD (eds). Scientific American Medicine. Section 3, subsection III. New York: Scientific American, 1978–1993, p 10. © 1993 Scientific American, Inc. All rights reserved.)

source has similar clinical manifestations. It has been postulated that PCOS represents the most severe expression of a spectrum of disorders of androgen excess, starting with hirsutism and normal menses and progressing to the full-blown clinical syndrome of hirsutism, obesity, and irregular anovulatory cycles (Table 19–3). As such, it has been postulated that the clinical abnormalities seen in these disorders represent the response of the normal ovary to androgen or insulin excess, or both. The clinical syndrome of PCOS thus appears to have multiple etiologies, which may have adrenal, ovarian, or other origins.

The late-onset congenital adrenal hyperplasias are disorders that are clinically indistinguishable from PCOS, manifesting as hirsutism, estrogen-sufficient amenorrhea or oligomenorrhea, and obesity. However, the etiology of these disorders is clearly adrenal, due to a partial deficiency of one of the adrenal enzymes. In their complete form, these enzyme deficiencies appear at birth as congenital adrenal hyperplasia with salt wasting or ambiguous genitalia. The partial forms of congenital adrenal hyperplasia are not evident until puberty or later in women; thus, the term "late-onset." Although these disorders occur with equal frequency in men and women, they are undetected in men because they are not clinically apparent. The three most common disorders are 21-hydroxylase deficiency, 3β-hydroxysteroid dehydrogenase deficiency, and 11β-hydroxylase deficiency (Fig. 19–3). The enzyme deficiency in each case results in diversion of the product pathway toward excess adrenal androgen production. Cortisol production levels are usually normal. The excess androgen has the same pathophysiologic effects as those described earlier for PCOS, with the same clinical consequences. Despite the name, enlargement of the adrenals does not usually occur. These disorders and their evaluation are also discussed in the chapter on hirsutism. The population prevalence of these disorders depends in part on the racial or ethnic group surveyed. Among persons of Ashkenazic Jewish origin who do not complain of amenorrhea or hirsutism, the prevalence of partial 21-hydroxylase deficiency is 3 to 5%. Among all whites, the prevalence is about 1%. Among women with hirsutism, 3β-hydroxysteroid dehydrogenase deficiency may be at least as common, and possibly more common, than 21-hydroxylase

TABLE 19–3. Hormonal Profiles in Normal Women and Patients with Idiopathic Hirsutism, Polycystic Ovary Syndrome, and Obesity*

		PATIENTS		
PLASMA HORMONES	**NORMAL WOMEN** **(N = 29)**	**Idiopathic Hirsutism** **(N = 30)**	**Polycystic Ovary Syndrome** **(N = 19)** *mean ± SD*	**Obesity and Amenorrhea** **(N = 8)**
Testosterone: SHBG ratio†	3.1 ± 1.3	5.6 ± 2.9‡	9.1 ± 6.8‡	5.4 ± 4.2‡
Estradiol: SHBG ratio†	5.2 ± 4.7	5.6 ± 3.5	7.5 ± 5.4	8.2 ± 6.9
Androstenedione (nmol/L)†	6.0 ± 1.7	7.7 ± 2.6‡	9.8 ± 3.3‡	5.7 ± 3.0
Estrone (pmol/L)	178 ± 71	175 ± 87	293 ± 136‡	251 ± 123‡
Estrone: androstenedione ratio	34 ± 16	26 ± 15	31 ± 13	50 ± 24‡
Basal LH:FSH ratio	1.1 ± 0.5	1.3 ± 0.7	2.7 ± 1.3‡	1.7 ± 0.7‡
LH (mI/U/L) after LH-RH§	12.3 ± 11.3	30 ± 55	51 ± 39‡	37 ± 32‡

*Data are derived from previous studies by the author and his co-workers. SHBG, Sex hormone–binding globulin; LH, luteinizing hormone; FSH, follicle-stimulating hormone; LH-RH, luteinizing hormone–releasing hormone.
†Ratios provide an index of the fraction of the steroids not bound to sex hormone–binding globulin.
‡Significantly different from values in normal women ($P < 0.05$. Student's t-test).
§Maximal increment after 200 μg of luteinizing hormone–releasing hormone was administered intravenously.
From McKenna TJ. Pathogenesis and treatment of polycystic ovary syndrome. New Engl J Med 1988;318:559. Reprinted by permission of the New England Journal of Medicine. Copyright 1988, Massachusetts Medical Society.

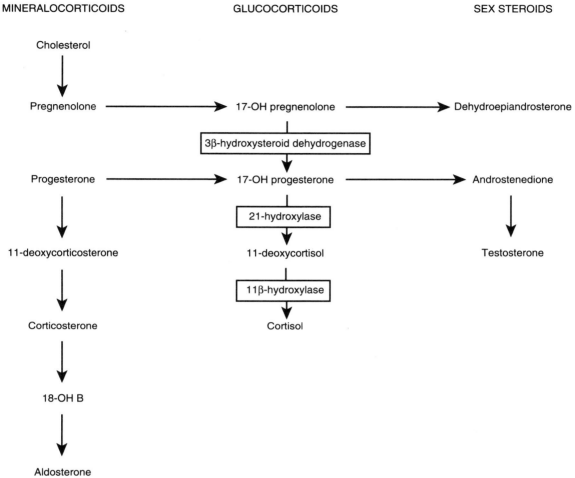

MINERALOCORTICOIDS　　　　　　　GLUCOCORTICOIDS　　　　　　　SEX STEROIDS

Figure 19–3. Sites of adrenal enzyme defects causing late onset congenital adrenal hyperplasias.

deficiency. In one group of hirsute U.S. women, many of whom had irregular menses, 61% had an identifiable enzyme defect. Almost 50% of those with a defect had 3β-hydroxysteroid dehydrogenase deficiency, and under 20% had 21-hydroxylase deficiency. Corresponding figures among Israeli women with hirsutism and oligomenorrhea were 12% and 10%, respectively, in another study.

Other endocrine disorders associated with estrogen-sufficient chronic anovulation can include adrenal or ovarian tumors, some variants of Cushing's syndrome, hyperthyroidism, and hypothyroidism. In Cushing's disease, which is Cushing's syndrome due to an adrenocorticotropic hormone–secreting tumor of the pituitary, the stimulation of adrenal androgen production by adrenocorticotropic hormone results in a PCOS-like syndrome. However, the clinical findings usually have a more sudden onset and a more rapid progression. In hypo- and hyperthyroidism, anovulation occurs due to altered sex steroid metabolism. Hyperprolactinemia also causes anovulation, amenorrhea, or both, but this is due to its antiestrogen effect.

Inadequate Estrogen Production

Once anatomic problems have been excluded, lack of withdrawal bleeding in response to progesterone implies that the endometrium is atrophic from inadequate estrogen levels. To confirm the absence of anatomic abnormalities, cyclic estrogen with progesterone can be administered and bleeding should occur. Other symptoms of estrogen deficiency, such as hot flashes or vaginal dryness, may be present in women with estrogen-deficient amenorrhea. There is also a substantial risk of osteoporosis, which is usually asymptomatic. Gonadotropins may be elevated, normal, or low. Low or normal gonadotropin levels suggest that the diagnosis is hypothalamic or pituitary insufficiency.

High gonadotropin levels are consistent with primary ovarian failure. Estrogen deficiency may not be absolute in many of these conditions; thus, some women have withdrawal bleeding following progesterone administration but still have a disorder in this category.

HYPOTHALAMIC AMENORRHEA. Hypothalamic amenorrhea may be due to midline cerebral tumors, infiltrative disorders, malnutrition, weight loss, chronic disease, anorexia nervosa, strenuous exercise, or psychological stress. The most common midline cerebral tumors are craniopharyngioma or germinoma. Clues to the presence of such tumors include concurrent diabetes insipidus, mild prolactin elevations (from hypothalamic-pituitary stalk interruption), visual disturbances, and deficiency of other pituitary hormones. Infiltrative disorders such as tuberculosis and sarcoidosis can affect the hypothalmus and have a similar manifestation, although usually without visual disturbances.

In hypothalamic amenorrhea due to psychological stress, termed functional hypothalamic amenorrhea, there is reduced or erratic hypothalamic pulsatile Gn-RH secretion, leading to abnormal LH dynamics. The postulated mechanism for the Gn-RH abnormality is an inappropriate elevation of hypothalamic β-endorphin and dopamine, both of which normally function as modulators of Gn-RH neuron secretory activity. Also observed in this type of amenorrhea are increased hypothalamic corticotropin-releasing factor levels, with resultant increased cortisol levels. It is known that corticotropin-releasing factor can inhibit Gn-RH, so the elevated corticotropin-releasing factor may also contribute to the loss of Gn-RH pulsatile secretion. Additional hormonal changes that have been noted in this disorder include increased nocturnal growth hormone and melatonin secretion and low total T4 and T3 despite normal thyroid-stimulating hormone levels. The mechanisms for these latter changes and their role in the pathophysiology of the amenorrhea are unknown.

Strenous exercise as a cause of amenorrhea appears to be related to both the intensity and type of athletic activity. In runners, there is a positive correlation between weekly mileage and incidence of amenorrhea. Among all types of athletes, high-intensity runners are much more likely to experience amenorrhea than swimmers with similar degrees of training intensity. In addition, up to a 3-year delay in the onset of menarche has been reported in runners, ballet dancers, and swimmers who begin training before the onset of menses.

A variety of mechanisms have been postulated to explain the loss of ovarian function. As in stress-induced amenorrhea, Gn-RH secretion is ab-

normal, with the resultant reduced frequency or amplitude, or both, of LH pulses. β-endorphins may again play a role. Exercise has been demonstrated to increase β-endorphin levels acutely, and higher resting levels of β-endorphins have been measured in amenorrheic athletes. As in stress-related amenorrhea, corticotropin-releasing factor and cortisol levels are elevated, as is nocturnal melatonin, and thyroid hormone levels are low. When sedentary women are subjected to an exercise regimen of progressively increasing intensity, they develop luteal phase defects and anovulation despite continued regular menstrual cycles, suggesting a progressive decline in ovarian function. However, it has not been possible to induce amenorrhea in such women, suggesting that other features may have to be present for amenorrhea to occur. Dietary composition and absolute body weight may be factors. Amenorrheic runners weigh less and eat less protein than eumenorrheic runners of similar levels of training intensity, and they also have a higher prevalence of eating disorders. Absolute body weight may be more important than body fat content, which was previously thought to be the primary causal factor. Swimmers have higher body fat contents (~20%) and less amenorrhea than runners (~15%) or ballet dancers (15%), so it has been suggested that a body fat content of at least 22% may be necessary for normal reproductive function. It may be, however, that total body fat is associated with factors that may be more causal, such as total body weight, diet composition, and caloric intake.

In malnutrition and anorexia nervosa, similar abnormalities in Gn-RH and LH pulsatile secretion have been documented to occur. In anorexia nervosa, a prepubertal pattern of nocturnal LH secretion has been shown. The resumption of normal eating habits with weight gain usually reverses these abnormalities. However, anorectics who return to a normal body weight but continue to have eating-disordered patterns of food consumption may not have resolution of their amenorrhea.

Even a modest weight loss of 10 to 15% has been documented to temporarily lower estradiol levels and induce anovulation. These responses to food deprivation may represent an adaptive biologic mechanism to prevent pregnancy in times of food scarcity.

PITUITARY DISORDERS. The most common pituitary disorder associated with amenorrhea is hyperprolactinemia, which may be a factor in up to 30% of cases of secondary amenorrhea. Because hyperprolactinemia is common, prolactin levels should always be measured as part of the initial evaluation, even if there is no galactorrhea. In about 50% of cases, the hyperprolactinemia is due to a secondary cause or is idiopathic, whereas the other 50% are found to be associated with a pituitary adenoma. The prevalence of pituitary lesions of greater than 3 mm in the absence of any endocrine disorder is high, reported in 4 to 20% of normal women studied by computed tomography scan (pituitary "incidentaloma"). Thus, care must be taken to exclude all secondary causes of hyperprolactinemia before proceeding to pituitary imaging. Even if a microadenoma is found, other causes of hyperprolactinemia should be excluded before assuming that the microadenoma is the source of excess prolactin. Causes of nonphysiologic hyperprolactinemia are summarized in Table 19–4. The mechanism of amenorrhea in hyperprolactinemia is most likely interference with hypothalamic function, as decreased gonadotropin pulsatility is known to occur. There may also be a direct effect on the ovary, as prolactin appears to make the ovary less responsive to gonadotropins. If estrogen deficiency is severe enough to result in amenorrhea, osteoporosis is a risk. Vertebral bone density is reduced by 20% in women with hyperprolactinemia and amenorrhea, whereas bone density remains normal in women who have hyperprolactinemia but normal menses. Bone density is at least partially restored with treatment.

The clinical presentation of prolactinoma, or prolactin-secreting pituitary adenoma, is most often limited to amenorrhea or oligomenorrhea. About a third of patients have galactorrhea as well. Headache and visual field defects may occur if there is a larger lesion, known as a macroadenoma (>1.0 cm), which is compressing the optic chiasm or other structures. However, in women, the cessation of menstrual periods leads to earlier detection than in men, usually at the microadenoma (<1.0 cm) stage. Less than 25% of women present with visual field defects, whereas up to 70% of men with prolactinoma present with this finding. Prolactin levels are usually greater than 250 ng per ml at the time of presentation in women with prolactinoma, higher than those seen with idiopathic hyperprolactinemia.

Other causes of hyperprolactinemia include medications, hypothyroidism, renal failure, and disruption of the hypothalamic pituitary stalk by tumor, head injury, or infiltrative disorders (see Table 19–4). Medications include those that interfere with dopamine, which is the primary inhibitor of prolactin. The phenothiazines and related drugs are dopamine receptor blockers, whereas methyldopa and reserpine deplete central dopamine stores. Estrogens stimulate prolactin secretion. In drug-induced hyperprolactinemia, prolactin levels are usually under 200 ng per ml and return to

TABLE 19–4. Conditions Associated with Inappropriate Prolactin Secretion

PHARMACOLOGIC CAUSES	PATHOLOGIC CAUSES
Estrogen Therapy	**Hypothalamic Lesions**
Anesthesia	Craniopharyngioma
DA Receptor Blocking Agents	Glioma
Phenothiazines	Granulomas
Haloperidol	Histocytosis disease
Metoclopramide	Sarcoid
Domperidone	Tuberculosis
Pimozide	Stalk transection
Sulpiride	Postsurgical or head injury
DA Reuptake Blocker	Irradiation damage of the hypothalamus
Nomifensine	Pseudocyesis (functional)
CNS-DA Depleting Agents	**Pituitary Tumors**
Reserpine	Cushing's disease
α-methyldopa	Acromegaly
Monoamine oxidase inhibitor	Prolactinoma
Inhibition of DA Turnover	Mixed GH, or ACTH- and PRL-secreting adenomas
Opiates	"Nonfunctional" adenomas
Stimulation of Serotoninergic System	**Reflex Causes**
Amphetamines	Chest wall injury and herpes zoster neuritis
Hallucinogens	Upper abdominal surgery
Histamine H$_2$-Receptor Antagonists	**Hypothyroidism**
Cimetidine	**Renal Failure**
	Ectopic Production
	Bronchogenic carcinoma
	Hypernephroma

DA, Dopamine; CNS, central nervous system; GH, growth hormone; ACTH, adrenocorticotropic hormone; PRL, prolactin.
From Yen SSC, Jaffe RB. Reproductive Endocrinology. 3rd ed. Philadelphia: WB Saunders, 1991, p 364.

normal when the medication is discontinued. If the medication must be continued (e.g., psychiatric medications) and the patient is amenorrheic, estrogen therapy should be instituted. Primary hypothyroidism is associated with hyperprolactinemia due to thyrotropin-releasing hormone stimulation of prolactin release. It is reversed with treatment of the hypothyroidism. In renal failure, the prolactin clearance rate is diminished. Any midline cerebral tumor or infiltrative disorder can cause mild hyperprolactinemia due to hypothalamic pituitary stalk compression, even if the tumor does not extend into the pituitary sella. The hyperprolactinemia is usually in the 100 to 150 ng per ml range, milder than that seen with prolactin-secreting adenomas.

Other pituitary disorders that can result in amenorrhea include panhypopituitarism or isolated acquired gonadotropin deficiencies. These can be due to compression or destruction of pituitary tissue by pituitary tumors other than prolactinomas, or to pituitary necrosis, hemorrhage, infarct, or autoimmune destruction. In most of these disorders, there is concurrent loss of multiple pituitary hormones, so that amenorrhea occurs in conjunction with findings of secondary hypothyroidism, adrenal insufficiency, or both. Isolated acquired gonadotropin deficiency is extremely rare.

Sheehan's syndrome, or postpartum pituitary necrosis, is panhypopituitarism due to necrosis of the pituitary during severe postpartum hemorrhage with hypotension. Major blood loss with hypotension from any cause can cause pituitary necrosis, but it is more likely to occur during postpartum hemorrhage, suggesting that the pituitary during pregnancy is uniquely susceptible to this phenomenon. Pituitary infarction or hemorrhage can result from trauma or interruption of the blood supply. Autoimmune hypophysitis, or destruction of pituitary tissue due to an autoimmune lymphocytic infiltration, is most common in young women and may occur in association with a pregnancy. Thus, it can be easily confused with Sheehan's syndrome. The diagnosis may be suggested by the presence of other autoimmune disorders.

PRIMARY (PREMATURE) OVARIAN FAILURE. This may be more properly referred to as hypergonadotropic amenorrhea, in which the ovaries are unresponsive to stimulation by gonadotropins. By definition, this is present when there is amenorrhea associated with a follicle-stimulating hormone level greater than 40 mIU per ml on at least two occasions in a woman younger than 40 years of age. Symptoms of estrogen deficiency such as hot flashes and dyspareunia are present in most of these women, and spinal bone density is decreased in more than half. A family history of

premature ovarian failure may be described in some women, suggesting a hereditary component.

Occasionally, premature ovarian failure is due to a genetic defect. Women with trisomy X, or 47, XXX, have normal pubertal development and menarche but develop ovarian failure early in life. Women with galactosemia develop premature ovarian failure as well.

More common causes of ovarian failure include treatment with chemotherapeutic agents or radiation for malignancy. The dose of chemotherapy that causes ovarian failure varies inversely with age, with younger women being less susceptible. Radiation-induced ovarian failure is dose dependent but not age dependent. Fifty percent of women treated for Hodgkin's disease with 400 to 500 rad of irradiation develop ovarian failure, and a dose of 800 rad induces ovarian failure in virtually all women. Cases of premature ovarian failure following viral infections such as mumps have been described, but causality has been difficult to establish.

An autoimmune etiology, as evidenced by antiovarian antibodies, is found in 20% of women with idiopathic premature ovarian failure. In 75% of these women, evidence for other autoimmune disorders is present. These include alopecia, diabetes mellitus, Addison's disease, hypoparathyroidism, idiopathic thrombocytopenic purpura, lupus, thyroid disease, vitiligo, and others. Although ovarian biopsy may reveal lymphocytic infiltrates, biopsy is not indicated to establish a diagnosis, as it is invasive and the results do not alter the prognosis or treatment plan.

Despite the previously mentioned diagnostic possibilities, in most cases of premature ovarian failure, no specific etiology is identified, and treatment must be pursued without identification of a specific causal factor.

DIAGNOSTIC EVALUATION OF AMENORRHEA

History and Physical Examination

A history of the present illness begins with detailed questioning regarding age of menarche and frequency, duration, and amount of menstrual flow (Table 19–5). Presence or absence of premenstrual symptoms or menstrual cramps should be established, as their absence is suggestive of anovulatory cycles. Alternately, the presence of such monthly symptoms without menstruation in women with primary amenorrhea might suggest an anatomic obstruction. Onset of oligomenorrhea or amenorrhea should be carefully verified by con-

TABLE 19–5. History and Physical Examination in Amenorrhea

HISTORY
Primary Amenorrhea
Childhood growth and development
Adult stature as compared with that of parents
Age of onset of breast and pubic hair development
Secondary Amenorrhea
Menstrual history: age of menarche, frequency, duration and
  amount of flow, molimina, dates of last menstrual period
  and previous menstrual period
Hirsutism: age and rapidity of onset, location, severity
Weight: any major loss, rapidity of loss; if obese, age and
  rapidity of onset of obesity
Exercise habits: frequency, intensity
Eating habits: any history or signs of eating disorders
Emotional stress, recent major life events
History of other endocrine or autoimmune disorders
Obstetric history, including duration of unprotected
  intercourse before conception
Gynecologic surgical procedures
Pelvic infections or venereal disease
Head trauma
Galactorrhea
Chemotherapy or radiation therapy
Family history of obesity, hirsutism, infertility, menstrual
  irregularity
Medications

PHYSICAL EXAMINATION
Height and weight
Skin changes: rule out vitiligo, hyperpigmentation
Body hair: Tanner stage and distribution pattern of any
  hirsutism
Breast development, breast discharge
External genitalia, including size of clitoris (should not exceed
  35 mm² length by width)
Presence of estrogen effect: quality of cervical mucus,
  lubrication of vaginal mucosa
Ovarian size or masses
Uterine or pelvic masses

firming the dates of the last several menstrual periods. Often women who perceive their periods as irregular or infrequent have normal menstrual intervals when menses are charted. Women with primary amenorrhea should also be asked about childhood growth and development, stature in relation to parents, and time of onset of breast and pubic hair development, if any. Complete absence of pubic or axillary hair might suggest testicular feminization. A history of growth delay or short stature might be suggestive of Turner's syndrome.

If hirsutism is a complaint, detailed questioning regarding its rapidity of onset, location, and severity should be pursued. Coarse terminal hair growth on the upper back or upper abdomen is a particularly sensitive sign of severe androgen excess. If weight gain is reported, the rapidity of onset and pattern of distribution should be established. In disorders such as adrenal or ovarian tumor, the

onset of hirsutism and weight gain can occur rapidly, within a few months and at any age, whereas in PCOS or adrenal hyperplasia there is usually a more gradual onset of hirsutism and obesity starting in late adolescence or early adulthood. A detailed history of exercise and eating habits, weight gain and loss patterns, emotional stress, and recent major life events should be taken in all patients to determine risk factors for hypothalamic amenorrhea. The review of systems should also include questions to elicit any symptoms of other endocrine or autoimmune disorders, such as hypothyroidism, or rheumatologic diseases.

Because pregnancy is a frequent cause of amenorrhea, patients should also be questioned regarding likelihood of pregnancy, including any recent pregnancy-related symptoms. Past medical history should include obstetric history (including duration of unprotected intercourse before pregnancy occurred) to determine if absolute or relative infertility has been present. It should include any gynecologic surgical procedures (including cesarean section) or pelvic infections to determine whether any risk factors are present for Asherman's syndrome. A history of head trauma might suggest pituitary or hypothalamic dysfunction due to infarct or hemorrhage. Failure to lactate following pregnancy might suggest Sheehan's syndrome. A family history of menstrual dysfunction, infertility, or hirsutism may be present in patients with adrenal hyperplasia. A family history of early menopause may be present in patients with premature ovarian failure. A history of chemotherapy or irradiation treatment should be elicited as well to determine risk for premature ovarian failure. A review of current and prior medications with attention to those that might cause hyperprolactinemia is essential (see Table 19–4 for a list of medications).

The physical examination should include a general examination to look for evidence of hypothyroidism, anemia, vitiligo, adrenal insufficiency, or stigmata of genetic disorders such as Turner's syndrome. It should include a measurement of height and weight and a determination of the distribution and extent of body hair (see Fig. 19–1 for the Tanner stages of pubic hair development and Chapter 20 for a grading scale of hirsutism). It should also include the stage of breast development (see Fig. 19–1) and the presence or absence of galactorrhea. Pelvic examination should include inspection of external genitalia with estimation of the size of the clitoris. The product of the vertical and horizontal dimensions of the clitoris should not exceed 35 mm². Enlargement is evidence of excess androgen effect. In women with primary amenorrhea, anatomic abnormalities such as imperforate hymen, transverse vaginal septum, or vaginal atresia should be evident on pelvic examination. Women with a normal uterus with anatomic outflow obstruction may have a palpable pelvic mass consisting of retained menstrual blood.

In women with intact anatomy, the bimanual examination should include assessment of the presence and size of both ovaries to rule out ovarian tumor, absence of ovaries, or enlarged ovaries suggestive of polycystic ovary syndrome. Normal-sized ovaries on palpation does not rule out PCOS, however. The size and position of the uterus should be assessed, and the cervix should be inspected for pregnancy-related changes. Evidence of adequate estrogenization can be sought by evaluating the vaginal mucosa, which should be moist, with a rugated appearance. Abundant cervical mucus that can be stretched is another manifestation of adequate estrogen effect.

Evaluation Algorithm

The algorithm for the diagnostic evaluation is outlined in Figure 19–4. The first step is to perform a pregnancy test, unless the patient is clearly prepubertal, suggesting a genetic abnormality, or

the vagina or pelvic organs have been documented to be absent. As hyperprolactinemia accounts for 30% of secondary amenorrhea, measurement of a serum prolactin level should be performed if the pregnancy test results are negative. Simultaneously, progesterone should be administered (medroxyprogesterone, 10 mg per day orally for 5–7 days) to assess estrogen adequacy. If withdrawal bleeding occurs within a week of completing the progesterone and prolactin levels are normal, the patient most likely has a disorder of chronic anovulation such as PCOS or late-onset congenital adrenal hyperplasia. If prolactin levels are elevated, a review of possible causes of hyperprolactinemia should be conducted and magnetic resonance imaging (MRI) should be considered. If there is no withdrawal bleeding and prolactin levels are normal, plasma gonadotropins should be measured. If they are elevated (FSH >40 mIU/ml), primary ovarian failure is confirmed. If they are normal or low, cyclic estrogen and progesterone should be administered (one cycle of an oral contraceptive or 1.25 mg per day of conjugated estrogens for 25 days with medroxyprogesterone added on days 11 through 25). If no withdrawal bleeding occurs within a week following this regimen, anatomic abnormalities causing outflow obstruction should

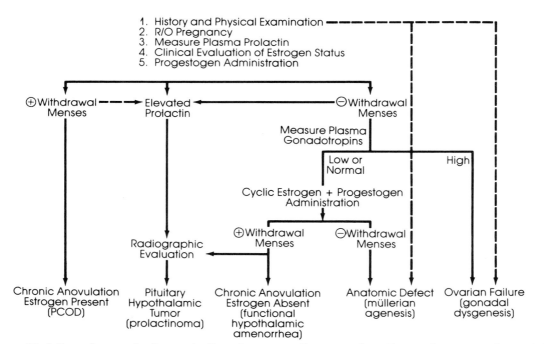

Figure 19–4. Flow diagram for the evaluation of women with amenorrhea. The most common diagnosis for each category is shown in parentheses. The dotted lines indicate that in some instances a correct diagnosis can be reached on the basis of history and physical examination alone. (Reproduced with permission from Carr BR, Wilson JD. Disorders of the ovary and female reproductive tract. In: Wilson JD, et al. (eds). Harrison's Principles of Internal Medicine. 12th ed. New York: McGraw-Hill, p 1788.)

be reconsidered, such as Asherman's syndrome in women with secondary amenorrhea. If there is withdrawal bleeding, the diagnosis is hypothalamic or pituitary amenorrhea. Although functional hypothalamic amenorrhea is most likely, particularly in women with risk factors such as eating disorders or intense exercise programs, MRI of the pituitary-hypothalamic area should be considered in all women with hypothalamic or pituitary amenorrhea to rule out midline lesions such as tumors.

Further Diagnosis and Treatment

DISORDERS OF ANOVULATION. Further diagnostic evaluation should include measurement of LH and FSH to determine the LH to FSH ratio, measurement of androgens to look for clues to PCOS or late-onset adrenal hyperplasia, and measurement of thyroid-stimulating hormone to rule out thyroid dysfunction. A fasting glucose measurement should be obtained because of the high prevalence of insulin resistance in disorders of androgen excess. Specific androgens to measure are testosterone and dehydroepiandrosterone sulfate (DHEAS). Testosterone levels above 200 ng per ml are suggestive of ovarian tumor, and pelvic ultrasound should be performed. Dehydroepiandrosterone sulfate levels above 7.0 μg per dl are suggestive of adrenal tumor, and an abdominal computed tomography scan should be performed. Intermediate elevations of testosterone are suggestive of PCOS, especially if the LH to FSH ratio is greater than 2. Intermediate elevations of DHEAS suggest late-onset congenital adrenal hyperplasia, and referral to an endocrinologist for stimulation testing with short-acting synthetic adrenocorticotropic hormone (Cortrosyn) is recommended. A simpler screen can also be performed that will rule out one of the three most common enzyme defects resulting in late-onset congenital adrenal hyperplasia. A 17-hydroxyprogesterone level, if drawn before 10 A.M., is usually elevated in 21-hydroxylase deficiency. If the results are normal, Cortrosyn testing will still have to be performed to screen for the other two enzyme defects.

The role of pelvic ultrasound is controversial in PCOS. A finding of multiple ovarian cysts is suggestive of the diagnosis but can also be seen in other conditions, such as during recovery from hypothalamic amenorrhea. Alternately, the absence of ovarian cysts does not rule out the diagnosis of PCOS. The diagnosis is based primarily on clinical and biochemical criteria and is often a diagnosis of exclusion in patients with clinical evidence of androgen excess and anovulation.

Treatment of amenorrhea of various origins is listed in Table 19–6. The amenorrhea of PCOS or late-onset congenital adrenal hyperplasia is critically important to treat, as the endometrial lining in both disorders is under constant unopposed stimulation by estrogen and is at increased risk of malignant transformation. Regular withdrawal bleeding helps to prevent this process. In PCOS, this can be accomplished by oral contraceptive therapy. Oral contraceptives are also helpful in the treatment of the hirsutism, acne, and other effects of excess androgen, because they suppress ovarian production of testosterone. If the patient does not wish to take oral contraceptives, monthly or bimonthly medroxyprogesterone therapy to induce withdrawal bleeding should be sufficient to allow shedding of the proliferative endometrium and minimize cancer risk. Weight reduction is also an important component of the treatment of PCOS. Significant weight loss in obese patients results in the resumption of ovulatory cycles in many cases.

Treatment of late-onset congenital adrenal hyperplasia depends on the severity of the syndrome. For those in whom a specific adrenal enzyme deficiency is identified, low-dose daily dexamethasone is sometimes used (0.5–0.75 mg every day at bedtime) to suppress adrenal androgen overproduction. Unfortunately, suppression of cortisol production may also occur. Patients must therefore be instructed to increase their dexamethasone dose in response to illness and to wear a medical bracelet identifying themselves as potentially adrenally insufficient should a medical emergency occur. Shorter-acting glucocorticoids (prednisone, cortisol) can also be used, which may not be as effective but do incur less risk of suppression of adrenal cortisol production. Many women resume ovulatory cycles on dexamethasone therapy. Alternately, treatment can be symptomatic, with use of oral contraceptives or medroxyprogesterone to induce regular withdrawal bleeding and spironolactone to treat hirsutism. In either PCOS or late-onset congenital adrenal hyperplasia, ovulation induction may be necessary if pregnancy is desired and the previously mentioned treatments have not restored ovulatory cycles.

HYPERPROLACTINEMIA. Treatment of medication-induced hyperprolactinemia consists of discontinuing the offending medication. This often poses a dilemma for psychiatric patients, who may not be able to discontinue their phenothiazines safely owing to the severity of their psychiatric illness and the lack of effective alternative medications. Those in whom discontinuation is not an option and who have not shown evidence of withdrawal bleeding following a medroxyprogesterone challenge should be treated with estrogen therapy

TABLE 19-6. Treatment of Amenorrhea

DISORDERS OF ANOVULATION, ESTROGEN SUFFICIENT
Polycystic Ovary Syndrome
(LH:FSH ratio >2, testosterone elevated but <200)
Oral contraceptive formulations containing low-androgenic progesterones
or
medroxyprogesterone 10 mg per day × 7 days monthly or bimonthly
and/or
spironolactone 25 mg t.i.d. starting dose
and
weight loss

Late-Onset Congenital Adrenal Hyperplasia
(DHEAS elevated but <7 μg/dl; specific enzyme abnormality identified by synthetic adrenocorticotropic hormone stimulation testing)
Low-dose glucocorticoids (dexamethasone .025 mg h.s. or prednisone 2.5–5.0 mg h.s. or q.o.h.s.)
or
oral contraceptive formulations containing low-androgenic progesterones
or
medroxyprogesterone 10 mg per day × 7 days monthly or bimonthly
and/or
spironolactone 25 mg t.i.d. starting dose

Adrenal or Ovarian Tumor
(DHEAS >7 μg/dl, or testosterone >200 are suggestive of adrenal or ovarian tumor respectively)
Image appropriate organ
and
refer for surgical and oncologic management

Anatomic Defects
(Vaginal atresia, cervical stenosis, Asherman's, others)
Refer for surgical management

DISORDERS OF ANOVULATION, ESTROGEN DEFICIENT
Hyperprolactinemia
(All values <50 should be repeated to confirm)
If due to hypothyroidism, treat with thyroxine
or
if medication related, discontinue offending medication or institute hormone therapy with oral contraceptives or conjugated estrogens and progesterone
or
if no secondary cause identified, get pituitary MRI scan
and
if microadenoma or idiopathic, start bromocriptine at 1.25–2.5 mg h.s.
or
if macroadenoma, refer for formal visual field testing and start bromocriptine

Hypothalamic Amenorrhea
(Low FSH and LH, no response to progesterone challenge, negative results on pituitary-hypothalamic MRI scan)
Reverse inciting behaviors (decrease exercise, increase caloric intake and weight)
and/or
psychiatric counseling if necessary
or
hormone therapy with oral contraceptives or conjugated estrogens and progesterone if behavioral modification is unsuccessful

Turner's Syndrome
(Primary amenorrhea, XO or related karyotype)
Growth hormone therapy if short stature and epiphyses not fused
and
hormone therapy with oral contraceptives or conjugated estrogens and progesterone

Testicular Feminization
(Primary amenorrhea and XY karyotype)
Remove testes
and
administer hormone therapy

Premature Ovarian Failure
(Elevated FSH >40 mIU/ml and no response to progesterone challenge)
Hormone therapy

LH, Luteinizing hormone; FSH, follicle-stimulating hormone; t.i.d., three times a day; DHEAS, dehydroepiandrosterone sulfate; h.s., at bedtime; q.o.h.s., every other night (bedtime).

(oral contraceptives or conjugated estrogens with cyclic progesterone). In those who do experience withdrawal bleeding following a progesterone challenge, there is probably sufficient estrogen to maintain bone density and cardiovascular benefits, and estrogen therapy is not necessary. Regular induction of withdrawal bleeding should be done to allow shedding of proliferative endometrium. If at any time estrogen deficiency becomes manifest, estrogen therapy should be instituted.

If there is no obvious secondary cause of the hyperprolactinemia, thyroid-stimulating hormone should be measured to rule out hypothyroidism. If the prolactin level is only slightly elevated, in the 20 to 50 ng per ml range, it should be repeated to confirm the result, as mild prolactin elevations may occur in response to stress, eating, sleep, or other mild stimuli. If the level of thyroid-stimulating hormone is normal and the prolactin elevation is confirmed, imaging of the pituitary with MRI should be performed. Although a prolactin-secreting microadenoma is unlikely if the prolactin level is under 250 ng per ml, imaging with MRI may still be appropriate for persons with prolactin levels in this range to rule out stalk compression by another type of midline tumor. Sella tomograms are no longer considered appropriate, as most tumors are microadenomas and do not distort the bony sella. If a microadenoma is identified or if the hyperprolactinemia is termed idiopathic, the treatment of choice to restore cyclic menses is oral bromocriptine, starting at 2.5 mg at bedtime and increasing as tolerated until hyperprolactinemia is resolved and menses resume. Because of the high recurrence rates, surgery is no longer considered the treatment of choice for prolactinoma. Even macroadenomas with visual field compromise usually respond promptly to bromocriptine therapy. The treatment must be continued indefinitely in many patients, as the bromocriptine does not induce permanent remission, and the spontaneous remission rate is only approximately 25% over time. If the patient has hyperprolactinemia but continues to menstruate regularly or responds promptly to progesterone challenge, bone density is probably not compromised. In hyperprolactinemic women who are menstruating regularly, observation without bromocriptine therapy may be appropriate as long as fertility is not an issue. Although only 25% of patients experience remission, the natural history of the disorder is fairly benign in those who do not remit, with only one third experiencing further elevations in prolactin levels and only a few showing evidence of an increase in tumor size. Thus, observation without treatment is a reasonable alternative in those in whom bone density is not compromised and fertility is not an issue.

Hypothalamic amenorrhea must be treated by removal of the inciting factors. If weight gain, decreased exercise, or counseling to reduce stress and address eating disorders is ineffective, then estrogen therapy should be instituted. If fertility is desired, continuous pulsatile infusion of Gn-RH has been shown to be effective in inducing ovulation. A single MRI examination of the hypothalamus and pituitary should be performed at diagnosis to rule out a midline tumor.

In disorders of pituitary gonadotropin deficiency, such as panhypopituitarism or Sheehan's syndrome, estrogen therapy and replacement of other pituitary hormones are necessary. Again, pituitary imaging with MRI should be performed initially to rule out tumor as the cause of the hypofunction.

ANATOMIC DEFECTS. Congenital anatomic defects of the vagina are usually amenable to surgical reconstruction to allow normal menstruation. If the uterus or endometrial lining is absent, however, menstruation cannot occur, although continued ovarian function ensures protection from osteoporosis and symptoms of estrogen deficiency. Acquired anatomic defects, such as Asherman's syndrome or cervical stenosis, can also be treated surgically to allow resumption of menstruation.

The presence of Turner's syndrome requires treatment in early adolescence with estrogen replacement to induce growth and development of secondary sex characteristics. Growth hormone is sometimes used as well to achieve a more normal adult height. Cyclic estrogen and progesterone are required permanently to prevent the complications of estrogen deficiency and to induce monthly bleeding.

Testicular feminization must be treated with surgical removal of the testes and permanent estrogen replacement.

Premature ovarian failure also requires estrogen therapy, together with progesterone, to induce monthly bleeding. If an autoimmune etiology is identified, immune supression with prednisone is sometimes successful at restoring ovarian function at least temporarily. Most patients remain infertile, but the occasional patient ovulates and conceives following a few months of estrogen therapy for as yet unexplained reasons.

Appropriate treatment of all types of amenorrhea must always include consideration of potentially serious health risks, which are too often ignored: The risk of endometrial cancer in those with anovulation and unopposed estrogen stimulation of the endometrial lining and the risk of osteoporosis and accelerated cardiovascular disease in those with estrogen deficiency are all quite significant and must be addressed as a routine part of the evaluation and treatment plan.

Hirsutism

Mary Lally Delaney

The diagnosis of hirsutism requires consideration of patient perceptions and cultural norms. Hirsutism is defined as excessive growth of terminal hair in a male distribution. It can be scored by the Ferriman and Gallwey system with the degree of hair growth graded from 0 (none) to 4 (frankly virile) in nine areas (upper lip, chin, chest, upper and lower abdomen, upper and lower back, upper arms, and thighs) (Fig. 20–1). Seven or fewer points on a scale of 0 to 36 is considered normal. Hirsutism is graded as mild with 8 to 12 points, moderate with 13 to 18 points, and severe with 19 or more points.

Virilization is a more severe abnormality than hirsutism and may involve male pattern baldness, clitoral hypertrophy, deepening of the voice, and increased muscularity in addition to excess terminal hair. A woman with rapid onset of hirsutism or with virilization should be investigated for a possible hormone-secreting tumor.

Hypertrichosis should be distinguished from hirsutism because it is not androgen dependent. It involves increased vellus, smooth hairs with uniform shaft diameters that are prominent in nonsexual areas. It may be congenital, metabolic, or related to medications.

PREVALENCE

In a study of women presenting to a medical clinic without endocrine disease or complaints of hirsutism, 4.3% had a Ferriman-Gallwey score higher than 7, which is consistent with at least mild hirsutism; 1.2% scored higher than 10.

Hirsutism is common among women in Mediterranean populations and is uncommon among women in Asian populations. Estimates of the prevalence of one cause of hirsutism, congenital adrenal hyperplasia, have ranged from 0.3% in whites to 1.9% in Hispanics and 3.7% in Eastern European (Ashkenazi) Jews.

In postpubertal women, normal androgen levels transform vellus hairs to terminal hairs in areas with androgen-responsive hair follicles such as the pubis and axilla. Many normal women also develop terminal hair on the face, lower abdomen, and chest. Most women with moderate to severe hirsutism or associated menstrual abnormalities choose to be evaluated.

ETIOLOGIES

In clinical practice, idiopathic hirsutism and polycystic ovary syndrome (PCOS) are the most common causes of hirsutism. With idiopathic hirsutism, pilosebaceous units containing hair follicles are felt to have increased sensitivity to androgens and to be more apt to develop terminal hairs despite normal androgen levels. There may be increased androgen binding or increased conversion of testosterone to dihydrotestosterone, the primary nuclear androgen in the pilosebaceous unit, by 5α-reductase in women with idiopathic hirsutism. Menses are characteristically normal with idiopathic hirsutism but are often irregular with PCOS. Idiopathic hirsutism is a diagnosis of exclusion.

Polycystic ovarian disease is a collection of heterogeneous disorders. Varying criteria have been applied to the diagnosis of PCOS. Sometimes the presence of ovarian cysts has been felt to be sufficient. Often clinical criteria including oligoamenorrhea, hirsutism, and obesity have been applied. Biochemical criteria including elevated luteinizing hormone (LH) to follicle-stimulating hormone (FSH) ratios, elevated androgens, hyperglycemia, or insulin resistance have been used. Combinations of anatomic, clinical, and biochemical criteria probably allow a better diagnosis of PCOS.

Some studies of women with PCOS have included women with congenital adrenal hyperplasia because of clinical similarities. Generally hirsutism is classified according to the primary cause. Some women with PCOS are felt to have defects of ovarian steroid biosynthesis. Interactions between ovarian and adrenal hyperandrogenism have been suggested in women with PCOS.

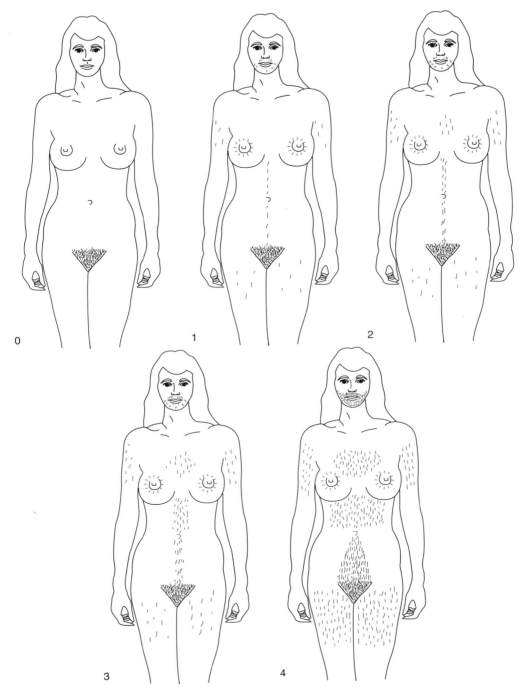

Figure 20–1. Hirsutism is graded from 0 (absent) to 4 (virile) based on severity in nine areas: upper lip, chin, chest, upper abdomen, lower abdomen, arm, thigh, upper back, and lower back. A total of 0–7 points is normal; 8–12 points signifies mild hirsutism; 13–18 points signifies moderate hirsutism; 19–36 points signifies severe hirsutism.

Late-onset congenital adrenal hyperplasias can appear after menarche with hirsutism. Irregular menses or anovulation may also occur. Classical adrenal hyperplasias are more serious disorders that may occur with ambiguous or virilized genitalia in genetic females at birth; salt-wasting forms may be associated with life-threatening adrenal insufficiency.

Three enzyme defects with autosomal recessive inheritance have been recognized in congenital adrenal hyperplasia. A 21-hydroxylase deficiency is the most common enzyme deficiency (>90% of cases) and leads to buildup of 17α-hydroxyprogesterone, which is a precursor for 11-deoxycortisol and subsequent cortisol synthesis. Aldosterone synthesis may also be decreased. Late-onset 21-hydroxylase deficiency has been estimated to occur in perhaps 1% of white women.

An 11β-hydroxylase deficiency is the second most common cause of congenital adrenal hyperplasia and is commonly associated with hypertension and hypokalemia in its classical form because of excess production of the mineralocorticoid deoxycorticosterone. Late-onset 11β-hydroxylase deficiency may cause hirsutism without signs of mineralocorticoid excess. Carmina and colleagues found that 2.2% of 182 hirsute Italian women had biochemical evidence of this enzyme deficiency on adrenocorticotropic hormone (ACTH) testing without associated hypertension. 11-Deoxycortisol is usually measured to assess suspected 11β-hydroxylase deficiency.

Congenital adrenal hyperplasia due to 3β-hydroxysteroid dehydrogenase defects results in decreased conversion of steroids with double bonds at the 5 to the 4 position (i.e., dehydroepiandrosterone to androstenedione, pregnenolone to progesterone, or 17α-hydroxypregnenolone to 17α-hydroxyprogesterone).

The glucocorticoid pathway is impaired by late-onset forms of congenital adrenal hyperplasias by increased androgen biosynthesis from overabundant precursors leading to hirsutism. The adrenal glands hypertrophy owing to excess secretion of ACTH by the pituitary, which attempts to overcome the steroidogenic block to cortisol production.

These enzyme deficiencies can be assessed by evaluating steroid responses to ACTH stimulation. A difficulty with the criteria established by some investigators is the lack of an independent test to verify or disprove the putative diagnosis of 11β-hydroxylase or 3β-hydroxysteroid dehydrogenase deficiency established by ACTH testing. By using statistical methods to establish abnormal results, some women with very mild biosynthetic defects may be labeled as having a disease when they are normal.

Several drugs can cause increased hair. Norgestrel, norethindrone, metronidazole, corticosteroids, anabolic or androgenic steroids, and cyclosporin are potential contributors to hirsutism. Drugs such as phenytoin, minoxidil, and diazoxide can cause hypertrichosis or increased vellus hairs rather than the terminal hairs characteristic of hirsutism. Metabolic diseases that can cause hirsutism include hypothyroidism, hyperprolactinemia, acromegaly, anorexia nervosa, and porphyria.

Ovarian and adrenal tumors can cause virilization. About 7% of ovarian tumors are functional with the production of estrogens or androgens. Arrhenoblastomas are the most common virilizing ovarian tumors. Hormone-producing ovarian tumors should be considered when the testosterone level is elevated to greater than twice normal. Adrenal tumors are in the differential diagnosis of hirsute women, especially with dehydroepiandrosterone sulfate (DHEAS) levels that are greater than two times normal. Virilization can also be a prominent feature of Cushing's syndrome.

Ovarian hyperthecosis may cause virilization in postmenopausal women. Hypertrophy of ovarian stroma occurs that is due to high levels of gonadotropins; the ovaries synthesize excess androgen in this condition. Some women have hyperthecosis premenopausally, which may be an extreme variant of PCOS.

DIAGNOSTIC EVALUATION

Evaluation should be based on the severity of the hirsutism, its duration, and the presence or absence of menstrual irregularities. The rapid development of severe hirsutism, virilization, or menstrual irregularities portends serious disease (Fig. 20–2).

History

The history should include the onset of the hirsutism (gradual or sudden), involved locations, associated acne or oily skin, types and frequency of use of hair control techniques, menstrual patterns, changes in voice timbre or muscularity, frontal or temporal scalp hair loss, galactorrhea, thyroid symptoms, and history of hypertension or hyperglycemia.

Physical Examination

The physical examination should include an assessment of the severity and distribution of the

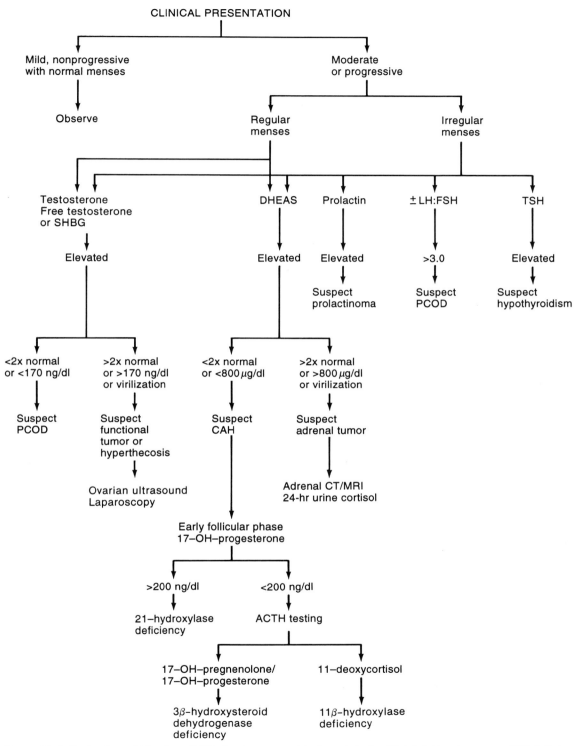

Figure 20–2. Evaluation of hirsutism. SHBG, Sex hormone–binding globulin; LH, luteinizing hormone; FSH, follicle-stimulating hormone; TSH, thyroid-stimulating hormone; DHEAS, dehydroepiandrosterone sulfate; PCOD, polycystic ovarian disease; CAH, congenital adrenal hyperplasia; CT, computed tomography; MRI, magnetic resonance imaging; ACTH, adrenocorticotropic hormone.

excess terminal hair. It may be helpful to standard-ize the evaluation of the patient's hirsutism by comparing it with a drawing that suggests grading of hirsutism. In general, 0 = none, 1 = sparse, 2 = mild, 3 = moderate, and 4 = severe (virile) (see Fig. 20–1).

For the upper lip:

0 = no terminal hairs
1 = few terminal hairs at the periphery
2 = small moustache at the periphery
3 = moustache extending halfway from periphery to midline
4 = full moustache to midline

Calculation of a Ferriman-Gallwey score is helpful in assessing the severity of the hirsutism and pro-vides a means of following clinical changes over time.

Signs of hirsutism should be evaluated, includ-ing male-type (diamond- rather than triangular-shaped) escutcheon, clitoral enlargement, deep voice, increased musculature out of proportion to exercise, male pattern baldness, and acne. A pelvic examination may detect an ovarian tumor. A clitoral index (the product of the vertical and hor-izontal dimensions of the glans) of <35 mm² is normal, and one of >100 mm² signifies viriliza-tion. Hypertension, striae, thin skin, easy bruising, and centripetal obesity suggest Cushing's syn-drome or disease in hirsute or virilized women. Women with acromegaly often have coarse fea-tures, large hands and feet, and possible increased spacing between teeth and may sweat more easily than others.

Laboratory Testing

Laboratory tests to evaluate hirsutism tend to be expensive. Clues from the history and physical examination can be used to direct the evaluation. If a woman has regular menses and mild hirsutism of gradual onset, a serious underlying disease is unlikely to be found. If the rest of her history and physical examination are unrevealing, she may not need any laboratory tests unless the hirsutism pro-gresses. She likely has a benign condition such as idiopathic hirsutism. Cosmetic measures are prob-ably best for treatment.

If the hirsutism is moderate or progressive or if menses are irregular, screening tests should in-clude testosterone, DHEAS, and free testosterone or a measure of sex hormone–binding globulin. 17β-OH-steroids (testosterone, dihydrotestoster-one, and estradiol) are highly bound to this pro-tein. Sex hormone–binding globulin levels rise with rising estrogen levels and hyperthyroidism

and decrease with elevated androgens, glucocorti-coids, and growth hormone and obesity. In a woman with elevated androgen levels, the amount of sex hormone–binding globulin may be low and the amount of free testosterone high even with a normal total testosterone level. An elevated level of urinary androstanediol glucuronoside has been suggested to correlate well with hirsutism, but sev-eral studies dispute an advantage over other meas-ures of androgens.

Women with irregular menses and hirsutism may have hyperprolactinemia or hypothyroidism, so measurement of prolactin levels or thyroid tests such as free thyroxine and thyroid-stimulating hor-mone levels may diagnose treatable disease. Women with PCOS usually have irregular menses and hirsutism. Their testosterone levels may be moderately elevated, and their DHEAS values are sometimes also above normal. The LH to FSH ratio may be above 3, and an ovarian ultrasound may reveal polycystic ovaries, but normal results on these tests do not exclude the diagnosis. A woman presenting with oligomenorrhea and hir-sutism after menarche who does not have evidence of virilization or a separate reason for hirsutism (hyperprolactinemia, thyroid disease, or congenital adrenal hyperplasia) can be classified clinically as having PCOS. Hyperglycemia may be associated with PCOS, Cushing's disease or syndrome, or acromegaly.

Elevated plasma DHEAS levels are indicative of adrenal hyperandrogenism. Testosterone levels may be elevated in either adrenal or ovarian hy-perandrogenism. A 17-ketosteroid measurement is helpful in women with episodic adrenal androgen secretion because it gives an integrated assessment of adrenal androgens, but it requires a 24-hour urine collection.

Women with hirsutism and elevated (but less than twice normal) DHEAS levels should be tested for congenital adrenal hyperplasia. The most cost-effective screening test is a morning, early follicu-lar 17α-OH-progesterone level, which evaluates possible 21-hydroxylase deficiency, the most com-mon form of congenital adrenal hyperplasia. Al-though this test could be done on hirsute women as an initial screening test, it is usually checked when the DHEAS is elevated or when the woman is from a population with an increased prevalence of congenital adrenal hyperplasia.

The full complement of tests used to investigate all three forms of congenital adrenal hyperplasia is described under special testing. Because of the ex-pense and limited yield of full ACTH testing, ACTH testing with cortisol and 17α-OH-proges-terone levels is probably sufficient unless a woman is moderately to severely hirsute, hypertensive, or hypokalemic or has a strong family history of hirsutism, early neonatal deaths, or ambiguous genitalia.

Women with virilization or rapid progression of hirsutism need a thorough evaluation for possible malignancy. Functioning ovarian and adrenal tumors are possible causes. Women found on screening tests to have high testosterone levels (often >170 ng/dl or 6 nm) may have virilizing ovarian tumors and should have their ovaries visualized by transvaginal ultrasound. Women with high DHEAS levels (often >800 μg/dl or 18.5 μM) who may have androgenic adrenal tumors should have computed tomography or magnetic resonance imaging scans to view their adrenal glands. Women with markedly elevated adrenal androgen levels should also be tested for the excess cortisol production of Cushing's disease or syndrome. If a tumor is suspected clinically or biochemically but not found with visualization of the adrenals or ovaries, venous catheterization can be done to localize the source of the hyperandrogenism. Laparoscopy may also be helpful in some patients.

Special Testing

A 24-hour urinary free cortisol by radioimmunoassay after chromatography or by high-pressure liquid chromatography can be used when Cushing's syndrome or disease is suspected clinically. Overnight, low-dose, and high-dose dexamethasone tests, corticotropin-releasing hormone tests, and inferior petrosal sinus sampling are sometimes used to diagnose hypercortisolism and help distinguish pituitary Cushing's disease from adrenal or ectopic Cushing's syndromes.

ACTH TESTING. Women with elevated adrenal androgens and hirsutism may have congenital adrenal hyperplasia. The most common enzyme deficiency can be screened for by measuring the follicular-phase morning 17α-hydroxyprogesterone level. Formal ACTH testing can detect more subtle enzyme defects and can screen for all three abnormalities by measuring cortisol, 17α-hydroxyprogesterone, 17α-hydroxypregnenolone, and 11-deoxycortisol before and after the administration of ACTH in women with possible congenital adrenal hyperplasia.

Adrenocorticotropic hormone testing is a simple office procedure that requires drawing baseline blood tubes followed by immediately administering 0.25 mg Cortrosyn (synthetic ACTH) intravenously or intramuscularly. If a butterfly needle or an intravenous catheter is used to draw the baseline blood, the ACTH can be given through the same needle. One hour after the ACTH is given, the post-ACTH blood samples are collected and labeled appropriately.

It is preferable to do this test in the follicular phase of the menstrual cycle and in the morning. During the luteal phase of the menstrual cycle, progesterone levels are high and could interfere with the 17α-hydroxyprogesterone assay.

If a woman has oligomenorrhea and the phase of her cycle cannot be determined clinically, the test can be performed, an aliquot of the pre-ACTH sample can be sent to the laboratory for assay of progesterone, and the rest can be frozen. If the progesterone level suggests that the patient is in the follicular phase, the rest of the hormone assays can be done. If the progesterone level suggests the luteal phase, the test can be rescheduled after the next menses. This approach is reasonable given the cost of checking expensive hormone assays in duplicate.

With 21-hydroxylase deficiency, 17α-hydroxyprogesterone is often elevated at baseline, and the level may rise dramatically after the exogenous ACTH amplifies the effects of the steroidogenic block.

Levels of 11-deoxycortisol may be elevated at baseline and rise in response to the administration of ACTH with 11β-hydroxylase deficiency.

With 3β-hydroxysteroid dehydrogenase deficiency, the ratio of 17α-hydroxypregnenolone to 17α-hydroxyprogesterone is typically elevated, especially after the administration of ACTH. Ratios of other pairs of steroids that differ only in the position of the double bond being at the 5 or 4 position of the steroid nucleus can be used. Measurement of the ratio of this pair of steroids (rather than that of dehydroepiandrosterone to androstenedione or pregnenolone to progesterone) is useful because the 17α-hydroxyprogesterone needs to be measured to test for 21-hydroxylase deficiency, and it is less expensive to add only one more steroid measurement with the laboratory.

TREATMENT

Treatment of hirsutism involves specific therapy for any underlying conditions as well as cosmetic management (Table 20–1). Tumors may need surgery for resection when possible and for establishing a pathologic diagnosis and directing further therapy. Hypothyroidism is readily treated with L-thyroxine replacement therapy. Women with hyperprolactinemia and normal results on thyroid tests who are not breast-feeding or taking medications known to elevate prolactin need pituitary evaluation for possible prolactinoma and, usually,

TABLE 20–1.   Treatment of Hirsutism

Treat Specific Etiologies:
   Adrenal or ovarian tumors
   Hypothyroidism
   Prolactinoma
   Acromegaly
   Porphyria
   Anorexia nervosa
Physical or Cosmetic Measures:
Temporary: Bleaching
          Shaving
          Depilatories
          Waxing
          Plucking
Permanent: Electrolysis
Systemic Measures:
  I. Dexamethasone 0.25–0.5 mg orally every bedtime to
    every other night:
      Late-onset congenital adrenal hyperplasia
      Risk of adrenal suppression
 II. Spironolactone 50–200 mg orally every day:
      Polycystic ovarian disease
      Idiopathic hirsutism
      Late-onset congenital adrenal hyperplasia
      Monitor blood pressure, renal function, potassium
      May cause irregular menses
      Teratogen, requires effective contraception
III. Ovarian suppression:
    A. Oral contraceptives:
        For polycystic ovary syndrome
        Cyproterone acetate and estradiol
    B. Gonadotropin-releasing hormone agonists:
        Not recommended
IV. Investigational antiandrogens:
      Flutamide, ketoconazole, finasteride
      Not currently recommended

dopamine agonist therapy. Prolactin can be elevated in primary hypothyroidism because thyrotropin-releasing hormone stimulates release of both thyroid-stimulating hormone and prolactin from the anterior pituitary. Some obese women with polycystic ovarian disease have decreased hirsutism with weight loss.

Physical or cosmetic methods of coping with hirsutism may be the mainstay of therapy for many women. Bleaching can make the hair less noticeable. Other choices include temporary removal with shaving, depilatories, waxing or plucking, or permanent removal with electrolysis.

Systemic methods of therapy have variable success rates with hirsute women. Usually they need to be used for at least 3 to 4 months to determine whether they are effective. Once a terminal hair has developed, it remains a differentiated, androgenized hair until it falls out at the end of its life span. Even if fewer hair follicles are being androgenized, the effects are not seen until the old group of terminal hairs is gone. Some women notice they

need to use local hair removal methods less often when the systemic therapy begins to take effect.

Congenital adrenal hyperplasia can be treated specifically with adrenal suppressive therapy. A typical regimen is dexamethasone 0.25 to 0.5 mg by mouth at bedtime, although some clinicians use every other night dosing. Dexamethasone with its long half-life is used to suppress the usual rise in adrenal hormones that occurs in the early morning. The lowest dose of dexamethasone that suppresses adrenal androgen levels should be used to decrease the extent of adrenal suppression that may occur in times of stress.

Women who are offered steroid suppression for late-onset congenital adrenal hyperplasia should understand the risk-benefit considerations involved. If they have a brisk cortisol response to ACTH testing, they are unlikely to have adrenal insufficiency before beginning steroid therapy, but this may develop with steroid use. Women taking even ''replacement'' doses of glucocorticoids to suppress adrenal androgens should wear a MedicAlert bracelet or necklace. Also, women offered steroid therapy should be aware that the effects of the steroids may be delayed for a few months after beginning therapy and that hirsutism will likely recur after the steroids are discontinued.

When women who have congenital adrenal hyperplasia are planning to become pregnant, their partners can be screened for evidence of congenital adrenal hyperplasia. Some women have taken suppressive doses of steroids beginning during early pregnancy to try to avoid ambiguous or virilized genitalia in potential female fetuses (with variable success and side effects), and this course of therapy would not be an option in a woman whose congenital adrenal hyperplasia is undiagnosed.

Spironolactone is an antiandrogen that acts at various levels to decrease hirsutism. It is felt to block peripheral 5α-reductase activity, increase peripheral conversion of testosterone to estradiol, block androgen receptors, and inhibit testosterone synthesis. It works well for many women with idiopathic hirsutism or PCOS. It is an alternative for many women with late-onset congenital adrenal hyperplasia that does not cause adrenal suppression.

Spironolactone is a potassium-sparing diuretic, so blood pressure should be monitored with therapy. Renal function should be assessed with creatinine and potassium values before and after beginning therapy. The dose needed can vary from 50 to 200 mg by mouth daily, often given in divided doses with meals to reduce stomach irritation.

Spironolactone can feminize a male fetus, so it needs to be used in conjunction with effective contraception. Irregular menses can occur on spirono-lactone therapy, especially with higher doses. This symptom can be troubling enough for women to stop taking it even when it decreases their hirsutism. The combination of an oral contraceptive and spironolactone is often effective and well tolerated.

Oral contraceptives can decrease ovarian hyperandrogenism by decreasing gonadotropin secretion and the subsequent ovarian response. They would be a good choice to treat a woman who desires contraception, especially if her testosterone level is mildly to moderately elevated, suggesting ovarian hirsutism.

In Europe, cyproterone acetate, which is an antiandrogenic progestational agent, is available with estradiol in a contraceptive formulation that is used frequently for hirsute women. Oral contraceptives with desogestrel can also be helpful for treatment of hirsutism. Ethinodiol diacetate is considered to be a progestational agent low in androgenic properties and is recommended in oral contraceptives used for hirsute women. Norethindrone and norgestrel are considered to be androgenic progestational agents, but Schriock and Schriock have reported that norgestrel may still be effective for treatment of hirsutism.

Gonadotropin-releasing hormone agonists, used for long periods, can decrease gonadotropin secretion and ovarian androgen production. Oral contraceptive therapy is preferable because the gonadotropin-releasing hormone agonists decrease estrogen production and can lead to decreased bone mass and to increased risk of osteoporosis and fractures. They are not currently recommended therapy for hirsutism. A combination of a gonadotropin-releasing hormone agonist and hormone therapy is possible but offers no advantage over oral contraceptive therapy.

Newer Antiandrogenic Agents

Flutamide, ketoconazole, and finasteride are not currently recommended for the treatment of hirsutism but may be possible therapies in the future. Flutamide is a nonsteroidal antiandrogen that may be effective for hirsutism. The mean Ferriman-Gallwey score for nine hirsute women given flutamide 250 mg orally three times a day for 3 months fell from 28.1 to 24.5 without a change in hormonal parameters. Flutamide may work through blockade of the androgen receptor. One problem with the therapy is that menstrual irregularities worsened with development of oligomenorrhea or amenorrhea in four out of nine women given flutamide.

Ketoconazole is an imidazole derivative usually used as an antifungal agent that can also decrease gonadal and adrenal steroid synthesis.

Significant improvement occurred in the Ferriman-Gallwey scores of nine women given ketoconazole in a 6-month placebo-controlled, double-blind, crossover study. The mean score fell from 28.3 to 27.7 with placebo and to 16.6 with 600 mg daily of ketoconazole. The DHEAS and testosterone levels fell, but the 17-OH-progesterone level rose on therapy. An assessment of the hormonal changes suggests that certain cytochrome P450 enzymes were inhibited by the ketoconazole. At high doses of ketoconazole adrenal suppression may occur, but Cortrosyn testing did not reveal abnormalities in these women. Seven of the nine women had frequent menstrual bleeding during the therapy, which would make it difficult to tolerate. Some women who have taken ketoconazole (up to 1200 mg per day) in studies of hirsutism have developed elevated transaminase levels. Many women have headaches or nausea, and some have pruritus or scalp hair loss.

Finasteride is a 5α-reductase inhibitor that blocks formation of 5α-dihydrotestosterone from testosterone. It is being studied in benign prostatic hypertrophy. Data are not available regarding possible applications in hirsutism. The U.S. Food and Drug Administration has not approved any drugs for use as systemic therapies for hirsutism. Caution is recommended in using newer antiandrogens for hirsutism until more research has been published regarding their safety.

SUMMARY

The most important clinical determination to be made in a woman with hirsutism is whether she appears to be at risk for a hormone-secreting tumor. This decision can be made with clinical, biochemical, and possibly radiographic data.

Once a tumor has been excluded, some clinicians propose a minimal testing approach because therapy is often nonspecific for nontumorous hirsutism. An advantage to more thorough testing is that some causes of hirsutism such as hypothyroidism, acromegaly, and hyperprolactinemia respond to specific therapy, and they may have systemic effects if untreated. Also congenital adrenal hyperplasia is an autosomal recessive disorder, and genetic counseling is possible after diagnosis. Many women with hirsutism respond to cosmetic measures. Systemic measures for hirsutism are nonspecific, and several months are needed to see their full effects. If one type of systemic treatment is unsuccessful or not well tolerated in a particular woman, other methods can be tried. Use of cosmetic hair removal methods is often helpful adjunctive therapy in women on systemic therapy for hirsutism.

REFERENCES

Reviews

Aiman J. Virilizing ovarian tumors. Clin Obstet Gynecol 1991;34 (4):835.

Ehrmann DA, Rosenfield RL. Clinical review 10. An endocrinologic approach to the patient with hirsutism. J Clin Endocrinol Metab 1990;71:1.

Ehrmann DA, Rosenfield RL. Hirsutism—Beyond the steroidogenic block. N Engl J Med 1990;323:909.

Kessel B, Liu J. Clinical and laboratory evaluation of hirsutism. Clin Obstet Gynecol 1991;34(4):805.

McKenna TJ. Pathogenesis and treatment of polycystic ovary syndrome. N Engl J Med 1988;318:558.

Rittmaster RS. Hyperandrogenism—What is normal? N Engl J Med 1992;327:194.

Schriock EA, Schriock ED. Treatment of hirsutism. Clin Obstet Gynecol 1991;34(4):852.

Congenital Adrenal Hyperplasia

Carmina E, Malizia G, Pagano M, et al. Prevalence of late-onset 11β-hydroxylase deficiency in hirsute patients. J Endocrinol Invest 1988;11:595.

Eldar-Geva T, Hurwitz A, Vecsei P, et al. Secondary biosynthetic defects in women with late-onset congenital adrenal hyperplasia. N Engl J Med 1990;323:855.

Siegel SF, Finegold DN, Lanes R, et al. ACTH stimulation tests and plasma dehydroepiandrosterone sulfate levels in women with hirsutism. N Engl J Med 1990;323:849.

Hirsutism Scoring Scale

Ferriman D, Gallwey JD. Clinical measurement of body hair growth in women. J Clin Endocrinol Metab 1961;21:1440.

Newer Antiandrogenic Agents

Akalin S. Effects of ketoconazole in hirsute women. Acta Endocrinol (Copenhagen) 1991;124:19.

Marcondes JA, Minnani SL, Luthold WW, et al. Treatment of hirsutism in women with flutamide. Fertil Steril 1992;57:543.

Premenstrual Syndrome

Joseph F. Mortola

HISTORICAL CONTEXT

Premenstrual syndrome (PMS) has been recognized since the ancient Greek civilization.[1] Hippocrates noted that women had more headaches and experienced a generalized feeling of ''heaviness'' prior to menses. The first modern description of PMS is credited to Frank in 1931, who reported that many women in the latter part of their menstrual cycle experienced a state of ''indescribable tension.''[2] Over the next several decades a variety of psychological explanations were offered for this anxiety state, including claims that women who experienced PMS had more difficulty with the feminine role and were more neurotic.[3] Psychological treatments were advocated based on Freudian or neo-Freudian constructs of the development of psychopathology. Unfortunately, many of these deeply entrenched concepts of the neurotic woman persist today and have impeded scientific research in the area of PMS.

In the 1950s, PMS began to receive greater attention through the writings of an English physician, Dr. Katrina Dalton. Based on the temporal association of PMS with the decline in ovarian progesterone production during the last week of the menstrual cycle, Dalton hypothesized that administration of progesterone would ameliorate symptoms. She published dramatic effects of this treatment.[4] The doses of progesterone used in some women were extremely high (up to 2400 mg/day). According to the Dalton hypothesis, only the native progesterone molecule would be effective in treating symptoms. Because native progesterone is not orally active, the treatment was administered as vaginal or rectal suppositories. Progesterone became the major pharmacologic intervention for PMS for the next 20 to 30 years. In the United States, after the treatment achieved popularity, clinics devoted to the treatment of PMS with progesterone became commonplace.

This work was supported in part by NIH/NICHD grant HD 12303.

Unfortunately, it was not until many years later that the treatment was subjected to a number of double-blind placebo-controlled trials. Taken together, these studies resulted in the conclusion that progesterone was no more effective than placebo in treating PMS.[5] It is only within the past 3 years that the end of the progesterone era in treating PMS has occurred. Despite the paucity of scientific evidence for its efficacy, many patients who have been treated for some time with progesterone are still convinced of its benefits. Physicians under this pressure from patients continue to prescribe it occasionally. Although it remains possible that an as yet uncharacterized subset of patients with PMS respond to progesterone, the use of progesterone for PMS cannot be advocated until this group is identified.

In the past 8 years there has been an explosion of information regarding the diagnosis, pathophysiology, and treatment of PMS. For the first time studies of PMS have been subjected to rigorous scientific methodology. Still, the diagnostic entity of PMS remains controversial. Significant social forces perpetuate the view that PMS is not a valid medical diagnosis. From a feminist perspective, PMS is a difficult dilemma. On the one hand, to legitimize PMS could be construed to indicate some biologic inferiority of women compared with men. On the other hand, to deny its existence is to ignore evidence of biologic correlates of the syndrome and to imply that women who are symptomatic are simply neurotic.

PREVALENCE

Much of the controversy surrounding PMS has been due to inadequate delineation of the syndrome. Accurate prevalence estimates have been difficult to obtain and have ranged from 2.5 to 80% of reproductive-aged women.[6] The prevalence of the syndrome is primarily a matter of definition. If women who experience any degree of fatigue, depression, sadness, breast tenderness,

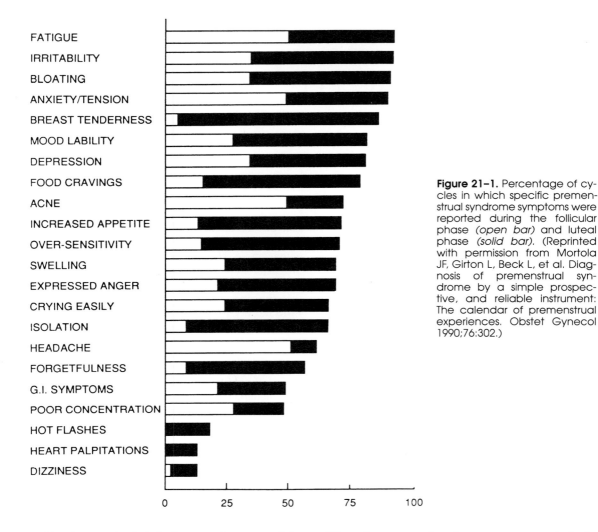

FATIGUE
IRRITABILITY
BLOATING
ANXIETY/TENSION
BREAST TENDERNESS
MOOD LABILITY
DEPRESSION
FOOD CRAVINGS
ACNE
INCREASED APPETITE
OVER-SENSITIVITY
SWELLING
EXPRESSED ANGER
CRYING EASILY
ISOLATION
HEADACHE
FORGETFULNESS
G.I. SYMPTOMS
POOR CONCENTRATION
HOT FLASHES
HEART PALPITATIONS
DIZZINESS

0   25   50   75   100

Figure 21–1. Percentage of cycles in which specific premenstrual syndrome symptoms were reported during the follicular phase *(open bar)* and luteal phase *(solid bar)*. (Reprinted with permission from Mortola JF, Girton L, Beck L, et al. Diagnosis of premenstrual syndrome by a simple prospective, and reliable instrument: The calendar of premenstrual experiences. Obstet Gynecol 1990;76:302.)

or bloating are included, the prevalence certainly exceeds 80%. However, disabling physical and emotional changes occur with much less frequency.

Thus, premenstrual symptoms represent a continuum from mild to incapacitating. Even among women who do not recognize symptoms, prospective recording has shown the majority to have menstrual cycle–related fluctuations in mood, despite their never having been aware of the phenomenon.

DIAGNOSTIC CRITERIA

More than 150 symptoms have been ascribed to PMS. Largely, this high number was the result of poor methodology and lack of attention to those symptoms that actually show consistent cyclic changes during the course of the menstrual cycle.

When these are taken into account, a relatively confined list of symptoms are recognized (Fig. 21–1). Of interest, one of the most common complaints in women with PMS is fatigue. The lack of specificity of this symptom alerts the clinician to the large number of entities that constitute the differential diagnosis of PMS. Despite the prevalence of fatigue, tension and depression are the most common primary complaints in women who present for PMS treatment.

A select group of other symptoms occur with sufficient frequency to merit inclusion in the syndrome. The behavioral symptoms include labile mood with alternating sadness and anger (81%), oversensitivity (69%), crying spells (65%), social withdrawal (65%), forgetfulness (56%), and difficulty concentrating (47%). The common physical symptoms include acne (71%) and gastrointestinal upset (48%). Appetite changes and food cravings are seen in 70% of women with PMS. Vasomotor flushes (18%), heart palpitations (13%), and dizziness (13%) are less commonly observed.[7]

None of the symptoms of PMS is unique to the syndrome. What is diagnostic of the disorder is the marked fluctuations of symptoms with the menstrual cycle. During the time from the fourth day after the onset of menses, until at least cycle day 12, symptoms, if they occur at all, are sporadic and no more frequent than those seen in the general population. This criterion is applicable to the vast majority of reproductive-aged women, although women with cycles that are typically shorter than 26 days in length may have the onset of symptoms slightly earlier than day 12.

Diagnosis of PMS also requires assessment of symptom severity. Therefore, a measurement of the degree of impairment should be ascertained. Because there is no gold standard by which to compare the severity of a self-reported symptom in one individual with that in another, more objective external manifestations of the disorder are required. This permits differentiation of PMS as a distinct syndrome at one end of the continuum between women who discern no physical and emotional differences during the course of the menstrual cycle and those who become incapacitated during the luteal phase. The assessment using functional status provides objective criteria for impairment. Identifiable disruption in performance can be ascertained by (1) marital or relationship discord, (2) poor work or school performance, (3) increased social isolation, or (4) seeking medical attention for a somatic symptom.

In addition to the application of criteria for symptom timing and degree of impairment, the diagnosis of PMS can be made only in the presence of spontaneous menstrual cycles. Frequently, oral contraceptive pills may mimic the symptoms of PMS. In such patients, accurate diagnosis depends on discontinuation of the oral contraceptive and assessing symptoms in the absence of any pharmacologic intervention. Moreover, self-prescribed substances such as alcohol or marijuana may obscure the ability to assess the progression of symptoms during the course of the menstrual cycle. Using these criteria, the diagnosis of PMS is made in approximately 2.5% of reproductive-aged women (Table 21–1).

DIFFERENTIAL DIAGNOSIS

The differential diagnosis of PMS includes a rather large number of medical and psychiatric disorders. A study of 263 women presenting for the complaint of PMS elucidates the differential diagnosis of this disorder: 10.2% were found to be

TABLE 21–1.   University of California, San Diego, Diagnostic Criteria for Premenstrual Syndrome

1. The presence by self-report of at least one of the following somatic *and* affective symptoms during the 5 days before menses in each of the three prior menstrual cycles:

Affective	Somatic
Depression	Breast tenderness
Angry outbursts	Abdominal bloating
Irritability	Headache
Anxiety	Swelling
Confusion	
Social withdrawal	

2. Relief of the above symptoms within 4 days of the onset of menses, without recurrence until at least cycle day 12.
3. The symptoms are present in the absence of any pharmacologic therapy, hormone ingestion, drug or alcohol use.
4. The symptoms occur reproducible during two cycles of prospective recording.
5. Identifiable dysfunction in social or economic performance by one of the following criteria:

Marital or relationship discord confirmed by partner
Difficulties in parenting
Poor work or school performance, poor attendance, tardiness
Increased social isolation
Legal difficulties
Suicidal ideation
Seeking medical attention for a somatic symptom(s)

From Mortola JF, Girton L, Beck L, et al. Depressive episodes in premenstrual syndrome. Am J Obstet Gynecol 1984; 161:1682. Reprinted with permission from The American College of Obstetricians and Gynecologists.

experiencing early menopausal symptoms, 20.5% admitted having no symptom-free interval or were found to have no such interval on prospective recording, 11% had affective or personality disorders, 10.6% were using hormonal contraceptives, 5.3% had eating disorders, 3.8% were alcohol or other substance abusers, and 8.4% complained of symptoms that could also be attributed to a previously diagnosed medical disorder such as diabetes or hypothyroidism. An additional 16.6% of subjects were noted to have menstrual irregularities with cycles less than 26 or more than 34 days in length. Thus, more than 75% of patients with PMS either had another diagnosis that was able to account for symptoms or were noted to have another complaint that required correction before an accurate diagnosis of PMS could be made.

Several reports have indicated a high incidence of affective disorder in patients with PMS. Premenstrual exacerbations of anxiety disorders have been observed.[8–10] Such cases should be managed by treating the underlying psychiatric disorder.

The primary care physician who treats women often is confused by the overlap between premenstrual symptoms and those that have been ascribed to a number of other diseases, including chronic fatigue syndrome, Epstein-Barr virus, and fibromyalgia. The most important difference between these syndromes and PMS is the absence of a clear symptom-free interval during the menstrual cycle.

PROSPECTIVE SYMPTOM INVENTORIES

Because of the inability to diagnose PMS based on the symptoms themselves as opposed to the timing of the symptoms, the importance of prospective recording has become apparent. Although many of the scales used most frequently in research to measure PMS symptoms are retrospective in nature,[11, 12] these have not had acceptance in clinical practice. Little information is afforded beyond that which can be learned during the clinical interview. Differences between prospective inventories and retrospective measures have been demonstrated.[13]

Several prospective rating scales are available.[13–16] One such scale, the Calendar of Premenstrual Experiences, has been tested in both PMS populations and asymptomatic controls.[17] It provides a valid, reliable, and simple to use measure (Fig. 21–2). A follicular phase score is tabulated rapidly by summing the total points obtained on this inventory on days 3 to 9 of the menstrual cycle and a luteal phase score by summing the total points on the last 7 days of the cycle. The diagnosis of PMS is based on the following criteria: (1) the luteal phase score is at least twice that of the follicular phase score, (2) the luteal phase score is at least 42, and (3) the follicular phase score is less than 40. A follicular phase score of greater than 40 should alert the clinician that the patient has a disorder other than PMS, because in well-selected populations, women with PMS only do not achieve higher follicular phase scores on this inventory.

Management of the patient who presents with the complaint of PMS but does not meet criteria for the syndrome is among the most difficult dilemmas in the office practice of the primary care physician. Initial management should include a serum follicle-stimulating hormone and a thyroid-stimulating hormone. Appropriate estrogen or progestin therapy should be instituted in symptomatic perimenopausal women and thyroid replacement therapy in individuals with hypothyroidism. Women with irregular menses should also be evaluated for hyperprolactinemia with a serum prolactin level and for stress-induced menstrual irregularity. Measurement of testosterone levels, ultrasonographic evidence of polycystic ovaries, a serum dehydroepiandrosterone sulfate, and 17α-hydroxyprogesterone levels may provide a diagnosis of chronic anovulation due to either polycystic ovary syndrome or late-onset congenital adrenal hyperplasia. A thorough physical examination, complete blood count, chemistry, and screening for rheumatologic disorders are important to consider in patients who do not show evidence of endocrinologic disturbances.

The majority of women who present with the complaint of PMS but fail to meet criteria for the diagnosis have a normal medical evaluation. Such women almost always demonstrate enhanced reactivity to premenstrual moliminal symptoms. Such sensitivity may be the result of an underlying affective disorder, personality disorder, or posttraumatic stress disorder. Antidepressant therapy should be instituted if a major depression is diagnosed. Personality and posttraumatic stress disorders are treated initially by a supportive relationship with the primary care provider. Often the patient is initially unwilling to consider the possibility of an emotional component to the disorder. However, more than 80% of patients accept psychological counseling after a period of time.

Dietary changes and elimination of salt and caffeine have been advocated for many of these patients. Unfortunately, these measures have little more than a placebo effect.

PATHOPHYSIOLOGY OF PREMENSTRUAL SYNDROME

Ovarian Steroids

Premenstrual symptoms invariably occur during the last week of the menstrual cycle. During the first half of the menstrual cycle (follicular phase), estrogen is produced in increasing concentrations. Progesterone production is negligible during the majority of the follicular phase, until just before ovulation. At the time of ovulation (midcycle), estrogen levels transiently drop and then begin to rise again during the third week after ovulation. During the third week of the menstrual cycle, both estrogen and progesterone levels increase, so that by the end of the third week, high levels of both hormones are achieved. During the last week of the cycle, estrogen and progesterone levels decline. Because of the association of the worst symptoms of PMS with the last week of the menstrual cycle (late luteal phase), the progesterone withdrawal hypothesis of PMS became popular. It has been found, however, that PMS symptoms actually begin to occur before the decline in progesterone. In fact, evidence suggests that the symptom pattern of PMS mimics the rise and fall in progesterone levels, with a time lag. This lag has been

CALENDAR OF PREMENSTRUAL EXPERIENCES

Name _____ Month/Year _____ Age _____ Unit ≠ _____

Begin your calendar on the *first* day of your menstrual cycle. Enter the calendar date below the cycle day. Day 1 is your *first* day of bleeding. Shade the box above the cycle day if you have bleeding. ■ Put an X for spotting. ☒

If more than one symptom is listed in a category, i.e., nausea, diarrhea, constipation, you do not need to experience all of these. Rate the most disturbing of the symptoms on the 1-3 scale.

Weight: Weigh yourself before breakfast. Record weight in the box below date.
Symptoms. Indicate the severity of your symptoms by using the scale below. Rate each symptom at about the same time each evening.

    0 = **None** (symptom not present)   2 = **Moderate** (interferes with normal activities)
    1 = **Mild** (noticeable but not troublesome)   3 = **Severe** (intolerable, unable to perform normal activities)

Other Symptoms: If there are other symptoms you experience, list and indicate severity.
Medications: List any medications taken. Put an X on the corresponding day(s).

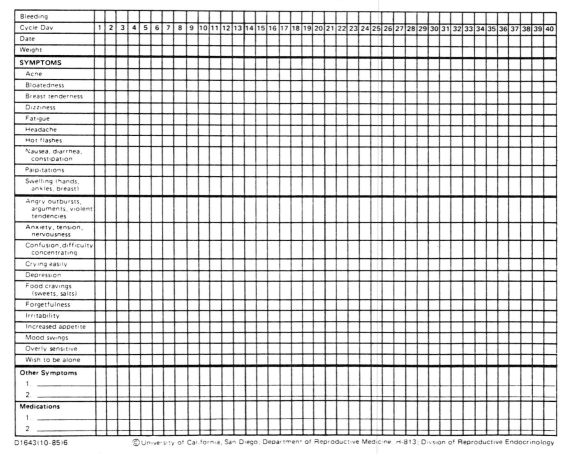

D1643(10-85)6   ©University of California, San Diego; Department of Reproductive Medicine, H-813; Division of Reproductive Endocrinology

Figure 21–2. The calendar of premenstrual experiences. (From Mortola JF, Girton L, Beck L, et al. Diagnosis of premenstrual syndrome by a simple prospective, and reliable instrument: The calendar of premenstrual experiences. Obstet Gynecol 1990;76:302. Reprinted with permission from The American College of Obstetricians and Gynecologists.)

found to be 4 days. Thus, if it is assumed that progesterone levels do not exert their maximal biologic effects until 4 days after exposure, the symptoms of PMS may be caused by progesterone.

Despite the importance of estrogen and progesterone levels in PMS symptoms, attempts to find differences in ovarian steroid levels in women with PMS have failed to yield consistent results. At the present time, the preponderance of evidence suggests that women with PMS do not have levels of estrogen or progesterone (or an estrogen to progesterone ratio) that are significantly different from those of asymptomatic women.[18, 19] It is more likely that there is a biologic predisposition such that some women manifest increased susceptibility to normal ovarian steroid fluctuations throughout the menstrual cycle. Whether this predisposition is genetically endowed or subject to environmental contingencies, however, remains to be determined.

Environmental Factors

A large number of factors that may predispose to the exaggerated responses to normal ovarian steroid fluctuations have been considered. Personality factors have been considered and largely excluded because there is evidence that personality profiles of women with PMS are remarkably similar to those of controls.[20] Stress, which was previously touted to be key in the etiology of PMS and has led to the widespread recommendation of psychological counseling for women with PMS, has been shown not to influence PMS severity.[21] It is more likely that PMS causes stress than that stress causes PMS.

In the absence of a clear psychological variable that predisposes an individual to PMS symptoms, a variety of environmental causes have been considered. Among these, the most prominent has been dietary. The elimination of sweet and salty foods has been widely recommended in the absence of a sound scientific foundation. A large epidemiologic study on the severity of PMS symptoms was conducted at a public university in Oregon. Of the 1419 female students who resided in the university's dormitories, 869 (61%) responded to a questionnaire asking them to rate premenstrual symptoms and to record a complete self-assessment of dietary intake.[22] Results indicated that students who reported high consumption of chocolate (but not other junk foods in general) had a higher prevalence of PMS (prevalence ratio 3.3). Similar results were found among women who consumed between four and 12 alcoholic beverages per week (prevalence ratio 2.5). These results remained statistically significant after controlling for the consumption of caffeinated beverages. Also found to be associated with PMS symptoms were the consumption of one to two caffeine-free colas per day and three or more cups of fruit juice per day.

Although the results of this study suggested that consumption of chocolate may be associated with PMS, the researchers were careful to point out that this is merely an association and does not imply causality. In fact, there is evidence that eating chocolate is a result of PMS rather than a cause. Moreover, there are several methodologic prob-

lems with the study, including very liberal criteria for determining statistical significance. Despite this attempt to clarify the issue, the role of chocolate, alcohol, and dietary intake in PMS symptomatology remains controversial.

Among other dietary considerations has been the role of vitamin B_6 in PMS. At the present time, the role of this vitamin in both the etiology and the treatment of PMS is undetermined.[23, 24]

Of interest is the well-done study by Facchinetti and colleagues demonstrating an improvement in total PMS symptom scores, including affective symptoms, with the administration of oral magnesium.[25] In a randomized double-blind prospective study, 360 mg of magnesium pyrrilidone carboxylic acid or placebo was administered three times a day in the second half of the menstrual cycle. The rationale of the study was based on the finding of lowered magnesium levels in both the erythrocytes and the lymphocytes of women with PMS and fluctuations of these levels during the menstrual cycle.[26–28] This study requires replication but may prove that magnesium is a simple and effective treatment for this disorder.

Neurotransmitter Hypotheses

Marked fluctuations in a variety of potent neurotransmitters occur during the menstrual cycle. Among the most attractive current hypotheses on the cause of PMS is the model that proposes that cyclic changes in ovarian steroids, which influence these central neurotransmitters, are responsible for most PMS symptoms. Substantial in vitro data and results of animal studies support this contention. Among the most prominent changes in neurotransmitters that occur as a result of estrogen and progesterone fluctuations are those involving the opioidergic system.[29]

Increasing levels of estrogen during the first 3 weeks of the menstrual cycle result in increasing levels of central β-endorphin. This β-endorphin rise is further potentiated by the rising levels of progesterone during the week following ovulation (week 3). Although β-endorphin contributes to a sense of well-being, it may also add to the general fatigue experienced by many women with PMS. Subsequently, during the fourth week of the cycle, as estrogen and progesterone levels decline, an acute β-endorphin (opiate) withdrawal occurs. Thus, many of the anxiety symptoms experienced may be a miniopiate withdrawal phenomenon. This hypothesis remains to be tested further, although support for it has been provided by Chuong and associates.[30]

It has been shown that progesterone is also a

partial agonist of the γ-aminobutyric acid–receptor complex. Since γ-aminobutyric acid is in general an inhibitory transmitter, rising progesterone levels in the third week may have a diazepam-like effect, contributing to fatigue, and later as progesterone falls, may produce an anxiety state similar to benzodiazepine withdrawal.[31]

At the present time, however, the greatest attention is being focused on serotonin changes that occur throughout the menstrual cycle. In subjects with PMS, whole blood serotonin levels and platelet serotonin reuptake are diminished during the last week of the menstrual cycle.[32, 33] Serotonin changes may be responsible for dysphoria, anxiety, and appetite changes. Taken together, these neurotransmitter changes are likely to be the major factor in PMS symptomatology.

TREATMENT

Nonspecific Treatments

In the absence of a complete understanding of the pathophysiology of PMS, attempts at alleviating symptoms through nonspecific interventions have achieved popularity. These include exercise, dietary modification, and vitamin and mineral supplements (Table 21–2).

TABLE 21–2. Efficacy of Treatments for Premenstrual Syndrome

Definitely Effective
Fluoxetine (Prozac)
Alprazolam (Xanax)
Gn-RH agonists

Probably Effective
Aerobic exercise
High carbohydrate diet

Equivocal
Vitamin B$_6$
Diuretics (for bloating)
Magnesium
Moderate chocolate (for mood)
Decreased chocolate (for mastalgia only)
Decreased caffeine (for mastalgia only)

Probably Ineffective
Evening primrose oil
Decreased sweet and salty food
Tricyclic antidepressants
Oral contraceptive pills
Lithium
Over-the-counter formulations for premenstrual syndrome

Definitely Ineffective
Progesterone

Exercise

Exercise constitutes the first-line treatment for patients with PMS. A variety of studies have shown that exercise has beneficial effects on PMS symptoms, although placebo-controlled studies are difficult to design. Women who exercise a great deal have been shown to decrease their luteal phase progesterone levels. Because PMS is likely to be a disorder mediated by luteal phase progesterone, studies showing a beneficial effect of exercise have a physiologic basis in support of their findings. The level of exercise utilized in these studies is 45 minutes per day and should include an aerobic component.

Dietary Modifications

An increase in appetite, particularly with desires for sweet and salty foods, is a prominent symptom of PMS. As a result, dietary modification by elimination of sweet and salty foods has been advocated widely. To my knowledge, no study has attempted to control for the placebo effect of a dietary treatment intervention. Such a study that might compare, for instance, diet modification with exercise or diet modification with the administration of a placebo drug has not been done. To recommend restriction of carbohydrates and salt has no basis in sound scientific evidence. On the contrary, recent evidence suggests that eating high carbohydrate meals may reduce symptoms of depression, tension, and fatigue in women with PMS.[34] Although at the present time no clear consensus exists as to which dietary changes might help women with PMS, the recommendation of higher carbohydrate meals is the most sound.

Vitamin and Mineral Supplements

A variety of dietary supplements have been utilized in treating PMS. Among the most commonly prescribed are vitamin B$_6$ and multivitamin regimens. Vitamin B$_6$ has been shown to be more effective than placebo in one double-blind study[35] but not in another.[36] Moreover, attempts to find deficiencies in vitamin B$_6$ levels or other vitamins in PMS patients have been unsuccessful.[37] At the present time, therefore, although vitamin B$_6$ is unlikely to be harmful when prescribed in 50 to 100 mg daily doses, proven efficacy is lacking. Several nutritional supplements have been claimed to be effective in treating PMS. However, the lack of adequate study design in tests of these commercially available, nonprescription products should discourage health professionals from prescribing them.

Oral Contraceptive Pills

The effect of oral contraceptive pills on PMS symptoms has been variable. One study reported that women who take oral contraceptive pills report fewer PMS symptoms than nonusers.[38] However, many women in the study had discontinued oral contraceptive pills precisely because of a worsening of premenstrual symptoms. One study demonstrated that women on oral contraceptives demonstrated a more prolonged pattern of negative mood during the menstrual cycle than nonusers.[39] Earlier studies have shown variable results of oral contraceptive pill use, with one study showing improvement in PMS symptoms in older but not younger women.[40] The only placebo-controlled study to date failed to demonstrate that the oral contraceptive pill was effective in treating PMS.[41]

Fluoxetine

The serotonin uptake inhibitor fluoxetine has been shown in double-blind, placebo-controlled studies to be effective in treating symptoms of PMS.[42, 43] Given data that serotonin levels are altered by ovarian steroids and that serotonin metabolism may differ in women with PMS, fluoxetine should be considered the first-line drug for PMS treatment, beginning at a dose of 20 mg each morning. Approximately 15% of women are unable to tolerate the medication primarily because of jitteriness, nausea, or headache and less commonly because of sedation. In those who experience sedation, an evening regimen may be considered. Of those who are able to tolerate the medication, approximately 75% experience a reduction of symptoms greater than 50%. Attempts to discontinue fluoxetine after 6 to 9 months, as is done in depression, have not been effective in uncontrolled studies. Thus, more prolonged therapy may be indicated.

It has been demonstrated that the beneficial effects of fluoxetine are not due to the generalized antidepressant effects.[44] Women treated with fluoxetine were compared with women treated with the tricyclic antidepressant imipramine, and a significant response was noted in 70% of subjects with fluoxetine as compared with only 25% of those treated with imipramine. A uniformly high response to fluoxetine was noted in women presenting with either anxious or depressed symptoms or with premenstrual appetite and sleep disturbance.

Alprazolam

A second effective treatment is based on data demonstrating an interaction of progesterone with the γ-aminobutyric acid receptor and therefore a potential influence of benzodiazepines on PMS symptoms. Smith and associates have demonstrated the efficacy of such a benzodiazepine, alprazolam, in PMS.[45] This finding has been replicated.[46] The addictive potential of this agent, however, makes it unsuitable for use in many patients. The effective dose is generally 0.25 mg four times a day. Patients should be cautioned regarding decreased reaction time, which may occur on this medication.

Diuretics

The efficacy of diuretics in treating premenstrual syndrome remains to be conclusively established. There have been some reports that both spironolactone in doses of 25 to 50 mg per day and hydrochlorothiazide in doses of 25 mg per day may be beneficial. In the carefully monitored patient, there are few contraindications to these treatments when limited to the luteal phase of the cycle. Such treatments are indicated when fluid retention symptoms predominate.

Gonadotropin-Releasing Hormone Analogues

Based on the association of PMS symptoms with the amount of progesterone in the luteal phase of the cycle, an ideal treatment for PMS would be one in which the progesterone levels could be decreased or eliminated. This assumption led to the hypothesis that symptoms of PMS would be relieved by the administration of a gonadotropin-releasing hormone (Gn-RH) agonist. These agonists work by first stimulating pituitary Gn-RH receptors and subsequently, after a period of 2 weeks, result in a down regulation of these receptors. In the down-regulation phase, luteinizing hormone and follicle-stimulating hormone production is markedly decreased and ovarian function ceases. Thus, a menopausal state (including hot flashes) is induced. The first report of the efficacy of this treatment was by Muse and co-workers in 1984.[47] These investigators were able to show a more than 75% reduction in PMS symptoms during the second month of Gn-RH agonist treatment, once down regulation of pituitary receptors had been achieved. This work using the Gn-RH analogue D-His[6] Pro[9] NEt-Gn-RH has subsequently been replicated by Hammarback and Backstrom with a similarly excellent outcome using another Gn-RH analogue.[48] As a result, the use of Gn-RH analogues constituted the first clearly successful hormonal treatment for PMS.

Until recently, the use of Gn-RH analogues as long-term treatments for PMS was limited by the development of osteoporosis and the potential for increased cardiovascular disease, which results from long-term estrogen deprivation. A study of a Gn-RH agonist plus estrogen-progestin has shown a similarly beneficial effect and represents an advance in the treatment of PMS. Low-dose steroid hormone therapy may maintain the beneficial effects achieved by, and circumvent the unacceptable consequences of, the use of a Gn-RH agonist.[49] At present, use of a Gn-RH agonist plus low-dose estrogen-progestin is experimental, and further study is required to document a sustained beneficial effect of this regimen over repeated treatment cycles.

SUMMARY

Advances in research have provided insights into the pathophysiology and treatment of PMS. Despite this, PMS has been a poorly understood syndrome, and controversy surrounding the diagnosis persists. Objective criteria for the diagnosis of PMS have been established, and it can be distinguished by prospective recording from a variety of other medical and psychiatric syndromes that have similar symptoms. In mild cases of PMS, dietary and exercise changes may be beneficial. In more severe cases, the serotonin uptake inhibitor fluoxetine has been shown to be effective. When this is not adequate, alprazolam or Gn-RH agonists can be considered.

REFERENCES

1. Simon H. Mind and Madness in Ancient Greece. Ithaca, NY: Cornell University Press, 1978, p 273.
2. Frank RT. The hormonal causes of premenstrual tension. Arch Neurol Psychiatry 1931;26:1053.
3. Coppen A, Kessel N. Menstruation and personality. Br J Psychiatry 1963;109:711.
4. Dalton K. The Premenstrual Syndrome and Progesterone Therapy. London: William Heineman Medical Books, 1984.
5. Rapkin A, Chang LH, Reading AE. Premenstrual syndrome: A double blind placebo controlled study of treatment with progesterone vaginal suppositories. J Obstet Gynecol 1987;7:217.
6. Hamilton JA, Parry BL, Alagna S, et al. Premenstrual mood changes: A guide to evaluation and treatment. Psychiatr Ann 1984;14:426.
7. Mortola JF, Girton L, Beck L, et al. Depressive episodes in premenstrual syndrome. Am J Obstet Gynecol 1984;161:1682.
8. Endicott J, Halbreich U, Schacht S, Nee J. Premenstrual changes and affective disorders. Psychosom Med 1981;43:519.
9. Kashiwagi T, McClure JH, Wetzel RD. Premenstrual affective syndrome and psychiatric disorder. Dis Nerv Syst 1981;37:116.
10. DeJong R, Rubinow DR, Roy-Byrne P, et al. Premenstrual mood disorder and psychiatric illness. Am J Psychiatry 1985;142:1359.
11. Moos RH. The development of menstrual distress questionnaire. Psychosom Med 1968;30:853.
12. Stout AL, Steege J. Psychological assessment of women seeking treatment for premenstrual syndrome. J Psychosom Res 1985;29:621.
13. Endicott J, Halbreich U. Retrospective report of premenstrual depressive changes: Factors affecting confirmation by daily ratings. Psychopharmacol Bull 1982;18:109.
14. Sampsom JA, Prescott P. The assessment of symptoms of the menstrual cycle and their response to therapy. Br J Psychiatry 1981;138:399.
15. Steiner M, Haskett RF, Carroll BJ. Premenstrual tension syndrome: The development of diagnostic criteria and new rating scales. Acta Psychiatr Scand 1980;62:229.
16. Taylor JW. The timing of menstruation-related symptoms assessed by a daily rating scale. Acta Psychiatr Scand 1974;60:87.
17. Mortola JF, Girton L, Beck L, et al. Diagnosis of premenstrual syndrome by a simple prospective and reliable instrument: The calendar of premenstrual experiences. Obstet Gynecol 1990;76:302.
18. Taylor JW. Plasma progesterone, oestradiol-17-beta and premenstrual symptoms. Acta Psychiatr Scand 1979;60:76.
19. Andersch B, Abrahamson L. Hormone profile in premenstrual tension: Effects of bromocriptine and diuretics. Clin Endocrinol (Oxf) 1979;11:657.
20. Trunnell ED, Turner CW, Keye WR. A comparison of the psychological and hormonal factors in women with and without premenstrual syndrome. J Abnorm Psychol 1988;97:429.
21. Beck LE, Gevirtz R, Mortola JF. The predictive role of psychosocial stress on symptom severity in premenstrual syndrome. Psychosom Med 1990;52:536.
22. Rossignol AM, Bonnander H. Prevalence and severity of the premenstrual syndrome: Effects of foods and beverages that are sweet or high in sugar content. J Reprod Med 1991;36:131.
23. Steward A. Vitamin B$_6$ in the treatment of premenstrual syndrome: Review. Br J Obstet Gynecol 1991;98:329.
24. Kleijnen J, Terriel G, Knipschild P. Vitamin B$_6$ in the treatment of premenstrual syndrome: Review reply. Br J Obstet Gynecol 1991;18:339.
25. Facchinetti F, Borelia P, Sances G, et al. Oral magnesium relieves premenstrual mood changes. Obstet Gynecol 1991;78:177.
26. Sherwood RA, Rocus BF, Steward A, Saxton RS. Magnesium and the premenstrual syndrome. Ann Clin Biochem 1986;23:667.
27. Facchinetti F, Borella P, Valentini M, et al. Premenstrual increase of intracellular magnesium levels in women with ovulatory, asymptomatic menstrual cycles. Gynecol Endocrinol 1988;2:249.
28. Faschinetti F, Borella P, Fioroni L, et al. Reduction of monocyte's magnesium in patients affected by premenstrual syndrome. J Psychosom Obstet Gynecol 1990;11:221.
29. Wardlaw SL, Wehrenberg WB, Ferin M, et al. Effect of

sex steroids on β-endorphin in hypophyseal portal blood. J Clin Endocrinol Metab 1986;63:323.

30. Chuong CJ, Coulam CB, Koo PC, et al. Neuropeptide levels in premenstrual syndrome. Fertil Steril 1985;44:760.

31. Majewska MD, Harrison NL, Schwartz RD, et al. Steroid hormone metabolites are barbiturate like modulators of the GABA receptor. Science 1986;232:1004.

32. Rapkin AJ, Edelmuth E, Chang LC. Whole blood serotonin in premenstrual syndrome. Am J Obstet Gynecol 1987;10:533.

33. Taylor DL, Matthew RH, Ho BT. Serotonin levels and platelet uptake during premenstrual tension. Neuropsychobiology 1984;12:16.

34. Wurtman JJ, Brzezinski A, Wurtman RJ, Laferrere B. Effects of nutrient intake on premenstrual depression. Am J Obstet Gynecol 1989;161:1228.

35. Stokes J, Medels J. Pyridoxine in premenstrual tension. Lancet 1972;1:1177.

36. Doll H, Brown S, Thurston A, Vessey M. Pyridoxine (vitamin B₆) and the premenstrual syndrome: A randomized crossover trial. J R Coll Gen Pract 1989;39:364.

37. Mira M, Stewart PM, Abraham SF. Vitamin and trace element status in premenstrual syndrome. Am J Clin Nutr 1988;47:636.

38. Graham GA, Sherwin BB. The relationships between retrospective symptom reporting and present oral contraceptive use. J Psychosom Res 1987;31:45.

39. Bancroft J, Rennie D. The impact of oral contraceptives on the experience of premenstrual mood, clumsiness, food cravings and other symptoms. J Psychosom Res 1993;37:195.

40. Andersch B, Hahn L. Premenstrual complaints. II: Influence of oral contraceptives. Acta Obstet Gynecol Scand 1981;60:579.

41. Talwar PP, Berge GS. A prospective randomized study of oral contraceptives: The effect of study design on repeated rates of symptoms. Contraception 1979;20:329.

42. Stone AB, Perlstein TB, Brown WA. Fluoxetine in the treatment of premenstrual syndrome. Psychopharm Bull 1990;26:331.

43. Wood SH, Mortola JF, Chen YF, et al. Treatment of premenstrual syndrome with fluoxetine: A double blind placebo controlled crossover study. Obstet Gynecol 1992;80:339.

44. Mortola JF, Moossazadeh F. A randomized trial of fluoxetine and imipramine in the treatment of premenstrual syndrome (abstract). 37th annual meeting of the Society for Gynecologic Investigation. San Antonio, Texas, 1991.

45. Smith S, Rinehart JS, Ruddick VE, Schiff I. Treatment of premenstrual syndrome with alprazolam: Results of a double-blind, placebo-controlled, randomized crossover clinical trial. Obstet Gynecol 1987;70:37.

46. Harrison WH, Endicott J, Rabkin JG, et al. Treatment of premenstrual dysphoria with alprazolam and placebo. Psychopharm Bull 1987;23:150.

47. Muse KN, Cetel NS, Futterman LA, Yen SSC. The premenstrual syndrome: Effects of medical ovariectomy. N Engl J Med 1984;311:1345.

48. Hammarback S, Backstrom T. Induced ovulation as treatment of premenstrual tension syndrome—A double blind crossover trial of LRH agonist versus placebo. Acta Obstet Gynecol Scand 1988;67:159.

49. Mortola JF, Girton L, Fischer U. Successful treatment of severe premenstrual syndrome by use of gonadrophin-releasing hormone agonist and estrogen/progestin. J Clin Endocrinol Metab 1991;71:252A.

Thyroid Disorders

Audrey B. Miklius and Gilbert H. Daniels

Disorders of the thyroid are among the most common endocrine abnormalities in women, with a prevalence exceeding that of diabetes. Thyroid function tests account for more than $1 billion spent on health care each year.[1] The primary care physician must be skilled in the evaluation and management of thyroid disorders.

This chapter begins with guidelines for examining the thyroid gland. A brief review of thyroid physiology is followed by a discussion of thyroid function tests and their interpretation. An algorithm for thyroid function testing is presented. Signs and symptoms of hypothyroidism and the most common causes of hypothyroidism are reviewed in detail, followed by general principles of thyroid hormone therapy. The clinical manifestations and differential diagnosis of hyperthyroidism are discussed as are treatment options for hyperthyroidism. A brief discussion of nonthyroidal illness concludes this chapter.

EXAMINATION OF THE THYROID

Systematic examination of the thyroid gland should be part of every complete physical examination. Palpation is the only way to detect certain diseases of the thyroid. An appreciation of the size, consistency, nodularity, and tenderness of the thyroid is often necessary to interpret the historical and laboratory findings.

The thyroid gland consists of two lateral lobes connected by an isthmus at the level of the cricoid cartilage. The lateral lobes are partially covered by the sternocleidomastoid muscles. The normal gland weighs 15 to 20 gm in adults. Each lateral lobe is about 4 cm long and 2 to 3 cm wide. The right lobe is normally larger than the left.

The thyroid can best be inspected by tilting the patient's head backward. This position brings the thyroid up from the supraclavicular region and throws it into relief against the superficial structures of the neck. The gland is fixed to the pretracheal fascia and therefore rises with the trachea and larynx with swallowing. This movement distinguishes the thyroid from other masses in the neck. Many goiters and nodules are visible when the patient swallows in this position.

The trachea should be palpated carefully because lateral deviation could suggest a large thyroid nodule or substernal goiter. This is done by placing the thumb and index finger on either side of the trachea and following the path of the trachea to the suprasternal notch. In the normally placed midline trachea, the fingers descend to the middle of the suprasternal notch. Lymph nodes in the neck should also be palpated carefully.

Thyroid palpation may be more easily learned when facing the patient. The patient's neck should be slightly flexed to relax the sternocleidomastoid muscles. The first step is to locate the cricoid cartilage. The isthmus of the thyroid gland lies horizontally beneath the cricoid cartilage. The isthmus can be examined by placing the thumb in a horizontal position with its upper edge along the lower margin of the cricoid cartilage. The thumb then applies moderate pressure while rolling down over the isthmus. The normal isthmus has the consistency of felt and is a few millimeters in length. An enlarged, firm, or nodular isthmus is often an indication of thyroid pathology.

The thumb should be used to locate the pyramidal lobe if one is present. The pyramidal lobe is a remnant of thyroglossal duct tissue. It has a vertical orientation and most often arises from the isthmic border of the left lobe; it is most easily palpated by moving the thumb back and forth in the horizontal plane. An easily palpable pyramidal lobe is often an indication of a general abnormality of the thyroid gland such as Hashimoto's thyroiditis or Graves' disease.

To examine the left lobe, the examiner steps to the patient's right and places two fingers of the right hand along the left lateral aspect of the trachea. The fingers meet the trachea at a 45-degree angle and point in a lateral direction. Starting high in the neck and working down, the fingers massage the trachea with a circular rubbing motion, applying firm pressure as they examine the patient's left lobe. Some examiners use their left thumb to stabilize the right side of the trachea. The right lobe is examined from the patient's left side using the left hand. Alternatively the right thumb can be used to palpate the right lobe and the left thumb to palpate the left lobe. It is very helpful for the patient to hold and swallow small sips of water during this part of the examination because swallowing causes the thyroid to rise. Size, texture, and consistency of the thyroid lobe can be appreciated. If nodules are present, they can be examined as the patient swallows, then trapped by the fingers beneath the nodule, and palpated again on the way down. The mobility of a nodule refers to the ease of movement of the nodule as a whole within the neck. Texture is best appreciated by squeezing the nodule between the fingers.

If nodules are found, it is essential to measure them in two or three dimensions if possible. A ruler, tape measure, or caliper is placed next to the patient's neck, and the measurements are recorded. Or several pieces of tape are placed directly on the patient's neck, and an outline of the nodule is traced directly onto the tape; this tape is then placed in the patient's permanent file.

Auscultation of the gland should be performed in patients with goiter, particularly in those with hyperthyroidism. A continuous low-pitched sound (venous hum) or a systolic or diastolic murmur (bruit) suggests the hypervascularity of a Graves' thyroid gland.

THYROID PHYSIOLOGY

Iodine is required for the synthesis of thyroid hormones. Dietary iodide is absorbed in the stomach, circulates in the blood stream, is trapped by the thyroid follicular cell, and is ultimately cleared by the kidneys. In the thyroid gland, the iodide is oxidized and combines with the tyrosine residues of an acceptor protein, thyroglobulin. Iodotyrosines are formed, which then couple to form the thyroid hormones triiodothyronine (T_3) and thyroxine (T_4) on the thyroglobulin. This organification reaction is catalyzed by the enzyme thyroid peroxidase and is inhibited by the antithyroid drugs propylthiouracil and methimazole. The thyroid hormones are stored in the form of thyroglobulin (colloid) in the follicular lumen. Proteolytic digestion of thyroglobulin releases T_4 and T_3 into the circulation. Thyroxine is the major secretory product of the thyroid. Peripheral conversion of T_4 to T_3 by the action of tissue 5'monodeiodinases accounts for more than 80% of T_3 production.[2]

The thyroid-stimulating hormone (TSH) thyrotropin is secreted by the anterior pituitary gland and is the major modulator of thyroid activity. Thyroid-stimulating hormone stimulates most of the processes required for thyroid hormone synthesis and secretion: iodide trapping, iodide organification, thyroglobulin production, and secretion of thyroid hormones. The secretion of TSH by the pituitary is inhibited by T_4 and T_3 and stimulated by thyrotropin-releasing hormone secreted by the hypothalamus. The secretion of TSH is also inhibited by glucocorticoids and stimulated by cortisol deficiency.

THYROID FUNCTION TESTS

Assessment of Thyroid Function by Measuring Thyroid-Stimulating Hormone

An inverse logarithmic relationship exists between thyroid function and serum TSH concentration; for example, a 50% decrease in free T_4 results in an 80-fold increase in serum TSH concentration. Serum TSH is therefore exquisitely sensitive to small changes in thyroid hormone.

The early TSH assays were able to detect the increased TSH values in hypothyroidism but were not sensitive enough to detect the suppressed levels in hyperthyroidism. The second- and third-generation TSH assays now available can measure TSH concentrations below the normal range, clearly distinguishing between the low or undetectable concentration of hyperthyroid patients from the normal concentration of euthyroid patients.[3] These tests have largely replaced the thyrotropin-releasing hormone test in the diagnosis of hyperthyroidism.

The normal range of TSH when using the sensitive TSH assay varies from laboratory to laboratory but is generally in the range of 0.5 to 5.0 mU per liter. Patients with primary hypothyroidism have TSH concentrations greater than 5 mU per liter. Patients with hyperthyroidism have concentrations less than 0.5 mU per liter and generally below the detection limits of the assay (e.g., <0.1 in second-generation and <0.01 in third-generation assays.)

Measurement of Thyroid Hormones

T_4 and T_3 are transported in the serum bound to three transport proteins. Thyroxine-binding globulin (TBG) represents the major binding protein. An

$$T_4 \times THBI \text{ (normalized } T_3 \text{ resin)} = \text{free } T_4 \text{ index}$$

Hyperthyroid	↑	↑	Increased
Hypothyroid	↓	↓	Decreased
TBG Increase	↑	↓	Normal
TBG Decrease	↓	↑	Normal

Figure 22–1. Distinguishing T_4 production abnormalities from thyroxine-binding globulin (TBG) alterations.

equilibrium exists between bound and unbound hormone, but only free or unbound hormone can enter cells to produce its biologic actions. Only 0.03% of T_4 and 0.3% of T_3 circulate in free form. Because the free or unbound fraction is metabolically active it would be most useful to measure free T_4 or T_3. However, direct measurement of the free hormones is costly and time consuming. A low-cost and reliable radioimmunoassay for total T_4 is available that measures circulating levels of thyroid hormone bound to serum proteins. Because it measures only bound hormone and not free hormone, it is only accurate in reflecting a patient's thyroid status 80% of the time.

Abnormal concentrations of TBG or altered thyroid hormone–binding protein affinity for thyroid hormone can alter total hormone levels (serum T_4) in clinically euthyroid patients, thus causing confusion. Although screening with the use of TSH measurements circumvents many of the problems of abnormal protein binding, understanding these abnormalities remains clinically important. An excess of TBG (due to estrogens in oral contraceptives or during pregnancy, drugs such as 5-fluorouracil, or a hereditary condition) causes an increase in serum T_4 concentration. Conversely, a decrease in serum TBG (e.g., due to a hereditary condition or states of protein loss) causes a decrease in serum T_4 concentration. Patients with such decreases do not have a thyroid disease. They are euthyroid with normal free or unbound T_4 concentrations.

The free T_4 index is a simple, inexpensive alternative to free T_4 measurements. The free T_4 index,

the product of the T_4 multiplied by the THBI (thyroid hormone–binding index) is proportional to the free T_4. The thyroid hormone–binding index is the new term given to the (normalized) T_3 resin test (T_3R). The T_3 resin test measures the protein-binding sites unoccupied by thyroid hormone. The greater the number of unoccupied sites, the lower the T_3 resin test or the thyroid hormone–binding index. In patients with thyroid disease, the T_4 and this index "move in the same direction" (Fig. 22–1); in patients with TBG abnormalities the T_4 and the thyroid hormone–binding index "move in the opposite direction." The free T_4 index is generally normal in euthyroid patients with abnormalities of TBG, however it may be slightly high or low in patients whose TBG is extremely high or low. In familial dysalbuminemic hyperthyroxinemia, an abnormal albumin has a high affinity for T_4 but not for T_3. These patients have high total T_4 concentrations and high free T_4 index but normal free T_4 using the dialysis method.[4] It is important to remember that despite changes in binding protein concentrations or affinities, the hypothalamic-pituitary-thyroid axis maintains the normal concentrations of free thyroid hormones. The TSH concentration is normal in individuals with binding protein abnormalities alone. If TSH is used as the initial screening study, patients with binding protein abnormalities are not a source of confusion.

Tests for Thyroid Dysfunction

Serum Hormone Tests

The sensitive TSH assay is the best outpatient screening test for thyroid dysfunction. An algorithm for testing thyroid function in outpatients is shown in Figure 22–2. The earliest sign of a failing thyroid gland is a rise in TSH concentration. When the TSH is elevated, a free T_4 index is

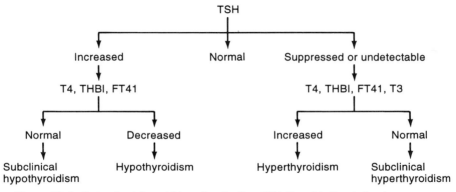

Figure 22–2. Outpatient thyroid function testing. TSH, Thyroid-stimulating hormone.

obtained to assess the degree of hypothyroidism. As TSH concentration rises, the failing gland secretes relatively more T_3 than T_4 to maintain the euthyroid state as long as possible. Therefore, T_3 measurements are not useful in hypothyroid patients. Patients with an increased TSH but a normal free T_4 index are said to have subclinical or biochemical hypothyroidism.

A subnormal TSH concentration suggests hyperthyroidism. When the TSH is subnormal or undetectable using a sensitive TSH assay, the free T_4 index and the total T_3 are measured to assess the degree of hyperthyroidism. Elevated T_3 concentration with normal free T_4 or free T_4 index occurs in 10 to 15% of hyperthyroid patients. This "T_3 toxicosis" is due to increased thyroidal T_3 secretion rather than increased peripheral conversion of T_4 to T_3. Patients with subnormal TSH concentrations but normal free T_4 and T_3 concentrations are said to have subclinical hyperthyroidism.

The TSH test does have limitations. Early in pregnancy, the TSH test results may be slightly subnormal owing to human chorionic gonadotropin–induced stimulation of the thyroid gland.[5] This abnormality is exaggerated in patients with hyperemesis gravidarum. The ability of the TSH assay to reflect thyroid function depends on an intact hypothalamic-pituitary axis. Measurements of TSH are misleading for diagnosis or therapy in patients with hypothalamic or pituitary disease.[6] For example, a low serum TSH due to pituitary destruction is associated with hypothyroidism; an elevated serum TSH due to a thyrotropin-secreting tumor of the pituitary results in hyperthyroidism. Furthermore, TSH of low biologic potency may be secreted in hypothalamic disease, resulting in a normal or slightly high serum TSH concentration despite hypothyroidism.[7] Severely ill patients in the hospital may have low serum TSH concentrations; high serum TSH may be noted during recovery from these illnesses.[8, 9] Lastly, TSH concentration may be misleading during the treatment of hyper- or hypothyroidism.[10] After therapy for hyperthyroidism, the free T_4 and T_3 concentrations become normal, whereas TSH concentrations may remain undetectable or suppressed for weeks. The response to therapy of hyperthyroidism should therefore be assessed by monitoring the free T_4 index and T_3 concentrations. In treating hypothyroidism, 5 to 6 weeks of equilibration is required after a change in thyroid hormone dose before TSH reaches its nadir.[11]

Antithyroid Antibodies

Antithyroid antibodies (primarily antimicrosomal) are found in more than 95% of patients with Hashimoto's thyroiditis.[12] The microsomal antigen has been identified as the thyroid peroxidase.[12, 13] Test results of commercially available thyroid peroxidase antibodies are positive in 98% of patients with Hashimoto's thyroiditis, including half of those who test negative for antimicrosomal antibodies. Antimicrosomal, anticolloid, and antithyroid peroxidase antibodies are also present in more than half of the patients with Graves' disease.[12] Antibodies for TSH receptor are positive in 95% of patients with Graves' hyperthyroidism but are generally unnecessary in clinical practice.[14] They may be useful in euthyroid pregnant patients who were treated previously with radioactive iodine or surgery to assess the risk for fetal or neonatal Graves' disease.

Thyroglobulin

Thyroglobulin, the precursor of thyroid hormone, is stored in the thyroid and released with thyroid hormone into the circulation. Unlike patients with other hyperthyroid disorders, patients with factitious hyperthyroidism have low serum thyroglobulin concentrations.[15] Thyroglobulin is also an important tumor marker for patients with well-differentiated (papillary and follicular) cancer of the thyroid. Antithyroglobulin antibodies can cause false high thyroglobulin readings and should be screened for in thyroglobulin assays.

Radioactive Iodine Uptake

Although not useful as a test of thyroid function, the 24-hour radioactive iodine uptake (RAIU) is an essential part of the evaluation of almost all nonpregnant hyperthyroid patients. A small amount of ^{123}I is administered by mouth. The RAIU in the thyroid is measured at 24 hours (normal 10–30%). The uptake is proportional to the thyroid's avidity for iodine and inversely proportional to the iodine pool in the body.

HYPOTHYROIDISM

Hypothyroidism is the clinical syndrome that results from thyroid hormone deficiency. The diagnosis of primary hypothyroidism is confirmed by the finding of an increased TSH and low free T_4 index. The signs and symptoms of hypothyroidism are listed in Table 22–1. The causes of hypothyroidism are listed in Table 22–2. Hashimoto's thyroiditis is the most common cause of spontaneous hypothyroidism. Hypothyroidism due to iodine deficiency is of major significance worldwide but does not exist in the United States. Iatrogenic

TABLE 22–1.   Signs and Symptoms of Hypothyroidism

SYMPTOMS	
General	Weakness, fatigue, lethargy
	Cold intolerance
	Modest weight gain despite decreased appetite
Skin and hair	Dry skin
	Puffy eyelids
	Hair loss
Respiratory	Exertional dyspnea
	Sleep apnea
Gastrointestinal	Constipation
Neuromuscular	Decreased memory
	Hearing impairment
	Paresthesias
	Vertigo
	Muscle cramps
	Unsteady gait
	Joint pain
Reproductive	Menorrhagia
	Amenorrhea
	Infertility
SIGNS	
General	Slow moving and speaking
Vital signs	Bradycardia
	Diastolic hypertension
	Hypothermia
Skin	Cool, dry, coarse
	Nonpitting edema
	Carotenemia
	Vitiligo*
	Coarse hair
	Loss of lateral eyebrows
Eyes	Exophthalmos*†
Mouth	Enlarged tongue
Thyroid	Diffuse goiter‡
	Not palpable§
	Nodular goiter*‖
Lungs	Pleural effusions
Heart	Quiet heart
	Cardiomegaly
Abdomen	Decreased bowel sounds
	Ileus
	Ascites
Extremities	Carpal tunnel syndrome
	Joint effusions, chondrocalcinosis
Neuromuscular	Myoedema
	Ataxia
	Delayed relaxation phase of deep tendon reflexes
Other	Galactorrhea

LABORATORY ABNORMALITIES IN HYPOTHYROIDISM

Anemia
Hyponatremia
Elevated cholesterol
Increased serum glutamic-oxaloacetic transaminase
Increased creatine phosphokinase
Increased CEA and CA-125
Elevated carotene
Prolonged partial thromboplastin time
Hyperprolactinemia
Abnormal results on electrocardiogram—low voltage, nonspecific ST and T wave
   abnormalities
Abnormal chest radiograph findings—increased cardiac silhouette

*Hashimoto's thyroiditis.
†Postradioactive iodine for Graves' disease.
‡Hashimoto's thyroiditis, lymphocytic thyroiditis, subacute thyroiditis.
§Postradioactive iodine for Graves' disease, thyroid agenesis, atrophic thyroiditis.
‖Biosynthetic defects, iodine deficiency.
CEA, Carcinoembryonic antigen.

TABLE 22–2. Causes of Hypothyroidism

GOITROUS	ATROPHIC
Hashimoto's thyroiditis	Surgery
Painful subacute thyroiditis	Radioactive iodine
Silent lymphocytic thyroiditis	External radiation
Biosynthetic defects	Atrophic thyroiditis
Iodine deficiency	Agenesis
Drugs (lithium, iodine, immunotherapy)	

hypothyroidism due to surgery, radioactive iodine therapy, and external radiation are all common. Central hypothyroidism due to hypothalamic or pituitary disease, although rare, has significant implications for treatment. Biosynthetic defects in thyroid hormone synthesis are very rare. Transient hypothyroidism due to painful or silent subacute thyroiditis is discussed in detail in the section on hyperthyroidism.

Hashimoto's Thyroiditis (Autoimmune Thyroiditis, Chronic Lymphocytic Thyroiditis)

Hashimoto's thyroiditis is a common genetic disorder with a strong female predominance, affecting at least 5% of all women.[16, 17] After age 60, 15 to 20% of the population has an elevated serum TSH concentration, often in conjunction with positive antithyroid antibodies.[18–20] The histologic features include diffuse lymphocytic infiltration of the thyroid with oxyphil changes in the follicular epithelium. In experimental animals, iodine deficiency prevents its expression;[21] worldwide, Hashimoto's thyroiditis is most common in countries with high iodine intake (e.g., United States and Japan). When exposed to excess iodine, euthyroid patients with Hashimoto's thyroiditis become hypothyroid.[22] Although normal thyroid glands show a slight decrease in function when exposed to excess iodine, hypothyroidism does not occur.

Hashimoto's thyroiditis is thought to be an autoimmune disorder. Antithyroid peroxidase antibodies are present in 98% of patients.[12] It is uncertain whether these antibodies actually cause hypothyroidism. Further evidence for its autoimmune nature is its association with other autoimmune disorders such as pernicious anemia, vitiligo, primary biliary cirrhosis, myasthenia gravis, polymyalgia rheumatica, temporal arteritis, Addison's disease, and type I diabetes mellitus.

Hashimoto's thyroiditis most commonly manifests as an incidentally found goiter on routine examination. The gland is diffusely enlarged on examination, with a texture that varies from rubbery to firm to stony hard. The surface of the gland is often bosselated or pebbly in texture. A pyramidal lobe is often palpable. If only one lobe is palpated, a ''nodule'' is commonly misdiagnosed. When a normal-sized thyroid is easily palpated, Hashimoto's thyroiditis should be suspected. Pain or tenderness on palpation may occur, but these are uncommon. Hypothyroidism occurs on presentation in 20%.[23] A thyroid scan provides little useful information; the RAIU can be low, normal, or high, and the scan pattern is often patchy and may mimic either hot or cold nodules. Patients with hypothyroidism should be treated with replacement thyroid hormone therapy. There is considerable controversy over whether patients with subclinical hypothyroidism (elevated TSH, normal free T_4, and total T_3) should be treated. In general, it reasonable to treat such patients when the TSH is greater than 10 and positive antimicrosomal antibodies are present. When the TSH concentration is elevated and antibodies are present, patients develop hypothyroidism at a rate of 5.0 to 7.5% per year.[24, 25] Levothyroxine suppressive therapy may be useful in the minority of patients with tenderness or pressure symptoms secondary to Hashimoto's thyroiditis.

Secondary Hypothyroidism

Postpartum pituitary necrosis (Sheehan's syndrome) and tumors of the pituitary, hypothalamus, or adjacent structures can lead to a deficiency of TSH with subsequent thyroid gland atrophy and secondary or central hypothyroidism. Gonadal or adrenal insufficiency commonly accompanies central hypothyroidism due to a deficiency of other pituitary hormones. Neurologic compromise due to a mass or infiltrating lesion may produce headaches or visual field defects.

Differentiation of central from primary hypothyroidism has important implications for the treatment of hypothyroidism. Thyroid hormone increases the metabolism of cortisol; treatment of secondary hypothyroidism with thyroid hormones may therefore precipitate adrenal insufficiency. Thyroid function tests generally distinguish primary from central hypothyroidism. In central hypothyroidism the TSH concentration is usually low in the presence of a low T_4. At times, however, the TSH concentration may be normal or even increased, due to the secretion of a form of TSH that has increased immunoreactivity but low bioactivity.[7, 26] A normal or increased TSH concentration is more likely to occur in patients with hypothalamic rather than pituitary lesions and occurs only when the serum T_4 is very low.

Patients with a low or normal TSH concentration and low free T_4 need careful assessment of pituitary function before initiating therapy. If adrenal insufficiency is suspected or found, glucocorticoids should be administered before treatment with thyroid hormone. With central hypothyroidism, the adequacy of thyroid hormone therapy cannot be determined by measuring TSH; clinical assessment and measurement of T_4 and free T_4 index are necessary.

Thyroid Hormone Therapy

The treatment of choice in patients with hypothyroidism is levothyroxine sodium. Eighty-five percent of circulating T_3 is derived from T_4 in the peripheral tissues; only T_4 needs to be given as replacement therapy. The biologic half-life of thyroxine is 7 days; therefore, only a single daily dose is necessary. The goal of thyroid hormone therapy is to give the minimum dosage of thyroxine needed to normalize the TSH. The mean replacement dose is 0.112 mg per day or 1.6 μg per kg per day.[27]

In older patients, particularly those with underlying heart disease, slow replacement therapy is wise, beginning with 12.5 to 25.0 μg per day and increasing the dose in increments of 12.5 to 25.0 μg at 4- to 6-week intervals. Younger patients are given a dose just short of 1.6 μg per kg per day. The mean thyroxine requirement is roughly proportional to the magnitude of the serum TSH elevation. Patients with mild hypothyroidism may require only 25 to 50 μg per day to normalize serum TSH. Once the patient has started thyroid hormone therapy, changes in dosage need not be made more often than every 4 to 6 weeks. The nadir of TSH may take 6 weeks to occur. A TSH measurement alone can be used to monitor thyroxine therapy in patients with primary hypothyroidism.[11]

The dose requirement can be altered by a host of factors. Pregnancy increases the requirement for thyroxine. This may occasionally occur early in pregnancy, and the increased requirement may be as much as 40 to 100%.[28, 29] Thyroid function tests should be checked at 8 weeks and again at 20 weeks of gestation (see Chapter 38). Phenytoin, carbamazepine, and rifampin increase the clearance of levothyroxine, often leading to a 50% increase in drug requirement.[8] Other drugs such as cholestyramine,[30] aluminum hydroxide, iron, sucralfate, activated charcoal, and possibly lovastatin (Mevacor)[31] decrease absorption of levothyroxine.

Patients taking these medicines should not take thyroxine at the same time of day.

Some generic preparations vary greatly in their levothyroxine content.[32] It is advisable to keep patients on the same brand if possible. The mean absorption of thyroxine in normal individuals is 80%. Absorption may be as low as 18% in patients with regional enteritis, sprue, pancreatic deficiency, and other diseases leading to malabsorption.[8] Patients with jejunal ileal bypass require three times their previous levothyroxine dosage.[33] Protein-losing states such as nephrotic syndrome and protein-losing enteropathy increase thyroid hormone requirement. Dose requirements in older patients may be 25% less than in younger patients[34] but should be titrated to TSH.

Hospitalized patients who are unable to take pills by mouth may safely miss a few days of levothyroxine. If they are unable to take anything by mouth for more than 3 days, thyroxine can be given by nasogastric tube or administered by the intravenous route at 80% of the oral dose.

At times, patients are placed on thyroid hormone without adequate documentation of hypothyroidism. In these cases, if the TSH is elevated while on therapy, the thyroid hormone is necessary and should not be stopped. If the patient has a goiter and has positive antithyroid antibodies, it is likely that the treatment is required. In other patients, it is safe to discontinue thyroid hormone or halve the dosage for 4 to 6 weeks and then to measure the TSH and the free T_4 index.

Surgery in Hypothyroid Patients

Elective surgery should be delayed if possible in patients with profound hypothyroidism until they are restored to a euthyroid state. One study reported that patients with mild to moderate hypothyroidism (mean T_4 around 2 μg/dl) tolerate surgery well without excess mortality, intensive care unit stays, or increased duration of hospitalization, although they have lower postoperative temperatures, a longer time to extubation, and more bleeding complications than euthyroid patients.[35] Hypothyroid patients undergoing cardiac surgery (mean T_4 2.2 μg/dl) are more likely to experience neuropsychiatric problems, mild congestive heart failure, constipation, and delayed recovery from anesthesia.[36] They are less likely to have a postoperative fever or to mount a fever with infection. The decisions about the timing of cardiovascular surgery must weigh the need for immediate surgery versus the risks and benefits of preoperative hormone therapy. If emergency surgery is required, it should not be delayed to treat with thyroid hormone.

HYPERTHYROIDISM

Hyperthyroidism is a syndrome characterized by excess thyroid hormone and its clinical manifestations. The diagnosis of hyperthyroidism is confirmed by the finding of a suppressed or undetectable TSH and an increased free T_4 index or total T_3, or both. The signs and symptoms of thyrotoxicosis are listed in Table 22–3. Hyperthyroidism may be caused by autonomy of the thyroid gland, excessive stimulation of the gland, exogenous intake of thyroid hormones, or excessive release of thyroid hormones from a damaged gland. Table 22–4 categorizes the causes of hyperthyroidism according to these mechanisms. Once the diagnosis of thyrotoxicosis is confirmed, the etiology may be unraveled by the patient's clinical characteristics and by the RAIU and radionuclide scan. The RAIU scan categorizes patients with hyperthyroidism into those whose thyroids trap iodine avidly and those whose thyroids do not (Table 22–5).

Graves' Disease

Graves' disease is the most common cause of hyperthyroidism in patients younger than 40. The prevalence of the disorder is 1 to 2 per 1000 persons. Women are affected eight times more frequently than men. A familial predisposition is present, with family members commonly having either Graves' disease or Hashimoto's thyroiditis.

The hyperthyroidism is due to the presence of autoantibodies that bind to the TSH receptor and trigger excess hormone production. Graves' disease is associated with other autoimmune disorders such as type I diabetes mellitus, Addison's disease, myasthenia gravis, Sjögren's syndrome, pernicious anemia, and idiopathic thrombocytopenic purpura.

Graves' disease is also known as diffuse toxic goiter. The majority of patients have some degree of exophthalmos; pretibial myxedema and thyroid acropachy (clubbing) are rare. The thyroid gland is usually diffusely enlarged, but having a normal-sized thyroid does not exclude the diagnosis. The texture of the thyroid gland varies and may be soft, rubbery, or firm. A thrill and bruit may be present. A disproportionate amount of T_3 may be secreted compared with that of T_4 owing to less efficient iodination of thyroglobulin in the hyperthyroid gland.

Graves' ophthalmopathy is an inflammatory disorder of the retro-orbital tissues and may be due to an autoimmune attack on retro-orbital fibroblasts. Although all patients with hyperthyroidism may have lid lag, lid retraction, and stare, inflammation of the orbital structures occurs only in Graves' disease. Swelling of retro-orbital tissue, particularly extraocular muscles and retro-orbital fat, may lead to exophthalmos, chemosis, periorbital edema, proptosis, and eyelid retraction. Exposure keratitis may occur owing to an inability to shut the eyelids. Diplopia, when present, is due to restriction of extraocular muscle movement. Compression of the optic nerve by the muscle cone at the orbital apex may lead to optic neuropathy. Approximately 25% of patients with Graves' disease have exophthalmos on clinical examination by objective measurement with an exophthalmometer. More sensitive studies reveal retro-orbital abnormalities in at least 75% of patients with Graves' disease.[37] Cigarette smoking is an important risk factor, as are male sex and age greater than 50.

Infiltrative dermopathy or pretibial myxedema occurs in 5 to 10% of patients and is almost always accompanied by ophthalmopathy.[38] It is characterized by pinkish to purplish-brown orange peel induration of the skin over the pretibial area and over the dorsa of the feet. Thyroid acropachy, or clubbing of the digits, is present in less than 1% of patients.

Assays for TSH receptor antibodies are now commercially available but generally are not necessary. However, pregnant women with high titers of thyroid-stimulating immunoglobulins are at risk for having babies with neonatal hyperthyroidism that is due to the transplacental passage of the antibodies.[39] Patients previously treated with surgery or radioactive iodine are at particular risk, as their own thyroids no longer serve as an endogenous bioassay for the TSH receptor antibodies.

Toxic Multinodular Goiter

Toxic multinodular goiter is a common cause of hyperthyroidism in the middle-aged and elderly. It is often associated with long-standing goiter and occurs when the nodules autonomously produce excess thyroid hormone. It is more common in women than in men. The severity of hyperthyroidism is variable but is usually less than in Graves' disease. Because of the older population at risk, cardiovascular symptoms predominate. In one series of 85 patients between 60 and 82 years of age, two out of three experienced heart failure and 20% reported angina.[40] The constellation of anorexia, apathy, weight loss, and constipation are more commonly seen in elderly patients with hyperthy-

TABLE 22–3.   Signs and Symptoms of Hyperthyroidism

SYMPTOMS	
General	Nervousness, fatigue, emotional lability
	Heat intolerance, increased sweating
	Weight loss despite increased appetite
	Anorexia
	Insomnia
Skin	Friable nails and hair
	Hair loss
Cardiovascular	Palpitations
	Angina
Respiratory	Dyspnea
Gastrointestinal	Nausea and vomiting
	Abdominal pain
	Frequent or loose bowel movements, or both
Neuromuscular	Tremor
	Muscle weakness
Genitourinary	Urinary frequency
	Nocturia
Reproductive	Oligomenorrhea
	Amenorrhea
	Infertility
SIGNS	
General	Hyperkinetic
Vital signs	Rapid pulse
	Increased systolic blood pressure
	Decreased systolic blood pressure
	Increased temperature
Skin	Warm and moist
	Hyperpigmentation
	Pretibial myxedema*
	Vitiligo*
	Fine hair
Eyes	Stare, lid lag
	Soft tissue swelling*
	Exophthalmos*
	Impaired motility*
	Loss of vision*
Mouth	Tongue tremor
Thyroid	Diffuse goiter
	Single or multiple nodules
	Not palpable†
Heart	Hyperdynamic precordium
	Increased first heart sound
	Atrial arrhythmias
Abdomen	Active bowel sounds
Neuromuscular	Proximal muscle weakness
	Tremor
	Brisk tendon reflexes
Extremities	Edema
	Onycholysis (Plummer's nails)
	Clubbing*

LABORATORY ABNORMALITIES IN HYPERTHYROIDISM

Increase in serum glutamic-oxaloacetic transaminase, serum glutamate pyruvate transaminase, alkaline phosphatase, and indirect bilirubin
Hypercalcemia
Decreased neutrophils*
Decreased cholesterol
Increased angiotensin-converting enzyme
Increased ferritin
Decreased parathyroid hormone
Decreased 1,25 dihydroxyvitamin D
Increased gastrin

*Graves' disease.
†Factitious hyperthyroidism, struma ovarii, occasionally Graves' disease or lymphocytic hyperthyroidism.

TABLE 22–4. Mechanisms of Hyperthyroidism

	AUTONOMY	EXCESS STIMULATION	EXOGENOUS	EXCESS RELEASE
Common	Toxic adenoma Toxic multinodular goiter	Graves' disease	Factitious thyroiditis	Painful thyroiditis Silent thyroiditis
Rare	Struma ovarii Follicular cancer	TSH-induced Trophoblastic disease (hCG-induced)	"Hamburger toxicosis"	

TSH, Thyroid-stimulating hormone; hCG, human chorionic gonadotropin.

roidism than in younger patients.[40, 41] Symptoms due to obstruction of the trachea, esophagus, or neck vessels are more common in this disorder than in Graves' disease. Exophthalmos and dermopathy are not present. On examination, the thyroid is generally large, and discrete nodules are palpable. However, substernal goiter may be evident only on computed tomography (CT) scan or chest radiograph. Euthyroid patients with multinodular goiters and low TSH concentrations are at particular risk for the development of hyperthyroidism when they are exposed to excess iodine (e.g., during CT with contrast, angiography, administration of amiodarone).[42] Consider prophylactic therapy with antithyroid drugs in such patients before exposure to iodine.

Toxic Adenoma ("Hot Nodule")

Single autonomously functioning thyroid nodules may lead to hyperthyroidism. This disorder is far less common than either Graves' disease or multinodular goiter. A long history of a slowly growing lump in the neck and a gradual onset of symptoms of hyperthyroidism are typical, although the onset of hyperthyroidism may be sudden after iodine exposure. Most patients are middle-aged or elderly, and cardiovascular symptoms may predominate. On examination, a single pal-

TABLE 22–5. Differential Diagnosis of Hyperthyroidism Based on Radioactive Iodine Uptake (RAIU)

INCREASED RAIU	DECREASED RAIU
Graves' disease	Subacute granulomatous thyroiditis
Toxic multinodular goiter	Silent lymphocytic thyroiditis
Toxic adenoma	Struma ovarii
Pituitary adenoma	Factitious (exogenous)
Trophoblastic disease	Hamburger toxicosis
	Iodine prophylaxis
	Metastatic follicular thyroid cancer

pable nodule may be appreciated, but the contralateral lobe is usually functionally suppressed and difficult to palpate. Hyperthyroidism may be mild or severe; T_3 may be preferentially elevated.

Trophoblastic Diseases

Trophoblastic diseases, including hydatidiform mole and choriocarcinoma, have rarely been associated with hyperthyroidism. Human chorionic gonadotropin secreted by these tumors can bind to the TSH receptor and stimulate the production of thyroid hormone.[5] Patients exhibit mild hyperthyroidism and generally do not require treatment other than removal of the tumor. Biochemical changes consistent with hyperthyroidism are common in patients with hyperemesis gravidarum. This illness usually occurs during the first trimester of pregnancy when the concentration of human chorionic gonadotropin is at its highest. The laboratory abnormalities are usually mild and resolve by the eighteenth week of pregnancy.

Thyroid-Stimulating Hormone–Producing Pituitary Adenoma

Pituitary tumors that produce TSH are very rare. Secretion of TSH in patients with these tumors leads to hyperthyroidism and a diffuse goiter in the presence of a normal or an elevated TSH concentration.[43] Do not exclude the diagnosis of hyperthyroidism with a normal TSH concentration if the clinical picture fits. Management requires control of hyperthyroidism with antithyroid drugs followed by surgical removal of the tumor.

Painful Subacute Thyroiditis (Subacute Granulomatous Thyroiditis, de Quervain's Thyroiditis)

Subacute thyroiditis causes thyroid pain and hyperthyroidism. Although genetically entrained, it seems to follow viral illnesses, particularly upper respiratory infections.

Symptoms are due to hyperthyroidism (50% of patients) as well as thyroid inflammation.[23] Eighty percent of cases occur in women, most often women between the ages of 35 and 50. Patients experience the fairly abrupt onset of anterior neck pain. Initially the pain is unilateral but may become bilateral and radiate to the ear or jaw. Hyperthyroidism results from leakage of preformed thyroid hormone into the circulation. The thyroid gland is exquisitely tender, hard, and at times nodular. Fever may be mild to marked.

The white blood cell count may be increased slightly and anemia may develop. The erythrocyte sedimentation rate is usually greater than 50 mm per hour; the finding of a normal erythrocyte sedimentation rate makes the diagnosis very unlikely. Because the intrathyroidal content of T_4 exceeds that of T_3 by 10:1, T_4 is disproportionately elevated relative to T_3. Hyperthyroidism inhibits the release of TSH, which results in a low RAIU; in addition, the inflammation may impair iodine uptake.

The clinical course consists of four phases. The initial phase (3–6 weeks) is characterized by a painful thyroid and often hyperthyroidism. Once all preformed thyroid hormone is depleted, patients may be euthyroid for several weeks. During the third phase, hypothyroidism develops and may last for a few weeks or months. Thyroid hormone therapy may be necessary when thyroid function becomes low and is generally required for 6 months. Thyroid function returns to normal in the fourth phase. The entire duration of the illness can last 4 to 6 months or up to a year. An individual patient may not experience all four of the classic phases.

Salicylates and nonsteroidal anti-inflammatory drugs are most useful in controlling the pain of subacute thyroiditis; glucocorticoids, although effective, are rarely necessary. To relieve symptoms of hyperthyroidism, β-blockers can be prescribed; antithyroid drugs and radioactive iodine are not effective.

Silent Lymphocytic Thyroiditis

Silent lymphocytic thyroiditis is an autoimmune inflammatory disease of the thyroid characterized by hyperthyroidism, a zero RAIU, and a painless thyroid. About 60 to 80% of cases occur in women.[23] Silent thyroiditis follows pregnancy in 5% of all women.[44] This disorder may account for 5 to 20% of all hyperthyroidism.[23] The mean age at diagnosis is 30 to 35 years. Patients note the

relatively abrupt onset of symptoms of hyperthyroidism. The gland is nontender and modestly firm. Only 50% of patients have a goiter.[45] As in painful subacute thyroiditis, there is a disproportionate rise in T_4 relative to T_3. The erythrocyte sedimentation rate, however, is normal or only slightly increased. Antimicrosomal antibodies are positive in 50% of patients.[23] The RAIU is suppressed owing to TSH suppression by thyroid hormone leakage from the thyroid. The course parallels that of painful thyroiditis; however, recurrent episodes and persistent thyroid abnormalities such as goiter and hypothyroidism are more likely.[45] β-Blockers can control the symptoms of hyperthyroidism. Although glucocorticoids shorten the time to euthyroidism, they are generally not required.[46]

When silent lymphocytic thyroiditis occurs in the postpartum period (5% of pregnancies) it is called postpartum thyroiditis. The onset of symptoms occurs about 6 weeks after delivery, and the course is similar to that in the sporadic form of lymphocytic thyroiditis. The prevalence of positive antimicrosomal antibodies is higher in the postpartum form,[47] and many patients have recurrences after each successive pregnancy.

Other Causes of Hyperthyroidism

In the very rare syndrome of struma ovarii, a teratoma of the ovary contains thyroid tissue that becomes hyperactive and leads to thyrotoxicosis. Radioactive iodine uptake in the neck is suppressed, but scanning over the pelvis reveals RAIU over the ovary. Rarely does metastatic follicular thyroid cancer produce sufficient thyroid hormone to cause hyperthyroidism.[48] Virtually all patients with this type of cancer have undergone total thyroidectomy; hence, the uptake of radioactive iodine (RAI) in the neck is low.

Factitious (exogenous) hyperthyroidism results from the surreptitious, inadvertent, or excessive ingestion of thyroid hormone. In this situation the thyroid gland is difficult to palpate, and thyroglobulin levels are low. Hyperthyroidism due to contamination of ground beef with thyroid gland tissue resulted from the inappropriate use of neck strap muscles in certain meat preparations.[49, 50] Neck trimmings are no longer used in the preparation of ground beef.

Iodine prophylaxis in areas of endemic goiter may result in jodbasedow hyperthyroidism. Such iodine-induced hyperthyroidism may occur in iodine-sufficient areas when patients with euthyroid hot nodules or multinodular goiters are exposed to excess iodine.[42] When the pool of iodine is high (for weeks or occasionally months after iodine exposure), the RAIU will be low.

TREATMENT OF HYPERTHYROIDISM

Beta-Blockers

Beta-blockers provide prompt temporary control of the hyperadrenergic symptoms of hyperthyroidism such as tachycardia, tremor, anxiety, weakness, and hyperkinetic behavior. In high doses propranolol may also block the conversion of T_4 to T_3. Because they do not interfere with hormone synthesis or secretion, β-blockers may be given to control symptoms while awaiting definitive diagnosis and therapy. The adequacy of the dose is determined by monitoring the resting and exercise heart rate and the degree of symptomatic relief.

Antithyroid Drugs

Methimazole (Tapazole) and propylthiouracil (PTU) are the two antithyroid drugs or thionamides available in the United States. Both block the synthesis but not the release of thyroid hormone. Clinical improvement does not occur until thyroid hormone stored in the gland is depleted, often 4 to 12 weeks. Propylthiouracil (but not methimazole) inhibits the conversion of T_4 to T_3, and this effect can be clinically significant in the treatment of thyroid storm.

Methimazole has a longer half-life, which allows a single daily dosage. Common adverse side effects of both PTU and methimazole include rash, fever, arthralgias, and nausea. If these minor adverse reactions occur with one of the drugs, the other can be substituted, but cross-sensitivity occurs in up to 50% of patients. Lupus-like reactions and hepatic necrosis are more common with PTU.[51] Cholestatic jaundice may occur with methimazole.

A rare but potentially fatal complication is agranulocytosis. This occurs in 0.1 to 0.5% of patients.[52] It occurs more commonly in patients older than 40 and in women. Onset is usually within 3 months of starting or restarting the drug but may occur at any time. Patients should be instructed to discontinue the drug and notify their physician if symptoms of agranulocytosis (fever, chills, mouth ulceration, or sore throat) occur. How often to check the white blood cell count is controversial. A baseline white blood cell count before initiating therapy and testing with each follow-up visit at 4- to 6-week intervals is sufficient.

A low baseline white blood cell count is common in Graves' disease and should not preclude the use of antithyroid drugs.

Methimazole crosses the placenta easily and can induce hypothyroidism and goiter in the fetus.[53] The more limited transfer of PTU and its lower potency makes PTU the drug of choice during pregnancy.[53, 54] Methimazole concentrations in breast milk are high, and therefore it is contraindicated in women who are breast-feeding. Propylthiouracil crosses into milk only one tenth as well, and many women have breast-fed while on PTU without apparent effect on their babies.[55]

Methimazole is started as a single daily dose of 30 mg. Starting doses of PTU vary from 100 to 150 mg every 6 to 8 hours. Symptomatic improvement in hyperthyroidism may occur as early as 2 weeks, but 6 to 12 or more weeks are necessary to achieve the euthyroid state. Once this state has been reached, two alternative approaches may be followed: The antithyroid drugs can be tapered to the lowest amount necessary to maintain euthyroidism, or, alternatively, levothyroxine can be added in a "block-replace" regimen. This is particularly helpful when follow-up visits are infrequent (e.g., with college students going away to school) or when wide swings between hyper- and hypothyroidism have been present.

Methimazole or PTU are often prescribed for young patients with Graves' disease to control hyperthyroidism while waiting for a remission to occur. Remission rates vary between 9 and 80% after 1 year of therapy but average 50%.[38] Antithyroid drugs are generally continued for at least 1 year, after which the drug may be discontinued to see if a remission has occurred. Patients are often misinformed that the drugs can be used for only 1 year. The decision to discontinue antithyroid drugs at 1 year is a mutual one made by the physician and patient depending on the current circumstances. Most immediate relapses occur in the first 3 to 4 months after discontinuing the drug. Remission is more likely in women; in patients with small glands, mild hyperthyroidism, and high antimicrosomal antibody titers; and in patients whose goiters rapidly shrink after beginning therapy.

A Japanese study reported higher remission rates in patients given levothyroxine in addition to their methimazole.[56] After 6 months of therapy, methimazole was tapered to 10 mg and levothyroxine or placebo was given with methimazole for 1 year. Thyroxine or placebo was continued for an additional 1.5 years after methimazole was discontinued. Remission rates of 99% were achieved with levothyroxine and 67% with placebo. Although of unproven benefit, the addition of thyroxine to methimazole after tapering to 5 to 10 mg and continuation after methimazole is discontinued might be considered. Other data suggest that the addition of thyroxine during pregnancy to euthyroid Graves' patients in remission may prevent postpartum recurrence of Graves' disease.[57]

Thionamides are also used to render patients euthyroid before surgery. Hyperthyroidism due to solitary toxic adenoma and toxic multinodular goiter can be controlled with thionamides, but lifelong therapy is generally required. Thionamides also block new hormone synthesis in iodine-induced hyperthyroidism.

Radioactive Iodine

Radioactive iodine, or ^{131}I, is safe, convenient to administer, and effective. After oral administration, ^{131}I is concentrated in the thyroid cells and causes thyroid cell death by beta emission. Control of hyperthyroidism takes several weeks to several months. Hypothyroidism is an expected result of RAI therapy in patients with Graves' disease.[58, 59] At least 50% are hypothyroid at 1 year; ultimately at least 75% will become hypothyroid. Radioactive iodine therapy of toxic adenomas causes hypothyroidism in 5% or less.[60] Patients with toxic multinodular goiters have variable rates of hypothyroidism.

[131]I is remarkably simple and safe. Rarely, radiation-induced thyroiditis causes thyroid pain, which is easily treatable with salicylates or nonsteroidal anti-inflammatory drugs. Exacerbation of hyperthyroidism, due to release of preformed hormone, may occur 7 to 14 days after RAI therapy. It is therefore prudent to pretreat high-risk patients (e.g., older patients and those with heart disease) with antithyroid drugs until euthyroid to deplete thyroid hormone stores. Antithyroid drugs are generally withdrawn 2 to 3 days before RAI therapy and are often resumed 4 to 7 days later.

[131]I therapy for hyperthyroidism exposes the ovaries to a rad dose equivalent to a barium enema or an intravenous pyelogram.[61] A dose of ^{131}I is thought to be 20 times safer than an equivalent x-ray dose. The ovarian rad dosage from ^{131}I is far lower than that from a hysterosalpingogram. There is no increased risk of cancer, leukemia, or birth defects in patients treated with [131]I.[61] Therapy with RAI is contraindicated in pregnancy as it concentrates in the fetal thyroid. A pregnancy test is generally performed before the administration of RAI. Women planning to become pregnant are usually advised to postpone pregnancy for 6 months after RAI therapy to ensure that their thyroid function has stabilized.

Surgery

Surgery plays a much smaller role in the treatment of hyperthyroidism now than in the past. Surgery is recommended for patients with large goiters that are causing obstructive symptoms, neck obstruction, poor compliance, contraindication to antithyroid medication, and refusal to take [131]I. The prevalence of hypothyroidism following surgery is related to the size of the thyroid remnant and varies from 4 to 49%.[62] Recurrent hyperthyroidism can also occur if the remnant size is too large. Risks include anesthesia itself, bleeding into the operative site, recurrent laryngeal nerve injury, and hypoparathyroidism. Patients should be rendered euthyroid with thionamides before surgery. Iodides are added 10 days preoperatively to reduce gland vascularity in patients with Graves' disease. Propranolol can control tachycardia and should be continued for 1 week after surgery. Graves' disease patients who cannot tolerate thionamides can be prepared for surgery with large doses of β-blockers alone or in combination with iodides.

Drugs That Alter the Function of the Thyroid Gland

Iodine serves as the substrate for thyroid hormone biosynthesis and as a modulator of thyroid function. When given in high doses, iodine decreases the organification of iodine, the release of thyroid hormone, and the iodine trapping process. Minimal temporary decreases in thyroid function are noted in normal individuals. In contrast, the damaged thyroid gland is very sensitive to these iodine effects, and decreased thyroid function results. Euthyroid patients with Hashimoto's thyroiditis often become hypothyroid when exposed to excess iodine. After RAI therapy for Graves' disease, saturated solution of potassium iodide (SSKI) can be administered to accelerate the return to euthyroidism.[63] Iodine is an important adjunct to antithyroid drug therapy in critically ill patients with hyperthyroidism (''thyroid storm'') because of its effect on inhibition of thyroid hormone release. The fetal thyroid is particularly sensitive to iodine; maternal iodide therapy has been associated with asphyxiating fetal goiters. However, nodular goiters and autonomous functioning adenomas overproduce thyroid hormone when exposed to excess iodine.

Amiodarone, an important antiarrhythmic, contains 37% iodine by weight.[8] Iodine-induced hypothyroidism may occur in patients with underlying Hashimoto's thyroiditis. Amiodarone-induced hyperthyroidism occurs in three forms: typical iodine-induced hyperthyroidism in patients with multinodular goiters (more common in areas of relative iodine deficiency), Graves' disease, and a spontaneously resolving form of hyperthyroidism that is similar to silent thyroiditis.[8, 64] In addition amiodarone blocks the conversion of T_4 to T_3, leading to an increased serum T_4 (and often free T_4) concentration; in euthyroid individuals TSH remains normal or is only slightly elevated.

Lithium inhibits the release of thyroid hormone from the thyroid gland. Transient TSH elevation occurs in about one third of patients treated with lithium.[65, 66] In some patients, presumably those with underlying Hashimoto's thyroiditis, profound hypothyroidism develops with lithium use. Goiter, presumably induced by TSH, is also common. When patients on lithium develop hyperthyroidism, silent lymphocytic thyroiditis is the most common cause. Lastly, lithium has rarely been used to treat Graves' hyperthyroidism and thyroid storm.

THYROID FUNCTION TESTS IN NONTHYROIDAL ILLNESS

Severe illness causes dramatic changes in thyroid hormone economy and a confusing array of changes in thyroid function testing. Hospitalized patients with nonthyroidal illness often (40–70%) have one or more abnormal results on thyroid function testing.[8] With rare exceptions, these abnormalities do not represent true hypo- or hyperthyroidism.

In severely ill or starving patients, the peripheral conversion of T_4 to T_3 is impaired owing to inhibition of the 5'-deiodinase enzyme.[9] The decreased metabolic rate that results is presumed to be a protective adaptation, preventing excess catabolism. In most situations, reverse T_3 (an inactive degradation product) concentration increases as serum T_3 decreases. Although these findings are regularly observed in ill patients, neither T_3 nor reverse T_3 are usually ordered as thyroid screening studies.

With more severe illness, serum T_4 may decline.[8, 9] The fall in T_4 may be due to decreased levels of binding proteins or displacement of T_4 from its binding proteins by circulating inhibitors. Although the free T_4 or free T_4 index should remain normal, these test results are often low in severely ill patients as well. Concentrations of TSH are often abnormal, further confusing the situation. Serum TSH concentration may fall with severe illness and be lowered further by the use of glucocorticoids or dopamine.[67] Illness alone generally does not lower the TSH to undetectable lev-

els in third-generation assays.[68] The finding of a low free T_4 (or free T_4 index) and a low TSH level suggests central hypothyroidism. Although a functional central hypothyroidism may exist in these patients, therapy with thyroid hormone does not change the outcome and is not indicated.[69] As patients recover from severe illness, the serum TSH rises and may rise above the normal range. Minimal TSH elevations (<20 mU/L) are generally not treated, whereas levothyroxine replacement is given when the TSH is above this value.[6, 8] Thyroid function tests should be used selectively in severely ill patients. In general T_4, free T_4 (or free T_4 index), and TSH tests are required to assess the situation.

In a small proportion of patients, total and free T_4 concentrations are elevated during the acute phase of an illness. This appears to be especially common in patients admitted for acute psychiatric illnesses. In one large series, 33% of these patients exhibited elevated total T_4 levels, and 18% had high free T_4 levels.[70] Levels of T_3 are not increased, and TSH levels are normal. The hyperthyroxinemia is usually transient, returning to normal within 2 weeks after admission.

Patients with liver disease may have characteristic abnormalities in thyroid function tests. In acute hepatitis and biliary cirrhosis, an increase in thyroxine-binding globulin levels leads to high total T_4 and normal free T_4. Patients with cirrhosis have diminished T_4 binding to thyroxine-binding globulin; total T_4 levels are therefore low. In nephrotic syndrome, urinary losses of thyroxine-binding globulin may lead to low total T_4 and T_3 levels. Patients with acquired immunodeficiency syndrome are unusual in that T_4 and T_3 commonly remain normal except in the most severely ill patients.[71] Reverse T_3 does not increase but remains normal or low.

REFERENCES

1. Nolan JP, Tarsa NJ, DiBenedetto G. Case-finding for unsuspected thyroid disease: Costs and health benefits. Am J Clin Pathol 1985;83:346.
2. Kaplan MM. Thyroid hormone therapy: What, when, and how much. Postgrad Med 1993;93:249.
3. Ross D. New sensitive immunoradiometric assays for thyrotropin. Ann Intern Med 1986;104:718.
4. Ruiz M. Familial dysalbuminemic hyperthyroxinemia: A syndrome that can be confused with thyrotoxicosis. N Engl J Med 1982;306:635.
5. Hershman JM, Lee HY, Sugawara M, et al. Human chorionic gonadotropin stimulates iodide uptake, adenylate cyclase, and deoxyribonucleic acid synthesis in cultured rat thyroid cells. J Clin Endocrinol Metab 1988;67:74.
6. Nicoloff JT, Spencer CA. The use and misuse of the sensitive thyrotropin assays. J Clin Endocrinol Metab 1990;71:553.
7. Eskildsen PC, Kruse A, Kirkegaard C. The pituitary-thy-

roid axis in patients with pituitary disorders. Horm Metabol Res 1989;21:387.

8. Cavalieri RR. The effects of nonthyroid disease and drugs on thyroid function tests. Med Clin North Am 1991;75:27.

9. Chopra IJ, Hershman JM, Pardridge WM, Nicoloff JT. Thyroid function in nonthyroidal illnesses. Ann Intern Med 1983;98:946.

10. Ross DS, Daniels GH, Gouveia D. The use and limitations of a chemiluminescent thyrotropin assay as a single thyroid function test in an out-patient endocrine clinic. J Clin Endocrinol Metab 1990;71:764.

11. Helfand M, Crapo LM. Monitoring therapy in patients taking levothyroxine. Ann Intern Med 1990;113:450.

12. Mariotti S, Caturegli P, Piccolo P, et al. Antithyroid peroxidase autoantibodies in thyroid diseases. J Clin Endocrinol Metab 1990;71:661.

13. Portmann L, Hamada N, Heinrich G, DeGroot LJ. Antithyroid peroxidase antibody in patients with autoimmune thyroid disease: Possible identity with antimicrosomal antibody. J Clin Endocrinol Metab 1985;61:1001.

14. McKenzie JM, Zakarija M. Clinical review 3. The clinical use of thyrotropin receptor antibody measurements. J Clin Endocrinol Metab 1989;69:1093.

15. Mariotti S, Martino E, Cupini C, et al. Low serum thyroglobulin as a clue to the diagnosis of thyrotoxicosis factitia. N Engl J Med 1982;307:410.

16. DeGroot LJ, Mayor G. Admission screening by thyroid function tests in an acute general care teaching hospital. Am J Med 1992;93:558.

17. Sawin CT, Castelli WP, Hershman JM, et al. The aging thyroid. Thyroid deficiency in the Framingham study. Arch Intern Med 1985;145:1386.

18. Livingston EH, Hershman JM, Sawin CT, Yoshikawa TT. Prevalence of thyroid disease and abnormal thyroid tests in older hospitalized and ambulatory persons. J Am Geriatric Soc 1987;35:109.

19. Sawin CT, Chopra D, Azizi F, et al. The aging thyroid. Increased prevalence of elevated serum thyrotropin levels in the elderly. JAMA 1979;242:247.

20. Sawin CT, Bigos ST, Land S, Bacharach P. The aging thyroid. Relationship between elevated serum thyrotropin level and thyroid antibodies in elderly patients. Am J Med 1985;79:591.

21. Allen EM, Appel MC, Braverman LE. The effect of iodide ingestion on the development of spontaneous lymphocytic thyroiditis in the diabetes-prone BB/W rat. Endocrinology 1986;118:1977.

22. Safran M, Paul TL, Roti E, Braverman LE. Environmental factors affecting autoimmune thyroid disease. Endocrinol Metab Clin North Am 1987;16:327.

23. Singer PA. Thyroiditis. Acute, subacute, and chronic. Med Clin North Am 1991;75:61.

24. Tunbridge WMG, Brewis M, French JM, et al. Natural history of autoimmune thyroiditis. BMJ 1981;282:258.

25. Rosenthal MJ, Hunt WC, Garry PJ, Goodwin JS. Thyroid failure in the elderly. Microsomal antibodies as a discriminant for therapy. JAMA 1987;258:209.

26. Samuels MH, Ridgway EC. Central hypothyroidism. Endocrinol Metab Clin North Am 1992;21:903.

27. Mandel SJ, Brent GA, Larsen PR. Levothyroxine therapy in patients with thyroid disease. Ann Intern Med 1993;119:492.

28. Kaplan MM. Monitoring thyroxine treatment during pregnancy. Thyroid 1992;2:147.

29. Mandel SJ, Larsen PR, Seely EW, Brent GA. Increased need for thyroxine during pregnancy in women with primary hypothyroidism. N Engl J Med 1990;323:91.

30. Northcutt RC, Stiel JN, Hollifield JW, Stant EG. The influence of cholestyramine on thyroxine absorption. JAMA 1969;208:1857.

31. Utiger R. Therapy of hypothyroidism—When are changes needed. N Engl J Med 1990;323:126.

32. Sawin C, Surks M, London M, et al. Oral thyroxine: Variation and biologic action in tablet content. Ann Intern Med 1984;100:641.

33. Azizi F, Belur R, Albano J. Malabsorption of thyroid hormones after jejunoileal bypass for obesity. Ann Intern Med 1979;90:941.

34. Rosenbaum RL, Barzel US. Levothyroxine replacement dose for primary hypothyroidism decreases with age. Ann Intern Med 1982;96:53.

35. Weinberg AD, Brennan MD, Gorman CA, et al. Outcome of anesthesia and surgery in hypothyroid patients. Arch Intern Med 1983;143:893.

36. Ladenson PW, Levin AA, Ridgway EC, Daniels GH. Complications of surgery in hypothyroid patients. Am J Med 1984;77:261.

37. Bahn RS, Garrity JA, Gorman CA. Diagnosis and management of Graves' ophthalmopathy. 1990;71:559.

38. McDougall IR. Graves' disease current concepts. Med Clin North Am 1991;75:79.

39. McKenzie JM, Zakarija M. Fetal and neonatal hyperthyroidism and hypothyroidism due to maternal TSH receptor antibodies. Thyroid 1992;2:155.

40. Davis PJ, Davis FB. Hyperthyroidism in patients over the age of 60 years. Clinical features in 85 patients. Medicine 1974;53:161.

41. Hurley JR. Thyroid disease in the elderly. Med Clin North Am 1983;67:497.

42. Martin FIR, Tress BW, Colman PG, Deam DR. Iodine-induced hyperthyroidism due to nonionic contrast radiography in the elderly. Am J Med 1993;95:78.

43. Wynne AG, Gharib H, Scheithauer BW, et al. Hyperthyroidism due to inappropriate secretion of thyrotropin in 10 patients. Am J Med 1992;92:15.

44. Amino N, Mori H, Iwatani Y, et al. High prevalence of transient post-partum thyrotoxicosis and hypothyroidism. N Engl J Med 1982;306:849.

45. Nikolai TF, Coombs GJ, McKenzie AK. Lymphocytic thyroiditis with spontaneously resolving hyperthyroidism and subacute thyroiditis. Long-term follow up. Arch Intern Med 1981;141:1455.

46. Nikolai TF, Coombs GJ, McKenzie AK, et al. Treatment of lymphocytic thyroiditis with spontaneously resolving hyperthyroidism (silent thyroiditis). Arch Intern Med 1982;142:2281.

47. Learoyd DL, Fung HY, McGregor AM. Postpartum thyroid dysfunction. Thyroid 1992;2:73.

48. Paul SJ, Sisson JC. Thyrotoxicosis caused by thyroid cancer. Endocrinol Metab Clin North Am 1990;19:593.

49. Hedberg CW, Fishbein DB, Janssen MD, et al. An outbreak of thyrotoxicosis caused by the consumption of bovine thyroid gland in ground beef. N Engl J Med 1987;361:993.

50. Kinney JS, Hurwitz ES, Fishbein DB, et al. Community outbreak of thyrotoxicosis: Epidemiology, immunogenetic characteristics, and long-term outcome. Am J Med 1988;84:10.

51. Vitug AC, Goldman JM. Hepatotoxicity from antithyroid drugs. Horm Res 1985;21:229.

52. Cooper DS. Which antithyroid drug? Am J Med 1986;80:1165.

53. Cooper DS. Antithyroid drugs. N Engl J Med 1984;311:1353.

54. Momotani N, Noh J, Oyanagi H, et al. Antithyroid drug therapy for Graves' disease during pregnancy. N Engl J Med 1986;315:24.

55. Kampmann JP, Johansen K, Hansen JM, Helweg J. Propylthiouracil in human milk: Revision of a dogma. Lancet 1980;1:736.

56. Hashizume K, Ichikawa K, Sakurai A, et al. Administration of thyroxine in treated Graves' disease: Effects on the level of antibodies to thyroid-stimulating hormone receptors and on the risk of recurrence of hyperthyroidism. N Engl J Med 1991;325:947.

57. Hashizume K, Ichikawa K, Nishii Y, et al. Effect of administration of thyroxine on the risk of postpartum recurrence of hyperthyroid Graves' disease. J Clin Endocrinol Metab 1992;75:6.

58. Sridama V, McCormick M, Kaplan EL, et al. Long-term follow-up study of compensated low dose ^{131}I therapy for Graves' disease. N Engl J Med 1984;311:426.

59. Farrar JJ, Taft AD. Iodine-131 treatment of hyperthyroidism: Current issues. Clin Endocrinol 1991;35:207.

60. Ross DS, Ridgway EC, Daniels GH. Successful treatment of solitary toxic thyroid nodules with relatively low dose iodine-131 with a low prevalence of hypothyroidism. Ann Intern Med 1984;101:488.

61. Graham GD, Burman KD. Radioiodine treatment of Graves' disease. An assessment of its potential risks. Ann Intern Med 1986;105:900.

62. Cusick EL, Krukowski ZH, Matheson NA. Outcome of surgery for Graves' disease re-examined. Br J Surg 1987;74:780.

63. Ross DS, Daniels GH, De Stefano P, et al. Use of adjunctive potassium iodide following radioactive iodine treatment of Graves' hyperthyroidism. J Clin Endocrinol Metab 1983;57:250.

64. Keidar S, Palant A, Grenadier E. Amiodarone-induced thyrotoxicosis: Four cases and a review of the literature. Post Grad Med J 1980;56:356.

65. Emerson CH, Dyson WL, Utiger RD. Serum thyrotropin and thyroxine concentration in patients receiving lithium carbonate. J Clin Endocrinol Metab 1973;36:338.

66. Transbol I, Christiansen C, Baastrup PC, et al. Endocrine effects of lithium. 1. Hypothyroidism, its prevalence in long-term patients. Acta Endocrinol 1978;87:759.

67. Wehmann RE, Gregerman RI, Burns WH, et al. Suppression of thyrotropin in the low-thyroxine state of severe nonthyroidal illness. N Engl J Med 1985;312:546.

68. Boles JM, Morin JF, Garre MA. Ultrasensitive assay of thyroid stimulating hormone in patients with acute nonthyroidal illness. Clin Endocrinol 1987;27:395.

69. Brent GA, Hershman JM. Thyroxine therapy in patients with severe nonthyroidal illnesses and low serum thyroxine concentration. J Clin Endocrinol Metab 1986;63:1.

70. Spratt DI, Pont A, Miller MB, et al. Hyperthyroxinemia in patients with acute psychiatric disorders. Am J Med 1982;73:41.

71. LoPresti JS, Fried JC, Spencer CA, Nicoloff JT. Unique alterations of thyroid hormone indices in the acquired immunodeficiency syndrome (AIDS). Ann Int Med 1989;110:970.

Management of Thyroid Nodules

Audrey B. Miklius and Gilbert H. Daniels

Thyroid nodules are among the most common endocrine abnormalities requiring evaluation. The prevalence of thyroid nodules, as reported in the Framingham population study, is higher than 6%.[1] Ultrasound data suggest that this figure substantially underestimates the frequency of nodules.[2] Fortunately, thyroid cancer is uncommon in the clinical setting, with an annual incidence of 50 new patients per million.[3] The primary goal in the evaluation of thyroid nodules is to distinguish between nodules that require surgery because they suggest the presence of malignancy and those that can be safely followed.

Nodularity of the thyroid can be a nonspecific manifestation of a variety of other thyroid diseases including multinodular goiter, Hashimoto's thyroiditis, and even Graves' disease. This chapter reviews the clinical and diagnostic evaluation of patients who are found to have thyroid nodules. A rational plan for the management of nodular thyroid disease is outlined. Techniques of thyroid palpation are reviewed in Chapter 22.

THYROID CANCER

The main concern when identifying a thyroid nodule is the rare but important possibility that this represents a thyroid cancer. Well-differentiated thyroid cancers (papillary and follicular) comprise 80% of the clinically detected thyroid cancer in the United States.[4] In addition, microscopic (occult) papillary carcinoma occurs in more than 10% of thyroid glands; this should be considered an incidental finding of no clinical significance. Most patients with well-differentiated thyroid cancer have a good prognosis. However, a small percentage of papillary cancers and a higher percentage of follicular cancers do behave in an aggressive fashion, with pulmonary and bony metastases. Anaplastic thyroid carcinoma develops in

older patients, often in preexisting benign or low-grade malignant lesions, and carries a dismal prognosis. Thyroid lymphoma develops in the setting of preexisting Hashimoto's thyroiditis. Medullary thyroid carcinoma may be inherited, requiring careful family screening. Pheochromocytomas and hyperparathyroidism may be associated findings (multiple endocrine neoplasia II). Thyroid lymphoma and medullary carcinoma have a variable prognosis.

How often is a thyroid nodule malignant? The true prevalence is unknown and varies between 1.5 and 38% depending on the study.[5] The highest prevalence is reported in surgical series. Selection bias makes these numbers difficult to interpret; nodules that are deemed suspicious are more often selected for surgery. In one hospital in which nodule excision was the general rule, only 6.5% of excised nodules were malignant.[6] This may represent a more accurate cancer risk, although subtle selection bias cannot be excluded.

Which clinical features increase the likelihood of a thyroid malignancy in a patient with a thyroid nodule (Table 23–1)? A prior history of head or neck irradiation predisposes to both benign and malignant nodules, particularly in women.[7] Radiation therapy was given for tonsillar or thymic enlargement, acne, birthmarks, or ringworm. Although radiation therapy for these benign conditions was uncommon after 1958, patients who have received radiation therapy for Hodgkin's disease or laryngeal carcinoma may be at similar risk. In two large series in which patients received predominantly tonsillar or nasopharyngeal irradiation, nodules were found in 20 to 27% of patients; approximately one third of patients had a thyroid malignancy.[8, 9] A nodule in a patient younger than 20 years is more likely to be malignant than a nodule in an older patient. Although women have a higher prevalence of nodules than men, a nodule in a man is more likely to be malignant. A family

TABLE 23–1. Risk Factors and Clinical Features of a Malignant Nodule

	MALIGNANT	BENIGN
Risk factors	Head and neck radiation	No irradiation
	Age <20	Age >20
	Male sex	Female sex
	Family history medullary carcinoma MEN II	Negative family history
Clinical features	Hard nodule	Soft nodule
	Irregular texture	Regular texture
	Fixed to surrounding tissue	Mobile
	Hoarseness	

MEN II, Multiple endocrine neoplasia II.

history of medullary thyroid carcinoma or multiple endocrine neoplasia II dramatically increases the risk of malignancy in a thyroid nodule.

Certain physical characteristics also suggest malignancy. A hard nodule is more apt to be malignant that a soft one. Nodule texture is determined by side-to-side compression of the nodule; posterior mobility of a nodule with pressure is often misinterpreted as a soft texture. Although large nodules are not necessarily more likely to be malignant than small nodules, the stakes are increased with large nodules; in general, the larger the thyroid cancer, the worse the prognosis. Nodules that are irregular in texture or fixed to surrounding tissues are of concern. Hoarseness due to vocal cord palsy, stridor, or rapid growth of a nodule is also a worrisome finding.

It should be apparent that the vast majority of patients with thyroid nodules have none of the features described above. Therefore, additional diagnostic tests are used to select for surgery patients whose nodules are most likely to be malignant. These techniques include thyroid function testing, thyroid scintigraphy, fine needle aspiration biopsy (FNAB), and thyroid ultrasound. Before discussing the application of these techniques, alternative causes of the nodular thyroid are discussed.

MULTINODULAR GOITERS

Multiple nodules are far more common than solitary ones. Autopsy studies show that more than one third of patients older than 50 years harbor multiple nodules.[10] Furthermore, 20 to 40% of patients with solitary nodules on physical examination are found to have multiple nodules during thyroid ultrasound.[11, 12] Multinodular goiters appear to be more common in women than in men. With the increasing prevalence of radiologic evaluations, incidental thyroid nodules are commonly discovered by ultrasound, computed tomography

scanning, or magnetic resonance imaging. Whether these incidentally discovered nodules pose the same risk as palpable nodules is uncertain but likely.

Why are multiple nodules in the thyroid gland so common? The answer is not certain. Patients with multiple nodules seem to inherit or develop groups of thyroid cells with accelerated growth potential. In areas of the world with iodine deficiency, increased concentrations of thyroid-stimulating hormone (TSH) further accelerate the growth of these cells. However, iodine deficiency does not exist in the United States.

Problems associated with multinodular goiters are summarized in Table 23–2. Hyperthyroidism may develop spontaneously in patients with multinodular goiters. In general there is an inverse relationship between concentration of TSH and thyroid volume, suggesting gradual development of autonomous thyroid function.[13] With time, the goiters tend to enlarge and concentration of TSH tends to decline. More than 20% of these patients have evidence of thyroid gland autonomy (low TSH concentration or failure of radioactive iodine uptake to decline with thyroid hormone administration).[13] These patients are at risk for the development of hyperthyroidism after iodine exposure.

Multinodular goiters can become quite large or can be strategically located (at the thoracic inlet), causing shortness of breath or stridor due to tra-

TABLE 23–2. Problems Associated with Multinodular Goiter

1. Hyperthyroidism
2. Tracheal compression
3. Esophageal compression
4. Substernal goiter
5. Cosmetic issues
6. Malignancy

cheal compression. The shortness of breath may be attributed to pulmonary or cardiac disease unless tracheal narrowing is appreciated on chest radiograph, by computed tomography scanning, or by performing pulmonary function tests (flow-volume loop). Symptoms may be exacerbated by raising the arms over the head (Pemberton's maneuver). Although difficulty swallowing food may occur with goiter, globus (discomfort with swallowing saliva) is far more common and requires only reassurance. Goiters that are primarily substernal are often discovered with routine chest radiographs. Substernal goiters and those causing obstructive symptoms often require surgical removal. Goiters that are large enough to cause cosmetic problems may require surgery as well.

The likelihood of malignancy appears to be lower in multinodular goiters than in solitary nodules. However, suspicious or dominant nodules should be evaluated as though they were solitary.[14] Patients who have previously received head or neck irradiation are of particular concern.

HASHIMOTO'S THYROIDITIS AND GRAVES' DISEASE

Autoimmune thyroiditis (Hashimoto's thyroiditis) may be confused with an isolated nodule or a multinodular goiter. The firmness of the lobes that makes these glands easy to palpate may cause confusion with nodular thyroid glands. Hypothyroidism or elevation of TSH is rare in patients with multinodular goiter; when either is present, the diagnosis is most likely Hashimoto's thyroiditis. The presence of strongly positive antithyroid (or antithyroid peroxidase) antibodies help confirm the diagnosis of Hashimoto's thyroiditis. The surface of the thyroid gland in Hashimoto's thyroiditis is bosselated, pebbly, or undulating, but frank nodules are uncommon. When discrete nodules are present, further evaluation is necessary. Mild to moderate tenderness may accompany Hashimoto's thyroiditis but is uncommon. The sudden growth of a lobe or part of the thyroid in a patient with known Hashimoto's thyroiditis raises the specter of thyroid lymphoma. Asymmetric thyroid enlargement in Graves' disease may mimic a nodule. The presence of ophthalmopathy, hyperthyroidism, and typical thyroid scan appearance confirms the diagnosis of Graves' disease.

SINGLE NODULES

Most single thyroid nodules prove to be benign adenomas. Autonomously functioning nodules are virtually always benign adenomas. These "hot" nodules produce increased amounts of thyroid hormone; when hormonal output is excessive, concentrations of TSH decline as does the function of the surrounding normal thyroid tissue. Hyperthyroidism may result. With the suppression of TSH, the contralateral side of the thyroid is no longer palpable. The majority of patients with hot nodules are euthyroid and can be followed clinically. Only 10% of these patients develop hyperthyroidism within 6 years.[15] However, elderly patients with hot nodules and patients with nodules greater than 3 cm in diameter have a higher likelihood of developing hyperthyroidism.

Many benign adenomas degenerate, causing liquefaction or hemorrhage; these partially cystic nodules are often incorrectly identified as thyroid cysts. True thyroid cysts may occur in the thyroid but are rare. The sudden appearance of a painful thyroid nodule is usually due to hemorrhage into a benign thyroid nodule. Unfortunately, thyroid malignancies may also be partially cystic or may cause pain.

NODULE EVALUATION

Blood Tests

A screening TSH (using an ultrasensitive TSH assay) is a valuable initial study. In patients with multinodular thyroids, a low concentration of TSH points to thyroid autonomy or frank hyperthyroidism. Suppressed TSH in a patient with a solitary nodule suggests that the nodule may be a hot nodule. An elevated concentration of TSH may indicate the presence of Hashimoto's thyroiditis rather than a multinodular goiter. Positive antithyroid (or antithyroid peroxidase) antibodies are compatible with Hashimoto's thyroiditis, particularly when found in high titer. However, the presence of positive antibodies should not dissuade the physician from further evaluation of a suspicious nodule.

Patients with a history of head and neck irradiation should also have a screening calcium performed because of the increased prevalence of hyperparathyroidism in this population.[16]

Thyroid Scintigraphy

Thyroid scans are useful for thyroid imaging and evaluating the functional characteristics of thyroid nodules; in addition, they are valuable in differentiating among the various causes of hyperthyroidism. It is important to palpate and mark thyroid abnormalities at the time of the thyroid scan. Thyroid scans are performed with radioiodine or technetium (in the form of pertechnetate). Iodine is concentrated by the thyroid gland and rapidly converted into organic form. The radioiodine of choice, ^{123}I, is administered orally, and the thyroid is scanned with a gamma counter 24 hours after administration. [123]I scans may give lower background, provide greater clarity, and easily allow a measurement of 24-hour radioactive iodine uptake. Pertechnetate is also trapped by the thyroid gland but is not converted into organic form or stored. Technetium-99m pertechnetate is administered intravenously, and scans are performed 20 minutes after administration. Technetium scans can be done the same day, are more readily available, have lower isotope cost, and can be performed on patients receiving drugs that block iodine organification (e.g., methimazole or propylthiouracil). Quantitative technetium uptakes require more sophisticated equipment. Occasionally nodules that are cold on iodine scanning are hot when scanned with technetium (see following discussion).

Hot nodules or hyperfunctioning nodules concentrate radioiodine better than normal thyroid tissue; they are virtually always benign. Unfortunately, only 5% of all thyroid nodules are "hot."[15] Rarely, malignant nodules concentrate iodine but do not convert it to organic form. Such nodules appear hot on technetium scans but cold on iodine scans. Nodules that are hot on technetium scanning require additional confirmation: either a suppressed concentration of TSH or a radioiodine scan.

Virtually all thyroid cancers concentrate iodine less well than normal thyroid tissue, leading to the maxim "thyroid cancers are cold." Most benign nodules also concentrate iodine less well, leading to the corollary "most cold nodules are benign." However, many thyroid nodules are indeterminate on scan, appearing neither hot nor cold. This occurs when cold or hot nodules are surrounded and obscured by normal thyroid tissue. Although such nodules are often called warm, they should be considered indeterminate.

A suppression scan allows equivocal nodules to be separated into cold or hot categories. Hot nodules are considered benign; cold nodules require further evaluation. Sufficient thyroid hormone is given to suppress TSH concentrations (e.g., levothyroxine (L-T_4), 1.8 to 2.0 μg per kg per day for 4 to 6 weeks, or levotriiodothyronine (L-T_3) (cytomel), 25 μg three times a day for 10 days). When TSH is suppressed in this manner, hot nodules continue to function and can easily be distinguished from background; normal thyroid tissue and cold nodules are not seen. Several caveats are important. Patients should be warned about the possible development of hyperthyroid symptoms during this test. Adverse cardiac effects are more likely with L-T_3; we prefer to use L-T_4. If the suppression scan shows areas of uptake not related to the nodule, TSH should be measured to ensure adequate suppression. Nodules occasionally shrink dramatically or even disappear during this time, suggesting benignity.

When the entire "nodule" corresponds to the lobe of the thyroid (or when two "nodules" are palpated and each corresponds to an entire lobe), then Hashimoto's thyroiditis should be considered.

Fine Needle Aspiration Biopsy

Fine needle aspiration biopsy represents a major advance in the evaluation of thyroid nodules.[17] Cutting needle biopsies performed with Vim-Silverman or Tru-Cut needles remove a core of thyroid tissue; these tests were restricted to a handful of surgeons and never gained popularity because of the difficulty of the method. In contrast, FNAB withdraws thyroid cells for cytologic diagnosis. The procedure is safe, simple, and relatively inexpensive and can be performed in an office setting by endocrinologists, primary care physicians, and surgeons. The quality of the specimen is dependent on experience; when performing more than 50 aspirations per year, an adequate specimen is obtained in 85 to 90% of cases.[18, 19]

Many techniques of FNAB have been employed. A local anesthetic is used to anesthetize the overlying skin, and then a 25-gauge needle is introduced into the nodule and specimens are obtained by capillarity (rotating the needle or moving the needle up and down) or by suction (attaching the needle to a syringe). The suction technique is greatly facilitated by using a "gun," which allows the syringe to be employed using one hand. Five or six separate aspirates are performed in an attempt to sample different parts of the nodule. The sample is expelled onto a slide, smeared, fixed, and stained for cytologic examination. Larger needles may also be employed with tissue fragments obtained from the needle washings.

Four cytologic results are possible: nondiagnostic, malignant, benign, and suspicious (Table 23–3). Nondiagnostic results are obtained 10 to 15% of the time and indicate that the FNAB needs to be repeated to obtain an adequate sample. Approximately 6 to 10% of FNAB results indicate a malignancy. Patients with malignant lesions are referred for surgery. An FNAB finding of malignancy proves to be malignant 96% of the time.[18, 19]

TABLE 23–3. Fine Needle Aspiration Biopsy Diagnoses

---

1. Nondiagnostic: Repeat specimen
2. Malignant: Surgery recommended
3. Benign (generally macrofollicular or colloid adenomas, occasionally Hashimoto's thyroiditis): Follow patient; reaspirate or operate if continued growth is noted
4. Suspicious (cellular or microfollicular adenomas, also called follicular neoplasms): Operate to exclude follicular carcinoma

---

Benign nodules are generally macrofollicular adenomas (colloid adenomas). The false negative rate in this situation may be as low as 1%, with reports varying between 0 and 5%.[20] The lowest rates occur in centers with the greatest cytodiagnostic expertise.

The suspicious category requires some explanation. When the thyroid follicles are organized into small compact groups with little or no colloid, the lesion is considered a microfollicular (cellular) lesion, also known as a follicular neoplasm. Both benign lesions (microfollicular adenomas) and malignant lesions (follicular carcinomas) may have a similar appearance on biopsy; the distinction can be made only when the entire nodule is analyzed by a pathologist. Capsular or vascular invasion is required to diagnose a follicular carcinoma. In the absence of these findings, the lesion is considered benign. For this reason, surgery is generally recommended for suspicious lesions. Ten to 20% of nodules fall into the suspicious category; 10 to 20% of persons who have surgery because of suspicious results on cytologic testing have malignant nodules.[21] In general, the larger the suspicious nodule, the higher the risk of its being malignant.

"Cystic" thyroid nodules pose a special problem as adequate cytologic material may not be obtainable. Small (1 cm or less) cystic nodules, those that contain clear fluid, and those that disappear after aspiration, are likely to be benign. Cysts that are large (>3 cm), that contain hemorrhagic fluid, that recur after aspiration, or that have a large (>1 cm) solid component should be regarded with suspicion.[22, 23] Patients with a history of head or neck irradiation, hoarseness, obstructive symptoms, or lymphadenopathy are more likely to have malignant cystic lesions.

Biopsy results may be misleading in two situations. Hot nodules, although benign, are often microfollicular in pattern and would therefore be considered suspicious if a biopsy were performed.[24] A radioiodine scan is therefore required for patients with a suspicious result on biopsy, if it has not been performed previously. Second, many patients with benign Hashimoto's thyroiditis are misdiagnosed as having suspicious microfollicular lesions or a possible lymphoma after FNAB. It is therefore important to distinguish between a true nodule and a typical case of Hashimoto's thyroiditis before FNAB, if possible, to avoid unnecessary and potentially misleading results.

Thyroid Ultrasound

Thyroid ultrasound is noninvasive and avoids radiation exposure. Unfortunately, there is no specific sonographic picture of thyroid malignancy.[25] Ultrasound may be useful in determining multinodularity, following the size of nodules, screening patients with a history of head or neck irradiation, and monitoring patients after surgery for thyroid cancer. Ultrasound-guided needle biopsies may be useful when nodules are small, have a sizable solid component after nondiagnostic aspiration of a partially cystic nodule, are difficult to palpate, or are in a high-risk location.

Many clinicians obtain ultrasounds to determine whether a nodule is cystic. This approach may be misguided. True cysts are rare, occurring in approximately one in 500 nodules.[26] These lesions are entirely sonolucent with a thin, discrete, smooth wall. Partially cystic nodules represent degenerated solid lesions with uneven thick walls and solid components. Approximately 20% of nodules have this appearance. Unfortunately, this appearance does not exclude malignancy. The ultrasound is useful in determining the size of the solid component after a nondiagnostic FNAB of a cystic-like lesion.

EVALUATION OF THE THYROID NODULE

It is not surprising that there is disagreement about the correct approach to evaluate a thyroid nodule. One approach is to perform a biopsy on all single or dominant thyroid nodules (Fig. 23–1). Patients with malignant nodules will be referred for surgery, and those with benign nodules can be followed. Patients with suspicious lesions require thyroid scans to exclude hot nodules and possibly Hashimoto's thyroiditis. This is the obvious approach when nuclear medicine facilities are unavailable, when the nodule is almost certainly malignant, or when a pregnant woman has a suspicious nodule. Whether this is the correct approach in all other patients is less certain.

A second approach (Fig. 23–2) is to perform thyroid function tests (screening TSH) and a thyroid scan in all patients with nodules. Only pa-

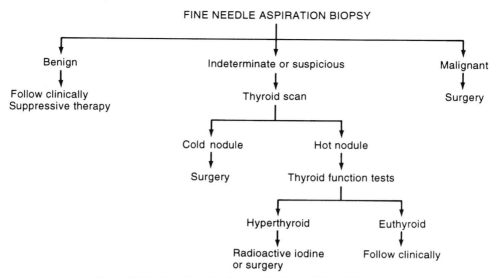

Figure 23–1. Algorithm for the evaluation of thyroid nodules.

tients with cold nodules are referred for FNAB. This approach avoids biopsies in patients with autonomous nodules, those with Hashimoto's thyroiditis, and possibly those with multiple nondominant nodules. Unfortunately, a normal TSH test result cannot exclude Hashimoto's thyroiditis or an early hot nodule.

Although the first approach appears to be more cost-effective, the difference in cost per nodule evaluated is not great. Occasionally a patient with a suspicious result on biopsy is not reassured by a scan that demonstrates a hot nodule and opts for surgery. Surgery may be the inevitable result of an avoidable biopsy in a patient with Hashimoto's thyroiditis. The cost of surgery in a few patients far outweighs the cost of scans for many. For these reasons, the second approach is generally pre-

ferred. An ultrasound is rarely helpful as part of either initial evaluation.

MANAGEMENT OF PATIENTS WITH THYROID NODULES

Solitary "Benign" Nodules

When the cytologic findings are benign (macrofollicular or colloid adenoma), solitary nodules can be safely followed. Whether these patients should be merely observed or should be followed with ultrasounds or serial biopsies, or both, remains controversial. The size of the nodules should be measured carefully in all dimensions. Placing paper tape over the nodule or nodules, tracing the

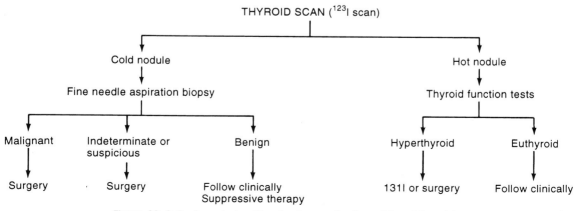

Figure 23–2. Preferred algorithm for the evaluation of thyroid nodules.

nodule, and archiving the tape in the patient record is an alternative approach. Serial ultrasounds are unnecessary when the size of the nodule is easily measurable. If nodules remain the same or decrease in size, repeat aspiration biopsies are also not needed. Continued growth of a nodule (not due to cystification), neck symptoms from a nodule, or continued patient anxiety about a nodule are all valid indications for surgery.

Should these patients be treated with thyroid hormone (levothyroxine) suppressive therapy? L-T_4 has been used in patients with thyroid nodules in an attempt to reduce the size of these lesions. Sufficient L-T_4 is given to decrease TSH, thus removing one potential growth stimulus. Is this therapy effective? Postsurgical patients with prior radiation exposure are less likely to develop new nodules if they are treated with suppressive therapy.[27] Patients with sporadic multinodular goiter show a decreased thyroid volume compared with that of placebo-treated patients.[28] The efficacy of thyroid hormone suppression in patients with solitary nodules remains controversial. Many uncontrolled studies have shown a greater than 50% reduction in diameter in 9 to 69% of cases.[5] Two double-blind placebo-controlled trials using ultrasound evaluation showed no difference between the small numbers of patients treated with levothyroxine versus placebo.[29, 30] Both of these trials were of short duration.

How to reconcile the consistent data from uncontrolled trials with the contrary data from controlled trials is a dilemma. Prevention of further growth of nodules by suppressive therapy is also a desirable goal, one not addressed by these studies. Approximately 10% of patients treated with suppressive therapy demonstrate continued nodule growth. When the increased size is not due to cystic degeneration, surgery is recommended. Approximately 10% of these nodules prove to be malignant.[5] It is unknown whether more patients will require surgery if they are not treated with suppressive therapy. Many clinically uninodular goiters are multinodular when assessed by ultrasound. It is possible that thyroid hormone suppression might prevent growth of other nodules in a uninodular gland.

Is suppressive therapy safe? It has been known for many years that hyperthyroidism results in increased bone resorption, negative calcium balance, and reduced bone density; some of the effects may be permanent. Decreased bone density has been recognized as a potential adverse effect of supraphysiologic L-T_4 replacement.[31] A cross-sectional study of premenopausal women taking suppressive therapy for thyroid nodules noted significant decrease in radial bone density in those on therapy for 5 years, with a larger decrease in those taking L-T_4 for more than 10 years. Bone density measurements were not obtained before beginning L-T_4 therapy. Other studies have shown similar effects.[32] Many of the patients in these studies were treated before the advent of sensitive TSH assays. Consequently, the doses of L-T_4 were higher than necessary to reduce TSH, and many patients had frankly elevated free T_4 concentrations. One study suggests that the risk of osteoporosis can be minimized if the dose of L-T_4 is carefully titrated to maintain a normal free T_4 concentration.[33] In addition to adverse effects on bone density, excess L-T_4 may have cardiac effects, including exacerbation of angina or cardiac arrhythmias.

Suppressive therapy is probably useful in many patients. The L-T_4 dosage should be the minimum required to lower the TSH below normal (but not to undetectable) values or to achieve the desired clinical effect. If the TSH measurement has a detection limit of 0.01 μU per ml (normal 0.5 to 5.0), the goal is generally a suppressed TSH between 0.1 and 0.5 μU per ml. In general, one should avoid suppressive therapy in older, sicker, or cardiac patients or in patients who have small nodules. Suppressive therapy is recommended for younger patients with larger, clinically worrisome, or symptomatic nodules.

The approach to the cystic nodules has already been discussed. Those nodules with a large solid component after aspiration are treated as solid nodules.

Autonomous Nodules

Patients with hot nodules require therapy when in a state of hyperthyroidism. Therapeutic options include radioiodine (^{131}I), surgery, or antithyroid drugs. Radioiodine is the usual therapy of choice. Hypothyroidism is uncommon (5%) because the radioiodine is concentrated by the nodule but not by the suppressed contralateral lobe.[34] Surgery is an effective alternative but does require general anesthesia; only half the thyroid is removed. Antithyroid drugs can control the hyperthyroidism but need to be given indefinitely. In elderly hyperthyroid patients or those with underlying cardiac disease, antithyroid drugs are often administered before definitive therapy with radioiodine or surgery.

What should be done with asymptomatic patients with low or undetectable TSH concentrations but normal concentrations of T_4, free T_4, and T_3? Patients older than 50, those with cardiac disease, or those at risk for osteoporosis should be treated with radioiodine. Younger patients can be followed, as occasionally thyroid function returns to normal. Patients with normal TSH concentrations and hot nodules can be observed, with thyroid function tests checked once or twice yearly or when symptoms develop.

Multinodular Goiters

Multinodular goiters require careful, long-term follow-up. Suppressive therapy may be indicated in those patients who have normal concentrations of TSH. All patients should be followed for the development of biochemical hyperthyroidism or compressive symptoms. With large goiters, the neck circumference should be recorded. Periodic computed tomography examination (preferably without contrast agents) may be necessary with large goiters to exclude progressive enlargement or tracheal compression. Patients with continued growth or symptoms from a goiter require surgery. If only one nodule enlarges, it should be aspirated for cytologic examination and to determine if cystification has occurred. As with a single nodule, continued growth of a nodule in a multinodular goiter requires surgery. Substernal goiters should be removed surgically, barring major medical contraindications.

Hyperthyroidism may be treated with radioiodine or with surgery; pretreatment with antithyroid drugs may be necessary (see Chapter 22). Iodide exposure should be avoided in patients with large multinodular goiters, particularly those with low TSH concentrations. Prophylactic treatment with antithyroid drugs before unavoidable iodine exposure may be considered particularly in patients with severe coronary disease. Treatment may need to be continued for 4 to 6 weeks after exposure. Although such therapy is of unproven benefit, life-threatening hyperthyroidism may be prevented in some patients.

Postradiation Patients

Patients with a history of neck irradiation should be examined carefully for thyroid nodules and other head and neck malignancies. The risk appears to continue for the life of the patients, although peak incidence of thyroid abnormalities occurs at about 25 years. Hyperparathyroidism is more common in this population; serum calcium and albumin should be measured periodically.[16] These patients may be at increased risk for breast cancer as well.[35]

Although of unproven benefit, some recommend periodic thyroid ultrasound examination in these patients. If the ultrasound results are normal, no therapy is indicated. Small (less that 1 cm) nodules should be suppressed with levothyroxine. Larger nodules should be scanned, and biopsies should be performed on cold nodules, with ultrasound guidance if necessary. If adequate cytologic reassurance cannot be obtained, surgery is recommended. Patients who have received high-dose radiation for Hodgkin's disease or laryngeal carcinoma are at risk for both thyroid nodularity and hypothyroidism.[36] Some researchers recommend prophylactic thyroid hormone therapy in these patients.[37]

REFERENCES

1. Vander JB, Gaston EA, Dawber TR. The significance of nontoxic thyroid nodules. Final report of a 15-year study of the incidence of thyroid malignancy. Ann Intern Med 1968;69:537.
2. Carroll BA. Asymptomatic thyroid nodules: Incidental sonographic detection. AJR 1982;138:499.
3. Hay ID. Thyroid carcinoma. In: Brain MC, Carborne PP (eds). Current Therapy in Hematology-Oncology-3. Burlington, Ontario: BC Decker, 1988, pp 339–345.
4. Robbins J, Merino MJ, Boice JD, et al. Thyroid cancer: A lethal neoplasm. Ann Intern Med 1991;115:133.
5. Molitch ME, Beck JR, Dreisman M, et al. The cold thyroid nodule: An analysis of diagnostic and therapeutic options. Endocr Rev 1984;5:185.
6. Werk EE, Vernon BM, Gonzalez JJ, et al. Cancer in thyroid nodules. A community survey. Arch Intern Med 1984;144:474.
7. Schneider AB, Shore-Freedman E, Weinstein RA. Radiation-induced thyroid and other head and neck tumors: Occurrence of multiple tumors and analysis of risk factors. J Clin Endocrinol Metab 1986;63:107.
8. Cerletty JM, Guansing AR, Engbring NH, et al. Radiation-related thyroid carcinoma. Arch Surg 1978;113:1072.
9. Favus MJ, Schneider AB, Stachura ME, et al. Thyroid cancer occurring as a late consequence of head-and-neck irradiation. Evaluation of 1056 patients. N Engl J Med 1976;294:1019.
10. Mortensen JD, Woolner LB, Bennet WA. Gross and microscopic findings in clinically normal thyroid glands. J Clin Endocrinol Metab 1955;15:1270.
11. Solbiati L, Volterrani L, Rizzatto G, et al. The thyroid gland with low uptake lesions: Evaluation by ultrasound. Radiology 1985;155:187.
12. Scheible W, Leopold GR, Woo VL, et al. High-resolution real-time ultrasonography of thyroid nodules. Radiology 1979;133:413.
13. Berghout A, Wiersinga WM, Smits NJ, et al. Interrelationships between age, thyroid volume, thyroid nodularity, and thyroid function in patients with sporadic nontoxic goiter. Am J Med 1990;898:602.
14. McCall A, Jarosz H, Lawrence AM, et al. The incidence of thyroid carcinoma in solitary cold nodules and in multinodular goiters. Surgery 1986;100:1128.
15. Hamburger J. Evolution of toxicity in solitary nontoxic autonomously functioning thyroid nodules. J Clin Endocrinol Metab 1980;50:1089.
16. Cohen J, Gierlowski TC, Schneider AB. A prospective study of hyperparathyroidism in individuals exposed to radiation in childhood. JAMA 1990;264:581.
17. Lowhagen T, Granberg P, Lundell G, et al. Aspiration biopsy cytology (ABC) in nodules of the thyroid gland suspected to be malignant. Surg Clin North Am 1979;59:3.

18. Nishiyama RH, Bigos ST, Goldfarb WB, et al. The efficacy of simultaneous fine-needle aspiration and large-needle biopsy of the thyroid gland. Surgery 1986;100:1133.

19. Gershengorn MC, McClung MR, Chu EW, et al. Fine-needle aspiration cytology in the preoperative diagnosis of thyroid nodules. Ann Intern Med 1977;87:265.

20. Grant CS, Hay ID, Gough IR, et al. Long-term follow-up of patients with benign thyroid fine-needle aspiration cytologic diagnoses. Surgery 1989;106:980.

21. Gharib H, Goellner JR, Zinsmeister AR, et al. Fine-needle aspiration biopsy of the thyroid. The problem of suspicious cytologic findings. Ann Intern Med 1984;101:25.

22. de los Santos ET, Keyhani-Rofagha S, Cunningham JJ, et al. Cystic thyroid nodules: The dilemma of malignant lesions. Arch Intern Med 1990;150:1422.

23. Rosen IB, Provias JP, Walfish PG. Pathologic nature of cystic thyroid nodules selected for surgery by needle aspiration biopsy. Surgery 1986;100:606.

24. Walfish PG, Strawbridge HT, Rosen IB. Management implications from routine needle biopsy of hyperfunctioning thyroid nodules. Surgery 1985;98:1179.

25. Van Herle AJ, Rich P, Ljung BE, et al. The thyroid nodule. Ann Intern Med 1982;96:221.

26. Simeone JF, Daniels GH, Mueller PR, et al. High-resolution real-time sonography of the thyroid. Radiology 1982;145:431.

27. Fogelfeld L, Wiviott MB, Shore-Freedman E, et al. Recurrence of thyroid nodules after surgical removal in patients irradiated in childhood for benign conditions. N Engl J Med 1989;320:835.

28. Ross D. Thyroid hormone suppressive therapy of sporadic nontoxic goiter. Thyroid 1992;2:263.

29. Reverter JL, Lucas A, Salinas I, et al. Suppressive therapy with levothyroxine for solitary thyroid nodules. Clin Endocrinol 1992;36:25.

30. Gharib H, James EM, Charboneau JW, et al. Suppressive therapy with levothyroxine for solitary thyroid nodules. N Engl J Med 1987;317:70.

31. Ross DS, Neer RM, Ridgway EC, et al. Subclinical hyperthyroidism and reduced bone density as a possible result of prolonged suppression of the pituitary-thyroid axis with L-thyroxine. Am J Med 1987;82:1167.

32. Ross D. Monitoring L-thyroxine therapy: Lessons from the effects of L-thyroxine on bone density. Am J Med 1991;91:1.

33. Greenspan SL, Greenspan FS, Resnick NM, et al. Skeletal integrity in premenopausal and postmenopausal women receiving long-term L-thyroxine therapy. Am J Med 1991;91:5.

34. Ross DS, Ridgway EC, Daniels GH. Successful treatment of solitary toxic thyroid nodules with relatively low-dose iodine-131, with low prevalence of hypothyroidism. Ann Intern Med 1984;101:488.

35. Hildreth NG, Shore RE, Dvoretsky PM. The risk of breast cancer after irradiation of the thymus in infancy. N Engl J Med 1989;321:1281.

36. Hancock SL, Cox RS, McDougall IR. Thyroid diseases after treatment of Hodgkin's disease. N Engl J Med 1991;325:599.

37. DeGroot LJ. Diagnostic approach and management of patients exposed to irradiation to the thyroid. J Clin Endocrinol Metab 1989;69:925.

REPRODUCTIVE ISSUES
Birth Control

24

Hormonal Contraception

Joan Bengtson

Contraceptive practices are ancient, but reliable hormonal contraceptives have been available only since the 1960s. Since its introduction, the birth control pill has evolved into one of the safest and most effective pharmacologic agents currently in use. A wealth of clinical experience confirms this assertion. It is estimated that 10 million women in the United States alone are currently taking the pill, and as many as 50 million have used it at some point in their lives.[1] Worldwide, the number of women who have used the pill exceeds 150 million. However, despite our vast experience, enormous misunderstanding exists about the pill, precluding its even more effective use. All practitioners in women's health must be familiar with the available hormonal contraceptive options to counsel and care for our patients most effectively.

Several types of hormonal contraceptives are currently available and are reviewed in this chapter. The combination oral contraceptive pill is the most familiar. Also available are progestin-only pills and parenterally administered progestin-only preparations. Some formulations are administered postcoitally as morning-after contraceptives. Investigational hormonal contraceptives are also considered in this chapter.

Most women of reproductive age (15–44 years) are sexually active. About two thirds are fertile yet not currently trying to conceive.[2] Among women at risk of unintended pregnancy, about 28% use hormonal contraceptives. As many as 10% of sexually active couples do not practice regular contraception at all.

High rates of abortion and teenage pregnancy imply that contraceptive practices in this country are inadequate. One reason may be a reluctance to use hormonal contraceptives because of unfounded fears and misperceptions. In a 1985 Gallup poll, 76% of women considered the pill to be a high-risk medication and 46% thought the risks of pill use exceed those of childbearing.[3] The same poll also showed that women consider the pill to be unreliable. Although the birth control pill is not ideal, it is certainly better than its reputation suggests.

The advantages of the birth control pill are as follows:

1. It is one of the most effective means of pregnancy prevention.

2. Its effects are readily reversible.

3. It is safe in most users, and high-risk patients can generally be identified so that use can be avoided by them.

4. Its use confers significant noncontraceptive benefits.

5. Its use is fairly well accepted and convenient; use is not coitally related.

The disadvantages are as follows:

1. Pill use is not risk free; serious life-threatening complications can occur.

2. Some users experience unacceptable side effects.

3. Its use requires significant user motivation to remember to ingest a pill daily.

4. It is not available without a prescription.

5. The cost is prohibitive for some patients.

PHARMACOLOGY

The pharmacology of hormonal contraceptives has evolved considerably during the past 3 decades. Current pills have distinct advantages over their earlier counterparts. At first, it may seem as though an impossibly large and confusing number of hormonal contraceptives are available (Table 24–1), but they are all one of two types, the com-bination pill or the progestin-only preparation. The combination pill contains both an estrogen com-ponent and a progestin component. All hormones in oral contraceptives are synthetic.

The estrogen component is either ethinyl estra-

TABLE 24–1. Hormone Contraceptive Preparations

MONOPHASIC ORAL CONTRACEPTIVES

Estrogen (μ)	Progestin (mg)	Product Names
Mestranol 50	Norethindrone 1	Genora 1/50 Nelova 1/50M Norethin 1/50M Norinyl 1 + 50 Ortho-Novum 1/50
Ethinyl estradiol 50	Norethindrone 1	Ovcon 50
Ethinyl estradiol 50	Norethindrone acetate 1	Norlestrin 1/50 Norlestrin Fe 1/50
Ethinyl estradiol 50	Ethynodiol diacetate 1	Demulen 1/50
Ethinyl estradiol 50	Norethindrone acetate 2.5	Norlestrin 21 2.5/50 Norlestrin Fe 2.5/50
Ethinyl estradiol 50	Norgestrel 0.5	Ovral
Ethinyl estradiol 35	Norethindrone 1	Genora 1/35 N.E.E. 1/35 Nelova 1/35E Norcept-E 1/35 Norethin 1/35E Norinyl 1 + 35 Ortho-Novum 1/35
Ethinyl estradiol 35	Norethindrone 0.5	Brevicon Genora 0.5/35 Modicon Nelova 0.5/35E
Ethinyl estradiol 35	Norethindrone 0.4	Ovcon 35
Ethinyl estradiol 35	Ethynodiol diacetate 1	Demulen 1/35
Ethinyl estradiol 35	Norgestimate 0.25	Ortho-Cyclen
Ethinyl estradiol 30	Desogestrel 0.15	Desogen Ortho-Cept
Ethinyl estradiol 30	Norethindrone acetate 1.5	Loestrin 21 1.5/30 Loestrin Fe 1.5/30
Ethinyl estradiol 30	Norgestrel 0.3	Lo/Ovral
Ethinyl estradiol 30	Levonorgestrel 0.15	Levlen Nordette
Ethinyl estradiol 20	Norethindrone acetate 1	Loestrin 21 1/20 Loestrin Fe 1/20

MULTIPHASIC ORAL CONTRACEPTIVES

Biphasic oral contraceptives	Nelova 10/11 Ortho-Novum 10/11
Triphasic oral contraceptives	Ortho-Novum 7/7/7 Triphasil Tri-Levlen Tri-Norinyl

PROGESTIN-ONLY PRODUCTS

Progestin (mg)	Product Names
Norethindrone 0.35 mg	Micronor Nor-QD
Norgestrel 0.075 mg	Ovrette
Levonorgestrel implants	Norplant
Medroxyprogesterone acetate	Depo-Provera

diol or mestranol. Mestranol is activated in the liver by demethylation to ethinyl estradiol. In some bioassays, ethinyl estradiol is more potent than mestranol, but there are no significant clinical differences in effect.[4, 5] Therefore, the type of estrogen is not important in selecting a formulation, and in fact, ethinyl estradiol is used in all of the available low-dose preparations (20–35 μg doses). However, the estrogen dose is an important consideration in pill choice. Serious side effects, including cardiovascular events, are dose related. Earlier formulations contained up to 150 μg of estrogen, but today only pills containing 50 μg and less are manufactured.[6]

Five progestins have traditionally been used in combination oral contraceptive pills in the United States. They are structurally related to androgens but lack a methyl group at the 19 position (19 norprogestins). The progestins exhibit androgenic activity and antiestrogenic activity in addition to progesterone-like effects. In general, the potencies of these drugs for androgenic effects parallel their potencies for progestin effects. Approximate equivalent doses for progesterone-like effects are as follows[7]:

Levonorgestrel	0.1 mg
d,l-Norgestrel	0.2 mg
Ethynodiol diacetate	0.36 mg
Norethindrone acetate	0.43 mg
Norethindrone	0.5 mg

The androgenic activity of the progestin may influence some of the risks associated with oral contraceptives. Measurable differences have been noted in the impact of the progestin component on blood lipid levels.[8] However, it has not been demonstrated that this effect translates into clinically significant differences in disease risk.[9] Nevertheless, these concerns have prompted the development of newer progestins (desogestrel, gestodene, norgestimate) that lack androgenic activity yet retain progesterone-like effects.[10] Two formulations containing the progestins have been introduced in the United States. Preliminary trials suggest that efficacy and side effects are comparable to those of older preparations, and the metabolic impact with respect to carbohydrates and lipids is negligible.[11]

Combination pills are administered cyclically. A pill is taken daily for 21 days. It is omitted for the next 7 days, and then the cycle repeats. Combination pills with a fixed daily dose of estrogen and progestin are called monophasic. Multiphasic preparations vary the dose during the course of a month of therapy. The progesterone-only pill is taken every day at a fixed dose.

Oral contraceptive effects are mediated by interactions with steroid hormone receptors. The synthetic estrogens stimulate the cytoplasmic estrogen receptor and promote the synthesis of progesterone receptors. The progestin not only stimulates progesterone and androgen receptors but also functions as an antiestrogen. Thus, the ultimate biologic effects result from a complex interaction of direct effects, potentiating effects, and antagonistic effects. At the level of many end-organs, however, the progestin effect is dominant.[12]

Oral contraceptives prevent pregnancy by several mechanisms of action. The primary effect is estrogen-mediated suppression of ovulation. Continuous high levels of circulating estrogen inhibit the midcycle surge of follicle-stimulating hormone and luteinizing hormone[13] by direct inhibition of pituitary function and indirectly by inhibition of gonadotropin-releasing hormone secretion from the hypothalamus. In the absence of the stimulating effect of the gonadotropins, the ovary fails to release an egg.

The progestin component also contributes contraceptive effects. Progestins induce the production of thick, viscid cervical mucus that is relatively impermeable to sperm. The endometrial lining is rendered atrophic and therefore not optimal for implantation. Progestins also adversely affect tubal motility, thus disrupting gamete transport.

The pharmacologic effects outlined earlier are exploited for therapeutic purposes other than contraception. Inhibition of ovarian function by gonadotropin suppression decreases formation of recurrent functional ovarian cysts. Dysmenorrhea is also effectively treated by ovarian suppression. The progesterone-like effects can induce atrophy of endometriosis implants, especially by administering the pill in a daily, noncyclic fashion.

CONTRACEPTIVE EFFECTIVENESS

The tendency has been to focus on the risks of hormonal contraceptives at the expense of highlighting their effectiveness. Patients should be aware that compared with other means of available contraception, oral contraceptives are the most effective reversible method (Table 24–2).[14] The level of effectiveness sought by a patient depends on personal as well as medical considerations. For example, patients seeking to delay pregnancy may not require as high a level of effectiveness as patients seeking to avoid pregnancy. Also, patients for whom pregnancy is medically risky should use methods less likely to fail.

Effectiveness is usually measured by the annual failure rate or the number of pregnancies occurring

TABLE 24–2. Failure Rates for Different Methods of Contraception

METHOD	FAILURE RATE PER 100 WOMAN-YEARS (95% CONFIDENCE LIMITS)
Female sterilization	0.13 (0.07–0.21)
Combination oral contraceptive	
50 μg estrogen	0.16 (0.12–0.21)
<50 μg estrogen	0.27 (0.17–0.41)
Progestin-only pill	1.2 (0.7–1.8)
Copper-T intrauterine device	1.2 (0.4–2.7)
Diaphragm	1.9 (1.8–2.1)
Condom	3.6 (3.3–3.9)
Coitus interruptus	6.7 (4.9–8.9)
Rhythm	15.5 (10.0–22.9)

From Vessey M, Lawless M, Yeates D. Efficacy of different contraceptive methods. Lancet 1982;1:841–842 © The Lancet, 1982.

among users during 1 year. Failure rates vary in different populations because pregnancy may result from both intrinsic failures of the method and failures due to incorrect use of the method. The theoretic effectiveness is the antifertility action when a method is used under ideal conditions with no omissions or errors in use. The actual use effectiveness is measured empirically when a technique is used under the realistic conditions of life. The difference between the two increases for techniques that are user dependent, difficult to use, and inconvenient (usually meaning coitally dependent). The actual use effectiveness can be improved by educational efforts by health care professionals to ensure proper use.

NONCONTRACEPTIVE BENEFITS

Although the risks of pill use have been overemphasized, a positive aspect of pill use has been largely ignored. The noncontraceptive benefits of oral contraceptives are rarely cited as a reason for women to select them from among the alternatives. These benefits are significant and range from modifying conditions that interfere with quality of life through prevention of life-threatening diseases.

The progestin-dominant effect of oral contraceptives induces a relative atrophy of the endometrium. As a result, patients taking the pill can anticipate predictable, light withdrawal flows instead of menses. In addition, because oral contraceptive cycles are anovulatory, levels of endometrial prostaglandins are diminished, resulting in reduction or elimination of dysmenorrhea.[15] The incidence of iron deficiency anemia is reduced by about 50% in pill users.[16]

The incidence of functional ovarian cysts is lower in oral contraceptive users compared with that in nonusers, owing to the inhibition of ovulation.[17] Ovarian cysts may necessitate hospital admission or surgical intervention in symptomatic patients; therefore, reducing their frequency is a significant benefit. Benign breast disease, another potential cause of hospitalization, is also reduced in users.[18]

Current oral contraceptive use reduces the risk of pelvic inflammatory disease or salpingitis by about 50%.[19] The mechanism of action may be the thickening of cervical mucus, rendering it more impervious to ascending bacteria from the lower genital tract. Salpingitis is an important cause of infertility and is a risk factor for ectopic pregnancy as well. Despite the decreased risk of upper genital tract disease, the risk of chlamydial cervicitis may be increased with oral contraceptive use.[20]

Pill use can also reduce the risk of two important gynecologic cancers, endometrial and ovarian. Birth control pills are the only prescription drug for which one can make this claim. The prognosis for ovarian cancer is poor because this carcinoma often becomes evident only after metastasis has occurred. Therefore, prevention is an important element of disease management. Oral contraceptive users have a 40% reduction in incidence compared with that of those who have never used them.[21] The protective effect increases with duration of use and persists for at least 15 years after discontinuation. It is estimated that about 2000 cases are averted each year in the United States because of pill use.

Endometrial cancer risk is also decreased in oral contraceptive users.[22] The relative risk is about 0.5, compared with that of nonusers. Although less lethal than ovarian cancer, endometrial cancer is far more prevalent: About 33,000 new cases are diagnosed each year. The mechanism of protection appears to be progestin-mediated prevention of excessive estrogen stimulation of the endometrium.

MINOR SIDE EFFECTS

Minor side effects do not represent significant threats to a patient's health and usually resolve after an adjustment period of 1 to 3 months. If a symptom does not resolve, then another formulation might be better tolerated. Although these effects are minor, they may contribute to discontinuation of the pill. Effectiveness requires compliance, which can be improved by anticipating annoying side effects and advising patients about them.

The common side effects are often designated estrogen mediated or progestin mediated (Table 24–3).[23] A distinction is not always possible, but it may assist in selecting one formulation over another. The estrogen component is likely to be responsible for headaches, nausea, leukorrhea, and telangiectasias. The progestin component causes breast tenderness, moodiness, acne, and hirsutism. A patient with one of these complaints may improve on a formulation with a lower dose or a less potent progestin.

One of the most common complaints is breakthrough bleeding, which is any bleeding that occurs before the week of the expected withdrawal flow. Endometrial integrity is maintained by a balance of estrogen and progestin. A deficiency of either relative to the other can result in breakdown of the lining and consequent bleeding. If a pill cycle is compared with the physiologic ovarian cycle (note that this analogy should not be pressed too far, however, because pill use is clearly a pharmacologic state), then breakthrough bleeding in the first half of the cycle (days 1–9) may be due to a relative estrogen lack. The endometrial tissues are primarily dependent on estrogen at this phase, and too little estrogen results in bleeding. During the second half of the cycle (days 10–21), progesterone stabilizes the estrogen-primed endometrium. If the progestin content of the pill is insufficient, bleeding may result in this part of the cycle.

Multiphasic preparations adjust the ratio of estrogen to progestin during the course of the cycle in an attempt to balance the endometrial needs and avoid breakthrough bleeding at a lower total monthly dose of progestin. However, irregular bleeding occurs in less than 5% of patients even with monophasic preparations after the initial adjustment.[6]

MAJOR SIDE EFFECTS

Cardiovascular diseases associated with oral contraceptive use include myocardial infarction, thromboembolic disease, and cerebrovascular accidents. The studies linking hormonal contraceptives with cardiovascular disease have significantly contributed to the perception that the pill is unsafe. However, a modern perspective requires a critical review of the older studies that originally defined the problem. Older studies evaluated patients using high-dose pills and have little applicability to today's low-dose formulations. Also, older studies sometimes failed to account for confounding factors such as age, other cardiovascular risk factors, and especially smoking history.

Healthy young nonsmokers appear to face no increased risk of mortality from cardiovascular disease due to current or past use of low-dose pills.[24, 25] Despite these encouraging reports, some factors define subgroups of women who face significant risk of cardiovascular disease in association with oral contraceptive use. They include abnormal lipid metabolism, chronic hypertension, diabetes, and advancing age.[26] However, the most important risk factor is smoking history. Even among young pill users (younger than 30 years), smokers have a higher risk of myocardial infarction than nonsmokers who use the pill. The effect is so pronounced after age 35 that pill use is contraindicated in smokers.[27]

Attention is being focused on the mechanism of cardiovascular disease in oral contraceptive users and on distinguishing contributions from the estrogen versus the progestin components. Thrombosis due to estrogen-mediated alterations in blood coagulability is probably an important pathophysiologic mechanism.[28] Thrombotic events may occur in both the arterial and venous sides of the vascular tree.

Alternatively, atherosclerotic disease may mediate the increased risk of cardiovascular events in pill users. It is well established that the risk of atherosclerosis is influenced by plasma lipid levels and composition.[29] Both estrogens and progestins can alter the lipid profile. Estrogens enhance the secretion of high-density lipoprotein and lower the level of low-density lipoprotein, whereas proges-

---

TABLE 24–3. **Side Effects of Oral Contraceptives and Their Relationship to Hormone Content**

Side effects associated with relative estrogen deficiency:
  Bleeding and spotting
  Hypomenorrhea/amenorrhea
  Atrophic vaginitis
  Vasomotor flushes
Side effects associated with relative estrogen excess:
  Breast tenderness
  Hypermenorrhea
  Nausea
  Headache
  Leukorrhea
  Weight gain
Side effects associated with relative progestin deficiency:
  Bleeding and spotting
  Hypermenorrhea
Side effects associated with relative progestin excess:
  Breast tenderness
  Acne
  Hirsutism
  Bloating
  Weight gain

From Dickey RP. Managing Contraceptive Pill Patients. 5th ed. Durant, Okla: Creative Informatics, 1987, pp 222–223.

tins, especially those with marked androgenic effects, have the opposite effects.[30] The changes associated with estrogen are protective, whereas those of progestin increase the atherogenic index. Because the net effect of the combination oral contraceptive pills tends to be progestin dominant, it is theorized that progestin-induced lipid changes may mediate the increased risk of cardiovascular disease in users. However, the progestin-induced changes tend to remain within physiologic limits, and no clinical data associate oral contraceptive use with promotion of atherosclerotic disease.[31] Also, the increase in cardiovascular risk is not correlated with duration of use, an effect one would expect if atherosclerosis were the mechanism.[32]

Hypertension occasionally complicates oral contraceptive use, and all patients should be monitored for it. It was previously thought to be due primarily to the estrogen component via an adverse effect on the renin-angiotensin system.[33] However, it now appears that the progestin component contributes to the risk as well.[28] In most cases, the blood pressure reverts to baseline with discontinuation of the pill. Oral contraceptives are relatively contraindicated in patients with chronic hypertension, even patients whose hypertension is well controlled on medication. However, they are a reasonably safe alternative in patients with a history of pregnancy-induced hypertension.[34]

Although women often cite fear of cancer as a reason to avoid hormonal contraceptive use, the data supporting a clear association are lacking. Some studies have suggested an association between pill use and cervical cancer and premalignant cervical lesions.[35] However, several potential confounding variables render the results unreliable. Cervical cancer is increased in women who initiate sexual activity before age 18 years, have multiple sexual partners, smoke, and are infected with the human papillomavirus. Studies have not always controlled adequately for these factors.[36] Furthermore, control patients may be using barrier methods of contraception. Positive results then may reflect only the protective effect of barrier methods against cervical cancer, not the harmful influence of oral contraceptives. Nevertheless, patients using hormonal contraceptives should be regularly screened with Papanicolaou smears.

More controversial is the relationship between oral contraceptive use and breast cancer. Epidemiologic studies do not support an aggregate increase in breast cancer risk.[37] However, some suggest that subsets of patients may have a higher likelihood of developing breast cancer with use.[38, 39] Specifically, women who initiate oral contraceptive use at a young age or who start before their first term pregnancy and use the pill for at least 5 years may be more likely to develop breast cancer before menopause. The methodology of these studies has been criticized, and the Food and Drug Administration has decided that the evidence is insufficient to warrant a change in labeling.[40] However, oral contraceptives have not been used long enough to resolve this concern, especially considering the average age for developing breast cancer. Therefore, this issue warrants ongoing attention.

Oral contraceptives are associated with a short-term increase in the risk of cholecystitis, but data from the Royal College of General Practitioners' study suggest that use may merely accelerate the onset of symptoms in women already predisposed.[41] No overall increase in incidence is noted among users monitored for 4 to 5 years.

The liver metabolizes and conjugates estrogen for excretion. Liver diseases that compromise this function may result in a hyperestrogenic state. Prolonged hyperestrogenism may in turn cause endometrial hyperplasia and may predispose to endometrial cancer. Patients with active liver disease, therefore, should not use oral contraceptives.

Data suggest an increase in the incidence of adenomas and focal nodular hyperplasia of the liver in oral contraceptive users.[42] However, these conditions are so rare that the attributable risk is only about 3 to 4 per 100,000 users per year.[43] Although these tumors are considered benign, they are very vascular, and death due to rupture and hemorrhage may occur.

MANAGING PATIENTS ON HORMONAL CONTRACEPTIVES

Initiating therapy with hormonal contraceptives requires comprehensive counseling and a thorough medical evaluation. Counseling includes discussion of all of the elements of informed consent— risks, benefits, and alternatives. Discussion of the alternatives should include consideration of the risks associated with an undesired pregnancy should a less effective method of birth control be chosen and fail. On reviewing the risks, the health care provider must exclude absolute contraindications and fully discuss relative contraindications. Absolute and relative contraindications are listed in Table 24–4.

Patients should undergo a physical examination, including blood pressure assessment and breast, abdominal, and pelvic examinations. Papanicolaou smears should be obtained, and a screening urine analysis should be checked for glucose intolerance. After the pills are begun, patients should be seen for a blood pressure check in 3 months and

TABLE 24–4. Absolute and Relative Contraindications to Oral Contraceptives

Absolute contraindications
   History of atherosclerotic disease
   History of deep vein thrombophlebitis
   Known or suspected estrogen-dependent neoplasm
   Undiagnosed abnormal vaginal bleeding
   Known or suspected pregnancy
   Significantly impaired liver function
   Insulin-dependent diabetes mellitus with complications
   Hypercholesterolemia
   Cigarette smoking in women older than 35 years
Relative contraindications
   Migraine headaches
   Hypertension
   Diabetes mellitus without complications
   Cigarette smoking
   Obesity
   Use of drugs that may interact with the pill

then for annual visits including Papanicolaou smears. Monitoring plasma lipids is not routine, because the changes associated with hormonal contraceptives remain within physiologic limits.[31]

Therapy should be initiated with a preparation containing 30 or 35 μg of ethinyl estradiol. Monophasic formulations are simplest and are tolerated by most patients. Almost all patients experience at least some mild side effects during the first 2 to 3 months of treatment. Patients should be warned of this and encouraged not to change pills until the adjustment period elapses. If a patient continues to have problems, changes can then be made according to considerations outlined later.

Conveniently packaged calendar dispensers assist patients with compliance. Packages contain only 21 hormone pills or 28 pills that include seven placebos to be taken during the off week. A patient is instructed to begin a package on the Sunday after the first day of her menstrual period. One pill is taken daily for 21 days, preferably at the same time each day. She then omits the pill or takes a placebo for 7 days before resuming the hormones again on Sunday. She is advised to use a backup method of contraception during the first month.

If side effects are intolerable or persist beyond 3 months, a change in formulation is indicated. Changes are made by determining whether the side effect is estrogen mediated or progestin mediated and adjusting accordingly (see Table 24–3).

As discussed previously, breakthrough bleeding occurring during the first half of the cycle (days 1–9) results from relative estrogen deficiency. Rather than switch to a pill with a higher estrogen dose, a formulation with a lower dose or a less potent progestin can be tried. Bleeding during the second half of the cycle (days 10–21) results from a relative progestin deficiency. A higher dose or a more potent progestin should be effective.

Amenorrhea may also result from a relative lack of estrogen. Patients should be reassured that menstrual flow is not necessary and that the lack of bleeding simply reflects atrophy of the endometrial lining due to the progestin-dominant hormonal milieu. However, amenorrhea may create so much anxiety about possible pregnancy that a patient may find it intolerable, in which case a less potent or lower-dose progestin should be tried.

Other side effects of estrogen deficiency include atrophic vaginitis and occasionally vasomotor symptoms. Patients with these complaints may benefit from a 50-μg formulation. Side effects caused by relative estrogen excess include nausea, headaches, leukorrhea, and weight gain. A preparation with only 20 μg of ethinyl estradiol is available. Alternatively, patients may elect a progestin-only preparation.

Insufficient progestin may result in heavy withdrawal bleeding. Symptoms associated with excessive progestin effect include weight gain, breast tenderness, acne, hirsutism, and bloating. A less potent progestin or a lower dose may be prescribed.

Patients occasionally forget to take a pill. If that happens regularly, a patient should reassess the appropriateness of this method of birth control for her, because efficacy is severely impaired. Whenever a pill is forgotten, the couple should immediately begin to use a backup contraceptive and continue to do so for the remainder of the cycle. If one pill is missed, the patient should take it as soon as the omission is discovered and should continue to take the rest of the pack on schedule. If two pills are missed, she should take both as soon as possible, then two on the next day, and subsequently complete the pack normally. If more than two pills are missed, the pack should be discarded and a new pack begun in 7 days.

Antibiotics, barbiturates, and benzodiazepines may reduce the effectiveness of hormone contraceptives by altering their metabolism.[44] If patients are prescribed a short-term course of these drugs, a backup contraceptive should be used. An alternative contraceptive is recommended for long-term users.

If a pill failure occurs and a patient becomes pregnant, she should be counseled about options for pregnancy termination, prenatal care, and issues of teratology. Patients should be informed that a 2 to 3% risk of birth defects exists for all pregnancies. Exposure to hormonal contraceptives does not appear to increase this risk.[45]

PROGESTIN-ONLY PREPARATIONS

Preparations containing only a progestin are also effective contraceptives. They offer a hormonal alternative to women who cannot or should not take estrogen. Included are lactating women and women who cannot tolerate the estrogen-mediated side effects of the combination pill. Unique methods of administration may provide an advantage of convenience in their use. Because the exposure to estrogen is eliminated, it is thought that the overall safety of these preparations is improved. However, data to confirm this are lacking, and similar contraindications apply.

Progestin-only preparations include pills (the mini-pill), long-acting injections (Depo-Provera, Upjohn, Kalamazoo, MI), and subdermal implants (Norplant, Wyeth-Ayerst, Philadelphia, PA). In all cases, patients are exposed to continuous rather than cyclic progestin. Ovulation is inhibited in most women by suppression of the midcycle gonadotropin surges. Other mechanisms of action include changes in cervical mucus, induction of an atrophic endometrium, and alteration in tubal motility.[46]

Progestin-only pills currently available in the United States consist of either 0.075 mg norgestrel or 0.35 mg norethindrone. Failure rates are about 1.2 per year.[14] A significant problem with the mini-pill relates to its continuation rate. Only about half the women who start remain on the pill after 1 year.[47]

Norplant is a new system of subdermal administration of levonorgestrel. It consists of six Silastic drug-filled capsules that are inserted into the superficial tissues of the upper arm. The system is designed to remain in place for 5 years, delivering a daily dose of progestin by diffusion through the wall of the capsule. Once the capsules are inserted, efficacy does not depend on a patient's compliance.[48]

Depo-Provera is a long-acting injectable preparation of medroxyprogesterone acetate. It has been approved for use as a contraceptive in the United States. A dose of 150 mg is injected every 3 months. The pregnancy rate is about 0.4.[49]

The most frequent side effect of progestin-only preparations is irregular uterine bleeding. To avoid discontinuation, it is important to counsel patients carefully about this. Many different bleeding patterns occur, from amenorrhea to prolonged spotting throughout the month. Over time, patients tend to develop more regular bleeding.[50] Other side effects include breast tenderness, bloating, and mood changes.

POSTCOITAL CONTRACEPTIVES

Synthetic estrogens and progestins have also been used as postcoital contraceptives. It is difficult to determine efficacy, because patients using this method have varying risks of pregnancy based on the regularity of the menstrual cycle and the timing of exposure. However, when these drugs are taken within 72 hours of unprotected intercourse, the pregnancy rate appears to be decreased from that expected on the basis of statistical considerations.[51] Postcoital contraceptives may be administered as ethinyl estradiol, 50 μg, plus norgestrel, 0.5 mg, two tablets immediately and two tablets in 12 hours. The main side effects are nausea and vomiting, experienced by about half of patients. If the method fails, a patient should be offered termination, although the teratogenic risks are probably small. Contraindications include severe hypertension.

INVESTIGATIONAL METHODS

The currently available hormonal contraceptives have enjoyed considerable success and acceptance. However, investigations continue to improve methods. One of the more controversial is mifepristone, or RU 486, a synthetic steroid that competitively inhibits the progesterone receptor. In early pregnancy, it causes sloughing of the endometrium and disruption of implantation. The precise mechanism of action is unknown, although it may work via prostaglandin mediators. Its use should substantially reduce the morbidity of surgical abortion. However, it has met with considerable political resistance in the United States and remains unapproved at this time.

The efficacy of mifepristone depends on the dose and the gestational age at which it is administered. A single 600-mg oral dose results in complete termination of pregnancy at a rate of 86% when administered before 42 days from the last menstrual period.[52] When a prostaglandin is administered 36 to 48 hours after mifepristone, the efficacy is improved to about 95%.[53] Complications and side effects include failure to complete pregnancy termination, bleeding, and uterine cramping.

Other newer methods of administration of hormone contraceptives are also being studied. Skin patches and transvaginal preparations may obviate the need for daily pill ingestion or surgical implantation. Vaccines that block the action of steroid hormones may provide another novel approach.[54]

REFERENCES

1. American College of Obstetricians and Gynecologists. Oral Contraceptives. ACOG Technical Bulletin 106. Washington, DC: American College of Obstetricians and Gynecologists, 1987.
2. Harlap S, Kost K, Forrest JD. Preventing Pregnancy, Protecting Health: A New Look at Birth Control Choices in the United States. New York: Alan Guttmacher Institute, 1991, p 19.
3. Gallup Organization. Attitudes Toward Contraception. Princeton, NJ: Gallup Organization, 1985, pp 1–11.
4. Chihal HJW, Peppler RD, Dickey RP. Estrogen potency of oral contraceptive pills. Am J Obstet Gynecol 1975;121:75.
5. Goldzieher JW, Pena A, Chenault CB, Woutersz TB. Comparative studies of the ethynyl estrogens used in oral contraceptives. II. Antiovulatory potency. Am J Obstet Gynecol 1975;122:619.
6. Stubblefield PG. Choosing the best oral contraceptive. Clin Obstet Gynecol 1989;32:316.
7. Dickey RP. Managing Contraceptive Pill Patients. 5th ed. Durant, OK: Creative Informatics, 1987, p 53.
8. Lipson A, Stoy DB, La Rosa JC, et al. Progestins and oral contraceptive-induced lipoprotein changes: A prospective study. Contraception 1986;34:121.
9. Consensus Committee. Consensus Development Meeting: Metabolic aspects of oral contraceptives of relevance for cardiovascular diseases. Am J Obstet Gynecol 1990;162:1335.
10. Rebar RW, Zeserson K. Characteristics of the new progestogens in combination oral contraceptives. Contraception 1991;44:1.
11. Chez RA. Clinical aspects of three new progestogens: Desogestrel, gestodene and norgestimate. Am J Obstet Gynecol 1989;160:1296.
12. Baxter FR. Measurements of androgenicity: The spectrum of progestogen activity. J Reprod Med 1986;31(Suppl):848.
13. Mishell DR, Kletzky OA, Brenner PF, et al. The effect of contraceptive steroids on hypothalamic-pituitary function. Am J Obstet Gynecol 1977;128:60.
14. Vessey M, Lawless M, Yeates D. Efficacy of different contraceptive methods. Lancet 1982;1:841.
15. Drife J. The benefits of combined oral contraceptives. Br J Obstet Gynaecol 1989;96:1255.
16. Mishell DR. Noncontraceptive health benefits of oral steroidal contraceptives. Am J Obstet Gynecol 1982;142:809.
17. Ory HW. Functional ovarian cysts and oral contraceptives. JAMA 1974;228:68.
18. Ory HW, Cole P, MacMahon B, Hoover R. Oral contraceptives and reduced risk of benign breast diseases. N Engl J Med 1976;294:419.
19. Rubin GL, Ory HW, Layde PM. Oral contraceptives and pelvic inflammatory disease. Am J Obstet Gynecol 1982;144:630.
20. Washington AE, Gove S, Schachter J, Sweet RL. Oral contraceptives, *Chlamydia trachomatis* infection, and pelvic inflammatory disease. JAMA 1985;253:2246.
21. Cancer and Steroid Hormone Study of the Centers for Disease Control and the National Institute of Child Health and Human Development. The reduction in risk of ovarian cancer associated with oral contraceptive use. N Engl J Med 1987;316:650.
22. Cancer and Steroid Hormone Study of the Centers for Disease Control and the National Institute of Child Health and Human Development. Combination oral contraceptive use and the risk of endometrial cancer. JAMA 1987;257:796.
23. Dickey RP. Managing Contraceptive Pill Patients. 5th ed. Durant, OK: Creative Informatics, 1987, pp 222–223.
24. Vessey MP, Villard-Mackintosh L, McPherson K, Yeates D. Mortality among oral contraceptive users: 20 year follow up of women in a cohort study. Br Med J 1989;299:1487.
25. Stampfer MJ, Willett WC, Colditz GA, et al. Past use of oral contraceptives and cardiovascular disease: A meta-analysis in the context of the Nurses' Health Study. Am J Obstet Gynecol 1990;163:285.
26. Breckwoldt M, Wieacker P, Geisthovel F. Oral contraception in disease states. Am J Obstet Gynecol 1990;163:2213.
27. Harlap S, Kost K, Forrest JD. Preventing pregnancy, protecting health: A new look at birth control choices in the United States. New York: Alan Guttmacher Institute, 1991, p 76.
28. Meade TW. Risks and mechanisms of cardiovascular events in users of oral contraceptives. Am J Obstet Gynecol 1988;158:1646.
29. Castelli WP. Cardiovascular disease in women. Am J Obstet Gynecol 1988;158:1553.
30. Knopp RH. Cardiovascular effects of endogenous and exogenous sex hormones over a woman's lifetime. Am J Obstet Gynecol 1988;158:1630.
31. Hoppe G. The clinical relevance of oral contraceptive pill-induced plasma lipid changes: Facts and fiction. Am J Obstet Gynecol 1990;163:388.
32. Rosenberg L, Palmer JR, Lesko SM, Shapiro S. Oral contraceptive use and the risk of myocardial infarction. Am J Epidemiol 1990;131:1009.
33. Laragh JH. Oral contraceptive-induced hypertension. Nine years later. Am J Obstet Gynecol 1976;126:141.
34. Pritchard JA, Pritchard SA. Blood pressure response to estrogen-progestin oral contraceptive after pregnancy-induced hypertension. Am J Obstet Gynecol 1977;129:733.
35. Vessey MP, Lawless M, McPherson K, Yeates D. Neoplasia of the cervix uteri and contraception: A possible adverse effect of the pill. Lancet 1983;2:930.
36. Swan SH, Brown WL. Oral contraceptive use, sexual activity and cervical carcinoma. Am J Obstet Gynecol 1981;139:52.
37. Romieu I, Berlin JA, Colditz G. Oral contraceptives and breast cancer: Review and meta-analysis. Cancer 1990;66:2253.
38. Miller DR, Rosenberg L, Kaufman DW, et al. Breast cancer before age 45 and oral contraceptive use: New findings. Am J Epidemiol 1989;129:269.
39. UK National Case-Control Study Group. Oral contraceptive use and breast cancer risk in young women. Lancet 1989;1:973.
40. Barber HRK. Are oral contraceptives safe? (editorial). The Female Patient 1989;14:10.
41. Royal College of General Practitioners' Oral Contraception Study. Oral contraceptives and gallbladder disease. Lancet 1982;2:957.
42. Kinch R, Lough J. Focal nodular hyperplasia of the liver and oral contraceptives. Am J Obstet Gynecol 1978;132:717.
43. Rooks JB, Ory HW, Ishak KG, et al. Epidemiology of hepatocellular adenoma: The role of oral contraceptive use. JAMA 1979;242:644.
44. Fraser IS, Jansen RPS. Why do inadvertent pregnancies occur in oral contraceptive users? Contraception 1983;27:531.
45. American College of Obstetricians and Gynecologists. Contraceptives and congenital anomalies. ACOG Committee Opinion No. 62, September 1988.
46. Kaunitz AM. Injectable contraception. Clin Obstet Gynecol 1989;32:356.

47. Hatcher RA, Guest F, Stewart F, et al. Contraceptive Technology 1988–1989. 14th ed. New York: Irvington, 1988, p 253.
48. Shoupe D, Mishell DR. Norplant: Subdermal implant system for long-term contraception. Am J Obstet Gynecol 1989;160:1286.
49. Said S, Omar K, Koetsawang S, et al. A multicentered phase III comparative clinical trial of depot-medroxyprogesterone acetate given three-monthly at doses of 100 mg or 150 mg: 1. Contraceptive efficacy and side effects. Contraception 1986;34:223.
50. Shoupe D, Mishell DR, Bopp BL, Fielding M. The significance of bleeding patterns in Norplant implant users. Obstet Gynecol 1991;77:256.
51. Dixon GW, Schlesselman JJ, Ory HW, Blye RP. Ethinyl estradiol and conjugated estrogens as postcoital contraceptives. JAMA 1980;244:1336.
52. Grimes DA, Mishell DR, Shoupe D, Lacarra M. Early abortion with a single dose of the antiprogestin RU-486. Am J Obstet Gynecol 1988;158:1307.
53. Silvestre L, Dubois C, Renault M, et al. Voluntary interruption of pregnancy with mifepristone (RU 486) and a prostaglandin analogue. N Engl J Med 1990;322:645.
54. Mishell DR. New and better methods of contraception. Contemp Obstet Gynecol 1992;37:15.

Nonhormonal Contraception

Paulette Thabault and Phyllis L. Carr

Barrier methods of contraception are one of few effective alternatives to hormonal contraception. These methods include the diaphragm, cervical cap, condom, and vaginal spermicides. Studies suggest that in addition to their contraceptive benefit, these methods decrease the rate of transmission of sexually transmitted diseases (STDs). The spermicidal agent nonoxynol 9, which is recommended for use with these methods, is also effective in decreasing the risk of human immunodeficiency virus (HIV) transmission. Additionally, use of the diaphragm and the condom are associated with a decreased risk for developing cervical dysplasia. The intrauterine device (IUD) is another alternative that is suitable for some women.

DIAPHRAGM

A diaphragm is a shallow rubber dome-shaped device with a flexible rim. Sizes range from 55 to 100 mm. A diaphragm is used with a spermicidal jelly or cream and is placed in the vagina up to 2 hours before intercourse. The diaphragm creates a barrier to the sperm and holds the spermicidal agent in place close to the cervix. It must remain inserted for 6 to 8 hours after intercourse. Additional spermicide is recommended for repeated intercourse.

Contraceptive failure rates associated with diaphragm use are highest among younger women and range from 2 to 18%. The effectiveness of the diaphragm as well as other contraceptive methods correlates with both age and socioeconomic status. Failure rates are lowest for women who are older than 30 years and who have a higher socioeconomic status, more years of education, and greater motivation. A cohort study of married women using a diaphragm for more than 5 months before enrollment revealed pregnancy rates of 4.1 per 100 woman-years for women 25 to 29 years of age and

1.1 for women 35 to 39 years of age. Both increasing duration of use and increasing age were associated with declining failure rates.

Fitting the diaphragm is easily accomplished in the office. The goal for proper fitting is to select the largest rim size that is comfortable for a patient. The posterior rim should reach to the posterior fornix, and the anterior rim should fit behind the pubic arch notch. A patient should be fitted with the same type of diaphragm prescibed, because there is some variation among different manufacturers. Use of a spermicide is recommended to prevent pregnancy and is helpful in decreasing sexual disease transmission including human papilomavirus and HIV.

A common problem associated with diaphragm use is an increase in the incidence of urinary tract infections, which is thought to be the result of a combination of factors including urethral obstruction, urinary stasis, increased vaginal colonization of *Escherichia coli,* and alteration of the vaginal flora by the spermicide. Encouraging frequent urination (especially postcoitally), limiting use to no longer than 8 hours, or refitting the diaphragm for a smaller rim size may help alleviate this problem. Other problems that may arise with the diaphragm include sensitivity to the latex or spermicide, pelvic discomfort or abdominal cramping, and vaginal discharge associated with prolonged use.

Toxic shock syndrome is a more serious complication that has been reported in association with prolonged diaphragm retention and with diaphragm use during menses. To minimize this risk, women should be advised against prolonged use and use during menses.

CERVICAL CAP

The Prentiff cavity-rim cervical cap, a thimble-shaped latex device smaller than the diaphragm, was approved by the U.S. Food and Drug Administration for contraceptive use in May of 1988. The cervical cap is available in the United States and Canada from Cervical Cap (CxC), Ltd, P.O. Box 38003-292, Los Gatos, CA 95031. The cap is available in four sizes ranging from a 22- to 31-mm diameter and a 1¼- to 1½-inch length and must be fitted by a trained clinician. It is used with a small amount of spermicide placed in the cap, creating a mechanical and chemical barrier to sperm.

A cervical cap is more difficult to fit and use than a diaphragm. Patients must be able to locate their cervix and accurately place and remove the cap. To be effective, the cap must fit snugly over the cervix and must not be dislodged by intercourse. For this reason, patients should be instructed to use a backup method during initial use and to check for proper placement after each act of intercourse. Effectiveness rates for the cervical cap are similar to those of the diaphragm and range from 85 to 95%.

Advantages of the cervical cap are that it may be left in place for as long as 48 hours and additional spermicide is not necessary for repeated intercourse. Cervical cap users report that it is less messy and more comfortable than a diaphragm. Because the rim is smaller and the cap sits farther back, urethral irritation is less and urinary tract infections are reported to be fewer. In addition, the cervical cap may be inserted as early as 40 hours before intercourse. Like the diaphragm, it should remain in place for at least 8 hours after intercourse.

The most common problems associated with the cervical cap are vaginal odor and discharge, particularly with prolonged use. Vaginal and cervical lacerations and abrasions have also been reported. Pain during intercourse may be more common in women who use the cervical cap, and a higher percentage may be infected with *Candida* or bacterial vaginosis. Some users have reported that their partners also experience discomfort. Finally, because of variations in cervical size and shape and the limited cap sizes available, only 80% of women can be fitted accurately.

In contrast to the diaphragm, which has been found to lower the rates of cervical neoplasia, the cervical cap has been suspected of possibly causing cervial cellular changes. In an unpublished multicenter trial, about 4% of cap users compared with 1.7% of diaphragm users developed abnormal findings on Papanicolaou (PAP) smears after 3 months of use. For this reason, a patient considering a cervical cap should have normal PAP smear results before beginning use and a follow-up PAP smear in 3 months. If results of the follow-up PAP

TABLE 25–1.   Contraindications to Cervical Cap Use

> Abnormal results of Papanicolaou smear
> Current vaginal or cervical infection
> Use during menses
> Postpartum period 6–12 weeks
> Postabortion period 2–4 weeks
> History of toxic shock syndrome
> Endometriosis

test are abnormal, cervical cap use should be discontinued. The patient should be evaluated with colposcopy, and treatment should be initiated if indicated. Other contraindications to cervical cap use are listed in Table 25–1.

For both the cervical cap and the diaphragm, education of patients is essential for effective use. This should include instruction for proper insertion and removal, directions for use and care, and recommended follow-up. Examples of written patient education guidelines for supplementing diaphragm and cervical cap fittings are listed in Tables 25–2 and 25–3.

VAGINAL CONTRACEPTIVE SPONGE

The vaginal contraceptive sponge is a small, dome-shaped polyurethane device that is saturated

TABLE 25–2.   Instructions for Diaphragm Use

Use the diaphragm each time you have intercourse.
Check the diaphragm for tears or holes each time you use it, before inserting it to have intercourse.
Insert the diaphragm within 2 hours before having intercourse. It must remain in place for a minimum of 6 to 8 hours after intercourse. The maximum amount of time it should remain in place is 24 hours.
You must use spermicidal jelly or cream with the diaphragm. You should put about 1 teaspoon inside the cup and smear a small amount on the rim and around the outside of the diaphragm.
Insert the diaphragm by folding the edges together. Insert it like a tampon, upward and toward the backbone. Check to be sure the diaphragm has completely covered the cervix.
If you want to have intercourse again within 6 hours of last having intercourse, you must apply an applicator full of the spermicidal cream or jelly into your vagina. Do not disturb or remove the diaphragm. You can obtain an applicator at the drug store.
Do not douche or use a tampon while the diaphragm is in place.
The size of the diaphragm should be checked every 2 years, or if you gain or lose 10 to 15 lb, or after pregnancy.
You can wash the diaphragm after use with a mild soap and water. You can also dust it with cornstarch to ensure dryness until the next use. Avoid talc because it damages the rubber and has been associated with ovarian cancer.

TABLE 25–3. Cervical Cap Instructions

1. You should use the cervical cap each time you have intercourse, except that it should *not* be used during menses.
2. You may insert the cap up to 40 hours before intercourse.
3. Before insertion, locate the cervix. Fill the cap one-third full of spermicide. Do not overfill the cap, because this may prevent the necessary suction from forming.
4. Squeeze the rim of the cap and direct it into the vagina as far as it will go. Use your forefinger to press the rim around the cervix until the dome covers the cervix.
5. Check for proper placement—sweep your finger around the rim of the cap. You should not be able to locate your cervix outside the cap. You may be able to feel your cervix behind the cap. The cervix feels firm, much like the tip of your nose. This indicates proper placement.
6. To improve cap suction, feel for the small notch on the rim of the cap and use it to rotate the cap approximately one-fourth turn.
7. During the first 1 to 2 months of use, a backup method is recommended. The pill or condoms are acceptable. Do not use the diaphragm as your backup, because it may dislodge the cap. After each act of intercourse, check the cap for proper placement over the cervix.
8. You must wear the cap for at least 8 to 12 hours from the last time you have intercourse. The maximum amount of time the cap may be left in place is 48 hours.
9. You do *not* need extra spermicide if you have intercourse more than once while the cap is in place.
10. To remove the cap, use your finger to push the rim of the cap to one side. Once dislodged, reach into the bowl of the cap and remove it.
11. To care for your cap, wash it with mild soap and water after each use, dry it well, and store it in its container. Cornstarch may be used to ensure dryness.
12. Examine the cap frequently for tears or holes.
13. If your cap develops an offensive odor, contact your provider, because this may indicate a vaginal infection.
14. A vaginal delivery, abortion, or other cervical procedure may alter the size of the cervix, and you will need to have your cap resized.
15. You need to have a Papanicolaou smear and a cervical cap check after the first 3 months of cervical cap use.

with 1 gm of nonoxynol 9 spermicide. The sponge is available in one size and without a prescription. It is moistened with water and inserted into the vagina before intercourse and may remain for as long as 24 hours. It is disposed of after removal. The sponge absorbs sperm and creates both a chemical and mechanical barrier. Effectiveness of the sponge is in the range of 75 to 85%. It is probably more effective in nulliparous women and less effective in parous users, although some controversy surrounds these data. Vulvar irritation, allergic reactions, increased vaginal yeast infections, and bacterial overgrowth have been associated with sponge use. Toxic shock syndrome has also occurred in women using the contraceptive sponge, and women should be advised against using the sponge during menses and told not to leave the sponge in place for more than 24 hours. The overall incidence of toxic shock is low, with one infection per 2 million sponges used.

CONDOMS

Condoms are a readily accessible and effective means of contraception. When they are used consistently and correctly (Table 25–4), effectiveness rates approach 95%. This rate is even higher when a condom is used in conjunction with a spermicide. First-year failure rates for condom use range between 1 and 4% for women older than 30 years, but for women younger than 25, this rate is between 10 and 33%. Because failure rates are highest in younger users, condom use in combination with oral contraceptives has been advised. The noncontraceptive benefit of decreasing sexual disease transmission should be emphasized, particularly for women at risk. In vitro studies have shown prevention of viral transmission, including herpesvirus and HIV, as well as *Chlamydia trachomatis*. Epidemiologic studies also demonstrate lower rates of gonorrheal infection and a lower incidence of cervical neoplasia, perhaps because of decreased transmission of human papillomavirus. Condom use has also been associated with regression of cervical dysplasia.

Condoms are marketed without a prescription and by a number of manufacturers. They are available in various textures and in lubricated or nonlubricated forms. Condoms are also available with a spermicidal lubrication, which should be advised for women at risk for contracting STDs. The greatest protection occurs with joint use of a condom and a spermicide. Condoms are generally made

TABLE 25–4. Male Condom Instructions

1. Use a new condom with each act of intercourse.
2. Handle the condom carefully to avoid damaging it with your fingernails or other sharp objects.
3. Put on the condom after the penis is erect and before any genital contact with your partner.
4. Ensure that no air is trapped in the tip of the condom.
5. Ensure adequate lubrication during intercourse. If necessary, use exogenous lubricants.
6. Use only water-based lubricants (K-Y jelly or glycerine) with latex condoms. Oil-based lubricants (petroleum jelly, shortening, mineral oil, body lotions) can weaken latex and should never be used.
7. Hold the condom firmly against the base of the penis during withdrawal and withdraw while the penis is still erect to prevent slippage.
8. Condoms should be stored in a cool, dry place. Avoid direct sunlight. Do not use a condom after its expiration date.

from latex, which may present a problem if either partner has a latex allergy. In this case, a natural membrane condom may be recommended. However, it should be noted that these condoms, which are actually made from the caecum of lamb intestine, are less protective against infection. Viruses, including HIV, can pass through natural membrane condoms.

VAGINAL SPERMICIDES

Vaginal spermicides containing nonoxynol 9 are available in many forms and without a prescription. These include foam, creams, suppositories, jellies, and film. The primary mechanism of these agents is inhibition of sperm motility. Used alone, vaginal spermicides are generally not very effective in preventing pregnancy, with failure rates of greater than 20%. Their greatest benefit is reduction in the rate of sexual disease transmission. The antiviral action of nonoxynol 9 may be the reason why women who use spermicides have one third the rate of cervical cancer as that in a control group.

Nonoxynol 9 has been shown to be active against *Neisseria gonorrhoeae,* herpes simplex virus types 1 and 2, *Trichomonas vaginalis, C. trachomatis,* and *Gardnerella vaginalis.* Its action may be dualistic, affecting the microorganism directly or the target cell it infects by blocking cellular attachment or penetration. Human immunodeficiency virus has been shown to be exquisitely sensitive to nonoxynol 9 in vitro. Reduced rates of reinfection for gonorrhea and other STDs in high-risk groups have been documented in spermicide-treated groups. Reinfection rates ranged from from 3 to 19% in spermicide-treated patients versus 25 to 40% in controls. Spermicides in conjunction with a condom or diaphragm are more effective as a contraceptive method and have the highest rates of prevention against STDs. Although earlier studies linked the use of a spermicide at the time of conception with an increased risk of congenital malformations, subsequent well-performed studies do not show such an increase.

FEMALE CONDOM

The latest barrier contraceptive method that has been developed is the female condom. This method provides a woman with a nonprescription means to prevent unwanted pregnancy and to greatly reduce the risk of contracting an STD. The condom contains two rings. A flexible ring at the pouched end is inserted into the vagina much like a diaphragm. The outer flexible ring remains outside of the vagina and offers some protection to the vulva.

This type of barrier method has several advantages. It may be inserted at the convenience of the woman several hours before intercourse and may be easily removed some time after intercourse. It offers some protection of the vulva, where infection can occur via entry by the urethra or through small tears on the vulva. Male erection is not a factor for proper use, as with a traditional condom. Because it is available in polyurethane and latex, persons with latex sensitivity remain able to use this device.

INTRAUTERINE DEVICE

The intrauterine device has been the subject of some controversy in the United States during the past 2 decades. The association of the Dalkon shield with pelvic inflammatory disease and the resultant lawsuits compelled many other companies to remove their products from the market, even though their IUDs did not pose the same high risk of infection. Despite the negative publicity, the IUD remains a safe and effective method of contraception for many women. Two types of IUDs are currently available in the United States: the ParaGard (a copper-containing device) and the Progestasert T (a progesterone-releasing device).

Although several theories have been proposed, the exact mechanism of action of the IUD is not known. One theory is that the IUD causes an inflammatory response due to the presence of a foreign body in the uterus, thus stimulating an accumulation of white blood cells and thereby phagocytosis of sperm. Another theory suggests that the IUD alters the suitability of the endometrium for implantation of the blastocyst. Alteration of the cervical mucus, immobilization of the sperm passing through the uterus, and alteration of ova development have also been described as possible mechanisms for the action of the IUD.

The IUD is a highly effective device, with a first-year failure rate ranging from 1.8 to 2.5 pregnancies per 100 woman-years for the Progestasert T and 0.5 to 1.0 per 100 woman-years during 4 years of use for the ParaGard. The Progestasert T currently has a Food and Drug Administration–approved life span of 1 year, and the ParaGard is approved for 8 years, although a British study suggests that this should be extended to 10 years. Contraindications to use of the IUD include pregnancy, prior pelvic inflammatory disease (PID) or ectopic pregnancy, uterine or cervical malignancy including abnormal findings on a PAP smear, and undiagnosed genital bleeding (Table 25–5).

The relationship between the IUD and the development of PID poses the most serious risk associated with IUD use. The health consequences of PID with resultant infertility caused by salpingitis and tubal occlusions must be considered before recommending the IUD. The most recent studies concerning this problem have identified other risk factors for the development of PID associated with IUD use. The most important factor is the risk for contracting an STD. Young nulliparous women also have a higher risk, which may reflect multiple sexual partners. Women without risks for developing STDs (those in stable, monogamous relationships) appear to have little risk for developing PID with IUD use. For these reasons, before recommending the IUD, a primary care provider should assess a patient's risks for contracting an STD.

Nulliparous women should be advised against using this method unless they have no prior history of pelvic infections and have a single stable sexual partner. The first 20 days after insertion is the most likely time for infection and perforation associated with insertion to occur. Prophylactic antibiotic use has been shown to reduce the risk of infection. A single dose of 200 mg of doxycycline has been shown to reduce the rate of infection from 1.9 to 1.3% and to decrease the number of unplanned clinic visits from 13 to 8.9%. Follow-up must be readily available during this postinsertion period.

Long-term IUD use has been associated with *Actinomyces israelii* infection. This is usually diagnosed on a PAP smear. Evidence for any pelvic infection should be sought, and the IUD removed if it is found. If active infection is not found, the patient may be treated with penicillin G, 500 mg four times a day for 10 days. If *Actinomyces* persists on PAP smear after treatment, the IUD should be removed.

A less serious but more common side effect of IUD use is irregular bleeding. Increased cramping and increased menstrual blood loss are also frequently reported. An associated clinical anemia has been documented in as many as 10% of users of copper IUDs, and iron deficiency determined by low ferritin levels in 20% of users after 12 months of observation. Some evidence, however, suggests that progesterone IUDs may decrease menstrual flow. Nonetheless, increased bleeding is often cited as a reason for IUD removal.

The most important factors related to the effectiveness of the IUD are the ease of insertion, the clinician's experience, the likelihood of expulsion, and the patient's ability to detect expulsion when this occurs. The rate of expulsion is higher in nulliparous women and is frequently a reason for discontinuing IUD use. Insertion during menstruation is associated with less discomfort because of cervical dilation during menses. Insertion during pregnancy is also thus avoided.

Indications for removal of an IUD include the presence of a tubo-ovarian abscess or PID, menorrhagia, excessive pain attributable to the IUD, menopause, pregnancy, or the Food and Drug Administration–approved life span of the IUD (1 year for the Progestasert T, 8 years for the ParaGard). Generally, the IUD can be easily removed in the office. If any difficulty is encountered, an ultrasonogram should be obtained to determine if the IUD is embedded in the uterus. If so, surgical removal may be required.

PERIODIC ABSTINENCE

Periodic abstinence, sometimes referred to as the rhythm method or natural family planning, is used as a contraceptive method by some women. Effective use of periodic abstinence requires that a woman abstain from intercourse for as much as half of the menstrual cycle for women with regular cycles. The method uses one or more techniques to predict ovulation or the fertile days of a woman's cycle. Intercourse is avoided during that phase of the cycle, or an alternative method, such as a barrier contraceptive method, is used. Failure rates for periodic abstinence are relatively high, with resultant low continuation rates. In one five-country study sponsored by the World Health Organization, the failure rate in the first year was 19.6%.

The three common methods used for predicting ovulation are the rhythm or calendar method, the cervical mucus method, and the symptothermal

TABLE 24–5. Contraindications to Insertion of an Intrauterine Device

Pregnancy
Uterine anomalies including cavity distortion
History of pelvic inflammatory disease
Postpartum endometritis or infected abortion within 3 months
Uterine or cervical malignancy including abnormal findings on Papanicolaou smear
Untreated acute cervicitis or vaginitis
Wilson's disease
Copper allergy
Multiple sexual partners
Increased susceptibility to infection (diabetes or immunodeficiency)
Genital actinomycosis
Prior ectopic pregnancy

TABLE 25–6. How to Calculate the Interval of Fertility

IF YOUR SHORTEST CYCLE HAS BEEN (NO. OF DAYS)	YOUR FIRST FERTILE (UNSAFE) DAY IS	IF YOUR LONGEST CYCLE HAS BEEN (NO. OF DAYS)	YOUR LAST FERTILE (UNSAFE) DAY IS
21*	3rd day	21	10th day
22	4th	22	11th
23	5th	23	12th
24	6th	24	13th
25	7th	25	14th
26	8th	26	15th
27	9th	27	16th
28	10th	28	17th
29	11th	29	18th
30	12th	30	19th
31	13th	31	20th
32	14th	32	21st
33	15th	33	22nd
34	16th	34	23rd
35	17th	35	24th

*Day 1, First day of menstrual bleeding.
From Hatcher RA, Guest F, Stewart F, et al. Contraceptive Technology, 1988–1989. 14th rev ed. New York; Irvington Publishers, 1988, p 356.

method. For the calendar method, a woman must first record the span of her menstrual cycles for a 6- to 8-month period. The earliest day a woman is fertile is calculated by subtracting 18 days from the length of the shortest cycle. The latest day on which fertility is likely is calculated by subtracting 11 days from the longest cycle (Table 25–6).

The cervical mucus method requires a woman to examine her cervical mucus daily and to become familiar with the characteristic changes associated with different phases of the cycle. The cervical mucus associated with ovulation is typically thin, abundant, and slippery. A drop of this mucus can be stretched between two fingers to a length of about 6 cm or more. A woman should be instructed to chart and record the mucus changes for several cycles before attempting to rely on it as a birth control method (Table 25–7).

A third method is the symptothermal method, which combines basal body temperature charting with the cervical mucus method discused earlier. The basal body temperature—the lowest body temperature of a healthy person while awake—is recorded daily. This temperature rises under the influence of progesterone produced by the corpus luteum. Therefore, the characteristic rise denotes

TABLE 25–7. Cyclic Characteristics of the Cervix and Cervical Mucus

TIME OF CYCLE	AMOUNT	VISCOSITY	APPEARANCE	SPINNBARKEIT	FERNING	CERVIX
Postmenstruation	Moderate	Thick	Cloudy	None	None	Firm, closed
Nearing ovulation	Increasing	Somewhat thick to thin	Mixed/cloudy and clear	Moderate	Moderate	Firm, closed
Ovulation	Maximum	Very thin and slippery	Clear	Maximum 2–3 or more inches	Well developed	Soft, open
Postovualation (about 3 days)	Decreasing	Thin	Mixed/cloudy and clear	Minimal or none	Minimal or none	Firm, closed
Nearing menstruation	Minimal	Thick	Cloudy	None	None	Firm, closed

Use this summary of characteristics of mucus to train patients and staff. Amount (volume) refers to the woman's subjective interpretation of what she feels with her finger at the introitus and/or inside her vagina. Viscosity means the consistency of mucus. Appearance can vary quite a bit, and clear mucus may be tinged with blood at the time of ovulation. Spinnbarkeit means elasticity: How much can you stretch a mucus sample before it breaks? Ferning means that a sample of mucus taken on a fertile day, smeared on a glass slide, and air dried will reveal a microscopic pattern resembling fern leaves.
From Hatcher RA, Guest F, Stewart F, et al. Contraceptive Technology 1988–1989. 14th rev ed. New York; Irvington Publishers, 1988, p 361. Adapted from Health Education Bulletin, July 1979, by the National Clearinghouse for family planning information. DHEW, Bureau of Community Health Services.

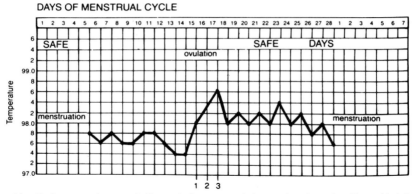

Figure 25-1. Basal body temperature variations during a model menstrual cycle. (From Hatcher RA, Guest F, Stewart F, et al. Contraceptive Technology, 1988–1989. 14th rev. ed. New York: Irvington Publishers, 1988, p 357.)

that ovulation has occurred. Many women, however, do not exhibit temperature fluctuations. One study found that six of 30 women had no identifiable basal body temperature pattern despite other confirmatory tests of ovulation (Fig. 25–1).

Women desiring to use periodic abstinence as a contraceptive method should be instructed by an experienced clinician. Education should include method use and drawbacks. The high failure rate and the length of required abstinence should be emphasized.

SUMMARY

In summary, the diaphragm and cervical cap are barrier methods of contraception that are reasonably effective and easy to use. In addition to their contraceptive benefit, they offer some protection against STDs. It is intended that they be used in conjunction with a spermicide. Proper fitting of the device and education of patients by a trained clinician are essential. Condoms and spermicidal agents are also very effective contraceptive agents and should be recommended to women at risk for developing STDs. The IUD remains an effective contraceptive method that can be safely recommended to parous women without risk factors for contracting STDs. Periodic abstinence is less effective but may be an option for some women motivated to practice this method of contraception.

BIBLIOGRAPHY

Burkman RT. Intrauterine devices. Curr Opin Obstet Gynecol 1991;3:482.

Burkman RT, Lee NC, Org HW, Rubin GL. Response to the intrauterine device and pelvic inflammatory disease: The Women's Health Study reanalyzed. J Clin Epidemiol 1991;44(2):123.

Cagen R. The cervical cap as a barrier contraceptive. Contraception 1986;33(5):487.

Farley TM, Rosenberg MJ, Rowe PJ, Chen JH, Meirik O. Intrauterine devices and pelvic inflammatory disease: An international perspective. Lancet 1992;339:785.

Gregersen E, Gregersen B. The female condom—a pilot study of the acceptability of a new female barrier method. Acta Obstet Gynecol Scand 1990;69:73.

Haslett S. Barrier methods of contraception. Nurs Stand 1990;4(50):24.

Hatcher RA, Guest F, Stewart F, et al. Contraceptive Technology, 1988–1989. 14th rev. ed. New York: Irvington Publishers, 1988.

Kronmal RA, Whitney CW, Mumford SD. The intrauterine device and pelvic inflammatory disease: The Women's Health Study reanalyzed. J Clin Epidemiol 1991;44(2):109.

Kulig JW. Adolescent contraception: Nonhormonal methods. Pediatr Clin North Am 1989;36(3):717.

Ladipo OA, Farr G, Otolorm E, et al. Prevention of IUD-related pelvic infection: The efficacy of prophylactic doxycycline at IUD insertion. Adv Contracept 1991;7:43–54.

Mishell DR. Contraception. N Engl J Med 1989;320:777.

North BB. Vaginal contraceptives—effective protection from sexually transmitted diseases for women? J Reprod Med 1988;33(3):307.

Petersen KR, Brooks L, Jacobsen B, Skouby SO. ESC meeting—intrauterine devices in nulliparous women. Adv Contracept 1991;7:333.

Secor RMC. The cervical cap. NAACOGS—Clinical Issues in Perinatal and Women's Health Nursing. 1992;3(2):236.

Weiss BD. The cervical cap. Am Fam Physician 1991;43(2):517.

The cervical cap. Med Lett Drugs Ther 1988;30:93–94.

Update: Barrier protection against HIV infection and other sexually transmitted diseases. JAMA 1993;270:933.

Intervention for Unintended Pregnancy

26

Counseling the Patient with an Unintended Pregnancy

Terry Beresford

A woman who has become pregnant unintentionally may decide to continue her pregnancy and have a child, even though this was not her original plan or desire. She needs information about pregnancy, prenatal care, and delivery and may also welcome the opportunity to express her concerns about the unexpected changes occurring in her life as a result of the unanticipated pregnancy. Another woman or the same woman at a different time in her life may decide against continuing the pregnancy and will need information about how to obtain abortion services. For a woman who finds herself unable to decide quickly and comfortably among the alternatives—(1) continuing the pregnancy and keeping the child, (2) continuing the pregnancy and placing the child for adoption, or (3) terminating the pregnancy—brief counseling centered on her feelings and her values and assistance with the decision-making process are appropriate.

OBJECTIVES OF COUNSELING

"The goals of problem pregnancy counseling are (1) to help the woman face the need for decision; (2) to provide her information about each of the options and the decision-making process; (3) to help her examine her feelings and values so that her decision can be consonant with them; (4) to assist her in anticipating the impact the consequences of her decision will have on herself and relevant others; (5) to provide her a referral to

appropriate services so she can implement her decision or obtain additional counseling if needed."[1]

ACCEPTANCE OF PREGNANCY TEST RESULTS

When a patient finds the news of her pregnancy particularly upsetting and hard to accept, she may have trouble focusing on decision-making until she has had the opportunity to express her feelings. She may cry or deny that intercourse has taken place or has occurred in a way that could lead to pregnancy or may insist that the test results are not accurate. Acceptance may be facilitated by acknowledging her feelings, for example, by saying, "You seem to be feeling overwhelmed at the idea of being pregnant just now. Let's talk about that." When a woman expresses no immediate feelings about her pregnancy, you can usually determine whether she needs time to accept the news and to express feelings about it by following your assumptions with a nonleading question such as "How do you feel about being pregnant?" or "Can you tell me about how you're feeling at hearing this news?"

FEELINGS, VALUES, AND PLANS

A respectful beginning to the counseling process can be made by contracting verbally and informally with a patient for discussion of her feelings.

For example, you might say, "Many women have mixed feelings on hearing that they're pregnant. We can discuss how *you* are feeling about being pregnant and your feelings about the alternatives available to you. Would you like to do that?" Common feelings about being unintentionally pregnant include these:

- Worry about being able to manage having a baby and rearing a child
- Fear of having to give up important goals and plans
- Concern about the reactions of her partner, family, and friends
- Happiness on learning that she is fertile
- Excitement at the significance of the event
- Pleasure to see herself as a potential mother
- Worry about the ethical or religious conflicts involved

A woman who says she does not know what to do may be helped to explore her feelings and values by guiding her through an examination of the three alternatives:

- What would be good for you about having a baby at this time? About adoption? About abortion?
- What would be the disadvantages of having a baby? Of adoption? Of abortion?
- How do you think you would feel if you chose to continue the pregnancy? If you placed a child for adoption? If you had an abortion?

Another useful approach is to help a woman focus on her plans and dreams to see how each of the alternatives would affect them. Helpful questions include the following:

- What are two or three things that matter most to you in your life right now?
- What are two or three things you hope to have or to achieve in the next 5 or 10 years?
- To have or to achieve those things, how would having a baby help? How would adoption help? How would abortion help?
- What would you lose or have to give up right now if you had a baby? If you place a baby for adoption? If you have an abortion?
- How would each of those choices affect you during the next 5 to 10 years?
- How does your financial situation affect these choices?
- How would other people who matter to you (such as partner, parents, family, friends) react to your choice of parenting? Adoption? Abortion?

Some additional and more specific questions about each of the alternatives may help a woman who continues to have difficulty making a choice:

- In what ways do you feel ready to take on the tasks of parenting? In what ways unready?
- Who has offered to give you help? If you are managing alone, what is your plan for doing so?
- How much do you want a child? When do you think would be the best time to have one?
- What are your partner's feelings about this pregnancy?
- What have others told you or shown you about rearing a child?
- What additional information do you need about pregnancy, childbirth, parenting, well-baby care, and financial support?
- How would you feel about having someone else rear your baby?
- What satisfactions do you think you would get from giving someone else the baby she cannot create for herself?
- How do you think you would handle the feelings involved in carrying a baby for 9 months, giving birth, and then giving it up for adoption?
- Do you know anyone who has adopted a child or placed a child for adoption? What have they told you about their experiences?
- What have you heard about abortion? What worries you most about having one?
- How does abortion fit with your personal beliefs? Your family's beliefs? The beliefs of your church?

After exploring their feelings, values, and plans, many women are able to decide which of the three options seems best to them at the present time. The choice is often made in terms of which option seems "least bad," because none may feel positive to a woman who wishes she had not become pregnant in the first place. The clinician can affirm for a woman that having leftover mixed feelings about both the choice she has made and the choices she has rejected is normal. A useful concluding question is, "Do you think you can handle those feelings?"

AMBIVALENCE

Nearly everyone experiences ambivalence, or mixed feelings, in connection with an unintended or unwanted pregnancy. The clinician can acknowledge those feelings, affirming their normalcy and helping a woman to understand that most major life decisions are accompanied by ambivalence. This is particularly true for decisions about reproduction because of the complexity of peoples' sexual and relational lives and the powerful values most people have internalized about life and death. For some women, extreme ambivalence with accompanying feelings of fear, guilt, or generalized anxiety may prevent decision-making. In these circumstances, a woman may find that even passing consideration of each of the alternatives arouses so much anxiety that she immediately rejects each one, unable to imagine herself making a choice or managing the mixed feelings that threaten to overwhelm her. The following steps may be helpful:

1. Alleviate anxiety by telling her that she does not have to decide at this moment. It will be important for her to have an accurate estimate of the length of gestation so that she can be realistic about time limits.

2. Allow her to focus at first on all the reasons that none of the alternatives seems possible to her. Continue to reiterate for her the nature of the conflict she feels—for example, "You're feeling torn because none of the options open to you seems acceptable" or "Having an unintended pregnancy puts you in a bind because you don't want to choose any of the alternatives."

3. Ask her what she needs to help her make a decision—for example, to talk with her husband, partner, or parent; to acquire more factual information about her options; to have time alone to gather her thoughts; to talk with a therapist or reproductive health counselor. Provide her with take-home materials that can help her with the decision process.[2]

4. If she expresses feelings of guilt about violating social, religious, or family norms, help her to understand the source of those feelings and to reaffirm for herself her own values and her own caring for those significant others whose values she feels she is violating. Help her to see that although she may not be able to serve all of her own values with her present decision, she need not give up any of those values permanently; ask her how she means to serve those values in the future.

5. Reaffirm for her that after considering the alternatives carefully, learning what she needs to know, and examining her own feelings and values, she will make the best decision she is able to make at the time and that no one else is in a position to make a better decision for her. Reassure her that although it is hard to decide and that giving up alternatives causes pain, this does not mean she is bad or that her choice is wrong.

6. Share with her any knowledge you have acquired about her health or the health of the fetus, which she needs to take into account in making her decision (e.g., human immunodeficiency virus status or results of amniocentesis or chorionic villus sampling), but avoid making the decision for her.[3]

SEXUAL ABUSE

Pregnant adolescent girls frequently report at least one incident of sexual abuse before age 18 years. Studies of young mothers in parenting programs suggest that 50 to 68% of the adolescents surveyed reported molestation or rape before their first pregnancy.[4] The pregnancy may be an unplanned result of an abusive incident or may in fact be intended by the adolescent, an example of decision-making influenced by factors stemming from earlier abusive incidents that have adversely affected her gender and sexual socializazation, her self-image, and her decision-making competence in sexual and reproductive matters. An abusive situation may also motivate a desire to escape through pregnancy. Because of the prevalence of sexual victimization and abuse in this population, a clinician dealing with an adolescent pregnancy may want to explore the patient's sexual history in greater detail. For a young woman to make a considered decision about the outcome of her pregnancy, she will need help in sorting out the emotional factors stemming from current or past abuse from those relating to her present values and plans. Questions about this sensitive area need to be formulated carefully and asked in a nonthreatening manner. Because many states have laws governing the reporting of sexual abuse of minors, the clinician must also caution patients about the limits of confidentiality in the doctor-patient relationship when discussing this topic.

COERCION AND FORCED CHOICE

Pregnancy that results from rape, particularly from rape by a stranger, usually produces intense conflict for a woman. Although she may feel doubly violated and unwilling to bear the rapist's child, the idea of abortion may never have been considered before, particularly if she is young. In some cases, the idea of being pregnant by the rapist is so repugnant to the woman that she wants an abortion immediately on learning that she is pregnant. She needs information about the advisability of waiting until the optimum time for abortion, at about 7 weeks from her last menstrual period, and she should be given supportive counseling to help her through the waiting period. Counseling for a rape victim should include an opportunity for her to discuss in detail the circumstances of the rape, including the sexual details; a realistic appraisal of her own role in the situation and affirmation of the unacceptability of rape regardless of circumstances; information about her alternatives; information about reporting the rape to the authorities if she so chooses; and an offer of referral to a rape crisis center or other women's support group.

A woman may strongly desire a child but feel forced to choose abortion because of a fetal abnormality or a social-psychological reason, such as the departure, incarceration, or death of the partner. In such cases, the woman may have a strong sense of victimization, feeling unable to make the choice she most desires for reasons beyond her control. Similarly, a woman who does not want a child but who has delayed seeking assistance until her gestational age is too advanced for abortion often feels victimized and out of control. In both types of cases, the woman is likely to be suffering from powerful feelings such as grief and loss, anger, helplessness, and depression. Although she may realize intellectually that she is forced to accept an alternative she does not want, she may have so much unresolved feeling about her circumstances that additional counseling is needed before she can act on the decision.

CONTRACEPTION

Unintended pregnancies may occur because of failure of a birth control method; because of careless, inconsistent, or incorrect use by the patient; or because of nonuse. When the cause is technical failure, a woman may feel anger or a sense of betrayal because she was attempting to control her fertility in an acceptable manner. When the failure lies with the patient, she may feel shame or embarrassment at what she sees as her mistake, or she may feel frustration at the need for constant fertility management by methods that are less than perfect. A woman who uses no birth control method may have issues related to her religious beliefs, to her inability to see herself as intentionally sexually active, to a present inability to plan and manage her sexual-relational life, or to a belief that she is unable or unlikely to conceive. It is rarely the case that the woman did not know of the existence of birth control methods, although she may be unfamiliar with the range of methods available or may have misinformation that deters her from using them.

When a woman's method of birth control has failed her, an affirmation of her feelings can be given—for example, "It's upsetting to have your method of birth control let you down" or "It's frustrating that we don't have a perfect method of birth control." After that acknowledgment, she may be ready to focus on her current problems: (1) What will she decide to do about this pregnancy, and (2) what method of birth control will she use in the future. She may wish to use the same method again, despite the failure, if she strongly prefers it over other methods, or she may want additional information about other methods to try. For a woman whose use was inconsistent or incorrect, some reassurance about her ability to try again may be most helpful—for example, "Even though you had trouble using your method this time, you can try it again if you want to." This patient may be particularly sensitive to judgmental attitudes of the clinician, because she is often condemning herself and concerned that she not be perceived by others as stupid or irresponsible. A supportive manner and reassurance that fertility management is often difficult and complicated may enable her to explore more fully the reasons she is having difficulty and may enable her to plan to change her behavior.

For a woman who does not use birth control, some exploration of her circumstances is more helpful than a lecture about being sexually responsible. "Can you tell me about your reasons for not using a method of birth control?" or "What kinds of problems have you had using contraception?" Information can be shared in a nonjudgmental way—for example, "A woman who is fertile and sexually active and who does not use contraception has about an 80% chance of a pregnancy during a year" or "Most women who have had an unintended pregnancy want to minimize the chances of that happening again. Let's look at the methods of birth control available to you."

In choosing a method of contraception, most women consider a number of factors:

- Effectiveness in preventing pregnancy
- Absence of medical risks
- Effectiveness in preventing sexually transmitted diseases
- Absence of unpleasant side effects
- Noninterference with spontaneity in sex
- Absence of messiness
- Low cost
- Congruence with her partner's attitudes
- Ability to use it secretly
- Availability without prescription

The first three factors are most often named by clinicians as being of primary importance, but patients frequently rank other factors as being of greater significance for them. Because no one method satisfies all requirements, a woman may be helped to choose if she can identify the factors of greatest importance to her at the present time and to select the method that comes closest to satisfying those. Following only the clinician's bias about a "best" method may lead to initial patient acceptance but subsequent discontinuation or incorrect use. A woman can be helped to anticipate what problems her chosen method may present her and can be given assurance that she can change her method whenever she wishes. A sense that her physician has faith in her competence and does not condemn her human errors is likely to have a positive effect on her contraceptive behavior in the future.[5]

For a patient with repeated unintended and unwanted pregnancies, more extensive exploration of her feelings and circumstances may be necessary before behavior change can occur. The woman may find being pregnant a desirable state, even though she does not want a child. She may consciously or unconsciously want a child but may be able to assess the situation realistically only after becoming pregnant. She may have trouble negotiating contraceptive behavior with her partner or with multiple partners. She may have unresolved conflicts about her sexuality and sexual behavior or about intimacy, her family, or her career. After exploring issues with her, a useful question can be, "Is this a time you'd like to make a change?" If she is so motivated, information, support, and help with decision-making are appropriate. If she is not motivated, the physician can state in a simple, straightforward manner the health implications of her current behavior and can offer to be of assistance when she feels ready to initiate change.

CLINICIAN BIAS

Sexual behavior has implications for a patient far beyond the issues of health; not only her relationships but her very sense of personhood is intimately bound up with her sexuality and her sexual and reproductive behavior. Although advice from a physician about the health aspects of pregnancy and fertility management can be of great value to a patient, other aspects may be of equal or greater importance to her and to her physician as well. A physician needs to be clear about the difference between values issues and health-related issues and to separate clearly for a patient advice offered on health and medical issues from comments or suggestions on lifestyle and values. Biases stemming from a physician's own value system or from inadequate or faulty information that results from adherence to that value system can influence the decision process about unintended pregnancy and contraceptive choice and can damage the physician-patient relationship of mutual respect. No professional person can be expected to be without values and therefore without biases; self-knowledge about bias and honesty in acknowledgment of bias are the professional standard. For additional examination of family planning issues and alternatives, consult manuals published by organizations that provide or refer for all alternatives, such as Planned Parenthood.[3, 6, 7]

REFERENCES

1. Beresford T. Pregnancy counseling. In: Rothman BK (ed). Encyclopedia of Childbearing. Phoenix: Oryx Press, 1992.
2. Beresford T. Unsure about Your Pregnancy. Washington, DC: The National Abortion Federation, 1991.
3. Beresford T, Pawlowski W, Garrity J. AIDS-HIV Information and Counseling in Family Planning Practice. Washington, DC: Planned Parenthood of Metropolitan Washington, 1988.
4. Boyer D, Fine D. Sexual abuse as a factor in adolescent pregnancy and child maltreatment. Fam Plann Perspect 1992;24:4.
5. Joos S, Hickam D. How health professionals influence behavior. In: Glanz K, Lewis FM, Rimer B (eds). Health Behavior and Health Education. San Francisco: Jossey Bass, 1990.
6. Saltzman L, Policar MS. The Complete Guide to Pregnancy Testing and Counseling. San Francisco: Planned Parenthood of Alameda/San Francisco, 1985.
7. Beresford T. Short Term Relationship Counseling. Baltimore: Planned Parenthood of Maryland, 1988.

Elective Termination of Pregnancy: What the Primary Care Physician Should Know

Donnica L. Moore

For many years, abortion has been a subject embroiled in fierce emotional, political, and philosophic debate. This debate is not the subject of this chapter, however. Since the 1973 Supreme Court decision in Roe v. Wade,[1] first-trimester elective termination of pregnancy has been legal in the United States and is considered to be the personal choice of a pregnant woman. Although subsequent state laws have restricted women's reproductive rights to various extents (particularly those of emancipated minors), therapeutic and elective abortions remain legal medical procedures.

Despite numerous contraceptive options, unintended pregnancy remains a condition of epidemic proportion. Although many women confronted with this situation choose to continue their pregnancies, all primary care physicians who treat women of reproductive age should be able to counsel women who choose to terminate their pregnancies; to advise them about the various procedures available to them; to refer them to a qualified abortion provider if requested; to provide adequate follow-up treatment, including contraceptive counseling; and to identify related complications. With the exception of specific counseling issues, these principles, practices, and even procedures are identical for patients who have had elective, therapeutic, or spontaneous abortions. Therefore, this is important knowledge for all primary care physicians to master, regardless of any personal views held about elective termination of pregnancy.

DEFINITIONS OF ABORTION

Abortion is generally defined by physicians as termination of a pregnancy before the age of fetal viability. Although this pregnancy loss may be spontaneous or induced, to the layperson, the term abortion is used to refer to an elective termination of pregnancy for any one of several reasons; miscarriage is the preferred term for a spontaneous abortion. Medical terminology further categorizes spontaneous abortions as threatened (vaginal bleeding without cervical dilation or extrusion of fetal tissue); inevitable (vaginal bleeding in the presence of abdominal cramping with cervical dilation); complete (all products of conception expelled; no dilation and curettage [D&C] required); incomplete (some products of conception retained; D&C required); missed (asymptomatic intrauterine fetal demise within the first trimester); or habitual (a history of more than three spontaneous abortions).

Whether spontaneous or induced, abortions that occur during the first 12 weeks of gestation are termed early abortions; those that occur from the end of week 12 through week 20 are late abortions. Any abortion complicated by infection is termed a septic abortion. Early spontaneous abortions are recognized in 10 to 15% of pregnancies, although the unrecognized rate may make this number much higher.[2]

Medical terminology further categorizes elective terminations as either therapeutic or medical abortions (those performed for one of a host of maternal or fetal indications) or elective abortions. These are considered legal abortions if performed by a physician in an approved facility; they are illegal abortions if performed by an individual not approved by the law. Medical indications for therapeutic abortion are illnesses or conditions that make continued pregnancy hazardous to the mother (e.g., severe uncontrolled diabetes, renal disease, advanced heart disease, acquired immunodeficiency syndrome); fetal conditions that interfere with normal growth and development (e.g., maternal rubella, teratogenic exposure, lethal hereditary conditions, certain chromosomal and metabolic abnormalities); and severe psychiatric conditions. Decisions about elective abortion are often based on the recommendation of the physician and have a major impact on maternal or fetal health. When pregnancy is terminated because of a chronic condition such as heart disease or diabetes, sterilization should be considered because there is little hope that the condition will improve enough to permit pregnancy in the future.

Nonmedical indications for elective abortion are primarily social or economic in character. The decision about abortion in these cases is made by an individual woman in consideration of her particular circumstances.

PREABORTION WORK-UP

Once a patient has requested elective termination of pregnancy, a complete history and physical examination should be performed as part of the preabortion work-up. This is necessary to select the safest abortion procedure, and findings may affect the choice of abortion facility or provider. The primary objectives of the preabortion evaluation are to confirm pregnancy, to estimate gestational age, to identify any relevant medical or surgical problems that require preabortion treatment, to rule out treatable sexually transmitted diseases, and to discuss postabortion contraception. As with any medical examination, this should be performed in a supportive, nonjudgmental fashion. Any ambivalence or reservations expressed by a patient should be further explored. True ambivalence toward the procedure should be considered a contraindication to abortion[3] and is an absolute indication for recommending further counseling.

History

The history should be complete, focusing on obstetric, gynecologic, medical, and surgical information. The estimated gestational age is dated from the first day of the last normal menstrual period; this is reliable only if the patient is sure of the date, if she has regular menses, and if her pregnancy did not result while continuing to take oral contraceptives. Because light bleeding at the time of implantation is not uncommon, if a patient reports that the last period was not normal (1–2 weeks late; very light), it is helpful to note the first date of the previous menstrual period. A patient's contraceptive history is critical information in best advising her about postabortion contraception. If she was using a contraceptive method that failed, it is appropriate to discuss other options with her because she may not have confidence in this method in the future. If her use of her contraceptive method was inappropriate, any misunderstandings should be identified, clarified, and discussed. Backup barrier options should also be discussed, in regard to both contraception and prevention of sexually transmitted diseases, if appropriate.

The obstetric history solicits information about all previous pregnancies and their outcome. Previous cesarean deliveries or complications related to excessive bleeding should be highlighted. As with any complete history, all medical problems should be explored, all previous operations noted (particularly pelvic), all allergies noted, and all medications or other drugs (including nonprescription preparations, alcohol, and illicit drugs) noted and reviewed. The teratogenic effects of any medications a patient has been taking should be explained to her and documented in the event that she decides to continue her pregnancy. This is particularly important with therapeutic classes of drugs for which safer alternatives are available (e.g., antiepileptics).

Physical Examination

A complete physical examination should be performed, including breast and rectal examinations, which are often overlooked without justification. The speculum examination should note any abnormalities suggestive of infection; tests for gonorrhea and chlamydial infection are considered routine by many practitioners. Common cervical changes include Chadwick's sign (a bluish or purplish coloration); nabothian cysts may also be seen. A Papanicolaou smear should be performed at this time if indicated (i.e., if she has not had one in the past year, if any cervical lesions are present, or if genital warts are noted for the first time). The bimanual examination should confirm the estimated gestational age. This may be difficult in early pregnancy, particularly if a patient is obese, if she has a full bladder, or if she has a retroverted uterus. Cervical softening (Goodell's sign) is usually pronounced in early pregnancy, even before uterine enlargement is felt. Note that the uterus should not be palpable abdominally until 12 weeks of gestation, when it can be palpated at the pubic symphysis. After this point, the fetal heart can usually be heard with a Doppler ultrasound device. It is considered inadvisable to have a patient listen to the fetal heart sounds if she has already decided to terminate her pregnancy.

All of this information is useful in determining the estimated gestational age. If the uterine size differs significantly from the estimated gestational age by the last menstrual period (size greater than dates), pelvic ultrasonography may be warranted. This is usually only the case when uterine size is greater than 12 weeks and the information is needed to determine the appropriate procedure, if the findings on physical examination are not consistent with pregnancy despite a positive pregnancy test, or if an ectopic pregnancy is suspected.

Laboratory Evaluation

Standard laboratory tests before any abortion procedure include hemoglobin or hematocrit, blood type and Rh factor, and a urine human chorionic gonadotropin or *qualitative* serum β–human chorionic gonadotropin. A *quantitative* serum β–human chorionic gonadotropin test is indicated only if ectopic pregnancy is suspected. As described earlier, a Papanicolaou smear is recommended if indicated; screening for gonorrhea and chlamydial infection is also recommended. In some high-risks areas, syphilis screening is routinely performed; screening for human immunodeficiency virus should be recommended for patients in a high-risk category.

Given that 74.4% of infants have severe congenital malformations if their mother contracts rubella in the first 4 months of pregnancy,[4] the preabortion screening offers a good opportunity to check the patient's rubella antibody titer if not previously documented. If negative, the patient should be offered a rubella vaccination after her abortion. Patients should be advised to use reliable contraception for 3 months after receiving this vaccine.[2]

All other tests should be selected on the basis of the individual circumstances. For example, if general anesthesia will be used, a chest radiograph and electrocardiogram should be considered for patients who are older than 35 years or who have cardiac or respiratory problems. Patients taking medications that must have adequate blood levels titrated should have these assessed before any operative procedure.

All preabortion laboratory results should be forwarded to the abortion provider to alert her or him to any risks, as well as to avoid needless duplication.

Preabortion Assessment

After taking the preabortion history and performing the physical examination, the physician should discuss that assessment with the patient. This includes recommending an abortion provider and an appropriate procedure, discussing anesthesia, recommending any necessary preabortion consultations, and discussing postabortion contraception. Although smoking is not specifically related to any increased abortion risk, aside from complications associated with general anesthesia, any patient who smokes should be counseled regarding the health benefits of stopping smoking.

Many physicians prescribe maternal vitamins for all pregnant patients, regardless of whether they decide to continue the pregnancy or to abort it. Vitamin supplementation is advisable to compensate for the additional metabolic demands on the patient, particularly if she reverses her decision and continues her pregnancy. The amount of time that these vitamins are continued after abortion depends on a patient's nutritional status and duration of pregnancy at the time of her abortion; no formal guidelines exist, however.

TERMINATION PROCEDURES

A number of abortion techniques are available; selection depends on the estimated gestational age, the individual patient profile, and the provider's preference. The risks, complications, and cost of the abortion also vary according to gestational age, provider experience, type of procedure, setting for the procedure, geographic location, and choice of anesthesia (general, local, sedation, or none).

Postcoital Contraception

It is controversial whether postcoital contraception should be considered an abortion technique. This technique is used within 72 hours after unprotected intercourse, which may be considered to be the result of a known contraceptive failure (e.g., broken condom); rape; or, most commonly, failure to use contraceptive. The goal of this method is to intercept implantation of a possible conception. Postcoital contraception (the morning-after pill) may be administered by any primary care physician. It should be considered emergency therapy only, not a primary means of contraception. The closer to the time of coitus in which the method chosen is administered, the more effective it is. All such therapies must be administered within 72 hours after coitus. None is 100% effective; if menses is delayed by more than 2 weeks, a pregnancy test should be performed.

DIETHYLSTILBESTROL. The first hormonal formulation used for postcoital contraception was diethylstilbestrol (DES), a synthetic estrogen. Patients who request treatment within 72 hours of unprotected intercourse are given 25 mg of DES orally twice daily for 5 days. This regimen is highly effective, although side effects are experienced by 50% of women. These primarily include nausea and vomiting; rarely reported are headaches, dizziness, diarrhea, bloating, breast discomfort, mild lower abdominal cramping pain, rash, and depression. Because maternal ingestion of DES is associated with teratogenic and other serious side effects in babies of both sexes (vaginal adenosis and adenocarcinoma particularly), DES should not be used as a postcoital contraceptive in women who do not agree to an abortion should pregnancy result.

COMBINATION THERAPY. A more commonly used alternative is administration of two oral contraceptive pills (containing a total of 1 mg of norgestrel and 100 μg of ethinyl estradiol) within 24 hours of unprotected intercourse, followed by a repeat dose 12 hours later. Patients should be warned that they may experience severe nausea and vomiting as a result of this regimen, although such symptoms are less than those experienced by patients using DES. They should also be informed that the length of their menstrual cycle will be affected. If treatment is given at or before midcycle, that cycle may be shorter than normal; treatment after midcycle tends to delay menses.

INTRAUTERINE DEVICE. The intrauterine device has also been used as a postcoital contraceptive; it has the advantage of then serving as an ongoing contraceptive. The association with possible increased risk of pelvic infections makes the intrauterine device unsuitable for young nulliparous women who may have more than one sexual partner.

First Trimester

In 1984, 90% of all abortions were performed at or before 12 weeks of gestation.[5]

VERY EARLY TERMINATION OF PREGNANCY. This technique refers to an abortion performed up to the sixth week after the last menstrual period and is also referred to as menstrual extraction, menstrual regulation, menstrual induction, or endometrial aspiration. The term originally referred to a procedure performed before pregnancy could be reliably diagnosed; thus, abortion may or may not have taken place. Reliable β–human chorionic gonadotropin assays now remove this uncertainty. This relatively simple outpatient procedure involves the use of a hand suction device and a small flexible cannula; mild analgesia or a paracervical block may be used to minimize cramping discomfort. The major disadvantage of this procedure is a relatively high failure rate of 2.5 continued pregnancies per 1000 abortions performed at 7 weeks estimated gestational age or earlier[6] to as high as 6%.[7] Side effects are mild and transient and include cramping, nausea, diaphoresis, and syncope.[8]

Aspiration of uterine contents may also be performed using a technique similar to the curettage described later. Significant differences are that cervical dilation is rarely required at this early gestation and that the time for the procedure is a few minutes less.

Antiprogesterone compounds (e.g., RU 486—mifepristone) have also been used successfully in other countries to terminate very early pregnancies. This class is discussed under investigational therapies because these compounds were not approved for treatment or research in the United States until recently.

SUCTION DILATION AND CURETTAGE. This technique is generally used up until 13 weeks gestation and is the most commonly performed abortion procedure, representing 85% of all abortions in the United States. When available, it is considered the pregnancy termination method of choice.[8] The procedure usually takes about 15 minutes to perform and may be administered in an outpatient setting under local (intracervical) anesthesia; general anesthesia may also be used in a hospital setting. Although the latter may be more emotionally appealing to a patient, it does subject her to the additional risks of general anesthesia, even though very short-acting anesthetics can be used. Local anesthesia costs less, has fewer side effects (particularly a lower risk of uterine perforation), and requires shorter administration and recovery time than general anesthetics.

The procedure is similar to menstrual extraction but usually requires some dilation of the cervix, after which a disposable curet with attached vacuum suction is used to empty the uterine contents; these should be collected and sent for pathologic examination to confirm that products of conception were obtained.

Oxytocic drugs are not generally necessary when local anesthesia is used; they are often used after general anesthesia because many of these agents potentiate uterine bleeding by relaxing the uterus. Patients who are Rh negative should receive an injection of anti-D immunoglobulin within 72 hours after the procedure. Patients may be sent home within a relatively short time after the procedure (1–2 hours; more if general anesthesia is used) with instructions for follow-up. Generally, only small doses of nonprescription nonsteroidal anti-inflammatory medications are required for pain relief.

In addition to the risks associated with anesthesia, possible early complications include uterine perforation (either as a result of the cervical dilator or additional, sharp curettage) and excessive bleeding as a result of cervical lacerations or retained products of conception. Long-term complications include cervical incompetence and consequent spontaneous abortions as a result of traumatic cervical dilation (can only be diagnosed in a subsequent pregnancy) and subfertility or infertility as a result of Asherman's syndrome (formation of uterine scarring), usually resulting from repeated D&C procedures. These are discussed at greater length later.

Second Trimester

Although performing abortions in the first trimester is far preferable, second-trimester abortions may be indicated for several reasons: as a result of earlier ambivalence on the part of the patient or her partner, changes in social circumstances, or unfavorable results of amniocentesis, which are usually unavailable before 18 to 20 weeks of gestation. The increasing availability of first-trimester chorionic villus sampling may decrease the number of second-trimester abortions performed for this reason.[8] Physiologically, the second trimester is the ''least physiologic time during pregnancy for the uterus to empty itself,''[9] because the uterus does not respond well to oxytocic drugs, the cervix is not easily dilated, and the fetus is larger.

There is no second-trimester method of choice; what has evolved is a combination of various medical and surgical techniques,[8] which are generally selected on the basis of the provider's preference and the estimated gestational age.

DILATION AND EVACUATION. This is the predominant method of termination in the early second trimester and the safest method through 20 weeks of gestation.[10] It requires adequate cervical dilation, often using the insertion of preoperative laminaria tents or prostaglandin suppositories after 15 weeks of gestation. This procedure can be performed under local or general anesthesia. Patients should fast before the procedure, and intravenous hydration is usually given. Curettage or ultraso-

nography may be performed after the procedure to ascertain that the uterus is satisfactorily emptied; many clinicians administer intravenous oxytocin either during the procedure or immediately afterward to facilitate uterine contractility and to limit blood loss.

Benefits to the patient are that this is a relatively quick (approximately 30 minutes) and safe procedure that can be performed on an outpatient basis, thus decreasing costs. Unlike with amnioinfusion, patients do not experience prolonged labor and do not experience fetal expulsion. There are no medical contraindications.[11] When correctly performed, this method has a low complication rate (0.69 per 100 cases)[12]; complications include all of those mentioned for D&C, with a greater risk of severity. Disadvantages to a patient are the limited availability of this procedure because more of a physician's time is required than for amnioinfusion methods and because many abortion providers object to the procedure.[11]

LAMINARIA. Laminaria tents are small sticks of dried, compressed seaweed. When several are inserted into the cervix, they readily absorb secretions and swell to four times their original diameter, depending on the length of time they are left in place. The cervix softens and dilates, thus facilitating subsequent manual dilation in dilation and evacuation procedures. This greatly increases the safety of the procedure, reducing the risk of uterine perforation[13] and the risk of incompetent cervix in subsequent pregnancies.[9]

Patients may experience some cramping pain when several laminaria are inserted together; this usually resolves within a few minutes and can be treated with oral analgesics. It is not uncommon for laminaria to be inserted as long as 12 hours before the termination procedure; a patient may then leave the office and return at the designated time for her evacuation procedure. Theoretically, the risk of infection is greater with this practice, although this has not been clinically documented.[14, 15]

AMNIOINFUSION. This procedure involves injecting solutions of hypertonic (20%) saline or prostaglandins directly into the amniotic sac (using local anesthesia) to induce abortion by inducing labor. Intravenous oxytocin may also be given to decrease the time for the subsequent labor period, and laminaria tents may also be inserted before the infusion. This method is usually used after 16 weeks of gestation; before this time, the sac is difficult to enter. It is generally performed as an inpatient procedure, although some facilities offer outpatient amnioinfusion, instructing patients to return when they are in active labor.

Disadvantages to patients include prolonged labor and experiencing the expulsion of the dead fetus and placenta. Increasingly, amnioinfusions are combinations of solutions intended to augment efficacy while decreasing complications.[16] Significant risks are associated with both infusions but are higher with prostaglandin infusions. Although prostaglandins have the advantage of inducing a shorter injection-to-abortion time, they are not fetocidal in as many as 7% of cases.[11] Other disadvantages include a higher incidence of nausea, vomiting, diarrhea, cervical trauma, blood loss, fever, endometritis, retained products of conception requiring D&C, and higher cost.[8] Prostaglandins are contraindicated in patients with a history of asthma, pulmonary hypertension, glaucoma, epilepsy, and hypertension.[17]

The advantages of the hypertonic saline infusions are their effectiveness, the relatively low rate of retained tissue, and the lower cost. The disadvantages are the association with potentially fatal risks of hypernatremia and disseminated intravascular coagulation syndrome if the saline solution is extravasated.[8] Hypertonic saline infusion is contraindicated in patients with a bloody tap (unless the clinician chooses to wait and attempt the procedure again after a few hours) and those with cardiac diseases.[8]

It should be noted that the death rate for infusion procedures overall was found to be 19.5 per 100,000; this is approximately eight times higher than that reported with D&C or dilation and evacuation procedures.[18]

HYSTEROTOMY. Hysterotomy involves surgical removal of the fetus through a uterine incision, similar to a cesarean section. It requires the same preparation and recovery as any major abdominal surgery and may be performed under regional or general anesthesia. Hysterotomy is rarely performed since the availability of prostaglandins; many investigators believe that this procedure has no place in contemporary abortion practice.[8] Possible indications include a failed second-trimester abortion or another need to enter the pelvic cavity. Maternal mortality is relatively high, representing 48 per 100,000 women between 10 and 29 years old and 70 per 100,000 women between the ages of 30 and 49.[19]

HYSTERECTOMY. Hysterectomy is rarely performed in conjunction with an abortion. Indications are mainly those of coexistent large fibroids or cervical carcinoma.[19] Hysterectomy is also rarely necessary as a result of uterine perforation sustained during a dilation and evacuation.

Patient Discharge Instructions

Although the complications for each of these procedures vary, the symptoms are similar, varying only in degree and duration. Patients generally experience some vaginal bleeding and cramping, not much heavier than their normal menstrual period, which lasts from a few days to 2 weeks. After an uncomplicated first-trimester abortion, patients should be instructed to avoid strenuous exercise and to put nothing into their vagina until the bleeding subsides: no douching, no tampons, and no coitus. After a second-trimester abortion, this recommendation is generally extended to 4 weeks.

Most patients may resume their normal activities, guided by their individual feelings of well-being. Patients should be advised to check their oral temperature twice daily and to call a physician if they experience any of the following symptoms: increasing rather than decreasing bleeding, vaginal bleeding heavier than their heaviest period, temperature greater than 100°F orally, or foul-smelling vaginal discharge. If antibiotics have been prescribed, a patient should be alerted to possible adverse reactions and advised to call if she experiences them.

Before leaving the abortion facility, all patients should be given an appointment for a postabortion checkup within 2 to 3 weeks after the procedure.

Prevention of D Isoimmunization

Abortion can cause Rh_0D sensitization. This occurs more frequently after induced abortion than after spontaneous abortion and more frequently after late abortion than after early abortion.[20] Before discharge from the abortion facility, all patients with Rh-negative blood types should be treated with Rh_0D immunoglobulin unless the father is known to be Rh_0D negative. The recommended dose depends on the gestational age. For early abortions, a dose of 50 μg of Rh_0D immunoglobulin should be adequate; for late abortions, the standard 300-μg dose is recommended.[20]

Prophylactic Antibiotics

The literature supports the practice of prescribing perioperative prophylactic antibiotics to reduce the incidence of postabortion infection.[16, 21–23] Few studies have been conducted to evaluate the advantages and disadvantages of routine postabortion antibiotics. Data regarding an optimal regimen are not available, but typically, a broad-spectrum antibiotic with coverage for vaginal and fecal flora (e.g., tetracycline or doxycycline) is administered for 24 hours.[8] Because adolescents have been shown to have a higher incidence of postabortion endometritis than women age 20 to 29 years, prophylactic antibiotics may be of greater benefit in this group.[24]

GENERAL COMPLICATIONS

Abortion generally is a safe procedure when performed correctly by a well-trained provider in a controlled setting. Both morbidity and mortality increase with increasing gestational age[19]; however, the overall risk of death resulting from complications of pregnancy and childbirth is nearly 12 times greater than the risk of death due to an induced abortion. In 1985, the maternal mortality rate was 4.7 deaths per 100,000 live births; the legal abortion mortality rate when performed before 21 weeks of gestation was 0.4 deaths per 100,000 abortions.[25]

Morbidity can be categorized as early or late complications.

Early Complications

Overall risk of early complications during first-trimester abortions is 1 to 2 per 100,000 for women of all ages.[2] Because the most serious early complications cannot be anticipated (hemorrhage and uterine perforation), it is essential that providers have the capabilities to treat them promptly if they occur.

RETAINED PRODUCTS OF CONCEPTION. This complication presents as heavy vaginal bleeding; it may be associated with lower abdominal cramping or pain. The incidence varies from 0.4 to 2.9%.[26–29] Treatment involves repeat curettage and is usually covered by prophylactic antibiotics.

HEMORRHAGE OR ANEMIA. Excessive bleeding may be due to retained products of conception as described earlier. It may also be due to cervical trauma, uterine perforation (described later), or uterine atony (postabortion syndrome). Blood loss increases with gestation; losses of 500 ml or greater are considered significant.[19] If bleeding does not respond to conservative treatment, laparotomy or rarely hysterectomy may need to be performed.

UTERINE PERFORATION. Uterine perforation is the most feared complication of abortion. Although occurring infrequently (0.9 per 1000 abortions), it greatly increases the associated morbidity and mortality, subjecting patients to infection, hemorrhage, trauma to abdominal organs (particularly the bowel), shock, and possibly hysterectomy.[30] If uterine perforation is suspected, di-

agnostic laparoscopy may be performed before laparotomy. If uterine perforation is documented, laparotomy is usually indicated; the management and postoperative course depend on the perforation site, the instrument used, and the likelihood and extent of bowel involvement

POSTABORTION SYNDROME. This is the name given to the unexplained uterine atony that may occur after an uncomplicated abortion. Patients may complain of severe pain within a few hours of the procedure. Physical examination reveals a tender, enlarged, boggy uterus that is filled with blood; however, vaginal bleeding is usually minimal. Prompt reaspiration or curettage followed by intravenous oxytocin is indicated.[8]

INFECTION OR SEPSIS. Most cases of postabortion infection are related to retained products of conception; treatment is to give a broad-spectrum antibiotic, to inspect the cervix for retained products of conception, and to re-evacuate the uterus if necessary. If visible in the cervix, retained placental membranes can usually be easily removed from the cervical canal with a ring forceps without significant discomfort to the patient, thus avoiding curettage. Endometritis may also occur in the absence of retained products of conception, resulting from ascending vaginal or cervical infection. Preabortion screening and treatment of chlamydial infection, gonorrhea, and severe cervicitis has reduced this incidence. Patients with uterine perforation should also be given broad-spectrum antibiotic therapy.

Because pelvic infections are associated with subsequent infertility, early treatment is advisable. Any patient who complains of persistent, worsening, or severe cramping or abdominal pain, fever, or malodorous discharge needs immediate care and should be treated aggressively with hospitalization or parenteral antibiotics if indicated.

Hypotension or oral temperature greater than 102°F puts patients in a high-risk category for septic shock, as does generalized peritonitis, anemia, or leukopenia.[2] Cervical, endometrial, and blood cultures should be obtained before starting broad-spectrum antibiotic coverage.

FAILED TERMINATION OF PREGNANCY. Rarely, the decidua only may be evacuated, especially in the case of termination very early in pregnancy, thus accentuating the importance of checking the pathology report and recommending a postabortion pelvic examination.[19] The findings may also suggest a missed ectopic pregnancy, a circumstance becoming increasingly common. The incidence of ectopic pregnancies varies throughout the world, from 1 in 28 pregnancies to 1 in 200 pregnancies.[31]

Late Complications

CERVICAL INCOMPETENCE. Cervical incompetence can cause future midtrimester spontaneous abortions and results from complications related to cervical dilation or lacerations. This is a greater risk for primigravidas.[19]

CHRONIC PELVIC INFLAMMATORY DISEASE. Chronic pelvic inflammatory disease may further result in decreased fertility and may occur without symptoms. It may also increase the risk of subsequent ectopic pregnancy.[32]

ASHERMAN'S SYNDROME. Asherman's syndrome is characterized by formation of intrauterine adhesions, usually as a result of multiple or overvigorous curettage procedures. This diagnosis is suspected if a nonpregnant patient does not resume menses within 8 weeks after abortion. Referral to a gynecologist is necessary; treatment consists of D&C or hysteroscopic examination with lysis of adhesions. Asherman's syndrome can cause infertility (which may be the cause for discovery) but is often asymptomatic.

Rh ISOIMMUNIZATION. This complication has been virtually eliminated as a problem for Rh-negative patients with the practice of routine preabortion Rh screening and postabortion anti-D immunoglobulin. This must be double-checked in all Rh-negative patients.

INVESTIGATIONAL AND FUTURE TECHNIQUES

RU 486 (Mifepristone; Synthetic Antiprostaglandin)

This controversial product is currently being sold and further investigated in France, Great Britain, Sweden, and China as a highly effective morning-after pill (postcoital contraceptive), which works by interfering with embryonic implantation when administered within 72 hours of intercourse. It also serves as an abortifacient that induces abortion as late as 9 weeks of gestation.[33] Despite the compound's potential role in the treatment of breast cancer, Cushing's syndrome, and other serious diseases, mifepristone is only recently available for research in the United States because the manufacturer is concerned about the current antiabortion political climate there.

Some investigators are evaluating the role of RU 486 as a possible monthly contraceptive to be taken at the time of expected menses, without knowing whether fertilization has or has not occurred.[34] Advantages include its availability in oral form; disadvantages include prolonged or heavy menstrual bleeding and gastrointestinal side effects. Efficacy rates vary according to the studies and the gestational age.

Prostaglandin Suppositories

These may offer a noninvasive early termination option for self-administration[35]; use is limited by the frequency and severity of gastrointestinal side effects.[36, 37] Prostaglandin vaginal suppositories have been used for cervical dilation before abortion.[38]

FOLLOW-UP

History

A thorough interval history should be elicited, focusing on a patient's general feelings (emotional and physical), the duration and amount of cramping and bleeding, and any signs or symptoms of infection or continued pregnancy. Other significant questions concern the resumption of sexual relations, review of postabortion contraceptive choice, and resumption of menses (this should usually occur within 4 weeks of the abortion or after the first package of oral contraceptives is completed). Any complications should be discussed and the treatment reviewed.

Physical Examination

Examination should be based on the history. Vital signs should be normal. In addition, the cervix should be inspected for lacerations and signs of infection. The uterus should be palpated for signs of involution; it should be of normal size and nontender.

Laboratory Tests

No routine laboratory tests are indicated at the postabortion follow-up visit. However, if preexisting abnormalities were noted, this is an appropriate time for follow-up and further evaluation. If gonorrhea or chlamydial infection was treated before the procedure, a test of cure should be performed.

Although it is the responsibility of the abortion provider to check the pathology report, the follow-up visit offers an opportunity to confirm that this was done. Although unusual, it is possible for no products of conception to have been obtained, in which case the patient should be evaluated to rule out an ectopic pregnancy. Even more unusual is the diagnosis of hydatidiform mole. In the event of this diagnosis, the patient should be referred to a gynecologic oncologist for further evaluation, treatment, and follow-up.

Postabortion Contraception

To provide an abortion without adequate contraceptive counseling and a voluntarily selected acceptable birth control method is to provide an incomplete health care service and ultimately is a disservice to the patient. Birth control should ideally be thoroughly discussed in the preabortion visits so that a patient may begin using her contraceptive choice after abortion. If her choice is oral contraception, the pills should be started immediately after the abortion, because ovulation may occur within 2 to 4 weeks after a first-trimester abortion. If the abortion occurs after 21 weeks, however, oral contraceptives should not be started until a week after the abortion, because the normally increased risk of postpartum thromboembolism may be further increased by oral contraceptives.[31]

Emotional and Psychological Issues

A common belief is that patients who undergo elective termination of pregnancy may experience negative emotional and psychological sequelae, referred to as the abortion trauma syndrome. The existence of this syndrome is not supported by the medical literature[39–42]; neither negative nor positive mental health effects have been consistently demonstrated.[43] Abortion compares favorably with childbirth with respect to psychosis: One large study found the incidence of postpartum psychosis to be 1.7 cases per 1000 versus 0.3 cases per 1000 in patients having undergone abortion.[44] To evaluate depression, physicians must distinguish between the transient feelings of stress and sadness commonly described as depression and the clinical psychiatric syndrome. Although it is not unusual for women to report these feelings before and shortly after an abortion, most report relief afterward.[45] As with the outcome of any medical procedure, the way a patient may react emotionally or psychologically to abortion should be considered within the context of the general and individual social and psychological circumstances in which it is performed.[42]

REFERENCES

1. Roe v Wade, 410 US 113, 1973.
2. Mattox JH. Abortion. In: Wilson JR, Carrington ER (eds). Obstetrics and Gynecology. 8th ed. St Louis: CV Mosby, 1987.
3. Neubardt S, Schulman H. Techniques of Abortion. 2nd ed. Boston: Little, Brown & Co, 1977.
4. Swan C. Rubella in pregnancy, an etiologic factor in congenital malformations, stillbirths, miscarriages, and abortions. J Obstet Gynaecol Br Commonwealth 1949;56:591.
5. Centers for Disease Control. Abortion Surveillance: Preliminary Analysis: United States 1986 and 1987. MMWR, Vol. 38, No. 38 Sept. 29, 1989.
6. Fielding W, Lee S, Borten M, et al. Continued pregnancy after failed first trimester abortion. Obstet Gynecol 1984;63(3):421.
7. Derman R. Early diagnosis of pregnancy. J Reprod Med 1981;26(Suppl 4):149.
8. Lichtman R, Papera S. Gynecology: Well Woman Care. Norwalk, CT: Appleton & Lange, 1990.
9. Grimes D, Cates W. Dilatation and evacuation. In: GS Berger, Brenner WE, Keith L (eds). Second Trimester Abortion. Boston: John Wright, 1981.
10. American College of Obstetricians and Gynecologists. Methods of Midtrimester Abortion. ACOG Technical Bulletin 109. Washington, DC: American College of Obstetricians and Gynecologists, 1987.
11. Hern W. Abortion Practice. Philadelphia: JB Lippincott, 1984.
12. Centers for Disease Control. Abortion Surveillance. Atlanta: CDC, US Department of Health, Education and Welfare, Public Health Service, 1977.
13. Grimes D. Second-trimester abortions in the United States. Fam Plann Perspect 1984;16(6):260.
14. Altman A, Stubblefield P, Schlam J, et al. Midtrimester abortion with laminaria and vacuum evacuation on a teaching service. J Reprod Med 1985;30(8):601.
15. Stubbefield P. Laminaria and other adjunctive methods. In: Berger GS, Brenner WE, Keith L (eds). Second Trimester Abortion. Boston: John Wright, 1981.
16. Hatcher R, Guest F, Stewart F, et al. Contraceptive Technology 1984–1985, 12th rev ed. New York: Irvington, 1984.
17. Schneider T. Voluntary termination of pregnancy. J Obstet Gynecol Neonatal Nurs 1984;13(Suppl 2):77s.
18. Berger GS, Tietze C, Pakter J, et al. Maternal mortality in NY state: July 1, 1970, to June 30, 1972. Obstet Gynecol 1974;43(3)315.
19. Filshie M, Guillebaud J. Contraception: Science and Practice. London: Butterworth, 1989.
20. American College of Obstetricians and Gynecologists. Prevention of D Isoimmunization. ACOG Technical Bulletin 147. Washington, DC: American College of Obstetricians and Gynecologists, 1990.
21. American College of Obstetricians and Gynecologists. Antimicrobial Therapy for Gynecologic Infections. ACOG Technical Bulletin 153. American College of Obstetricians and Gynecologists, 1991.
22. Grimes D, Schulz K, Cates W. Prophylactic antibiotics for curettage abortion. Am J Obstet Gynecol 1984;150(6):689.
23. Levallois P, Rious JE. Prophylactic antibiotics for suction curettage abortion: Results of a clinical controlled trial. Am J Obstet Gynecol 1988;158(1):100.
24. Burkman R, Atienza M, King T. Morbidity risk among young adolescents undergoing elective abortion. Contraception 1984;30(2):99.
25. Council on Scientific Affairs, American Medical Association. Induced Termination of Pregnancy before and after

Roe v Wade: Trends in the Mortality and Morbidity of Women. Chicago: American Medical Association, 1992.

26. Hodgson JE, Portman KC. Complications of 10,453 consecutive first trimester abortions: A prospective study. Am J Obstet Gynecol 1974;120:802.

27. Loung KC, Buckle AER, Anderson MM. Results in 1000 cases of therapeutic abortion managed by vacuum aspiration. Br Med J 1971;4:477.

28. Pakter J, Harris D, Nelson F. Surveillance of abortion progress in New York City. Bull N Y Acad Med 1971;47(8):853.

29. Stone M, Morris N, Blair M. Factors influencing morbidity following termination of pregnancy. Eur J Obstet Gynecol Reprod Biol 1977;7:69.

30. Grimes D, Schulz D, Cates W. Prevention of uterine perforation during curettage abortion. JAMA 1984;251(16): 2108.

31. Mishell DR, Brenner PF (eds). Management of Common Problems in Obstetrics and Gynecology. 2nd ed. Oradell NJ: Medical Economics, 1988.

32. Beral V. An epidemiological study of recent trends in ectopic pregnancy. Br J Obstet Gynecol 1975;775.

33. Glaisier A, Thong KJ, Dewar M, et al. Mifepristone (RU486) compared with high dose estrogen and progestogen for emergency postcoital contraception. N Engl J Med 1992;327(15):1041.

34. Spitz I, Barden C. Antiprogestins: Prospects for a once-a-month pill. Fam Plann Perspect 1985;17(6):260.

35. Rosen A, von Knorring K, Bygdeman M, et al. Randomized comparison of prostaglandin treatment in hospital or at home with vacuum aspiration for termination of early pregnancy. Contraception 1984;29(5):423.

36. Borton M, Friedman E. Early pregnancy interruption with a single PGF2α 15-methyl-analogue vaginal suppository. J Reprod Med 1985;30(10):741.

37. Foster H, Smith M, McGruder C, et al. Postconception menses induction using prostaglandin vaginal suppositories. Obstet Gynecol 1985;65(5):682.

38. Kajanoja P, Mandelin M, Makila U, et al. A gemeprost vaginal suppository for cervical priming prior to termination of first trimester pregnancy. Contraception 1984; 29(3):251.

39. Adler NE, David HP, Major BN, et al. Psychological responses after abortion. Sciences 1990;248:41.

40. Dagg PKB. The psychological sequelae of therapeutic abortion—denied and completed. Am J Psychiatry 1991;148:578.

41. Osofsky JD, Osofsky JH. The psychological reaction of patients to legalized abortion. Am J Orthopsychiatry 1972;42:48.

42. Stotland NL. The myth of the abortion trauma syndrome. JAMA 1992;268(15):2078.

43. Koop CE. Unpublished letter to President Ronald Reagan, January 1989. Described in: Koop: The Memoirs of America's Family Doctor. New York: Random House, 1991.

44. Brewer C. Incidence of postabortion psychosis: A prospective study. Br Med J 1977;1:476.

45. Green HS, Lal S, Lewis SC, et al: Psychosocial consequences of therapeutic abortion. King's therapeutic study III. Br J Psychiatry 1976; 128:74.

BIBLIOGRAPHY

Association of Reproductive Health Professionals. To Plan a National Campaign to Reduce Unintended Pregnancy, 1992 Consensus Conference Highlights and Recommendations. Washington, DC: Association of Reproductive Health Professionals, 1992.

Council on Scientific Affairs, American Medical Association. Induced termination of pregnancy before and after Roe v. Wade. JAMA 1992;268(22):3231.

Gold RB. Abortion and Women's Health: A Turning Point for America? New York: Alan Guttmacher Institute, 1990.

Henshaw SK, Morrow E. Induced Abortion, A World Review: 1990 Supplement. New York, Alan Guttmacher Institute, 1990.

Henshaw SK, Van Vort J. Abortion Factbook 1992 Edition: Readings, Trends, and State and Local Data to 1988. New York: Guttmacher Institute, 1992.

Lauersen NH, Wilson KH, Beling CG, et al. Comparison of hypertonic saline for induction of mid-trimester abortion. Am J Obstet Gynecol 1974;120:875.

Wagatsuma T. Intra-amniotic injection of saline for therapeutic abortion. Obstet Gynecol 1965;93:743.

Infertility

28

Evaluation and Treatment of Infertility

Elizabeth S. Ginsburg

DEFINITIONS AND PREVALENCE OF INFERTILITY

It is estimated that 24% of couples in the United States will experience infertility at some point in their reproductive lives.[1] The incidence of infertility has risen, in part, because of later age at marriage and delayed childbearing during marriage.[2, 3] Infertility is defined as the absence of conception after 1 year of unprotected intercourse. Primary infertility is infertility in a woman who has never been pregnant. Secondary infertility is infertility in a woman who has been pregnant in the past, whether the pregnancy resulted in the birth of a child or not. The overall incidence of primary and secondary infertility is similar; in one study, 13% of infertility was primary and 17% secondary.[1] The incidence of infertility increases with maternal age older than 34 years,[4] low socioeconomic status,[5] and a history of sexually transmitted diseases.[6]

INFERTILITY EVALUATION

It is reasonable to encourage and pursue an infertility evaluation in couples who have had 1 year of regular sexual intercourse without conception. If a patient has not documented attempts at conception for 1 year but is anxious about a potential undiagnosed abnormality, it may be reasonable to initiate an earlier evaluation. Women older than 34 years have decreased fecundity or ability to conceive.[4] The physician should take a thorough history and initiate preliminary infertility testing after 6 months of unsuccessful attempts at conception (Table 28–1). In a younger woman, a history should be taken and a physical examination per-

formed. If there is no indication of an infertility factor and coital frequency and technique appear to be normal, she should be encouraged to wait a year before beginning testing. It is often helpful to explain that lack of conception does not necessarily imply an abnormality and that conception may take months to occur in normal couples. Studies have shown that 60% of couples who eventually conceive do so within 3 months, 75% by 6 months, 85% by 1 year, and 93% by 2 years.[7] Noninvasive preliminary testing is, however, perfectly safe and may be instituted at a patient's request. Both partners should be strongly encouraged to participate in the infertility evaluation. In

TABLE 28–1. Infertility Testing

	PRELIMINARY TESTING	SPECIALIZED TESTING
Male factor	Semen analysis	Hamster egg penetration test
Ovulatory defects	Hormonal: Follicle-stimulating hormone Thyroid-stimulating hormone Prolactin Basal body temperature charting	Midluteal progesterone Endometrial biopsy
Cervical factor	Postcoital test	Antisperm antibodies
Miscellaneous	Cervical *Chlamydia* culture Rubella screen Tay-Sachs screen Sickle trait screen Other screening as indicated	
Tubal disease		Hysterosalpingogram Laparoscopy
Uterine defect	Ultrasonography	Hysterosalpingogram Hysteroscopy

some instances, the male partner is reluctant to miss work to accompany his wife during the various testing procedures. He should be encouraged to be present for at least one office visit and to actively follow the progress of the investigation. Educating the couple as they proceed through the infertility evaluation maximizes the chances that testing will be carried out appropriately. Encouraging self-education with lay texts on infertility may help patients' adherence and gives patients perspective on the prevalence of their problem while preparing them for possible future therapies.

Infertility History

The history helps a physician identify infertility factors and educates patients, who may be unaware of the wide variety of factors that can affect fertility. During the history taking, myths about infertility may be discounted and patients' fears directly addressed. Myths surrounding infertility are discussed in greater depth later in this chapter.

Age of Partners

The age of the woman is of vital importance in predicting the outcome of infertility. Prompt, complete evaluation and early referral to a specialist are indicated in women older than 35 years. Women should be made aware of the increased risk of chromosomal abnormalities in a fetus as maternal age increases, and 35 years is the age at which amniocentesis is generally recommended.[8] Men older than 55 years also have an increased risk of trisomy 21 in their offspring.[9, 10] Couples who present for evaluation after 3 years of infertility may have a worse prognosis for achieving a pregnancy.[11]

Prior Pregnancies

Spontaneous and therapeutic abortions and ectopic, premature, and full-term pregnancies all should be recorded. A history of two to three consecutive first-trimester losses indicates a need for evaluation for recurrent abortion, as does a single second-trimester loss without a history of term delivery.

Coital Frequency and Technique

The physician must ask how frequently the couple has intercourse. Lack of an initial response may be due to embarrassment that frequency is low. It is not uncommon to find very infrequent coitus in couples with infertility because of stress associated with recurrent nonconception cycles. Coitus should optimally occur every other day in the midcycle period, during which ovulation occurs. Normal sperm are capable of fertilizing a human egg for 48 to 72 hours after ejaculation, during which time they remain motile in the cervical mucus.[12] The egg is thought to be fertilizable for 12 to 24 hours after ovulation.[13] Ejaculation more frequently than every other day may result in decreased sperm counts.[14] It is normal for a large part of the ejaculate to escape from the vagina. However, lying supine (in a woman with an anteverted uterus) or prone (in a woman with a retroverted uterus) after intercourse may aid in sperm-cervical mucus contact. Lubricating jellies have spermicidal properties and should be discouraged.[15] It is important to determine if the couple is aware that the woman ovulates approximately 14 days before the expected menstrual period.

Contraceptive History

The use of an intrauterine device, especially the Dalkon shield, is associated with tubal factor infertility.[16] Other birth control methods have not been implicated as causes of subsequent infertility.

Medications

The use of antihypertensive medications, antidepressants, digoxin, clofibrate, cimetidine, and many other medications is associated with male impotence.[17] Cimetidine, spironolactone, sulfasalazine, chemotherapeutic agents, and other medications may decrease sperm quantity and quality.[18] Medications causing elevations in serum prolactin levels, such as the phenothiazines, may cause anovulation in women.

Substance Abuse

Alcohol, marijuana, and cigarette use are associated with impaired semen quality. Cigarette smoking in women increases the incidence of primary infertility.[19] Couples should be counseled about these factors and assisted in stopping all substance use before conception. The infertility evaluation is generally not delayed to accomplish this.

Exposures

Radiation doses in excess of 800 rads are virtually always associated with ovarian failure,[20] which would be manifested by amenorrhea. Heat exposure, even one febrile episode, decreases sperm parameters for as long as 2 to 3 months. Saunas, hot tubs, hot baths, sitting for long periods of time, and wearing close-fitting briefs should be avoided. The effects of chemical exposures on fertility are not fully understood.

Specific Components of the Infertility History

Regular menses occurring every 21 to 35 days, with no more than 1 week's variation from cycle to cycle, is usually associated with ovulatory cycles. Premenstrual symptoms such as bloating, breast tenderness, and cramping with menstrual bleeding are also consistent with an ovulatory cycle. Irregular menses, or uterine bleeding occurring more frequently than every 21 days or less frequently than every 35 days, is associated with irregular ovulation (oligo-ovulation) or absent ovulation (anovulation).

A history of pelvic or abdominal infection such as a ruptured appendix, pelvic inflammatory disease, or Crohn's disease and a history of gonorrheal or chlamydial cervicitis or use of an intrauterine device all are risk factors for scarring and blockage of the fallopian tubes. Pelvic pain, especially in combination with uterine cramping (dysmenorrhea) of recent onset, suggests the presence of endometriosis. This can lead to infertility by inciting peritoneal fibrosis involving the ovaries and fallopian tubes, and immunologic mechanisms have been implicated as well.[21, 22]

Hormonal and metabolic abnormalities are also implicated in infertility. Subclinical hypothyroidism has been linked to menstrual irregularity and delayed endometrial maturation (luteal phase defect).[23] Milky or clear to greenish nipple discharge may represent hyperprolactinemia, which may lead to a luteal phase defect, irregular menses and ovulation, or complete anovulation and amenorrhea. Complete amenorrhea in the absence of pregnancy or recent uterine surgery suggests anovulation. Hot flashes, vaginal dryness, or dysuria may reflect hypoestrogenism and premature menopause. Increasing facial and body hair growth may signify androgen-producing tumors, adult-onset congenital adrenal hyperplasia, Cushing's disease, or chronic anovulation consistent with polycystic ovary syndrome. Systemic illness, physical stress such as that associated with intensive athletic training, and even emotional stress can cause hypothalamic dysfunction, which is manifested by anovulation with irregular or absent menses.

A history of cervical cone biopsy, laser therapy, or cryotherapy for cervical dysplasia may implicate deficient or abnormal cervical mucus production as an infertility factor. A history of prenatal exposure to diethylstilbestrol (DES) is associated with congenital cervical as well as uterine anomalies.

Men should be asked about a history of mumps, which can be complicated by orchitis and azoospermia (absent sperm production); hernia repair; bladder surgery; testicular trauma, which can interrupt testicular blood supply; and testicular pain, which may denote the presence of epididymitis or orchitis. Sexual function should be addressed. Difficulty obtaining or maintaining an erection and lack of ejaculation or difficulty ejaculating may reflect physiologic or psychological problems that warrant the attention of specialists. It may be difficult for a couple to assess ejaculate volume, but the presence of only a small amount of fluid after ejaculation may suggest retrograde ejaculation, which may be associated with the autonomic neuropathy of diabetes mellitus, surgical procedures, or the use of certain medications.

Physical Examination

Women

Thyromegaly may imply the presence of thyroid dysfunction. Hirsutism, or terminal hair growth on the chin, neck, upper lip, cheeks, sternum, back, or buttocks, is often associated with anovulation and irregular or absent menses. Acanthosis nigricans, which manifests with dark, thickened skin on the back of the neck and over the joints, is associated with insulin resistance, anovulation, and high serum androgen levels (a syndrome of hyperandrogenism, insulin resistance, and acanthosis nigricans).[24] Bilateral clear or milky nipple discharge (i.e., galactorrhea) in a woman who has never delivered a baby may be associated with an elevated serum prolactin level and oligo-ovulation or anovulation. A very short cervix may be associated with prior surgery or with maternal DES exposure. Exposure to DES may also cause an extra peak of tissue on the dorsal surface of the cervix, called a coxcomb, or it may cause a cervical hood, a fold of tissue in the same location. A hypoplastic uterus that is almost nonpalpable on bimanual examination might also increase suspicions about prenatal DES exposure. A large or irregularly shaped uterus suggests fibroids and may be associated with heavy or prolonged menstrual periods (menorrhagia). A uterus that is tender, fixed, and retroverted may reflect pelvic scarring secondary to endometriosis. Retroversion alone is not an abnormal finding and is not an infertility factor. Enlarged or unusually tender ovaries may signal ovarian cysts or endometriosis in women with dysmenorrhea and infertility. Suspicion of fibroids or ovarian masses should be confirmed by ultrasonography.

Men

If findings on the history and subsequent semen analysis are normal, it is unnecessary to examine the man specifically for the purpose of elucidating the cause of infertility. If results of the semen analysis are abnormal, the examination should focus on the presence of secondary sexual characteristics, testicular size and consistency, and the presence of a varicocele.

MAKING A DIAGNOSIS

Hormonal Evaluation

Women with irregular or absent menses have ovulatory dysfunction. A normal premenopausal serum follicle-stimulating hormone (FSH) level precludes premature ovarian failure (menopause). Similarly, normal serum thyroid-stimulating hormone and prolactin levels preclude thyroid disease and the presence of hyperprolactinemia, respectively. Mild hyperprolactinemia may be secondary to hypothyroidism and corrects with thyroid hormone replacement. Adrenal disease is a less common cause of ovulatory dysfunction. An elevated serum level of 17-hydroxyprogesterone suggests adult-onset 21-hydroxylase deficiency (congenital adrenal hyperplasia). Elevated dehydroepiandrosterone sulfate levels may signal an adrenal tumor. So-called polycystic ovarian disease or chronic oligo-ovulation or anovulation may occur in women who may or may not have characteristic obesity, hirsutism, acne, and the pathognomonic polycystic ovarian appearance on ultrasonography, which consists of numerous small cysts in the periphery of both ovaries. Serum levels of testosterone and dehydroepiandrosterone sulfate may be mildly elevated in polycystic ovarian syndrome. If results of pituitary hormone testing are normal in an amenorrheic woman, hypothalamic dysfunction with disordered pituitary stimulation is a diagnosis of exclusion. In general, women with irregular or absent menses require hormonal manipulation and

should be referred to a specialist with expertise in infertility.

Documentation of Ovulation

In normally menstruating women, basal body temperature charts are a noninvasive, inexpensive way to gain more information about their cycles. A woman must take her temperature before getting out of bed in the morning, because any exercise may elevate her temperature. A regular oral thermometer is perfectly acceptable, but some women may find a basal body temperature thermometer easier to use because it has wide separation in the markings; the thermometer registers a narrow range. The temperature should be plotted on a graph, starting with the first day after the end of the menstrual period (Fig. 28–1). A dip in temperature may occur at the time of the luteinizing hormone (LH) surge. A persistent temperature rise of at least 0.4°F implies that ovulation has occurred. Ovulation occurs during the temperature rise; however, the basal body temperature chart is able to predict ovulation within only 2 to 3 days.[25] The temperature elevation is due to the thermogenic effects of progesterone produced by the ovary after ovulation on the central nervous system. The postovulatory portion of the menstrual cycle is called the luteal phase. The temperature elevation should persist for at least 11 days before the onset of the next menstrual period. Temperature then falls, paralleling declining progesterone levels. The normal temperature rise is called a biphasic response. The lack of a temperature elevation may represent absent ovulation; however, monophasic temperature charts can occur during ovulatory cycles. A fall in temperature before 11 days (a short luteal phase) may signal a luteal phase defect, with subnormal progesterone production from the corpus luteum. The significance of luteal phase defect is that theoretically the endometrium may not be sufficiently developed to support embryo implantation and growth.

For women with irregularly biphasic temperature charts or those with monophasic charts, a serum progesterone level obtained after ovulation can confirm the presence or absence of ovulation. Progesterone levels peak approximately 7 days after ovulation (the midluteal phase). A progesterone level of 10 ng per ml suggests adequate progesterone production from the corpus luteum, the site in the ovary from which ovulation occurred.[26] A biphasic basal body temperature chart and even a serum progesterone level of 10 ng per ml do not necessarily mean that endometrial development is adequate.[27] If abnormalities in ovulation testing are

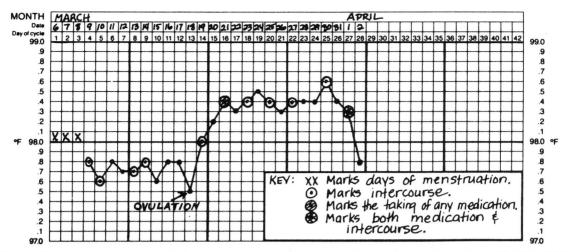

Figure 28–1. A sample basal body temperature chart. (Courtesy of Serono Laboratories, Inc., 100 Longwater Circle, Norwell, Mass. 02061.)

found, such as a luteal phase of less than 11 days or a low midluteal progesterone level, an endometrial biopsy should be performed. An endometrial biopsy specimen reveals the effect of progesterone on the endometrium and is the gold standard for the diagnosis of luteal phase defect.

Ovulation may also be documented by commercially available urine LH testing. The midcycle surge of pituitary LH is the impetus for ovulation and is detectable in the urine. Kits are relatively expensive, with 5 to 6 days of testing (one menstrual cycle) costing $15 to $30. They are less practical to use in women with irregular cycles, because several kits would be needed. Rapid serum LH testing with same-day results is available in many hospitals with infertility practices. The testing is expensive and is best used in conjunction with fertility therapies rather than merely to confirm ovulation. Daily ultrasonography in the follicular phase of the menstrual cycle can be used to monitor the development of a dominant (preovulatory) follicle but is extremely expensive ($150–$250 per study). It is used with infertility therapies when ovulation is induced with medication and monitoring follicular development is necessary.

Cervical Factor Infertility

Cervical factor infertility refers to an abnormal sperm-cervical mucus interaction. The postcoital test is a commonly performed but controversial test that assesses this interaction. The couple is instructed to abstain from intercourse (and the man should not ejaculate) for 48 hours before ovulation, with the timing of ovulation estimated by basal body temperature charting or urine LH testing. Abstaining for 5 days or more may decrease sperm parameters. The couple should have intercourse 2 to 12 hours before the scheduled postcoital test.

The postcoital test is performed by aspiration of cervical mucus from within the endocervical canal, often with an angiocatheter attached to a syringe. The mucus should be copious and clear. It should be capable of being stretched to at least 8 cm. Some of the mucus is ejected onto a microscope slide, and a portion of this is allowed to air-dry. A cover slip is placed on the remainder, and this portion is immediately inspected under the microscope and should not contain squamous cells, white blood cells, or bacteria. At least five sperm per high-power field should be seen to be actively moving forward. The number of motile sperm that constitutes a normal test result is extremely controversial, and even one motile sperm present in all high-power fields may be adequate.[28, 29] The air-dried portion should show ferning (Fig. 28–2A). Ferning is caused by crystallization of sodium chloride in the cervical mucus and is an effect of estrogen on cervical mucus. Cloudy or gummy cellular cervical mucus may be due to incorrect timing or cervicitis (Fig. 28–2B). A small amount of mucus may be due to incorrect timing or inadequate capacity of the cervix to produce mucus due to prior cervical surgery or an unexplained deficiency. Sperm shaking in place in the presence of good quality cervical mucus may signal the presence of antisperm antibodies in the semen, cer-

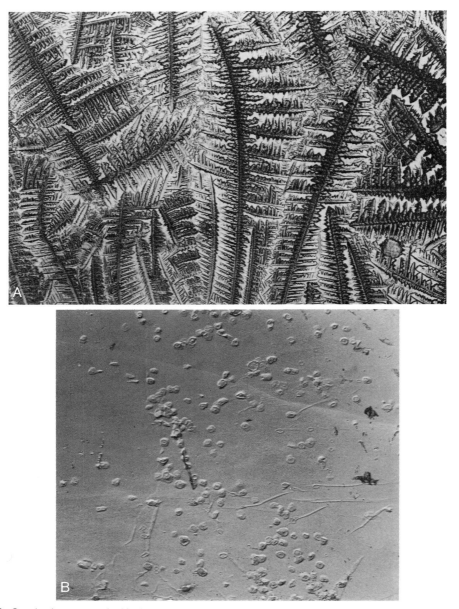

Figure 28–2. Cervical mucus, air-dried on a slide in the postcoital test. *A,* Ferning occurs in clear, acellular cervical mucus. *B,* Ferning is absent in thick or cellular cervical mucus.

vical mucus, or serum of the woman. Poorly motile or nonmotile sperm with good quality cervical mucus may represent poor sperm quality. Low numbers of sperm or absent sperm may imply low sperm counts, poor coital technique, or an excessively long period of time since coitus. In some cases, a poor postcoital test result remains unexplained. If the postcoital test result is abnormal on two occasions, the couple should be referred for further evaluation and therapy.

The cross-mucus test is an in vitro postcoital test using normal donor mucus with sperm from the male partner. This commercially available test can help identify whether poor or absent motility seen in vivo is due to abnormalities within the woman's mucus. A normal cross-mucus test result would signify that sperm function was normal and that the female partner had either poor quality cervical mucus or possibly antisperm antibodies.

Male Factor Infertility

Approximately 40% of infertility is due to abnormal semen parameters. The semen analysis is the primary test of male factor infertility. Semen samples should be produced by masturbation after 48 hours of abstinence, because more frequent ejaculation is associated with decreased semen parameters.[14] Normal values are listed in Table 28–2. A decreased volume, count, motility, or morphology warrants at least two repeat semen analyses to confirm a diagnosis of male factor infertility. A varicocele, which is a dilated testicular vein, is often associated with decreased sperm numbers (oligospermia), motility (asthenospermia), and morphology (teratospermia). Decreased sperm numbers may also be due to pituitary insufficiency with concomitantly decreased testosterone levels. An increase in the number of round cells (which represent immature sperm forms) and white blood cells may denote abnormal spermatogenesis or infection and is also an indication for repeat semen analysis.

The hamster egg penetration test is a test of fertilizing capacity. The percentage of hamster eggs penetrated by the male partner's sperm is compared with that of the fertile control sperm. At least 10% of the eggs should be penetrated.[30] The test is of limited use, because men whose sperm successfully fertilize human oocytes during in vitro fertilization may have abnormal hamster egg penetration results.[31] Referral to an infertility service is recommended for evaluation of male factor infertility.

Evaluation of Tubal Disease

Chlamydial infection is the most common sexually transmitted disease in the United States. It is also often silent and can cause pelvic inflammation with subsequent damage to the fallopian tubes without recognized symptoms.[32] Screening for chlamydial infection may have a role in infertile patients.[33] The initial infertility evaluation includes evaluation of tubal patency with a hysterosalpingogram. The patient lies in the lithotomy position, the cervix is visualized with a speculum, and a catheter or cannula is inserted into the cervix. The radiologist or gynecologist then injects radiopaque dye, and the internal contour of the uterus and fallopian tubes is seen. Free spill of dye into the peritoneal cavity denotes tubal patency. An abnormal internal uterine contour should be evaluated by a gynecologist hysteroscopically, and obstructed tubes should be evaluated by laparoscopy.

Additional Testing

When embarking on an infertility evaluation, it is prudent to ascertain whether the couple is at risk for transmitting common genetic diseases to their children. Screening for Tay-Sachs disease in a couple of Eastern European Jewish descent, sickle trait in black partners, and so forth is best performed at the outset. Immunity to rubella should also be ascertained early in the evaluation. Rubella vaccination should be discussed with the couple, with the understanding that birth control should be used for 3 months after vaccination to prevent infection in a fetus should pregnancy occur.

THERAPY

Therapy of infertility is based on the cause. Ovulatory defects are treated with clomiphene citrate or human menopausal gonadotropins. Luteal phase defect may be treated with clomiphene citrate during cycle days 5 to 9. Clomiphene citrate enhances follicular development and increases follicular progesterone production. Alternatively, progesterone vaginal suppositories may be used in the luteal phase of the cycle. Intrauterine inseminations are used for male factor, cervical factor, and unexplained infertility. Intrauterine insemination of washed sperm at the time of ovulation bypasses the cervical mucus and therefore places more sperm in closer proximity to the oocyte. Sperm must be washed to avoid an anaphylactoid reaction that can result from intrauterine placement of unwashed sperm containing prostaglandin-rich prostatic fluid. Intrauterine insemination has been shown to increase pregnancy rates in some[34] but not all studies,[35] and there is little consensus on its efficacy.[36] Intracervical insemination of the male partner's sperm does not enhance the chance of pregnancy.[37] The addition of ovarian stimulation

TABLE 28–2. Normal Semen Parameters

Volume	2–5 ml
pH	7.2–7.8
Fructose	Present
Viscosity	Nonviscous
Agglutination	None
Round cells/ml	Normal range not established
Sperm/ml	20–500 million/ml
Sperm motility	50–100%
Sperm velocity	Normal range not established (u/sec)
Linearity	Normal range not established (index/%)
Sperm morphology	50–100%

has been shown to increase pregnancy rates in combination with intrauterine insemination.[38]

In vitro fertilization (IVF) yields the highest pregnancy rates per cycle of therapy. In standard IVF, a woman is treated with human menopausal gonadotropins, which are LH and FSH, by daily intramuscular injections to stimulate the development and maturation of multiple oocytes within the ovaries. Many IVF programs also use subcutaneous gonadotropin-releasing hormone agonist therapy to improve control over the ovarian stimulation and to obtain greater oocyte numbers and quality. The development of the oocytes is monitored by ultrasonography and serum estradiol levels. Monitoring also helps avoid overstimulation of the ovaries (hyperstimulation). When the oocytes are mature but before ovulation, they are aspirated from a woman's ovaries using a transvaginally ultrasonographically guided needle. Each oocyte is inseminated with approximately 50,000 sperm in specially prepared media. Approximately 48 hours after insemination, three to five resulting embryos are returned to the endometrial cavity via a thin, flexible transfer catheter, which is passed through the cervical os. Excess embryos can be frozen for future use. Using fresh embryos, the clinical pregnancy rate varies from 15 to 25% per cycle, depending on the IVF program and patient population. Micromanipulation is an exciting development in IVF, involving placement of sperm inside the outer covering of the oocyte. Micromanipulation can result in successful fertilization in cases of extremely severe male factor infertility, in which standard IVF is unsuccessful or imprudent. Multiple birth rates from IVF vary widely in different programs but are in the range of 15 to 35%. Unfortunately, IVF is extremely time-consuming, inconvenient for patients, and expensive. A single cycle of standard IVF, from initiation of therapy to embryo transfer, costs from $10,000 to $12,000. The emotional price can also be very high because for most couples, IVF is the last chance of achieving a successful pregnancy.[39]

Ovulatory Defects

If oligo-ovulation or anovulation is diagnosed in a woman who is not hypoestrogenic, clomiphene citrate is the first therapy used to induce ovulation. It is administered orally for 5 days during the early part of the menstrual cycle. In anovulatory women, it is administered after progesterone-induced withdrawal bleeding. It works at the level of the hypothalamus and pituitary, increasing pituitary FSH production and thereby stimulating the ovaries. The dose is increased until ovulation occurs with

each cycle or a pregnancy results. If a woman has been found to have elevated adrenal androgens, glucocorticoids may be used in conjunction with clomiphene citrate.[40] Glucocorticoids alone may induce ovulation in women with adult-onset congenital adrenal hyperplasia. If ovulation does not occur on the maximum dose of clomiphene, human menopausal gonadotropins (LH and FSH) are used to stimulate ovarian oocyte development directly. In women with hypothalamic amenorrhea, intravenous gonadotropin-releasing hormone may be given through a pump, bypassing the abnormal hypothalamic output and stimulating endogenous pituitary LH and FSH production and secretion. If anovulation is due to premature menopause, there are no viable oocytes within the ovaries and ovulation induction is not possible. Oocyte donation is the only option in this situation. In this procedure, oocytes from another woman are combined with sperm from the male partner, and resulting embryos are transferred back into the infertile woman's uterus. The baby will be hers by gestation but genetically related to the male partner only.

Male Factor

Male factor infertility remains the most difficult infertility problem to treat. Daily treatment of an infertile man with clomiphene citrate therapy for a minimum of 3 months—the time that sperm require for development—has been used. However, its benefit in improving sperm parameters is unclear.[41] For a man with a varicocele, surgical correction may be indicated. Semen parameters have been reported to improve in approximately 70 to 80% of men treated.[42] No randomized trials have been performed, and it is controversial whether pregnancy rates improve after varicocele repair. Intrauterine inseminations, with or without ovarian hyperstimulation, and IVF are also used to treat male factor infertility.

Artificial insemination with donor sperm may be performed in cases of severe male factor infertility when IVF fails or is not undertaken. Fresh sperm is no longer used for insemination owing to the risks of acquired immunodeficiency syndrome and other sexually transmitted diseases. Many commercial sperm banks screen potential donors for sexually transmitted and inheritable diseases. After collection, sperm samples are frozen and then stored for 6 months, and the donor is then retested for sexually transmitted diseases. Couples select their donor, who remains anonymous, from a catalog that details the donor's physical characteristics, ethnic background, profession, and interests. Intracervical or intrauterine inseminations every 1 to 2 days are performed around the time of ovulation. Pregnancy takes longer to occur with frozen than with fresh sperm, and most women who conceive do so within 12 months.

Cervical Factor

Cervical factor infertility is relatively uncommon, responsible for approximately 5% of infertility in the United States. Estrogen administration for approximately 7 days before ovulation can be attempted to stimulate cervical mucus production, but this depends on the presence of functional endocervical glands. A trial of guaifenesin, the mucolytic component of cough syrups, can be tried if mucus is thick and acellular. Intrauterine insemination of washed sperm bypasses the abnormal or deficient cervical mucus. If results of antisperm antibody testing are positive, implying that the cause of the poor postcoital test results is immunologic, intrauterine inseminations of the male partner's sperm is undertaken.[43] In vitro fertilization is most successful in this group of patients.

Tubal Disease

Depending on the site of tubal occlusion, as documented by a hysterosalpingogram, surgery may result in tubal patency and pregnancy in as many as 80% of women.[44] If the tubal blockage is in the proximal end of the fallopian tube, pregnancy rates are lower. Blockage in two separate sites in the same tube is a relative contraindication to reparative surgery. Depending on the extent and type of tubal disease and the preference and expertise of the gynecologic surgeon, surgery can be performed by laparotomy or laparoscopy. If the occlusion is secondary to a prior tubal ligation, a basic infertility evaluation including evaluation of the male partner is still indicated. Repair is generally carried out using microscopic technique during laparotomy, with ensuing pregnancy rates of 20 to 80%, depending on the length and condition of the remaining fallopian tube. If tubal surgery fails to produce pregnancy within a year or if it is not undertaken owing to the extensive nature of the tubal disease, IVF is the next step and is very successful in this group of patients.

Endometriosis

Endometriosis is generally treated by either electrocautery or laser ablation at the time of diagnosis, during either laparoscopy or laparotomy. If disease is diffuse, with widespread speckling of the peritoneum or bowel, medical therapy for residual disease is begun postoperatively. Gonadotropin-releasing hormone agonists work by inhibiting pulsatile gonadotropin-releasing hormone output from the hypothalamus, thus preventing ovulation and inducing a hypoestrogenic state that withdraws estrogenic support from the endometriotic implants. Danazol is a synthetic androgenic hormonal compound that causes atrophy of endometrial implants. Medical therapy is equally successful with both types of medication and is given for 6 months[45] (see Chapter 8).

Unexplained Infertility

Several therapies are available for the 15 to 20% of couples in whom infertility remains unexplained. The least time-consuming and expensive is clomiphene citrate in conjunction with intrauterine insemination of the man's sperm. One randomized trial showed pregnancy rates of 9.5% per cycle, compared with 3.3% in untreated couples.[46] Human menopausal gonadotropins can be administered, often in conjunction with intrauterine insemination. Pregnancy rates of 19[47] to 26%[48] per cycle of therapy have been reported. If these therapies are unsuccessful, human menopausal gonadotropin therapy combined with oocyte retrieval and then laparoscopic replacement of oocytes and sperm into the fallopian tubes (gamete intrafallopian transfer, or GIFT) is often the next recommended procedure. Gamete intrafallopian transfer is very successful in patients with unexplained infertility, with pregnancy rates of approximately 30% per cycle. In selected cases, zygote intrafallopian transfer may be recommended. In this method, standard IVF is performed but embryos are transferred into the fallopian tubes instead of the uterus approximately 48 hours after oocyte retrieval. The intratubal transfer is performed laparoscopically, under general endotracheal anesthesia. The disadvantage of zygote intrafallopian transfer as compared with gamete intrafallopian transfer is the need for additional laboratory facilities for embryo culture and a second anesthetic for embryo transfer. The clinical pregnancy rate of the two techniques is equivalent.

SPECIAL CONSIDERATIONS

Psychology of Infertile Couples

Infertility inflicts tremendous stress on virtually all couples. Sexual intercourse becomes an act of necessity, and when infertility persists, intercourse becomes associated with feelings of stress and failure.[49] Women dread their menses, often becoming very tearful and angry with each menstrual period. They may find themselves avoiding friends or relatives who are pregnant or who have young children because of intense feelings of jealousy, sorrow, and frustration. Although women tend to have more social supports, they experience more stress than men during IVF.[50] This finding is not surprising in light of the fact that the woman undergoes the physical stresses in the majority of infertility therapies even when the underlying problem is male factor infertility. It is helpful to discuss available psychological supports, whether that support comes from friends, family, or local counseling services. This helps the couple realize that their problem is common and that psychological stress commonly accompanies infertility. RE-SOLVE, Inc. (1310 Broadway, Somerville, MA, 02144; [617] 623-1156), is a national support group that many couples find useful. The RE-SOLVE network can facilitate telephone contact with other infertile couples for patients living in relatively remote areas. Most important, the physician should acknowledge verbally the stresses infertility imposes and remain as available as possible for emotional support as well as medical advice.

Adoption is an issue the physician should mention as a routine part of a discussion of infertility. For many couples, having an overall plan in mind can be comforting, and having their names on an adoption list may act as a safety net, decreasing their feelings of anxiety. Other couples are not comfortable with adoption and may not wish to discuss it. If either member of the couple is older than 45 years, adoption may be difficult because of age requirements of adoption agencies. As the work-up progresses, identifying a problem may relieve some anxiety by giving the couple a physiologic reason for their infertility. They can then have some control over their situation by deciding what course of action they want to pursue, whether it is therapy, nonintervention, or adoption.

MYTHS

It is important to dispel myths. Couples are often concerned that anxiety about their infertility is preventing conception. To produce infertility, psychological stress would have to be severe enough to inhibit ovulation in the woman or erection or ejaculation in the man, and this is almost never encountered. Some studies do show that semen parameters are worsened by stress; however,

no studies to date have proved that emotional stress can cause infertility.[51] Many women with secondary infertility after a therapeutic abortion fear that their infertility is punishment. However, uncomplicated therapeutic abortion is not associated with infertility.[52]

AGE AS A FACTOR IN INFERTILITY

Fecundity declines with increasing age, with the most rapid decline occurring after age 35 years. A woman in her late thirties may take longer to conceive in the absence of diagnosed infertiltiy factors, presumably because of the age of her oocytes, because fertility declines with increasing age.[4]

If a woman is in her thirties, especially if she is older than 35 years, it is appropriate to complete the infertility evaluation as rapidly as possible. Referral to a gynecologist who is interested and experienced in infertility diagnosis and treatment is appropriate in areas where such services are available. The initial evaluation, including semen analysis, documentation of ovulation, hormonal testing, postcoital test, and test of tubal patency, can be completed during two menstrual cycles. An outline of the evaluation can be presented to the couple during the initial visit. Giving patients control over the sequence and pace of the evaluation is helpful in easing their feelings of frustration and helplessness.

PROGNOSIS

Success in the treatment of infertility depends on its duration, diagnosis, the woman's age, and what therapies the couple is willing or able to undergo. Overall, 35% of couples undergoing therapy for infertility ultimately conceive independently of therapy and 41% conceive after therapy.[53] A physician's guidance and support help them identify the causes of their infertility, guide them toward appropriate specialists and therapy, and ultimately help them achieve a pregnancy.

REFERENCES

1. Greenhall E, Vessey M. The prevalence of subfertility: A review of the current confusion and a report of two new studies. Fertil Steril 1990;54:978.
2. Mosher W, Pratt W. Fecundity and infertility in the United States, 1965–1988. Advance data from vital and health statistics. Hyattsville, Md: National Center for Health Statistics, No. 192, December 4, 1990.
3. Mosher W, Pratt W. Fecundity and infertility in the United States: Incidence and trends. Fertil Steril 1991;56:192.
4. Stovall DW, Toma SK, Hammond MG, Talbert LM. The

effect of age on female fecundity. Obstet Gynecol 1991;77:33.

5. Howe G, Westhoff C, Vessey M, Yeates D. Effects of age, cigarette smoking and other factors on fertility: Findings of a large prospective study. Br Med J (Clin Res Ed) 1985;290:1697.

6. Mosher WD, Aral SO. Factors related to infertility in the United States, 1965–1976. Sex Transm Dis 1985;12:117.

7. Guttmacher AF. Factors affecting normal expectancy of conception. JAMA 1956;161:855.

8. Simpson JL, Golbus MS, Martin JR, et al (eds). Genetics in Obstetrics and Gynecology. New York: Grune & Stratton, 1982, p 58.

9. Matsunaga E, Tonamura A, Oishi H, et al. Reexamination of paternal age effect in Down's syndrome. Hum Genet 1978;40:259.

10. Stene J, Fischer G, Stene E, et al. Paternal age effect in Down's syndrome. Ann Hum Genet 1977;40:299.

11. Barnea ER, Holford TR, McInnes DRA. Long-term prognosis of infertile couples with normal basic investigations: A life-table analysis. Obstet Gynecol 1985;66:24.

12. Hanson FW, Overstreet JW, Katz DF. A study of the relationship of motile sperm numbers in cervical mucus 48 hours after artificial insemination with subsequent fertility. Am J Obstet Gynecol 1982;143:85.

13. Oehninger S, Acosta AA, Veeck LL, et al. Delayed fertilization during in vitro fertilization and embryo transfer cycles: Analysis of causes and impact on overall results. Fertil Steril 1989;52:991.

14. Hornstein MD, Cohen JN, Thomas PP, et al. The effect of consecutive day inseminations on semen characteristics in an intrauterine insemination program. Fertil Steril 1992; 58:433.

15. Goldenberg RL, White R. The effect of vaginal lubricants on sperm motility in vitro. Fertil Steril 1975;26:872.

16. Cramer DW, Schiff I, Schoenbaum SC, et al. Tubal infertility and the intrauterine device. N Engl J Med 1985; 312:937.

17. Abramowitz M (ed). Drugs that cause sexual dysfunction: An update. The Medical Letter 1992;34:73.

18. Speroff L, Glass RH, Kase NG (eds). Male Infertility in Clinical Gynecologic Endocrinology and Infertility. 4th ed. Baltimore: Williams & Wilkins, 1989, p 569.

19. Laurent SL, Thompson SJ, Addy S, et al. An epidemiologic study of smoking and primary infertility in women. Fertil Steril 1992;57:565.

20. Asch P. The influence of radiation on fertility in man. Br J Radiol 1980;53:271.

21. Meek SC, Hodge DD, Musich JR. Autoimmunity in infertile patients with endometriosis. Am J Obstet Gynecol 1988;158:1365.

22. Osterlynck DJ, Meuleman C, Waer M, et al. The natural killer activity of peritoneal fluid lymphocytes is decreased in women with endometriosis. Fertil Steril 1992;58:290.

23. Gerhard I, Becker T, Eggert-Kruse W, et al. Thyroid and ovarian function in subfertile women. Hum Reprod 1991;6:338.

24. Barbieri RL, Ryan KJ. Hyperandrogenism, insulin resistance and acanthosis nigricans syndrome: A common endocrinopathy with distinct pathophysiologic features. Am J Obstet Gynecol 1983;147:90.

25. Quagliarello J, Arny M. Inaccuracy of basal body temperature charts in predicting urinary luteinizing hormone surges. Fertil Steril 1986;45:334.

26. Hull MGR, Savage PE, Bromham DR, et al. The value of a single progesterone measurement in the midluteal phase as a criterion of a potentially fertile cycle (''ovulation'') derived from treated and untreated conception cycles. Fertil Steril 1982;37:355.

27. Shoupe D, Mishell DR, LaCarra M, et al. Correlation of endometrial maturation with four methods of estimating day of ovulation. Obstet Gynecol 1989;73:88.

28. Quagliarello J, Arny M. Intracervical versus intrauterine insemination: Correlation of outcome with antecedent postcoital testing. Fertil Steril 1986;46:870.

29. Collins JA, So Y, Wilson EH, et al. The postcoital test as a predictor of infertility among 355 infertile couples. Fertil Steril 1984;41:703.

30. Rogers BJ. The sperm penetration assay: Its usefulness reevaluated. Fertil Steril 1985;43:821.

31. Margalioth EJ, Navot D, Laufer N, et al. Zona-free hamster ovum penetration assay as a screening procedure for in vitro fertilization. Fertil Steril 1983;40:386.

32. Mardh PA. An overview of infectious agents of salpingitis, their biology, and recent advances in methods of detection. Am J Obstet Gynecol 1980;138:933.

33. Hodgson R, Driscoll GL, Dodd JK, et al. *Chlamydia trachomatis*: The prevalence, trend and importance in initial infertility management. Aust N Z J Obstet Gynecol 1990;30:251.

34. Kerin JFP, Kirby C, Peek J, et al. Improved conception rate after intrauterine insemination of washed spermatozoa from men with poor quality semen. Lancet 1984;1:533.

35. te Velde ER, van Kooy RJ, Waterreus JJH. Intrauterine insemination of washed husband's spermatozoa: A controlled study. Fertil Steril 1989;51:182.

36. Speroff L, Glass RH, Kase NG (eds). Male Infertility in Clinical Gynecologic Endocrinology and Infertility. 4th ed. Baltimore: Williams & Wilkins, 1989, pp 574–576.

37. Nachtigall RD. Indications, techniques and success rates for AIH. Seminars Reprod Endocrinol 1987;5:5.

38. Sigman M, Vance ML. Medical treatment of idiopathic infertility. Urol Clin North Am 1987;14:459.

39. Collins A, Freeman EW, Boxer AS, Tureck R. Perceptions of infertility and treatment stress in females as compared with males entering in vitro fertilization treatment. Fertil Steril 1992;57:350.

40. Daly DC, Walters CA, Soto-Albors CE, et al. A randomized study of dexamethasone in ovulation induction with clomiphene citrate. Fertil Steril 1984;41:844.

41. World Health Organization. A double-blind trial of clomiphene citrate for the treatment of idiopathic male infertility. Int J Androl 1992;15:299.

42. Dhabuwala CB, Hamid S, Moghissi KS. Clinical versus subclinical varicocele: Improvement in fertility after varicocelectomy. Fertil Steril 1992;54:854.

43. Gregoriou O, Vitoratos N, Papadias C, et al. Intrauterine insemination as a treatment of infertility in women with antisperm antibodies. Int J Gynecol Obstet 1991;35:151.

44. Schlaff WD, Hassiakos DK, Damewood MD, Rock JA. Neosalpingostomy for distal tubal obstruction: Prognostic factors and impact of surgical technique. Fertil Steril 1990;54:984.

45. The Nafarelin European Endometriosis Trial Group. Nafarelin for endometriosis: A large scale, danazol-controlled trial of efficacy and safety, with 1-year followup. Fertil Steril 1992;57:514.

46. Deaton JL, Gibson M, Blackmer KM, et al. A randomized, controlled trial of clomiphene citrate and intrauterine insemination in couples with unexplained infertility or surgically corrected endometriosis. Fertil Steril 1990;54:1083.

47. Dodson WC, Whitesides DB, Hughes CL, et al. Superovulation with intrauterine insemination in the treatment of infertility: A possible alternative to gamete intrafallopian transfer and in vitro fertilization. Fertil Steril 1987;48:441.

48. Serhal PF, Katz M, Little V, Woronowski H. Unexplained infertility—The value of pergonal superovulation combined with intrauterine insemination. Fertil Steril 1988; 49:602.

49. Mahlstedt PP. The psychological component of infertility. Fertil Steril 1985;43:335.
50. Collins A, Freeman EW, Boxer AS, Tureck R. Perceptions of infertility and treatment stress in females as compared with males entering in vitro fertilization treatment. Fertil Steril 1992;57:350.
51. Wright J, Allard M, Lecours A, Sabourin S. Psychosocial distress and infertility: A review of controlled research. Int J Fertil 1989;34:126.
52. Daling JR, Weiss NS, Voight L, et al. Fertil Steril 1985;43:389.
53. Collins JA, Wrixon W, Janes LB, Wilson EH. Treatment-independent pregnancy among infertile couples. N Engl J Med 1983;309:1201.

Spontaneous and Recurrent Abortion

Angela Palumbo and Elizabeth S. Ginsburg

INCIDENCE OF SPONTANEOUS ABORTION

Spontaneous abortion is a relatively frequent event, occurring in as many as 30 to 50% of all conceptions.[1] In many cases, the pregnancy loss occurs before the time of the expected menses, and thus it is not recognized clinically and is interpreted as a late menstrual period. The rate of clinically recognized spontaneous abortion is in the range of 10 to 15%.[2] The rate of recurrent abortion is more difficult to assess. According to one study,[3] the risk of repetitive abortion is 24%, 26%, and 32% after one, two, and three consecutive abortions, respectively.

DEFINITION OF SPONTANEOUS ABORTION

In the majority of cases, spontaneous abortions are sporadic, isolated events in the reproductive history of a couple and are followed by successful pregnancies. However, the incidence of spontaneous abortion does increase progressively after one or more abortions, and in some couples spontaneous abortions occur repetitively. Recurrent or habitual abortion is defined as the occurrence of three or more pregnancy losses before the twentieth week of gestation. Recurrent abortion affects 1 to 3% of couples.[2, 3] According to Poland and colleagues, the incidence of recurrence is 19% after one spontaneous abortion and 47% after three spontaneous abortions,[4] suggesting that it may be worthwhile to start investigating for the cause of recurrent abortion after the second miscarriage.

MANIFESTATION OF SPONTANEOUS ABORTION

Spontaneous abortion usually manifests with vaginal bleeding and uterine cramping, followed by passage of fetal and placental tissue. When the pregnancy loss occurs in the first 2 or 3 weeks after conception, the miscarriage may remain undiagnosed because the menstrual period is not missed. In this scenario, the bleeding with associated cramping might be more severe and a serum pregnancy test (β-human chorionic gonadotropin [β-hCG]) would be positive.

Threatened abortion is diagnosed when bleeding during early pregnancy occurs without cervical dilation. Cramps are usually mild or absent. When the cervical os dilates, abortion is inevitable: The cramping and bleeding increase, and clots are usually passed. With further progression, the cramps become more severe and the bleeding becomes heavier and is accompanied by passage of tissue, which appears gray-white. Incomplete abortion occurs when the uterus does not expel all of the products of conception and is associated with prolonged cramping and bleeding. In some cases, most commonly between the fourth and eighth week of gestation, all of the uterine contents are eventually expelled. After what a patient usually describes as an episode of heavy bleeding with passage of tissue and severe cramping, the bleeding and cramping subside, and the abortion is complete. In incomplete abortions, the cervix may remain open, leading to an increased risk of uterine infection. Less commonly, in the second trimester of pregnancy, a patient may experience watery vaginal discharge that is followed by cramping and then delivery of the fetus. In this type of miscarriage, painless cervical dilation occurs.

ACUTE EVALUATION OF SPONTANEOUS ABORTION

Vaginal bleeding during pregnancy is always an anxiety-provoking event, particularly for patients who have had previous miscarriages and who may recognize the symptoms and anticipate the outcome. In this situation, it is extremely important for a physician to provide psychological support as well as medical care.

History

When a patient first presents with vaginal bleeding, it is important to ask the date of the last normal period as well as the date of the first positive pregnancy test, whether the patient has started prenatal care, and whether ultrasonography has confirmed an intrauterine pregnancy. The most important differential diagnosis is between threatened abortion and ectopic pregnancy. In some cases, patients have to be carefully monitored for several days with serial β-hCG measurements and ultrasonography before a definite diagnosis can be made.

The history should include the gravidity (number of pregnancies), parity (number of prior deliveries of at least 20 weeks' gestation), previous spontaneous or therapeutic abortions, or ectopic pregnancies. Risk factors for ectopic gestations, such as a history of pelvic inflammatory disease, pelvic surgery, or prior use of an intrauterine device, are also important.

Physical Examination

At the time of the initial physical examination, vital signs determine whether a patient is stable or hypovolemic as a result of blood loss, in which case immediate therapeutic intervention such as intravenous fluids and uterine evacuation is necessary. The amount of vaginal bleeding is also helpful in assessing blood loss.

The vaginal examination is essential in the differential diagnosis. The first thing to determine, by both a speculum and a bimanual examination, is whether the cervical os is open or closed. The ability to easily insert a finger through the internal os into the uterus during the bimanual examination indicates that the os is open. If the cervix is closed in a woman who is pregnant and is experiencing vaginal bleeding and cramps, then the most likely diagnosis is threatened abortion. However, the possibility of an ectopic or molar pregnancy must be considered. A carefully taken history, with special attention to the ectopic risk factors, is helpful. In ectopic pregnancy, the pain is often located to one side and is sharp and intermittent but can also be continuous. In threatened abortion, the pain is usually crampy and in the midline, in the suprapubic area. These characteristics, however, are by

no means universal, and in some cases patients may have minimal complaints of pain even in the presence of hemoperitoneum. The uterine size is also important and often is larger than expected from the date of the last menstrual period in cases of molar pregnancies, equal to or less than dates in threatened abortions, and often less than dates in ectopic pregnancies. The presence of an adnexal mass or adnexal tenderness on physical examination is strongly suggestive of an ectopic pregnancy. The definitive diagnosis, however, is made by serial measurements of the β-hCG and ultrasonography. In a normal pregnancy, the β-hCG should increase by at least 66% every 48 hours. The absence of an intrauterine pregnancy on transabdominal ultrasonography when the serum β-hCG is greater than or equal to 6000 MIU per ml or on transvaginal ultrasonography when the serum β-hCG is approximately 1800 MIU per ml, especially in the presence of abnormally rising β-hCG levels, establishes the probable diagnosis of ectopic pregnancy. Before the era of transvaginal ultrasonography and sensitive β-hCG assays, culdocentesis was the gold standard for the diagnosis of ectopic pregnancy. It is now used much less commonly, but it still has a place in situations when transvaginal ultrasonography is not readily available or when the diagnosis is unclear. Culdocentesis involves the insertion of a 20-gauge spinal needle attached to a 10- to 20-ml syringe through the apex of the vagina, posterior to the cervix (the posterior vaginal fornix), into the peritoneal cavity. Aspiration of at least 5 ml of nonclotting blood denotes the presence of hemoperitoneum and is consistent with a leaking or ruptured ectopic pregnancy.

In some cases, ultrasonography shows an empty sac in the uterus. This condition, known as a blighted ovum, has the same natural history as other miscarriages in which an embryo is actually present. Once the diagnosis is made, the patient can be observed for spontaneous bleeding and expulsion of uterine contents. However, because this may take several weeks to occur, uterine dilation and suction curettage are usually performed. In other cases, the uterus may be smaller than dates and ultrasonography may show fetal demise, called a missed abortion.

If the cervical os is open, the abortion is inevitable or incomplete. At this stage, the bleeding can be heavy and a curettage may need to be performed. In cases of complete abortion, patients report a history of heavy bleeding and cramping with passage of clots and tissue. At the time of the examination, bleeding is minimal or absent, the cervical os is closed, and the uterus is of normal size. Ultrasonography may be helpful to rule out the presence of retained tissue within the uterus if some cramping and bleeding persist. If ultrasonography shows retained tissue, the uterus must be evacuated to avoid infection and further blood loss.

Diagnostic Tests

Laboratory tests should include a complete blood count, determination of blood type, and antibody screen.

Ultrasonography is useful to document an intrauterine pregnancy, to check fetal viability, to rule out retained products after a complete abortion, or to evaluate the characteristics of an adnexal mass.

ACUTE TREATMENT OF SPONTANEOUS ABORTION

All Rh-negative patients with bleeding in early pregnancy, including those with ectopic and molar pregnancies, must receive RhoGAM to prevent isoimmunization in future pregnancies.

Patients with threatened abortion may usually be discharged home and instructed to abstain from intercourse and to call if the bleeding or pain increases. They should also be asked to retrieve any passed tissue for pathologic evaluation. As discussed earlier, in an incomplete abortion, evacuation of the uterus is performed on an emergency basis. After 12 weeks of gestation, some physicians perform the procedure in the operating room, because the risk of uterine perforation is higher and a laparotomy may be needed.

The retained tissue or fetus should always be sent for pathologic confirmation of villi to rule out an ectopic pregnancy, and for the diagnosis of molar pregnancy. In cases of recurrent abortion, a chromosomal evaluation should be performed. In this case, the tissue must be placed in saline rather than in formalin so that the cells can grow in tissue culture.

Serial β-hCG testing is important when no villi are seen in the tissue obtained from uterine evacuation because of the association with an ectopic pregnancy. It is also important to monitor β-hCG levels down to zero in patients with a molar pregnancy.

Most patients can be discharged a few hours after instrumentation of the uterus. In most cases, they should receive antibiotics (doxycycline is usually sufficient, unless there is evidence of chorioamnionitis). In some cases, methylergonovine is given to promote uterine contractility and decrease bleeding. Patients should be instructed to be alert for signs of infection (pelvic pain or fever) or retained tissue (bleeding and cramping).

THE ETIOLOGY OF RECURRENT ABORTION

Chromosomal Abnormalities

More than 50% of first-trimester spontaneous abortions result from chromosomal abnormalities in the fetus,[5] and the most common is monosomy 45X (Turner's syndrome). In the majority of cases, parental karyotypes are normal[6] and the fetal chromosomal abnormalities are the result of sporadic errors in gametogenesis. If a chromosomal defect of the aborted fetus is identified, the couple is at increased risk for subsequent pregnancy losses. Possible causes of recurrent errors in gametogenesis include advanced parental age,[7,8] delayed fertilization,[9] infection,[10] radiation, and toxic substances.[11]

Balanced translocations have been found in about 6% of all couples[12] and account for 6 to 7% of recurrent spontaneous abortions.

Endocrine Abnormalities

A luteal phase defect reflects the inability of the corpus luteum to produce a sufficient amount of progesterone to maintain normal luteal phase endometrium and therefore early pregnancy. Diagnosis of a luteal phase defect is based on two endometrial biopsy specimens that are out of phase by 3 days or more. Luteal phase defect may cause infertility or recurrent abortions. The incidence of luteal phase defect in patients with habitual abortion has been estimated to range between 18[13] and 35%[14–16] in various studies. Hyperprolactinemia may be associated with luteal phase defects, with subsequent infertility and recurrent abortions.

Hypothyroidism, both clinical and subclinical, has been associated with both infertility and recurrent pregnancy losses.[17] Modern sensitive thyroid-stimulating hormone radioimmunoassays allow identification of a great number of patients with compensated hypothyroidism, manifested by an elevated level of thyroid-stimulating hormone with a normal T_4 value.

Higher rates of abortion due to congenital anomalies are observed in women with poorly controlled diabetes mellitus (see Chapter 37).

Anatomic Abnormalities of the Uterus

Congenital

A unicornuate and a didelphic uterus are associated with midtrimester pregnancy losses and premature deliveries. However, septate and bicornuate uterus may cause early pregnancy losses, because the septum is often the site of implantation.[18] Most but not all studies show that the uterine abnormalities associated with diethylstilbestrol (DES) exposure, including hypoplastic and T-shaped uteri, may also be associated with recurrent abortion.[19]

Acquired

The presence of intrauterine synechiae (Asherman's syndrome), scarring that usually follows a postpartum or postabortal curettage, may cause habitual abortion either by decreasing the size of the uterine cavity or by causing defective endometrial vascularization.[20]

Uterine fibroids are thought to be associated with as many as 18% of recurrent pregnancy losses,[21–23] possibly as a result of mechanical factors or abnormal vascularization and development of the endometrium.

Systemic Diseases

Systemic lupus erythematosus (SLE) is associated with recurrent abortion, mainly owing to immunologic factors.[25] In SLE, immune complexes are deposited on the trophoblastic basement membrane and in blood vessels, possibly contributing to the pathogenesis of recurrent abortion in these patients.[25] Another possible pathogenetic mechanism is the occurrence of fetal cardiac anomalies.[26] Maternal cyanotic congenital cardiac disease may cause recurrent pregnancy losses by impairing fetal oxygenation.[27] Chronic renal insufficiency is associated with increased risk of abortion, especially in the presence of hypertension.[28] In general, the more severe the renal dysfunction, the poorer the prognosis.[29]

Infections

Viral infections such as genital herpes[30] and cytomegalovirus[31] are associated with early pregnancy losses. The role of *Chlamydia, Mycoplasma,* and toxoplasmosis as causes of recurrent abortion has been proposed but not firmly demonstrated.

TORCH titers, however, are not useful in the evaluation of the cause of recurrent abortion.

Environmental Factors

Exposure to numerous chemical wastes such as carbon tetrachloride and benzene as well as anesthetic gas has been associated with a high incidence of spontaneous abortion.[32] Exposure to radiation may cause chromosomal abnormalities; however, studies in humans linking irradiation to recurrent abortion are lacking. Cigarette smoking, alcohol abuse, and several drugs such as folate antagonists have been associated with pregnancy losses.[33] The association of video display terminals with spontaneous abortion remains controversial (see Chapter 75).

Immunologic Factors

In about 50% of cases, none of the previously mentioned potential etiologic factors are detected. Immunologic mechanisms may be involved in these apparently unexplained recurrent abortions. The following immunologic theories have been proposed.

Antiphospholipid antibodies, including the lupus anticoagulant, are immunoglobulin G antibodies directed against the phospholipid portion of the prothrombin activator complex.[34] They have been found in women with and without SLE. These antibodies prolong the partial thromboplastin time and, paradoxically, cause thromboembolic phenomena, possibly interfering with placental perfusion.

Blocking antibodies may also have a role in the etiology of recurrent abortion. According to this theory, the capability of the embryo and fetus, which is antigenically foreign to the mother, to grow within the uterus without being rejected depends on the production of a blocking serum antibody. This blocking antibody, coupled with the immunosuppressive effects of progesterone, may prevent rejection of fetal tissue and therefore abortion. Some women suffering recurrent abortions have been found to lack this blocking antibody.[35] Some evidence also suggests that major histocompatibility antigen homozygosity between the two partners may prevent the formation of blocking antibodies by the mother, thus causing recurrent pregnancy losses.[36]

An embryo or trophoblastic toxic factor has been isolated from the the serum of many women with recurrent pregnancy losses.[37] It has been postulated that this embryotoxic factor is a potential cause of recurrent abortion in couples with otherwise normal findings.

EVALUATION OF RECURRENT ABORTION

Evaluation of a couple with recurrent abortion starts with a carefully taken history. This must include a detailed description and sequence of the previous pregnancy losses, the gestational age at which they occurred, and any available information about the products of conception or aborted fetus whenever genetic studies or pathologic examination was performed. Patients should also be specifically asked whether any elective abortions were performed in the past, information that is often not volunteered. It is important to know whether any pregnancies were carried to fetal viability or to term. Any history of infections, chronic diseases, in utero DES exposure or exposure to drugs, and radiation or toxic environmental agents should be elicited.

The diagnosis of recurrent abortion is made after three pregnancy losses, and in most patients, a complete work-up is not indicated after only one or two abortions. However, each case must be considered separately, taking into consideration the age of the couple, the presence of concurrent infertility, and the degree of anxiety experienced by the couple.

A general physical examination can detect signs of metabolic diseases. The pelvic examination can reveal cervical abnormalities, such as anatomic defects associated with DES exposure. Anomalies related to DES exposure include a very short cervix, a coxcomb with extra tissue on the dorsum of the cervix, a hood or circumferential extra fold of tissue, or a hypoplastic, tiny uterus that may be difficult to palpate. Other cervical abnormalities include lacerations or infections. Uterine abnormalities consistent with fibroids, such as increased size or irregular shape, may also be noted on pelvic examination.

Laboratory tests (Table 29–1) should include a complete blood count and chemistry profile to rule out systemic diseases. Thyroid function tests and a prolactin measurement assess the endocrine status. An endometrial biopsy aids in the diagnosis of luteal phase defects. To confirm the presence of a luteal phase defect, the biopsy specimen must show a developmental endometrial delay of 3 days or more on two separate cycles. It is best to perform the biopsy just before the expected menses (i.e., on day 26 or 27 of a 28-day cycle). Antinuclear antibodies are useful for the diagnosis of SLE, if clinical evidence suggests this disease. Anticardiolipin antibody and lupus-like anticoagulant disclose a potential immunologic cause. Depending on the method used in any particular laboratory, a prolonged partial thromboplastin time may be a useful screening test to indicate the presence of a lupus-like anticoagulant. A karyotypic analysis should be performed in both partners to rule out cases of balanced translocations or mosaicism. A hysterosalpingogram or hysteroscopy should be performed to disclose uterine factors. Cervical cultures for *Chlamydia* and *Ureaplasma* may be useful to document infectious factors.

Despite extensive investigation, no cause is detected in approximately 50% of couples with recurrent abortion. Experimental immunologic testing has become available in some institutions for patients with recurrent unexplained pregnancy losses. Such tests, still experimental, include detection of the so-called embryotoxic factor.[37]

When a woman with a history of recurrent abortion conceives, early pregnancy should be carefully monitored by serial β-hCG measurements and ultrasonography. This often allows early diagnosis of an impending miscarriage (e.g., a very slow heart rate or absent growth of a gestational sac), avoiding the trauma of acute hemorrhage and severe cramping. If the pregnancy proceeds well, the couple's anxiety is thus relieved.

TREATMENT

Luteal phase defect may be treated with progesterone supplementation, starting after the midcycle basal body temperature rise. Progesterone is usually administered as 25- or 50-mg vaginal suppositories, given twice daily. If the patient becomes pregnant, this therapy is continued until 10 weeks of pregnancy, when the placenta has adequate production of progesterone. Intramuscular injections of progesterone in oil are also available. Clomiphene citrate is an alternative treatment. Clomiphene probably acts at the level of the hypothalamus and pituitary, increasing ovarian stimulation and thereby increasing ovarian estradiol and pro-

---

TABLE 29–1. Laboratory Tests

Complete blood count and chemistry profile
Thyroid function tests
Prolactin
Anticardiolipin antibody and lupus anticoagulant
Karyotypic analysis of both partners
Endometrial biopsy
Hysterosalpingogram and/or hysteroscopy
Cervical cultures for *Chlamydia* and *Ureoplasma*

gesterone production. Clomiphene itself, however, may cause a luteal phase defect in as many as 20% of cases.

Clinical or subclinical hypothyroidism, even if compensated (elevated thyroid-stimulating hormone level with normal T_4) should be treated to achieve normalization of the level of thyroid-stimulating hormone.

Hyperprolactinemic patients should be treated with bromocriptine. Treatment must be started slowly to avoid orthostatic hypotension, with 1.25 mg (½ tablet) daily for 1 week, then 2.5 mg a day the next week. If the prolactin level remains elevated, the dose should be increased to 2.5 mg twice a day.

Surgical removal of fibroids, or myomectomy, may be indicated in cases of uterine fibroids in which no other etiologic factor for miscarriage is identified. When intrauterine synechiae are detected, they may be lysed hysteroscopically. Some cases of müllerian anomalies, especially uterine septa, also warrant surgical correction. If the history suggests painless delivery of a fetus in the second trimester, in the next pregnancy a cerclage suture should be placed around the cervical os at around 13 to 14 weeks to prevent recurrent cervical incompetence.

Whenever a chromosomal cause is detected (i.e., a chromosomal abnormality was identified in one or more of the previous abortuses) or a balanced translocation is found in one of the partners, any subsequent pregnancy carried beyond 15 weeks should be evaluated by amniocentesis to ensure the presence of a normal fetal karyotype. Alternatively, chorionic villus sampling may be performed for karyotypic analysis in the first trimester; however, some studies show that this may carry a greater risk of pregnancy loss and some congenital abnormalities.

Experimental therapies include corticosteroids in the management of patients with SLE or the lupus anticoagulant, injections of white blood cells from male partners in cases of HLA homozygosity,[36] and high-dose progesterone in women with positive embryotoxic factors. The efficacy of such therapies is still under investigation.

PROGNOSIS

After a miscarriage or dilation and evacuation for an abnormal pregnancy, it is prudent to encourage a patient to have a normal menstrual period (not the menses immediately following the procedure or pregnancy loss) before attempting to conceive again. The next menstrual period usually occurs within 4 to 6 weeks after the miscarriage.

Couples who are having difficulties dealing with or accepting the loss should be referred for counseling. If a couple has a history of recurrent abortion and desires to pursue a medical evaluation, they should be advised to use barrier methods of birth control.

Fortunately, in most cases the prognosis is favorable. The risk of miscarriage is only 2% in an unselected group of patients who have had ultrasonography documenting fetal viability before 12 weeks of gestation.[38] Couples who have had only one miscarriage have a 95% chance of a successful outcome in the next pregnancy.[39] Approximately 75% of couples achieve a live birth even after three previous miscarriages.[40] Recurrent pregnancy loss is stressful for a couple, and a physician can minimize this stress by providing or referring the couple for emotional support and, if indicated, proceeding with an evaluation in a timely fashion. It is reasonable for the primary practitioner to refer couples with recurrent miscarriages to a gynecologist with expertise in this area or to a center with specialists in infertility and recurrent pregnancy loss.

REFERENCES

1. Miller JF, Williamson EM, Glu J. Fetal loss after implantation. Lancet 1981;1:553.
2. Roth DB. The frequency of spontaneous abortion. Int J Fertil 1963;8:431.
3. Warburton D, Fraser F. Spontaneous abortion risks in man: Data from reproductive histories collected in a medical genetics unit. Am J Hum Genet 1964;16:1.
4. Poland BJ, Miller JR, Jones DC, et al. Reproductive counseling in patients who have had a spontaneous abortion. Am J Obstet Gynecol 1977;27:685.
5. Strobino BR, Kline J, Shrout P, et al. Recurrent spontaneous abortion: Definition of syndrome. In: Porter I, Hook EB (eds). Human Embryonic and Fetal Death. New York: Academic Press, 1980, p 315.
6. Elias S, Simpson JL. Evaluation and clinical outcome of patients at apparent increased risk for spontaneous abortion. In: Porter I, Hook EB (eds). Human Embryonic and Fetal Death. New York: Academic Press, 1980, p 331.
7. Hook EB. Rates of chromosome abnormalities at different maternal ages. Obstet Gynecol 1981;58:282.
8. Matsunaga E, Tonomura A, Oishi H, et al. Reexamination of paternal age effect in Down's syndrome. Hum Genet 1978;40:259.
9. Simpson JL. Genetic consequences of aging sperm or aging ova: Animal studies and relevance to humans. In: Sciarra J, Zatuchni GI, Spiedel JJ (eds). Risks, Benefits and Controversies in Fertility Control. Hagerstown, MD: Harper & Row, 1978, p 506.
10. Kundsin RB, Ampola M, Streeter S, Neurath P. Chromosomal aberrations induced by T strain mycoplasmas. J Med Genet 1971;8:181.
11. Simpson JL. What causes chromosomal abnormalities and gene mutations? Contemp Obstet Gynecol 1981;17:99.
12. Simpson JL. Repeated suboptimal pregnancy outcome. Birth Defects 1981;17:113.
13. Tulppala M, Bjorses UM, Stenman UH, et al. Luteal phase

defects in habitual abortion: Progesterone in saliva. Fertil Steril 1991;56:41.

14. Balasch J, Creus M, Marquez M, et al. The significance of luteal phase deficiency on fertility: A diagnostic and therapeutic approach. Hum Reprod 1986;1:145.

15. Vanrell JA, Balasch J. Luteal phase defects in repeated abortion. Int J Gynaecol Obstet 1986;24:111.

16. Jones GES, Delfs E. Endocrine patterns in term pregnancies following abortion. JAMA 1951;146:1212.

17. Jones WS, Man E. Thyroyd dysfunction in human pregnancy. Am J Obstet Gynecol 1969;104:909.

18. Jones HW Jr, Jones GES. Double uterus as an etiologic factor for repeated abortion: Indication for surgical repair. Am J Obstet Gynecol 1953;65:325.

19. Haney AF, Hammond CB, Soules MR, Creasman WT. Diethylstilbestrol induced upper genital tract anomalies. Fertil Steril 1979;31:142.

20. Polishuk WZ, Siew FP, Gordon R, Lebenshart P. Vascular changes in traumatic amenorrhea and hypomenorrhea. Int J Fertil 1977;22:189.

21. Robins SA. In: Robin LL (ed). Golden's Diagnostic Roentgenology. Vol 4. Baltimore: Williams & Wilkins, 1972.

22. Kerr MG. Infertility in women clinically attributed to uterine factors. J Reprod Fertil 1969;8(suppl):1.

23. Rosati P, Bellati U, Exacoustos C, et al. Uterine myoma in pregnancy: Ultrasound study. Int J Gynecol Obstet 1989;28:109.

24. Fraga A, Mintz G, Orozco J. Systemic lupus erythematosus: Fertility, fetal wastage and survival rate with treatment: A comparative study. Arthritis Rheum 1973;16:541.

25. Crennan DM, McCormick JN, Wojtacha D, et al. Immunological studies of the placenta in systemic lupus erythematosus. Ann Rheum Dis 1978;37:129.

26. Chameides L, Truex RC, Vetter V, et al. Association of systemic lupus erythematosus with congenital complete heart block. N Engl J Med 1977;297:1204.

27. McAnulty JH, Metcalfe T, Veland K. Cardiovascular disease. In: Burrow GN, Ferris TF (eds). Medical Complications During Pregnancy. Philadelphia: WB Saunders, 1982, p 145.

28. Felding C. Pregnancy following renal diseases. Clin Obstet Gynecol 1968;11:579.

29. Bear RA. Pregnancy in patients with renal disease. Obstet Gynecol 1976;48:13.

30. Nahmias AJ, Josey WE, Naib ZM, et al. Perinatal risk associated with maternal herpes virus infection. Am J Obstet Gynecol 1971; 110:825.

31. Kriel RL, Gates GA, Wulff H, et al. Cytomegalovirus isolations associated with pregnancy wastage. Am J Obstet Gynecol 1970;106:889.

32. Munson RR. Occupational hazards and fetal death. In: Porter I, Hook EB (eds). Human Embryonic and Fetal Death. New York: Academic Press, 1980, p 159.

33. Rush D. Cigarette smoking, nutrition, social status, and perinatal loss: Their interactive relationship. In: Porter I, Hook EB (eds). Human Embryonic and Fetal Death. New York: Academic Press, 1980, p 207.

34. Lubbe WF, Graham C, Liggins MB. Lupus anticoagulant and pregnancy. Am J Obstet Gynecol 1985;153:322.

35. Rocklin RE, Kitzmiller JL, Carpenter CB, et al. Maternal-fetal relation: Absence of an immunologic blocking factor from the serum of women with chronic abortions. N Engl J Med 1976;295:1209.

36. Komlos L, Zamir R, Josua H, Halbrecht I. Common HLA antigens in couples with repeated abortions. Clin Immunol Immunopathol 1977;7:330.

37. Hill JA, Polgar K, Harlow BL, Anderson DJ. Evidence of embryo- and trophoblastic-toxic cellular immune response(s) in women with recurrent spontaneous abortion. Am J Obstet Gynecol 1992;166:1044.

38. Mackenzie WE, Holmes DS, Newton JR. Spontaneous abortion rate in ultrasonographically viable pregnancies. Obstet Gynecol 1988;71:81.

39. Regan L, Braude PR, Trembath PL. Influence of past reproductive preformance on risk of spontaneous abortion. Br Med J 1989;299:541.

40. Warburton D, Fraser F. On the probability that a woman who has had a spontaneous abortion will abort in subsequent pregnancies. J Obstet Gynaecol Br Commonw 1961;68:784.

ISSUES IN PREGNANCY

30

Preconceptional Care and Management of Early Pregnancy

Dale K. Weldon and Karen M. Freund

Early pregnancy and the transition to prenatal care is often a time of fragmented medical care for women.[1] Many primary care providers, including family practitioners and gynecologists, do not provide obstetric services and require that a woman transfer her care to another provider. Internists and other primary care providers who do not provide obstetric care may still be asked questions from patients wishing to conceive. More important, these physicians may see patients who are not using contraception who would benefit from a discussion of their plans should they conceive. Many women are unaware of pregnancy until the middle of the first trimester and do not begin prenatal care until after 10 weeks of gestation when major organogenesis is complete and the greatest risk of spontaneous abortion has passed. The window of intervention to provide counseling and care in these areas is often best provided by the primary care provider. Therefore, in addition to addressing the need for contraception in women of childbearing potential, addressing plans for children should be part of an initial evaluation. Most women are eager for information when they attempt to conceive. Diet, nutrition, weight, anticipated weight gain, exercise, and habits such as smoking and drinking, drug use, and other general health concerns are important areas to address.

DIET AND NUTRITION

Routine review of dietary intake, including both deficiencies of minerals and vitamins and overin-

take of caloric nutrients has special relevance for women planning to conceive. Specific dietary counseling should address the increased need for calcium and ensure that current calcium intake is adequate. The risk of iron deficiency should be assessed (see Chapter 3). Ideally, weight reduction for women who are overweight should be initiated before conception. With weight reduction, fertility may actually be enhanced for obese women with irregular cycles due to anovulation. Providers should assess for past and current bulimia and anorexia. Pregnancy in a patient with an eating disorder is associated with an increased risk of complications. Women with a prior eating disorder may also experience greater distress with the changes in body habitus that occur during pregnancy, leading to difficulty with appropriate weight gain. It is therefore helpful to address these issues before conception and in the first trimester.

In general, pregnancy requires an average of 200 to 300 kcal more per day to provide for the changes occurring in the woman's body and to promote appropriate growth of the fetus.[2] A diet history should be taken from the patient to elicit information about deficiencies that may be present. It is important to know whether the patient restricts her diet in any way because of cultural or religious beliefs or because of intolerance to certain foods. Eating a well-balanced diet should be encouraged, and supplements can be recommended if needed.

In the guidelines set forth by the Food and Nutrition Board of the Institute of Medicine in 1990, recommendations for weight gain are given in ranges based on prepregnant weight for height.[3] The guidelines were based on studies of maternal and fetal morbidity and mortality in relation to weight and weight gain during pregnancy. Underweight women are encouraged to gain more, and overweight women should strive for less gain. Weight loss programs are contraindicated in pregnancy. For underweight patients, a total weight gain of 28 to 40 pounds is recommended. For normal weight women, a total weight gain of 25 to 35 pounds is suggested. Overweight women should gain 15 to 25 pounds. A 15-pound weight gain is recommended for obese women (Table 30–1).

The use of folic acid supplements during the months before conception and in the early weeks of pregnancy has been shown to reduce the risk of neural tube defects (spina bifida and anencephaly) by 50% or more.[4–10] This marked risk reduction has been noted in women at higher risk for neural tube defects as well as in women in the general population. Clinical trials for women at high risk of neural tube defects utilized a folate dose of 4 mg daily, which is 10 times greater than the current recommended daily allowance of 0.4 mg for folate.[4, 5] Case-control studies have shown a similar magnitude of benefit from folate doses of 0.4 mg in normal risk women.[8–11] It is interesting to note that the benefit of folate in at least some of the studies[11] was seen from supplementation, not from high dietary folate intake. Based on this evidence, the U.S. Public Health Service has recommended folate supplementation of 0.4 mg daily, the dose in most daily multivitamin supplements,[12] for all women capable of becoming pregnant.[13] The decision to recommend folate supplementation for all women of childbearing potential was based on the fact that 50% of all pregnancies in the United States are unplanned.[14] For women with a previous fetus with a neural tube defect, current guidelines recommend the consumption of 4 mg daily of folate from 1 month before conception and for the first 3 months of pregnancy.[5] Because

higher doses of folate are not well studied and are known to complicate the diagnosis of vitamin B_{12} deficiency, the recommendation for their use is limited to these higher risk women.

An additional 30 mg of ferrous iron is required daily during the second and third trimesters. Other than the specific needs for folate and iron, the current recommendation of the Institute of Medicine is that women eating a well-balanced diet do not need additional vitamin supplementation.[3] However, because a daily multivitamin with iron provides both additional folate and iron needs, most providers continue to recommend this as the easiest method to meet all supplemental needs throughout pregnancy.

MEDICATION USE

Providers treating women of childbearing potential should review all over-the-counter and prescription medications in use. Consideration should be given to potential fetotoxic effects of medication in the event of an unplanned pregnancy. For patients attempting to conceive, explicit discussion on plans to taper or discontinue medications with potential fetal effects should occur before pregnancy. Particular attention should be given to antiseizure medications (see Chapter 43), antihypertensives (see Chapter 36), isotretinoin, anxiolytics, antidepressants (see Chapter 42), acetylsalicylic acid, iodine-based cough preparations (see Chapter 42), and bromide-containing antihistamines. Recommendations for alternatives such as acetaminophen for fever or hydralazine for hypertension should be provided.

SUBSTANCE USE

A careful review of tobacco, alcohol, and other substance use should be addressed around the time of conception. The risks of smoking during pregnancy are discussed in Chapters 34 and 65. Tobacco use is also associated with reduced fertility. Ideally, women who smoke should try to quit before conceiving. The use of nicotine replacement systems is not approved during pregnancy, and given that nicotine may have direct toxic effects on the fetus, the use of nicotine replacement systems to quit smoking is best accomplished before pregnancy. The risks of alcohol use during pregnancy are discussed in Chapters 34 and 66. It is prudent to recommend that women minimize alcohol intake while trying to conceive. Similarly, treatment for addiction is best accomplished before pregnancy.

TABLE 30–1. Weight Gain During Pregnancy

Body Mass Index (BMI) = Weight (kg) ÷ (Height [m])^2
or
(Weight [lb] ÷ 2.2) ÷ ([Height (in) ÷ 39.4])^2

BASELINE BMI	RECOMMENDED WEIGHT GAIN (POUNDS)
<19.8	28–40
19.8–26.0	25–35
26.1–29.0	15–25
>29.0	15

Data on caffeine consumption before and during pregnancy remain controversial. Caffeine has been shown in many animal studies, including studies of primates, to increase the risk of miscarriage and stillbirth and possibly the risk of chromosomal abnormalities.[15] Most studies have shown intrauterine growth retardation with more than three cups of coffee daily.[16-18] However, the effect of lower amounts of caffeine before and following conception on chromosomal abnormalities and miscarriages is debated. One case-control study showed an association of miscarriage with caffeine consumption before as well as during pregnancy.[19] Another cohort study with prospective assessment of caffeine intake found no association between moderate caffeine intake equivalent to fewer than three cups of coffee daily and spontaneous abortion, intrauterine growth retardation, or microcephaly. In addition, the association between heavy caffeine use and low birth weight and microcephaly was no longer significant after adjusting for smoking and other risk factors.[20] Criticisms of the case-control studies showing a positive association include the retrospective nature of inquiry, which can lead to recall bias, in which women with poor pregnancy outcomes differentially remember higher caffeine use. Also decreased caffeine intake has been shown to be associated with nausea during early pregnancy, and because nausea is strongly associated with favorable outcomes, the association between caffeine intake may reflect the fact that women with nausea decrease caffeine consumption. Criticism of cohort studies showing no association include the difficulty in accurately estimating caffeine consumption and the power to detect differences for lower caffeine ranges.[21]

The U.S. Food and Drug Administration issued an advisory to pregnant women to limit caffeine consumption in 1980.[22] Most studies indicate that high levels of caffeine are harmful. Caffeine easily crosses the placenta and has been shown to decrease placental blood flow. Metabolism of caffeine by the fetus is reduced owing to lack of liver enzymes. Also, the half-life of caffeine increases from 3 to 10 hours during the course of pregnancy.[23, 24] Given the conflicting data for lower amounts, it is probably prudent to recommend that women limit caffeine intake beginning when they attempt to conceive to 100 mg daily or less (estimates of caffeine are 100 mg per cup of coffee, 40 mg per cup of tea or cola, and 13 mg per cup of cocoa).

EXERCISE

Women often request advice on the safety of exercise during pregnancy. In general, the benefits of regular exercise extend into pregnancy, in terms of cardiovascular health[25] and carbohydrate metabolism.[26] Mobility, strength, and balance may be of particular importance during the latter trimester of pregnancy when the center of gravity is shifted forward and balance requires readjustment. Although some studies suggest that physical activity during pregnancy has a number of beneficial effects, including a decrease in the duration and severity of labor and improved neonatal outcomes,[27-30] other studies do not confirm this.[31]

The concerns regarding exercise during pregnancy include the potential for raising body core temperature, which has been shown to have a toxic effect in the first trimester.[32] Jones and colleagues, however, found that core body temperatures in pregnant women who exercised did not rise above 39°C.[33] This is likely because of increased maternal blood volume allowing for more efficient cooling through the skin. Other concerns about exercise in the first trimester include the risk of miscarriage. Clapp looked at spontaneous abortion rates in patients who engaged in vigorous aerobic exercise before and during pregnancy and found their rate of miscarriage to be less than that for the controls.[34]

Another potential concern is the worry of injury during pregnancy. The shift in center of gravity coupled with sudden or rapid movement and the compensatory lumbar lordosis may make muscle and joint injury more likely. Later in pregnancy, increased joint laxity, particularly of the pubic symphysis, may alter ability to exercise.

Given these concerns, women who wish to exercise should build their cardiovascular conditioning before pregnancy and exercise to maintain existing conditioning during pregnancy. Aerobic routines should take into consideration joint laxity later in pregnancy. Standard sit-ups should be avoided when there is separation of the abdominal rectus muscles and should be replaced by diagonal sit-ups. Swimming is often considered ideal exercise during pregnancy, as weight is supported and external heat exchange is increased.

GENETIC COUNSELING AND TESTING

Genetic counseling and testing will become a more significant issue, as data from the Human Genome Project and other bimolecular research are able to identify gene markers of disease susceptibility and carrier gene status. Testing may soon be available to assess carrier status for a large number of conditions. To the extent that such testing is used to assist in reproductive choices for individuals and couples, primary care providers will play a greater role, because ideally such information is of greatest use in reproductive counseling if obtained before conception. The role of such testing on a population basis to identify carrier status is still being defined. For most conditions for which testing is available, it is recommended only for those with a family history of the condition of concern. A review has outlined both the ethical and medical concerns around widespread testing, including the costs and benefits to the individual and society, the psychological impact of testing, and the possibility of discrimination based on knowledge of carrier status.[35] The role of biotechnology companies, federal agencies, advisory groups, and professional organizations in determining the use of this technology remains to be defined. The following are examples of tests currently in use and the evolution of their applications.

Screening for Tay-Sachs disease in populations at risk (both men and women of Ashkenazic Jewish or French Canadian ancestry) has been advocated since the 1970s. Screening for sickle cell carrier trait with hemoglobin electrophoresis was also initiated in the 1970s and is advocated for all individuals of African American ancestry.

The gene for cystic fibrosis was first identified in 1989,[36] and by 1991, the technology was refined to identify 85 to 90% of mutations. However, testing for this gene is currently recommended only for those with a family history of the disorder. A number of advisory agencies strongly advocated against developing widespread population-based testing until pilot programs to determine the risks and benefits have completed their research. Such pilot testing programs are currently under way and, it is hoped, will provide important lessons on how best to use this new technology.[35]

Maternal serum alpha-fetoprotein as a screening method for neural tube defects also was initially developed in the 1980s. Although the medical committee of the American College of Obstetricians and Gynecologists felt that issues of laboratory quality control, patient counseling, and follow-up testing required further study before recommending this as a routine test, it is now considered standard medical care, in part owing to an 1985 alert issued by the College's Professional Liability Department.[35] The U.S. Preventive Task Force recommends the use of alpha-fetoprotein testing only when there is access to standardized laboratories, follow-up care and counseling, and skilled ultrasonography and amniocentesis capability.[37] Maternal serum alpha-fetoprotein is currently offered to all women at 16 to 18 weeks of gestation. Besides the detection of neural tube defects, maternal serum alpha-fetoprotein is also able to detect most abdominal wall defects such as omphalocele and gastroschisis, and low levels of maternal serum alpha-fetoprotein have been associated with trisomy 21 (Down's syndrome). The addition of estriol and human chorionic gonadotropin levels with maternal serum alpha-fetoprotein has been advocated, which can detect up to 60% of cases of trisomy 21.[38, 39]

Prenatal chromosomal analysis is offered to all women who will be 35 or older at the time of delivery, women with a previous history of a child with a chromosomal abnormality, and women with other specific risk factors for congenital abnormalities (Table 30–2). Prenatal testing can be done by targeted ultrasound evaluation, amniocentesis, or chorionic villus sampling. Amniocentesis is generally done at 16 weeks of gestation under ultra-

---

TABLE 30–2. Indications for Prenatal Diagnosis

GENERAL RISK FACTORS
Maternal age ≥35 years at the time of delivery
Elevated or reduced maternal serum alpha-fetoprotein concentration
Results of triple screening: elevated or reduced maternal serum alpha-fetoprotein, human chorionic gonadotropin, and unconjugated estriol concentrations

SPECIFIC RISK FACTORS
Previous child with a structural defect or chromosomal abnormality
Previous stillbirth or neonatal death
Structural abnormality in the mother or father
Balanced translocation in the mother or father
Inherited disorders: cystic fibrosis, metabolic disorders, sex-linked recessive disorders
Medical disease in the mother: diabetes mellitus, phenylketonuria
Exposure to a teratogen: ionizing radiation, anticonvulsant medicines, lithium, isotretinoin, alcohol
Infection: rubella, toxoplasmosis, cytomegalovirus

ETHNIC RISK FACTORS

Disorder	Ethnic or Racial Group	Screening Marker
Tay-Sachs disease	Ashkenazi Jewish, French Canadian	Decreased serum hexosaminidase A concentration
Sickle cell anemia	Black African, Mediterranean, Arab, Indian and Pakistani	Presence of sickling in hemolysate followed by confirmatory hemoglobin electrophoresis
Alpha- and beta-thalassemia	Mediterranean, Southern and Southeast Asian, Chinese	Mean corpuscular volume <80 μm³, followed by confirmatory hemoglobin electrophoresis

From D'Alton ME, DeCherney AH. Current concepts: Prenatal diagnosis. New Engl J Med 1993; 328:115. Reprinted by permission of the New England Journal of Medicine.

sound guidance. Chromosomal analysis is performed on cultured amniotic fluid cells and usually requires 10 to 14 days. The risk of fetal loss following amniocentesis is generally considered in the range of 0.5 to 1.0%.[40–43] Chorionic villus sampling is done by aspiration of placental or chorionic tissue between 9 to 12 weeks of gestation. The results are available in 1 to 2 days; therefore, the advantage of chorionic villus sampling is the availability of test results in a quicker time period and at an earlier gestational age. The risk of fetal loss from chorionic villus sampling is generally considered to range between 1.7 to 4.6%.[44–45] There has also been concern regarding limb-reduction defects in the children of patients who underwent early chorionic villus sampling.[46–53]

Carrier detection as well as prenatal diagnosis is now possible for a large number of neurogenetic and other hereditary disorders. Genetic counseling is recommended to assist in reproductive choices for those with a personal or family history of a genetic or hereditary disorder or a previous child with birth defects or mental retardation.

INFECTIOUS DISEASES

As part of counseling before pregnancy, immunity status and risk factors for a number of infectious diseases that can affect fetal development should be addressed, as management options are greater in this time period. This includes determining the status of rubella and measles immunity; assessing the risk factors and exposure status to human immunodeficiency virus, cytomegalovirus, and hepatitis viruses; and screening for sexually transmitted diseases (Table 30–3).

Rubella immunity should be documented for all women of childbearing potential. For women born after 1957, documentation of clinical measles or two vaccinations is recommended to ensure im-

munity. Both measles and rubella are live virus vaccines, available in combination with mumps virus vaccine. Rubella vaccine viruses can cross the placenta and infect the fetus, as evidenced by rubella-specific IgM titers in cord blood at birth. The Centers for Disease Control and Prevention have followed the cases of women who were given rubella vaccine inadvertently within 3 months before or after conception from 1971 to 1988. No cases of congenital rubella syndrome were documented in 538 women vaccinated with Cendehill and HPV-77 vaccine strains from 1971 to 1979 and none in 254 women who received the RA 27/3 vaccine from 1979 to 1988.[54] The risk of congenital rubella syndrome from vaccine is felt to be negligible, with a theoretic 95% confidence interval of 0 to 1.2.[55] Current recommendations are that women should receive the vaccine only if they are not pregnant and should be advised to use contraception for 3 months after vaccination. Vaccine use before or during pregnancy ordinarily should not be a reason to terminate pregnancy, given the negligible risk of vaccine-associated defects.

Women with a history of multiple sex partners, previous intravenous drug use or sex with a partner who is an intravenous drug user, immigration from endemic areas, and health occupation exposure to infectious fluids should be tested for immunity and carrier status to hepatitis B. Women without previous infection who are at risk should be offered vaccination both to protect themselves and to reduce the risk of vertical transmission to the fetus. This series can be continued safely during pregnancy. Women who are chronic carriers of hepatitis B can transmit the disease to their child at birth. Knowledge of antigen status can ensure that the child receives prompt vaccination and immunoglobulin at birth. Current data reveal that vertical transmission of hepatitis C is rare except in women coinfected with human immunodeficiency virus[56] or women with chronic hepatitis[57]; routine screening for hepatitis C of all women is not currently advocated. All women who are contemplating pregnancy should be counseled about the risks of the human immunodeficiency virus (see Chapter 48).

Cytomegalovirus can cause both primary and recurrent infection, although recent data suggest that congenital cytomegalovirus is more severe in primary infection and that the presence of maternal antibody provides substantial protection.[58] Women at greater risk of exposure are daycare workers and teachers. Preliminary data suggest that knowledge of cytomegalovirus antibody status and avoiding contact with toddlers' saliva and urine may be effective and that determination of cytomegalovirus antibody status before pregnancy is war-

---

TABLE 30–3. Screening Before or at the First Prenatal Visit

ABO and Rh blood typing and antibody screen
Rubella titer
Hepatitis B surface antigen
Rapid plasma reagin (RPR) or Venereal Disease Research Laboratories test (VDRL)
Hematocrit
Urine culture
Papanicolaou smear
Cultures or other testing for gonorrhea and chlamydia
Human immunodeficiency virus counseling
Purified protein derivative (PPD)
Toxoplasmosis (veterinarians and cat owners)

ranted.[59] Similarly, human parvovirus B19, the cause of erythema infectiosum, which is associated with adverse fetal outcomes, has also been shown to be transmitted in daycare and school settings.[60] Testing is not yet readily available, but the same recommendations for careful hygiene apply and may decrease transmission to adults working with ill children.[61] Acute toxoplasmosis infection can also cause fetal complications. The ability to distinguish acute from previous infection is difficult given currently available tests. It may be reasonable to screen veterinarians and those owning cats for previous exposure. Otherwise, patients should be counseled to avoid litter boxes and to garden with gloves to avoid soil contact during pregnancy.

Routine screening for sexually transmitted diseases including syphilis, gonorrhea, and chlamydial infection should be completed either before conception or during the first prenatal visit. A history of previous genital herpes infection, or recurrent symptoms to suggest herpes, should be sought. Because herpes is transmitted at the time of delivery when active infection is present, cesarean section is indicated when active lesions are present. One study found low neonatal morbidity when screening all women with a past history of herpes with weekly herpes cultures after the thirty-sixth week.[62] However, the study lacked controls. Neither the American College of Physicians[63] nor the U.S. Preventive Task Force[37] recommends screening cultures in asymptomatic women. Screening for exposure to tuberculosis using the standard purified protein derivative (PPD) should also be offered. Because the increased risk of fetal prematurity and low birth weight as well as maternal renal disease from urinary tract infection can be reduced with treatment, a screening urine culture is recommended at the first prenatal visit.[64]

OCCUPATIONAL AND ENVIRONMENTAL ISSUES

Heat exposure during the first trimester has been associated with neural tube defects. Causes of heat exposure include fever higher than 100°F, use of hot tubs and saunas, and possibly electric blankets.[32] Women planning to conceive should avoid these heat sources and should be advised to use acetaminophen for fevers as a means of decreasing risk.

Many women are concerned about workplace exposures to potential teratogens. Chapter 75 provides a detailed discussion and examples of how to evaluate for workplace hazards and management recommendations when such hazards are

identified. Some of the most common possible teratogens include lead, organic solvents, ionizing radiation, and anesthetic gases.

Exposure to lead has been associated with miscarriage and birth defects and should be discussed with women who work in metal smelting and battery manufacturing; who use lead solder, including in electronic assembly; and who use certain pottery glazes. Anesthetic gases have been associated with increased rates of spontaneous abortion, preterm labor, and low birth weight.[65] The exposure of dental assistants to nitrous oxide has been associated with reduced fertility.[66] The use of a scavenger system to capture unused gas should be in place, especially in dental offices, and maternal exposures should be limited. The danger of exposure to electromagnetic radiation from video display terminals continues to be controversial, with recent studies showing no association.[67] Ionizing radiation at levels above 20 rad have been shown to cause birth defects, and exposures between 1 and 10 rad have been associated with childhood leukemia. Current recommendations include protective shielding to reduce the potential fetal exposure to no more than 0.5 rad and frequent film badge monitoring during pregnancy.[68]

COMMON PROBLEMS IN EARLY PREGNANCY

Hyperemesis Gravidarum

Primary care providers may be asked for information regarding common first trimester problems. Most common of the first trimester problems is nausea and vomiting. This is generally not disabling and disappears by the thirteenth week. Patients have had limited success improving symptoms by avoiding strong odors, using sea bands (AccuPressure bands worn on the wrist), undergoing hypnosis, and a host of other remedies. Occasionally nausea and vomiting is so severe as to cause dehydration and weight loss. In these cases, intravenous fluid replacement and electrolyte correction may be necessary either short term in the hospital or longer term using home intravenous therapy. Antiemetic suppositories or injections may be of some use, keeping in mind that most of these have been insufficiently tested during pregnancy to ensure their safety. In the most severe, extended cases, hyperalimentation may be required.

Severe cases of hyperemesis should be evaluated for other causes of nausea and vomiting. Hepatitis, multiple gestation, and molar pregnancy may be associated with hyperemesis, as may other

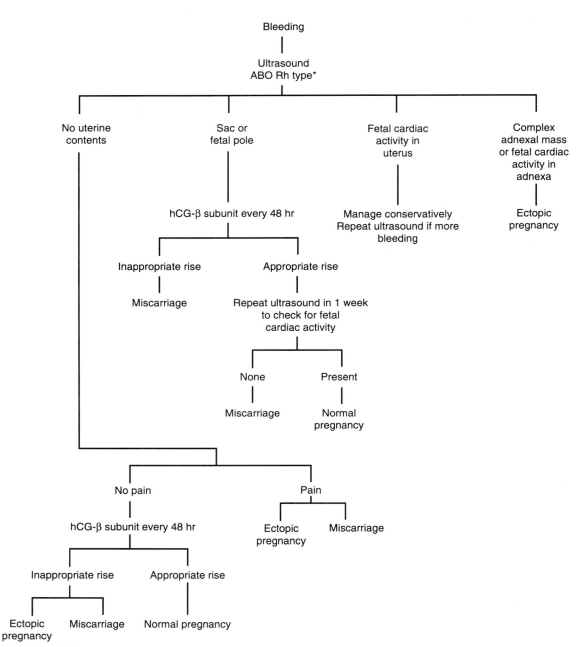

Figure 30-1. Management of bleeding in early pregnancy. *Rh$_o$ immune globulin is necessary to prevent Rh sensitization if the mother is Rh negative.

gastrointestinal disorders. There is also evidence that transient hyperthyroidism is associated with hyperemesis gravidarum.[69-71] The question of whether the change in the results of thyroid studies is the result or the cause of the hyperemesis has not been resolved, so whether to treat the hyperthyroidism remains controversial (see Chapter 38).

Headaches

Headaches are common in early pregnancy and are probably hormone related. Usual headache remedies including acetaminophen, caffeine, and rest are usually sufficient to treat them. Additional medication may be required for more severe headaches or for patients with a history of migraines. The usual guideline of selecting the medication with the least fetal risk, particularly during the period of organogenesis, should be followed. If headaches are persistent or severe, or both, further evaluation is warranted.

Vaginal Bleeding

Bleeding in early pregnancy may be normal and frequently occurs at implantation, which happens around the time of the first missed menses. Bleeding may also be related to a tiny separation of the placenta or a subchorionic hematoma, or may be an indication of an abnormal pregnancy (spontaneous abortion, blighted ovum, hydatidiform mole, or ectopic pregnancy). Other symptoms, such as the presence or absence of pain, may help in making the diagnosis, but any bleeding in early pregnancy should be evaluated with an ultrasound and possibly serial quantitative β-hCG (human chorionic gonadotropin) levels. Abdominal ultrasound should detect a gestational sac at 6 weeks of gestation (based on last menstrual period) or when the β-hCG is greater than 6000 MIU per ml.[72] A fetal pole should be noted at 7 weeks, and a fetal heart beat should be visible at 8 weeks. Vaginal ultrasound may detect an intrauterine gestational sac as early as 5 weeks at a β-hCG level of 1500 MIU per ml.[73] Fetal cardiac activity can be seen by vaginal probe around 7 weeks (β-hCG >17,000 MIU/ml).

Figure 30–1 illustrates the evaluation of first-trimester bleeding. In a normal pregnancy, quantitative β-hCG levels should at least double every 48 to 72 hours.[74] Inappropriately rising or falling levels indicate an abnormal pregnancy, and the patient should be referred to her obstetrician for further management. Bleeding in the face of appropriately rising levels of β-hCG and a normal result on ultrasound may be managed by discouraging intercourse and decreasing the patient's level of activity, although strict bedrest is not indicated. An Rh-negative patient who has bleeding should receive Rh$_o$ immune globulin to prevent Rh sensitization.

Pelvic Pain

Pain may occur normally in early pregnancy as the uterus enlarges. This may be midline suprapubic, crampy or constant, or bilateral symptoms in the inguinal area. Crampy pain accompanied by bleeding is seen with threatened abortion or spontaneous abortion. Unilateral pelvic pain may indicate an ectopic pregnancy. Suprapubic pain with dysuria, frequency, or hematuria may be a sign of a urinary tract infection. If severe, any pelvic pain in early pregnancy should be evaluated by the patient's obstetrician.

REFERENCES

1. Jack BW, Culpepper L. Preconception care. Risk reduction and health promotion in preparation for pregnancy. JAMA 1990;264:1147.
2. Nutrition during pregnancy. ACOG Technical Bulletin No. 179. April, 1993.
3. Institute of Medicine, Food and Nutrition Board, Committee on Nutritional Status during Pregnancy and Lactation, Subcommittee on Dietary Intake and Nutrient Supplements during Pregnancy and Subcommittee on Nutritional Status and Weight Gain during Pregnancy. Nutrition during Pregnancy: Part I, Weight Gain; Part II, Nutrient Supplements. Washington, DC: National Academy Press, 1990.
4. Laurence KM, Jamers N, Miller M, et al. Double blind randomized controlled trial of folate treatment before conception to prevent recurrence of neural-tube defects. BMJ 1981;282:1509.
5. Centers for Disease Control and Prevention. Use of folic acid for prevention of spina bifida and other neural tube defects, 1983–1991. MMWR 1991;40:513.
6. Smithells RW, Nevin NC, Seller MJ, et al. Further experience of vitamin supplementation for the prevention of neural tube defect recurrences. Lancet 1983;1:1027.
7. Vergel RG, Sanchez LR, Heredero BL, et al. Primary prevention of neural tube defects with folic acid supplementation: Cuban experience. Prenat Diagn 1990;10:149.
8. Werler MM, Shapiro S, Mitchell AA. Periconceptional folic acid exposure and risk of occurrent neural tube defects. JAMA 1993;269:1257.
9. Mulinare J, Cordero JF, Erickson JD, Berry RJ. Periconceptional use of multivitamins and the occurrence of neural tube defects. JAMA 1988;260:3141.
10. Bower C, Stanley FJ. Dietary folate as a risk factor for neural-tube defects: Evidence from a case-control study in Western Australia. Med J Aust 1989;150:613.
11. Milunsky A, Jick H, Jick SS, et al. Multivitamin/folic acid supplementation in early pregnancy reduces the prevalence of neural tube defect. JAMA 1989;262:2847.
12. Moss AJ, Levy AS, Kim I, et al. Use of Vitamin and Mineral Supplements in the United States: Current Users, Types of Products, and Nutrients. Hyattsville, MD: National Center for Health Statistics, 1989 (Advance data, No. 174).
13. Centers for Disease Control and Prevention. Recommendations for the use of folic acid to reduce the number of cases of spina bifida and other neural tube defects. MMWR 1992;41(No. RR-14):1.
14. Grimes DA. Unplanned pregnancies in the U.S. Obstet Gynecol 1986;67:438.
15. Dlugosz L, Bracken MS. Reproductive effects of caffeine: A review and theoretical analysis. Epidemiol Rev 1992;14:83.
16. McDonald AD, Armstrong BG, Sloan M. Cigarette, alcohol, and coffee consumption and prematurity. Am J Public Health 1992;82:87.
17. Martin TR, Bracken MB. The association between low birth weight and caffeine consumption during pregnancy. Am J Epidemiol 1987;126:813.
18. Kuzma JW, Sokol RJ. Maternal drinking behavior and decreased intrauterine growth. Alcohol Clin Exp Res 1982;6:396.

19. Infante-Rivard C, Fernandez A, Garthier R, et al. Fetal loss associated with caffeine intake before and during pregnancy. JAMA 1993;270:2940.

20. Mills JL, Holmes LB, Aarons JH, et al. Moderate caffeine use and the risk of spontaneous abortion and intrauterine growth retardation. JAMA 1993;269:593.

21. Eskenazi B. Caffeine during pregnancy: Grounds for concern? JAMA 1993;270:2973.

22. Goyan JE. Food and Drug Administration News Release No. P80-36. Washington, DC: Food and Drug Administration, September 4, 1980.

23. Aldridge A, Bailey J, Neims AH. The disposition of caffeine during and after pregnancy. Semin Perinatol 1981;5:310.

24. Knutti R, Rothweiler H, Schlatter C. The effect of pregnancy on the pharmacokinetics of caffeine. Arch Toxicol 1982;5:187.

25. Pivarnik JM, Ayres NA, Mauer MB, et al. Effects of maternal aerobic fitness on cardiorespiratory responses to exercise. Med Sci Sports Exerc 1993;25:993.

26. Jovanovic-Peterson L, Peterson CM. Is exercise safe or useful for gestational diabetic women? Diabetes 1991; 40:170.

27. Hatch MMC, Shu XO, McLean DE, et al. Maternal exercise during pregnancy, physical fitness, and fetal growth. Am J Epidemiol 1993;137:1105.

28. Botkin C, Driscoll CE. Maternal aerobic exercise: Newborn effects. Fam Pract Res J 1991;22:387.

29. Clapp JF. Exercise and fetal health. J Dev Physiol 1991;15:9.

30. Rice PL, Fort IL. The relationship of maternal exercise on labor, delivery and health of the newborn. J Sports Med Phys Fitness 1991;31:95.

31. Lokey EA, Tran ZV, Wells CL, et al. Effects of physical exercise on pregnancy outcomes: A meta-analytic review. Med Sci Sports Exerc 1991;23:1234.

32. Milunsky A, Ulcickas M, Rothman KJ, et al. Maternal heat exposure and neural tube defects. JAMA 1992;268:882.

33. Jones RL, Botti JJ, Anderson WM, et al. Thermoregulation during aerobic exercise in pregnancy. Obstet Gynecol 1985;65:340.

34. Clapp JF. The effects of maternal exercise on early pregnancy outcome. Am J Obstet Gynecol 1989;161:1453.

35. Wilfond BS, Nolan K. National policy development for the clinical application of genetic diagnostic technologies. Lessons from cystic fibrosis. JAMA 1993;270:2948.

36. Riordan JR, Rommens JM, Kerm BS, et al. Identification of the cystic fibrosis gene: Cloning and characterization of complementary DNA. Science 1989;245:1066.

37. U.S. Preventive Services Task Force. Guide to Clinical Preventive Services. Baltimore, Williams & Wilkins, 1989.

38. Maternal serum-alpha-fetoprotein measurement in antenatal screening for anencephaly and spina bifida in early pregnancy: Report of the U.K. collaborative study on alpha-fetoprotein in relation to neural-tube defects. Lancet 1977;1:1323.

39. Maddow JE, Palomaki GE, Knight GJ, et al. Prenatal screening for Down's syndrome with use of maternal serum markers. N Engl J Med 1992;327:588.

40. The NICHD National Registry for Amniocentesis Study Group. Midtrimester amniocentesis for prenatal diagnosis: Safety and accuracy. JAMA 1976;236:1471.

41. Simpson NE, Dallaire L, Miller JR, et al. Prenatal diagnosis of genetic disease in Canada: Report of a collaborative study. Can Med Assoc J 1976;115:739.

42. Working party on amniocentesis: An assessment of the hazards of amniocentesis. Br J Obstet Gynaecol 1978;85 (suppl):12.

43. Tabor A, Philip J, Madsen M, et al. Randomized controlled

trial of genetic amniocentesis in 4606 low-risk women. Lancet 1986;1:1287.

44. MCR Working Party on the Evaluation of Chorion Villus Sampling. Medical Research Council European Trial of Chorionic villus sampling. Lancet 1991;337:1491.

45. Canadian Collaborative CVS-Amniocentesis Clinical Trial Group. Multicentre randomized clinical trial of chorionic villus sampling and amniocentesis: First report. Lancet 1989;1:1.

46. Firth HV, Boyd PA, Chamberlain P, et al. Severe limb abnormalities after chorion villus sampling at 56–66 days' gestation. Lancet 1991;337:762.

47. Burton BK, Schulz CJ, Burd LI. Limb anomalies associated with chorionic villus sampling. Obstet Gynecol 1992;79:726.

48. Monni G, Ibba RM, Lai R, et al. Limb-reduction defects and chorion villus sampling. Lancet 1991;337:1091.

49. Mahoney MJ. Limb abnormalities and chorionic villus sampling. Lancet 1991;337:1422.

50. Jackson LG, Wapner RJ, Brambati B. Limb abnormalities and chorionic villus sampling. Lancet 1991;337:1423.

51. Schloo R, Miny P, Holzgreve W, et al. Distal limb deficiency following chorionic villus sampling? Am J Med Genet 1992;42:404.

52. Froster-Iskenius UG, Baird PA. Limb reduction defects in over one million consecutive live births. Teratology 1989;39:127.

53. Froster UG, Baird PA. Limb-reduction defects and chorionic villus sampling. Lancet 1992;339:66.

54. Centers for Disease Control and Prevention. Rubella vaccination during pregnancy—United States, 1971–1988. MMWR 1989;38:289.

55. Centers for Disease Control and Prevention. Rubella prevention. Recommendations of the Immunization Practices Advisory Committee (ACIP). MMWR 1990;39(RR-15):1.

56. Reinus JF, Leikin EL, Alter HJ, et al. Failure to detect vertical transmission of hepatitis C virus. Ann Intern Med 1992;117:881.

57. Ohto H, Terazawa S, Sasaki N, et al. Transmission of hepatitis C virus from mothers to infants. N Engl J Med 1994;330:744.

58. Fowler KB, Stagno S, Pass RF, et al. The outcome of congenital cytomegalovirus infection in relation to maternal antibody status. N Engl J Med 1992;326:663.

59. Yow MD, Demmler GJ. Congenital cytomegalovirus disease—20 years is long enough. N Engl J Med 1992; 325:702.

60. Gillespie SM, Cartter ML, Asch S, et al. Occupational risk of human parvovirus B19 infection for school and daycare personnel during an outbreak of erythema infectiosum. JAMA 1990;263:2061.

61. Pickering LK, Reves RR. Occupational risks of child-care providers and teachers. JAMA 1990;263:2096.

62. Grossman JH, Wallen WC, Sever JL. Management of genital herpes simplex virus infection during pregnancy. Obstet Gynecol 1981;58:1.

63. American College of Obstetricians and Gynecologists. Perinatal herpes simplex virus infection. ACOG Technical Bulletin No. 122. Washington, DC: American College of Obstetricians and Gynecologists, 1988.

64. Zinner SH, Kass EH. Long-term follow-up of bacteriuria of pregnancy. N Engl J Med 1971;285:820.

65. Vessey MP, Nunn JF. Occupational hazards of anaesthesia. BMJ 1980;281:696.

66. Rowland AS, Baird DD, Weinberg CR, et al. Reduced fertility among women employed as dental assistants exposed to high levels of nitrous oxide. N Engl J Med 1992;327:993.

67. Schnorr TM, Grajewski BA, Hornung RW, et al. Video

display terminals and the risk of spontaneous abortion. N Engl J Med 1991;324:727.

68. American College of Obstetricians and Gynecologists. Guidelines on Pregnancy and Work. Chicago, The American College of Obstetricians and Gynecologists, 1977.

69. Shulman A, Shapiro MS, Bahary C, Shenkman L. Abnormal thyroid function in hyperemesis gravidarum. Acta Obstet Gynencol Scand 1989;68:533.

70. Goodwin TM, Montoro M, Mestman JH. Transient hyperthyroidism and hyperemesis gravidarum: Clinical aspects. Am J Obstet Gyencol 1992;167:648.

71. Wilson R, McKillop JH, MacLean M, et al. Thyroid func-

tion tests are rarely abnormal in patients with severe hyperemesis gravidarum. Clin Endocrinol 1992;37:331.

72. Kadar N, DeVore G, Romero R. The discriminatory hCG zone: Its use in the sonographic evaluation for ectopic pregnancy. Obstet Gynecol 1981;58:156.

73. Fossum GT, Davajan V, Kletzky OA. Early detection of pregnancy with transvaginal ultrasound. Fertil Steril 1988;49(5):788.

74. Fritz MA, Guo S. Doubling time of human chorionic gonadotropin (hCG) in early normal pregnancy: Relationship to hCG concentration and gestational age. Fertil Steril 1987;47:584.

31

Delayed Childbearing

Linda J. Heffner

The decision of an increasing number of American women to delay childbearing into and beyond the third decade of life has resulted in an "epidemic" of pregnancies in older women. It is estimated that at least 8.6% of total births in the United States by the year 2000 will be to women older than 35.[1] Unfortunately for some of these women, the obstetric term "elderly primigravida," used to define a woman delivering her first child at age 35 years or older, conjures up a picture of a fragile pregnancy in a woman near the end of her reproductive lifespan. This image may make both the physician and the patient fearful—the physician because he or she does not know where the real risks may lie and the patient because she fears a loss of control over a very important life event.

Although there are no formal studies of the reasons why women delay childbearing until their mid to late thirties, several reasons leading to their choice can be hypothesized (Table 31–1). Involuntary infertility and the previous lack of a suitable partner may leave many women with no choice as to the timing of their childbearing. In contrast to the relatively small number of reasons why childbearing might be delayed is a long list of purported risks that physicians may quote. Careful review of the more recent data indicates that many of the risks are perceived rather than real and that careful medical attention can minimize the impact of the others on pregnancy outcome. The focus of this chapter is a critical examination of the risks of delayed childbearing and the formulation of an approach to counseling women older than 35 who are contemplating pregnancy.

RISKS OF DELAYED CHILDBEARING

Infertility

Although actual fertility rates (the number of live births per 1000 women of the same age) have been increasing since the 1970s for women older than 35 years of age, this increase results directly from the decision of a larger number of women to delay childbearing until the third and fourth decades.[2] Fecundity, which is the true measure of the ability of a couple to establish a pregnancy within a fixed time period, does decline with age.[3] In combination with the clinical definition of infertility (the inability of a couple to conceive within 1 year of actively trying to do so), this age-related decline in fecundity results in a threefold increase in infertility rates in women older than 35.[4] The decline in fecundity seen with advancing maternal age appears to result from a decline in oocyte quality rather than a decline in endometrial responsiveness to steroid hormones.[5] Other factors influencing fertility such as sexually transmitted diseases and occupational and environmental exposures may also explain some of the increase in age-specific infertility rates.[6]

Older couples often feel a tremendous pressure to conceive within the short time they feel remains of their reproductive years. Most infertility specialists recommend that older couples who have been trying unsuccessfully for 6 months to establish a pregnancy see a health care professional

TABLE 31–1. Delayed Childbearing

RISKS	BENEFITS
Increased rates of	Greater financial stability
Infertility	Earlier opportunities for
Miscarriage	career development
Chromosomal abnormalities	More life experiences prior
Abnormal birth weight	to parenting (maturity)
Large infants	
Small infants	
Stillbirth	
Medical complications	
Hypertension	
Diabetes	
Obstetric complications	
Abnormal bleeding	
Labor difficulties	

skilled in the evaluation of infertility. Although a full infertility evaluation may not be started initially, several simple tests of ovulatory capacity and sperm quality can be performed. Encouraging results have been obtained with ovum donation programs for women older than 40 with ovarian failure, providing an option for women whose ovum quality has deteriorated to the point at which conception no longer seems possible.[7]

Miscarriage

Miscarriage, or spontaneous abortion, is a very common event in pregnancy, even among young women. Population studies suggest that at least 15% of all recognized pregnancies miscarry within the first 3 months of pregnancy.[8] At least 50% of miscarried pregnancies have a chromosomal abnormality.[9] Because older women have an increased risk of chromosomal abnormalities, it is not surprising that the miscarriage rate rises as a woman ages.[8] Unfortunately, there may also be a modest increase in risk of miscarrying a chromosomally normal fetus in women older than 35.[10] This fact has not been clearly established because of the lack of control for gravidity, pregnancy order, and history of prior miscarriages in the previously mentioned study. A nonchromosomal decline in oocyte quality might be responsible for the observed increase in miscarriages among older women, just as it appears to diminish fecundity.

Although the majority of women who have miscarriages have little risk of repeated recurrences, a small proportion of women may have a specific disorder underlying their miscarriages. Examples of these problems include uterine malformations, unusual antibodies to phospholipids or to pregnancy tissues, and parental chromosomal translocations. It is important that all women who experience three or more consecutive miscarriages be evaluated for the possibility of an underlying disorder causing the recurrent miscarriages because some of these abnormalities are amenable to medical therapy. Although most of these problems occur independently of maternal age, women may add several years to their age during the period in which the recurrent miscarriages occur. Older women with recurrent miscarriages should be referred promptly to a specialist skilled in their evaluation.

Chromosomal Abnormalities

An increase in chromosomal abnormalities in the offspring of older women is a widely recog-

nized risk of delayed childbearing. An increased frequency of chromosomal abnormalities has been found among miscarried pregnancies, induced abortions, midtrimester fetal karyotypes, stillbirths, and livebirths from older women.

The risk of a chromosomal abnormality does not increase suddenly in the later reproductive years but increases steadily from the early years on. Most of the increase results from an increase in trisomies, both of autosomes and sex chromosomes,[11, 12] the best known of which is Down syndrome or trisomy 21. Table 31–2 lists the maternal age–specific risks for Down syndrome and for all chromosomal abnormalities in a format widely used in prenatal counseling.

Initially, it was also believed that the frequency of nonchromosomal congenital malformations increases among the offspring of older mothers; however, this impression has not been substantiated in studies in which chromosmally abnormal fetuses and maternal conditions known a priori to

TABLE 31–2.   Age-Specific Risks for Chromosomal Abnormalities in Liveborn Infants

MATERNAL AGE AT DELIVERY	RISK OF DOWN SYNDROME	RISK OF ANY CHROMOSOMAL ABNORMALITY*
20	1/1667	1/526
21	1/1667	1/526
22	1/1429	1/500
23	1/1429	1/500
24	1/1250	1/476
25	1/1250	1/476
26	1/1176	1/476
27	1/1111	1/455
28	1/1053	1/435
29	1/1000	1/417
30	1/952	1/385
31	1/909	1/385
32	1/769	1/322
33	1/602	1/286
34	1/485	1/238
35	1/378	1/192
36	1/289	1/156
37	1/224	1/127
38	1/173	1/102
39	1/136	1/83
40	1/106	1/66
41	1/82	1/53
42	1/63	1/42
43	1/49	1/33
44	1/38	1/26
45	1/30	1/21
46	1/23	1/16
47	1/18	1/13
48	1/14	1/10
49	1/11	1/8

*Excludes 46,XXX for ages 20–32 because data are not available.
Data have been modified from the maternal age-specific rates derived by Hook and colleagues (Hook EB. Rates of chromosome abnormalities at different maternal ages. Obstet Gynecol 1981;58:282–285; and Hook EB, Cross PK, Schreinemachers DM. Chromosomal abnormality rates at amniocentesis and in live-born infants. JAMA 1983;249:2034–2038).

be associated with birth defects are excluded. In the largest study of more than 26,000 liveborn children with birth defects, no increase could be found in 43 categories of birth defects for mothers older than 35.[13] Rates for patent ductus arteriosus, hypertrophic pyloric stenosis, and congenital dislocated hip were actually decreased among the children of the older women.

Because of the increased risk of chromosomal abnormalities, all women who will be 35 years of age or older at delivery should be offered a fetal karyotype as part of their prenatal care. The currently available methods for obtaining fetal cells for karyotype include amniocentesis and chorionic villus sampling. Amniocentesis is most often performed between 12 and 16 weeks of gestation using menstrual dates, with procedure-related loss rates of 2.3% and 0.5%, respectively, for the two extremes of fetal age.[14, 15] Chorionic villus sampling may be done slightly earlier than the earliest amniocentesis with a 2.5% procedure-related loss rate;[16] concern has been raised about an increased incidence of limb defects among newborns whose mothers underwent chorionic villus sampling.[17] Some care providers now restrict the use of chorionic villus sampling to testing for genetic disorders with a high recurrence risk for carrier parents.

Abnormalities in Infant Birth Weight

Although mean birth weight for infants delivered by women older than 35 is the same as that for younger women, there is a modest offsetting increase in the numbers of both large and low birth weight babies in older women.[18, 19] There are several possible explanations for this redistribution of birth weights in the older mothers.

Although most large infants develop without any known explanation, maternal obesity and diabetes both are associated with increased infant birth weight. Both of these conditions occur with increased frequency among older women and probably explain at least some of the increase in numbers of large infants born to older mothers. Women older than 35 are approximately 1.5 times more likely to bear an infant weighing more than 4000 gm than are younger women.[20–22]

Low infant birth weight (<2500 gm) can result from either prematurity or from diminished intrauterine growth. Prematurity has not been shown consistently to be increased among the offspring of older mothers[20, 23–26]; thus, it appears that most of the increase in low birth weight among the offspring of older mothers results from inadequate intrauterine growth. Hypertension is a risk factor for diminished intrauterine growth and is seen in increased proportions among populations of older women. Cigarette smoking, which can diminish fetal growth, seems to have more of an effect on birth weight in older mothers than in younger ones.[27]

The impact of the modest splaying of the birth weight distribution among older women on the ultimate pregnancy outcome is uncertain. As will be discussed in more detail later, the cesarean delivery rate is elevated among older gravidas; the increased proportion of larger babies may be partly responsible for this observation. Small, chronically undernourished fetuses are at increased risk for fetal distress in labor and for intrauterine death due to asphyxia. Smaller infants who cannot tolerate the rigors of normal labor may contribute to the increase in cesarean delivery rates among older mothers. The stillbirth rate is elevated among older mothers, although birth weight and presumed cause of death have not been analyzed.

Liberal use of ultrasound when a fetus of abnormal size is suspected is appropriate at any maternal age. The presence of maternal hypertension or diabetes in older women poses sufficient risk that their pregnancies ideally should be managed by an obstetric specialist trained in high-risk pregnancies.

Increase in Stillbirths

As mentioned earlier, most studies of pregnancy outcomes in women older than age 35 have demonstrated an increase in stillbirths.[28] Women in their late thirties have about twice the risk of stillbirth than do women younger than 30; by age 45 stillbirths occur approximately four times more often. There appear to be several reasons for the increase. First, fetuses with chromosomal abnormalities are at increased risk for death in utero.[29] Most studies of pregnancy outcome in older women do not control for the expected increase in the number of chromosomally abnormal fetuses. Second, medical complications of pregnancy, notably hypertension and diabetes, are more frequent among older gravidas. Both these conditions can lead to fetuses of abnormal size that are at risk for antenatal asphyxia.

Several studies have divided their older parturients into lower- and higher-risk groups and have found that the increased risk of stillbirth is confined to the higher-risk groups with hypertension or obesity.[22, 24] The results of other studies have not been so encouraging.[21] No studies have controlled for fetal chromosomal abnormalities among the older mothers.

There have been no clinical trials of the utility

of routine fetal surveillance in reducing the still-birth rate among older gravidas. Nonetheless, it would seem prudent to watch fetal growth carefully among uncomplicated older gravidas and institute antepartum surveillance for unusually large or unusually small fetuses. Electronic fetal monitoring during labor of older gravidas is appropriate because some studies, although not all, have reported decreased 1-minute Apgar scores in the infants of older mothers, suggesting that they tolerate labor less well.[20-22, 24-26] As mentioned earlier, older women with underlying medical problems carry a disproportionate amount of the risk for a poor pregnancy outcome and should be under expert care throughout the pregnancy whenever possible.

Medical Complications

The incidence of both hypertension and diabetes is increased in older gravidas. Hypertension in pregnancy is classified as either preexisting or pregnancy induced; both categories show increases among women older than 35, although most studies group all hypertensive disorders together. In two large studies of more than 35,000 women each, preeclampsia rates were doubled in women older than 40 compared with rates for women younger than 30.[19, 30] Overall, hypertensive disorders in pregnancy appear to at least quadruple by age 40 from the baseline 2 to 3%.[22, 24]

Like hypertension, diabetes mellitus increases in prevalence with advancing age. Gestational diabetes also increases with age from 0.3 to 1.7% in the youngest age groups to 1.0 to 4.1% in older women.[20, 30]

Obesity also appears to be a marker for less than optimal pregnancy outcome among older women.[24] It is unclear how much of the effect is independent of the association of obesity with hypertension and diabetes.

Obstetric Complications

Several obstetric complications are increased among older women. These include increases in the incidence of third-trimester bleeding and delivery by cesarean section. Maternal mortality also increases with advancing maternal age but is a very rare complication, even with the age-related increase (current maternal mortality in the United States is less than 10 per 100,000 live births).[31]

Third-trimester bleeding results from either a placenta previa or a placental abruption. Both appear to occur more frequently among older primi-gravidas.[20, 22, 24, 32] Women of any age who are hypertensive are at increased risk for a placental abruption; no measurement has been made of the independent contribution of maternal age. Advancing maternal age is an independent risk factor for placenta previa, doubling the baseline risk of 4.4 per 1000 by age 35.[32] In addition, one study has demonstrated an increased risk of intrapartum or postpartum hemorrhage and transfusion that is independent of high parity.[21]

The most consistently demonstrated obstetric complication among older women is the significantly higher proportion who undergo cesarean delivery. All studies of women aged 35 years and older have demonstrated at least a 70% greater risk of delivery by cesarean section, regardless of their parity, over women in their twenties. Multiple attempts have been made to identify factors that lead to this increase. It may be explained partially by the redistribution of birth weight into increased proportions of both abnormally large and abnormally small babies; however, the association with age remains even when controlled for labor induction, epidural anesthesia, meconium in the amniotic fluid, and fetal distress.[33] Older gravidas appear to have an increased incidence of malpresentations[21, 22] and are also more likely to have an assisted vaginal delivery with forceps or vacuum extractor than younger women.[21, 25] A higher proportion of older women may have long second stages of labor.[26] It is likely that the strong positive association between advanced maternal age and the use of cesarean delivery results from a combination of the previously mentioned biologic factors along with multiple social factors. In one report, ''advanced maternal age'' was the primary indication written in the medical record in 31% of women older than 35 years of age undergoing cesarean section.[25]

PUTTING THE RISKS OF DELAYED CHILDBEARING IN PERSPECTIVE

Although the previous discussion has identified some discrete areas of risk for the woman who has delayed her childbearing, the likelihood of delivery of a healthy child by most older women is high. Although fecundity appears to decline substantially after age 40, the recent understanding that this represents a decline in ovulation or oocyte quality promises new therapies to enhance the pregnancy rates among older women who desire children. Once pregnant, the most signficant risk among healthy women is of a fetal chromosomal abnormality; this risk may rise as high as 2 to 3%

for women by their early forties. The availabiity of techniques for the detection of chromosomal abnormalities makes this a manageable problem for many. The relatively common problems of pregnancy-induced hypertension and gestational diabetes, which appear to double in frequency even among otherwise healthy gravidas over age 35, appear to have only a small impact on the ultimate delivery of a healthy child.

For older women who enter pregnancy with specific medical problems, the chances of a good pregnancy outcome are as much related to the underlying medical disorder as they are to advanced maternal age. These women should be strongly encouraged to seek preconceptual counseling by a qualified maternal-fetal medicine specialist so that disease-specific risks can be determined. Even among medically complicated patients, good pregnancy outcomes are possible for many.

In discussing pregnancy and delivery plans with older women, personal experience suggests that preparing them for more interaction with the medical system than that experienced by younger women prevents unrealistic expectations and later disappointments. At a minimum, they should anticipate genetic counseling for advanced maternal age and screening for gestational diabetes. The increased prevalence of pregnancy-induced hypertension and gestational diabetes, which may not ultimately affect their chances of having a healthy baby, may require substantial changes in their lifestyle during pregnancy. They may need to modify their work schedules or stop working entirely. For career-oriented women, such changes may be very difficult and a source of considerable conflict between patient and provider.

In summary, pregnancy outcome for most older women are good, provided attention is paid to the specific areas of increased risk. To optimize the pregnancy experience, older women should seek providers who are comfortable with pregnacies complicated by advanced maternal age and who can be supportive of the woman's choice.

REFERENCES

1. Spencer G. Projections of the population of the United States, by age, sex and race: 1983–2080. Current population reports—Population estimates and projections. Washington, DC: U.S. Department of Commerce (series P-25, no 952), 1984.
2. Centers for Disease Control and Prevention. Postponed childbearing—United States. 1970–1987. JAMA 1990; 263(3):360.
3. Stovall DW, Toma SK, Hammond MG, et al. The effect of age on female fecundity. Obstet Gynecol 1991;77(1):33.
4. The National Center for Health Statistics, 1989.
5. Navot D, Bergh PA, Williams MA, et al. Poor oocyte quality rather than implantation failure as a cause of age-related decline in female fertility. Lancet 1991; 337(8754):1375.
6. Aral SO, Cates W Jr. The increasing concern with infertility—Why now? JAMA 1983;250(17):2327.
7. Sauer MV, Paulson RJ, Lobo RA. Reversing the natural decline in human fertility. JAMA 1992;268(10):1275.
8. Harlop S, Shiono PH, Ramcharan S. A life table of spontaneous abortions and the effect of age, parity, and other variables. In: Porter IH, Hook EB (eds). Embryonic and Fetal Death. New York: Academic Press, 1980, pp 145–158.
9. Kajii T, Ferrier A, Niikawa N, et al. Anatomic and chromosomal anomalies in 639 spontaneous abortuses. Human Genet 1980;55(1):87.
10. Stein Z, Kline J, Susser E, et al. Maternal age and spontaneous abortion. In: Porter IH, Hook EB (eds). Embryonic and Fetal Death. New York: Academic Press, 1980, pp 107–127.
11. Hook EB. Rates of chromosomal abnormalities at different maternal ages. Obstet Gynecol 1981;58(3):282.
12. Hook EB, Cross PK, Schreinemachers DM. Chromosomal abnormality rates at amniocentesis and in live-born infants. JAMA 1983;249(15):2034.
13. Baird PA, Sadovnick AD, Yee IML. Maternal age and birth defects: A population study. Lancet 1991;337(8740): 527.
14. Penso CA, Sandstrom MM, Garber MF, et al. Early amniocentesis: Report of 407 cases with neonatal follow-up. Obstet Gynecol 1990;76(6):1032.
15. Katayama KP, Roesler MR. Five hundred cases of amniocentesis without bloody tap. Obstet Gynecol 1986;68(1): 70.
16. Jackson LG, Zachary JM, Fowler SE, et al. A randomized comparison of transcervical and transabdominal chorionic-villus sampling. N Engl J Med 1992;327(9):594.
17. Firth HV, Boyd PA, Chamberlain P, et al. Severe limb abnormalities after chorionic villus sampling at 56–66 days' gestation. Lancet 1991;337(8744):762.
18. Kaltreider F. The elderly multigravida. Obstet Gynecol 1959;13(2):190.
19. Kane SH. Advancing age and the primigravida. Obstet Gynecol 1967;29(3):409.
20. Grimes DA, Gross GK. Pregnancy outcomes in black women aged 35 and older. Obstet Gynecol 1981;58(5): 614.
21. Kirz DS, Dorchester W, Freeman RK. Advanced maternal age: The mature gravida. Am J Obstet Gynecol 1985; 152(1):7.
22. Lehmann DK, Chism J. Pregnancy outcome in medically complicated and uncomplicated patients aged 40 years or older. Am J Obstet Gynecol 1987;157(3):738.
23. Forman MR, Meirik O, Berendes HW. Delayed childbearing in Sweden. JAMA 1984;252(22):3135.
24. Spellacy WN, Miller SJ, Winegar A. Pregnancy after 40 years of age. Obstet Gynecol 1986;68(4):452.
25. Tuck SM, Yudkin PL, Turnbull AC. Pregnancy outcome in elderly primigravidae with and without a history of infertility. Br J Obstet Gynaecol 1988;95(3):230.
26. Berkowitz GS, Skrovon ML, Lapinski RH, et al. Delayed childbearing and the outcome of pregnancy. New Engl J Med 1990;322(10):659.
27. Cnattingius S, Axelsson O, Eklund G, et al. Smoking, maternal age, and fetal growth. Obstet Gynecol 1985: 66(4):449.
28. Hansen JP. Older maternal age and pregnancy outcome: A review of the literature. Obstet Gynecol Surv 1986;41(11):726.

29. Machin GA. Chromosome abnormality and perinatal death. Lancet 1974;1(874):549.
30. Tysoe FW. Effect of age on the outcome of pregnancy. Trans Pacif Coast Obstet Gynecol Soc 1970;38(1):8.
31. Atrash HK, Koonin LM, Lawson HW, et al. Maternal mortality in the United States, 1979–1986. Obstet Gynecol 1990;76(6):1055.

32. Zhang J, Savitz DA. Maternal age and placenta previa: A population-based, case-control study. Am J Obstet Gynecol 1993;168(2):641.
33. Martel M, Wacholder S, Lippman A, et al. Maternal age and primary cesarean section rates: A multivariate analysis. Am J Obstet Gynecol 1987;156(2):305.

Physiologic Adaptations to Pregnancy

Emily R. Baker

Although pregnant women are normal and healthy, their physiology differs radically from that of nonpregnant women. Physicians who care for pregnant women must always keep this in mind. The usual adult norms of laboratory values and physiologic function cannot always be applied. The changes that occur affect every organ system, some more dramatically than others. Some organ systems undergo changes that would otherwise be interpreted as disease states. In others, function becomes "super" normal. These changes often begin very early in pregnancy without obvious benefit to the mother or fetus. Some of them are clearly adaptations to the needs of the developing embryo and fetus or are preparations for parturition. Another remarkable feature of these physiologic and structural adaptations is their near complete reversibility after delivery.

This chapter reviews by organ system the maternal physiologic and structural adaptations to pregnancy. Only clinically important changes are discussed. Changes in normative laboratory values and maternal symptoms are presented as well.

HEMATOLOGIC CHANGES

Plasma Volume and Red Blood Cells

Plasma volume expands significantly, beginning at 6 to 8 weeks' gestation, and increases linearly until approximately 34 weeks, when it reaches a plateau or declines slightly. The mean increase is 50%, although it ranges from 20 to 100%. The absolute increase in the average healthy primigravida is from 2600 to 3900 ml.[1] Expansion of the plasma volume appears to be integral to the well-being of the pregnancy. Hemoconcentration is associated with hypertensive disorders of pregnancy and with fetal growth retardation. Birth weights are positively correlated with plasma volume ex-

pansion, and women with multiple gestations have proportionately larger increases in plasma volume.

Red blood cell volume also increases but not to the degree of plasma volume. This produces the so-called physiologic anemia of pregnancy. Substantial decline of hemoglobin and hematocrit values are expected and do not necessarily represent pathologic anemia. During a pregnancy, red blood cell volume increases 20% on average, from a 1400 ml prepregnancy level to 1650 ml at term. Up to a 30% increase in red blood cell volume can be observed in women who take iron supplements. Venous hematocrit values fall from the prepregnancy average of 40% to approximately 34% at 30 to 34 weeks' gestation. Serum iron and the percent saturation of total iron-binding capacity fall in pregnancy, making their application less useful. An iron-binding capacity of 15% or less is consistent with iron deficiency. Serum ferritin is likely the most useful test of iron stores.[2] Erythrocyte indices do not change in pregnancy.

The etiology of blood volume expansion is not well understood. The function of plasma volume expansion may be to decrease blood viscosity, to protect against hypotension, to dissipate fetal heat production, and to assist with renal filtration. The expansion of blood volume allows a woman to tolerate the average 500 ml blood loss from a vaginal delivery and 1000 ml blood loss from an uncomplicated cesarean section. Plasma volume contracts with the postpartum diuresis so that in the absence of pathologic anemia or massive hemorrhage, loss of 1000 ml of blood does not cause a significant fall in hemoglobin concentration.

Controversy exists over the need for iron supplementation in healthy pregnant women, although it is common practice currently in the United States. Ample evidence exists that the fall of hematocrit reflects beneficial hemodilution. Recent studies demonstrate a U-shaped relationship between hemoglobin concentration and rates of preterm birth, fetal growth retardation, and perinatal mortality, with increased rates of adverse outcome occurring at the extremes of hemoglobin concentration.[3] Studies of iron supplementation have not found significant beneficial or detrimental effects on fetal growth or pregnancy outcome.[4] The primary argument for supplementation is to prevent depletion of iron stores. Approximately 800 mg of iron are required for each pregnancy, which can deplete the total iron stores of 2.5 gm. Women coming to pregnancy with adequate stores can meet the needs of the current pregnancy but may not be able to replete iron stores between pregnancies, especially with iron-poor diets.

White Blood Cells and Platelets

A significant leukocytosis occurs in pregnancy, with the leukocyte count rising to a mean of 10,000 (5000–16,000) cells per mm[3] in late pregnancy.[5] This is predominantly accounted for by an increase in circulating polymorphonuclear cells. In labor, the white blood cell count can be as high as 20,000 to 30,000 cells per mm[3] in the absence of infection. The white blood cell count returns to prepregnancy levels within a week after delivery. Platelet counts fall slightly during pregnancy but in general remain within prepregnancy ranges. Results of studies of the incidence of thrombocytopenia in pregnancy vary from 7.6 to 24%.[6, 7] Some pregnant women with thrombocytopenia are found to have medical or obstetric disorders, but most have idiopathic mild thrombocytopenia attributed to the physiologic changes of pregnancy. The fall in platelets is due to increased peripheral destruction as demonstrated by shorter platelet life span and larger mean platelet size.[8] The appearance of thrombocytopenia in the third trimester should prompt an evaluation for preeclampsia, but aggressive medical evaluation for mild thrombocytopenia is unnecessary.

Coagulation Factors

Pregnancy is often referred to as a hypercoagulable state. Several plasma clotting factors do rise in pregnancy, and fibrinolysis decreases. The risk of thromboembolic disease increases. The risk of thromboembolism is most pronounced around delivery and for 6 weeks afterward. Fibrinogen demonstrates the most dramatic rise of the clotting factors, rising to 400 to 500 mg per dl. (The increase in fibrinogen causes the sedimentation rate to increase two- to sixfold.) Although some controversy exists, it appears that factors VII, VIII, X,

and fibrin increase as well.[9] It appears that levels of antithrombin III, which limits clot formation, are not altered in pregnancy. Despite these factor changes, clotting and bleeding times are not significantly altered by pregnancy.

CARDIOVASCULAR SYSTEM CHANGES

A large amount of research has gone into defining cardiovascular physiology during pregnancy. Controversy over conflicting results has been common. Study parameters have been found to vary considerably depending on maternal position and gestational age.[10] The maternal position most commonly used for baseline measurements is the left lateral recumbent position, which eliminates pooling of blood in the extremities and maximizes venous return to the heart by preventing compression of the vena cava. In general, the cardiovascular adaptations are felt to result in a hyperdynamic state, with increases in heart rate, cardiac output, and stroke volume and decreases in systemic vascular resistance and blood pressure. These adaptations return to normal after delivery but can take several months to return to prepregnancy values.[11] Studies that use patients who are 6-weeks' postpartum as controls will underestimate the degree of change.

Structural Changes

As the diaphragm rises during pregnancy, the heart is displaced superiorly, laterally, and anteriorly. This, along with a small amount of pericardial effusion, often gives the erroneous impression of cardiomegaly. On chest radiographs the border of the left side of the heart also appears straightened. Left axis deviation appears on electrocardiogram.

The heart and vessels must adapt to the volume load of pregnancy. Myocardial hypertrophy is demonstrated by histology and by electrocardiography. Some echocardiographic studies suggest increased myocardial contractility. Left and right ventricular end-diastolic volumes are increased without a significant change in left ventricular end-systolic size.[12, 13] Because end-diastolic pressures do not increase, this suggests increased compliance.

The entire vascular tree accommodates the increased volume and blood flow with a softening of collagen and with smooth muscle hypertrophy. As a result, the pulmonary artery and pulmonary vasculature appear prominent on chest radiographs.

Venous compliance also increases, with distention being most apparent in the lower extremities.

By 24 to 28 weeks' gestation, the size and weight of the uterus are capable of significant compression of the vena cava in the supine position. By term, the potential occlusion is likely complete, and venous return is accomplished through the paravertebral circulation. In the supine position, cardiac output falls up to 30% at term.[12] This does not result in hypotension in most women because blood pressure is maintained by an increase in peripheral resistance, which may have adverse effects on uterine blood flow. Up to 10% of pregnant women do experience a supine hypotension syndrome with dizziness, nausea, and syncope.

Signs and Symptoms

Several of the signs and symptoms of pregnancy are caused by cardiovascular changes and can mimic cardiac disease.[14] From early in pregnancy, many women experience dyspnea, fatigue, and decreased exercise tolerance. Syncope and dizziness in the upright position occur from early pregnancy in up to 10% of women, presumably due to vasodilation. Palpitations, or a general awareness of the heart beating, are not infrequent. The point of maximum impulse is displaced laterally and superiorly. Later in pregnancy, extremity edema from increased venous pressure and decreased plasma colloid oncotic pressure is extremely common, as is distention of the neck veins.

On auscultation the first heart sound is louder, and there is an exaggerated split of the mitral and triscupid components. The second heart sound is unchanged. Third heart sounds can be heard in up to 90% of pregnant women by 20 weeks of gestation. An early to midsystolic murmur is almost universally present, is best heard at the left sternal border, and is thought to be due to increased flow across the aortic and pulmonic valves. Up to 15% of women will have a murmur of mammary vessel origin, which is best heard in the second intercostal space and can be changed by pressure on the stethoscope head. Fourth heart sounds and diastolic murmurs are far less common and probably warrant investigation by a cardiologist.

Cardiac Output

Cardiac output increases 30 to 50% in pregnancy, beginning early in the first trimester.[15] By 10 weeks of gestation, cardiac output has reached 6 liters per minute. There is likely slight additional increase in the second trimester, with persistence of elevated cardiac output to term. This increase is facilitated by both a decrease in peripheral vascular resistance and the development of a low resistance shunt in the uteroplacental circulation. The increase in cardiac output is determined by increases in stroke volume and heart rate. The increase in stroke volume predominates early in pregnancy and then falls back toward normal at term. An increase in heart rate compensates for this fall in stroke volume and maintains cardiac output. By the third trimester, heart rate may have increased as much as 15 to 20 beats per minute over nonpregnant values. Both cardiac output and heart rate depend on maternal position. As discussed previously, cardiac output declines significantly in the supine position. The distribution of cardiac output changes and reflects the needs of the uteroplacental circulation (Fig. 32–1).

Vascular Resistance

Peripheral vascular resistance falls during pregnancy and is 20% lower at term than in the nonpregnant state. This is likely due to smooth muscle relaxation in vessel walls and to the low-resistance uteroplacental circulation acting like an arteriovenous fistula. Fetal heat production may also produce vasodilation. The decreased blood pressure and increased cardiac output in pregnancy both contribute to decreased peripheral resistance. As blood pressure rises toward term and cardiac output remains stable, systemic resistance must also rise somewhat, although the amount has not been quantified. Pulmonary vascular resistance has also been demonstrated to fall approximately 34% by term.[16] Other interesting alterations occur in the vasculature. Pregnant women without preeclampsia demonstrate refractoriness to the effects of pressor agents such as angiotensin. In contrast, pregnant women are very sensitive to autonomic blockade as produced by spinal or epidural anesthesia or by pharmacologic ganglionic blockade. This produces serious hypotension from loss of venomotor tone and venous pooling. The effect can be diminished by providing additional intravascular fluid and avoiding caval compression.

Arterial and Venous Pressures

Arterial blood pressure values also depend on maternal position, with the lowest values demonstrated in the left lateral recumbent position. The systolic blood pressure changes little during pregnancy, decreasing perhaps 5 mm Hg.[15] By 28 to

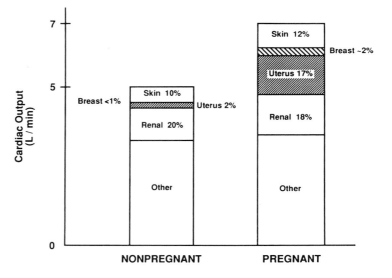

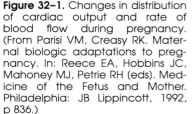

Figure 32–1. Changes in distribution of cardiac output and rate of blood flow during pregnancy. (From Parisi VM, Creasy RK. Maternal biologic adaptations to pregnancy. In: Reece EA, Hobbins JC, Mahoney MJ, Petrie RH (eds). Medicine of the Fetus and Mother. Philadelphia: JB Lippincott, 1992, p 836.)

32 weeks of gestation, supine diastolic blood pressures can be as much as 15 to 20 mm Hg below nonpregnant levels. Diastolic pressures rise slowly back toward normal levels at term. However, at any gestational age, a diastolic blood pressure greater than 90 mm Hg should be considered abnormal, and pressures greater than 80 mm Hg should prompt observation for hypertension and preeclampsia. Compared with systemic pressures, pulmonary artery pressures and pulmonary capillary wedge pressures differ little in pregnancy.[16]

Venous pressures are unchanged in the arms but in the legs increase from 10 cm H_2O to 25 cm H_2O at term. Portal venous pressures increase but not to a pathologic degree and may contribute to the development of hemorrhoids. Central venous pressures are not altered by pregnancy.

Hemodynamics of Parturition

Labor and the immediate postpartum period are a time of acute hemodynamic fluctuation and stress.[12] In labor cardiac output may be increased to 40% above the already elevated late pregnancy levels.[17] Much of this is mediated by increased stroke volume, but increased heart rate from pain and fear also have an effect. The use of regional anesthesia can ameliorate much of the increase in cardiac output. Each contraction causes an acute rise in preload with 300 to 500 ml of blood being shunted from the uterine to the systemic circulation. Systolic and diastolic blood pressure increases 20 to 30 mm Hg during contractions. The most stressful period for cardiac function is the immediate postpartum period when cardiac output

reaches a value approximately 60% above prelabor values. This is attributed in part to the autotransfusion of 500 ml of blood, the increased venous return, and the mobilization of extracellular fluid. A reflex bradycardia often occurs after delivery as well.

RESPIRATORY TRACT CHANGES

Several structural changes occur in the upper respiratory tract during pregnancy. The shape of the thoracic cage changes even before any mechanical influence from the enlarging uterus. The subcostal angle increases with the transverse diameter of the chest, increasing about 2 cm, and the chest circumference increases approximately 6 cm. The level of the diaphragm rises 4 cm during pregnancy, and excursion of the diaphragm increases 1 to 2 cm despite the enlarging uterus. There is increase in the vascularity and friability of the upper airway mucosa, leading to complaints of chronic nasal congestion and nasal bleeding.

Several lung volumes alter significantly during pregnancy (Fig. 32–2).[18, 19] The tidal volume (the volume of air exchanged per breath) increases 40% and accounts for the 40% increase in minute ventilation. This is thought to be due to central nervous system effects of progesterone. Respiratory rate changes little. The expiratory residual volume (amount of air that can be expired from resting expiratory level) and the residual volume (amount of remaining air in the lungs after maximal expiration) both decrease by 20%. The functional residual capacity (amount of air in the lungs at resting expiratory level) is therefore also de-

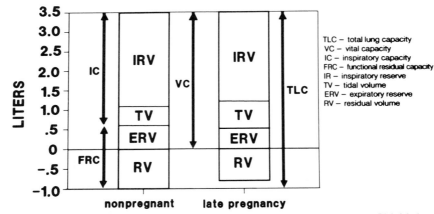

Figure 32-2. Changes in lung volumes during pregnancy. (From Cruikshank DP, Hayes PM. Maternal physiology in pregnancy. In: Gabbe SG, Niebyl JR, Simpson JL (eds). Obstetrics: Normal and Problem Pregnancies. 2nd ed. New York: Churchill Livingstone, 1991, p 128.)

creased by 20%. As a result, the pregnant woman is very susceptible to the rapid development of hypoxia with inadequate ventilation. There is little change in total lung volume (about 5% decrease) and no change in inspiratory reserve volume (maximum amount of air that can be additionally inspired after normal inspiration) or in vital capacity (maximum amount of air forcibly expired after maximal inspiration).

Pulmonary function is not diminished by pregnancy. Airway resistance is not altered significantly. Although oxygen consumption increases 20%, this need is easily met by the 40% increase in minute ventilation. As a result, P_{O_2} levels increase to 104 to 108 mm Hg. The increased ventilation also causes a significant decrease in P_{CO_2} levels to 27 to 32 mm Hg. The resulting respiratory alkalosis is compensated for by a metabolic acidosis with increased renal excretion of bicarbonate. Normal serum bicarbonate levels in pregnancy are 18 to 32 mEq per liter. Despite very adequate ventilation and respiratory function, many pregnant women complain of dyspnea. No satisfactory explanation exists for this symptom.

RENAL AND UROLOGIC SYSTEM CHANGES

Structural Changes

The most striking structural change is the development of mild collecting system dilation in most pregnant women.[20] The ureters above the pelvic brim, calyces, and pelves dilate by the middle of pregnancy. Ureteral diameters can reach 2 cm. The right side is more commonly dilated than the left,

which may be due to the cushioning effect of the sigmoid colon, the dextrorotation of the uterus, and the course of the right ovarian vein. Renal volume increases by up to 30%, possibly owing to increased renal blood volume and interstitial fluid.[21] Because of the collecting system dilation and urinary stasis, pregnant women with asymptomatic bacteriuria are predisposed to ascending infection. Another effect of the dilation is the impairment of interpretation of urologic and renal function tests.

Despite the ureteral dilation, peristalsis does not seem to be affected. Late in pregnancy, ureteral tone does appear to be increased. Urodynamic evaluations demonstrate decreased bladder capacity and increased bladder pressure. Although the anatomic and functional length of the urethra increases,[22] up to two thirds of women experience stress incontinence during pregnancy.

Functional Changes

Both renal plasma flow and glomerular filtration increase significantly in pregnancy beginning as early as 6 weeks' gestation.[23] Renal plasma flow increases up to 80% to a mean value of 840 ml per minute by 16 weeks. There is a small decrease in renal plasma flow in the third trimester. Glomerular filtration rates measured by studies of insulin clearance increase by about 50% in the first trimester and persist at this level through delivery. In pregnancy creatinine clearances of 120 to 200 ml per minute are normal.

Owing to increased filtration, serum levels of urea and creatinine decrease. Serum creatinine levels decrease from prepregnancy values of 0.8 to 1.0 mg per dl to 0.5 to 0.6 mg per dl in midgestation. A serum creatinine level of 0.9 mg per dl and greater in pregnancy is distinctly abnormal and warrants investigation for disease, primarily for preeclampsia. Urea levels are 8 to 9 mg per dl by the end of the first trimester. Serum uric acid levels fall approximately 25% in the first and second trimesters to levels of 2 to 3 mg per dl, then rise back to prepregnancy levels by term. Interpretation of third-trimester uric acid levels are often not useful without baseline nonpregnancy values.

Renal handling of sodium is significantly altered in pregnancy.[24] Despite an enormous increase in the filtered load of sodium and the natriuretic effect of progesterone, pregnant women remain in positive sodium balance, allowing transfer of sodium to the fetus and expansion of maternal extracellular fluid volume. Levels of aldosterone, desoxycorticosterone, and estrogen increase, all of which increases sodium reabsorption. Aldosterone levels rise from approximately 100 ng per ml to as high as 700 ng per ml by the end of pregnancy. The rise in aldosterone is partially attributable to similar rises in the renin-angiotensin system.[25] Plasma atrial natriuretic peptide levels are unchanged.[26] There is no clinically significant change of the serum level of sodium or of the other electrolytes other than bicarbonate, which is decreased to compensate for a respiratory alkalosis, as previously discussed. Plasma osmolality decreases to approximately 280 mOsm per liter without promoting a diuresis. Responses to sodium and water challenges are normal, so this change must represent a resetting of the "osmostat."[27]

Owing to the increased filtration rates and some changes in tubular function, urinary losses of some substances increase. Glucosuria occurs in up to 10% of pregnant women. This makes impossible the evaluation of glucose control in pregnant diabetics by urine glucose checks. There is also slight but not very significant increases in excretion of albumin and some amino acids. Up to 300 mg per day of proteinuria is considered normal. More than 500 mg of daily proteinuria is associated with adverse pregnancy outcome.[28] Folate and vitamin B_{12} losses are increased as well.

ENDOCRINE SYSTEM CHANGES

Placental Hormones

Human chorionic gonadotropin (hCG) is the first placental hormone product. It rises rapidly after implantation, peaks at day 60, then falls to a plateau at 18 weeks of gestation. Human chorionic gonadotropin supports the corpus luteum until the placenta is capable of taking over sex steroid hor-

mone production. In very high levels, as with molar pregnancy, human chorionic gonadotropin can have a stimulating effect on the thyroid gland.

Human placental lactogen is detectable by 8 weeks' gestation and then rises steadily throughout the rest of pregnancy. It has anabolic effects on metabolism that are similar to those of growth hormone.[29] It promotes lipolysis, protein sparing, and nitrogen retention. It also mediates increased peripheral insulin resistance. Another function is to stimulate breast growth and readiness for lactation.

Following the early part of the first trimester, estrogens and progesterone are produced primarily by the placenta. Production of estrogens including the major estrogen, estriol, requires cooperation of the mother, fetus, and placenta. The placenta is capable of producing progesterone independently.

Thyroid

Despite having changes in thyroid physiology and structure, pregnant women remain euthyroid, and the hypothalamic-pituitary-thyroid axis functions normally. The thyroid gland enlarges during pregnancy owing to follicular hyperplasia and increased vascularity. Plasma iodide levels fall because of renal losses that are due to increased filtration and decreased tubular reabsorption. The thyroid compensates by increasing absorption of iodide from the blood. Goiter does not occur unless the diet is deficient in iodine.

Thyrotropin-releasing hormone is unchanged by pregnancy and is the only thyroid hormone that can cross the placenta. Although some controversy exists, thyroid-stimulating hormone levels seem to be unchanged as well. Total thyroxine (T_4) and triiodothyronine (T_3) are increased significantly owing to the rise in thyroid-binding globulin levels. The amounts of free T_3 and T_4 are within normal limits. The high levels of thyroid-binding globulin also impair determination of thyroid-binding capacity by the resin T_3 uptake test. The free thyroxine index is therefore not as useful in pregnancy in estimating free hormone concentration.

Unlike the thyroid hormones other than thyrotropin-releasing hormone, iodide crosses the placenta freely. The fetus requires this supply to generate its own thyroid hormone. Pregnant women should not be given radioiodine or iodine-containing products that can produce fetal goiter and hypothyroidism.

Parathyroid

The fetus requires significant amounts of calcium and phosphorus for skeletal development. To avoid depletion of maternal calcium, adjustments are required in calcium homeostasis. Total serum calcium falls approximately 10% in pregnancy owing to the fall in serum albumin (about 1 gm/dl). Ionized calcium remains essentially unchanged despite increased renal filtration and transfer to the fetus. To provide needed calcium, levels of parathyroid hormone increase significantly over nonpregnant levels.[30] Parathyroid hormone acts to improve absorption of calcium from the gut, to decrease renal losses, and to mobilize bone. There is no loss of bone density despite the increases in parathyroid hormone activity. The skeleton appears to be protected by increased levels of calcitonin and by estrogen, which interferes with the action of parathyroid hormone on bone. There is increased activity of 1,25-dihydroxyvitamin D_3 that is due to increased stimulation of 1α-hydroxylase by parathyroid hormone and by the sex steroids. 1,25-Dihydroxyvitamin D_3 synthesis by the placenta has been demonstrated as well.

Pancreas and Metabolism

Pregnancy is marked by significant pancreatic beta-cell hyperplasia and hypertrophy. Fasting blood glucose falls 15 to 20 mg per dl by the first trimester under the influence of increased peripheral glucose use and decreased gluconeogenesis. Pregnancy is said to be a state of accelerated starvation due to the lower fasting blood glucose levels and the enhanced ketone production, which is thought to be caused by inadequate insulin production during starvation. Postprandial blood glucose levels rise to 130 to 140 mg per dl because of insulin resistance due to the effects of human placental lactogen, prolactin, progesterone, and cortisol. Tissue sensitivity to insulin falls as much as 80% by the end of pregnancy. Average blood glucose levels are normal (80–90 mg/dl).

The enhanced insulin production serves several purposes. Early in pregnancy, the extra insulin allows extra calories to be used for lipid storage and glycogen production. The fetus relies on glucose transfer for survival, although elevated levels of glucose in the first trimester are teratogenic. Later in pregnancy, as insulin resistance increases with increasing levels of human placental lactogen, more glucose is available for fetal energy needs. Some women are unable to mount a sufficient insulin response to overcome the tissue resistance and develop gestational diabetes.

Other Hormones

Free cortisol levels increase steadily, reaching twice nonpregnant levels by term. There is increased hepatic production of cortisol-binding globulin in response to estrogen stimulation. Despite having increases in corticosteroid levels, pregnant women do not experience hypercortisolism, with the possible exception of the formation of striae.

The pituitary gland enlarges in pregnancy mostly because of hyperplasia and hypertrophy of lactotrophs. Serum prolactin levels increase at least 10 times over nonpregnant levels but maintain diurnal variation. Prolactin prepares the breasts for lactation and affects maternal metabolism.

GASTROINTESTINAL SYSTEM CHANGES

Motility and tone throughout the gastrointestinal tract is decreased, which is attributable to the effects of progesterone on smooth muscle and to the decreased levels of motilin.[31] Decreased motility contributes to the symptoms of nausea, heartburn, gastric reflux, bloating, and constipation. Nausea is extremely common in the first trimester and occasionally persists into the second trimester. Recurrence of nausea and vomiting in the third trimester is a cause for concern and should prompt evaluation for diseases such as preeclampsia.

Esophagitis and hiatal hernia are more common in pregnancy. The incidence of peptic ulcer disease is decreased in pregnancy probably as a result of delayed gastric emptying, increased gastric mucous secretion, and decreased gastric acid production in the first and second trimesters. Gastric acid production reaches and even exceeds nonpregnant values by the third trimester, which increases the risks of aspiration at the time of delivery. The incidence of hemorrhoids is increased owing to venodilation, constipation, and increased portal venous pressures. The gallbladder is also affected by decreased motility and shows significant increases in fasting and residual volumes and decreased rates of emptying.[32] This decrease in motility and change of bile composition predisposes parous women to gallstone formation.

Appetite usually increases in pregnancy after first-trimester nausea abates with most women increasing their caloric intake by 200 to 300 kcal per day. Changes in food preference and cravings are common. Pica, the ingestion of nonnutritive substances such as paper or soap, is reported but is uncommon. There are few changes to the oral cavity other than hyperplasia and softening of the gums. Saliva production is unchanged, and there is no increase in cavity formation.

The liver does not increase in size nor does hepatic blood flow change in pregnancy. The physical findings of palmar erythema and spider angiomas can mimic liver disease but are due to increased estrogens. Laboratory values that appear abnormal include decreased serum albumin and total protein. Serum albumin averages 3 gm per dl at term. Alkaline phosphatase levels rise two to four times by term due to placental isoenzyme production. Estrogen-induced increases occur in the production of many proteins such as fibrinogen, several other clotting factors, and several binding proteins. Some lipids also increase, including cholesterol and triglycerides, which can double by term. Bilirubin levels are unchanged, as are the transaminase levels. Elevation of alanine aminotransferase and aspartate aminotransferase in the third trimester is abnormal and suggests the diagnosis of severe preeclampsia.

REPRODUCTIVE TRACT AND BREAST CHANGES

The uterus undergoes obvious and remarkable structural changes in pregnancy. In the first trimester, it softens considerably and doubles its weight. The size increase continues so that in primigravid women the uterus increases from a nonpregnant average of 40 gm to a term weight of 1200 gm. At 12 weeks of gestation the uterus is at the level of the pelvic brim, and at 20 weeks it is roughly at the level of the umbilicus. After that time the distance from the top of the uterus to the symphysis pubis measured in centimeters equals roughly the weeks of gestation. Uterine blood flow increases along with uterine size. By term uterine blood flow is 500 to 700 ml per minute, with the majority of the flow going to the placental circulation.

The entire lower genital tract has increased vascularity, edema, and connective tissue changes, making the tissues more pliable. The cervix produces more mucus owing to glandular hyperplasia. The vaginal mucosa thickens, and there is hypertrophy of underlying smooth muscle. The increased vascularity of the vulva occasionally results in the development of varicosities.

The breasts increase in size early in pregnancy because of vascular engorgement, which leads to complaints of breast heaviness and tenderness. After the first trimester, breast growth continues steadily owing to an increasing mass of glandular tissue. The increase in breast size is variable but averages 200 ml per breast. For unknown reasons, breast growth is considerably greater in primiparas younger than 20 years of age than in those older than 30 years. The nipples and areolae enlarge, and the nipples become more mobile. There is commonly increased pigmentation of the areolae. Small sebaceous glands under the areolae, Montgomery's glands or tubercles, become more prominent. Although the increase in size, glandularity, and tenderness of the breasts makes evaluation of breast masses more difficult, diagnosis of a breast mass should not be deferred because of pregnancy.

SKIN AND MUSCULOSKELETAL CHANGES

Increased pigmentation of the face, areolae, abdomen (linea nigra), axilla, and perineum is found in up to 90% of pregnant women in variable degrees. It is thought that this occurs under the influence of the sex steroids or melanocyte-stimulating factor. The changes generally regress after delivery. A few women experience melasma gravidarum ("mask of pregnancy") with noticeable pigment changes over the nose and cheeks. This entity is more common in women with dark complexions than in women with light complexions. Preexisting pigmented moles sometimes get darker, and some grow during pregnancy. Striae, linear tears in the dermis, occur in 50 to 90% of pregnant women. They initially appear purple or red and are most often located on the abdomen, buttocks, thighs, and breasts. After delivery, they take on a silver color. There is no known method of prevention. The etiology is not related to amount of weight gain, but there does seem to be a genetic component.

Estrogen increases the rate of hair growth throughout pregnancy. The proportion of hair in the resting phase, telogen, falls slightly toward the end of pregnancy and then increases significantly after delivery. The result is a sudden hair loss 2 to 4 months after delivery, with resumption of normal hair growth by approximately 6 months after childbirth. Estrogen also contributes to cutaneous vascular dilation and proliferation. Capillaries become dilated and may form angiomas, which regress after delivery. Palmar erythema is common as well.

Maternal posture changes to accommodate the altered center of gravity due to the enlarging uterus. An exaggerated lordosis develops to maintain balance. This contributes significantly to the common complaint of low back pain. Women also report pelvic discomfort from loosening and separation of the sacroiliac and symphysis pubis joints in preparation for parturition.

POSTPARTUM CHANGES

Functional and Structural Changes

Most of the structural and physiologic changes resolve steadily after delivery.[33] Plasma volume falls about 1 liter with delivery and then has a temporary increase of 900 to 1200 ml in the first 3 days after childbirth owing to mobilization of extracellular fluid. Many women report exacerbation of edema in the first few postpartum days. Measurements of the clotting factors are normal after 2 weeks. Most of the changes in cardiovascular dynamics initially resolve quickly, but some parameters such as stroke volume and systemic vascular resistance may take several months to return to normal. Ureteral diameters are normal by 6 weeks. Normal bladder function usually returns, but there can be long-lasting dysfunction due to perineal soft tissue and nerve damage in cases of long, difficult labors and perineal trauma. Glomerular filtration returns to prepregnancy levels by 8 weeks after delivery.

The uterus involutes to near prepregnancy size by 6 weeks after delivery. There is reversal of the vascular and glandular changes of the cervix and healing of delivery trauma by 6 weeks as well. Ovulation can occur as early as 27 days postpartum. In nonlactating women the mean time to ovulation is 70 to 75 days, and in lactating women it is 190 days. Menstruation resumes by 12 weeks in 70% of women who do not breast-feed. The delay in resumption of menstruation depends on the duration of breast-feeding, but in lactating women it takes 36 months for 70% to have begun menstruation.[33] Lactation suppresses ovulation by the continued presence of prolactin. There is no effect on gonadotropin levels, but low estrogen levels are detected in lactating women.

Symptoms

There are a number of common symptoms in the puerperium. A vaginal discharge (lochia) persists for 3 to 5 weeks. It is at first serosanguineous, then serous or mucopurulent. The perineal discomfort from delivery trauma takes up to 3 weeks to resolve depending on the amount of trauma and laceration. Effective treatment includes local measures such as sitz baths, topical anesthetics, and oral analgesics. Fatigue and lethargy are extremely common. If profound they could be due to thyroid dysfunction. In breast-feeding women, several complaints are due to hypoestrogenism. These include night sweats and dyspareunia from vaginal atrophy. The use of water-based lubricants eases symptoms from vaginal dryness. Although intercourse may be resumed as soon as the perineum has healed and the red vaginal discharge has ceased, many women experience decreased libido for several months after delivery.

Breast engorgement occurs a few days after delivery. For women who do not breast-feed, this state will persist for 2 to 3 days and then resolve, and breast size will decrease to that of the prepregnancy state. Pharmacologic suppression of lactation with either bromocriptine or estrogens is not commonly used currently owing to side effects and rebound engorgement. Breast binding or use of a well-fitting bra and modest fluid restriction are usually quite effective. Ice packs and oral analgesics are helpful for the discomfort.

Breast engorgement in lactating women is best treated by frequent round-the-clock nursing or breast pumping. Nipple soreness is commonly experienced and is primarily caused by poor positioning of the baby. Prompt correction of position and frequent position changes are important to prevent further nipple trauma. Mastitis is a common complication of breast-feeding and is manifested by an area of redness and tenderness accompanied by fever and myalgia. The initiating event is impairment of drainage of milk from a section of the breast, which causes local engorgement and tissue damage. Mastitis is not always infectious, although bacterial infection can supervene if the milk is not adequately expressed. Treatment includes continued breast-feeding, supplemental expression of milk and oral antibiotics such as ampicillin or dicloxacillin. Inadequate treatment may result in the formation of a breast abscess that requires surgical drainage.

Although mood swings are common during pregnancy, serious depressive symptoms often occur after delivery. Transient mild sadness—''postpartum blues''—is experienced by up to 60% of new mothers.[34] These feelings generally last up to 10 days. Clinical depression occurs in 10 to 15% of mothers after childbirth. Psychiatric consultation should be considered for long-lasting or severe depression. The recurrence rate of postpartum depression is 50% in subsequent pregnancies. Affected women often respond to antidepressants.

REFERENCES

1. Hytten FE, Leitch I. The Physiology of Human Pregnancy. 2nd ed. Oxford: Blackwell Scientific Publications, 1971.
2. Letsky EA. Blood volume, haematinics anaemia. In: de Swiet M (ed). Medical Disorders in Obstetric Practice. 2nd ed. Oxford: Blackwell Scientific Publications, 1989, p 48.
3. Murphy JF, Newcombe RG, O'Riordan J, et al. Relation of haemoglobin levels in first and second trimesters to outcome of pregnancy. Lancet 1986;1:992.
4. Hemminki E, Rimpelä U. Iron supplementation, maternal packed cell volume, and fetal growth. Arch Dis Child 1991;66(4):422.
5. Peck TM, Arias F. Hematologic changes associated with pregnancy. Clin Obstet Gynecol 1979;22(4):785.
6. Burrows RF, Kelton JG. Thrombocytopenia at delivery: A prospective survey of 6715 deliveries. Am J Obstet Gynecol 1990;162:731.

7. How HY, Bergmann F, Koshy M, et al. Quantitative and qualitative platelet abnormalities during pregnancy. Am J Obstet Gynecol 1991;164(1 part 1):92.

8. Tygart SG, McRoyan DK, Spinnato JA, et al. Longitudinal study of platelet indices during normal pregnancy. Am J Obstet Gynecol 1986;154:883.

9. Letsky EA. Coagulation defects. In: de Swiet M (ed). Medical Disorders in Obstetric Practice. 2nd ed. Oxford: Blackwell Scientific Publications, 1989, p 104.

10. Easterling TR, Schmucker BC, Benedetti TJ. The hemodynamic effects of orthostatic stress during pregnancy. Obstet Gynecol 1988;72(4):550.

11. Capeless EL, Clapp JF. When do cardiovascular parameters return to their preconception values? Am J Obstet Gynecol 1991;165(4 part 1):883.

12. Elkayam U, Gleicher N. Hemodynamics and cardiac function during normal pregnancy and the puerperium. In: Elkayam U, Gleicher N (eds). Cardiac Problems in Pregnancy: Diagnosis and Management of Maternal and Fetal Disease. 2nd ed. New York: Alan R. Liss, 1990, p 5.

13. Laird-Meeter K, Van de Lay G, Bom TH, et al. Cardiocirculatory adjustments during pregnancy—An echocardiographic study. Clin Cardiol 1979;2:328.

14. Elkayam U, Gleicher N. Changes in cardiac findings during normal pregnancy. In: Elkayam U, Gleicher N (eds). Cardiac Problems in Pregnancy: Diagnosis and Management of Maternal and Fetal Disease. 2nd ed. New York: Alan R. Liss, 1990, p 31.

15. Brinkman CR III. Biologic adaptations to pregnancy. In: Creasy RK, Resnik R (eds). Maternal-Fetal Medicine: Principles and Practice. 2nd ed. Philadelphia: WB Saunders, 1989, p 734.

16. Clark SL, Cotton DB, Lee W, et al. Central hemodynamic assessment of normal term pregnancy. Am J Obstet Gynecol 1989;161:1439.

17. Robson SC, Dunlop W, Boys RJ, et al. Cardiac output during labour. BMJ 1987;295:1169.

18. Baldwin GR, Moorthi DS, Whelton JA, et al. New lung functions and pregnancy. Am J Obstet Gynecol 1977;127:235.

19. Rees GB, Pipkin FB, Symonds EM, et al. A longitudinal study of respiratory changes in normal human pregnancy with cross-sectional data on subjects with pregnancy-induced hypertension. Am J Obstet Gynecol 1990;162(3):826.

20. Schulman A, Herlinger H. Urinary tract dilatation in pregnancy. Br J Radiol 1975;48(572):638.

21. Christensen T, Klebe JG, Bertelsen V, et al. Changes in renal volume during normal pregnancy. Acta Obstet Gynecol Scand 1989;68:541.

22. Iosif S, Ingemarsson I, Ulmsten U. Urodynamic studies in normal pregnancy and in puerperium. Am J Obstet Gynecol 1980;137(6):696.

23. Dunlop W. Serial changes in renal haemodynamics during normal human pregnancy. Br J Obstet Gynaecol 1981;88(1):1.

24. Dafnis E, Sabatini S. The effect of pregnancy on renal function: Physiology and pathophysiology. Am J Med Sci 1992;303(3):184.

25. Fagundes VG, Lamas CC, Francischetti EA. Renin-angiotensin-aldosterone system in normal and hypertensive pregnancy: Response to postural stimuli. Hypertension 1992;19(suppl II):1174.

26. Lowe SA, Macdonald GJ, Brown MA. Acute and chronic regulation of atrial natriuretic peptide in human pregnancy: A longitudinal study. J Hypertens 1992;10:821.

27. Davision JM, Schiells EA, Philips PR, et al. Serial evaluation of vasopressin release and thirst in human pregnancy. J Clin Invest 1988;81:798.

28. Stettler RW, Cunningham FG. Natural history of chronic proteinuria complicating pregnancy. Am J Obstet Gynecol 1992;167(5):1219.

29. Handwerger S. Clinical counterpoint: The physiology of placental lactogen in human pregnancy. Endocr Rev 1991;12(4):329.

30. Allgrove J, Adami S, Manning RM, et al. Cytochemical bioassay of parathyroid hormone in maternal and cord blood. Arch Dis Child 1985;60:110.

31. Christofides ND, Ghatei MA, Bloom SR, et al. Decreased plasma motilin concentrations in pregnancy. BMJ 1982;285:1453.

32. Braverman DZ, Johnson ML, Kern FJ. Effects of pregnancy and contraceptive steroids on gallbladder function. N Engl J Med 1980;302:362.

33. Bowes WA Jr. Postpartum care. In: Gabbe SG, Niebyl JR, Simpson JL (eds). Obstetrics: Normal and Problem Pregnancies. 2nd ed. New York: Churchill Livingstone, 1991, p 753.

34. Hamilton JA. Postpartum psychiatric syndromes. Psych Clin North Am 1989;12(1):89.

Emotional Aspects of Pregnancy and the Postpartum Period

Rochelle Rame Friedman

Women's lives are unique in being defined by biologic events: birth, menarche, pregnancy, menopause, and death. At these times physical changes take place at a rapid rate, and, not surprisingly, these are also times when major psychological struggles tend to occur. In contrast to the belief held by early practitioners of psychoanalysis, pregnancy is not a quiescent time when women turn inward and thus cannot be analyzed. Pregnancy is a time when most women rework their definition of who they are, a time when early issues resurface and must be resolved, a time of vulnerability, and a time when their hopes and fears for themselves and for their future children resurface.

PREGNANCY-RELATED CONCERNS

At this time in history, couples do not take fertility for granted. Everyone knows someone who has had trouble conceiving, because one in 10 couples encounter difficulty achieving a pregnancy. This means that for many couples the pregnancy experience begins with anxiety about whether they will have difficulty conceiving. Each month that passes without conception occurring increases the fear that they too may be infertile. For one in 10 couples this is the case, and for them the pursuit of pregnancy is difficult physically, emotionally, and financially. When couples do become pregnant, anxiety shifts from concern about conception to fear that something might go wrong during the 9 months ahead. Concerns range from worry about having an ectopic pregnancy or a miscarriage to anxiety about amniocentesis or ultrasound results, worries about having a premature delivery, as well as fears about the outcome of labor and delivery.

The ability to control one's destiny is a central concern for many people. Increasingly, people see control over the outcome of all endeavors as their birthright. Because pregnancy once initiated follows a course that is for the most part not controllable, many find it a very difficult and anxiety-provoking time. Those who expect that if they follow their physician's directions all will go well feel cheated if they encounter difficulty anywhere along the way. They expect a perfect pregnancy, a smooth labor and delivery, and, ultimately, a perfect child.

Fortunately, the overwhelming majority of pregnancies go well and result in healthy babies and happy parents. However, even successful pregnancies are not necessarily uneventful. The pregnancy experience may begin with one or both parents feeling a variety of conflicting emotions: delight at being pregnant; anxiety about whether it is what they want; and worry about the effect having a child will have on their lives and on the lives of their existing children.

THE PREGNANCY EXPERIENCE

Attachment

For many prospective parents the first psychological task of pregnancy is that of resolving their ambivalence and dealing with the anxiety evoked by this major life change. The second psychological task of pregnancy is that of forming an attachment to their future child. For women who want a child this attachment usually occurs early on in the pregnancy and grows as the pregnancy progresses. Because the experience of pregnancy is more remote for men, it is not unusual for them to form an attachment later in the pregnancy than their wives do—or not to form an attachment until the baby is actually born. When the outcome of the pregnancy is in question, it is not unusual for prospective parents to hold off on forming an attachment. This is often the case for couples who have experienced a previous pregnancy loss or stillbirth and who fear another poor outcome as well as for those who are awaiting the results of prenatal diagnostic tests whose outcome will determine whether or not the pregnancy will be carried to term.[1] In what is an effort to spare themselves pain if the outcome is poor, they hold off on forming an attachment until they know that everything is all right. This is not always easy to do as the pregnancy may intrude into the parent's consciousness despite their attempts to keep this from happening. This may occur because the symptoms of early pregnancy are bothersome and cannot be ignored; because the results of ultrasound examination graphically demonstrate that there is, indeed, a baby developing inside; or because quickening has occurred before the results of prenatal diagnostic testing are available. Research is under way whose purpose it is to develop earlier and better means of detecting genetic abnormalities; this should prove helpful in making termination possible at an earlier stage in pregnancy. As a rule, the earlier in pregnancy that test results can be made available, the less severe the physical and emotional trauma should abortion be necessary.

When a pregnancy is not successful, either because it is ectopic, because it is not viable and ends in miscarriage, or because the results of prenatal testing indicate severe problems necessitating interruption of the pregnancy, the attachment that parents have formed is disrupted. The way in which parents experience the loss of a pregnancy depends on the intensity of the attachment that they have formed. This loss is commonly experienced by prospective parents as similar to a death; their wished-for child has been lost. The grief that parents experience after losing a pregnancy resembles the grief reaction that follows the death of a loved one in both intensity and duration, as well as in the kinds of feelings that are experienced. This reaction may be poorly understood by family, friends, colleagues, or caregivers. When others do misunderstand, they may urge prospective parents to suppress their grief and get on with their lives.[2]

At the other end of the spectrum are some mothers and many fathers who do not form a significant attachment to their future child during the course of the pregnancy. Infrequently, the failure to form an attachment may be an ominous sign that indicates a pathologic level of ambivalence about the pregnancy. More often parents' failure to form an attachment results from their difficulty believing that the pregnancy will result in the birth of a viable baby. This phenomenon is seen most often among women who are expecting their first child and who because of their lack of prior experience have trouble believing that pregnancy actually produces a child, among women who have experienced prior pregnancy loss or stillbirth, and among men who by virtue of not carrying the child themselves do not have a first-hand knowledge of it.

Most often parents who have not formed an attachment during the pregnancy are able to form an attachment to their infant within a day or two of delivery. Whatever disbelief or ambivalence they experienced during the pregnancy is usually dispelled by the actual presence of the newborn child. However, difficulty in forming an attachment may occur when pregnancy results in the birth of a child with significant congenital difficulties. In this situation parents mourn the loss of the hoped-for ''ideal'' child that they were anticipating, and they must find a way to accept and love a child that is not perfect. Often this is a painful process, which entails grieving for a loss and at times living with uncertainty, as it may not be apparent at the time of birth or even for a year or more what the full extent of the infant's difficulties may be or what effect the child's problems may have on the child's or the parents' lives.

Body Image

Pregnancy is a time of extremely rapid bodily change. Even when pregnancy is desired, a woman may have negative feelings about the effect it will have on her body. In the 1990s, the ideal female body is slender and boyish; small hips and breasts, a flat stomach, and long legs are valued. This androgenous ideal is the antithesis of what the pregnant body looks like. Women worry that pregnancy will make them fat, that it will cause their breasts to sag, that it will cause stretch marks, and that afterward their stomach will not be as flat as it was previously. Some women have difficulty accepting the ways in which pregnancy affects their bodies; they experience the changes in their body as frightening and disgusting. Women who have had an eating disorder may find that pregnancy raises old concerns about gaining weight or becoming fat, while others may find that during pregnancy they are able to temporarily put aside their anxiety. Similarly, husbands may have their own issues about what body type they do or do not find attractive. Men who find the changes wrought by pregnancy unappealing make it more difficult than it otherwise might be for their wives to accept the ways in which their body has been altered.

Control Issues

Women who are used to being in control of most aspects of their lives may find it difficult to deal with the fact that once a pregnancy is initiated there is little that they can do to affect the outcome. Once a couple decides that they want to try to have a child, they enter a universe over which they have a very limited amount of control. They cannot choose how long it will take them to conceive—whether conception will happen quickly, whether it will take months of trying, or whether they will encounter fertility problems. Once conception occurs, they have no control over whether the embryo will implant in the uterus or ectopically, whether it will develop normally, or whether miscarriage will occur. Most troubling, they cannot control whether the pregnancy will result in the birth of a healthy infant or in the birth of one who has congenital difficulties.

Most women have some worry about whether the baby they are carrying will be normal. Typically anxiety is most severe at times in the pregnancy when there is concern that something could go wrong. Women who have lost a previous pregnancy or had a stillbirth tend to experience significant anxiety as the time approaches when the first loss occurred. For those awaiting the results of prenatal testing, anxiety tends to intensify as the time when results are expected grows near. Similarly, almost all pregnant women find that their concern that something will go wrong becomes more intense as their due date approaches. Some pregnant women have nightmares about delivering an abnormal child; others are plagued by frightening daytime fantasies. Some women find that it is relieving to talk about their worst fears, whereas others feel no need to talk or that it is tempting fate to do so. It is not unusual for anxiety to mount with each subsequent pregnancy. This seems to be because the more parents and children one knows, the more one accumulates information about problem pregnancies and poor outcomes. It is not unusual for parents to feel betrayed when their child is born with difficulties. Some parents feel that because they tried to do everything right, that is, did not smoke, did not drink alcohol or consume caffeine, ate only healthy foods, gained the recommended amount of weight, took their prenatal vitamins, and abstained from taking other medication, they should have been assured of having a healthy baby. When this does not happen they are at a loss to make sense of things. They find it hard to accept that doing everything one can does not necessarily guarantee good results.

THE EMOTIONAL EXPERIENCE

It is common to feel very vulnerable during pregnancy. Even those who are intellectually aware that normal activities are not harmful to a healthy pregnancy tend to worry that something they did might disrupt the pregnancy or harm the baby. In addition to feeling physically vulnerable many pregnant women also feel psychologically vulnerable. Not infrequently they report feeling that their boundaries have been violated by people who feel free to comment on how they look, to ask intrusive questions, or even to touch them. They find that there is no way to hide the fact that they are pregnant and no good way to avoid the unwanted attention it brings. Hearing about other women's pregnancy and birth experiences may be frightening, particularly when what is shared are tales about bad outcomes. An accumulation of these may cause a woman to have difficulty believing that things are most likely to go well for her.

It is difficult to assess what role the high hormone levels of pregnancy play in affecting a woman's psychological state. It is not unusual for pregnant women to feel more easily hurt or slighted than usual, to experience periods when they feel anxious or depressed, or to experience mood shifts that do not seem to be in response to anything of which they are aware. Feelings of happiness and well-being are also commonly reported.

Much has been said about what role emotional factors play in women's reproductive functioning. The following have been attributed to poor psychological adjustment: dysmenorrhea, dyspareunia, infertility, miscarriage, difficult or prolonged labor, newborn colic, and difficulty breast feeding.[3] Psychoanalytic theory, when it dealt with this issue at all, tended to blame the woman for causing her own troubles. Case reports as well as retrospective studies were cited to support the belief that a woman's conflicts about her femininity or about her wish to become a mother, or about both, may have resulted in the aforementioned ills. However, there is no evidence that this is true for the majority of women who experience reproductive difficulties.

Counselors who have worked with women who have experienced reproductive difficulties have found that this population experiences a significant amount of anger, frustration, and sadness about what they have been through. Some women experience these feelings for a long period of time;

others find that the grief they experience as a result of infertility or a pregnancy loss dominates their lives at first and then becomes less consuming as time passes. There is no doubt that women who have experienced reproductive problems are more upset as a group than those who have not; however, their distress is most often a consequence of what they have experienced and not the cause.

THE PHYSICAL EXPERIENCE

The physical effects of pregnancy seem to contribute to the vulnerability that women experience. Normally a young woman can live her life almost oblivious of her body. Not so during pregnancy. A pregnant body intrudes into consciousness because it keeps changing, because of its size, because it may feel awkward or uncomfortable, and because it does not function in quite the same way that it used to. The symptoms of pregnancy—nausea, vomiting, fatigue, and frequent urination—may interfere with feelings of well-being and contribute significantly to feeling vulnerable.

Most women are quite awed by how physical an experience pregnancy is. During the 9 months of pregnancy one is almost always aware of one's biology. Many women are aware of mood changes as well as changes in various organ systems. As pregnancy progresses and one's body changes in more and more dramatic ways, these changes intrude into awareness more and more. Similarly, as the fetus increases in size and becomes more active, these sensations become more intrusive. Complications in the pregnancy may be silent or they may express themselves through physical symptoms such as cramping, bleeding, dizziness, lightheadedness, or swelling. One of the challenges that all pregnant women face is that of differentiating between physical changes that are a normal consequence of being pregnant and those that indicate that something is wrong. At no time during pregnancy is one as aware of the power of the biologic process as during labor and delivery. The usual progression is that contractions occur closer and closer together and that they are more and more forceful. As labor progresses, it tends to dominate. Whoever else one may be is temporarily irrelevant; during labor one is a body struggling to deliver the fetus to the outside world. It is not unusual for women to find the experience of being overwhelmed by this biologic process quite disconcerting.

TRANSITION FROM CHILDHOOD TO ADULTHOOD

Pregnancy is a time of psychological transition from childhood to adulthood, from being parented to being a parent. This is an enormous developmental step and one that is fraught with anxiety for some soon-to-be parents. They worry about being able to manage, if they will be good parents, if they will love their child, and if they will be able to be the giving person in the relationship for as long as it is necessary. Expectant parents are anxious about what they have taken on and about whether they will be up to the task. Those whose own parents were poor role models worry that they might repeat their parents' mistakes. Prospective parents also are concerned about how having a child will affect their lives. During childhood, adolescence, and young adulthood one usually has the luxury of attending to one's own needs and wants first. Putting aside or delaying one's own gratification to attend to one's child's needs comes easily to some new parents. Others may experience difficulty doing this. They may resent the child for taking their time, for crying so much, for waking up at night, or for always needing something. Teenaged parents and parents whose own needs were not met adequately when they were children seem to have particular difficulty putting their own needs aside.

Being a parent changes one's relationship to one's own parents. One's primary identification shifts from being a child to being the parent of one's own child. This is usually accompanied by a shift in primary affiliation from one's family of origin to a new nuclear family consisting of oneself, one's spouse, and one's child or children and by corresponding psychological adjustments. As a parent, one is the person who is ultimately responsible. As a parent, one has to provide not only for oneself but also for the needs of one's spouse and child or children.

SOCIAL CIRCUMSTANCES

Myriad social factors may affect the pregnancy experience. Whether the pregnancy is desired has an enormous effect on how one feels about it. Whether the child has been conceived inside or outside of marriage may affect how parents feel, as does whether the parents' relationship is a happy one. Number and spacing of other children in the family may be important, along with the cumulative level of stress the prospective parents are feeling. When there are significant economic worries, health concerns, or multiple demands on time and energy, the pregnancy may feel like one burden too many. One factor that has an enormous effect on how an individual or a couple feels about being pregnant has to do with previous reproductive histories. Some people worry that they will be punished and be unable to conceive for having been sexually active, for having been promiscuous, or for having had an abortion. Pregnancy can be reassuring for those with such concerns.

Whether the pregnancy was planned, whether it was desired, and the circumstances under which it occurred are all important factors. Women who have concerns about the identity of the father often have a difficult time dealing with the pregnancy and deciding what to do about it. Those who were forced to have intercourse and those whose birth control failed to be effective are likely to have negative feelings. Those who have conceived through one of the assisted reproductive technologies may regard the pregnancy as something akin to a miracle.

EMOTIONAL FACTORS AND OBSTETRIC COMPLICATIONS

When the cause of an illness or condition is poorly understood, there is a tendency to ascribe a causal relationship to associated factors. For example, emotional factors are often blamed when the etiology of a malady is not known. Because the mind-body connection is not well understood and because there is much that we do not know about causation, we should be careful about assuming what role, if any, emotional factors play in the etiology of a particular condition.

Pseudocyesis, or false pregnancy, is a syndrome that is believed to be wholly psychoneurotic in origin. Women who develop pseudocyesis experience all or many of the symptoms of pregnancy: amenorrhea, abdominal enlargement, breast engorgement, nausea, vomiting, and weight gain. When this diagnosis is suspected, ultrasound examination and a pregnancy test should be ordered to confirm that the woman is not, in fact, pregnant. Psychoanalytic theory explains pseudocyesis as the physical expression of a woman's conflict about being pregnant. It is theorized that the conflict between the wish to become pregnant and the fear of it is resolved by developing hysterical symptoms of pregnancy. The population believed to be at risk for developing this condition are women who want to be pregnant but who are unable to for some reason and those who are approaching menopause.

Hyperemesis gravidarum, or pernicious vomiting, is a syndrome of uncontrollable and severe nausea and vomiting. A great deal of debate has concerned whether this condition is caused by physical factors (i.e., sensitivity to high hormone levels) or emotional factors. The theory of emotional causation holds that vomiting is the expression of the unconscious wish to reject the pregnancy. Although this theory has at times been taken for fact, it has not been demonstrated that emotional factors play a role. However, women with this syndrome have been found to be ambivalent about being pregnant. Whether this ambivalence is the cause or the effect of having hyperemesis has not been explored, nor has the possibility that this population is no more ambivalent about being pregnant than are women in general. Because hyperemesis can be a life-threatening condition, it must be taken seriously and treated promptly and aggressively. The patient may require hospitalization to manage the vomiting and the resulting dehydration, the electrolyte imbalance, and the poor nutrition. Psychiatric evaluation may be of value in addressing issues of ambivalence, whether they are a cause or a result of hyperemesis. A combination of supportive and insight-oriented psychotherapy may be of use.

Other obstetric syndromes that were believed to have been caused by emotional factors are habitual abortion, toxemia, pain in labor, difficult labor, the need for cesarean section, and premature birth. As we have learned more about these conditions and as other etiologic factors have been discovered, the link between these syndromes and a woman's emotional state has been questioned. An alternative hypothesis is that women who have complications during pregnancy experience more anxiety than do women with uncomplicated pregnancies and that, here again, the increased emotionality of those who have complications is a result and not a cause of their difficulties.

EMOTIONAL DIFFICULTIES DURING PREGNANCY

To assess a woman's risk of developing psychiatric difficulties during pregnancy, one must consider biologic, social, and psychological factors. The more predisposing or stress factors a woman has in various aspects of her life, the more likely she is to experience problems.[4] Therefore, it is important to take a comprehensive history and to inquire periodically about how things are going. A complete evaluation should include an inquiry into the patient's own history as well as family members' histories of psychological difficulties; her experience during previous pregnancies; and her course during previous postpartum periods. It is also necessary to determine whether vegetative symptoms diagnostic of depression are present; whether the patient is experiencing significant or disturbing changes in mood; and whether anxiety, panic, or obsessive-compulsive symptoms are a problem.

There is a tendency for clinicians to miss or underdiagnose psychological difficulties during pregnancy because pregnancy is thought of as a time when women are at peace with themselves. Because this is not true of all women, the possibility that emotional difficulties may occur or recur should always be considered.

TREATING PREGNANT WOMEN WITH UNDERLYING PSYCHIATRIC DISORDERS

The physician faced with treating a pregnant woman who has an underlying psychiatric disorder must deal with a dilemma. Medication that might be necessary or helpful to the mother may cause harm to the fetus. It is always necessary to weigh the costs of treating or not treating the pregnant patient against the potential risk to the fetus. Psychotropic drugs may affect the fetus negatively by causing teratogenesis, by having gross or subtle effects on the neonatal nervous system, or by having direct toxic effects.[5] Therefore, psychotropic medication should be avoided if at all possible, especially during the first trimester. Although some medications may not, at present, have been demonstrated to affect the fetus adversely none has been shown to be completely safe. As a general rule it is a good idea, whenever possible, to discontinue psychotropic medication several months before a woman attempts to become pregnant. If this is not done in advance and the patient conceives while on medication, it should be withdrawn gradually or stopped. Patients who become significantly symptomatic when medication is tapered as well as those who in the course of their pregnancy develop symptoms that significantly impair or even endanger their lives should be referred to a psychopharmacologist for an evaluation.

Lithium

Patients on lithium should, whenever possible, be withdrawn from this medication before conception. If a woman on lithium therapy becomes pregnant, gradual withdrawal is advised, and the patient should be informed about possible teratogenic effects. Babies born to women who are on lithium are at significant risk for having Ebstein's anomaly, a defect of the tricuspid valve. There is also a significant incidence of reversible lithium-induced neonatal goiter among babies born to

mothers who were maintained on lithium during pregnancy.[6–9]

Tricyclic Antidepressants

There is no clear evidence linking the use of tricyclic antidepressants with congenital malformations of the fetus. Nevertheless, if at all possible, their use should be avoided, especially during the first trimester. It is recommended that patients taper and then stop antidepressant medication several months before trying to conceive because many of these medications have a long half-life.[10]

If it is necessary to use a tricyclic medication during the last two trimesters it should always be stopped 5 to 10 days before delivery so that the newborn does not develop tricyclic withdrawal symptoms.

Benzodiazepines

Benzodiazepines should not be used during the first trimester of pregnancy and should be avoided whenever possible during the second and third trimesters. It is fairly well established that the use of benzodiazepines during the first trimester is associated with an increased incidence of cleft lip and cleft palate. It is also advised that benzodiazepines should not be used by nursing mothers, as they may be excreted into the breast milk.[10]

Antipsychotic Medication

Studies have failed to demonstrate an increased incidence of congenital malformations in the children of women who were treated with phenothiazines during pregnancy. Nevertheless, it is recommended that antipsychotic agents not be used, especially during the first trimester.

When phenothiazines are used during the last two trimesters it is necessary to stop medication 5 to 10 days before the due date. This is because some children born to mothers treated with phenothiazines have exhibited extrapyramidal symptoms that have persisted up to 6 months. It has been suggested that when treating a psychotic patient who is pregnant electroconvulsive therapy should be considered as an alternative to antipsychotic medication.[11]

Psychological Issues in Labor and Delivery

Emotional factors have been implicated as causative or contributing to pain in labor—failure of labor to progress and failure to deliver vaginally. Although there is little real evidence to support these notions, they have been slow to die. Women who require a cesarean section and those who need medication to control the pain of labor and delivery may feel that they have failed in some way or that their bodies have let them down. The extent to which these attitudes arise, on the one hand, from their own self-doubt or their need to prove themselves through their reproductive competence and, on the other, from an internalization of what society and the medical establishment define as success and failure is unclear.

The majority of women find that the anticipation of labor and delivery is fraught with anxiety. Everyone has heard about long and extremely painful labors, precipitous labor, difficult deliveries, maternal deaths, and stillbirths. In addition, these frightening occurrences cause anxiety because they are out of the individual's control, because they are painful, and because they might result in a baby who has a birth defect. The two most common fears that women have about labor and delivery are that they might die or that something might go wrong that will cause harm to the baby. When dealing with a pregnant woman, especially one who is nearing term or one who is in labor, it is reasonable to assume that she is feeling a significant amount of distress whether or not she openly expresses anxiety.

THE POSTPARTUM PERIOD

Despite the pain and exertion of labor and delivery, most women experience a feeling of exhilaration at the first sight of their child. Many describe this time as the happiest time in their lives. Some women fall in love with their baby at first sight; others take somewhat longer to establish a bond. Particularly for first-time parents, this is a period of enormous psychological adjustment. The tasks that face parents in the postpartum period are those of forming a mutually gratifying relationship with their child; establishing successful nursing or bottle feeding; coping with sleep deprivation and fatigue; dealing with the physical sequelae of pregnancy, labor, delivery, and the postpartum period; integrating these experiences; forming an attachment to their child; and giving up the fantasy formed during pregnancy of what their baby would be like. This reconciliation is most easily accomplished when the actual baby is similar to the one for which they wished. Parents who must deal with a child with birth-related complications or congenital defects face the difficult task of mourning the loss of the child they had wished for and of learning to love and accept the child they do have. The more significant the child's problems and the more unknown its prognosis, the more difficult this adjustment is.

In addition to adjusting to being a parent, bonding with one's newborn, and coping with fatigue, discomfort, and sleeplessness, new mothers must adjust to shifts in hormone levels and to a body that has been altered by pregnancy, delivery, and nursing. Some women adjust easily to these changes, but others have difficulty with one or the other. Women who have had an eating disorder or who have had body image problems may have particular difficulty with the persistence of weight gain and the altered body contours characteristic of the postpartum period.

Another issue that frequently arises in the postpartum period is whether one is an adequate parent. Women tend to blame themselves for every difficulty they encounter. It is their fault if the baby has trouble nursing, if the baby has colic, or if their milk supply is not adequate. Well-meaning friends and relatives may inadvertently exacerbate this tendency by giving advice or by voicing concern about the baby or about parenting practices.

The postpartum period is a time of enormous physical, social, and psychological adjustment. As a result, many new parents feel overwhelmed and exhausted. New parents should be advised to seek help. A friend, a family member, or a baby nurse who can share the burden can be invaluable, as can help with cleaning or meal preparation. Several support groups exist to help new parents during this very stressful time (La Leche League, C' Sec, and COPE).* Many factors play a role in determining what a woman's postpartum experience will be like: her genetic makeup; whether she has a predisposition to depression; whether she has a history of severe premenstrual syndrome, major mental illness, or previous postpartum syndrome; her particular physiology; whether labor and delivery were traumatic; whether the birth resulted in a baby with or without difficulties; and whether adequate social, financial, and medical resources are available to her.

From the obstetric point of view, the postpartum period begins at delivery and ends 6 weeks later when the reproductive organs have returned to normal. From the psychological perspective, the postpartum period is considered to end 9 months to 1 year after birth. The postpartum period is the time in a woman's life when she is at the greatest

---

*COPE, 530 Tremont Street, Boston, MA 02116, (617) 357-5588; La Leche League International, 1400 North Meacham Road, Schaumburg, IL 60173, 1-800-525-3243 or (708) 519-7730.

risk of having emotional problems severe enough to warrant admission to a psychiatric hospital.

Postpartum Blues

The most benign of the postpartum syndromes is known as "the blues" or "the baby blues." Between 50 and 75% of women experience the blues. Typically, onset occurs on the third or fourth day after delivery. Symptoms tend to be most severe between the seventh and tenth day and usually subside at about day 14. No treatment is required, as the blues resolve spontaneously. Common symptoms include sadness, crying, anxiety, irritability, impatience, restlessness, and hypersensitivity. Less often women experience sleep disturbance and poor appetite. If symptoms are severe, if they fail to resolve spontaneously, or if they resolve and then recur, the patient should be evaluated to rule out a more severe postpartum syndrome.

Postpartum Depression

Postpartum depression is not an infrequent problem and may occur at any time in the first year after birth, with the highest incidence at 6 to 8 weeks. A woman who is suffering from a postpartum depression has some or all of the following symptoms: depressive, obsessive, or racing thoughts; agitation; anger; irritability; fear; insomnia; decreased appetite; poor concentration; and thoughts of harming herself or her baby. The disturbance may begin insidiously or acutely, may range from mild to severe, and may fluctuate in intensity.

The predisposition to having a postpartum depression seems to be genetically transmitted. Women who have had a prior postpartum depression have a 10 to 50% chance of having another in a subsequent pregnancy; women who have had a nonpregnancy-related affective illness are at greater than usual risk. Postpartum depression may take a variable course and should be followed closely. Because a woman who is suffering from a postpartum depression may become acutely suicidal, she should not be left alone, and hospitalization should be considered.[12]

Postpartum Panic Disorder

Postpartum panic disorder is a rare problem, with onset usually occurring within the first 3 months after delivery. It may occur in women who

have no prior history of having panic attacks as well as in those who have had them. Women with a history of panic attacks have an increased risk of becoming symptomatic after delivery. Symptoms tend to be intense and frightening and characteristically include feelings of dread, severe anxiety, panic, terror, heart palpitations, shortness of breath, ringing in the ears, and numbness and tingling of the perioral area and of the extremities.[13]

Postpartum Obsessive-Compulsive Disorder

Women with postpartum obsessive-compulsive disorder experience, intrusive, repetitive thoughts or behaviors, or both. Characteristically, they report overwhelming, frightening, intrusive thoughts and mental images of harming the baby, as well as horror at having these thoughts. Intrusive thoughts or images may occur constantly or intermittently. Although women who have postpartum obsessive-compulsive disorder are not psychotic and are not suffering from a primary depression, they may fear that they are becoming crazy and they may become depressed as a reaction to their symptoms. Women present as extremely agitated as well as anxious and fearful. They should not be left alone, and they should not be the caretaker of their child because of their anxiety about acting on their thoughts.

This rare syndrome typically begins 2 to 3 weeks after childbirth and may affect those who have never experienced obsessive-compulsive symptoms as well as those who have. It is believed that women who have a prior history of having had obsessive-compulsive disorder are at increased risk of developing it after childbirth.

Postpartum Psychosis

This syndrome typically occurs in the first 2 weeks after delivery and is characterized by the acute onset of psychotic thinking, extreme agitation, insomnia, confusion, hallucinations, and delusions. Because symptoms tend to worsen at a rapid rate and because behavior may get out of control, evaluation and treatment should take place immediately. Hospitalization is required as is treatment with antipsychotic medication, and, when indicated, with lithium.[14]

Postpartum psychosis occurs following 1 to 2 out of 1000 deliveries. Women with a past history of bipolar illness have a 40% chance of developing a postpartum psychosis after their first pregnancy.

All women who have had one postpartum psychosis experience recurrence of the syndrome with subsequent pregnancies. Repeat episodes tend to be increasingly severe.

During pregnancy, reproductive hormone levels are 50 times greater than normal. At the time of delivery, hormone levels fall abruptly. In addition, major changes occur in amino acid, neurotransmitter, and thyroid hormone levels. All of these have been implicated as contributing to the etiology of postpartum disorders. Some physicians in the United States and Great Britain are administering estrogen and progesterone to high-risk women. Included in this high-risk group are women with a prior history of having had affective illness, severe premenstrual syndrome, a postpartum disorder, or a family history of postpartum difficulty. The protocol is to administer fairly high doses of both estrogen and progesterone at the time of delivery, and to decrease the dose gradually over a 2-month period. Those at risk may also be started on antidepressant medication immediately after delivery.

Women who experience a first occurrence of postpartum depression or panic disorder should be treated with both psychotherapy and antidepressant medication at the onset of symptoms. Women with postpartum obsessive-compulsive disorder, like others with this syndrome, do best if treated with an antidepressant that is specifically a serotonin reuptake inhibitor. Those with psychotic disorders should be treated with antipsychotic medication and, if indicated, with lithium. The national support network, Depression after Delivery (DAD), which provides support and information to women, families, and professionals, can be invaluable in helping women and their families manage postpartum distress.*

REFERENCES

1. Friedman RR, Gradstein B. Surviving Pregnancy Loss. 2nd ed. Boston: Little, Brown & Company, 1992, pp 109–110.
2. Friedman RR, Gradstein B. Surviving Pregnancy Loss. 2nd ed. Boston: Little, Brown & Company, 1992, pp 7–19.
3. Lennae KJ, Lennae R. Alleged psychogenic disorders in women: A possible manifestation of sexual prejudice. N Engl J Med 1973;288:1.
4. Sichel DA. Psychiatric issues of the postpartum period. Curr Affect Ill 1992;11(10):5.
5. Kellogg C, Tervo D, Ison J, et al. Prenatal exposure to diazepam alters behavioral development in rats. Science 1980;207:205.
6. Linden S, Rich CL. The use of lithium during pregnancy and lactation. Clin Psych. 1983;44(10):358.
7. Lithium-related congenital cardiac abnormalities: Prenatal screening. Bio Ther in Psych 1983;6(2):7.
8. When a woman taking lithium wants to have a baby. Bio Ther in Psych 1983;6(5):19.
9. Pregnancy in the bipolar patient. Bio Ther in Psych 1988;11(11):41.
10. Calabrese JR, Gulledge AD. Psychotropics during pregnancy and lactation: A review. Psychosomatics 1985;26(5):416.
11. Psychotropic drugs and the fetus. Bio Ther in Psych 1984;7(4):13.
12. Sichel DA. Psychiatric issues of the postpartum period. Curr Affect Ill 1992;11(10):5.
13. Metz A, Sichel DA. Postpartum panic disorder. J Clin Psychiatry 1988;49(7):278.
14. Lithium in postpartum psychosis. Psych Drug Alerts 1991;5(9):65.

*Depression after Delivery, P.O. Box 1282, Morrisville, PA 19067. Phone 1-800-944-4PPD or (215) 295-3994.

Medication and Substance Use in Pregnancy

Phyllis L. Carr

EPIDEMIOLOGY AND SCOPE OF THE PROBLEM

The majority of women take at least one prescription drug during pregnancy. The Collaborative Study on Drug Use in Pregnancy reported in 1990 that drug use in 17 countries varied from 61 to 100% of women ingesting at least one medication during pregnancy, with a mean of 2.2 drugs per person. Another overview of drug use studies in pregnancy reported that women took a mean of 4.7 drugs, with a range of 2.9 to 5.5. Iron and vitamins were the most commonly prescribed drugs, followed by analgesics, antiemetics, antiinfective agents, psychotropic agents (minor tranquilizers), antihistamines, and diuretics. Most studies found that self-administered medication use had declined in recent years.

Five times more stillbirths and deformed children were reported between 1956 and 1965 than between 1941 and 1950—the latter being a period felt to have less medication generally available. Although only 25 human teratogens are known, insufficient data are available on many substances and medications to ensure that they are safe in pregnancy. It is uniformly agreed that a comprehensive surveillance program of medications in pregnancy is needed to allow physicians and patients greater knowledge of potential complications associated with the use of medications in pregnancy.

This chapter reviews the types of studies that are helpful in determining an association between medications and congenital anomalies. General concepts to be considered before prescribing medication in pregnancy, based on the physiology of pregnancy and the timing in gestation, are also presented. Commonly used substances and medications in pregnancy also are reviewed.

STUDY DESIGN AND ASSESSMENT OF RISK

Assessing the cause and effect relationship between medications taken during pregnancy and congenital abnormalities is difficult. In general, three types of studies have provided data on medications and congenital malformations. The first type, the case study, is helpful when both the malformation and the exposure are rare and can implicate a drug as a teratogen. Diethylstilbestrol and the occurrence of vaginal carcinoma in the female offspring of mothers who ingested this medication during pregnancy is an example. Case studies, however, provide no data on the risk for birth defects.

The second form, the case-control study, is generally retrospective and measures the occurrence of an exposure among cases and controls. The relative risk for a birth defect cannot be estimated directly from a case-control study. However, an odds ratio can be an accurate estimate of the relative risk when the birth defect is rare, as most are. This is simply a ratio of exposure in the cases divided by the same ratio in the controls.

The third cohort study is the only type of study that can provide a direct estimate of the relative risk. This form of study evaluates a group exposed to the drug and one that is not exposed, usually in a prospective manner. Because birth defects are rare, these studies are large and expensive. The absolute risk depends on the prevalence of the birth defect. Even a high relative risk for a rare defect still has a low absolute risk for that defect.

Other difficulties in the methodology of studies relating drug use to birth defects include confounders, recall bias, and misclassification. A confounder is a variable that is independently associated with both the exposure and the disease, such as high parity, maternal age, and Down's syndrome.

Stratification of the data with independent analysis of each stratification and summing of the stratified data can control for confounding variables. Recall bias refers to the fact that women who had a bad outcome from their pregnancy may recall the events of their pregnancy in greater detail than mothers with a normal pregnancy. This problem is normally dealt with by using an unrelated birth defect as a control for the congenital anomaly under study. Misclassification refers to the fact that a woman classified as not taking a medication may inadvertently have taken the drug without being aware of it. This frequently happens with combination, over-the-counter medications that may include a drug in the study. Misclassification tends to be random, affecting both the exposed and unexposed proportionately.

EMBRYOLOGY AND DRUG EFFECTS

The effect of any drug on the fetus depends on the stage of fetal development. During the preimplantation phase (days 0 to 14), teratogens have little effect. Drug levels that affect the blastocyst tend to be lower than maternal serum levels. If the teratogen is very toxic, the ovum dies, or the affected part regenerates so completely that no noticeable postnatal effect occurs. From implantation until day 60, the period of organogenesis, the embryo is maximally sensitive to teratogens. Even after this period, the fetus continues to develop and remains sensitive to teratogens until the end of intrauterine life. In the neonatal period, the transport of drugs is affected by uterine contractility and the change from maternal metabolization of medication to that of the fetus, with its immature liver and kidney function.

MATERNAL PHYSIOLOGY

There are also physiologic changes in pregnancy that affect the pharmacokinetics of medication. Maternal gastrointestinal motility decreases with advancing gestation. This may increase or decrease absorption of a drug, depending on whether greater absorption of the drug occurs because of the greater transit time or decreased absorption occurs because of binding of the drug to substances that prevent absorption. The plasma protein concentration also decreases during pregnancy, which allows a greater amount of bioactive, unbound drug. This is countered by an increase in the volume of distribution for the drug, which lowers serum levels. The increase in renal blood flow also results in an elevated creatinine clearance.

Drugs that are excreted renally are cleared more quickly in pregnancy until the last 6 weeks, when the creatinine clearance again falls.

The placental circulation is established by the fourth to fifth week after conception. Most drugs cross the placenta by simple diffusion, depending on the molecular weight, lipid solubility, protein binding, and concentration gradient of the particular drug. As the placenta matures, the distance between the maternal and fetal circulation is reduced, the capillaries enlarge, and the amount of connective tissue diminishes, further facilitating diffusion.

Congenital Anomalies

Roughly 3% of newborns require medical attention for a birth defect, and an additional 3% of children are discovered to have a malformation in the next several years that is thought to have been present from birth. Only 3 to 5% of these anomalies are the result of a known teratogen, which is a drug, chemical, virus, physical agent, or deficiency state that, by acting during the embryonic or fetal period, alters morphology or subsequent function in the postnatal period. Fewer than 25 agents are known to be teratogenic in humans. Many teratogens are species specific; this makes the assessment and extrapolation of congenital anomalies from animal models difficult. Other important factors that influence the effects of a teratogen include the dose of the drug, the gestational age of the fetus, the duration of administration of the drug, the maternal-fetal blood pH gradient, the differences in maternal and fetal protein binding, the variations in absorption and transplacental transfer of the drug, and the rate of placental metabolism of the drug.

SUBSTANCES RELATED TO SOCIAL HABITS AND CUSTOMS

Caffeine

There has been controversy regarding the effects of caffeine during gestation. Several retrospective studies from the early 1980s related coffee consumption to birth defects and fetal wastage. Animal studies indicated a decrease in intrauterine fetal growth, lower birth weight, and skeletal abnormalities with increased ingestion of caffeine. In the fall of 1980, as a result of these studies, the U.S. Food and Drug Administration advised pregnant women to use caffeine sparingly. A large cohort study by Linn and colleagues in 1982 found that the malformation rate was not increased among newborns of coffee drinkers. There was also no difference in the incidence of low birth weight babies and no evidence of shortened gestation. These results were confirmed in a multicenter study in 1993. Most obstetricians advise moderate use of caffeine (one cup of coffee per day) during pregnancy (Table 34–1).

Tobacco

Despite an overall decrease in cigarette consumption in the 1980s and early 1990s, women of childbearing age have actually increased their consumption. Smoking causes a number of adverse effects in women in addition to the well-known pulmonary and cardiovascular effects. Women who smoke have higher rates of infertility: 21% of women who smoked were infertile compared with 14% of women who never smoked. Early pregnancy loss is also associated with smoking. There is an increased frequency of spontaneous abortion in smokers, possibly due to interference with implantation. The conceptus appears to be chromosomally normal. In a case-control study by Kline and associates that controlled for age, number of previous spontaneous abortions, induced abortions, and live births, 41% of the women who had had a spontaneous abortion smoked compared with 28% of the controls.

Placental problems are also related to smoking. Higher rates of abruptio placenta and placenta previa are reported. Placentas of women who smoke have fewer fetal capillaries, thickened basement membranes, and increased collagen content of the villose stroma. This results in decreased placental blood flow, which could account for the frequency of low birth weight babies in smokers. Nicotine is vasospastic, which can also cause placental ischemia. The serum thiocyanate level varies directly with the number of cigarettes smoked and is inversely related to birth weight, implying a direct dose-related effect independent of caloric intake. Reduction in smoking during pregnancy increases the birth weight of the infant.

Nicotine also causes a reduction in the frequency of fetal breathing movements. Herbal cigarettes do not affect fetal breathing movements despite equivalent carboxyhemoglobin levels. Nicotine gum, however, also inhibits fetal breathing activity. Sudden infant death syndrome occurs twice as frequently in infants of mothers who smoke compared with infants of those who never smoked. Elevated levels of epinephrine and norepinephrine in the fetus are felt to be secondary to fetal hypoxia or a direct effect on the adrenergic system, or both.

No clearly defined patterns of malformation have been described in relation to tobacco use, but there are reports of cleft lip, cleft palate, and anencephaly. Children whose mothers smoked 10 or more cigarettes per day during pregnancy were on the average 1.0 cm shorter and 3 to 5 months retarded in reading, mathematics, and general ability as compared with the offspring of nonsmokers.

Alcohol

Alcohol ingestion during pregnancy has been reported to cause a number of complications in addition to the fetal alcohol syndrome. Ethanol retards intrauterine growth and reduces birth weight, resulting in babies that are small for gestational age and that have a perinatal mortality rate of 17%. It also causes delays in postnatal growth and development. The devastating effects of alcohol on the fetus are likely related to its quite prolonged exposure to the substance. Levels of fetal alcohol dehydrogenase are very low. Because of this, the amniotic fluid serves as a reservoir for the alcohol. At 3½ hours after a fixed dose of alcohol, levels were present in the amniotic fluid even though they were absent from the maternal serum at 1 hour.

The fetal alcohol syndrome generally occurs in the offspring of women with high alcohol consumption; however, it is unclear what amount of alcohol in pregnancy is necessary to result in the appearance of this syndrome. Abnormalities in each of four categories, define the fetal alcohol syndrome: (1) central nervous system dysfunction, including retardation, microcephaly, hypotonia, and hyperactivity; 44% of infants with this syndrome have an IQ of less than 80; (2) growth deficiencies below 2 standard deviations for length and height and decreased adipose tissue; (3) facial abnormalities, including short palpebral fissures, short and upturned nose, and hypoplastic maxilla; (4) variable major and minor malformations, including joint abnormalities (subluxations, abnormal palmar creases, and thoracic cage abnormalities) and congenital heart disease (atrial septal defect, ventricular septal defect, and tetralogy of Fallot).

Methadone

Although methadone is not reported to be teratogenic in humans, it is responsible for behavioral and neurodevelopmental dysfunction in infants

TABLE 34–1.   Medications in Pregnancy

DRUG	TOXICITY	RECOMMENDATION
Acetaminophen	?Rare Gastroschisis	Analgesic of choice in pregnancy
Acne		
Benzoyl peroxide	None reported	?Safe
Erythromycin	None known	Avoid estolate, safe
Isotretinoin	Teratogenic	Contraindicated
Topical	Not known	?Safe
Tetracycline	Tooth and bone abnormalities	Contraindicated
Topical	No data	
Alcohol	Fetal alcohol syndrome	Contraindicated
Antacids	Not teratogenic	Safe, use low sodium content
Anticoagulants		
Heparin	Maternal osteoporosis	Anticoagulant of choice in pregnancy
Warfarin	Embryotoxic	Contraindicated
Anticonvulsants		
Phenobarbital	Multiple anomalies	If possible, discontinue for first trimester
Phenytoin	Multiple anomalies	or altogether; use 1 agent in lowest
Carbamazine	Fewer negative fetal cognitive effects c/w phenytoin	dose
Valproic acid	Multiple anomalies	
Primidone	Multiple anomalies	
Trimethadione		Contraindicated
Antihistamines	?Cleft palate	Tripelennamine (PBZ) probably safe
Antihypertensives		
ACE inhibitors	Neonatal renal problems	Contraindicated
α-β–Blocker	Hepatotoxicity; limited data	Weigh benefits
β-Blockers	?Growth retardation	Weigh benefits
Calcium channel blockers	Limited data; may inhibit labor	Weigh benefits
Diuretics	Pancreatitis	Use if required for blood pressure control prior to pregnancy; not in preeclampsia
Hydralazine	Most data	Drug of choice in pregnancy
Methyldopa	Most data	Drug of choice in pregnancy
Nitroprusside	Fetal cyanide poisoning	Contraindicated
Aspirin	?Rare gastroschisis, premature closure PDA, bleeding	Low dose safe prior to term
Asthma		
Beta agonists (inhaled)	None known	Probably safe
Inhaled steroids	None known	Probably safe
Oral steroids	None estabished	Probably safe
Theophylline	Tachycardia	Probably safe
Benzodiazepines	?Cleft palate, floppy infant syndrome, withdrawal	Avoid in first and third trimesters; weigh benefits in second
Caffeine	None established	Safe in moderation
Cocaine	Spontaneous abortion, abruptio placentae, premature delivery, malformations	Contraindicated
Cough preparations	See Narcotics	Weigh benefits, avoid iodine preparations, dextromethorphan
Codeine		
Decongestants	Most data	Drug of choice in pregnancy; avoid phenylephrine, phenylpropanolamine
Pseudoephedrine		
H₂ receptor antagonists	None reported to date	Weigh benefits
Marijuana	Impaired growth, ?childhood AML	Contraindicated
Narcotics	Behavioral and developmental dysfunction, withdrawal	Weigh benefits
Nonsteroidals	Premature closure PDA, bleeding and prolonged labor at term	Generally safe; weigh benefits
Oral hypoglycemics	Anomalies	Use insulin
Thyroid preparations		
Iodine	Congenital goiter, hypothyroidism, retardation	Contradindicated
Methimazole	Crosses placenta more readily than PTU, retardation	PTU preferred
Propylthiouracil	Retardation	Drug of choice in pregnancy
Radioactive ¹³¹I	Goiter, hypothyroidism, retardation	Contraindicated
Tobacco	Abruptio placentae, growth retardation, SIDS	Contraindicated
Tricyclics	?Malformations, neonatal withdrawal, prolonged labor	Avoid in first and third trimesters, weigh benefits in second

c/w, Compared with; ACE, angiotensin-converting enzyme; PDA, patent ductus arteriosus; AML, acute myelomonocytic leukemia; PTU, propyl-thiouracil; SIDs, sudden infant death syndrome.

who are exposed to it in utero. At delivery, the neonate exhibits acute signs of narcotic withdrawal. Methadone suppresses fetal rapid eye movement sleep and produces a hyperactive state with increased behavioral arousal. Hyperactivity and sleep disturbances have been shown to persist for up to 2 years in these children. Although mean developmental scores are within the normal range at 1 year, neurodevelopmental dysfunction is evident, with a clearly reduced attention span.

Even shorter periods of exposure to narcotics are associated with behavioral differences. Studies of babies of mothers who receive large doses of analgesia during labor reveal them to be less attentive for the first 4 days after delivery. Consolability and cuddliness scores, which affect maternal-infant bonding, were higher for babies of mothers who had not been premedicated. Although analgesia may be required during labor and delivery, it should be used as sparingly as possible.

Marijuana

Women who use marijuana during pregnancy have impaired fetal growth and deliver infants with lower birth weights and shorter lengths than those of women who do not. This is evident even after controlling for other confounding variables such as smoking. Delta-9-tetrahydrocannabinol, the main ingredient of marijuana, crosses the placenta more readily in early pregnancy than late pregnancy. The substance is fat soluble and has a large enterohepatic circulation. Because of this, a single maternal exposure may have a very prolonged fetal exposure—up to 30 days. Marijuana smoking is associated with up to five times the carboxyhemoglobin levels of smoking a cigarette, which may impair fetal oxygenation and growth. Marijuana also increases the maternal heart rate and blood pressure, which reduces placental blood flow to the fetus.

Although marijuana is not associated with any known congenital anomalies, it has been suggested that it has a role in the development of childhood acute nonlymphocytic leukemia. Maternal use of marijuana has been linked to the development of acute myelomonocytic and monocytic leukemia in the offspring.

Cocaine

Women who use cocaine during pregnancy have a higher rate of spontaneous abortion and abruptio placentae. The frequency of abruptio placentae in cocaine-using women ranged from 10 to 19%, compared with 3% in nonusing women. This has been thought to be secondary to the vasoconstriction and abrupt rise in blood pressure associated with cocaine use. The placental vasoconstriction decreases blood flow to the fetus, and the increased norepinephrine levels increase uterine contractility. Abruptio placentae accounts for the increased frequency of stillbirths in cocaine-using women and of maternal hemorrhage and fetal hypoxia.

Maternal cocaine use during pregnancy is also associated with premature delivery—31% before 38 weeks of gestation compared with 3% of non–drug-using controls—and with premature labor—21% compared with 1% of controls. The use of cocaine throughout pregnancy is also associated with impaired fetal growth, including lower birth weight and decreased length and head circumference. Infants that are small for gestational age are born to 15 to 36% of women who use cocaine during pregnancy but only to 7% of those who are nonusers. Cocaine is an appetite depressant, and women who use cocaine gain less weight during pregnancy. It has both an indirect effect mediated by maternal undernutrition and an independent direct negative effect on birth weight.

Teratogenicity

A number of malformations have been associated with in utero exposure to cocaine; however, a specific syndrome has not been identified. The alterations in fetal blood flow caused by the vasoconstriction and rebound vasodilation may disrupt morphogenesis by intermittent hypoxia. Cocaine-associated anomalies involve the genitourinary tract, the cranium and central nervous system, and the cardiovascular system and include limb reduction defects and ileal atresia.

Neonatal Complications

Behavioral changes are noted in 30 to 40% of the infants of women who use cocaine during pregnancy, including irritability, tremor, increased muscle tone, abnormal reflexes, tachypnea, poor feeding, and abnormal sleep patterns. Infants exposed to cocaine show patterns of depressed interactive behavior, a greater degree of tremulousness, and a greater degree of startle responses. It is unclear whether these behavioral changes are a manifestation of drug withdrawal, a direct effect of the cocaine, or a combination of both. Approximately 75% of neonates exposed to cocaine have developmental delays during the first year of life. Seizures are also described in cocaine-exposed infants but appear to decline in frequency with age. Some studies have reported an increase in sudden infant death syndrome in cocaine-exposed infants, although other studies have not found such an increase.

OVER-THE-COUNTER MEDICATIONS

There are more than 200 active ingredients present in over-the-counter medications in more than 500,000 available products. Manufacturers were not required to show the safety of their products until 1938, and efficacy was not required until 1962. Most studies reveal a decrease in use of over-the-counter medications during pregnancy over the past decade. Analgesics are the most frequently used over-the-counter medication during pregnancy.

Aspirin

Most studies of aspirin use during pregnancy have not found an increase in deformities, although one study did find a mildly elevated relative risk of gastroschisis, a rare but serious congenital defect of the abdominal wall. Large doses of aspirin taken regularly over a long period of time appear to reduce birth weights of neonates. Lower doses, however, appear to have no effect. Aspirin use during late pregnancy is associated with a prolonged duration of pregnancy, postmature babies, as well as a prolonged duration of labor, more blood loss during birth, and more prepartal bleeding. Aspirin use is also associated with premature closure of the ductus arteriosus. No significant increase in aspirin-induced mortality has been found. Cautious, symptom-related low-dose aspirin use is probably safe before the latter part of pregnancy.

Acetaminophen

Acetaminophen has not been associated with fetal malformations and has generally been considered safe in pregnancy. An increased risk for gastroschisis, however, has also been found with the use of acetaminophen. Most obstetricians recommend this as the drug of choice during pregnancy when an analgesic is necessary. However, acetaminophen lacks anti-inflammatory action, as it predominantly suppresses prostaglandin synthesis in the central nervous system, whereas aspirin acts peripherally as well.

Antihistamines

Antihistamines also appear to be relatively safe in pregnancy. Although animal studies have revealed an increase in cleft palate associated with meclizine, this has never been found in humans despite rather frequent use in pregnancy. If teratogenicity is present, it appears to be low.

GASTROINTESTINAL DRUGS

Antinauseants

Bendectin was first marketed for nausea in 1956. It is estimated that at one point up to 25% of pregnant women took this medication. It is a combination of dicyclomine (antispasmodic), doxylamine (antihistamine), and pyridoxine (antinauseant). A weak association with congenital heart defects was reported in 1979. A subsequent study free of recall bias, however, found no evidence of an increase in birth defects. The drug was withdrawn from the market because of the number of lawsuits brought against the manufacturer. No other antinauseant has been as well studied or is known to be as safe in pregnancy as bendectin.

Antacids

No teratogenic effects have been associated with the use of antacids during pregnancy. It is wise to use antacids with a low sodium content because of the difficulties with fluid retention and swelling during pregnancy.

H$_2$ Receptor Antagonists

Data on the H$_2$ receptor antagonists are limited. A study of 23 women exposed to these drugs in the first trimester revealed three premature births, but normal developmental milestones for all infants. One infant had a hemangioma of the eyelid. To date, cimetidine and ranitidine have not been reported to be teratogenic.

AGENTS FOR ACNE

Topical and oral agents for acne are common medications among women of childbearing age. Tetracycline administration during pregnancy increases the risk of fatty liver, especially if large doses are used, renal disease is present, or drug levels are above the therapeutic range. Its use during the second or third trimester is associated with staining and, less frequently, enamel hypoplasia of the deciduous teeth; the permanent teeth are unaffected. It also reversibly decreases bone growth rate in premature infants. Its use has not been associated with major congenital anomalies. Topical tetracycline has never been reported to cause any congenital abnormalities. Blood levels are generally less than 0.1 gm per ml or less. With such a small amount of systemic absorption, it is unlikely that topical tetracycline causes adverse effects on the fetus.

Erythromycin, both topical and oral, appears to be safe in pregnancy if the estolate form is avoided. Systemic absorption of the topical form is minimal, and it should be considered safe during pregnancy. Clindamycin has never been associated with any teratogenic effects; however, the side effect of pseudomembranous colitis has been reported with use of the topical form as well as the oral form. It is not more frequent in pregnancy than in the nonpregnant state.

Topical benzoyl peroxide is bactericidal for propionibacterium acnes. Approximately 5% of topically applied benzoyl peroxide is absorbed through the skin. Although no studies on the long-term use of the drug in pregnancy have been published, it appears to be safe.

Oral isotretinoin is contraindicated in pregnancy, as it is a potent teratogen. Reliable birth control is necessary when this medication is utilized. Malformations of the craniofacial area, heart, and thymus have been described. Topical tretinoin has not been associated with malformations of the offspring of mothers who applied it during pregnancy, and less than 5% of the agent is systemically absorbed. It may be safe in pregnancy; however, data are limited.

PSYCHOTROPIC DRUGS

Tricyclic Antidepressants

Although data are limited on the effects of tricyclic antidepressant use in pregnancy, association between congenital malformations and use of these antidepressants has not been proved. There have been isolated case reports of limb deformities, and animal studies are also suggestive of this. It is advisable to avoid the use of tricyclics in pregnancy, particularly in the first trimester. There has also been concern about the effects of tricyclics on the neurologic development of the fetus, and evidence exists that these agents may interfere with normal labor by decreasing muscle contractility. A

withdrawal syndrome in neonates has been described, including cyanosis, difficulty breathing, feeding difficulties, dystonic movements, and seizures. Because of the decreased muscle contractility, which could prolong labor, withdrawal from tricyclics before parturition has been advised. However, intrauterine withdrawal may not be as safe as extrauterine withdrawal. Fetal seizures with meconium passage and aspiration could result in fetal demise. Generally supportive measures and hospitalization for depression during pregnancy are often preferred to medication.

Benzodiazepines

The use of benzodiazepines in the first trimester has been associated with oral clefts in some studies, although others have not supported this finding. Generally it is best to avoid them if possible. Several large studies have failed to associate the use of benzodiazepines with an increase in congenital malformations. Adverse neonatal effects, referred to as the "floppy infant syndrome," have been reported both with long-term use and with relatively small amounts at parturition. This syndrome includes muscular hypotonicity, failure to feed, impaired temperature regulation, and low Apgar scores. A withdrawal syndrome consisting of tremors, irritability, and a hyperactive sucking reflex is also described. Concentrations of the drug are higher in the fetus throughout gestation and at term. Benzodiazepines should be avoided in the first trimester, are contraindicated in the third trimester, and should be used sparingly, if at all, in the second trimester.

Antimicrobial Agents

Antimicrobial agents, their toxicity in pregnancy, and recommendations regarding use can be found in Table 34–2.

CONCLUSION

A comprehensive review of medications in pregnancy is beyond the scope of this chapter. The methodologic considerations necessary to assess the cause and effect relationship between medications and congenital abnormalities are presented, as well as a summary of the physiologic variables that affect the interaction of the drug with the fetus. The effects of some of the most commonly used substances and medications in pregnancy are also reviewed.

TABLE 34–2. Antimicrobial Agents in Pregnancy

DRUG	TOXICITY IN PREGNANCY	RECOMMENDATION
Antibacterial		
Aminoglycosides*	Possible eighth-nerve toxicity in fetus	Caution†
Aztreonam (Azactam)	None known	Probably safe
Cephalosporins‡	None known	Probably safe
Chloramphenicol (Chloromycetin and others)	Unknown—gray syndrome in newborn	Caution†, especially at term
Cinoxacin (Cinobac)	Arthropathy in immature animals	Contraindicated
Clindamycin (Cleocin)	None known	Caution†
Dapsone (Aviosulfon and others)	None known; carcinogenic in rats and mice; hemolytic reactions in neonates	Caution†, especially at term
Erythromycin estolate (Ilosone and others)	Risk of cholestatic hepatitis appears to be increased in pregnant women	Contraindicated
Erythromycins, other	None known	Probably safe
Imipenem-cilastatin (Primaxin)	Toxic in some pregnant animals	Caution†
Methenamine mandelate (Mandelamine and others)	Unknown	Probably safe
Metronidazole (Flagyl and others)	None known—carcinogenic in rats and mice	Caution†
Nalidixic acid (NegGram and others)	Unknown—arthropathy in immature animals; increased intracranial pressure in newborn	Contraindicated
Nitrofurantoin (Furadantin and others)	Hemolytic anemia in newborn	Caution†; contraindicated at term
Norfloxacin (Noroxin)	Arthropathy in immature animals	Contraindicated
Penicillins§	None known	Probably safe
Spectinomycin (Trobicin)	Unknown	Probably safe
Sulfonamides	Hemolysis in newborn with G6PD deficiency; increased risk of kernicterus in newborn; teratogenic in some animal studies	Caution†; contraindicated at term
Tetracyclines	Tooth discoloration and dysplasia, inhibition of bone growth in fetus; hepatic toxicity and azotemia with intravenous use in pregnant patients with decreased renal function or with overdosage	Contraindicated
Trimethoprim (Proloprim and others)	Folate antagonism; teratogenic in rats	Caution†
Trimethoprim-sulfamethoxazole (Bactrim and others)	Same as sulfonamides and trimethoprim	Caution†; contraindicated at term
Vancomycin (Vancocin and others)	Unknown—possible auditory and renal toxicity in fetus	Caution†
Antituberculosis		
Capreomycin (Capastat)	None known	Caution†
Cycloserine (Seromycin and others)	Unknown	Caution†
Ethambutol (Myambutol)	None known—teratogenic in animals	Caution†
Ethionamide (Trecator-SC)	Teratogenic in animals	Caution†
Isoniazid (INH and others)	Embryocidal in some animals	Caution†
Pyrazinamide	Unknown	Caution†
Rifampin (Rifadin; Rimactane)	Teratogenic in animals	Caution†
Streptomycin	Possible eighth-nerve toxicity in fetus	Caution†
Antifungal systemic		
Amphotericin B (Fungizone and others)	None known	Caution†
Flucytosine (Ancobon)	Tertogenic in rats	Caution†
Griseofulvin (Fulvicin P/G and others)	Embryotoxic and teratogenic in animals; carcinogenic in rodents	Contraindicated
Ketoconazole (Nizoral)	Teratogenic and embryotoxic in rats	Caution†
Miconazole (Monistat i.v.)	None known	Caution†
Nystatin (Mycostatin)	None reported	Probably safe
Antiviral, systemic		
Acyclovir (Zovirax)	None known	Caution†
Amantadine (Symmetrel and others)	Teratogenic and embryotoxic in rats	Contraindicated
Ribavirin (Virazole)	Mutagenic, teratogenic embryolethal in nearly all species and possibly carcinogenic in animals	Contraindicated
Vidarabine (Vira-A)	Teratogenic in rats and rabbits	Caution†
Zidovudine (Retrovir)	Unknown—mutagenic in vitro	Caution†

TABLE 34–2.   Antimicrobial Agents in Pregnancy *Continued*

DRUG	TOXICITY IN PREGNANCY	RECOMMENDATION
Antiparasitic		
Chloroquine (Aralen and others)	None known with doses recommended for malaria prophylaxis	Probably safe in low doses
Crotamiton (Eurax)	Unknown	Caution†
Dehydroemetine	Not established, but known to be cardiotoxic	Contraindicated
Diloxanide (Furamide)	Safety not established	Caution†
Emetine	Not established, but known to be cardiotoxic	Contraindicated
Furazolidone (Furoxone)	None known; carcinogenic in rodents; hemolysis wih G6PD deficiency in newborn	Caution†; contraindicated at term
Hydroxychloroquine (Plaquenil)	None known with doses recommended for malaria prophylaxis	Probably safe in low doses
Iodoquinol (Yodoxin)	Unknown	Caution†
Lindane (Kwell and others)	Absorbed from the skin; potential central nervous system toxicity in fetus	Contraindicated
Mebendazole (Vermox)	Teratogenic and embryotoxic in rats	Caution†
Metronidazole (Flagyl and others)	None known—carcinogenic in rats and mice	Caution†
Niclosamide (Niclocide)	Not absorbed; no known toxicity in fetus	Probably safe
Oxamniquine (Vansil)	Embryocidal in animals	Contraindicated
Paromomycin (Humatin)	Poorly absorbed; toxicity in fetus unknown	Probably safe
Pentamidine (Pentam 300)	Safety not established	Caution†
Permethrin (Nix 1% Creme Rinse)	Poorly absorbed; no known toxicity in fetus	Probably safe
Piperazine (Antepar and others)	Unknown	Caution†
Praziquantel (Biltricide)	None known	Probably safe
Primaquine	Hemolysis in G6PD deficiency	Contraindicated
Pyrantel pamoate (Antiminth)	Absorbed in small amounts; no known toxicity in fetus	Probably safe
Pyrethrins and piperonyl butoxide (RID and others)	Poorly absorbed; no known toxcity in fetus	Probably safe
Pyrimethamine (Daraprim)	Teratogenic in animals	Caution†
Pyrimethamine-sulfadoxine (Fansidar)	Teratogenic in animals; increased risk of kernicterus in newborn	Caution†, especially at term
Quinacrine (Atabrine)	Safety not established	Caution†
Quinine	Large doses can cause abortion; auditory nerve hypoplasia, deafness in fetus; visual changes, limb anomalies, visceral defects also reported	
Suramin sodium (Germanin)	Teratogenic in mice	Caution†
Thiabendazole (Mintezol)	None known	Caution†

*Amikacin (Amikin), gentamicin (Garamycin and others), kanamycin (Kantrex and others), netilmicin (Netromycin), streptomycin, tobramycin (Nebcin).

†Use only for strong clinical indication in absence of suitable alternative.

‡Cefaclor (Ceclor), cefadroxil (Duricef; Ultracef), cefamandole (Mandol), cefazolin (Ancef and others), cefonicid (Monocid), cefoperazone (Cefobid), ceforanide (Precef), cefotaxime (Claforan), cefotetan (Cefotan), cefoxitin (Mefoxin), ceftazidime (Fortaz; Tazidime; Tazicef), ceftizoxime (Ceflzox), ceftriaxone (Rocephin), cefuroxime (Kefurox; Zinacef), cephalexin (Keflex and others), cephalothin (Keflin and others), cephapirin (Cefadyl and others), cephradine (Anspor and others), moxalactam (Moxam).

§Amdinocillin (Coactin), amoxicillin (Amoxil and others), amoxicillin-clavulanic acid (Augmentin), ampicillin (Polycillin and others), aziocillin (Azlin), bacampicillin (Spectrobid), carbenicillin (Geocillin; Geopen; Pyopen), cloxacillin (Tegopen and others), cyclacillin (Cyclapen-W), dicloxacillin (Dycill and others), hetacillin (Versapen), methicillin (Staphcillin), mezlocillin (Mezin), nafcillin (Nafcil; Unipen), oxacillin (Prostaphlin and others), penicillin G, penicillin V, piperacillin (Pipracil), ticarcillin (Ticar), ticarcillin-clavulanic acid (Timentin).

From Safety of antimicrobial drugs in pregnancy. Med Lett Drugs Ther 1987;29:61–63.

REFERENCES

Bauchner H, Zuckerman B, McClain M, et al. Risk of sudden infant death syndrome among infants with in utero exposure to cocaine. J Pediatr 1988;113:831.

Bonati M, Bortolus R, Marchetti F, et al. Drug use in pregnancy: An overview of epidemiological (drug utilization) studies. Eur J Clin Pharmacol 1990;38:325.

Bryant HE, Visser N, Love EJ. Records, recall loss, and recall bias in pregnancy: A comparison of interview and medical records data of pregnant and postnatal women. Am J Public Health 1989;79:78.

Butler NR, Goldstein H. Smoking in pregnancy and subsequent child development. BMJ 1973;4:573.

Chasnoff IJ, Burns KA, Burns WJ. Cocaine use in pregnancy: Perinatal morbidity and mortality. Neurotoxicol Teratol 1987;9:291.

Chasnoff IJ, Burns WJ, Schnoll SH, Burns KA. Cocaine use in pregnancy. N Engl J Med 1985;313:666.

Collaborative Group on Drug Use in Pregnancy. Drug use in pregnancy: A preliminary report of the International Co-operative Drug Utilization Study. Pharm Weekbl Sci 1990;12:75.

Cordero JF, Oakley GP. Drug exposure during pregnancy: Some epidemiologic considerations. Clin Obstet Gynecol 1983;26:418.

Finnegan LP. Drug Dependence in Pregnancy: Clinical Management of Mother and Child. Washington, DC: US Department of Health, Education, and Welfare, 1979.

Goyan JE. Food and Drug Administration news release no. P80-36. September 4, 1980.

Hill LM, Kleinberg F. Effects of drugs and chemicals on the fetus and newborn. Mayo Clin Proc 1984;59:707.

King JC, Fabro S. Alcohol consumption and cigarette smoking: Effect on pregnancy. Clin Obstet Gynecol 1983;26:437.

Kline J, Stein YA, Susser M, Warburton D. Smoking: A risk factor for spontaneous abortion. N Engl J Med 1977;297:793.

Koren G, Zemlickis DM. Outcome of pregnancy after first trimester exposure to H_2 receptor antagonists. Am J Perinatol 1991;8:37.

Lenz W. Epidemiology of congenital malformations. Ann NY Acad Sci 1965;123:228.

Linn A, Schoenbaum SC, Monson RR, et al. No association between coffee consumption and adverse outcomes of pregnancy. N Engl J Med 1982;306:141.

Mills JL, Holmes LB, Aarons JH, et al. Moderate caffeine use and the risk of spontaneous abortion and intrauterine growth retardation. JAMA 1993;269:593.

Mortola JF. The use of psychotropic agents in pregnancy and lactation. Psychiatr Clin North Am 1989;12:69.

Niederhoff H, Zahradnik HP. Analgesics during pregnancy. Am J Med 1983;75:117.

Robison LL, Buckley JD, Daigle AE, et al. Maternal drug use and risk of childhood nonlymphoblastic leukemia among offspring: An epidemiologic investigation implicating marijuana. Cancer 1989;63:1904.

Rothman KF, Pochi PE. Use of oral and topical agents for acne in pregnancy. J Am Acad Dermatol 1988;16:431.

Shepard TH. Teratogenicity of therapeutic agents. Curr Probl Pediatr 1979;10:5.

Weathersbee PS, Olsen LK, Lodge JR. Caffeine and pregnancy: A retrospective survey. Postgrad Med 1977;62:64.

Werler MM, Mitchell AA, Shapiro S. First trimester maternal medication use in relation to gastroschisis. Teratology 1992;45:361.

Wu T-C, Tashkin DP, Djahed B, Rose JE. Pulmonary hazards of smoking marijuana as compared with tobacco. N Engl J Med 1988;318:347.

Young SL, Vosper HJ, Phillips SA. Cocaine: Its effects on maternal and child health. Pharmacotherapy 1992;12:1.

Zuckerman B, Frank DA, Hingson R, et al. Effects of maternal marijuana and cocaine use on fetal growth. N Engl J Med 1989;320:762.

Legal Issues in Pregnancy and Abortion

Nancy R. Williams and Donna Poresky

This chapter identifies and reviews legal, ethical, philosophic, and social implications of medical issues related to pregnancy and fertility to better equip the physician to recognize and deal with them when they arise in the clinical setting. An opportunity for prior thought enables the physician to establish a personal approach to resolving these dilemmas and to compile a list of reliable resources to whom the physician can turn directly and without delay for assistance in dealing with issues that are beyond the realm of personal expertise. The urgency inherent in a crisis situation absorbs much energy and can distract from the reasoned focus that a more unhurried, distanced assessment allows. Often, if the legal and ethical parameters are identified and discussed early in treatment, more alternatives exist.

ABORTION

Historical Context

Historically, the focus of concern about abortion related to maternal health and safety owing to the fact that early abortions were usually accomplished either by administering dangerous poisons in an attempt to terminate the pregnancy without killing the woman or by utilizing rudimentary surgical techniques that very often resulted in infection caused by a lack of knowledge of sterile technique and asepsis.[1] Although there were a few early court cases, no legislation was enacted regulating abortion in the United States until 1821. That statute, passed in Connecticut, applied only to postquickening abortions, or those abortions performed after the pregnant woman was able to feel fetal movement, and it prohibited only the use of poisons. This is illustrative of the relative lack of emphasis on the fetus as a separate holder of rights, either in a legal or a moral sense. Abortions

were performed fairly frequently during the late eighteenth and early nineteenth centuries, owing in part, perhaps, to a liberalization of attitudes concerning sexuality.[2] Nevertheless, according to some, most of the abortions performed during this time were on unmarried women in an attempt to conceal the "illicit sexual activity"[3] that had led to an unwanted pregnancy. At this time having children, at least within a marriage, was viewed as being economically advantageous, because by a fairly early age, their labor contributed to the support of the family.[3]

In the mid 1800s abortion became more of a politically controversial issue. At about that time organized medicine began to mobilize as professional physicians attempted to "police their borders"[4] in an effort to regulate "irregular physicians and apothecaries promising miraculous abortional procedures."[4] At the same time, a more sophisticated understanding of the science of human reproduction and fetal development was emerging. It became increasingly difficult for some practitioners to accept quickening as a legitimate distinction and not just as an arbitrary point along the spectrum of fetal development. In 1857, the American Medical Association, led by obstetrician-gynecologist Dr. Horatio Storer, began a crusade to end the availability of abortion in the United States, focusing its platform on, among other things, the fetus' right to life.[4]

Antiabortionists used a number of arguments to gain support for their cause. One strategy was to accuse white, middle-class Protestant women, who were increasingly utilizing abortion services, of "race suicide,"[5] citing the fact that this group of women was giving birth to many fewer babies than were immigrant women of other races or ethnic backgrounds and religions. Another tactic was to attempt to portray access to abortion as a threat to traditional sex roles by claiming, accurately enough, that the ability to control reproduction freed women from the constraints of unwanted pregnancy and childrearing responsibilities and enabled them to make choices that were once not available to them.[6]

These efforts resulted in the passage of a number of state statutes strictly limiting a woman's access to abortion predominantly to cases in which her life was endangered by the continuation of the pregnancy. Many of these statutes cast the physician in the primary role of determining whether an abortion could be performed legally by framing the question as one of medical necessity[7] and then leaving the physician great discretion as to how to define medical necessity. Because laws prohibiting abortion were rarely enforced, many physicians interpreted the therapeutic exception to the ban on abortions so broadly as to include factors such as poverty as sufficient justification under the law.[8]

From 1950 to 1970 physicians performing abortions came under increased scrutiny. Critics argued that because medical advances had greatly decreased the dangers previously associated with childbirth, the number of medically necessary abortions should be diminished. The consequence of this heightened scrutiny was that, although the number of legally performed abortions dropped, the number of dangerous, "back alley" abortions rose.[9] Reformers urged lawmakers to create exceptions to the abortion ban in addition to circumstances in which abortion was necessary to save the life of the pregnant woman. Preservation of the woman's mental health, pregnancies resulting from rape or incest, and prenatal diagnosis of serious impairment of the fetus were all offered as valid justifications for abortion.[10] Reform efforts eventually focused on repeal, and garnered support from women's groups as well as from many other socially and politically active groups, including a large segment of organized medicine.[11] Opposition to the expansion of legal access to abortion remained vocal and firm among certain conservative religious and political groups.

In the midst of all of this legislative activity, a series of cases dealing with the use of contraceptives, led by *Griswold v Connecticut* in 1965,[12] came before the United States Supreme Court. *Griswold* involved a Connecticut state statute that made it a crime to use "a drug, medicinal article, or instrument for the purpose of preventing conception."[13] The Court reversed the criminal conviction of a Yale physician and a planned parenthood official who had been prosecuted for supplying a married couple with contraceptives. The Court held that there are certain guarantees in the Bill of Rights that create personal "zones of privacy"[14] around issues of marriage, childbearing, and family. The concurring justices based their support for this decision on the Ninth Amendment, which states that "the enumeration in the Constitution of certain rights will not be construed to deny or disparage others retained by the people."[14]

This right of privacy concerning the use of contraceptives within marriage was extended to unmarried people in 1972. In *Eisenstadt v Baird*,[15] the United States Supreme Court explained that "[i]f the right of privacy means anything, it is the right of the individual, married or single, to be free from unwarranted government intrusion into matters so fundamentally affecting a person as a decision whether to bear a child."[16] These cases articulated for the first time the concept of a right to personal privacy that is not found explicitly anywhere in the Constitution, and helped to set the stage for the United States Supreme Court's landmark 1973 decision on abortion.

In a 1972 survey article on the then current state of abortion law, Knecht noted inconsistency and contradiction at the state level.[17]

> The law regulating abortion is one of the most complex and widely discussed issues of our time. Literature on the subject is widespread and the increase in law review articles over the last four years has been extensive. Physicians complain that restrictive abortion laws place them in hypocritical positions. Some women complain that restrictive abortion laws deny them dignity. As mature human beings they feel they should have the right to decide whether or not to carry a pregnancy to term. Others complain that the liberalization of abortion laws is inconsistent with the inviolate right of every human being to be born. No other single topic so excites the emotions of society, for abortion involves women's rights, religious beliefs, sex, medicine, and a myriad of other concerns. Although there has been considerable state legislation since 1967, recent court decisions indicate this legislation is ineffective. These cases have emphasized increasing polarization and conflict and until the Supreme Court decides the issue, the abortion controversy will remain.[18]

Privacy

Roe v Wade, a landmark decision in the legal regulation of abortion, was delivered on January 22, 1973, by a 7 to 2 divided Supreme Court, after having been argued twice, first in 1971 and then again in 1972.[19] Unfortunately, contrary to Knecht's somewhat optimistic projection, the polarization and conflict continued unabated and are perhaps even more virulent now, some twenty years after the decision was handed down. The continued controversy does seem to substantiate Knecht's characterization of the unique complexity associated with issues related to abortion.

Roe involved a Texas statute that had remained essentially unchanged since 1857, and that made it a crime to procure an abortion except where it was "an abortion procured or attempted by medical advice for the purpose of saving the life of the mother."[20] The statute was challenged as an improper infringement on a pregnant woman's right to choose to terminate her pregnancy.

Justice Blackmun wrote the opinion for the Court, which held that a right to privacy exists in the Fourteenth Amendment concept of personal liberty and restriction on state action. That right of privacy encompasses personal procreative decisions, including a woman's choice to terminate a pregnancy.

Because *Roe* characterized this right to decide whether to terminate a pregnancy as a fundamental right, the state would need a compelling reason for interfering with a woman's decision to exercise that right. Note that this fundamental right is not absolute, only that the threshold for legitimate state intervention is relatively high. The opinion identified two state interests in limiting abortions, the protection of maternal health and the protection of fetal life. To balance these potentially competing interests, *Roe* established a schedule that loosely corresponded to a trimester framework.

According to *Roe,* states could only regulate abortions during the first trimester by requiring that the procedure be performed by a physician. The focus here was clearly on the state's interest in the protection of maternal health, and the rationale for this limited intervention was that at that point, early in the pregnancy, the risks to the pregnant woman involved in an abortion procedure were less than or equal to those that she might undergo in childbirth.

The *Roe* Court found that the risks to the pregnant woman associated with abortion increased as the pregnancy progressed. Thus, it was concluded that, during the second trimester, states could regulate abortion in ways "reasonably related to maternal health."[21]

Finally, the Court held that once the fetus had progressed to the point of viability, or that point at which the fetus is "potentially able to live outside the mother's womb, albeit with artificial aid,"[22] the state's interest in protecting "the potentiality of human life"[23] becomes so compelling that the state may regulate or proscribe abortions except those performed to "save the life or health of the mother."[21] Although the state's interest in potential life becomes compelling at the point of viability, the unborn fetus does not, until birth, achieve the status of "personhood," for purposes of the Fourteenth Amendment. It should also be noted that, although viability generally occurs toward the end of the second trimester, the question is not merely one of fetal age. Clearly the definition of viability is a functional one and involves a number of factors, including fetal weight and lung development.

Roe generated much controversy. Some criticized the concept of viability as arbitrary and argued that as technology advances, the point of viability will continue to be pushed back until it becomes meaningless. Justice O'Connor, in her dissenting opinion in *City of Akron Center for Reproductive Health,*[24] suggested that *Roe* was on a "collision course with itself."[25] Critics of *Roe* balanced the interests differently and accorded more status to the human fetus, viable or nonviable, at any stage of development based on religious or philosophic justifications. In any event, this decision triggered many attempts to modify or overturn the precedent it established. Fearing that *Roe* might be overturned, the forces interested in the protection of choice in reproductive decision-making unsuccessfully attempted to marshall support for a constitutional amendment that would codify the rights that *Roe* articulated. Others mobilized to attempt to limit or restrict *Roe* by working for passage of state statutes that would, if not lead to *Roe's* outright repudiation, gradually erode the holding so as to leave it without any practical impact.

State Restrictions on Abortion

Generally, state efforts to restrict abortion relate to limitations on funding, to requirements concerning consent or notification, and to attempts to regulate medical procedures for performing or for maintaining records on abortion or for obtaining informed consent.[26] Whether any specific restriction is constitutional depends on whether it "unduly burdens" the woman's right. The following cases provide information concerning this newly evolving standard.

Webster v Reproductive Health Services,[27] a 5 to 4 decision handed down in 1989, represents a plurality of the Supreme Court, which means that a majority was unable to agree on any single piece of reasoning. Although *Webster* did not overrule *Roe* in upholding certain state-imposed restrictions on abortion, it did signal for some the beginning of a judicial retreat from the protection of abortion rights that seemed to have been the trend for the prior 16 years.[28] The case arose from a challenge to a 1986 Missouri abortion statute, which attempted to establish the following:

● Life begins at conception, and an unborn child,

from conception, has a protectable interest in life, health, and well-being.[29]

- The attending physician is required to certify that she or he has personally obtained the woman's informed consent.[30]
- Any abortion after 16 weeks must be performed in a hospital.[31]
- Detailed testing for viability must be performed before any abortion later than 20 weeks of gestation.[32]
- The use of public funds, public employees, and public facilities "to perform or assist an abortion not necessary to save the life of the mother or for the purpose of encouraging or counseling the woman to have an abortion not necessary to save her life is prohibited."[33]

The Supreme Court ruling did not address all of the issues raised, but did hold that

- Missouri could constitutionally prohibit state-employed doctors from performing abortions not necessary to save the life of the woman.
- Missouri could prohibit abortions that were not necessary to save the life of the woman from being performed in a state institution.
- Missouri could require the doctor to determine fetal viability at or after 20 weeks.

In its analysis, the Court referred to what are known as the "funding cases," in which the Court has held that the state has no affirmative duty to fund abortions.[34] The right to have an abortion generally has been characterized as a negative right that translates into a right to be left alone or to be protected from "undue" state interference in making the decision. It generally has not been viewed as a positive right or one that could be exercised affirmatively to force the state to provide abortion as a service. The Court in *Webster* reasoned that it is not unconstitutional for Missouri to prohibit the performance of abortions by public employees and in public facilities because, "Missouri's refusal to allow public employees to perform abortions in public hospitals leaves a pregnant woman with the same choices as if the State had chosen not to operate any public hospitals at all."[35]

Critics charge that *Webster* is not internally consistent. One concern relates to some of the specific testing that was mandated by statute after 20 weeks. Because, for example, amniocentesis is considered to be of little or no value to assess fetal lung maturity before 28 to 30 weeks of gestation,[36] it would arguably present unjustifiable risks to the woman because it is of questionable benefit in the determination of fetal viability at that stage of pregnancy. One could argue that to perform this

testing at that time would be inconsistent with language, included in the same statute that mandates that the physician "us[e] and exercis[e] that degree of care, skill, and proficiency commonly exercised by the ordinarily skillful, careful and prudent physician engaged in similar practice under the same or similar conditions."[32]

Although not overruling *Roe, Webster* seemed to invite states to test how far they could go in regulating abortion without violating the "undue burden" test articulated by Justice O'Connor. The difficulty is, as Baron notes, that "[the] test is not only vague as to what constitutes an 'undue burden,' it is also puzzlingly incomplete."[37] Justice Blackmun, who wrote the opinion in *Roe,* wrote in his concurrence in *Webster,* "For today, the women of this Nation still retain the liberty to control their destinies. But the signs are evident and very ominous, and a chill wind blows."[38]

In 1992, in *Planned Parenthood of Southeastern Pennsylvania v Casey,*[39] the Supreme Court, in a 5 to 4 ruling, reaffirmed the core holding in *Roe,* the constitutional right to abortion, but at the same time expanded on the ways in which a state could regulate and limit the abortion decision.[40] At issue in this case were the provisions of the Pennsylvania Abortion Control Act of 1982,[41] which, except in an emergency, provided the following:

- Before obtaining an abortion, a pregnant woman must be given information about fetal development, childbirth, potential assistance available for medical care, potential paternal liability for support, and alternatives to abortion.[42]
- There must be a 24-hour mandatory waiting period between the receipt of this information by the pregnant woman and the performance of an abortion procedure.[42]
- The attending physician must keep records on each abortion performed, and some of these records would be subject to inspection.[43]
- An unmarried, financially dependent woman under 18 years would need the consent of one parent, a guardian, a certification of majority, or a judicial finding of best interest.[44]
- A married woman must give notice, certified in writing, to her husband of her decision to have an abortion unless the spouse is not the father, the father cannot be located, the father has criminally assaulted her, or she fears bodily injury as a result of such notice.[45]

A joint opinion by three justices upheld all of the provisions of the Pennsylvania law except the one requiring spousal notification. *Roe,* although not overruled, was redefined. Since *Casey,* a pregnant woman can be said to possess a "constitutional liberty"[46] right to choose to terminate her pregnancy before viability that the State cannot "undu[ly] burden."[47] An undue burden has been further defined in *Casey* as "a state regulation [that] has the purpose or effect of placing a substantial obstacle in the path of the woman seeking an abortion of a nonviable fetus."[47] Clearly, any state regulation that imposes an absolute prohibition on abortion of a nonviable fetus would fail, but the extent to which states can legislate so as to restrict access is still unsettled. Even *Casey,* which dealt with a Pennsylvania law that had not yet gone into effect, left open the possibility that the provisions that were upheld, like the 24-hour waiting period, when implemented, would, in fact, result in the kind of undue burden that the Court stated would be unacceptable. If the Court finds at some future date, based on new evidence, that certain provisions do confer an undue burden, then those provisions should be struck down.

The Future of the Right to Abortion in the United States

In *Casey* the Supreme Court reaffirmed the core principle in *Roe v Wade,* the right of a pregnant woman to decide to terminate her pregnancy before viability. The Court also seemed to emphasize that the pregnant woman's decision, and not the physician's right to practice medicine, is central. However, since recent decisions like *Webster* and *Casey* have supported increased state restrictions on abortion short of those that seem to "unduly burden" the pregnant woman before viability, it is fair to assume that efforts to foster the maximum level of state intervention will continue. Attempts to pass an amendment to the United States Constitution have stalled, at least for now, although Congress could pass some version of a Freedom of Choice Act. The current administration has professed to be in favor of reproductive choice, and, by executive order in early 1993, President Clinton removed a number of restrictions on abortion that had been implemented by prior administrations.[48] Also of note is the potential impact on *Roe* of changes in the composition of the United States Supreme Court.

In addition to the impact of legislative activity on the state and federal levels and the influence of the judiciary, advances in technology may well refocus some of the debate around abortion. Most notably, the use of the French abortion pill, RU 486, perhaps used in combination with some form of oral prostaglandin, may make it possible for a woman to terminate an early pregnancy in the privacy of the home, making her and her physician much less likely targets of antiabortion protesters.

FORCED MEDICAL OR SURGICAL INTERVENTION

Overview

The concept of forced treatment of an adult person of sound mind without consent invokes adversarial images that are inconsistent with the ideal model of the physician-patient relationship, a relationship that should be built on a foundation of mutual trust and respect. Historically, the physician's duty was clearly to the pregnant woman, who until relatively recently, was the only patient that could be treated directly. Over time, as more sophisticated methods evolved for evaluating and ultimately for accessing the fetus in utero, some physicians came to regard the fetus as a second patient, in some ways separate if not distinct from the pregnant woman. Clearly the interests of the two are not always identical and may even be incompatible. The following cases illustrate the dilemma that can arise in this context.

Forced Cesarean Section

In re AC involved an emergency petition for declaratory relief to determine whether a pregnant woman who suffered from terminal cancer in her twenty-sixth week of pregnancy should undergo a cesarean section to attempt to benefit the fetus.[49] AC had apparently decided to accept a course of palliative treatment aimed at increasing her comfort and extending her life until at least her twenty-eighth week of pregnancy, even though she was informed that the palliative treatment she sought might present her fetus with increased risk. As AC's physical condition began to deteriorate rapidly, she was intubated and her wishes apparently became increasingly difficult to ascertain. There is no evidence that AC ever consented to a cesarean section before the twenty-eighth week of pregnancy, a time after which she had been told that the likelihood of the survival of her fetus would improve. AC's family opposed performance of a cesarean section. Counsel were appointed by the court to represent the separate interests of AC and the fetus. In addition, the District of Columbia intervened on behalf of the fetus.

The trial court made the following findings of fact:

● AC was 26½ weeks pregnant.
● AC would be likely to die within 2 days of terminal cancer, although cesarean section could further shorten her life.
● The fetus was viable, and had a 50 to 60%

chance for survival if delivered as soon as possible by cesarean section.

Following the hearing, a court-ordered cesarean section was performed. The baby girl, who was born prematurely, died within 2½ hours. AC died after 2 days.

Although the case became moot as to AC and her baby once the cesarean section was performed, the appellate court recognized that the issues addressed were important ones and that the same questions were likely to arise in the future and so accepted the case for review. On appeal, the District of Columbia Court of Appeals addressed two issues. First, who has the right to decide what medical treatment should be performed on a patient who is pregnant with a viable fetus? The court held that " . . . in virtually all cases the question of what is to be done is to be decided by the patient—the pregnant woman—on behalf of herself and her fetus.''[50]

The second issue addressed by the court was the standard that should be used in determining whether medical treatment should be administered to the pregnant patient when that patient is no longer able to make this decision for herself. The court considered either a balancing of the mother's interests in privacy and bodily integrity against the interest of the state, under *parens patriae*, in protecting the potential life of the fetus or a scheme of substituted judgment that would be consistent with the usual preferred standard in surrogate decision-making involving once-competent adults. The court concluded that substituted judgment should have been used in this case and indeed should be used in most cases. Further, the court concluded that on the facts presented in this case, the cesarean section was properly ordered and performed.

Note that although the result might have been the same, that is, the cesarean section was performed, the analysis is very different under each approach. In this case, the court began with the paradigm of the adult person of sound mind who has a privacy-liberty interest in preserving bodily integrity and who, based on this, has a right to consent or to refuse to consent to medical-surgical intervention, even if that treatment is potentially lifesaving. Once a patient becomes incompetent to make an informed, voluntary decision, it is the court's duty ''as surrogate for the incompetent, to determine as best it can what choice that individual, if competent would make with respect to medical procedures.''[51] The opinion did not address under what circumstances, if any, a ''balancing of interests'' test should be administered.

State law can vary on the relative weight ac-

corded a particular interest, although clearly, under current law, viability is the point at which the state's interest in the ''potentiality'' of fetal life intensifies. It should be noted, however, that although the holding in *Roe* recognizes that after viability the state may intervene to regulate or proscribe abortions, that is, to prevent a pregnant woman from terminating her pregnancy except when necessary to preserve her life or health,[22] it does not necessarily follow that the state can therefore coerce a nonconsenting adult woman of sound mind to undergo an extremely invasive surgical procedure to benefit or even to save a viable fetus. Although the woman who elects to continue her pregnancy through viability may well possess a moral obligation to attempt to ensure the health and well-being of her unborn child, the basis of any legal duty is much less clear. This case is significant because it represents a determination by an appellate court that it was the pregnant woman's substituted judgment, or *what she would have wanted,* as best as could be determined, that was the appropriate standard on which to base a decision concerning her medical treatment. The fact that she was terminally ill and pregnant with a viable fetus did not undermine her right to decide.

More recently, when deciding *In the Interest of Baby Boy Doe, a Fetus v Mother Doe,*[52] the Appellate Court of Illinois was faced with the question of whether the right of a pregnant woman to avoid unwanted medical intervention should be balanced against the right of her fetus (if, in fact, such a right exists) to be born healthy. This court held, as did the *In re AC* court, ''that no such balancing test should be employed, and that a woman's competent choice to refuse medical treatment as invasive as a cesarean section during pregnancy must be honored, even in circumstances where the choice may be harmful to her fetus.''

Generally, the presumption is that an adult person of sound mind has a right to make decisions about treatment, including both decisions to consent or to refuse to consent to interventions. This right generally includes interventions that might be necessary to save the patient's life. To deprive the pregnant woman of this basic right seems to negate her interest in controlling her own body and seems to be, as Annas suggests, ''counterproductive, unprincipled, sexist, and repressive.''[53] Still, states differ in the protection accorded a viable fetus. Therefore, in complex cases involving a pregnant woman who is refusing consent for an intervention determined to be necessary to save the life of a viable fetus, it is prudent to seek the advice of knowledgeable counsel as to current legal parameters in that specific jurisdiction before proceeding.

Refusal of Life-Sustaining Blood or Blood Products

Similar issues can arise in cases of refusal of life-sustaining blood or blood products by a patient based on her religious beliefs. Again, although jurisdictions may vary, as a general rule, an adult person of sound mind may elect to refuse even life-sustaining treatment. It is obvious that this refusal should be voluntary, informed, and made by one who has the capacity to understand and process information relative to the risks and benefits associated with treatment alternatives and to communicate her decision. Faced with this situation, most courts have allowed the patient to forgo even "necessary" medical treatment.[54] In the obstetric context, it is clear that although a woman generally may refuse life-sustaining blood or blood products for herself after delivery, she may not block necessary medical interventions for her already born minor child.[55] Particularly difficult legal and ethical issues arise when the blood or blood product is needed to save the life of the woman who has not yet delivered and is pregnant with a viable fetus. The same arguments that were raised for recognizing the pregnant adult woman's right to consent to or to refuse to consent to surgical interventions like caesarean section could be made here, although again, when faced with this situation, the physician should seek the advice of knowledgeable counsel, because specific state law varies as to what protection is owed to the unborn viable fetus.

SUMMARY

In optimal situations, these issues should be explored early in the pregnancy so that decisions need not be made in a crisis, when little time exists for thoughtful analysis. In the vast majority of cases, no court intervention is required, and appropriate management decisions are made by the patient in consultation with her physician.

The following useful recommendations were adopted in 1990 by the American Medical Association Board of Trustees:

1. Judicial intervention is inappropriate when a woman has made an informed refusal of a medical treatment designed to benefit her fetus.

If an exceptional circumstance could be found in which a medical treatment poses an insignificant or no health risk to the woman, entails a minimal invasion of her bodily integrity, and would clearly prevent substantial and irreversible harm to her fetus, it might be appropriate for a physician to seek judicial intervention. However, the fundamental principle against compelled medical procedures should control in all cases that do not present such exceptional circumstances.

2. The physician's duty is to provide appropriate information, such that the pregnant woman may make an informed and thoughtful decision, not to dictate the woman's decision.

3. A physician should not be liable for honoring a pregnant woman's informed refusal of medical treatment designed to benefit the fetus.

4. Criminal sanctions or civil liability for harmful behavior by the pregnant woman toward her fetus are inappropriate. . . .

6. To minimize the risk of legal action by a pregnant patient or an injured child, the physician should document medical recommendations made, including the consequences of failure to comply with the physician's recommendations.[56]*

Early, open communication between the physician and the patient is often the most important factor in resolving these excruciating dilemmas. When a physician feels unwilling or unable to accept a competent patient's decision concerning treatment options, such as the Jehovah's witness who intends to refuse even life-sustaining blood or blood products, the physician should be honest in disclosing this to the patient as early in the relationship as possible and should attempt to arrange transfer of the patient to another physician who is in a position to honor the patient's wishes.

PRENATAL SUBSTANCE ABUSE

Overview

Prenatal substance abuse presents circumstances in which the behavior of the pregnant woman directly affects the health and well-being of the fetus she carries. Obviously, virtually any behavior in which a pregnant woman engages has the potential for direct or indirect impact on her fetus, and even legal activities, such as consuming alcohol or smoking, can result in significant, long-term negative consequences. Once again, potentially competing interests are involved, and the goal is to somehow identify and establish a framework for decision-making.

There is a consensus in society that substance abuse is a tragedy with many victims. In addition to the adult addict, babies who are born addicted present enormous costs, not just in terms of dollars but in lost potential and in apparently needless pain and suffering. A number of approaches have

---

*Used with permission from Cole HM. Legal interventions during pregnancy. JAMA 1990; 264:2663–2670. Copyright 1990, American Medical Association.

been implemented by different states in an attempt to address and to stem this problem. Public health initiatives that focus on treatment rather than punishment have been the models supported by an overwhelming majority of health care providers based on a rationale of efficacy.[57] If the goal is to help to foster healthy births, any mechanism that undermines access to prenatal care is counterproductive. Some efforts to use criminal or civil laws to address this problem have been attempted, but generally, at least on appeal, this approach has failed. One case is illustrative.

Utilization of Criminal Statutes

In *Johnson v Florida,* a pregnant woman who ingested cocaine on the morning that she went into labor with her second child was prosecuted under a Florida statute that made it illegal for an adult to deliver a controlled substance to a minor.[58] The prosecution alleged that the illegal delivery occurred during the estimated 30 to 90 seconds between the birth of the child and the severance of the umbilical cord.

Although the trial court found the defendant guilty, and her conviction was upheld by the appellate court, it was subsequently overturned by the Florida Supreme Court. The conviction was ultimately overturned based on the following factors. First, the court relied on the statute's legislative history, which failed to demonstrate that lawmakers intended that the statute be applied in this context. On the contrary, the court determined that the issue of explicitly including illegal drug delivery from mother to child during pregnancy as part of this specific legislation was apparently considered and rejected when the statute was drafted. From the legislative history it seemed clear that the intended application of this legislation was in the context of drug dealers. In addition, the court found that the medical and scientific evidence presented failed to establish that a significant amount of the illegal drug was actually transferred from mother to child during the short interval between delivery of the child and severance of the umbilical cord.

In overturning the woman's criminal conviction, the court relied on public policy and reason, as well as on law. *Johnson v Florida* seems representative of a national trend against the utilization of criminal statutes in an attempt to address the public health issues related to illegal substance abuse during pregnancy. This trend seems to reflect a recognition that attempts to enforce these laws in this context not only fail to deter drug use in these cases, but also have the unintended potential to discourage pregnant substance abusers, who are already considered to be at high risk, from accessing health care providers. This would place their already vulnerable fetuses at an even greater risk.

Termination of Parental Rights

Similar arguments have been offered in opposition to automatically terminating the parental rights of a pregnant substance abuser. Once again, state laws vary, and the prudent physician should keep abreast of current law in the jurisdiction in which she or he practices or should seek legal counsel from an attorney knowledgeable in health law for help in assessing a specific case. The Connecticut Supreme Court held, in part, in *In re Valerie D,* that a 23-year-old woman's prenatal drug use, while egregious, could not be the basis for a termination of her parental rights.[59] The court based its decision on a determination that the state's child abuse statute was not intended to embrace prenatal conduct. Some states have included language that explicitly includes unborn children in their child abuse statutes, and, in fact, the Connecticut attorney general is reported to have said that he may seek a similar change in that state's legislation.[60] Such a move would be ill-conceived. All of the public policy concerns that were raised in the previous section also apply here to make any intervention that diminishes a pregnant addict's access to prenatal care by discouraging her utilization of the health care system counterproductive to the goal of providing for healthier newborns. In addition, given the complexity of the process of gestation and the vulnerability of the fetus to legal as well as illegal toxins at different developmental points, it is extremely difficult to ascertain the direct and proximate cause of any injury.

SUMMARY

The American Medical Association Board of Trustees offered the following relevant recommendations in a 1990 statement:

4. Criminal sanctions or civil liability for harmful behavior by the pregnant woman toward her fetus are inappropriate.

5. Pregnant substance abusers should be provided with rehabilitative treatment appropriate to their specific physiological and psychological needs.[56]

Lynn Paltrow, who represented Jennifer Johnson in the Florida case, was reported as having credited the medical community consensus that drug use during pregnancy was a health issue rather than a concern for the criminal justice system with the fact that no state has passed specific legislation making it a crime to give birth to an infant exposed to drugs in utero.[60] In addition, creative attempts to use old statutes that were passed for other purposes, as in these two cases, have thus far been unsuccessful on final appeal.

HAZARDS IN THE WORKPLACE

Overview

In recent years growing concerns have surfaced related to issues pertaining to a safe work environment. These issues are complicated enough when focused on the appropriate level of safety that must be provided for the employee personally. However, the level of complexity mushrooms when the inquiry is extended to include issues related to the safety of an unborn fetus that might be exposed to health hazards encountered by the pregnant woman on the job. These issues have most frequently surfaced in the legal system when an employer, concerned about protecting the unborn children of its employees to avoid adverse publicity, increased insurance and medical costs, or potential costly tort litigation, attempts to exclude pregnant or nonpregnant but fertile women from the workplace.[61]

Fetal Protection Policies

The issue addressed in *Automobile Workers v Johnson Controls* was whether a fetal protection policy excluding fertile female employees from certain jobs because of an increased risk to an as yet unconceived fetus was constitutional.[62] The United States Supreme Court held that it was not.

Johnson Controls utilized lead in the manufacture of batteries. Exposure to lead can be harmful to employees, as well as to the fetus of a pregnant employee. Before 1977, Johnson Controls did not have any female employees in its battery manufacturing division. Between 1977 and 1982 the employer allowed women to perform these jobs but warned them of the potential risk of exposure to lead during pregnancy. In 1982, after several female employees became pregnant, Johnson Controls attempted to change its employment practices to exclude women from these jobs.

A class action suit was brought charging that Johnson Controls' fetal protection policy was in violation of Title VII of the Civil Rights Act of 1964[63] in that the policy illegally discriminated against women. The policy was reviewed to determine whether it was biased on its face, or although not biased on its face, whether it had a disparate impact on a protected group. In this case the U.S. Supreme Court found that the fetal protection policy at Johnson Controls was clearly on its face biased against women because it did not include fertile male employees. The only way for the policy to stand would be for the company to establish that the inability to become pregnant was a "bona fide occupational qualification"[64] or that infertility was "reasonably necessary to the operation of the business."[64] The Court found that in this case Johnson Controls had failed to demonstrate that a woman's fertility interfered with the performance of her job in the manufacture of batteries, and therefore the Court held that the policy was illegal.

One argument offered by Johnson Controls was that allowing women to work in positions that potentially placed their fetuses at risk of exposure to lead made the company vulnerable to costly tort liability. The Court rejected this argument, reasoning that, even though some states offer recovery on a cause of action for prenatal injury based either on negligence principles or wrongful death statutes, the possibility of a finding against Johnson Controls, absent negligence, was remote, because the employer claimed that it complied with Occupational Safety and Health Administration standards and warned its employees about the potentially damaging effects of lead exposure.

In addition, the Pregnancy Discrimination Act of 1978,[65] which states that "for the purposes of Title VII, discrimination on the basis of sex includes discrimination because of or on the basis of pregnancy, childbirth or related medical conditions,"[66] explicitly rejects discrimination based on sex-specific fetal protection policies. Congress, the Court concluded, has left to the individual woman the right to choose which of her roles is more important, reproductive or economic.[67]

TREATMENT OF MINORS IN THE OBSTETRIC-GYNECOLOGIC CONTEXT

Overview

In general, medical treatment of a minor without parental consent gives rise to a cause of action by the parents for assault and battery, even if the outcome of the treatment was beneficial to the minor. This is consistent with the evolving doctrine of informed consent that is premised on a constitutional right to privacy and on the common law right to self-determination. The right to privacy and to bodily integrity is vested in the minor but is exercised on the minor's behalf by a surrogate. In our Anglo American legal system, the presumption is that parents generally act in the best interests of their minor children. In addition, a number of cases have acknowledged that parents have an interest in the well-being of their offspring and a right to participate in decisions related to the care and upbringing of their children.[68] In practice, then, parents are the usual surrogate decision-makers for their children. Generally, children are considered to be minors, and therefore legally incompetent, until they reach the age of majority, a milestone set by state statute, that marks the entry into legal adulthood.

Although a statutory age of majority sets a black line that for most purposes establishes a boundary that is useful because of its clarity, it is by some measures inherently arbitrary. Clearly, individuals develop at different rates physically as well as cognitively, and some children, even though under the age of majority, are indeed capable of making informed decisions about their own medical care. Consent, to be valid, must be voluntary, informed, and rendered by one with capacity. Competence is presumed once one attains the age of majority, and that presumption can only be formally overturned in court by a finding of incompetence.

In practice, the physician is charged with obtaining and documenting informed consent. This means that the physician must assess the patient and determine whether the patient has the capacity to give a voluntary, informed consent. This involves disclosure by the physician of information relative to diagnosis, prognosis, the risks and benefits of recommended treatment, other alternative treatments, the risks and benefits of these alternatives, and the consequences of no treatment. The patient with capacity must be able to understand the information disclosed, process it so as to make a decision concerning treatment or the refusal of treatment, and communicate that decision so that it can be implemented.

Emergency Treatment

In the event of a medical emergency, the general rule is that a minor may receive medical treatment without parental consent. Even if parental consent is lacking, not because the parent is unavailable but because the parent is intentionally refusing to allow what in the judgment of the attending physician is necessary medical treatment, the treatment may still proceed with a court order if time

permits. In a crisis, the focus is on saving the life of the minor, and necessary medical treatment can be initiated in good faith even without a court order. In these cases, it is important that the medical record reflect the nature of the medical emergency that justified the immediate intervention. As a general rule, even though they did not consent, parents are responsible financially for the necessary care of their children. This rule is based on a concept of implied consent that recognizes that on occasion the nature of the medical emergency requires urgent interventions to avert significant or permanent harm.

When the treatment sought is elective or non-emergency treatment, the general rule is that consent should be obtained from the parent or guardian of the minor. Some exceptions exist to this requirement, however, and under certain circumstances, a child under the age of majority may independently consent to medical treatment for herself without providing notice or obtaining consent from a parent or guardian.

Statutory Exceptions

Most state legislatures have, in one form or another, addressed the issue of the minor's ability to consent to medical treatment. Some states have passed general treatment statutes that simply lower the age of majority with regard to all health care decisions. In other jurisdictions, statutes are passed that focus on specific treatment situations. For example, many states have particular statutes that deal with a minor's access to treatment for drug and alcohol abuse, the diagnosis and treatment of sexually transmitted diseases, contraceptives, abortion, psychiatric treatment, and other specific health care interventions.

Although statutes in different states may address similar issues, the form as well as the substance can vary widely. It is crucial for the physician whose practice may involve the treatment of minors to remain aware of current legislation in the local jurisdiction. Some statutes explicitly allow treatment under certain circumstances, whereas others prohibit it. Although a public health rationale often underlies statutes that permit the minor access to health care without parental consent, other pressures for passage of legislation relevant to minor treatment statutes can come from lobbying groups with political or religious agendas.

Obviously, once a physician accepts a minor patient for treatment, the rules inherent in any good doctor-patient relationship should apply. The patient is entitled to the disclosure of information on which she can base an informed consent and is also entitled to an expectation of confidentiality. Financial considerations are generally not a justification for violating physician-patient confidentiality.

Emancipation

Emancipation is an attempt to take a practical approach to the real circumstances that contribute to a determination of a minor's ability to function as an adult. The law on emancipation varies widely from state to state and may be defined either by statute or by case law. In either situation, an emancipated minor is usually described as one who is financially independent, does not live with her parents, and, in general, is responsible for herself. Factors relevant to a determination of emancipation may be marriage, pregnancy, or military service.

Mature Minor

In this context, the mature minor is one who is capable of making health care decisions for herself. This determination is based on her functional ability to understand and to process information related to her diagnosis and prognosis—to the risks and benefits associated with any recommended treatment as well as with those associated with alternative treatments—and to communicate her decision concerning her choice of treatment. Generally, the mature minor is an older adolescent, often 15 years of age or older.[69] The focus is on the minor's ability to understand the ramifications of health care decisions rather than on outside factors that are used to indicate maturity in general. The Restatement of the Law of Torts (Second), which is compiled by the American Law Institute, supports the use of the mature minor exception to the general rule requiring parental consent and provides, in part, that there should be no liability for lack of consent of a parent or guardian attendant upon the treatment of a minor who "... is capable of appreciating the nature, extent and consequences of the invasion ..." and who consents to the intervention.[70] Generally, in these cases the treatment is intended to benefit the minor herself and not a third party, and although the intervention need not necessarily be defined as an emergency, it should be medically necessary.[71]

SUMMARY

Two things are key to feeling comfortable and responsible in this complicated area involving medicine, law, and ethics. First, a basic understanding of the fundamental issues involved and some method of analysis should be achieved before a crisis situation occurs. At the very least, the physician should attempt to determine whether she or he has a strong personal position on, for example, a competent Jehovah's witness's right to refuse life-sustaining blood transfusions either before or after delivery. Early disclosure of a firmly held view against respecting the patient's wishes presents the patient with more options and could avoid an unnecessary future confrontation. Although a court order may provide some protection from liability, the reality is that it is excruciating for all concerned when a competent adult is overpowered, either physically or pharmacologically, and forced to submit against her will to medical or surgical interventions. Some physicians are honestly uncertain as to how they would respond in an actual situation in which the patient was refusing interventions that could save her life. In that case, it is appropriate to inform the patient of the uncertainty and allow her to determine whether to remain a patient or to find another physician.

Second, the physician should identify resources that are immediately available and can assist in specific situations. Often, if the case involves an inpatient, institutional mechanisms exist, such as a hospital ethics committee, that can help to identify important issues and to offer a framework for decision-making. Other resources might be the patient advocate, social worker, or risk management specialist. If the question has legal dimensions, as many of these problems do, knowledgeable in-house or outside counsel can help to clarify the legal parameters, although those are often dependent on medical indications, like viability or capacity for decision-making. Sometimes a formal psychiatric consultation can provide more insight into effective communication with the patient as well as their competence. It is also helpful to learn in advance how any or all of these resources can be accessed on weekends, holidays, or off-hours, or even whether they can be utilized for issues that arise in the outpatient setting.

REFERENCES

1. Tribe LH. Abortion: The Clash of the Absolutes. New York: WW Norton & Co, 1990, p 29. *Roe v Wade,* 410 U.S. at 147, 93 S.Ct. at 724.
2. Tribe LH. Abortion: The Clash of the Absolutes. New York: WW Norton & Co, 1990, p 28.
3. Tribe LH. Abortion: The Clash of the Absolutes. New York: WW Norton & Co, 1990, p 29.
4. Tribe LH. Abortion: The Clash of the Absolutes. New York: WW Norton & Co, 1990, p 30.
5. Tribe LH. Abortion: The Clash of the Absolutes. New York: WW Norton & Co, 1990, p 32.

6. Tribe LH. Abortion: The Clash of the Absolutes. New York: WW Norton & Co, 1990, p 33.
7. Tribe LH. Abortion: The Clash of the Absolutes. New York: WW Norton & Co, 1990, p 34.
8. Tribe LH. Abortion: The Clash of the Absolutes. New York: WW Norton & Co, 1990, p 35.
9. Tribe LH. Abortion: The Clash of the Absolutes. New York: WW Norton & Co, 1990, p 43.
10. Tribe LH. Abortion: The Clash of the Absolutes. New York: WW Norton & Co, 1990, p 42.
11. Tribe LH. Abortion: The Clash of the Absolutes. New York: WW Norton & Co, 1990, p 46, 47.
12. 381 U.S. 470, 85 S.Ct. 1678, 14 L.Ed.2d 510 (1965).
13. 381 U.S. at 479, 85 S.Ct. at 1678.
14. 381 U.S. at 484, 85 S.Ct. at 1681.
15. 405 U.S. 438, 92 S.Ct. 1029, 31 L.Ed.2d 349 (1972).
16. 405 U.S. 438,453, 92 S.Ct. 1029,1038, 31 L.Ed.2d 349.
17. Knecht JA. Comment: A survey of the present statutory and case law on abortion: The contradictions and the problems. 1972, University of Illinois Law Forum, 183.
18. Knecht JA. Comment: A survey of the present statutory and case law on abortion: The contradictions and the problems. 1972, University of Illinois Law Forum, 177.
19. 410 U.S. 113, 93 S.Ct. 705, 35 L.Ed.2d 147 (1973).
20. 410 U.S. at 118, 93 S.Ct. at 709.
21. 410 U.S. at 163, 93 S.Ct. at 732.
22. 410 U.S. at 159, 93 S.Ct. at 730.
23. 410 U.S. at 163, 93 S.Ct. at 731.
24. 462 U.S. 416, 103 S.Ct. 2481, 76 L.Ed.2d 687 (1983).
25. 462 U.S. at 459, 103 S.Ct. at 2507.
26. Furrow BR. Bioethics: Health Care, Law and Ethics. St Paul, Minn: West Publishing Co, 1990, pp 84–85.
27. 492 U.S. 490, 109 S.Ct. 3040, 106 L.Ed.2d 410 (1989).
28. Tribe LH. Abortion: The Clash of the Absolutes. New York: WW Norton & Co, 1990, pp 20–21.
29. V.A.M.S. ss 1.205, 1.205, subds. 1(1,2).
30. V.A.M.S. s 188.039.
31. V.A.M.S. s 188.025.
32. V.A.M.S. s 188.029.
33. Annas GJ. Standard of Care: The Law of American Bioethics. New York: Oxford University Press, 1993, p 51; V.A.M.S. ss 188.205, 188,210, 188.215.
34. *Harris v McRae,* 448 U.S. 297, 100 S.Ct. 2671, 65 L.Ed.2d 784 (1980); *Maher v Roe,* 432 U.S. 464, 97 S.Ct. 2366, 53 L.Ed.2d 484 (1977); *Poelker v Doe,* 432 U.S. 519, 97 S.Ct. 2391, 53 L.Ed.2d 528 (1977).
35. 109 S.Ct. at 3052.
36. Tribe LH. Abortion: The Clash of the Absolutes. New York: WW Norton & Co, 1990, p 21, citing *Webster v. Reproductive Health Services,* 851 F.2d 1071, 1075 n.5 (8th Circ. 1988).
37. Baron CH. Law, medicine and health care. Abortion and Legal Process in the United States: An Overview of the Post-Webster Legal Landscape. 1989;17,370.
38. 109 S.Ct. 3079.
39. 505 U.S.—, 112 S.Ct. 2791, 120 L.Ed.2d 674 (1992).
40. 505 U.S.at—112 S.Ct. at 2804, 120 L.Ed.2d at 694.
41. 18 Pa. Cons. Stat. ss 3203–3220 (1990).
42. 18 Pa. Cons. Stat. s 3205.
43. 18 Pa. Cons. Stat. s 3207.
44. 18 Pa. Cons. Stat. s 3206.
45. 18 Pa. Cons. Stat. s 3209.
46. 505 U.S. at—, 112 S.Ct. at 2816, 120 L.Ed.2d at 709.
47. 505 U.S. at—, 112 S.Ct. at 2820, 120 L.Ed.2d at 714.
48. Time Magazine, February 1, 1993, p 17.
49. 573 A.2d 1235 (D.C. App. 1990).
50. 573 A.2d at 1237.
51. 573 A.2d at 1249, citing *In re Boyd,* 403 A.2d at 750 (D.C. 1979).
52. 1994 WL 111529 (Ill. App. 1 DIST.).
53. Annas GJ. Foreclosing the use of force: A.C. reversed. Hastings Center Report, July/August 1990, p 29.
54. *In re Brooks' Estate,* 32 Ill.2d.361, 205 N.E. 2d 435 (1965); *In re Osborne* 294 A.2d 372 (D.C. App. 1972); *Mercy Hospital, Inc. v. Jackson,* 62 Md. App. 1972, 489 A.2d 1130 (App. 1985), vacated on other grounds, 306 Md. 556, 510 A.2d 562 (1986) (affirming denial of petition to appoint a guardian to consent to Jehovah's Witness blood transfusion during C-section); Public Health Trust of Dade County v. Wons, 541 So.2d 96 (Fla.1989).
55. State v. Perricone, 37 N.J. 463, 181 A.2d 751, cert denied, 371 U.S. 890 (1962). See also Southwick AF. The Law of Hospital and Health Care Administration. 2nd ed. Ann Arbor, Mich: Health Administration Press, 1988, p 405.
56. Cole HM. Legal interventions during pregnancy: Court ordered medical treatments and legal penalties for potentially harmful behavior by pregnant women. JAMA 1990;264:2670.
57. The Hartford Courant (editorial), September 19, 1992, p C.9. See also Cole HM. Legal interventions during pregnancy: Court ordered medical treatments and legal penalties for potentially harmful behavior by pregnant women. JAMA 1990; 264:2667; ACOG Committee Opinion, Committee on Obstetrics: Maternal and Fetal Medicine. 9/92; 114:2–3; Mariner WK, Glantz LH, Annas GJ. Pregnancy, drugs and the perils of prosecutions. Criminal Justice Ethics 1990:37.
58. 602 So.2d 1288 (Fla. 1992).
59. *In re Valerie D.,* 223 Conn. 492 (1992).
60. Hansen M. Developments: Courts side with moms in drug cases. ABA Journal 1992:18.
61. Furrow BR. Bioethics: Health Care, Law, and Ethics. St. Paul, Minn: West Publishing Co, 1990, p 158.
62. 111 S.Ct. 1196 (1991).
63. 78 Stat. 255, as amended, 42 U.S.C. s 2000e-2(a).
64. 111 S.Ct. at 1204, 42 U.S.C. s 2000e-2(e)(1).
65. 92 Stat. 2076, 42 U.S.C. s 2000e(k).
66. 111 S.Ct. 1203.
67. 111 S.Ct. at 1210.
68. *Pierce v Society of Sisters,* 268 U.S. 510, 45 S.Ct. 571, 69 L.Ed. 1070 (1925); *Meyer v Nebraska,* 262 U.S. 390, 43 S.Ct. 625, 67 L.Ed. 1042 (1923).
69. Holder AR. Legal Issues in Pediatric and Adolescent Medicine. 2nd ed. New Haven and London: Yale University Press, 1986, p 134.
70. Holder AR. Legal Issues in Pediatric and Adolescent Medicine. 2nd ed. New York and London: Yale University Press, 1986, p 135.
71. Holder AR. Legal Issues in Pediatric and Adolescent Medicine. 2nd ed. New York and London: Yale University Press, 1986, pp 134–135.

MANAGEMENT OF MEDICAL PROBLEMS IN PREGNANCY

Hypertension in Pregnancy

Phyllis August

Hypertension in pregnancy is a challenging and serious clinical problem. It may be associated with considerable maternal and fetal morbidity and mortality; thus, those caring for pregnant women should be familiar with the pathophysiology, diagnosis, and treatment of the hypertensive disorders of pregnancy.

Normal pregnancy is associated with profound alterations in cardiovascular, renal, and endocrine physiology. Knowledge of these changes is helpful in understanding the pathophysiology of the hypertensive disorders.

HEMODYNAMIC CHANGES

During pregnancy, the cardiac output rises 30 to 40% relative to the nonpregnant resting state.[1, 2] The increase in cardiac output occurs as early as the twelfth week and is a result of increased heart rate, decreased afterload, and increased stroke volume.[1] The decreased afterload is a result of vasodilation, and the increased stroke volume is believed to be due to the increase in plasma volume (up to 50%) that occurs during gestation.

Despite the increased cardiac output and increased plasma volume, blood pressure falls during normal pregnancy in association with a decrease in peripheral vascular resistance. The decrease in blood pressure is apparent by the end of the first trimester, and it reaches a nadir in the second trimester. Blood pressure then increases gradually in the third trimester and often approaches prepregnancy levels at term. The reasons for the fall in peripheral vascular resistance are not established, but they are presumed to be associated with increased vasodilatory substances such as prostaglandins, estrogens, and possibly progesterone.[3, 4] The possibility that endothelial-derived relaxing factor (nitric oxide) may have a role in the increased vasodilation in pregnancy is an attractive hypothesis that is currently being investigated.

RENAL CHANGES

Both glomerular filtration rate (GFR) and renal blood flow increase dramatically in pregnancy.[5] Midpregnancy increments are as great as 50 to 60%, with a slight fall apparent in the third trimester. Significant elevation of the creatinine clearance is apparent as early as 4 weeks after conception.[6] The basis for these striking changes is not known, but they have been attributed to the increased cardiac output and fluid volume as well as concurrent endocrine changes, although many of these changes are apparent only after GFR has

335

already risen. Micropuncture studies of single-nephron GFR in pregnant rats demonstrate that the increase in GFR is due to increased glomerular plasma flow, which in turn is a result of renal vasodilation.[7] Clinically, the alterations in renal hemodynamics result in a lowering of the normal values for blood urea nitrogen and serum creatinine, compared with nonpregnant levels.

In addition to the alterations in renal hemodynamics, many other renal adaptations to pregnancy have been reported, including increased uric acid clearance, decreased plasma osmolality, increased urinary calcium excretion, and a cumulative retention of sodium.

ENDOCRINE CHANGES

The endocrine adaptations to pregnancy are the most dramatic physiologic adjustments that occur. The fetus, placenta, and maternal ovaries and adrenal glands participate in the production of large amounts of estradiol-17β, estriol, progesterone, aldosterone, deoxycorticosterone, human placental lactogen, and human chorionic gonadotropin, as well as other pregnancy-specific peptide hormones and prostaglandins.[8] Although considerable progress has been made in our understanding of the synthesis and metabolism of these substances, less is known about the precise ways in which these hormones maintain a normal pregnancy. Both estrogen and progesterone have been shown to have hemodynamic and renal effects; therefore, it is likely that these hormones interact with other regulatory systems in the control of blood pressure during pregnancy.

Normal pregnancy is characterized by marked stimulation of the renin-angiotensin-aldosterone system.[9, 10] All components of the system that have been measured are elevated as early as the first trimester, and these elevations are sustained until term. The basis for the stimulation of this system during pregnancy is not known, although in view of the lower blood pressure and decreased systemic vascular resistance, it is likely that the stimulation of the renin-angiotensin-aldosterone system is secondary to these hemodynamic alterations. It is also likely that the renin-angiotensin-aldosterone system is stimulated in response to natriuretic stimuli, because despite extremely high levels of aldosterone in pregnancy, serum electrolyte values and blood pressure are normal. Thus, the preponderance of data suggests that the high levels in pregnancy are physiologic. In association with increased levels of all components of the renin-angiotensin-aldosterone system in normal pregnancy is refractoriness to the pressor effects of angiotensin II.[11] The basis for this decrease in pressor sensitivity is not known; however, it presumably is at least in part due to the marked increase in circulating angiotensin II levels. Studies of platelet angiotensin II binding have demonstrated that early in pregnancy, there is a fall in platelet angiotensin II binding that parallels the decrease in pressor response to angiotensin II.[12]

It is against this background of the dramatic alterations in physiology during normal pregnancy that the pathophysiology of the hypertensive disorders in pregnancy must be considered.

TERMINOLOGY AND DEFINITIONS

It is helpful to classify the different entities associated with hypertension in pregnancy because it is important to identify preeclampsia. This disorder is associated with great maternal and fetal morbidity and mortality, especially when compared with uncomplicated chronic hypertension. Many classification schemes have been proposed for the hypertensive disorders of pregnancy.[13–15] The Committee on Terminology of the American College of Obstetricians and Gynecologists' 1972 report[13] has been the most practical. In this nosology, hypertension in pregnancy is classified into four groups: (1) chronic hypertension, (2) preeclampsia-eclampsia, (3) chronic hypertension with superimposed preeclampsia, or (4) transient hypertension. This classification has also been endorsed by a Working Group Report on High Blood Pressure in Pregnancy, published by the National High Blood Pressure Education Program at the National Institutes of Health.[16]

Preeclampsia occurs primarily in primigravidas after the twentieth week of gestation and is characterized by elevated blood pressure, proteinuria, generalized edema, and at times coagulation or liver function abnormalities. Preeclampsia is characterized by vasospasm, at times severe, which may lead to reduced perfusion of multiple organs, including the uterus, placenta, kidneys, brain, and liver. Indeed, although elevated blood pressure and proteinuria are clinically useful ways of diagnosing preeclampsia, they are usually late manifestations of a subclinical process that has been present since early pregnancy. Preeclampsia may evolve rapidly, at times without warning, to a convulsive phase, eclampsia, a life-threatening complication.

Chronic hypertension complicating pregnancy is usually essential hypertension and is mild to moderate in severity. In many patients, blood pressure decreases substantially during gestation, and their pregnancies proceed uneventfully to parturition. However, these women may have an increased incidence of superimposed preeclampsia,[17] which is diagnosed when blood pressure suddenly increases in late pregnancy, often associated with the onset of proteinuria or hyperuricemia, thrombocytopenia, and liver function abnormalities. Some women with chronic hypertension manifest proteinuria early in pregnancy owing to intrinsic renal disease, and in these women, superimposed preeclampsia may be difficult to diagnose. In some women, mild or moderate elevations of blood pressure occur in late pregnancy or the immediate puerperium, normalizing postpartum. This entity, termed transient hypertension, usually has a benign course and probably occurs in women destined to develop essential hypertension later in life.

PREECLAMPSIA-ECLAMPSIA

Epidemiology

The true incidence of preeclampsia is difficult to determine, given the variable diagnostic criteria used by different investigators. It has been demonstrated with the use of renal biopsy specimens that many multiparous women given a diagnosis of preeclampsia have either other underlying diseases such as essential hypertension or primary renal disease.[18–20] In nulliparous women, the group in whom the diagnosis is most likely to be correct, the incidence is approximately 6%.[17]

Most pregnancy complications relating to hypertension are associated with preeclampsia, and women who have high blood pressure before conception and who develop superimposed preeclampsia have the highest incidence of maternal and fetal morbidity, including prematurity, growth retardation, and fetal and maternal death.[21]

It is important to recognize factors that predispose to the development of preeclampsia, because identification of high-risk patients singles out those who need closer surveillance during pregnancy and those who may be candidates for the newer therapeutic and preventive strategies. The factors that predispose to preeclampsia are discussed next.

NULLIPARITY. Primigravidas are from six to eight times more likely to develop preeclampsia.[17, 22] Previous pregnancy has a protective effect on the incidence of preeclampsia, even if it is incomplete. A second- but not a first-trimester abortion appears to afford some protection for subsequent pregnancies.[23] Such observations and evidence that multiparous women who have been impregnated by a new partner have an increased risk of preeclampsia have led to the speculation that preeclampsia may result from an altered maternal immune response to paternal or fetal antigens.[24]

FAMILY HISTORY OF PREECLAMPSIA. Chesley and Cooper[25] have shown that mothers and sisters of women with preeclampsia are more likely to have had the disease. These investigators suggest that a single recessive gene may be responsible. The hypothesis that the condition may be a result of a maternal-fetal genotype has been set forth.[26] Thus, although it is suspected that preeclampsia may be a genetic condition, the genes involved or the mode of inheritance is not known.

MULTIPLE GESTATION. The incidence of preeclampsia is approximately four to five times greater with a twin gestation.[17]

CHRONIC HYPERTENSION. The incidence of superimposed preeclampsia in women with chronic hypertension is a subject of debate (published figures range from 5–86%), but most researchers agree that preeclampsia is more common in this setting. Using the criteria of the Committee on Terminology, the incidence is approximately 25%.[17]

DIABETES. Women with diabetes mellitus have a higher incidence of preeclampsia, although coexisting hypertension or renal disease may be mistaken for preeclampsia.[27]

HYDROPS FETALIS. The risk of preeclampsia in cases of nonimmune fetal hydrops is as high as 50%.

HYDATIDIFORM MOLE. Both preeclampsia and eclampsia have been reported with hydatidiform mole.[28] This form of preeclampsia tends to occur earlier in pregnancy, often in the second trimester.

EXTREMES OF AGE. The incidence of preeclampsia is reportedly higher in both adolescents and older women.[22, 29, 30] Although older women are more likely to have essential hypertension, it appears that preeclampsia is more common in older primigravidas than in multiparous women, supporting the belief that the incidence of preeclampsia truly is increased.[22]

Diagnosis of Preeclampsia

Although severe, fulminant preeclampsia or eclampsia may be easily diagnosed, in many instances it is difficult to distinguish between preeclampsia and either chronic or transient hypertension. Because preeclampsia may be life threatening even when the blood pressure is only mildly elevated, failure to recognize this entity can have serious consequences. In addition, early recognition permits close surveillance and appropriate decisions about the need to deliver.

BLOOD PRESSURE. The failure to appreciate that even normal levels (e.g., 120/85 mm Hg) of blood pressure may be abnormal in a pregnant woman is a common reason for underdiagnosing preeclampsia. A slight rise in blood pressure in the second trimester may be the initial sign of the disease, and if this is not recognized and the patient is scheduled for a revisit in 3 to 4 weeks, both she and the fetus may be in danger. Thus, any elevation in blood pressure must be evaluated, and it is prudent to overdiagnose rather than to miss mild cases. The standard criteria for diagnosing hypertension in pregnancy are (1) systolic blood pressure increases of 30 mm Hg or greater or (2) diastolic blood pressure (Korotkoff's phase 5) increases of 15 mm Hg or greater compared with the average of values before 20 weeks' gestation.[16] When prior blood pressure values are not known, a reading of 140/90 mm Hg is considered abnormal. However, as noted, a level of 120/80 mm Hg may be abnormal, especially in a woman who was previously recorded as having a pressure of 90/60 mm Hg. Moreover, the hypertension associated with preeclampsia is classically labile, and blood pressure readings may vary significantly from moment to moment.[31]

It should be pointed out that there is considerable controversy about whether Korotkoff's phase 4 (muffling of sounds) or phase 5 (disappearance of sounds) is the preferable estimate of diastolic blood pressure during pregnancy.[32] A review concluded that Korotkoff's phase 5 may more accurately reflect intra-arterial diastolic pressure.[33] Nevertheless, in some women, muffled sounds are heard to phase 0, and thus Korotkoff's 4 should be used in these instances. To avoid confusion, both phase 4 and phase 5 should be recorded throughout pregnancy.

PROTEINURIA. The Committee on Terminology of the American College of Obstetricians and Gynecologists defines abnormal proteinuria as greater than 300 mg in a 24-hour urine specimen. The magnitude of proteinuria in patients with preeclampsia may vary greatly, and some women with preeclampsia develop severe nephrotic syndrome.[34] The diagnosis of preeclampsia in the absence of proteinuria is uncertain; however, it is important to recognize that proteinuria may be a late manifestation of preeclampsia. Therefore, in the appropriate clinical setting, it is often necessary to treat women for preeclampsia before proteinuria develops. Because dipstick determination of proteinuria is associated with a high degree of error, it is advisable to obtain 24-hour urine collections to confirm the presence of proteinuria during pregnancy.[35]

EDEMA. Because edema frequently occurs during normal gestation, its presence alone is not a useful diagnostic criterion for preeclampsia.

However, this sign should not be ignored and must be taken in the clinical context in which it appears. For example, sudden and rapid weight gain is more likely to occur in women who develop preeclampsia.[17]

LABORATORY TESTS. Laboratory tests are necessary for establishing the diagnosis and assessing the severity of preeclampsia. It is often helpful to record baseline data in high-risk patients at an early stage of pregnancy. The standard laboratory evaluation for a woman suspected of having preeclampsia includes hematocrit, platelet count, urinalysis, serum creatinine, urea nitrogen, uric acid, and tests of liver function.

Several additional laboratory abnormalities have been identified in patients with preeclampsia. Many of these tests are not routinely performed, and their usefulness may thus be limited. However, they have helped to identify certain features of the pathogenesis of preeclampsia. Some of these assays have been proposed as useful predictors of preeclampsia when performed early in pregnancy.[36]

Among the measurements reported to be useful in the diagnosis or prediction of preeclampsia are plasma factor VIII–related antigen, plasma antithrombin III, plasma fibronectin, urinary calcium excretion, and platelet angiotensin II receptor number.

Disturbances in coagulation have been extensively investigated in patients with preeclampsia. Although most patients with preeclampsia do not demonstrate marked consumption of coagulation factors, in many cases some evidence suggests enhanced consumption of various clotting components, as well as platelet aggregation. Both a rise in the factor VIII–related antigen and a reduced antithrombin III concentration have been reported in women with preeclampsia.[36] It has been reported that factor VIII–related antigen activity rises early in pregnancy, before the development of preeclampsia,[37] and that blood levels correlate with disease severity and fetal outcome.[38]

Antithrombin III, the major serine-protease inhibitor of coagulation factors, is reported to be reduced in women with preeclampsia.[39–41] Weiner and co-workers, in a prospective study of 127 pregnant women, found the sensitivity of low antithrombin III activity levels to diagnose preeclampsia to be 76%, with a specificity of 91%.[41] In some instances, antithrombin III activity declined as early as 13 weeks before the development of clinical disease. Given the wide range of normal for this parameter, the investigators recommend an early baseline antithrombin III activity level, which may then be compared with values obtained when hypertension develops. Others have not found this test to be as reliable.[40]

Several investigators have reported that plasma levels of fibronectin are elevated in patients with preeclampsia.[42, 43] Fibronectins are large glycoproteins that are found in both a soluble form in plasma and a larger, nonsoluble form in the extracellular matrix. Both total plasma fibronectin, as well as a variant found predominantly in large vessel endothelial cells, Endothelin-1, are elevated in the blood of women with preeclampsia and in some studies have been shown to predict the disease.[43] It has been suggested that the elevated plasma levels of Enothelin-1 and fibronectin are a result of generalized endothelial cell injury, thus lending support to the concept of altered endothelial cell function as integral in the pathogenesis of preeclampsia (discussed later).[44]

Measurement of urinary calcium excretion has also been suggested as a diagnostic test to distinguish preeclampsia (pure and superimposed) from more benign hypertensive disorders of pregnancy.[45–47] Taufield and colleagues demonstrated that women with preeclampsia had markedly lower urinary calcium excretion than normotensive pregnant women or women with uncomplicated chronic hypertension.[45] Other groups have subsequently confirmed these observations[46–50] and have pointed out that the calcium-to-creatinine ratio in a single voided urine specimen may be as useful as a 24-hour sample.[51] The mechanism of hypocalciuria is unknown, although studies suggest that alterations in calcium regulatory hormones may have a role.[52]

Pathophysiology

Preeclampsia is a multisystem disorder characterized by vasospasm, reduced flow, and ischemia of the kidneys, liver, brain, and placenta. Activity of the coagulation cascade is increased as is platelet aggregation. Much of the investigation into the pathophysiology of preeclampsia in the past has focused on the mechanisms of hypertension, cardiovascular hemodynamics, renal function, and coagulation. However, new developments in the fields of molecular and cell biology have been applied to research concerning the pathophysiology and etiology of preeclampsia.

PLACENTA. The placenta has been considered to be the primary source for the pathophysiology of preeclampsia because delivery is the only definitive cure. Evidence now suggests that placental abnormalities occurring between 10 and 20 weeks' gestation are among the earliest developments leading to the disease,[53, 54] even though maternal signs of preeclampsia may not appear until the late third trimester.

In normal pregnant women, the maternal spiral arteries, the blood vessels that supply the placenta, are transformed from thick-walled muscular arteries into sac-like flaccid vessels. This transformation permits greater volumes of blood delivery at a lower pressure and flow rate and appears to be due to invasion of maternal vessels by trophoblasts, resulting in destruction of the elastic muscular walls and the endothelium of these vessels.[55, 56] In women destined to develop preeclampsia, trophoblastic invasion of maternal vessels is not as extensive, especially in the myometrial segments of the spiral arteries.[53, 54, 57–59] The result is that these vessels remain muscular and responsive to vasoactive stimuli.

A distinct morphologic lesion, acute atherosis, has also been described in the uteroplacental vessels in women with preeclampsia during the latter months of gestation. This lesion is characterized by fibrinoid necrosis of the arterial walls and deposition of fat-laden macrophages.[53, 54, 60]

The net result of these alterations in the uteroplacental vessels is ischemic changes in the placenta and, ultimately, morphologic damage and impairment of functional activity. It is not known what causes the failure of trophoblast invasion of the maternal spiral arteries in women destined to develop preeclampsia. Moreover, it is not clear how this process leads to maternal disease. It has been hypothesized that placental ischemia leads to release of circulating factors, such as lipid peroxides, that cause generalized endothelial cell damage in the maternal vasculature.[61] The observations that vascular prostacyclin production is diminished whereas thromboxane A_2 generation is increased in women with preeclampsia[62–64] are in accord with the notion that endothelial damage and platelet aggregation are involved in the pathogenesis of the disease (Fig. 36–1).

Additional supportive evidence for a role of altered prostaglandins in the pathophysiology of preeclampsia comes from reports of the efficacy of low-dose aspirin in preventing preeclampsia in susceptible individuals.[65–69]

Other products of endothelial cells such as endothelial-derived relaxation factor and endothelin may be involved in the pathogenesis of preeclampsia (see Fig. 36–1). Several reports describe increased plasma levels of the potent vasoconstrictor endothelin in women with preeclampsia,[70–72] although the physiologic relevance of these observations has been questioned because endothelin is thought to be a locally active peptide and the significance of plasma levels is not known. Several laboratories are currently investigating the role of

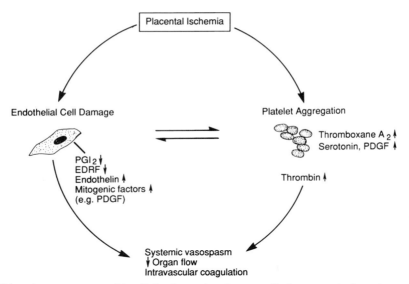

Figure 36-1. In this schema proposed by Roberts and colleagues,[61] decreased uteroplacental blood flow resulting in placental ischemia is hypothesized to lead to maternal disease (systemic vasospasm, decreased organ flow, and intravascular coagulation) by causing the release of toxic substances that mediate generalized endothelial cell damage and platelet aggregation. Damaged endothelial cells may produce less vasodilatory substances (prostacyclin (PGI₂) and endothelium-derived relaxing factor (EDRF)) and release mitogenic factors (platelet-derived growth factor (PDGF)). Platelet aggregation, a consequence of endothelial damage, in turn leads to increased thromboxane A₂. Platelet aggregation and endothelial damage in turn aggravate placental ischemia (see text).

endothelial-derived relaxation factor in the physiology of normal and hypertensive pregnancies,[73, 74] although no available data suggest it has an important role.

It is fairly well established that generalized vasospasm, increased intravascular coagulation, and decreased organ perfusion play a part in the multisystem clinical manifestations characteristic of preeclampsia that are summarized in Figure 36–2. The most dramatic are severe hypertension, renal dysfunction, seizures, intracerebral hemorrhage, pulmonary edema, and hepatic rupture. Short of these life-threatening complications, however, women with preeclampsia demonstrate deviations from almost all of the normal physiologic changes of pregnancy.

BLOOD PRESSURE. The hypertension of preeclampsia is characterized by marked lability, reversal of the normal circadian rhythm,[75] and increased sensitivity to several vasoconstrictors (e.g., norepinephrine, angiotensin II), which may precede clinical manifestations of the disease including frank hypertension.[76] Although in normal pregnancy, plasma renin activity is elevated compared with that in nonpregnant individuals, most investigators observe that renin and aldosterone are suppressed in women with preeclampsia.[77, 78]

CARDIAC FUNCTION. Controversy surrounds the cardiovascular hemodynamics in pre-

eclampsia. Several investigators have reported a wide spectrum of hemodynamic profiles using pulmonary artery (Swan-Ganz) catheters as well as noninvasive techniques.[1, 2, 79, 80] Studies of untreated women with carefully diagnosed preeclampsia have failed to conclusively establish a hemodynamic profile that is unique to preeclampsia. Cardiac outputs have been reported as high, normal, or low, usually with high systemic vascular resistance. This controversy has important therapeutic implications, because some clinicians recommend treating severe preeclampsia with a combination of volume expansion and vasodilator therapy[79] whereas others point out that such an approach may lead to pulmonary edema.[81]

PLASMA VOLUME. Numerous reports during the years have stated that plasma volume, as measured by Evans blue dye dilution, is reduced in women with preeclampsia and that in some cases, reduced plasma volume may precede the development of hypertension.[82] Controversy remains about whether the reduction in intravascular volume is a primary event or secondary to vasoconstriction and hypertension. The studies of central hemodynamic monitoring have not resolved this issue, because both low and normal wedge pressures have been reported in preeclampsia.

RENAL FUNCTION. Patients demonstrate proteinuria and reduced GFR and renal plasma

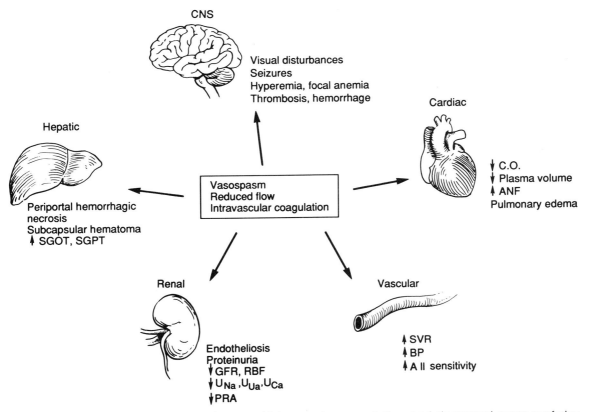

Figure 36-2. Generalized vasospasm, increased intravascular coagulation, and decreased organ perfusion lead to a panoply of clinical manifestations, which are summarized. C.O., Cardiac output; ANF, atrial natriuretic factor; SVR, systemic vascular resistance; BP, blood pressure; A II, angiotensin II; GFR, glomerular filtration rate; RBF, renal blood flow; U_{Na}, urinary sodium; U_{Ua}, urinary uric acid; U_{Ca}, urinary calcium; PRA, plasma renin activity; SGOT, serum glutamic-oxaloacetic transaminase; SGPT, serum glutamate pyruvate transaminase.

flow. Also notable are decreased urate clearance, hypocalciuria, and reduced sodium excretion.[83] These alterations in renal function are most likely due to a combination of structural changes in the kidneys (glomerular endotheliosis) as well as vasospasm and could reflect alterations in circulating hormones that affect renal hemodynamics.

LIVER. Liver dysfunction may occur in preeclampsia, and the clinical spectrum encompasses mild elevations of liver enzymes to liver rupture.[84] The mechanism of liver damage in preeclampsia has not been conclusively established, although the histologic finding of periportal hemorrhages and ischemic lesions as well as fibrin deposition suggests that endothelial cell damage and activation of the coagulation system maybe involved.[84–87] Liver dysfunction may be associated with abdominal pain, which has been postulated to be due to distention of Glisson's capsule.[84] Several researchers have emphasized that evidence of liver dysfunction in preeclampsia signals severe disease and fetal jeopardy. Other ominous features that

may be present along with abnormal liver function are microangiopathic hemolytic anemia and low platelet count, the so-called HELLP syndrome (hemolysis, elevated liver enzymes, and low platelets), which most consider to be an indication for urgent delivery.[88] The syndrome may appear without hypertension or proteinuria, making diagnosis difficult. Any woman with malaise and right upper quadrant pain should be evaluated with liver function tests, hematocrit, and platelet count.

CENTRAL NERVOUS SYSTEM. Eclampsia, the convulsive phase of the disorder and the most dreaded complication of preeclampsia, is the most frequent cause of death in women with this disease. The mechanisms leading to convulsions are not known. Cerebral edema, vasospasm leading to severe ischemia or hemorrhage, and hypertensive encephalopathy all have been postulated.[85, 89] It has been well established that eclampsia may occur with what would ordinarily be considered mild degrees of hypertension; thus, the relative importance of hypertension is not clear.[90] Although computed tomography scans of patients with eclampsia have often been reported as appearing normal, they may occasionally demonstrate edema, hypodense areas, or hemorrhage.[90, 91]

Therapy of Preeclampsia

PREVENTION. Through the years, many different dietary and pharmacologic strategies have been used with the hope of preventing preeclampsia. Until recently, none proved to be successful.

LOW-DOSE ASPIRIN. Encouraging preliminary data from several small clinical trials conducted in the mid-1980s suggested that low-dose aspirin administered to pregnant women may prevent preeclampsia by reversing the imbalance between prostacyclin and thromboxane that may be responsible for many of the manifestations of this disease.[65–69] Several small clinical trials have been completed, as well as some larger studies now published.[92–94] Although a meta-analysis supports the notion that aspirin is beneficial in pregnancy,[69] several questions remain unanswered. For example, which population should be targeted for therapy? Two studies came to different conclusions about the effectiveness of aspirin in preventing preeclampsia in relatively low-risk normotensive nulliparous women.[92, 93] A study of higher-risk patients did not find aspirin to be beneficial, although this was not a placebo-controlled trial.[94] The largest trial reported to date, the CLASP trial, failed to show a benefit of aspirin in low- to moderate-risk patients.[95] A large multicenter trial in high-risk patients is nearing completion. At present, although aspirin does seem to have beneficial effects in preventing preeclampsia and possibly in ameliorating some of the complications of hypertensive pregnancy, no consensus has been reached about which patients should be treated. Some physicians are prescribing aspirin to a few selected patients who appear to be at very high risk for preeclampsia, recurrent fetal death, or severe fetal growth retardation or whose previous pregnancies were complicated by preeclampsia of early onset and poor fetal outcome.

CALCIUM SUPPLEMENTATION. Based on epidemiologic evidence that the incidence of preeclampsia is lower in populations with a high dietary intake of calcium[96] and that calcium supplementation lowers blood pressure in normotensive and nonpregnant women, calcium supplementation during pregnancy has been proposed for the prevention of preeclampsia. A large trial performed in South America demonstrated a beneficial effect of calcium supplementation on hypertension in pregnancy.[97] A multicenter trial is currently under way in the United States to evaluate the efficacy of calcium supplementation in the prevention of preeclampsia.

Principles of Treatment of Preeclampsia

The ultimate goal of treating a patient with preeclampsia is to deliver a mature, healthy infant without compromising maternal health. When the disease manifests near term and fetal maturity is certain, the definitive treatment is delivery. Difficulties arise when preeclampsia develops when the fetus is still quite immature and its survival is in doubt; a decision must be made about whether it is safe for the mother to postpone delivery.

Important considerations in this regard are that preeclampsia is not likely to remit and the disease usually progresses to a severe state. Therefore, if signs of severe disease are already present—that is, persistent hypertension at levels exceeding 110 mm Hg (diastolic), abnormal results of liver function tests, low platelet count, oliguria, and deteriorating renal function—then delivery is virtually mandatory. Conservative management in such cases may not be associated with improved fetal outcome and may in fact result in serious maternal morbidity.[98]

In some situations, however, postponing delivery may be appropriate. A woman may occasionally develop preeclampsia remote from term with mild to moderate hypertension and no signs of deteriorating renal or hepatic function or coagulopathy. In such cases, valuable time may be gained for the fetus by temporizing. In some cases, it may be necessary to administer antihypertensive therapy to maintain maternal blood pressure in a safe range (e.g., < 110 mm Hg diastolic; discussed later). Such women should be treated in the hospital, where it is easier to monitor progression of the disease and intercede rapidly when complications arise. Also, such circumstances allow frequent antepartum testing, including nonstress testing, sonography, and biophysical profile, tests that help predict fetal jeopardy. The decision to continue the pregnancy can be made on a day-to-day basis. Indeed, one report of a conservative approach to women with preeclampsia presenting between 24 and 27 weeks suggested that such an approach resulted in improved perinatal survival.[99] It must be emphasized, however, that conservative treatment of early preeclampsia is appropriate only when aggressive monitoring of maternal and fetal status is possible.

ANTIHYPERTENSIVE THERAPY. The role of antihypertensive therapy in the management of preeclampsia is controversial. The basis for this

TABLE 36–1. Antihypertensive Drugs in Pregnancy

CLASS/DRUG	DOSE/ROUTE	ADVERSE EFFECTS	COMMENTS
Central adrenergic inhibitors (methyldopa)	Oral; 300–3000 mg in 2–4 divided doses	Fatigue, dry mouth	Well-documented safety for mother and fetus. Considered by many to be the drug of choice in pregnancy, especially for chronic hypertension
β-Blockers	Oral; dose dependent on agent	Fetal bradycardia, impaired fetal response to hypoxia, possibly intrauterine growth retardation	Growth retardation reported when used early in pregnancy
α-β–Blocker (labetalol)	Oral; up to 1200 mg in 2 divided doses IV; 20 mg IV then 20–80 mg every 20–30 min; up to 300 mg	Similar to β-blockers, hepatotoxicity has been reported in adults	May have advantages in pregnancy with respect to preservation of uteroplacental blood flow. IV has been used successfully in peripartum period.
Hydralazine	Oral 50–300 mg in 2–4 divided doses; 5 mg IV/IM, then 5–10 mg every 20–40 min, or constant infusion of 0.5–10 mg/hr	Headache, flushing, tachycardia	Drug of choice for parenteral therapy, broad experience of safety; however, IV may be unavailable in near future. Oral therapy ineffective when used alone
Calcium channel blockers	Oral, dependent on agent	Headache, flushing, constipation	Limited data in pregnancy. May inhibit labor
Diuretics	Dependent on agent used	May cause volume depletion, electrolyte imbalance, pancreatitis	Can be continued in salt-sensitive essential hypertension, renal or heart disease. Not recommended in preeclampsia
Nitroprusside	Relatively contraindicated because of fetal cyanide toxicity		
Angiotensin-converting enzyme inhibitors	Contraindicated because of neonatal renal problems after 2nd- and 3rd-trimester exposure		

IV, Intravenously; IM, intramuscularly.
Adapted from Barron WM. Hypertension. In: Barron WM Lindheimer MD: Medical Disorders During Pregnancy. St Louis: Mosby-Year Book, 1991, pp 1–41.

controversy is that it is still uncertain whether or not the uteroplacental circulation is autoregulated, and thus the impact of lowering maternal blood pressure on placental perfusion is of great concern, especially because diminished uteroplacental blood flow usually is already present in preeclampsia. Lowering maternal blood pressure does not cure or reverse preeclampsia, and it may not benefit the fetus; thus, reduction of pressure should be reserved for reasons of maternal safety.

There is disagreement about what level of blood pressure should be treated. In the peripartum period, many authorities would begin therapy when diastolic pressure is 105 mm Hg or greater. Excessive reduction of blood pressure should be avoided because it may compromise placental function or lead to placental abruption. If temporization is planned, treatment is started when diastolic levels approach 100 mm Hg (or 95 mm Hg before gestational week 30). When diastolic blood pressures are consistently greater than 105 mm Hg, the advisability of continuing the pregnancy for longer than 24 to 48 hours is questionable. In such cases,

parenteral agents are most frequently used, because delivery is imminent, unless blood pressure is rapidly controlled and temporization is important for fetal survival.

The drug most commonly used in management of hypertension in the peripartum period is intravenous hydralazine, a drug most obstetric staff know well and one with a long history of safe and effective use in women with preeclampsia (Table 36–1).[100] In addition to the well-known side effects of tachycardia, headache, tremulousness, nausea, and vomiting, some reports suggest that hydralazine administered in the setting of severe volume contraction may cause rapid and excessive decrements in blood pressure and may provoke oliguria as well as fetal distress.[101, 102] Therefore, treatment should commence with 5-mg doses, followed by 5- to 10-mg increments every 20 to 30 minutes. Parenteral labetalol has been administered to women with preeclampsia with favorable results.[103–106] This drug is a combined α$_1$- and β-blocker, and studies suggest that uteroplacental blood flow is maintained after parenteral use.[106, 107]

Several features of calcium channel blockers make them attractive agents for controlling hypertension in women with preeclampsia. These drugs have a rapid onset of action, rarely cause hypotension, and are relatively free of serious side effects. Unfortunately, only a few, uncontrolled studies have investigated the use of calcium channel blockers in pregnancy.[108–110] Although the results seem to show that these agents are effective in controlling blood pressure, the information about fetal effects is limited. A few anecdotal reports suggest that the interaction of magnesium sulfate and calcium channel blockade has led to precipitous reductions in blood pressure.[111] Therefore, it is advisable to await the results of additional trials in progress before using these agents on a routine basis.

Finally, an occasional patient with severe hypertension resistant to the antihypertensive agents previously discussed may require diazoxide or sodium nitroprusside. The latter drug has been associated with cyanide poisoning of sheep fetuses (albeit with large doses); however, when necessary, the mother's health should be considered first.

Prevention and Treatment of Convulsions

There is disagreement about the treatment and prophylaxis of eclamptic convulsions, especially among obstetricians and neurologists. In the United States, parenteral magnesium sulfate is routinely administered in the peripartum period to prevent convulsions,[100, 112] although some argue that it may not cross the blood-brain barrier and that it is not an established anticonvulsant.[113, 114] Use of magnesium sulfate is based on several large series, unfortunately all of them uncontrolled.[112] It must also be emphasized that magnesium sulfate is not an antihypertensive agent; however, it is of interest that in in vitro studies of cultured endothelial cells from human umbilical veins, magnesium has been reported to stimulate prostacyclin synthesis.[115]

Phenytoin,[116] phenobarbital, and diazepam[117] are most commonly used outside of the United States as alternatives to magnesium sulfate. Few controlled trials have investigated these agents in the prophylaxis of eclamptic seizures, and a consensus group at the National Institutes of Health found little reason to abandon magnesium therapy at this time.

HEMODYNAMIC MONITORING. In occasional severe or complicated cases, invasive hemodynamic monitoring may be useful, particularly when oliguria or respiratory difficulties arise. Criteria have been proposed for pulmonary catheterization in patients with severe preeclampsia.[118] However, many experts believe that these criteria are too broad and find the situations in which Swan-Ganz catheterization is necessary to be relatively uncommon.

POSTPARTUM ISSUES. Although delivery is the cure for preeclampsia, it is important to recognize that the disease may first become clinically apparent in the postpartum period, particularly the first week. Moreover, several of the clinical and laboratory abnormalities may worsen postpartum before they improve. This has been well documented in women with the syndrome of hemolysis, elevated liver enzymes, and low platelets (HELLP syndrome),[119] in whom thrombocytopenia usually is most severe 48 hours postpartum. Hypertension also persists into the postpartum period and may become more severe before it disappears, although little documentation of this phenomenon is found in the literature. This is particularly important in women who wish to breast-feed, because antihypertensive agents are likely to get into breast milk. It is also well known that eclamptic seizures may develop in the postpartum period as well, particularly in the first 48 hours.

RECURRENCE OF PREECLAMPSIA AND PROGNOSIS. Elegant studies by Chesley and colleagues have demonstrated that the development of preeclampsia or eclampsia is not predictive of the later development of essential hypertension.[120] The extent to which this is true seems to depend on the certainty of the diagnosis of preeclampsia (e.g., multiparous women, who are more likely to have chronic hypertension, are more likely to develop hypertension later in life).[19]

With respect to future pregnancies, the long-held view that preeclampsia is a disease of first pregnancy is, for the most part, true. However, certain points are worth making in this regard. In contrast to women who have had a previous normotensive pregnancy, nulliparous women with preeclampsia *are* at increased risk for having preeclampsia in subsequent pregnancies.[121] It appears that the risk of having preeclampsia in subsequent pregnancies is related to the time of onset of preeclampsia during the first pregnancy, with the highest risk being in those who had preeclampsia remote from term, particularly if preeclampsia developed in the second trimester.[122]

CHRONIC HYPERTENSION DURING PREGNANCY

As many as 50 million Americans have elevated blood pressure (>140/90).[123] The prevalence of chronic hypertension in pregnancy is not known and differs widely in different geographic areas but is probably between 3 and 10% of all pregnancies. Because preeclampsia is usually a disease of first pregnancy, many or most multiparous women with elevated blood pressure during pregnancy will have chronic hypertension.

Clinical Evaluation of Hypertensive Patients before Conception

Hypertensive women contemplating pregnancy should receive thorough evaluation before pregnancy. It is advisable to carefully rule out secondary hypertension, because patients with renal disease, pheochromocytoma, renovascular hypertension, or collagen disease frequently have a higher incidence of complications during pregnancy. Secondary hypertension (adrenal adenomas, renovascular hypertension) should be treated before pregnancy. Patients with intrinsic renal disease should be advised about the risks of pregnancy if they have azotemia (creatinine level >2 mg/dl) and hypertension.[124, 125] These risks include a high incidence of superimposed preeclampsia, a high incidence of perinatal morbidity and mortality, and the possibility that maternal renal function may deteriorate further as a result of the pregnancy.[126] These concerns are especially applicable to women with renal transplants, in whom pregnancy should be undertaken only after consultation with a nephrologist with expertise in this area. Although pheochromocytoma is rare, it is associated with a very high incidence of maternal and fetal mortality,[126] and it is important to make this diagnosis in a pregnant woman or a woman planning to become pregnant.

Hypertensive women considering pregnancy can be advised of the high likelihood of a favorable outcome in most cases of mild to moderate essential hypertension. They should be aware of the increased risk of superimposed preeclampsia. It is often helpful for women to be informed before pregnancy of possible adjustments in lifestyle that may be necessary during pregnancy if blood pressure is elevated—specifically, the possibility that restricted activity, bed rest, or even hospitalization may be advisable.

Certain antihypertensive agents are either contraindicated in pregnancy (e.g., angiotensin-converting enzyme inhibitors) or have not been used extensively (e.g., calcium channel blockers). Thus, it is advisable to prescribe medications that are believed safe for pregnancy even before conception (discussed later).

Rationale for Treatment

The majority of women with chronic hypertension in pregnancy have mild to moderate elevations in blood pressure, and therefore the risk of acute cardiovascular complications is extremely low. In the small percentage of women who have severe hypertension, the increased risk of cerebral hemorrhage, heart failure, and myocardial infarction necessitates close monitoring and aggressive treatment of these women during pregnancy.

Although perinatal morbidity and mortality are increased in women with chronic hypertension,[127, 128] most pregnancies in these women result in healthy term infants. Women with chronic hypertension are at increased risk of developing superimposed preeclampsia, and evidence suggests that most if not all of the increased perinatal morbidity and mortality associated with chronic hypertension is attributable to this complication.[129] The literature is conflicting, however, and some studies have shown that babies born to women who have chronic hypertension in pregnancy and who do not develop superimposed preeclampsia do as well as those born to normotensive women. Other studies report a higher perinatal loss in uncomplicated hypertensive pregnancy (compared with normotensive), especially with higher levels of blood pressure.

The objective in treating pregnant women with chronic hypertension is to minimize the short-term risk of elevated blood pressure to the mother while avoiding therapeutic maneuvers that compromise fetal well-being. The specific goals for the mother are to prevent cardiovascular complications of severe hypertension and, if possible, to prevent preeclampsia. When maternal hypertension is severe (diastolic blood pressure >110 mm Hg), treatment should be instituted to avoid hypertensive vascular damage.

The indications for treatment of mild to moderate hypertension during pregnancy are less clear. In nonpregnant individuals, treatment of mild to moderate hypertension is recommended for prevention of long-term cardiovascular consequences of elevated blood pressure.[123] For the duration of a pregnancy, these concerns are not relevant, whereas the prevention of preeclampsia and maintenance of fetal well-being are. At present, the available data do not support treatment of mild to moderate hypertension as a means of preventing preeclampsia.[130]

With regard to fetal well-being, several studies suggest but do not conclusively demonstrate benefits of treating mild to moderate hypertension during pregnancy.[131] Given the potential hazards of antihypertensive treatment during pregnancy (the possibility that medications may reduce placental blood flow and the possible adverse effects of drugs on a fetus), treatment of mild to moderate hypertension must be undertaken cautiously, weighing the risks and benefits of treatment for both the mother and fetus at all times. Excessive blood pressure reduction is to be avoided, and a conservative approach is recommended. If diastolic blood pressure in the first trimester is between 90 and 100 mm Hg, then it is reasonable to await the expected physiologic decrease in blood pressure in the second trimester before using antihypertensives. If diastolic blood pressure is less than 90 mm Hg in a patient already taking medication early in pregnancy, then a reduction in medication can be contemplated. Most authorities would begin treatment when diastolic blood pressures are consistently 100 mm Hg or greater.

Treatment of Chronic Hypertension: Nonpharmacologic Therapy

Close medical supervision is the mainstay of treatment of pregnant women with chronic hypertension. It is advisable to try to control the blood pressure without medication when possible, and in patients with mild hypertension this goal is not difficult to attain because blood pressure falls in most pregnant women during the first and second trimesters. Indeed, in women with preexisting hypertension, the decrement in blood pressure during pregnancy may be as great as 20 mm Hg.

The strategies for nonpharmacologic therapy of hypertension during pregnancy differ from those in nonpregnant individuals. Although weight reduction and exercise might benefit a nonpregnant individual, these measures are not advised during pregnancy.

RESTRICTION OF ACTIVITY. Bed rest is the only means available for maximizing uteroplacental blood flow during pregnancy and is considered established therapy in preeclampsia. In chronic hypertension, its effectiveness has not been well studied; however, it is an integral feature of management. Rest has been shown to reduce premature labor, lower blood pressure, and promote diuresis.[132, 133] Strict bed rest is rarely necessary. However, all pregnant women with elevated blood pressure, whatever the cause, should be advised to limit their activities when possible and to set aside time during the day when they can be off their feet. Although many women find it difficult to restrict their activity, it is helpful to explain the benefits to patients before pregnancy so that they can make adjustments in child care, job, and other responsibilities. In patients with mild to moderate

hypertension, restriction of activity may be effective in lowering blood pressure and antihypertensive medications may be avoided. In patients with severe hypertension, it is usually advisable to hospitalize them for bed rest and medications when necessary.

DIET. Weight reduction cannot be recommended during pregnancy. If a hypertensive woman is overweight and planning a pregnancy, then weight reduction before pregnancy is advisable.

Hypertensive pregnant women have lower plasma volume than normotensives, and some studies suggest that the severity of hypertension correlates with the degree of plasma volume contraction.[134] For this reason, sodium restriction is generally not recommended during pregnancy.[135] If, however, a pregnant women with chronic hypertension is known to have salt-sensitive hypertension and she has been successfully treated with a low-salt diet before pregnancy, then it is reasonable to continue this during pregnancy. Patients with renal disease and reduced creatinine clearance are more likely to require sodium restriction for blood pressure control, and this should be continued during pregnancy.

Preliminary studies have shown that dietary calcium supplements may lower blood pressure in pregnant and nonpregnant women; however, insufficient data are available to recommend calcium supplements for this indication.

HOME BLOOD PRESSURE MONITORING. The rationale for close observation of pregnant hypertensive women is that changes in clinical status (such as development of superimposed preeclampsia) can be recognized before they become severe. This is easier to accomplish if patients are instructed to measure their blood pressure at home and keep a record of the readings. They can then contact medical personnel if the blood pressure rises significantly, before a scheduled visit. Home monitoring of blood pressure is often helpful because it enables patients to determine how much limitation of activity is necessary to keep their blood pressure controlled. Preliminary data on home blood pressure monitoring during pregnancy suggest that it is a useful adjunct to the care of hypertensive women.[136]

Pharmacologic Therapy

When choosing antihypertensive therapy, it is important to consider both antihypertensive efficacy and short-term effects on the fetus. Methyldopa has been most extensively evaluated in pregnancy and is therefore recommended.[16, 137] β-

Blockers compare favorably with methyldopa with respect to efficacy and are considered safe in the latter part of pregnancy.[137–140] Of note is a report suggesting that use of β-blockers early in pregnancy may be associated with growth retardation of the fetus.[140] Labetalol has also been used successfully in pregnancy, although reports of rare hepatotoxicity in nonpregnant individuals are a cause for concern.[141]

Calcium channel blockers have not been studied sufficiently to recommend their use in pregnancy. Nevertheless, several anecdotal reports have documented that they are effective antihypertensive agents in pregnant women.[108–110] Adverse fetal effects have not been reported; however, the safety of calcium channel blockers has not been satisfactorily established.

Angiotensin-converting enzyme inhibitors have not been used extensively in pregnancy. However, serious neonatal problems including renal failure and death have been reported in pregnant women taking these agents[142]; therefore, they should be avoided. It is preferable to discontinue angiotensin-converting enzyme inhibitors on learning of conception, and it advisable to prescribe other agents in women trying to conceive.

The use of diuretics in pregnancy is controversial. The primary theoretic concern is that these agents may prevent the physiologic volume expansion of normal pregnancy. Extensive experience with prophylactic diuretics in nonhypertensive pregnant populations does not show clear-cut evidence of adverse effects. Therefore, pregnant women with chronic hypertension may be treated with diuretics if they were taking these agents before pregnancy or if they have a history of salt-sensitive hypertension.

SUMMARY

It is important to distinguish between hypertension brought on by pregnancy (preeclampsia) and elevated blood pressure present before conception, because the former condition may be life threatening to both mother and child whereas the latter is frequently benign. Lowering blood pressure in women with preeclampsia does not improve fetal outcome, nor does it cure the disease, but it should be attempted when maternal health is at risk. In women with chronic hypertension, severe hypertension should always be treated. There is no evidence that treatment of mild to moderate hypertension prevents superimposed preeclampsia. No consensus has yet been reached about whether lowering mild to moderate hypertension improves fetal outcome. Treatment of chronic hypertension generally begins with restricted activity when diastolic blood pressures reach 90 to 100 mm Hg. Antihypertensives become necessary when diastolic pressures exceed 100 mm Hg.

REFERENCES

1. Wallenburg Henk CS. Hemodynamics in hypertensive pregnancy. In: Rubin PC (ed): Handbook of Hypertension, Hypertension in Pregnancy. New York: Elsevier Science, 1988, pp 66–101.
2. Lang RM, Pridjian G, Feldman T, et al. Alterations in left ventricular mechanics in pregnancy induced hypertension (preeclampsia); increased afterload or cardiomyopathy. Am Heart J 1991;121:1768.
3. Terragno NA, McGiff JC, Murray S, Terragno A. Patterns of prostaglandin production in the bovine fetal and maternal vasculature. Prostaglandins 1978;16:847.
4. Tamai T, Matsuura S, Tatsumi N, et al. Role of sex steroid hormones in relative refractoriness to angiotensin II during pregnancy. Am J Obstet Gynecol 1984;149:117.
5. Davison JM, Dunlop M. Renal hemodynamics and tubular function in normal human pregnancy. Kidney Int 1980;18:152.
6. Davison JM, Noble MCB. Serial changes in 24 hour creatinine clearance during normal menstrual cycles and the first trimester of pregnancy. Br J Obstet Gynecol 1980;88:10.
7. Baylis C. Effects of early pregnancy on glomerular filtration rate and plasma volume in the rat. Renal Physiol 1980;2:333.
8. Pritchard JA, MacDonald PC, Gant NF (eds). Williams Obstetrics. 17th ed. East Norwalk, CT: Appleton-Century-Crofts, 1985.
9. Wilson M, Morganti AA, Zervoudakis I, et al. Blood pressure, the renin-aldosterone system and sex steroids throughout normal pregnancy. Am J Med 1980;68:97.
10. August P, Sealey JE. The renin-angiotensin system in normal and hypertensive pregnancy and in ovarian function. In: Laragh JH, Brenner BM (eds). Hypertension: Pathophysiology, Diagnosis and Management. New York: Raven Press, 1990, pp 1761–1778.
11. Abdul-Karim R, Assali NS. Pressor response to angiotensin in pregnant and nonpregnant women. Am J Obstet Gynecol 1961;82:246.
12. Baker PN, Pipkin FB, Symonds EM. Longitudinal study of platelet angiotensin II binding in human pregnancy. Clin Sci 1992;82:377.
13. Hughes EC (ed): Obstetric-Gynecologic Terminology. Philadelphia: FA Davis, 1972, pp 422–423.
14. Davey DA, MacGillivray I. The classification and definition of the hypertensive disorders of pregnancy. Am J Obstet Gynecol 1988;158:892.
15. World Health Organization. The hypertensive disorders of pregnancy. WHO Tech Rep Ser 1987;758:8.
16. National High Blood Pressure Education Program Working Group. Report on high blood pressure in pregnancy. Am J Obstet Gynecol 1990;163:1689.
17. Chesley LC. Hypertensive Disorders in Pregnancy. New York: Appleton-Century-Crofts, 1978.
18. Mc Cartney CP: Pathological anatomy of acute hypertension in pregnancy. Circulation 1964;30(suppl 2):37.
19. Fisher KA, Luger A, Spargo BH, et al. Hypertension in pregnancy: Clinical-pathological correlations and remote prognosis. Medicine 1981;60:267.

20. Katz AJ, Davison JM, Hayslett JP, et al. Pregnancy in women with kidney disease. Kidney Int 1980;18:192.

21. Dunlop JCH. Chronic hypertension and perinatal mortality. Proc R Soc Med 1966;59:838.

22. Taylor DJ. Epidemiology of hypertension during pregnancy. In Rubin: PC (ed): Handbook of Hypertension: Hypertension in Pregnancy. New York: Elsevier Science, 1988, pp 223–240.

23. Campbell DM, MacGillivray I, Carr-Hill R. Preeclampsia in second pregnancy. Br J Obstet Gynecol 1985;92:131.

24. Beer AE: Possible Immunologic bases of preeclampsia/eclampsia. Semin Perinatol 1978;2:39.

25. Chesley LC, Cooper DW. Genetics of hypertension in pregnancy: Possible single gene control of pre-eclampsia and eclampsia in the descendants of eclamptic women. Br J Obstet Gynaecol 1986;93(9):898.

26. Cooper DW, Brennecke SP, Wilton AN. Genetics of pre-eclampsia. Hypertens Pregnancy 1993;12(1):1.

27. White P. Pregnancy complicating diabetes. Surg Gynecol Obstet 1935;61:324.

28. Page WE. The relation between hydatid moles, relative ischemia of the gravid uterus, and the placental origin of eclampsia. Am J Obstet Gynecol 1939;37:291.

29. Butler NR, Alberman ED. Perinatal Problems. Second Report of the British Perinatal Mortality Survey. Edinburgh: ES Livingstone, 1958, p 108.

30. Shapiro S, Schlesinger ER, Nesbitt RE Jr. Infant, Perinatal, Maternal and Childhood Mortality in the United States. Cambridge, MA: Harvard University Press, 1968.

31. Sawyer MM, Lipshitz J, Anderson GD, et al: Diurnal and short-term variation of blood pressure: Comparison of pre-eclamptic, chronic hypertension and normotensive patients. Obstet Gynecol 1981;58:291.

32. Perry IJ, Wilkinson LS, Shinton RA, Beevers DG. Conflicting views on the measurement of blood pressure during pregnancy. Br J Obstet Gynecol 1991;98:241.

33. Johenning AR, Barron WM. Indirect blood pressure measurement in pregnancy. Korotkoff phase 4 versus phase 5. Am J Obstet Gynecol 1992;167:577.

34. Sarles HF, Herring ME, Watson TF, et al. The nephrotic syndrome due to preeclamptic nephropathy. Ann Intern Med 1964;61:300.

35. Kuo VS, Koumantiakis G, Mappl SC, Gallery EDM. Proteinuria and its assessment in normal and hypertensive pregnancy. Am J Obstet Gynecol 1992;167:723.

36. Dekker GA, Sibai BM. Early detection of preeclampsia. Am J Obstet Gynecol 1991;165:160.

37. Redman CWG, Beilin LJ, Denson KWE, et al. Factor VIII consumption in preeclampsia. Lancet 1977;2:1249.

38. Whigham KAE, Howie DW, Shah MM, Prentics CRM. Factor VIII related antigen/coagulant activity ratio as a predictor of fetal growth retardation: A comparison with hormones and uric acid measurements. Br J Obstet Gynecol 1980;87:797.

39. Weiner CP, Brandt J. Plasma antithrombin III: An aid in the diagnosis of preeclampsia-eclampsia. Am J Obstet Gynecol 1982;142:275.

40. Weenink GH, Borm JJ, ten Cate JW, et al. Antithrombin III levels in normotensive and hypertensive pregnancy. Gynecol Obstet Invest 1983;16:230.

41. Weiner CP, Kwaan HC, Xu C, et al. Antithrombin III activity in women with hypertension during pregnancy. Obstet Gynecol 1985;65:301.

42. Lazarchick J, Stubbs TM, Romein L, et al. Predictive value of fibronectin levels in normotensive gravid women destined to become preeclamptic. Am J Obstet Gynecol 1986;154:1020.

43. Lockwood CJ, Peters JH. Increased levels of ED1+ cellular fibronectin precede the clinical signs of preeclampsia. Am J Obstet Gynecol 1990;162:358.

44. Rodgers GM, Taylor RN, Roberts JM. Preeclampsia is associated with a serum factor cytotoxic to human endothelial cells. Am J Obstet Gynecol 1988;159:908.

45. Taufield PA, Ales K, Resnick L, et al. Hypocalciuria in preeclampsia. N Engl J Med 1987;316:715.

46. O'Hara N, Yamasaki M, Morikawa H, et al: Dynamics of calcium metabolism and calcium regulatory hormones in pregnancy-induced hypertension. Nippon Naibunpi Gakkai Zasshi 1986;62:882.

47. Rodriguez MH, Masaki DI, Mestman J, et al. Calcium/creatinine ratio and microalbuminuria in the prediction of preeclampsia. Am J Obstet Gynecol 1988;159:1452.

48. Hutchesson ACJ, Macintosh MC, Duncan SLB, Forrest ARW. Hypocalciuria and hypertension in pregnancy: A prospective study. Clin Exp Hypertens Pregnancy B9 1990;(2):15.

49. Sanchez-Ramos L, Sandroni S, Andres FJ, Kaunitz AM. Calcium excretion in preeclampsia. Obstet Gynecol 1991;77:510.

50. Sanchez-Ramos L, Jones DC, Cullen MT. Urinary calcium as an early marker for preeclampsia. Obstet Gynecol 1991;77:685.

51. Rodriguez MH, Masaki DI, Mestman J, et al. Calcium/creatinine ratio and microalbuminuria in the prediction of preeclampsia. Am J Obstet Gynecol 1988;159:1452.

52. August P, Maracaccio B, Gertner JM, et al. Abnormal 1,25 dihydroxyvitamin D (1,25 (OH_2D_3)) metabolism in preeclampsia. Am J Obstet Gynecol 1992;4:1295.

53. Fox H. The placenta in pregnancy hypertension. In: Rubin PC (ed). Handbook of Hypertension. Vol 10. Hypertension in Pregnancy. New York: Elsevier Science, 1988, pp 16–37.

54. Zuspan FP, O'Shaughnessy R. The uteroplacental bed: Its anatomic and neuroendocrine alterations. In: Laragh JH, Brenner BM, Kaplan NM (eds). Endocrine Mechanisms in Hypertension. New York: Raven Press, 1989.

55. Pijnenborg R, Bland JM, Robertson WB, et al. The pattern of interstitial trophoblastic invasion of the myometrium in early pregnancy. Placenta 1981;2:303.

56. Ramsey EM, Houston ML, Harris JW. Interactions of the trophoblast and maternal tissues in three closely related primate species. Am J Obstet Gynecol 1976;124:647.

57. Khong TY, De Wolf F, Robertson WB, et al. Inadequate maternal vascular response to placentation in pregnancies complicated by pre-eclampsia and by small-for-gestational age infants. Br J Obstet Gynaecol 1986;93:1049.

58. Robertson WB, Brosens I, Dixon HG. The pathological response of the vessels of the placental bed to hypertensive pregnancy. J Pathol Bacteriol 1967;93:581.

59. Gerretsen G, Huisjes HJ, Elema JD. Morphological changes of the spiral arteries in the placental bed in relation to pre-eclampsia and fetal growth retardation. Br J Obstet Gynaecol 1981;88:876.

60. Zeek PM, Assali NS. Vascular changes in the decidua associated with eclamptogenic toxemia of pregnancy. Am J Clin Pathol 1950;20:1099.

61. Roberts JM, Taylor RN, Musci TJ, et al. Preeclampsia: An endothelial cell disorder. Am J Obstet Gynecol 1989;161:1200.

62. Friedman SA. Preeclampsia: A review of the role of prostaglandins. Obstet Gynecol 1988;71(1):122.

63. Fitzgerald DJ, FiztGerald GA. Eicosanoids in the pathogenesis of preeclampsia. In: Laragh JH, Brenner BM (eds). Hypertension: Pathophysiology, Diagnosis, and Management. New York: Raven Press, 1990, pp 1789–1807.

64. Ylikorkala O, Makila VM. Prostacyclin and thromboxane in gynecology and obstetrics. Am J Obstet Gynecol 1985;152:318.

65. Beaufils M, Densimons R, Uzan S, et al. Prevention of preeclampsia by early antiplatelet therapy. Lancet 1985.840.

66. Wallenburg HCS, Dekker GA, Makovitz JW, et al. Low-dose aspirin prevents pregnancy-induced hypertension and pre-eclampsia in angiotensin-sensitive primigravidae. Lancet 1985;i:1.

67. Schiff E, Peleg E, Goldenberg M, et al. The use of aspirin to prevent pregnancy-induced hypertension and lower the ratio of thromboxane A2 to prostacyclin in relatively high risk pregnancies. N Engl J Med 1989;321:351.

68. Benigni A, Gregorini G, Frusca T, et al. Effect of low-dose aspirin on fetal and maternal generation of thromboxane by platelets in women at risk for pregnancy-induced hypertension. N Engl J Med 1989;321:357.

69. Collins R: Antiplatelet agents for IUGR and preeclampsia. In: Chalmers I (ed). Oxford Data Base for Perinatal Trials. Version 1.2. Disk issue 6, Autumn 1991, Record 4,000 (an electronic publication).

70. Nova A, Sibai BM, Barton JR, et al. Maternal plasma level of endothelin is increased in preeclampsia. Am J Obstet Gynecol 1991;165:724.

71. Schiff E, Gen-Baruch G, Peleg E, et al. Immunoreactive circulating endothelin-1 in normal and hypertensive pregnancies. Am J Obstet Gynecol 1992;166:625.

72. Clark BA, Halvorson L, Sachs B, Epstein FH. Plasma endothelin levels in preeclampsia: Elevation and correlation with uric acid levels and renal impairment. Am J Obstet Gynecol 1992;1566:962.

73. Molnar M, Hertelendy F. NW-Nitro-L-arginine, an inhibitor of nitric oxide synthesis, increases blood pressure in rats and reverses the pregnancy induced refractoriness to vasopressor agents. Am J Obstet Gynecol 1992;166:1560.

74. Baylis C, Engels K. Adverse interactions between pregnancy and a new model of systemic hypertension produced by chronic blockade of endothelial derived relaxing factor (EDRF) in the rat. Clin Exp Hypertens Pregnancy B11 1992;(2&3):117.

75. Ruff SC, Mitchell RH, Murnaghan GA. Long-term variations of blood pressure rhythms in normotensive pregnancy and pre-eclampsia. In: Sammour MB, Symonds EM, Zuspan FP, El-Tomi N (eds). Pregnancy Hypertension. Cairo: Ain Shams University Press, 1982, p 129.

76. Gant NF, Daley GL, Chand S, et al: A study of angiotensin II pressor response throughout primigravid pregnancy. J Clin Invest 1973;52:2682.

77. August P, Lenz T, Ales KL, et al. Longitudinal study of the renin-angiotensin-aldosterone system in hypertensive pregnant women: Deviations related to the development of superimposed preeclampsia. Am J Obstet Gynecol 1990;163:1612.

78. Broughton Pipkin F: The renin-angiotensin system in normal and hypertensive pregnancies. In: Rubin PC (ed). Handbook of Hypertension, Hypertension in Pregnancy. New York: Elsevier Science, 1988, pp 118–151.

79. Cotton DB, Lee W, Huhta JC, et al. Hemodynamic profile of severe pregnancy induced hypertension. Am J Obstet Gynecol 1988;158:523.

80. Easterling TR, Benedetti TJ. Preeclampsia. A hyperdynamic disease model. Am J Obstet Gynecol 1989;160:1447.

81. Mabie WC, Ratts TE, Sibai BM. The central hemodynamics of severe preeclampsia. Am J Obstet Gynecol 1989;161:1443.

82. Chesley LC, Lindheimer MD. Renal hemodynamics and intravascular volume in normal and hypertensive pregnancy. In: Rubin PC (ed). Handbook of Hypertension. Vol 10. Hypertension in Pregnancy. New York: Elsevier Science, 1988, pp 38–65.

83. Lindheimer MD, Katz AI. The kidney in pregnancy. In: Brenner BM, Rector FC Jr (eds). The Kidney. 3rd ed. Philadelphia: WB Saunders, 1986, pp 1253–1295.

84. Romero R, Vizoso J, Emamian M, et al. Clinical significance of liver dysfunction in pregnancy-induced hypertension. Am J Perinatol 1988;5:146.

85. Sheehan HL, Lynch JB. Pathophysiology of Toxaemia of Pregnancy. London, Churchill, 1973.

86. Rolfes DB, Ishak KG. Liver disease in toxemia of pregnancy. Am J Gastroenterol 1989;81:1138.

87. Manas KJ, Welsh JD, Rankin RA, et al. Hepatic hemorrhage without rupture in preeclampsia. N Engl J Med 1985;312:424.

88. Weinstein L. Syndrome of hemolysis, elevated liver enzymes and low platelet count; a severe consequence of hypertension in pregnancy. Am J Obstet Gynecol 1982;142:159.

89. Donaldson JO. Neurology of Pregnancy. 2nd ed. Philadelphia: WB Saunders, 1989.

90. Sibai BM. Eclampsia. In: Rubin PC (ed). Handbook of Hypertension. Vol 10. Hypertension in Pregnancy. New York: Elsevier Science, 1988, pp 320–340.

91. Brown CEL, Purdy P, Cunningham FG. Head computed tomographic scans in women with eclampsia. Am J Obstet Gynecol 1988;159:915.

92. Hauth JC, Goldenberg RL, Parker CR, et al. Low-dose aspirin therapy to prevent preeclampsia. Am J Obstet Gynecol 1993;168:1083.

93. Sibai B, Caritis S, Phillips E, et al. Prevention of preeclampsia: Low-dose aspirin in nulliparous women: A double-blind, placebo-controlled trial. Am J Obstet Gynecol 1993;168(2):286.

94. Italian Study of Aspirin in Pregnancy. Low-dose aspirin in prevention and treatment of intrauterine growth retardation and pregnancy-induced hypertension. Lancet 1993;341:396.

95. CLASP Collaborative Group. CLASP: A randomized trial of low-dose aspirin for the prevention and treatment of preeclampsia among 9364 pregnant women. Lancet 1994;343:619.

96. Belizan JM, Villar J, Repke J. The relationship between calcium intake and pregnancy-induced hypertension: Up-to-date evidence. Am J Obstet Gynecol 1988;158:898.

97. Belizan J, Villar J, Gonzalez L, et al. Calcium supplementation to prevent hypertensive disorders of pregnancy. N Engl J Med 1991;325(20):1399.

98. Sibai BM, Taslimi M, Abdella TN, et al. Maternal and perinatal outcome of conservative management of severe preeclampsia in midtrimester. Am J Obstet Gynecol 1985;152(Suppl 1):32.

99. Sibai BM, Akl S, Fairlie F, Morett M. A protocol for managing severe preeclampsia in the second trimester. Am J Obstet Gynecol 1990;163:733.

100. Pritchard JA, Cunningham FG, Pritchard FA. The Parkland Memorial Hospital protocol for treatment of eclampsia: Evaluation of 245 cases. Am J Obstet Gynecol 1984;148(7):951.

101. Belfort M, Uys P, Dommisse J, et al. Hemodynamic changes in gestational proteinuric hypertension: The effects of rapid volume expansion and vasodilator therapy. Br J Obstet Gynaecol 1989;96:634.

102. Vink GJ, Moodley JH, Philpott RH. Effect of dihydralazine on the fetus in the treatment of maternal hypertension. Obstet Gynecol 1980;55:519.

103. Walker JJ, Greer I, Calder AA. Treatment of acute pregnancy-related hypertension: Labetalol and hydralazine compared. Postgrad Med J 1983;59(Suppl 3):168.

104. Davey DA, Dommisse J, Garden A. Intravenous labetalol and intravenous dihydralazine in severe hypertension in

pregnancy. In: Riley A, Symonds EM (eds). The Investigation of Labetalol in the Management of Hypertension in Pregnancy. Amsterdam, Excerpta Medica, 1982, pp 51–61.

105. Ashe RG, Moodley J, Richards AM, et al. Comparison of labetalol and dihydralazine in hypertensive emergencies of pregnancy. S Afr Med J 1987;71:354.

106. Lunell NO, Nyllund L, Lewander R, et al. Acute effect of an antihypertensive drug, labetalol, on uteroplacental blood flow. Br J Obstet Gynaecol 1982;89:640.

107. Jouppila P, Kirkinen P, Koivula A, et al. Labetalol does not alter the placental and fetal blood flow or maternal prostanoids in pre-eclampsia. Br J Obstet Gynaecol 1986;93:543.

108. Walters BNJ, Redman CWG. Treatment of severe pregnancy-associated hypertension with the calcium antagonist nifedipine. Br J Obstet Gynaecol 1984;91:330.

109. Constantine G, Beevers DG, Reynolds AL, et al. Nifedipine as a second line antihypertensive drug in pregnancy. Br J Obstet Gynaecol 1987;94:1136.

110. Sibai BM, Barton JR, Akl S, et al. A randomized prospective comparison of nifedipine and bed rest versus bed rest alone in the management of preeclampsia remote from term. Am J Obstet Gynecol 1992;167:879.

111. Snyder SW, Cardwell MS. Neuromuscular blockade with magnesium sulfate and nifedipine. Am J Obstet Gynecol 1989;161:35.

112. Sibai BM. Magnesium sulfate is the ideal anticonvulsant in preeclampsia-eclampsia. Am J Obstet Gynecol 1990;162:1141.

113. Dinsdale HB. Does magnesium sulfate treat eclamptic seizures? Arch Neurol 1989;45:1360.

114. Kaplan PW, Lesser RP, Fisher RS, et al. No, magnesium sulfate should not be used in treating eclamptic seizures. Arch Neurol 1988;45:1361.

115. Nadler JL, Goodson S, Rude RK. Evidence that prostacyclin mediates the vascular action of magnesium in humans. Hypertension 1987;9:379.

116. Slater RM, Smith WD, Patrick J, et al. Phenytoin infusion in severe preeclampsia. Lancet 1987.1417.

117. Cree JE, Meyer J, Hailey DM. Diazepam in labour: Its metabolism and effect on the clinical condition and thermogenesis of the newborn. BMJ 1973;4:251.

118. Clark SL, Cotton DB. Clinical indications for pulmonary artery catheterization in the patient with severe preeclampsia. Am J Obstet Gynecol 1988;158:453.

119. Martin JN, Blake PG, Perry KG, et al. The natural history of HELLP syndrome: Patterns of disease progression and regression. Am J Obstet Gynecol 1991;164:1500.

120. Chesley LC, Annitto JE, Cosgrove RA. The remote prognosis of eclamptic women. Sixth periodic report. Am J Obstet Gynecol 1976;124:446.

121. Sibai BM. Management and counseling of patients with preeclampsia remote from term. Clin Obstet Gynecol 1992;35(2):426.

122. Sibai BM, Mercer B, Sarinoglu C: Severe preeclampsia in the second trimester: Recurrence risk and long-term prognosis. Am J Obstet Gynecol 1991;165:408.

123. Joint National Committee for the Detection and Treatment of Hypertension. V. Arch Intern Med 1993;153:154.

124. Packham DK, Fairley KR, Ihle BU, et al. Comparison of pregnancy outcome between normotensive and hypertensive women with primary glomerulonephritis. Clin Exp Hypertens Preg 1987–1988;[B]6:387.

125. Hou SH, Grossman SD, Madias NE. Pregnancy in women with renal disease and moderate renal insufficiency. Am J Med 1985;78:185.

126. Schenker JG, Chowers I. Pheochromocytoma and pregnancy. Review of 89 cases. Obstet Gynecol Surg 1971;25:739.

127. Page EW, Christianson R. The impact of mean arerial blood pressure in middle trimester upon the outcome of pregnancy. Am J Obstet Gynecol 1976;125:740.

128. Friedman EA, Neff RK. Pregnancy hypertension: A systematic evaluation of clinical diagnostic criteria. Littleton, MA: PSP Publishing, 1977.

129. Dunlop JCH. Chronic hypertension and perinatal mortality. Proc R Soc Med 1966;59:838.

130. Redman CWG: Therapy of non-preeclamptic hypertension in pregnancy. Am J Kidney Dis 1987;9:324.

131. Fletcher AE, Bulpitt CJ. A review of clinical trials in pregnancy. In: Rubin PC (ed). Hypertension in Pregnancy. New York, Elsevier, 1988, pp 102–117.

132. Chesley LC, Sloan DM. The effect of posture on renal function in late pregnancy. Am J Obstet Gynecol 1964;89:754.

133. Papiernik E, Kaminski M. Multifactorial study of the risk of prematurity at 32 weeks of gestation. 1. A study of the frequency of 30 predictive characteristics. J Perinat Med 1974;2:30.

134. Gallery EDM, Hunyor SN, Gyory AZ. Plasma volume contraction: A significant factor in both pregnancy-associated hypertension and chronic hypertension in pregnancy. Q J Med 1979;48:593.

135. Palomaki JF, Lindheimer MD. Sodium depletion simulating deterioration in toxemic pregnancy. N Engl J Med 1979;252:88.

136. Rayburn WF, Zuspan FP, Pichl EJ. Self-monitoring of blood pressure during pregnancy. Am J Obstet Gynecol 1984;148:159.

137. Lowe SA, Rubin PC. The pharmacologic management of hypertension in pregnancy. J Hypertens 1992;10:201.

138. Barron WM: Hypertension. In: Barron WM, Lindheimer MD (eds). Medical Disorders in Pregnancy. 2nd ed. St. Louis, Mosby Year Book, 1994.

139. Gallery E. Chronic and secondary hypertension. In: Rubin PC (ed). Handbook of Hypertension: Hypertension in Pregnancy. New York: Elsevier Science, 1988, pp 202–223.

140. Bulters L, Kennedy S, Rubin PC. Atenolol in essential hypertension during pregnancy. BMJ 1990;301:587.

141. Douglas DD, Yang RD, Jensen P et al. Fatal labetalol-induced hepatic injury. Am J Med 1989;87:235.

142. Hanssens M, Kierse MJNC, Vankelecom F, Van Assche FA. Fetal and neonatal effects of treatment with angiotensin-converting enzyme inhibitors in pregnancy. Obstet Gynecol 1991;78:128.

Diabetes in Pregnancy

Lois Jovanovic-Peterson and Charles M. Peterson

Before the advent of insulin, few infants of diabetic mothers survived.[1] A review of the literature relating mortality rates to mean maternal glucose levels reveals that the perinatal mortality rate of 100% before 1922 decreased in parallel with the decrease in maternal glucose levels.[2–5] However, the perinatal mortality rate by the 1970s plateaued at 8%, correlating with a mean maternal blood glucose level of 120 mg per dl (6.66 mmol/L).[5] The literature after the mid-1970s is conflicting in terms of the relationship between further lowering of the mean maternal blood glucose and the mortality rate. Many reports claim that when maternal glucose levels are normalized, the mortality rate of the offspring is equal to that in the general population.[3, 6–10] Others claim that the mortality rate still is twice the rate in the general population.[11–13]

The problem appears in part to be that it is impossible to normalize blood glucose levels in an insulin-dependent diabetic woman after pregnancy is diagnosed and to affect the malformation rate (Table 37–1). Organogenesis is completed by the eighth gestational week.[14] Thus, hyperglycemia in the first few weeks of pregnancy increases the probability that a diabetic woman may have a malformed child.[15, 16] Those women documented to have hyperglycemia greater than 6 standard deviations above the mean of a normal population have a risk of up to 23%.[3] Improvement in the infant mortality rate can occur only if women are enrolled in blood glucose normalization programs before they become pregnant.

Growth and development of the fetus after organogenesis are also affected by hyperglycemia. Maternal glucose freely crosses the placenta. Maternal insulin does not cross the placenta. The fetus, which does not have diabetes, responds appropriately to hyperglycemia from the mother by secreting large quantities of insulin. Over time, the fetal pancreas becomes autonomous. Fetal hyperinsulinemia causes not only fetal adiposity but also metabolic aberrancy. A neonate born to a diabetic mother who has been in poor diabetic control typically is big (macrosomic), hypoglycemic, erythremic, hyperbilirubinemic, and hypocalcemic and may develop respiratory distress syndrome.[16] This "big sick baby" syndrome can be prevented if maternal euglycemia is sustained throughout pregnancy.[17]

Most women experience pregnancy only two or three times in their lives. For diabetic women, a pregnancy must be planned to ensure that mothers and their infants will be healthy. Prepregnancy planning means choosing a form of contraception that is effective yet does not affect glucose metabolism. In addition, for all women who become pregnant, a concerted effort must be made to diagnose pregnancy-induced hyperglycemia or gestational diabetes, to ensure that growth and development of the fetus are normal. This chapter

TABLE 37–1. Percentage of Malformed Infants Related to the Number of Standard Deviations Above the Mean First-Trimester Glycosylated Hemoglobin of a Normal Population of Mothers from the Same Country

| STUDY | NORMAL | DIABETIC WOMEN | | |
		≤4 SD	4–6 SD	>6 SD†
Leslie et al[9]	—	0	—	6.0
Miller et al[3]*	2.1	0	5.1	24.4
Ylinen et al[15]	—	—	—	23.5
Steel[6]*	1.7	1.4	3.3	12.7
Greene et al[13]	2.1	—	3.0	2.2
Goldman et al[10]	—	0	—	—
Fuhrmann et al[12]	0.8	1.6	—	15.8
Damm and Molsted-Pedersen[7]*	1.7	1.0	2.7	7.4
Kitzmiller et al[8]*	2.1	1.4	0	10.8
Mills et al[11]	2.1	4.9	4.5	9.0

*Studies in which the diabetic women who had glycosylated hemoglobin levels <2 SD above normal had a lower malformation rate than the normals.

†Or undocumented because of late enrollment.

SD, Standard deviations.

summarizes the causes of hyperglycemia during pregnancy, the rationale for normalizing glucose levels, and one protocol that has proved to be successful in achieving and maintaining euglycemia before and during pregnancy.

EARLY PREGNANCY-RELATED HORMONES PROMOTE INCREASED FUEL FOR A FETUS WITHOUT SACRIFICE OF MATERNAL GLUCOSE HOMEOSTASIS

With (and perhaps antecedent to) implantation of a trophoblast, the production of pregnancy-related hormones begins. These hormones immediately alter the metabolism of nutrients to shift the priority of metabolic products toward the growing fetus. A buffering mechanism must be initiated early in pregnancy to prevent a mother from suffering deleterious hypoglycemia between feedings as her fuel reserves continue to flow to her unborn child. Maternal glucose homeostasis is sustained by a delicate interplay of maternal hormones designed to increase fat storage, decrease energy expenditure, and delay glucose clearance. In addition, fetal needs are met through the fetal control of nutrients mediated by various fetal hormones. Hormonal messages from the conceptus can affect metabolic processes, uteroplacental blood flow, and cellular differentiation.

Immediately after ovulation, the corpus luteum is converted into a structure that makes 17OH-progesterone. Lutenizing hormone from the pituitary is necessary to keep the corpus luteum functioning. Once conception and subsequent implantation occur, human chorionic gonadotropin stimulates the corpus luteal production of 17OH-progesterone until placental production of steroids is adequate. Thus, human chorionic gonadotropin is needed for only the first 12 weeks of gestation because the corpus luteum is needed only during these early phases of placental growth.[18] Human chorionic gonadotropin does not seem to affect glucose homeostasis. Other hormones that do promote production of glucose are therefore urgently needed early in pregnancy.

The adult ovary is capable of making steroids directly from acetate, but this capability is not true of the placenta. Estrogen formation by the placenta is dependent on precursors that reach it from both fetal and maternal compartments. To form estrogens, the placenta aromatizes the androgens coming primarily from the fetus. The fetal adrenal gland provides dihydroepiandrosterone, which proceeds through a series of hydroxylations and then double-bond formation or aromatization into estrone and estradiol-17β. In addition, some of the fetal dihydroepiandrosterone undergoes 16α-hydroxylation in the fetal liver or fetal adrenal gland to become 16α-hydroxydihydroepiandrosterone sulfate, which is cleaved in the placenta to 16α-OH-hydroxydihydroepiandrosterone and aromatized to estriol.[19] The estrogen rise occurs within 35 days of conception, just in time to provide a glucose-producing stimulus when the conceptus begins to siphon glucose from the mother.

Estrogens have weak anti-insulin properties. Thus, another hormone is needed to potentiate the glucose production rate before the fetus grows much larger. Estrogens act in concert with glucocorticoids to promote further glucose production. Estrogens stimulate liver production of cortisol-binding globulin. As cortisol-binding globulin is increased, the maternal adrenal gland secretes more cortisol to saturate the elevated level of cortisol-binding globulin and to produce enough cortisol to increase the level of free cortisol. Hypercortisolemia causes insulin resistance, delayed glucose clearance, and thus more glucose for fetal use. The appearance of cortisol is timed to contribute to the rising fetal demand for glucose and provides the strongest diabetogenic property of any of the pregnancy-related hormones.

In contrast to estrogen, progesterone production by the placenta is independent of the quantity of precursor available, uteroplacental perfusion, fetal well-being, or even the presence of a live fetus. Thus, progesterone is not useful as a marker of impending abortion.[20] Most placental progesterone is derived directly from cholesterol. The placenta does not make 17OH-progesterone until week 32 of gestation, when it starts to metabolize progesterone. Once the corpus luteum deteriorates, progesterone is the major form of the hormone. Progesterone has a direct effect on glucose metabolism.[21] When progesterone is administered to normal fasting women, the serum insulin concentration rises while glucose remains unchanged. Progesterone does not peak until week 32 of gestation. Those women who screen negative on a glucose screening test for gestational diabetes at 26 weeks may not pass the test at 32 weeks, partly because of the diabetogenic properties of progesterone. Thus, progesterone is second to cortisol in anti-insulin potency.

Two other pregnancy-related peptide hormones warrant discussion. The first hormone is prolactin, and the second human chorionic somatomammotropin (hCS). Barberia and associates[22] showed that the initial rise in prolactin level in pregnancy occurs within a few days after estradiol increases above nonpregnant levels (30–33 days after the luteinizing hormone peak), whereas the rise in prolactin levels above the nonpregnant luteal phase level occurs 32 to 36 days after the luteinizing hormone peak. The estrogen level seems to initiate the secretion of prolactin. Without a rise in estrogen followed by a rise in prolactin, spontaneous abortion seems imminent.[20]

What is the function of prolactin so early in pregnancy? Prolactin is so named because it is necessary for lactation, a third-trimester event. What is a lactation-promoting hormone doing in the first few weeks of pregnancy? Some believe that prolactin is "luteotropic" and works in concert with human chorionic gonadotropin to sustain the corpus luteum.[23] Others[24] have suggested that prolactin enhances cell-to-cell communication among the beta cells in pancreatic islets. These investigators have shown a tenfold increase in beta-cell coupling, independent of glucose stimulation in response to prolactin. Thus, prolactin may be necessary early in pregnancy to stimulate both maternal and fetal beta-cell hypertrophy.

Human chorionic somatomammotropin is a protein hormone with immunologic epitopes and biologic properties similar to pituitary growth hormone. The original name, human placental lactogen, was derived from its lactogenic properties in animals; however, such properties in women have not been confirmed. Josimovich[25] found that hCS has luteotropic properties, which would explain a rise early in pregnancy. Similar to prolactin, hCS has an effect on glucose metabolism.

The effects of hCS on fat and carbohydrate metabolism are similar to those following treatment with growth hormone: inhibition of peripheral glucose uptake and stimulation of insulin release. A comparable maximal increase in plasma free fatty acids occurs after administration of hCS or human growth hormone in hypopituitarism. In addition, infusion of hCS into an hypophysectomized, diabetic man caused the blood glucose to rise fourfold above baseline.[26]

In summary, the hormonal changes early in pregnancy can be viewed teleologically as a serial rise in hormones intended to maintain a constant glucose supply to the fetus. As fetal metabolic requirements increase, the gluconeogenic hormones rise. The order of hormonal presentation in pregnancy is inverse to their relative gluconeogenic property. The earliest hormone, human chorionic gonadotropin, has no gluconeogenic effect, and cortisol, a late hormone, is the most potent.

DEVELOPMENT OF PREGNANCY-INDUCED GLUCOSE INTOLERANCE

During the course of pregnancy, the insulin requirement rises progressively.[27] Carbohydrate tolerance is minimally perturbed in normal pregnant women because the pancreas can increase insulin production to compensate for the diabetogenic stresses of pregnancy. Kuhl and Hornnes[28] investigated the cause of hyperglycemia in the 1% of their population who failed to maintain normoglycemia during pregnancy. They found that the insulin response of hyperglycemic pregnant women differed from that of normoglycemic pregnant women in two pertinent ways: (1) insulin response to a carbohydrate load was delayed, and (2) insulin response per unit of glycemic stimulus was significantly lower. Insulin degradation was unaffected by pregnancy, and the proinsulin share of the total plasma insulin immunoreactivity did not increase during pregnancy. They concluded that the main cause of gestational diabetes, or diabetes that is uncovered in pregnancy, is insulin resistance. Gestational diabetes occurs when a pregnant woman has a compromised insulin secretory capacity and thus cannot produce enough insulin to compensate for the hormone-induced insulin resistance.

Screening for gestational diabetes should take place at that moment in pregnancy when the occurrence of gestational diabetes is most common yet should provide sufficient time to correct the metabolic imbalance before the fetus has any untoward effect from the hyperglycemia. The recommended screening and diagnostic protocol[29] is shown in Table 37–2. Screening is recommended for all pregnant women at 26 ± 2 weeks' gestation. Earlier testing is warranted if a woman has a strong family history of gestational diabetes or has had a previous pregnancy complicated by gestational diabetes or resulting in the delivery of a macrosomic infant. Women who require repeat

---

TABLE 37–2. Glucose Tolerance Test (100-gm Load) Criteria for Diagnosis and Treatment

Diet controlled	A fasting level <105 mg/dl and two or more values above
	1 hr: 190 mg/dl
	2 hr: 165 mg/dl
	3 hr: 145 mg/dl
Treatment	Trial of diet. Initiate insulin if fasting level >105 on the glucose tolerance test or fasting on self-monitoring of blood glucose >90 mg/dl and/or 1 hr postprandial on self-monitoring blood glucose level >140.

TABLE 37–3. Definition of Normoglycemia in Pregnancy

Based on a 24-hour profile of normal, nondiabetic pregnant women:
Fasting plasma glucose: 55–65 mg/dl (3.06–3.61 mmol)
One-hour postprandial plasma glucose: <140 mg/dl (<7.78 mmol)
Mean plasma glucose over 24 hr: 80–84 mg/dl (4.4–4.7 mmol)

testing at 32 weeks of gestation include those who had a positive screen but a negative glucose tolerance test result at 24 to 28 weeks of gestation and women older than 33 years and greater than 130% above ideal body weight.

PROTOCOLS FOR ACHIEVING AND MAINTAINING HEALTH IN PREGNANCIES

One result of maternal loss of glucose and gluconeogenic substrate to the fetus is a decline in maternal fasting glucose levels to 55 to 65 mg per dl.[30] Simultaneously, plasma ketone concentrations are several times higher and free fatty acid levels are elevated after an overnight fast. The second half of pregnancy is characterized by further lowering of glucose levels.

Although maternal fasting glucose levels remain below nonpregnant levels, insulin levels increase markedly during pregnancy. This rise occurs in part because of the increasing anti-insulin hormonal activity discussed earlier. A normal pancreas can adapt to these factors by increasing insulin secretion. If the pancreas fails to respond adequately, gestational diabetes results. The earliest effect of these changes is a rise in the postprandial glucose levels, which tend to be highest 1 hour after breakfast. The definition of normoglycemia in pregnancy is presented in Table 37–3.

In a woman with maternal hyperglycemia, the fetus is exposed to either sustained or intermittent pulses of hyperglycemia, both of which are mutagenic and teratogenic in the first trimester. Both situations also prematurely stimulate fetal insulin secretion. Pedersen's hypothesis[31] links maternal hyperglycemia to fetal morbidity. Thus, fetal hyperinsulinemia may result in (1) increased fetal body fat (macrosomia) and therefore a difficult delivery; (2) inhibition of pulmonary maturation of surfactant and therefore respiratory distress of the newborn; (3) changing serum potassium concentration secondary to the elevated insulin and glucose levels and thus a predisposition toward

cardiac arrhythmias and death; and (4) neonatal hypoglycemia with potential neurologic damage. Hyperglycemia leads to maternal complications such as polyhydramnios, hypertension, urinary tract infections, candidal vaginitis, and recurrent spontaneous abortions. Thus, a vigorous effort to achieve and maintain normoglycemia before and throughout pregnancy is warranted.

DIET PRESCRIPTION FOR PREGNANT DIABETIC WOMEN

The mainstay of therapy for gestational diabetic women is dietary management to maintain adequate nutrition and normoglycemia. The euglycemic diet, which is designed to prescribe enough calories to meet the nutritional needs of a pregnant woman but not cause postprandial hyperglycemia, is shown in Table 37–4.[32]

A closer look at Table 37–4 reveals that less than 40% of the calories are prescribed in the form of carbohydrate because the carbohydrate content of foods is responsible for the peak postprandial glucose level. The breakfast meal must be small and the carbohydrate portion minimal. Pregnancy produces severe morning carbohydrate intolerance. Later in the day, more carbohydrate can be tolerated. This diet of frequent small feedings is designed to avoid postprandial hyperglycemia and starvation ketosis. It promotes an average weight gain of 12.5 kg during pregnancy. In the first 8 to 10 weeks, a pregnant woman needs 25 kcal per kg per 24 hours; thereafter, she needs 30 kcal per kg per 24 hours (present pregnant weight). For women who are more than 120% of ideal body

TABLE 37–4. Diet Calculation for Women 80% to 120% of Ideal Body Weight

TIME	MEAL	FRACTION (kcal/kg)	% OF DAILY CARBO-HYDRATES
8:00 A.M.	Breakfast	2/18	10
10:30 A.M.	Snack	1/18	5
12:00 P.M.	Lunch	5/18	30
3:00 P.M.	Snack	2/18	10
5:00 P.M.	Dinner	5/18	30
8:00 P.M.	Snack	2/18	10
11:00 P.M.	Snack	1/18	5

kcal × weight in kilograms:
<80% ideal body weight: 40 kcal/kg/day
80–120% ideal body weight: 30 kcal/kg/day
120–150% ideal body weight: 24 kcal/kgday
>150% ideal body weight: 12–20 kcal/kg/day

weight, the diet should be calculated as 24 kcal per kg per 24 hours or less (present pregnant weight). Morbidly obese pregnant women usually require only 12 kcal per kg of present pregnant weight to keep them above the ketonuric threshold. These dietary prescriptions apply to both gestational diabetic women and to pregestational (type I and type II) diabetic women.[33]

No matter how educated a pregestational woman is about diabetes management, metabolism is changed so greatly during pregnancy that reinforcement is always necessary. Ideally, this education to achieve and maintain normoglycemia should begin before conception. The education program usually requires 5 to 7 days to teach the requisite goals and skills to normalize blood glucose throughout gestation with insulin and food adjustments. The training process is best achieved in specialized centers for diabetes self-care or in the hospital.

CRITERIA FOR INITIATING INSULIN IN A GESTATIONAL DIABETIC WOMAN

Once a diagnosis of gestational diabetes is made, a woman should immediately be referred to a dietitian who can translate the recommended dietary prescription into a meal plan. The woman should next be instructed on the technique of blood glucose self-monitoring and told to check and chart her blood glucose levels when fasting and 1 hour after meals. Based on these glucose results, insulin should be started if the fasting level is greater than 105 mg per dl or the 1-hour postprandial is greater than 120 mg per dl if stillbirth is to be avoided.[29] If the treatment goals also include prevention of macrosomia, then insulin should be started when the fasting level exceeds 90 mg per dl or the 1-hour postprandial is greater than 120 mg per dl.[34] To normalize an elevated fasting blood glucose level, NPH insulin given before bed is recommended; to normalize the postprandial glucose levels, premeal regular insulin is recommended.[32]

UTILITY OF EXERCISE AS A TREATMENT STRATEGY FOR GESTATIONAL DIABETES

Gestational diabetes is considered to be in part a disease of glucose clearance, although it has been shown that this disorder is a heterogeneous entity.[35] Initiation of insulin therapy per se is palliative but does not speak to the primary defect(s), which may include hyperinsulinemia.

Cardiovascular conditioning exercise facilitates glucose use, among other ways, by increasing insulin binding to and affinity for its receptor.[36] Although exercise therapy during pregnancy has been gaining acceptance,[37] it remains controversial.[38–41] Specifically, maternal exercise on a bicycle ergometer has been associated with fetal bradycardia.[38, 39] Arm ergometry has not been associated with either uterine activity or fetal bradycardia.[42]

We found[43] that women with gestational diabetes can train using arm ergometry and that such a program of cardiovascular conditioning exercise results in lower levels of glycemia than a program of diet alone. The effects of exercise on glucose metabolism became apparent after 4 weeks of training and appeared to affect both hepatic glucose output (as reflected by fasting glucose levels) and glucose clearance (as reflected by glucose values after a 50-gm oral glucose challenge).

The implications of this study for the health care of women with gestational diabetes remain to be determined. Compliance with the protocol was excellent, and no maternal or infant morbidity was associated with the training program in this small series. The study may also imply that a cardiovascular conditioning program could obviate insulin treatment in many women with gestational diabetes.

STEPS IN A GLUCOSE NORMALIZATION PROGRAM FOR PREGESTATIONAL DIABETIC WOMEN (TYPES I AND II)

Preconceptional Programs

Optimal Birth Control for Diabetic Women

The risk of malformations in a diabetic pregnancy increases as the blood glucose level rises in the first few weeks of pregnancy. Thus, the normalization program needs to be started before conception. The fact that hyperglycemia during organogenesis increases the risk of malformations underscores the need for safe and effective birth control for a diabetic woman. Unless she is in the best health and achieves the best glucose control, the pregnancy becomes high risk. Her method of birth control should be effective yet not deteriorate her metabolic status. Four types of birth control are used: (1) barrier methods, (2) intrauterine devices, (3) hormonal manipulation, and (4) sterilization. Barrier methods such as the diaphragm and cervical cap are excellent choices for diabetic women who are highly motivated. These methods do not affect glucose control; however, they have the highest failure rate unless used meticulously. Combining the barrier method with the rhythm method (abstinence during the 4 days surrounding ovulation) increases the effectiveness of the barrier method.

Intrauterine devices, although reported to be highly effective in preventing pregnancy, are not recommended in the United States because of the risk of uterine perforation, infection, pelvic inflammatory disease, and tubal pregnancies. In addition, intrauterine devices may be less effective in women with diabetes.[44]

Oral contraceptives may be an effective method of birth control in young women with diabetes. Oral contraceptives are relatively contraindicated in women who have high blood pressure, vascular disease, retinopathy, neuropathy, nephropathy, or high levels of cholesterol or triglycerides and in women who smoke. The advantage of using oral contraceptives is that they are 97 to 98% effective. If oral contraceptives are chosen as a method of birth control, the low-dose (estrogen- or progestin-only) pills are recommended for women with diabetes. Although the combination pill (estrogen and progestin) is slightly more effective in preventing pregnancy, it can interfere with diabetes control and may require an increasing insulin dose to maintain normal blood glucose levels in women with type I diabetes. Progestin-only pills avoid the estrogen-related risks of vascular problems, including high blood pressure. However, this type of pill may result in irregular menstrual periods and weight gain. In addition, some women experience problems controlling blood glucose levels with high-dose progestin oral contraceptives.[45] If a woman develops hypertension while taking oral contraceptives, she is at increased risk for retinopathy or nephropathy.

It is usually advisable for young diabetic women who wish to use oral contraceptives to wait until 6 months after the onset of menstruation to begin use; however, blood lipids (cholesterol and triglycerides) and vascular status should be checked before starting and should be monitored periodically during use. The short-term risks (1–2 years) of taking oral contraceptives appear to be low, although the long-term risks are uncertain. One report describes an increased breast cancer rate in women who started the pill before the age of 30 and continued its use for more than 8 years.[45]

Although much effort has gone into developing new methods of birth control in the past 20 years, variations on hormone preparations are the only birth control options that will become available in this country in the near future. In addition to the low-dose estrogen and progestin-only pills mentioned earlier, preparations that release small amounts of hormones over a long period of time have been developed. Injections of hormones at 8-week to 3-month intervals are effective, although they may result in severe menstrual problems. Some preparations result in fewer bleeding abnormalities, but they must be administered at shorter (1-month) intervals. The long-acting contraceptive methods are currently widely used in China and Latin America. A long-acting progesterone injection, Depo-Provera, has been approved in the United States for use as a birth control method.

Another variation on this method uses hormone capsules inserted under the skin; it provides effective contraception for up to 5 years. This contraceptive method is reversible, because fertility returns on removal of the implants. To date, no published reports have described their use in diabetic women.

Insertable hormone-containing vaginal devices have also been developed. One such device, a silicone rubber ring, is inserted into the vagina for a period of 3 weeks, then removed for 1 week to allow regular menstrual bleeding. An intrauterine device that releases hormones has also been developed and is currently available. Experience with these devices in diabetic women is limited. No satisfactory male contraceptives are on the horizon, despite extensive research in this area.

Genetic Counseling for Diabetic Women

The chances that a type I insulin-dependent diabetic woman will have a diabetic child are 1.6%. The chances that a diabetic father will have a diabetic child are 6.0%.[46] Of course, the chances that a diabetic mother and a diabetic father will have a diabetic child are greater. Such couples should be reassured that their child probably will not be born with diabetes. It is rare for a child younger than 2 years to develop diabetes.

Type II diabetes may pass to a child in 25% of cases. Type II diabetes usually presents after the age of 40 years and usually occurs if a person becomes overweight and unfit.

Planning Pregnancy

The first step in a prepregnancy normalization program is to measure a woman's glycosylated hemoglobin. If her glycosylated hemoglobin value is greater than 2 standard deviations above the mean for a normal population, then her insulin program needs adjusting until her glycosylated hemoglobin level is in the normal range. In most cases, this process requires at least six blood glucose checks a day (before and 1 hour after each meal) and three injections a day of insulin. The insulin program should be designed to normalize the premeal and postmeal blood glucose levels. The target prepregnancy blood glucose levels are premeal levels in the 80 to 90 mg per dl range and postmeal levels in the less than 140 mg per dl range. Once pregnancy is documented, target blood glucose levels are premeal values of 55 to 70 and continued postmeal blood glucose levels less than 120 mg per dl. A normalization program is facilitated by a team approach that includes nurse educators, dietitians, and physicians.[47]

The second step in the self-care program is to teach self-monitoring of blood glucose levels and to ensure (through a quality control program) that the values are accurate to within 10% of a laboratory standard. Most women prefer systems using reflectance meters because of the perceived accuracy over visually read reagent strips.

The diet is maintained as described earlier for the gestational diabetic women while insulin is administered to mimic normal pancreatic function. A normal pancreas secretes 50% of the insulin as mealtime boluses. This delivery may be mimicked by four injections a day of combinations of NPH and regular insulin; however, it is possible to decrease the number of injections to three if a patient is willing to time lunch to coincide perfectly with the morning NPH insulin midday peak. The total daily dose of insulin is based on gestational week and the woman's current pregnant body weight (Table 37–5). The division of the insulin into three injections a day is also shown in Table 37–5. After the initial insulin calculation, the dose is tailored to fit each woman by adjusting the dose until all the blood glucose levels before and 1 hour after each meal are normal (Table 37–6).

Monitoring of blood glucose levels (six per day: before and 1 hour after each meal), plus the use of

TABLE 37–6. Insulin Adjustment Based on a Patient's Self-monitoring of Blood Glucose Levels

TIME	INSULIN ANALYZED	ADJUSTMENT PROCEDURE
7:30 A.M.	Bedtime NPH	If BG >90 mg/dl Check an HS and 3 A.M. BG. If HS high, increase dinner regular or decrease evening snack. If HS normal but 3 A.M. high (>100 mg/dl), then increase bedtime NPH by 2. If 3 A.M. is low (<60 mg/dl), then decrease bedtime NPH by 2. If 7:30 A.M. is <60 mg/dl, decrease bedtime NPH by 2.
10:00 A.M.	A.M. Regular	If 1-hr PC >140 mg/dl, increase tomorrow's A.M. regular by 2. If 1-hr PC <110 mg/dl, decrease tomorrow's A.M. regular by 2.
1:00 P.M.	Lunch regular	If 1-hr PC >140 mg/dl, increase tomorrow's lunch regular by 2. If 1-hr PC <110 mg/dl, decrease tomorrow's lunch regular by 2.
4:30 P.M.	P.M. NPH	If BG >90 mg/dl, then increase A.M. NPH by 2. If BG <60 mg/dl, then decrease A.M. NPH by 2.
6:00 P.M.	Dinner regular	If 1-hr PC >140 mg/dl, increase dinner regular by 2. If 1-hr PC <110 mg/dl, decrease dinner regular by 2.

BG, Blood glucose; PC, postprandial; HS, hour of sleep; NPH, neutral protamine Hagedorn (insulin).

TABLE 37–5. Initial Calculation of Insulin Therapy for Four Injections a Day*

	FRACTION OF TOTAL DOSE	
TIME	NPH	Regular
Prebreakfast	5/18	2/9
Prelunch		1/6
Predinner		1/6
Bedtime	1/6	

*Total insulin requirement =
0.7 U/kg for weeks 6–18
0.8 U/kg for weeks 18–26
0.9 U/kg for weeks 26–36
1.0 U/kg for weeks 36–41

titration procedures, ensures a smooth increase of insulin as the pregnancy progresses to a higher insulin requirement (up to 1 U/kg/24 hours at term) (see Table 37–5).[17] Twin gestations result in a doubling of the insulin requirement.[1]

Each patient must also be taught her personal lag time between the injection and the initiation of the meal. Simultaneous injection of insulin and ingestion of glucose results in brittle diabetes. The simple sugars in food raise the blood glucose level before the subcutaneous insulin peaks in the bloodstream. The quickly metabolized glucose will be gone when the insulin levels are at their maximum in 3 hours. To correct this problem, the insulin should be injected at least 30 to 45 minutes before the meal to allow the insulin and the food to peak together.

Once the glycosylated hemoglobin is in the target range and the other criteria are met (Table 37–

7), a patient may then try to conceive. Education on the use of a basal body temperature thermometer facilitates the process of timing conception. Frequent contact with the health care team is then necessary to maintain normoglycemia as the luteal phase hormones rise. A pregnancy test should be performed 1 day after the missed period. If the test is positive, then 9 months of careful titration of the doses of insulin to the increasing hormones of pregnancy is necessary.

TABLE 37–7. Preconceptional Control Protocol

1. Assess the patient's medical fitness for pregnancy with particular attention to retinopathy, nephropathy, hypertension, and ischemic heart disease. The preconception medical evaluation should include:
   a. Ophthalmologic consultation
      Diagnosis: Fundus photography
      Treatment: Laser therapy, if necessary
   b. Blood pressure
      Diagnosis: Blood pressure ideally should be 130/80 mm Hg off any antihypertensive medications that may be teratogenic.
      Treatment: Only methyldopa and hydralazine should be used if blood pressure cannot be maintained below 130/80 mm Hg, because these are the only antihypertensive medicines that have proved over time not to increase the risk for congenital anomalies.
   c. Kidney status
      Diagnosis: 24-hr urine for creatinine clearance, total proteinuria, and microalbuminuria.
      Treatment: Although the literature is conflicting, a creatinine clearance >50 ml/min is sufficient to adequately sustain a pregnancy.
   d. Cardiac status
      Diagnosis: The high prevalence of maternal mortality in some series mandates a cardiac assessment with a treadmill stress test in all patients with evidence of nephropathy and/or hypertension.
      Treatment: If the stress test reveals evidence of atherosclerotic heart disease, the woman should be advised against becoming pregnant.
2. Assess the patient's gynecologic fitness for pregnancy.
   The preconception gynecologic examination should include:
   Diagnosis: Anatomically and hormonally normal female
   Treatment: Either advise against pregnancy or correct the problem.
3. Assess the emotional status of a woman to be able to take on the metabolic, physical, and financial burden of a pregnancy.
   Diagnosis: Mentally, emotionally, and financially fit
   Treatment: Contraception is necessary until all is in order and a woman is ready to conceive.
4. Obtain maximum cooperation on committment from patients and their partners.
   Treatment: Programs of intensive insulin delivery require time, effort, and shared efforts. Unless a couple is aware of the major effort for these programs, compliance and metabolic control are in jeopardy.
5. Identify and treat infertility.
   Diagnosis and treatment: In light of the increasing risk to the pregnancy with increasing age and duration of diabetes, infertility problems should be diagnosed and treated as soon as feasible in concert with metabolic control programs.
6. Obtain diabetic control before conception.
   Diagnosis: If the glycosylated hemoglobin level is >4 standard deviations above a normal mean glycosylated hemoglobin for women without diabetes, then an intensive insulin delivery program is warranted.
   Treatment: Normalization programs require 3–4 injections a day of subcutaneously injected insulin (NPH and regular) or an insulin infusion pump. Self-monitoring of blood glucose is performed at least six times a day (before and 1 hr after each meal). Repeat the glycohemoglobin measurement 1 mo after initiation of the program. Depending on how high the baseline value, the glycohemoglobin now may be within the normal range. If it is still elevated, then it is retested every month. Once the result is in the target range, permission is granted to become pregnant on the next cycle. During this crucial cycle, the woman is encouraged to pay closer attention to her blood glucose levels after she ovulates. Pregnancy tests do not turn positive until 1 day after the missed period. Thus, for 2 wk after ovulation, the woman pretends she is pregnant and steps up her efforts to correct every blood glucose level. A pregnancy test 1 day after the missed period will confirm pregnancy and set the stage for the woman to maintain close watch on her blood glucose levels for 9 mo. If the pregnancy test is negative, then she has to maintain her glucose levels stable to maintain her target glycohemoglobin. Each cycle should have a repeat glycohemoglobin test performed by day 5 to allow the woman to receive permission to become pregnant by the time she usually ovulates.
7. Identify time of conception.
   Diagnosis: Pregnancy dating is exquisitely important in making delivery decisions. The plan outlined in number 6 clearly identifies conception and dates the pregnancy with a pregnancy test 1 day after the missed period.
   Treatment: A preconception program should include asking the woman to keep a menstrual calendar. If the period is missed, a pregnancy test should be performed.
8. Check immune status against rubella, toxoplasmosis, syphilis, hepatitis, and human immunodeficiency virus.
9. Encourage patients to stop smoking before pregnancy and to refrain from any medications while attempting to become pregnant.

Follow-up Visits

The visits on an outpatient basis and by telephone should be frequent enough to provide the needed consultation, guidance, and emotional support to facilitate compliance. In addition, tests and therapy should be appropriate for gestational age (Table 37–8). The health care delivery team should give the impression that they, too, put forth an extra effort for this precious pregnancy. Therefore, each patient should have phone access to the team on a 24-hour basis for questions, and visits should be spaced not longer than 2 weeks apart. A glycosylated hemoglobin level should be drawn at monthly intervals to confirm that the home blood glucose diary reflects maternal glycemia.

Prevention of Hypoglycemia

Each patient should be taught to respond to symptoms of hypoglycemia (tingling sensations, diaphoresis, palpitations) by first checking blood glucose. If the blood glucose level is less than 70 mg per dl, she should drink 240 ml (8 ounces) of milk and recheck her blood glucose value 15 minutes later. This protocol is designed to return the blood glucose level to normal without rebound hyperglycemia.[48]

In addition, patients and their families should be taught to inject glucagon subcutaneously to treat insulin reactions that cannot be corrected with food. During times of morning sickness or vomiting, judicious use of glucagon can be used to prevent hypoglycemia. In general, 0.15 mg (15 units in a U-100 insulin syringe) of glucagon will raise blood glucose values 30 mg per dl within 15 minutes and maintain the levels for about 3 hours.

MATERNAL COMPLICATIONS AND PREGNANCY

Chronic diabetes is associated with a higher prevalence of retinopathy, nephropathy, and cardiovascular disease. Pregnancy poses the highest risk in diabetic women with atherosclerotic heart disease, with a maternal mortality rate in some series greater than 50%.[49] Clearly, diabetic women with evidence of vascular disease need a cardiac assessment including an electrocardiogram, chest radiograph, and even a stress test to document cardiac status before undertaking the risk of pregnancy.

The prevalence of pregnancy in women with diabetic nephropathy is increasing, mainly because of the current philosophy that improved glucose control improves the outcome of pregnancies complicated by diabetes. The current prevalence of diabetic nephropathy during pregnancy at the Joslin Clinic is reported to be 9.6%. The perinatal survival of infants born to these mothers at the Joslin Clinic has also continued to improve; for the years 1938 to 1958, the survival rate was 59%;

TABLE 37–8. Flow Chart for the Management of Pregestational Diabetes, Types I and II, and Pregnancy

Week of gestation		
−6	GHb	Normalization of GHb levels
−2	GHb	Recheck GHb to ensure normality before conception.
		Teach how to measure basal body temperature.
+2	GHb	Reinforce diet plan:
	Self-monitoring of blood glucose: 6 per day	25 kcal/kg/day
	TFT	Insulin plan:
	Kidney function	0.7 U/kg/day
	Eye examination	
	Physical examination	
	Routine prenatal care	
+8–41	GHb every 2–4 wk	Increase diet up to 30 kcal/kg/day
	Self-monitoring of blood glucose: 6 per day	
	Ultrasonography at 8, 20 and 32 wk	At 18 weeks:
	Repeat tests at wk 22–24 and 32–34 wk:	increase insulin: 0.8 U/kg/day
	Kidney function	
	TFT	
	Eye examination	Admit for bed rest if pressure up
	Physical examination	
+32–41	Obstetric surveillance protocol to assess fetal well-being	At 32 weeks:
		increase insulin: 0.9–1.0 U/kg/day

GHb, Glycosylated hemoglobin; TFT, thyroid function tests.

for 1963 to 1975, the rate rose to 71%; and for 1975 to 1978, the rate was up to 89%.[49]

Our study reported 100% survival of infants born to nephropathic diabetic mothers who were maintained under intensive glucose control for the entire pregnancy.[50] In those mothers maintained with normal hemoglobin A_{1cs} and blood pressure, renal function tended to improve with gestation.[51] A study by Kitzmiller and co-workers[52] concluded that "pregnancy is not associated with permanent worsening of renal function in the majority of diabetic patients." In several studies, however, coexisting hypertension has been associated with poor perinatal outcome and deterioration of kidney function. Thus, as more nephropathic diabetic women become pregnant, it is imperative that clinicians target not only glucose and insulin management strategies but also optimal blood pressure control to ensure the best possible outcome of these pregnancies.

The diagnosis of diabetic nephropathy during pregnancy is made on the basis of persistent proteinuria of greater than 300 mg per 24 hours occurring in the *first* half of pregnancy in the absence of urinary tract infection. This latter point is important because the prevalence of urinary tract infection in the first trimester of pregnancy at the Karlsburg Diabetes Institute in the German Democratic Republic was reported to be 25%.[53] Readers should note that the definition of diabetic nephropathy during pregnancy is based on the degree of proteinuria, not creatinine clearance. The creatinine clearance is an important prognostic indicator for prepregnancy counseling. A creatinine clearance less than 50 ml per minute before pregnancy has been associated with a high prevalence of pregnancy-induced hypertension and fetal wastage.

In normal pregnancy, by 10 weeks of gestation, increased cardiac output has increased the creatinine clearance by 20%. As pregnancy progresses, creatinine clearance continues to rise into the third trimester and reaches a plateau at 140 ± 20 standard deviations ml per minute. Normal pregnancy is not associated with proteinuria. Although levels up to 150 to 300 mg of protein per 24 hours of urine excreted are elevated, complications are only associated with levels greater than 300 mg per 24 hours.

In pregnancies complicated by diabetic nephropathy with maternal glucose and blood pressure maintained in the normal ranges, renal function is not worsened. Kitzmiller's series[52] confirmed that creatinine clearance does not deteriorate with pregnancy, but the women in this series did not show the expected increase in creatinine clearance noted in normal gestation. We did

find an increase in creatinine clearance if nephropathic patients were maintained normotensive and normoglycemic.[51] Of note, despite the increase in creatinine clearance, protein excretion continued to increase throughout pregnancy. Although massive proteinuria was associated with troublesome edema, no effect on the fetal-placental unit was noted as long as the blood pressure was maintained in the normal range. Those women who had subclinical evidence of hypothyroidism in the first trimester (thyroid-stimulating hormone > 5.0 μU/ml) tended to become hypothyroid if their protein excretion increased in the second trimester to more than 4 gm per 24 hours. Fifty percent of the nephropathic patients reached this level of proteinuria. Thus, it is prudent to measure thyroid-stimulating hormone monthly throughout pregnancy in patients with diabetic nephropathy.

In addition to hypothyroidism, anasarca, and hypoalbuminemia, proteinuria during pregnancy is also associated with anemia, perhaps also because of loss of erythropoietin into the urine. Studies are now in progress to evaluate the therapeutic potential for recombinant erythropoietin in this clinical situation. Whether the rise in blood pressure associated with erythropoietin administration will preclude its utility in nephropathic diabetic pregnancies remains to be determined.

For diabetic women with hypertension, pregnancy is a hazardous undertaking. As gestation proceeds, the most frequent threat is a precipitous rise in blood pressure that may compromise the well-being of the mother and the fetus. Fetal death is more common in pregnant hypertensive women than in those with normal blood pressure. Nevertheless, the chances of having a viable baby have been markedly enhanced in recent years by better fetal monitoring, better blood pressure control, and improvements in neonatal intensive care. A decision to attempt pregnancy in these circumstances remains difficult for most women and requires careful planning, if possible, by all concerned.

It would be best to eliminate all antihypertension medications during the critical time of fetal organogenesis or weeks 0 to 8 of fetal development. If the blood pressure is less than 140/80 mm Hg in a woman taking antihypertensive medications before pregnancy, then the medication can be safely discontinued in order for her to become pregnant, if she is willing to be compliant with a low-salt diet and fluid restriction to less than 2 liters a day of oral intake. Withholding blood pressure medications until after organogenesis is ideal; however, if the blood pressure rises above 140/80 mm Hg despite the low-salt and fluid-restricted diet, then more aggressive strategies must be attempted. Generally, pregnancy is associated with a decline in systolic blood pressure to weeks 12 to 24 of gestation. Thereafter, in nondiabetic women, blood pressure gradually rises to levels at term that are similar to prepregnant values.

Although there is no clear dividing line between hypertension and normotension in pregnancy, it is customary in studies of pregnancy to use a limit of 140/90 mm Hg to define mild hypertension. This figure is three standard deviations above normal mean diastolic and systolic blood pressure at week 6 of gestation.[54] In pregnancies complicated by diabetes, the cutoff of 140/90 mm Hg may be too high. The majority of patients with diabetic nephropathy also have diabetic retinopathy. It has been shown that a blood pressure exceeding 140/80 mm Hg is associated with deterioration of retinal status. In addition, it has been reported that pregnancy per se deteriorates retinal status. We would thus advise a target blood pressure below 130/80 mm Hg.[54]

The only treatment strategy for hypertension associated with improved fetal growth is bed rest. Lying on the left side should be encouraged to facilitate venous return from the lower extremities. Venous flow is impaired when the gravid uterus is blocking the inferior vena cava. Bed rest increases uterine blood flow and therefore is associated with improved fetal growth. Thus, a concerted trial of bed rest should be made as the first line of therapy (Table 37–9).

If the blood pressure continues to be elevated despite absolute bed rest and salt restriction, medication should then be added. Only two antihypertensive medications have stood the test of time and have not been associated with congenital anomalies: methyldopa and hydralazine.

Methyldopa has the advantageous side effect of drowsiness. It thus aids in enforcing bed rest. It has a short half-life; thus, to be used effectively, it should be given at least every 6 hours. A starting dose of 250 mg every 6 hours can be increased up to 500 mg every 6 hours, and blood pressure should be monitored at least twice daily. If the patient is at home, she will require a self-testing blood pressure device.

If her blood pressure is persistently greater than 130/80 mm Hg, then hydralazine can be added. Hydralazine, too, should be prescribed every 6 hours and is ideal as an addition to methyldopa. Beginning doses can be 10 mg every 6 hours, increased to 25 mg every 6 hours.

Diuretics are used sparingly because of their association with reduced uterine perfusion. Clonidine has not been adequately evaluated in pregnancy but has been associated with an embryopathy in animals. Converting enzyme inhibitors have been associated with fetal death and renal abnor-

TABLE 37–9. Treatment Strategies for Patients with Hypertension due to Diabetic Kidney Disease

Preconception
Step 1:
- Normalize blood glucose.
- Maintain blood pressure <130/80 mm Hg.
- Document that creatinine clearance is >50 ml/min.

Step 2:
- Cautiously stop blood pressure medicines.
- Document that blood pressure is <130/80 mm Hg.
- Start low-salt (3 gm) restricted-fluids (<2 quarts/day) diet.

Postconception
- Document that blood pressure is <130/80 mm Hg.
- If >130/80 mm Hg, begin strict bed rest.
- If blood pressure is still >130/80, begin methyldopa, 250 mg PO every 6 hr.
- If blood pressure is still >130/80 mm Hg, increase to 500 mg PO every 6 hr.
- If blood pressure is still >130/80 mm Hg, add hydralazine, 10 mg PO every 6 hr.
- Increase to 25 mg PO every 6 hr if blood pressure is still >130/80 mm Hg.
- Alternative antihypertensives, beginning with the safest: labetalol and nifedipine.

Drugs useful for a hypertensive crisis
Hydralazine, 25–50 mg IM
Nifedipine, 10 mg every 4 hr increased by 10-mg increments up to 30 mg every 4 hr
Diazoxide, 50 mg IV every 2 min

PO, Orally; IM, intramuscularly; IV, intravenously.

malities, although they have been used late in pregnancy. The β-blockers have had variable success and are only rarely associated with fetal death. A newer β-blocker, labetalol, has received the best reviews. Experience with calcium channel blockers such as nifedipine has also been limited. Thus, if the old standbys methyldopa and hydralazine do not lower blood pressure, the choice of other agents is difficult.

Up to 1983, 1200 gestations in 789 patients who had previously undergone renal transplantation were reported. Of these women, 308 had diabetes as the cause of their kidney disease. Seventy-one percent of these women delivered a live term infant. Kidney rejection episodes occurred in 9% of these pregnancies. Other major maternal complications included severe hypertension and proteinuria. The neonatal complications included intrauterine growth retardation and prematurity. Immunosuppression therapy occasionally caused thymic atrophy, transient leukopenia, active cytomegalovirus infection, bone marrow hypoplasia, chromosome aberrations, hypoglycemia, and hypocalcemia. Most researchers recommend that pregnancy be attempted by transplant recipients only if the blood pressure and renal status have been normal for at least 2 years on low-dose maintenance immunosuppression.[49]

Diabetic nephropathy is not a contraindication to pregnancy. Severe hypertension is a contraindication. Pregnancies maintained normotensive (<130/80 mm Hg) and normoglycemic can be predicted to result in a healthy infant without deterioration of the mother's kidney function. In our experience,[50] mothers who have sustained euglycemia and normotension throughout pregnancy have continued improvement in their kidney function after the pregnancy. Eight women who have later had a second baby have continued to have further improvement in their kidney function, which has remained stable for more than 7 years, suggesting that if hypertension and hyperglycemia are avoided, pregnancy may actually be associated with an improvement in kidney function in women with diabetic renal disease.

Maternal eye status requires comprehensive evaluation before planning a pregnancy. Normal findings on retinal examination usually suggest that retinopathy will not occur during a pregnancy. Even one microaneurysm, however, may mean that the retinal status may deteriorate during pregnancy. Proliferative retinopathy could evolve to malignant retinopathy. In addition, aggressive programs to normalize the blood glucose level may aggravate the predisposed retina to accelerate the retinopathic process. The best plan is to have an ophthalmologist examine patients before pregnancy. If retinopathy exists, even background retinopathy, a program to normalize blood glucose levels should be targeted to bring the blood glucose into the normal range over 3 to 6 months. Pregnancy can then be planned, with the ophthalmologist maintaining surveillance monthly throughout pregnancy. Laser therapy is not contraindicated during pregnancy and should be used judiciously if new vessel growth occurs. Retinopathy usually regresses postpartum, but breast-feeding, which sustains salt- and water-retaining hormones (specifically prolactin) in an elevated range, may exacerbate retinopathy.[55]

All diabetic women who are planning to become pregnant need a comprehensive work-up as outlined in Table 37–7.

TIMING OF DELIVERY

When pregnancy is complicated by hyperglycemia, the risk of stillbirth increases as term approaches. In an attempt to decrease these losses, obstetricians have electively induced delivery in such pregnancies between 35 and 38 weeks' gestation. However, this approach may have resulted in significant neonatal morbidity because of prematurity and hyaline membrane disease.[56]

Neonatal morbidity can be markedly reduced if delivery is delayed until pulmonary maturity is documented. Therefore, watchful waiting is warranted and should be continued as long as maternal normoglycemia is maintained and the fetus is stable. Because programs of normoglycemia are relatively new and tools for fetal surveillance are improving rapidly, a protocol for optimal fetal surveillance is yet to be validated.

In pregnancies in which glucose control has been less than optimal, the lecithin-to-sphingomyelin ratio of the amniotic fluid should be assessed at 36 to 37 weeks' gestation.[57] The presence of phosphatidylglycerol in the fluid also implies pulmonary maturity. A fetus with documented pulmonary maturity and poor results on fetal surveillance protocols should be delivered. In a pregnancy in which glucose control is documented to be normal by six blood glucose determinations a day and normal glycosylated hemoglobin tests monthly, the woman should expect a term delivery.

LABOR AND DELIVERY

With improvement in antenatal care, intrapartum events play an increasingly crucial part in the outcome of pregnancy. Before active labor, insulin requirements are present as noted previously, and glucose infusion is not necessary to maintain a blood glucose level of 70 to 90 mg per dl. With the onset of active labor, insulin requirements decrease to zero and glucose requirements are relatively consistent at 2.55 mg per kg per minute. From these data, a protocol for supplying the glucose needs of labor has been developed.[58] The goal is to maintain maternal blood glucose levels between 70 and 90 mg per dl. The protocol for a planned induction is outlined in Table 37–10. In cases of the onset of active spontaneous labor, insulin is withheld and intravenous dextrose infusion is begun at a rate of 2.55 mg per kg per minute (10 gm/hour in a 60-kg woman). If labor is latent, normal saline is usually sufficient to maintain normoglycemia until active labor begins, at which time dextrose is infused at 2.55 mg per kg per minute. The blood glucose level is then monitored hourly, and if it is less than 60 mg per dl, the infusion rate is doubled for the subsequent hour. If the blood glucose value rises to greater than 140 mg per dl, 2 to 4 U of regular insulin is given intravenously or subcutaneously each hour until the blood glucose level is 70 to 90 mg per dl. In the case of an elective cesarean section, the

TABLE 37–10. Protocol for Planned Induction of Labor and Delivery in Women with Insulin-Dependent Diabetes or Insulin-Requiring Gestational Diabetes

1. The evening before the planned induction of labor and delivery, give the usual dose of NPH before bed.
2. Nothing to eat (NPO) after midnight.
3. If blood glucose is <60 mg/dl throughout the night, hard candy and frozen sweetened ices are permissible to bring the blood glucose back up to >60 mg/dl (3.3 mmol).
4. On the morning of the induction, no more subcutaneous insulin is necessary.
5. Start the intravenous with a solution of normal saline and infuse at a rate of 75 ml/hr.
6. Measure the blood glucose by finger-stick determination and switch the intravenous solution based on the blood glucose measured such that:
   - Blood glucose <60 mg/dl = $D_{10}W$ at 75 ml/hr for 20 min, recheck blood glucose and continue to infuse for as long as it takes to bring blood glucose to >60 mg/dl.
   - Blood glucose 60–110 mg/dl = D_5W.
   - Blood glucose >110 mg/dl = normal saline.
   - Blood glucose >140 mg/dl = normal saline and give 2–4 U of regular insulin for every hour that the blood glucose is >140 mg/dl.

bedtime dose of NPH insulin is repeated at 8 A.M. on the day of surgery and every 8 hours thereafter if the surgery is delayed. A dextrose infusion as described may be started if the blood glucose level falls below 60 mg per dl.[59]

NEONATAL CARE

If the blood glucose level of a diabetic woman is normalized throughout pregnancy, there is no evidence that unusual attention needs to be paid to her child. However, if a normal blood glucose level has not been documented throughout pregnancy, it is wise to monitor the infant in an intensive care unit for at least 24 hours postpartum. The blood glucose level should be monitored hourly for 6 hours. If the neonate shows no signs of respiratory distress, hypocalcemia, or hyperbilirubinemia at 24 hours after delivery, he or she is discharged to the nursery.[60]

POSTPARTUM INSULIN REQUIREMENTS

Maternal insulin requirements usually decline precipitously postpartum and can be decreased for up to 48 to 96 hours postpartum. Insulin requirements should be recalculated at 0.6 U kg per 24 hours based on the postpartum weight and should be started when the postprandial glucose level exceeds 150 mg per dl or the fasting glucose level is greater than 100 mg per dl. The postpartum caloric requirements are 25 kcal per kg per day, based on postpartum weight.

BREAST-FEEDING

Those who advocate breast-feeding say that the advantages include a passive immunity against infection for the infant, better tooth development, convenience for the mother, and increased bonding. In addition, one report suggests that when cow's milk is given to infants before the ninth month of age, antibodies to the bovine albumin may cross-react to the pancreas in predisposed infants and initiate the development of diabetes.[61] Now that diabetic women are succeeding in becoming pregnant and delivering normal, healthy infants, they too want the option of nursing their infants.

Human milk is composed of protein, fat, and carbohydrate in the form of lactose. Maternal serum glucose and insulin are present in such small quantities that under normal circumstances, neither of these are detected in maternal milk.[62]

A woman with diabetes often has high levels of circulating insulin, a result of either the doses she injects or type II diabetes and insulin resistance. A high circulating insulin level can result in significant insulin levels in milk. These levels peak about 1 hour after the peak in serum and are about equal to the serum levels.

Insulin is not absorbed from the gut but is degraded in the stomach by digestive enzymes. Neonates do not have well-developed digestive enzymes, and thus insulin in milk may be absorbed across the neonatal gut into the baby's bloodstream. It has been postulated but not proved that elevated levels of insulin in maternal milk may contribute to neonatal adiposity, especially if the mother is spilling glucose into the milk.

Glucose spills become detectable in maternal milk when maternal blood glucose level is approximately 140 mg per dl.[62] Added glucose in maternal milk may cause tooth decay, produce a preference for sweetness, and add an extra 2% of the total calories in 24 hours, an increase sufficient to cause obesity if sustained over 20 years. Although few data are available to substantiate the preceding hypothesis, it would appear prudent for a nursing woman with diabetes to maintain her blood glucose level as near to normal (<140 mg/dl) as possible.

Nutritionists have traditionally suggested that a nursing woman add 200 to 300 calories per day to her diet to compensate for the calories lost by breast-feeding. It has been shown that the caloric needs of a nursing mother may not be higher than in women who are not nursing. Nursing apparently alters fuel maintenance so that calories are used efficiently and metabolism slows to compensate for the calories lost. Thus, a nursing woman can eat to satiety rather than force-feed extra calories, making weight gain less likely during breast-feeding. Water and calcium intake do need to be increased.

Because nursing women may not need more calories than other women, there is no need to increase the insulin requirement.[63] On the contrary, because the body loses carbohydrates to produce breast milk, the insulin requirement may drop. When a baby nurses in the middle of the night, a time when most women do not eat, the baby acts as a siphon, drawing off milk and calories, in turn increasing the risk of hypoglycemia. Most nursing mothers with diabetes find that their overnight insulin requirement (bedtime NPH) can easily be cut in half. In instances when the baby nurses twice in a night, mothers have been able to discontinue their nighttime NPH. The daytime insulin requirement appears not to change. If a woman has difficulty with middle-of-the-night low blood glucose levels, then the NPH dose before bed should be discontinued and the other insulin doses should be distributed as needed in the prebreakfast injection and the predinner injection.

Diabetic women may be encouraged to breast-feed their infants. Not only is maternal milk better than formula feeding, but also nursing provides motivation to continue the work it takes to maintain euglycemia.[62]

REFERENCES

1. White P. Pregnancy complicating diabetes. JAMA 1945;128:181.
2. Jovanovic L, Peterson CM. Management of the pregnant diabetic women. Diabetes Care 1980;3:63.
3. Miller E, Hare JW, Cloherty JP, et al. Elevated maternal hemoglobin Alc in early pregnancy and major congenital anomalies in infants of diabetic mothers. N Engl J Med 1981;304:1331.
4. Adashi EY, Pinto H, Tyson JE. Impact of euglycemia on the outcome in diabetic pregnancy. Am J Obstet Gynecol 1979;133:268.
5. Day R, Insley J. Maternal diabetes and congenital malformations. Arch Dis Child 1976;51:935.
6. Steel JM. Prepregnancy counseling and contraception in the insulin-dependent diabetic patient. Clin Obstet Gynecol 1985;28:553.
7. Damm P, Molsted-Pedersen L. Significant decrease in congenital malformations in newborn infants of an unselected population of diabetic women. Am J Obstet Gynecol 1989;161:1163.
8. Kitzmiller JL, Gavin LA, Gin GD, et al. Preconceptional

9. Leslie RDG, Pyke DA, John PN, White JM. Hemoglobin Alc in diabetic pregnancy. Lancet 1978;2:958.
10. Goldman JA, Dickerd D, Feldberg D. Pregnancy outcome in patients with insulin-dependent diabetes mellitus with preconceptual diabetic control: A comparative study. Am J Obstet Gynecol 1986;155:193.
11. Mills JL, Knopp RH, Simpson JL, et al. Lack of relation of increased malformation rates in infants of diabetic mothers to glycemic control during organogenesis. N Engl J Med 1988;318:671.
12. Fuhrmann K, Ruher H, Semmler K, et al. Prevention of congenital malformations in infants of insulin dependent diabetic mothers. Diabetes Care 1983;6:219.
13. Greene MF, Hare JW, Cloherty JP, et al. First trimester hemoglobin A1 and risk of major malformation and spontaneous abortion in diabetic pregnancy. Teratology 1989;39:225.
14. Mills JL, Baker L, Goldman AS. Malformations in infants of diabetic mothers occur before the seventh gestational week: Implications for treatment. Diabetes 1979;28:292.
15. Ylinen K, Aula P, Stenmen UH, et al. Risk of minor and major fetal malformations in diabetics with high hemoglobin Alc values in early pregnancy. Br Med J 1984;289:345.
16. Miodovnik M, Mimouni F, Dignam PS. Major malformations in infants of IDDM women; vasculopathy and early first trimester poor glycemic control. Diabetes Care 1988;11:713.
17. Jovanovic-Peterson L, Peterson CM, Saxena BB, et al. Feasibility of maintaining normal glucose profiles in insulin-dependent pregnant women. Am J Med 1980;68:105.
18. Csapo AL, Pulkkinen MO, Wiest WG. Effects of luteectomy and progesterone replacement in early pregnant patients. Am J Obstet Gynecol 1973;115:759.
19. Jaffe RB, Yen SSC. The endocrinology of pregnancy. In: Reproductive Endocrinology: Physiology, Pathophysiology and Clinical Management. Philadelphia: WB Saunders, 1978, pp 521–536.
20. Jovanovic-Peterson L, Dawood MY, Landesman R, Saxena BB. Hormonal profile as a prognostic index of early threatened abortion. Am J Obstet Gynecol 1978;130:274.
21. Hiriis-Nielsen J, Nielsen V, Molsted-Pedersen L, Deckert T. Effects of pregnancy hormones on pancreatic islets in organ culture. Diabetes 1986;III:336.
22. Barberia JR, Whu-Fadil S, Kletzky OA, et al. Serum prolactin patterns in early human gestation. Am J Obstet Gynecol 1975;121:1107.
23. Ho Yuen B, Cannon W, Lewis J, et al. A possible role for prolactin in the control of human chorionic gonadotropin and estrogen secretion by the fetoplacental unit. Am J Obstet Gynecol 1980;136:286.
24. Michaels RL, Sorenson RL, Parsons JA, Sheridan JD. Prolactin enhances cell-to-cell communication among beta-cells in pancreatic islets. Diabetes 1987;36:1098.
25. Josimovich JB. Endocrinology of Pregnancy Placental Lactogenic Hormone. New York: Harper & Row, 1971, pp 184–196.
26. Gaspard VJ, Sandront HM, Luyckx AS, et al. The control of human placental lactogen (HPL) secretion and its interrelation with glucose and lipid metabolism in late pregnancy. In: Early Diabetes in Early Life. New York: Academic Press, 1975, pp 273–278.
27. Jovanovic-Peterson L, Druzin M, Peterson CM. Effect of euglycemia on the outcome of pregnancy in insulin-dependent diabetic women as compared with normal control subjects. Am J Med 1981;71:921.
28. Kuhl C, Hornnes PJ. Endocrine pancreatic function in

women with gestational diabetes. Acta Endocrinol 1986;277:19.

29. Summary and recommendations of the third international workshop/conference on gestational diabetes. Diabetes 1990 (Suppl 2);40:197.

30. Gillmner MDG, Beard RW, Oakley NW, et al. Diurnal plasma free fatty acid profiles in normal and diabetic pregnancies. Br Med J 1977;2:670.

31. Pedersen J. The Pregnant Diabetic and Her Newborn. Copenhagen: Munksgaard International Publishers, 1977, pp 1–280.

32. Jovanovic-Peterson L, Peterson CM. Dietary manipulation as a primary strategy for pregnancies complicated by diabetes. J Am Coll Nutr 1990;9:320.

33. Jovanovic-Peterson L, Peterson CM, Wilkins M. Management of the obese gestational diabetic pregnant woman. Diabetes Professional Fall 1990:6.

34. Jovanovic-Peterson L, Peterson CM, Reed GF, et al. Maternal postprandial glucose levels and infant birth weight: The diabetes in early pregnancy study. Am J Obstet Gynecol 1991;164:103.

35. Freinkel N, Metzger BE, Phelps RL, et al. Gestational diabetes mellitus: Heterogeneity of maternal age, weight, insulin secretion, HLA antigens, and islet cell antibodies and the impact of maternal metabolism on pancreatic B-cell and somatic development in the offspring. Diabetes 34 1985;(Suppl 2):1.

36. Jovanovic-Peterson L, Peterson CM. Is exercise safe or useful for gestational diabetic women. Diabetes 1991;(Suppl 2)40:179.

37. American College of Obstetrics and Gynecology. Home exercise Program. Washington, D.C.: American College of Obstetrics and Gynecology, 1986.

38. Jovanovic-Peterson L, Kessler A, Peterson CM. Human maternal and fetal response to graded exercise. J Appl Physiol 1985;58:1719.

39. Mittelmark RA, Wiswell RA, Drinkwater BL. Fetal responses to maternal exercise. In: Mittelmark RA, Posner MD (eds). Exercise in Pregnancy. Baltimore: Williams & Wilkins; 1991, pp 213–224.

40. Paolone AM, Shangold M, Paul D, et al. Fetal heart rate measurements during maternal exercise—avoidance of artifact. Med Sci Sports Exerc 1987;19(6):605.

41. Jovanovic-Peterson L, Peterson CM. Fuel metabolism in pregnancy—clinical aspects. In: Artal R (ed). Exercise in Pregnancy. Baltimore: Williams & Wilkins; 1990, pp 45–60.

42. Durak EP, Jovanovic-Peterson L, Peterson CM. Comparative evaluation of five aerobic machines and their effect on uterine activity during pregnancy. Am J Obstet Gynecol 1990;162:754.

43. Jovanovic-Peterson L, Durak EP, Peterson CM. Randomized trial of diet versus diet plus cardiovascular conditioning on glucose levels in gestational diabetes. Am J Obstet Gynecol 1989;161:415.

44. Kimmerle R, Kurz KH, Weiss R, Berger M. Effectiveness, Safety and Acceptability of a Copper Intrauterine Device (CU safe 300R) in 58 Type 1 Diabetic Women. New York: American Diabetes Association, 1992.

45. Mischell DR. Medical progress: Contraception. N Engl J Med 1989;320:777.

46. Warram JH, Krolewski AS, Gottlieb MS, Kahn CR. Differences in risk of insulin-dependent diabetes in offspring of diabetic mothers and diabetic fathers. N Engl J Med 1984;311:149.

47. Jovanovic-Peterson L. Summary and comment on expanded care in obstetrics for the 1980's: Preconception and early post conception counseling. Diabetes Spectrum 1990;3:179.

48. Jovanovic-Peterson L, Peterson CM. Optimal insulin delivery for pregnant diabetic patients. Diabetes Care 1982;(Suppl 1)5:24.

49. Hare JW. Diabetes Complicating Pregnancy: The Joslin Clinic Method. New York: Alan R Liss, 1989.

50. Jovanovic-Peterson L, Peterson CM. Is pregnancy contraindicated in women with diabetic nephropathy? Diabetic Nephropathy 1984;3:36.

51. Jovanovic-Peterson L, Peterson CM. De novo hypothyroidism in pregnancies complicated by type 1 diabetes and proteinuria: A new syndrome. Am J Obstet Gynecol 1988;159:441.

52. Kitzmiller JL, Brown ER, Phillippe M, et al. Diabetic nephropathy and perinatal outcome. Am J Obstet Gynecol 1981;141:741.

53. Fuhrmann K, Reiher H, Semmler K, et al. Congenital anomalies: Etiology, prevention and prenatal diagnosis. In: Jovanovic L, Peterson CM, Fuhrmann K (eds). Diabetes and Pregnancy. New York: Praeger, 1986, pp 168–186.

54. Peterson CM, Jovanovic-Peterson L. Approach to hypertension in pregnancy complicated by diabetes. Diabetes Professional, Summer 1991:1.

55. Jovanovic-Peterson L, Peterson CM. Diabetic retinopathy. In: Coustan DR, Ritkin RM, Scott JR (eds). Clinical Obstetrics and Gynecology: Diabetes and Pregnancy. Philadelphia: JB Lippincott, 1991, pp 516–525.

56. Drury MI, Greene AT, Stronge JM. Pregnancy complicated by clinical diabetes mellitus: A study of 600 pregnancies. Obstet Gynecol 1977;49:519.

57. Huffaker J. Fetal pulmonary maturation in the infant of the diabetic mother. In: Jovanovic-Peterson L, Peterson CM, Fuhrmann K (eds). Diabetes and Pregnancy. Teratology, Toxicity and Treatment. New York: Praeger, 1986, pp 361–392.

58. Jovanovic-Peterson L, Peterson CM. Insulin and glucose requirements during the first stage of labor in insulin-dependent diabetic women. Am J Med 1983;75:607.

59. Jovanovic-Peterson L, Peterson CM. Insulin and glucose administration during labor and delivery. Diabetes Professional. Spring. 1991:20.

60. Cowett RM. The metabolic sequelae in the infant of the diabetic mother. In: Jovanovic L (ed). Controversies in Diabetes and Pregnancy. New York: Springer-Verlag, 1988, pp 149–171.

61. Jovanovic-Peterson L, Peterson CM. Maternal milk and plasma glucose and insulin levels: Studies in normal and diabetic subjects. J Am Col Nutr 1989;8:125.

62. Jovanovic-Peterson L. Women and diabetes: What you should know about breast-feeding. Diabetes Self-Management July/August 1991:14.

63. Behan E. Eat Well, Lose Weight While Breastfeeding. New York: Villard Books, 1992.

38

Thyroid Disease and Pregnancy

Caren G. Solomon and Ellen W. Seely

Thyroid disease is relatively frequent in young women and is not uncommonly diagnosed during or soon after pregnancy. The association of thyroid dysfunction with the pregnant or postpartum state in part reflects the fact that otherwise healthy women may not visit a physician before pregnancy. In addition, immunologic alterations characteristic of early pregnancy and the postpartum state may induce certain thyroid disorders.

Diagnosis of thyroid dysfunction in pregnancy may be complicated by changes in thyroid function test results characteristic of the normal pregnant state. Levels of T_4 are characteristically elevated related to the rise in thyroxine-binding globulin (TBG). This elevation can raise suspicions of hyperthyroidism. The newer supersensitive thyroid-stimulating hormone (TSH) assays have helped in distinguishing the TBG-related rise in T_4 (where TSH is in the normal range) from hyperthyroidism (where TSH is suppressed). However, with wider use of these newer assay, it has become clear that other pregnancy-related disorders (e.g., hyperemesis gravidarum) may be asso-

ciated with suppressed TSH levels, and therefore, thyroid function test results must be interpreted in the context of the clinical presentation.

Although potentially complicated, diagnosis of thyroid dysfunction in pregnancy is important because both hyperthyroidism and hypothyroidism may have deleterious effects on a mother and her fetus. This chapter describes thyroid disorders that may occur in pregnancy and postpartum and provides guidelines for their diagnosis and management.

EFFECTS OF PREGNANCY ON THE NORMAL THYROID

Pregnancy is associated with significant changes in thyroid function test results (Table 38–1). Levels of TBG increase early in gestation, an effect that is thought to be secondary to an estrogen-induced decrease in liver metabolism of this protein. Levels of TBG are measured and reported directly by some laboratories, but increases in this

TABLE 38–1. Thyroid Values in Pregnancy

	TSH	T_4	TBG	FT_4	T_3
Normal pregnancy	⇌ (May be low in 1st trimester)	↑	↑	⇌ (? ↑)	↑
Hyperthyroid	↓	↑ ↑	↑	↑	↑ ↑
Hyperemesis*	↓	↑ ↑	↑	↑	⇌
Molar pregnancy	↓	↑ ↑	↑	↑	↑ ↑
Postpartum thyroiditis†					
Hyperthyroid phase	↓	↑ ↑	⇌	↑	↑ ↑
Hypothyroid phase	↑	↓	⇌	↓	⇌
Hypothyroidism‡	↑	↓	↑	↓	⇌

*When hyperemesis is associated with signs of malnutrition, TBG can be low.
†In the early phase of hypothyroidism secondary to postpartum thyroiditis, the TSH can still be suppressed.
‡In severe hypothyroidism, total T_3 will fall but is usually preserved when mild.
TSH, Thyroid-stimulating hormone; TBG, thyroxine-binding globulin; FT_4, free T_4.

protein are more commonly reflected by a fall in T_3 resin uptake. Levels of T_4 and T_3 increase consistent with the rise in TBG; free T_4 and T_3 levels probably remain normal, although they may be slightly increased. Most helpful in evaluating thyroid function in pregnancy is the level of TSH, which should remain in the normal range in euthyroid pregnancy. However, one situation in which the TSH level may be confusing is in the first trimester of pregnancy, when the level can be low. This transient decline in TSH may result from the thyroid-stimulating effect of high levels of human chorionic gonadotropin (hCG), which has the same alpha chain as TSH. Even in this setting, though, TSH levels, as measured by the supersensitive assays now available, should be detectable, and levels should return to the normal range as hCG levels decline with progression of pregnancy.

It is often claimed that goiters are common in normal pregnancy. Although the thyroid gland may enlarge significantly in pregnant women living in regions of iodine deficiency,[1] thyroid size does not increase appreciably during pregnancy in iodine-replete areas such as the United States. Ultrasound examination may be able to pick up small increases in thyroid volume not detectable by physical examination,[2] but detection of an obviously enlarged thyroid in a pregnant woman is an indication for further evaluation to identify the cause.

FERTILITY AND THYROID DISEASE

Reproductive function may be adversely affected by thyroid disease. Hypothyroidism has been linked to luteal phase defects[3] and anovulation, in many cases as a result of associated hyperprolactinemia. Spontaneous abortion, usually in the first trimester, has also been reported with hypothyroidism, although hypothyroidism appears to account for only a small minority of pregnancy losses.[4] Early pregnancy losses have been noted to be more common in women with elevated titers of thyroid autoantibodies, even in the setting of normal results of thyroid function tests.[5] Hyperthyroidism may also inhibit ovulation and increase risk of miscarriage, but generally only when thyrotoxicosis is severe. Mild to moderate hyperthyroidism is thought to have minimal effect on fertility or ability to maintain a pregnancy.[4] However, the effect of mild thyroid dysfunction on reproductive function has not been well studied. Of note, a history of treatment with radioactive iodine antedating pregnancy appears to have no adverse impact on subsequent childbearing.[6]

HYPERTHYROIDISM IN PREGNANCY

Hyperthyroidism complicates 0.2% of pregnancies and is associated with maternal morbidity and both fetal and neonatal morbidity and mortality.[7] Complications in the mother include thyroid storm and inadequate weight gain; fetal and neonatal complications are discussed later.

Graves' disease, an autoimmune process in which thyroid-stimulating immunoglobulins (TSI) are directed against the TSH receptor, is the most common cause of hyperthyroidism in pregnancy. Hydatidiform mole, another cause of hyperthyroidism, is discussed later. Hyperthyroidism may also be caused by toxic nodules, either in isolation or within a multinodular goiter; because these disorders are more common with increasing age, they rarely underlie hyperthyroidism in pregnancy.

Diagnosis of hyperthyroidism may be complicated by the similarity of many of its symptoms to manifestations of normal pregnancy—for example, heat intolerance and palpitations. Furthermore, as noted earlier, elevations in T_4 and T_3 levels above the normal range are characteristic of normal pregnancy, reflecting the increased levels of TBG.

Nonetheless, clinical and biochemical data may raise suspicion of hyperthyroidism. For example, ophthalmopathy or subnormal weight gain or even weight loss is suggestive when present. Severe hyperemesis is an occasional manifestation. Biochemically, marked elevations in T_3 and T_4 and a suppressed or undetectable TSH level are generally diagnostic of hyperthyroidism. (A potential exception is hyperemesis gravidarum, discussed later.)

Once hyperthyroidism has been diagnosed, therapy is generally medical, although surgery is an option for severely hyperthyroid patients poorly controlled on medications or intolerant of them. Radioactive ^{131}I is strictly contraindicated during pregnancy. Uptake by the fetal thyroid can result in profound hypothyroidism with devastating effects on development.[8] Although the fetal thyroid does not generally begin to function until the twelfth week of gestation, and several reports describe radioactive iodine being administered inadvertently before this time without adverse effects,[9] this therapy is best avoided at all stages of pregnancy.

Medical treatment involves inhibition of thyroid hormone synthesis with propylthiouracil (PTU) or methimazole. Propylthiouracil is the preferred medication to treat hyperthyroidism in pregnancy. Because PTU crosses the placenta, it should be given in the smallest dose possible to control hyperthyroidism; the goal is to bring the mother's thyroid function test results into the slightly hyperthyroid to upper normal range while maintaining a euthyroid fetus.[10] It is generally recommended that PTU doses not exceed 400 mg daily, given in two to three divided doses. Overtreatment must be carefully avoided because it increases the risk of fetal hypothyroidism and goiter. Although high doses of PTU can block conversion of T_4 to T_3, the primary action of PTU in the dose range recommended during pregnancy is to block organification of thyroid hormone. Although PTU doses higher than those recommended are occasionally required to control severe maternal hyperthyroidism, risks to the fetus must be recognized, and surgery in the second trimester should probably be considered as a therapeutic alternative.

Methimazole may also be used to treat Graves' disease in pregnancy. However, because it crosses the placenta to a greater extent than PTU,[11, 12] it is more likely to induce fetal hypothyroidism. Furthermore, methimazole may be associated with a fetal scalp defect known as aplasia cutis,[13] although this association has been called into question.[14] As a result, methimazole is generally considered a second choice in the United States, although it is widely used in Europe.

Graves' disease often remits as pregnancy progresses.[15] Thus, the dose of PTU may be gradually decreased in the majority of cases and in many cases may be discontinued in the third trimester. Thyroid function test results therefore should be monitored at frequent intervals (i.e., every 4 to 6 weeks) to facilitate dose reduction as possible.

Beta-blockers may be used to help control symptoms of hyperthyroidism temporarily until antithyroid medication becomes effective. Propranolol is considered relatively safe in pregnancy although it has been associated with intrauterine growth retardation. Therefore, if needed to control symptoms, β-blockers should be tapered as symptoms are controlled so that the fetus is exposed for as short a period as possible.

Because iodide crosses the placenta and inhibits fetal thyroid hormone release, this therapy has been considered dangerous even for temporary treatment of hyperthyroidism, owing to the concern that the fetal thyroid is less able to escape the suppressive effects of this therapy. Although this effect has been questioned,[16] iodide therapy should be reserved for emergency situations such as thyroid storm and then used only temporarily.

Recurrence or exacerbation of hyperthyroidism after delivery is common,[15] occurring in as many as 70% of women with a history of Graves' disease. Follow-up of thyroid function test results within 2 to 3 months postpartum is thus important. Because antithyroid drugs cross into breast milk, concern has been expressed about breast-feeding

in women being treated with these medications. As compared with methimazole, PTU passes into breast milk only 10% as well and thus is preferred if a woman is breast-feeding.[11, 17–19] PTU doses less than 200 to 300 mg daily are considered relatively safe by many experts. However, in view of the deleterious effects of even mild hypothyroidism on mental and physical development, it is suggested that any infant who is breast-fed by a mother taking antithyroid medication have thyroid function checked regularly.

To decrease risk of exacerbation of previous Graves' disease during pregnancy or postpartum, it is often recommended that women diagnosed with Graves' disease be treated with radioactive iodine before becoming pregnant. In this case, a 6- to 12-month delay after therapy is recommended before conception to avoid any risk to the fetus. Of note, past therapy with radioactive iodine or thyroidectomy does not eliminate the risk of neonatal Graves' disease in offspring, because TSI may persist in high titer in the mother and be transferred to the fetus through the placenta.

Radioactive ^{131}I may not be attractive as a treatment option in the early postpartum period. Studies have shown that therapeutic doses of ^{131}I cross into breast milk and may be detectable for as long as 2 months, depending on the dose given.[20, 21] Therefore, cessation of breast-feeding is generally recommended. If a mother chooses to pump and discard milk during this time, in order to resume breast-feeding later, an expressed sample of milk should be checked for radioactivity before restarting. In addition to interfering with breast-feeding, the use of therapeutic doses of radioactive ^{131}I necessitates avoidance of close contact between mother and child for several days after therapy.

It has been suggested that treatment with thyroid hormone during and after pregnancy in women who have had remission of Graves' disease during pregnancy may markedly decrease risk of recurrence of hyperthyroidism postpartum.[22] The mechanism of this effect thus far remains unclear, but suppression of production of antibodies against the thyroid hormone receptor is apparent when thyroid hormone is given. It is interesting to speculate whether this therapy might decrease risk of neonatal Graves' disease as well, although this has yet to be evaluated.

FETAL AND NEONATAL COMPLICATIONS OF MATERNAL GRAVES' DISEASE

The Fetus

Fetal hyperthyroidism is a rare complication of maternal Graves' disease. Because TSI are of the immunoglobulin G class, these immunoglobulins can cross the placenta. Permeability of the placenta for immunoglobulins increases as pregnancy progresses, with a dramatic increase in fetal immunoglobulin G levels to approximate maternal levels after 26 weeks' gestation; this likely accounts for the usual presentation of fetal Graves' disease in the third trimester of pregnancy.[23]

Administration of antithyroid medication (e.g., PTU or methimazole) to a hyperthyroid woman during pregnancy usually results in concomitant control of maternal TSI-induced fetal hyperthyroidism, because these medications cross the placenta. However, if a woman has been treated for Graves' disease before pregnancy with radioactive iodine ablation or thyroidectomy, high TSI levels may persist despite resolution of hyperthyroidism. Transplacental passage of maternal TSI can lead to stimulation of the fetal thyroid and fetal hyperthyroidism, in the absence of any clinical manifestations in the mother. Thus, it is important that women with even a remote history of treated Graves' disease be made aware that this medical history may be important during pregnancy and should be conveyed to their caregivers.

Fetal hyperthyroidism can be associated with premature labor, craniosynostosis, and intrauterine fetal growth retardation and demise. Signs of fetal hyperthyroidism are tachycardia (heart rate > 160), increased fetal activity, fetal goiter on ultrasonography, and accelerated bone age. Fetal tachycardia can serve as a simple though not precise clinical marker to assess the need for initiating and adjusting therapy. Percutaneous umbilical blood sampling allows direct determination of fetal thyroid status and may be an alternative in centers with great expertise in the technology.[24]

Therapy of fetal Graves' disease has entailed treating the mother with PTU or methimazole, beginning in the late second or third trimester and titrating the dose to a fetal heart rate of 120 to 160.[4, 23]

The Neonate

Neonatal Graves' disease, symptomatic thyrotoxicosis in the newborn, results from transplacental passage of thyroid-stimulating antibodies. Manifestations include tachycardia, tachypnea, irritability, difficulty in feeding, and inadequate weight gain. A large goiter in a neonate may result in tracheal compression, asphyxia, and potentially death. Because PTU and methimazole cross the placenta, infants born to mothers taking these medications may not present with hyperthyroidism at birth because this may have been treated in

utero with the antithyroid medication. The neonate may therefore have normal thyroid test results at 2 to 3 days of life. However, because the transplacentally transferred TSI persist for as long as several months, the baby can present with hyperthyroidism after the antithyroid medication is cleared, usually 1 to 2 weeks postpartum. Characteristic symptoms are failure to thrive and irritability; this diagnosis should be kept in mind as a potential cause of such manifestations in the early postpartum period. Neonatal hyperthyroidism typically resolves within 2 to 3 months postpartum.[25]

In addition to frank thyrotoxicosis, infants born to mothers with Graves' disease may manifest other disturbances of thyroid function. Transient biochemical hyperthyroidism occurs in a small number of neonates. A greater percentage manifest temporary hypothyroidism, usually biochemical but occasionally symptomatic. This condition is generally attributable to transplacental passage of antithyroid drugs but may also result from transfer of maternal thyroid-inhibiting antibodies.[4]

Even in the absence of thyroid dysfunction, neonates born to mothers with Graves' disease have an increased propensity to be small for gestational age. Reported risk factors for this complication include longer duration of maternal Graves' disease before pregnancy, longer duration of thyrotoxicosis during pregnancy, and a TSI level of at least 30% at the time of delivery.[26]

HYPEREMESIS GRAVIDARUM

Hyperemesis gravidarum (i.e., intractable vomiting in pregnancy associated with weight loss and dehydration) is associated with abnormal thyroid function test results[27] in up to 75% of cases. Significant elevations in T_4, T_3 resin uptake, and free T_4 are characteristic. Suppression of TSH and TSH unresponsiveness to thyroid-releasing hormone stimulation have been reported often but not invariably. One large series using the supersensitive TSH assay reported suppressed or undetectable TSH levels in almost all patients with hyperemesis and T_4 elevations.[28]

Physical examination may help distinguish this disorder from hyperthyroidism. A goiter or exophthalmos is suggestive of hyperthyroidism. Hyperthyroidism is also suggested by persistent tachycardia after adequate hydration.

The pattern of changes in thyroid function test results may help to distinguish hyperemesis from true hyperthyroidism. Hyperemesis is frequently associated with an elevated T_4 but with a normal T_3 level and minimally elevated (<33% above normal range) free T_3 index. Hyperthyroidism, in contrast, is characterized by elevations in T_3 at least as marked as in T_4. Suppression of TSH to an undetectable range may occur in either condition but is more common with true hyperthyroidism.

The elevation in thyroid hormone levels noted with hyperemesis is generally attributed to stimulation of the thyroid gland by hCG, which, as noted previously, has an alpha chain identical to that of TSH. Levels of hCG tend to be higher in women with hyperemesis than in normal pregnancy, and a positive correlation between hCG, thyroid hormone levels, and vomiting has been found.[29] The role of hCG as stimulating the thyroid in this condition has been questioned by some investigators.[30]

Distinguishing the changes in thyroid function test results noted with hyperemesis from those of true hyperthyroidism may be difficult. Nonetheless, the distinction is important. Thyroid function changes with hyperemesis are transient and self-limited. Antithyroid drugs appear to hasten only slightly the return of thyroid test results to normal.[27] Although antithyroid drugs may occasionally result in marked amelioration of hyperemesis, this finding is inconsistent. Furthermore, no improvement in fetal outcome or birth weight has been demonstrated in offspring of women treated with antithyroid drugs for the transient thyroid changes associated with hyperemesis. Thus, the general recommendation is that hyperemesis in the absence of frank hyperthyroidism be treated with supportive therapy (fluids, antiemetics, peripheral nutrition if indicated), without antithyroid medications.

TROPHOBLASTIC DISEASE AND HYPERTHYROIDISM

Elevations in thyroid function test results are even more common with molar pregnancy or choriocarcinoma. T_3 levels are also typically elevated in the setting of trophoblastic disease. Nonetheless, levels of T_3 and ratios of T_3 to T_4 are much lower than those characteristic of Graves' disease.[31–33]

The typically high circulating levels of hCG with molar pregnancy or choriocarcinoma are believed to be responsible for thyroid stimulation. As in the case of normal pregnancy, however, this hypothesis continues to be controversial.[33]

Clinical hyperthyroidism is much less common than biochemical hyperthyroidism but is well reported. Its frequency has ranged from 0 to 60% of cases with biochemical hyperthyroidism.[31–33] In addition to common manifestations of hyperthyroidism such as sweating and tremor, pulmonary edema and cardiac failure have been reported in women with hyperthyroidism in the setting of trophoblastic disease.[32] The incidence of clinical disease has been noted to increase with increasing hCG levels.[32]

Hyperthyroidism attributable to hydatidiform mole is treated by evacuation of the uterus, with reported normalization of thyroid function within 1 week. In the setting of choriocarcinoma, reduction of tumor mass with chemotherapy markedly improves hyperthyroidism. Temporizing measures include treatment with potassium iodide to inhibit thyroid hormone secretion and β-blockade to decrease peripheral manifestations of hyperthyroidism.

HYPOTHYROIDISM DURING PREGNANCY

Hypothyroidism is more common than hyperthyroidism in pregnancy, as it is in the nonpregnant state. Because hypothyroidism is relatively common in young women, many pregnant women will have been diagnosed with hypothyroidism and maintained on thyroid hormone replacement before pregnancy. Others are diagnosed with hypothyroidism during pregnancy simply because they have not consulted a physician for years previously. Also, women with marginal thyroid reserve may not be able to meet increased demands for thyroid hormone that may be associated with pregnancy.

The most common cause of hypothyroidism during pregnancy, as in the nonpregnant state, is Hashimoto's thyroiditis, an autoimmune destruction of the thyroid gland virtually always associated with the presence of antibodies directed against thyroid peroxidase. Other causes include prior head or neck irradiation and prior radioiodine or surgical treatment for hyperthyroidism or other thyroid disease.

Complications reported in association with hypothyroidism during pregnancy include preeclampsia, placental abruption, postpartum hemorrhage, and anemia in the mother and low birth weight and increased mortality in the offspring.[34] In addition, the offspring may suffer impairment of long-term development.[35]

The symptoms of hypothyroidism in pregnant patients, as in nonpregnant patients, include fatigue, weight gain, and constipation. However, the similarity of these symptoms to those of normal pregnancy may complicate the diagnosis. Physical examination may be helpful in diagnosis if it reveals bradycardia, a goiter, dry skin, or delayed relaxation phase of reflexes. Elevation of serum

TSH level remains the best tool for confirming a diagnosis of hypothyroidism during pregnancy.

Thyroid hormone, a natural substance, is considered absolutely safe in pregnancy. Women should be treated with a dose sufficient to maintain TSH in the normal range. Doses outside of pregnancy are generally in the range of 0.8 μg per pound but are often somewhat higher in pregnancy. This increased requirement may be due to the estrogen-induced increase in TBG levels, resulting in a need for more thyroid hormone to fill more hormone-binding sites, or may possibly be due to placental metabolism of thyroid hormone. To ensure appropriate thyroid hormone replacement, TSH level should be checked approximately 4 weeks after any dose adjustment.

In women taking a stable dose of thyroid hormone before pregnancy or established on an appropriate dose in early pregnancy, it is important to remember that thyroid hormone requirements may increase with progression of pregnancy.[36] Increased requirements, as manifested by elevation in TSH, are generally noted early and have been reported at only 4 weeks' gestation.[37] Because requirements can continue to increase during pregnancy, however, it is reasonable to check levels of TSH each trimester. A return to prepregnancy thyroid doses postpartum is expected, and thus the dose can be decreased to prepregnancy levels after delivery.[37]

It was once believed that maternal thyroid hormone did not cross the placenta to any significant extent and therefore did not have a role in fetal development. However, a 1989 study demonstrating measurable serum T_4 levels in neonates unable to produce thyroid hormone, secondary to either thyroid agenesis or an organification defect, provided evidence for placental transfer of thyroxine.[38] At the same time, these data provided an explanation for the normal intrauterine development characteristic of these infants despite their lack of endogenous thyroid hormone production. Recognition that fetal thyroid hormone may be derived from the mother raises the question of an adverse effect of maternal hypothyroidism on fetal growth and development. Because the fetal thyroid does not generally produce thyroid hormone until the twelfth week of gestation, maternal thyroid hormone may have an important role in the first trimester. One study noted that offspring of insufficiently treated hypothyroid mothers may have impaired developmental, intellectual, and motor scores at 8 months and at 4 and 7 years.[35] Nonetheless, further studies are needed to define better the role of maternal thyroid hormone in fetal development and the fetal consequences, if any, of inadequately treated maternal hypothyroidism.

POSTPARTUM THYROIDITIS

Postpartum thyroiditis, also known as lymphocytic or painless thyroiditis, occurs in as many as 10% of postpartum women.[39–42] It is important to remember that postpartum thyroiditis may occur after a spontaneous abortion as well.[43] In its classic form, it is characterized by three phases: transient hyperthyroidism first, then transient hypothyroidism, and finally a return to euthyroidism. In actuality, one or more of these phases may be absent or inapparent. Some women become permanently hypothyroid.

Transient hyperthyroidism, which occurs in 70% of cases, begins approximately 1 to 3 months after delivery and persists for 1 to 2 months. Delay in diagnosis is common owing to the similarity of many of its manifestations to normal postpartum complaints, such as fatigue, difficulty sleeping, and anxiety. However, such symptoms as palpitations or tremor, or appearance of a goiter, noted in up to 90% of cases, may raise suspicion of the diagnosis. Thyroid function test results reveal elevated T_4 and T_3 levels with suppressed TSH levels.

Once hyperthyroidism is confirmed, the most important differential diagnosis is Graves' disease, which often flares 2 months or more postpartum after remission in late pregnancy and accounts for 10 to 15% of cases of postpartum hyperthyroidism. Graves' disease is suggested by a history of this condition before or during pregnancy, ophthalmopathy, a large goiter, onset of symptoms 3 or more months after delivery, and higher T_3 levels with T_3-to-T_4 ratio greater than 20. The diagnosis is often unclear at the time of presentation.

If symptoms are mild, a course of watchful waiting for improvement in hyperthyroidism or evolution to hypothyroidism consistent with thyroiditis is reasonable. Frequently, no treatment is necessary. When symptoms such as palpitations or tremor are more bothersome, a β-blocker (e.g., propranolol, 20 mg three to four times daily) can be used; this medication may be useful even when Graves' disease underlies hyperthyroidism. Rarely, prednisone (up to 40 mg daily) may have a role in severe thyroiditis, reducing inflammation and thus shrinking large goiters as well as inhibiting peripheral conversion of T_4 to T_3. Because hyperthyroidism in thyroiditis is caused by leakage of hormone from an inflamed thyroid rather than ongoing synthesis of thyroid hormone, medications that inhibit thyroid hormone synthesis have no role in treating this condition, in contrast to their integral role in treating Graves' disease.

When a precise diagnosis cannot be made clinically and is needed to dictate therapy, radioactive ^{123}I uptake may be measured. Uptake is typically high with Graves' disease and essentially zero with thyroiditis. However, radioactive ^{123}I readily crosses into breast milk and thus necessitates temporary discontinuation of breast-feeding for approximately 3 days after administration.[21] During this time, breast milk should be pumped and discarded. Iodine transport into the breasts in a lactating woman may markedly decrease thyroid iodine uptake, complicating the diagnosis of Graves' disease.[44]

A technetium scan, although not able to measure thyroid uptake, can at times help distinguish between thyroiditis and Graves' disease, and the shorter half-life of technetium allows resumption of breast-feeding in 24 to 48 hours.[20]

Hyperthyroidism is generally followed by a phase of hypothyroidism, attributable to depletion of hormone from the leaky gland and delay in resynthesis. Hypothyroidism generally begins 3 to 6 months postpartum and persists for 3 to 5 months. The hypothyroid phase is more often symptomatic, characterized by depression, difficulty in losing weight, and fatigue. As with symptoms of hyperthyroidism, though, manifestations may easily be confused with normal postpartum complaints. However, in postpartum thyroiditis, TSH level is elevated and T_4 level may fall well below the normal range. Once recognized, hypothyroidism should generally be treated with thyroid hormone replacement. Therapy is usually indicated when T_4 is frankly low, TSH level is greater than 10, or symptoms are present. When TSH level is only minimally elevated without other abnormalities, the need for treatment is controversial; some patients clearly feel better with therapy, but others note no benefit.

In most cases, a gradual return to euthyroidism follows the hypothyroid phase of thyroiditis. Thus, an attempt should be made to taper thyroid replacement beginning approximately 6 months after initiation of therapy, with close monitoring of thyroid function test results. In some cases, hypothyroidism persists, with lifelong requirement for thyroid hormone replacement. Even when hypothyroidism resolves initially, patients have an increased propensity to later development of permanent hypothyroidism, which may occur in as many as 25% of cases; high titers of antithyroid antibodies are predictive of this condition. In addition, a recurrence rate of at least 25% in subsequent pregnancies has been reported.[45]

Several risk factors for postpartum thyroiditis have been identified. Positive testing for antimicrosomal antibodies in pregnancy is prognostic. Thirty percent or more of women who test positive may develop thyroiditis postpartum, and the incidence increases with higher titers. In contrast, women who test negative are unlikely to manifest this condition postpartum.[46] Also predictive are a family history of autoimmune thyroid disease and a personal history of painless thyroiditis unassociated with pregnancy or in a previous pregnancy. For reasons that remain unclear, postpartum thyroiditis has also been noted to occur more frequently after delivery of a girl.[39]

THE THYROID NODULE IN PREGNANCY

Thyroid nodules are common, particularly in women, with a reported incidence in women of reproductive age of 1 to 2%. Nodules are not infrequently discovered during pregnancy, at least in part because otherwise healthy women may not visit a physician before this. Although 95% of nodules are benign, discovery of a nodule necessitates further evaluation. Because the work-up of a nodule in pregnancy is in many ways similar to that in the nonpregnant state, the following discussion is intended only to highlight aspects of the evaluation unique to pregnancy. Readers are referred to Chapter 23 for a more detailed discussion of thyroid nodules.

As noted previously, symptoms suggestive of hyperthyroidism, such as heat intolerance and palpitations, are also common in euthyroid pregnancy. Likewise, TSH suppression, which may be a clue to an autonomously functioning or hyperfunctioning nodule in the nonpregnant state, may occur in normal early pregnancy.

Radiologic evaluation of a thyroid nodule is also different in pregnancy. A thyroid scan, central to the work-up in many patients, is contraindicated during pregnancy because it relies on the use of radioactive tracers. Instead, ultrasound evaluation is a reasonable alternative. Although this test cannot provide the functional information available from a thyroid scan, it can distinguish between solid and cystic nodules. Wholly cystic nodules are almost never malignant. Furthermore, ultrasonography can be used to guide fine-needle aspiration, which can safely be performed in pregnancy.

THYROID CANCER AND PREGNANCY

It has been suggested that thyroid neoplasia may behave differently during pregnancy than in the nonpregnant state. An incidence of malignancy as high as 43% has been reported in thyroid nodules diagnosed during pregnancy, possibly reflecting referral bias but nevertheless of potential concern. Several reports, moreover, have noted a more aggressive course when thyroid cancer arises or recurs during pregnancy.[47]

Surgery is considered generally safe when performed in the second trimester by an experienced surgeon. Obviously malignant or very suspicious lesions are best resected at this time rather than waiting until after delivery. Some patients nonetheless prefer to delay surgery until after childbirth. Because many suspicious lesions at fine-needle aspiration will ultimately prove to be benign and many thyroid cancers are indolent, the choice must ultimately be left to the patient. However, a decision should be made with the full understanding of the risks of delay, particularly with respect to the possibility of especially aggressive disease related to the pregnant state.

REFERENCES

1. Burrow GN. Hyperthyroidism during pregnancy. N Engl J Med 1978;298:150.
2. Nelson M, Wickus GG, Caplan RH, Beguin EA. Thyroid gland size in pregnancy. An ultrasound and clinical study. J Reprod Med 1987;32:888.
3. Bohnet GH, Fiedler K, Leidenberger FA. Subclinical hypothyroidism and infertility (letter). Lancet 1981;11 (8258):1278.
4. Thomas R, Reid RL. Thyroid disease and reproductive dysfunction: A review. Obstet Gynecol 1987;70:789.
5. Freitas JE, Swanson DP, Sisson JC. Iodine-131: Optimal therapy for hyperthyroidism in children and adolescents? J Nucl Med 1979;20:847.
6. Stagnaro-Green A, Roman SH, Cobin RH, et al. Detection of at-risk pregnancy by means of highly sensitive assays for thyroid autoantibodies. JAMA 1990;2646:1422.
7. Burrow GN. The management of thyrotoxicosis in pregnancy. N Engl J Med 1985;313:562.
8. Green G, Gareis FJ, Shepard TH, Kelley VC. Cretinism associated with maternal sodium iodide I 131 therapy during pregnancy. Am J Dis Child 1971;122:247.
9. Stoffer SS, Hamburger JI. Inadvertent ^{131}I therapy for hyperthyroidism in the first trimester of pregnancy. J Nucl Med 1976;17:146.
10. Momotani N, Noh J, Oyanagi H, et al. Antithyroid drug therapy for Graves' disease during pregnancy. Optimal regimen for fetal thyroid status. N Engl J Med 1986; 315:24.
11. Cooper DS. Antithyroid drugs. N Engl J Med 1984; 311:1353.
12. Marchant B, Brownlie BEW, Hart DM, et al. The placental transfer of propylthiouracil, methimazole and carbimazole. J Clin Endocrinol Metab 1977;45:1187.
13. Mujtaba Q, Burrow GN. Treatment of hyperthyroidism in pregnancy with propylthiouracil and methimazole. Obstet Gynecol 1975;46:282.
14. Van Dijke CP, Heydendael RJ, De Kleine MJ. Methimazole, carbimazole and congenital skin defects. Ann Intern Med 1987;106:60.
15. Amino N, Tanizawa O, Mori H, et al. Aggravation of thyrotoxicosis in early pregnancy and after delivery in Graves' disease. J Clin Endocrinol Metab 1982;55:108.
16. Momotani N, Hisaoka T, Noh J, et al. Effects of iodine on thyroid status of fetus versus mother in treatment of Graves' disease complicated by pregnancy. J Clin Endocrinol Metab 1992;75:738.
17. Kampmann JP, Hansen JM, Johansen K, Helweg J. Propylthiouracil in human milk. Revision of a dogma. Lancet 1980;1(8171):736.
18. Cooper DS. Antithyroid drugs. To breast-feed or not to breast-feed. Am J Obstet Gynecol 1987;157:234.
19. Lamberg B-A, Ikonen E, Osterlund K, et al. Antithyroid treatment of maternal hyperthyroidism during lactation. Clin Endocrinol 1984;21:81.
20. Mountford PJ, Coakley AJ. A review of the secretion of radioactivity in human breast milk: Data, quantitative analysis and recommendations. Nucl Med Comm 1989;10:15.
21. Romney BM, Nicholoff EL, Esser PD, Alderson PO. Radionuclide administration to nursing mothers: Mathematically derived guidelines. Radiology 1986;160:549.
22. Hashizume K, Ichikawa K, Nishii Y, et al. Effect of administration of thyroxine on the risk of postpartum recurrence of hyperthyroid Graves' disease. J Clin Endocrinol Metab 1992;75:6.
23. Zakarija M, McKenzie JM, Hoffman WH. Prediction and therapy of intrauterine and late-onset neonatal hyperthyroidism. J Clin Endocrinol Metab 1986;62:368.
24. Porreco RP, Bloch CA. Fetal blood sampling in the management of intrauterine thyrotoxicosis. Obstet Gynecol 1990;76:509.
25. McKenzie JM, Zakarija M. Fetal and neonatal hyperthyroidism and hypothyroidism due to maternal TSH receptor antibodies. Thyroid 1992;2:155.
26. Mitsuda N, Tamaki H, Amino N, et al. Risk factors for developmental disorders in infants born to women with Graves' disease. Obstet Gynecol 1992;80:359.
27. Bouillon R, Naesens M, Van Assche FA, et al. Thyroid function in patients with hyperemesis gravidarum. Am J Obstet Gynecol 1982;143:922.
28. Goodwin TM, Montoro M, Mestman JH. Transient hyperthyroidism and hyperemesis gravidarum: Clinical aspects. Am J Obstet Gynecol 1992;167:648.
29. Goodwin TM, Montoro M, Mestman JH, et al. The role of chorionic gonadotropin in transient hyperthyroidism of hyperemesis gravidarum. J Clin Endocrinol Metab 1992; 75:1333.
30. Kennedy RL, Darne J, Davies R, Price A. Thyrotoxicosis and hyperemesis gravidarum associated with a serum activity which stimulates human thyroid cells in vitro. Clin Endocrinol 1992;36:83.
31. Nagataki S, Mizuno M, Sakamoto S, et al. Thyroid function in molar pregnancy. J Clin Endocrinol Metab 1977; 44:254.
32. Norman RJ, Green-Thompson RW, Jialal I, et al. Hyperthyroidism in gestational trophoblastic neoplasia. Clin Endocrinol 1981;15:395.
33. Amir SM, Osathanondh R, Berkowitz RS, Goldstein DP. Human chorionic gonadotropin and thyroid function in patients with hydatidiform mole. Am J Obstet Gynecol 1984;150:723.
34. Davis LE, Leveno KJ, Cunningham FG. Hypothyroidism complicating pregnancy. Obstet Gynecol 1988;72:108.
35. Man EB, Brown JF, Serunian SA. Maternal hypothyroxinemia: Psychoneurological deficits of progeny. Ann Clin Lab Sci 1991;21:227.
36. Mandel SJ, Larsen PR, Seely EW, Brent GA. Increased need for thyroxine during pregnancy in women with primary hypothyroidism. N Engl J Med 1990;323:91.
37. Kaplan MM. Monitoring thyroxine treatment during pregnancy. Thyroid 1992;2:147.
38. Vulsma T, Gons MH, De Vijler JJM. Maternal-fetal transfer of thyroxine in congenital hypothyroidism due to a total organification defect or thyroid agenesis. N Engl J Med 1989;321:13.
39. Amino N, Mori H, Iwatani Y, et al. High prevalence of

transient post-partum thyrotoxicosis and hypothyroidism. N Engl J Med 1982;306:849.

40. Jansson R, Bernander S, Karlsson A, et al. Autoimmune thyroid dysfunction in the postpartum period. J Clin Endocrinol Metab 1984;58:681.

41. Freeman R, Rosen H, Thysen B. Incidence of thyroid dysfunction in an unselected postpartum population. Arch Intern Med 1986;146:1361.

42. Nikolai TF, Turney SL, Roberts RC. Postpartum lymphocytic thyroiditis. Arch Intern Med 1987;147:221.

43. Stagnaro-Green A. Post-miscarriage thyroid dysfunction. Obstet Gynecol 1992;80:490.

44. Amino N, Mori H, Iwatani Y, et al. Post-partum thyroid dysfunction (reply to letters). N Engl J Med 1982; 307:1025.

45. Walfish PG, Farird NR. Postpartum thyroid dysfunction (letter). N Engl J Med 1982;307:1024.

46. Feldt-Rasmussen U, Hoier-Masden M, Rasmussen NG, et al. Anti-thyroid peroxidase antibodies during pregnancy and post-partum. Autoimmunity 1990;6:211.

47. Rosen IB, Walfish PG. Pregnancy as a predisposing factor in thyroid neoplasia. Arch Surg 1986;121:1287.

Thromboembolic Complications of Pregnancy and the Puerperium

James J. Heffernan

Thromboembolic disease is a major cause of pregnancy-associated maternal death and morbidity. Fetal wastage is also increased among women who experience thromboembolic complications, in part related to clinically apparent comorbid conditions and in part associated with the presence of antiphospholipid antibodies in the maternal circulation. Most episodes of thromboembolic disease during pregnancy or the puerperium involve iliofemoral deep vein thrombophlebitis (DVT) with or without associated pulmonary emboli (PE). Other thromboembolic complications include cerebral cortical vein or sinus thrombosis, ovarian vein thrombosis, and septic pelvic thrombophlebitis.

EPIDEMIOLOGY

Pulmonary embolism was identified as a major cause of pregnancy-associated death within only the past several decades. In the United States, PE currently is the leading cause of maternal mortality among women whose pregnancies end in a live birth, and it accounted for 27.1% of 1363 such deaths reported during the period 1979 to 1986 (Fig. 39–1).[1] Most such emboli are thrombotic in origin. Pulmonary embolism is also the leading cause of death among pregnant women who die undelivered and is the third leading cause of death among women whose pregnancies end in stillbirth or abortion (frequently amniotic fluid embolism). Overall, PE accounts for 23.4% of pregnancy-associated maternal deaths, ranking second behind hemorrhage. Moreover, PE is likely underrepresented, because it is not listed as a cause of maternal death in routine vital statistic reports.

As with most direct causes of obstetric mortality, PE-associated maternal deaths have decreased, with reductions of more than 50% reported for both black and white women during the period from 1970 to 1985.[2, 3] However, black women maintain a 2.5-fold higher risk. Age appears to be an even more important risk factor, with a 2.7-fold increased risk among patients 30 years of age or older and a tenfold increase in relative risk among women older than 40 years compared with those younger than 25 years.

Older, longitudinal data from the Tecumseh Community Health Study suggest that one half of first thromboembolic events in women younger than 40 years are pregnancy associated.[4] From these same data, DVT or PE was identified at a rate of 5.9 per 1000 pregnancies. Other older studies have identified DVT in 0.018 to 0.29% of all deliveries.[5, 6]

It has been a common belief that prepartum thrombophlebitis occurs most commonly in the third trimester. Although it is true that symptoms of leg swelling and pain occur most frequently in the third trimester, prospectively obtained data demonstrate that venous thrombosis documented by objective testing occurs with equal frequency in all three trimesters or possibly predominates in the first trimester.[7, 8] A striking increase in the concentration of symptomatic episodes of DVT and PE is noted in the immediate postpartum period, however, especially after cesarean delivery. Older data suggested a 3- to 5-fold excess of DVT in the puerperium compared with the antepartum period and a 3- to 16-fold excess after cesarean compared with vaginal delivery.[6, 9, 10] The striking preponderance of clinically observed left-sided il-

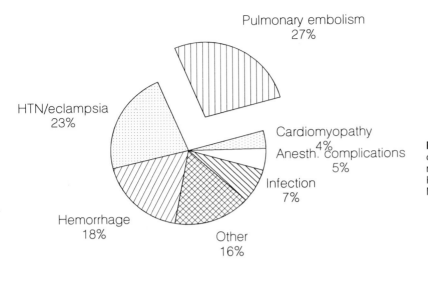

Figure 39–1. Pregnancy-associated maternal mortality (pregnancies resulting in live births. HTN, Hypertension. (Data from MMWR 1991;40:1–13.)

iofemoral DVT has been borne out by several studies using various diagnostic modalities.[7, 11, 12]

The presence of antiphospholipid antibodies in the maternal circulation, detected by either clotting assays (lupus anticoagulant) or immunoassays (anticardiolipin antibodies), has been associated with an increased risk of both thrombosis and pregnancy loss.[13] Other observed risks for DVT and PE include prior history of thromboembolism, immobilization, inherited deficiencies of coagulation inhibitors (especially antithrombin III, protein C, and protein S), pelvic or lower extremity trauma, and possibly higher parity.

PATHOPHYSIOLOGY

For the most part, pregnancy and the trauma of delivery fulfill Virchow's 150-year-old triad of risk factors for thromboembolic disease: (1) venous stasis, (2) hypercoagulable blood, and (3) venous intimal injury.

Venous blood flow from the lower extremities decreases during the course of pregnancy and especially during labor, in part related to dilation of capacitance vessels and expansion of blood and plasma volume in the first two trimesters and in part related to progressive extrinsic compression of pelvic veins by the enlarging uterine contents.[14] A sharp increase in venous pressure and a decrease in flow accompany engagement and descent of the fetal head during labor and delivery. The prepon-

derance of left iliofemoral DVT has been attributed to relative obstruction of the left iliac vein as it is crossed by the right iliac artery or a low bifurcating aorta in the setting of an overlying gravid uterus. Venous webs at this site may also contribute to the development of DVT.

During pregnancy, levels of clotting factors V, VII, VIII, IX, X, XII, and fibrinogen increase, levels of factors XI and XIII decrease, and platelet counts remain in the normal range.[9] The tendency toward increased activation of the coagulation system is generally offset by an increase in fibrinolytic activity. Anatomic factors, such as venous stasis or abnormalities of venous architecture from previous DVT, inherited or acquired deficiencies of coagulation inhibitors (especially antithrombin III, protein S, or protein C), and circulating antiphospholipid antibodies, all may readily tip the balance toward overt thromboembolic disease during pregnancy. The rapid decrease in fibrinolytic potential within 1 hour of delivery likely explains in part the increase in observed episodes of thromboembolic disease in the immediate puerperium.

Although no hard evidence demonstrates venous intimal injury related to pregnancy per se, such may exist at the microscopic level related to the increased set-points of the coagulation and fibrinolytic systems, especially in areas of venous pooling behind valve cusps in the lower extremities.

(See Chapter 32 for a more detailed discussion of the physiologic changes of pregnancy.)

CLINICAL FEATURES

Deep Vein Thrombophlebitis

In general but with several notable exceptions, the clinical features of venous thromboembolism in pregnancy are the same as those in nonpregnant patients. Deep vein thrombophlebitis is suggested by some combination of pain, tenderness, swelling, edema, change in skin color, and the presence of palpable cords in the affected limb. Of special note, the overwhelming majority of cases of DVT associated with pregnancy occur on the left. Pooled data from several studies have confirmed this observation, with 86 of 91 episodes of pregnancy-associated DVT localized to the left iliofemoral system (two bilaterally) by various objective modalities including venography, impedance plethysmography, and ultrasonography.[11–13] The diagnosis of DVT is also suggested if the midthigh circumference of the symptomatic leg (measured 15 cm above the superior pole of the patella) or the midcalf circumference (measured 8–10 cm below the tibial tubercle) exceeds that of the unaffected side by more than 2 cm or if Homans' sign (calf pain on dorsiflexing the foot of the affected side) or the Löwenberg's test (pain distal to a blood pressure cuff inflated rapidly to 180 mm Hg) is positive. A confounding issue is the fact that many if not most pregnant women experience some degree of leg swelling, edema, and often discomfort during the late stages of pregnancy. Phlegmasia cerulea dolens, the painful, blue, swollen leg of complete venous obstruction, occurs very rarely but may be associated with muscle compartment syndromes or secondary arterial compromise. A phenomenon noted among a significant minority of pregnant women ultimately diagnosed with DVT is disease originating in or limited to the iliac vein. Initial symptoms in this situation may be confined to the groin or lower abdominal quadrant, usually on the left. It is important to note that even in the more typical case, no physical finding is sufficiently accurate to establish the diagnosis of DVT without objective testing. Common diagnoses in the differential of DVT include cellulitis, postphlebitic syndrome, soft tissue injury, edema states (especially preeclampsia), and benign swelling of pregnancy.

Pulmonary Embolism

The clinical features of PE differ little between pregnant and nonpregnant patients but for the fact that pregnant women are, on the basis of age, overall condition, and comorbidity, generally healthier and have better physiologic reserve than most other categories of patients who experience PE. The most common symptoms and signs of PE among pregnant women are chest pain (usually but not always pleuritic), dyspnea, tachypnea, and tachycardia. Other clinical features include cough, fever, hemoptysis, diaphoresis, a sense of apprehension, pleural or pleuropericardial friction rubs, and cyanosis. Signs of consolidation with or without evidence of pleural effusion may be present in the setting of pulmonary infarct or hemorrhagic congestion from a submassive PE.

Syncope or profound hypotension may be the initial manifestation of massive PE. Signs of acute right-sided heart strain or failure may be present: an accentuated pulmonary component of the second heart sound; an exaggerated physiologic splitting, or fixed splitting, of the second heart sound; a right ventricular heave or gallop; and jugular venous distention, sometimes with hepato-jugular reflux.

Adjuncts to the physical examination that may reinforce the suspicion of PE include arterial blood gas measurements, chest radiographs, and an electrocardiogram. However, none of these studies alone or in combination is sufficiently discriminatory to diagnose or preclude PE without recourse to more specific diagnostic procedures. Because pregnant women are generally young and have good respiratory function, arterial hypoxemia (arterial partial pressure of oxygen <85 mm Hg) or an alveolar-arterial gradient exceeding 15 mm Hg lends weight to the suspicion of PE, especially when the chest radiograph appears normal or nearly so. Unfortunately, other diagnoses (e.g., pneumonia) may better explain hypoxemia in a given patient, and a significant subset of patients who experience PE may demonstrate arterial blood gases within a range considered normal. Chest radiographs may appear abnormal in as many as 75% of pregnant women with PE, but the findings are again usually nonspecific: atelectasis, infiltrate, volume loss, and pleural effusion. Focal oligemia (segmental areas of decreased vascular markings) and a Hampton's hump (a pleural-based consolidation from lung infarct or hemorrhagic congestion) are more helpful radiographic findings but occur at most in 2 to 3% of cases. Similarly, the classic electrocardiographic finding of an S1-Q3-T3 pattern in the setting of PE is noted extremely rarely. More commonly, one finds tachycardia with some combination of nonspecific ST-T changes, with or without evidence of right-sided heart strain, and occasionally right bundle branch block. Clinical entities in the differential diagnosis of PE include pneumonitis, amniotic fluid embolism, musculoskeletal chest wall pain, reactive airways diseases (especially asthma), viral pleurodynia, or myopericarditis, coronary heart disease (extremely uncommon), pneumothorax, and subdiagphragmatic processes such as cholecystitis.

EVALUATION

Establishing Likelihood

Although no combination of factors from the history, physical examination, and basic adjunctive tests (arterial blood gases, chest radiographs, or electrocardiogram) are sufficiently discriminatory to preclude or confirm the diagnosis of DVT or PE, establishment of prior probability (pretest likelihood) using clinical parameters is important in guiding the interpretation of more directed studies. Prospectively obtained data among nonpregnant patients suspected of having PE have demonstrated that a clinical assessment of an 80 to 100% likelihood of PE was correct in 68% of 91 instances, confirmed by pulmonary angiography, whereas a pretest clinical assessment of 0 to 19% likelihood was correct in ruling out PE in 91%.[15] Combining pretest clinical assessments with the results of ventilation-perfusion scans improves the predictive value when clinical and scan assessments are concordant: The positive predictive value of a high-probability scan increases from 88 to 96% if supported by a high-likelihood clinical assessment; the negative predictive value of a low-probability scan rises from 86 to 96% if accompanied by a clinical assessment of low likelihood. Unfortunately, such concordant high-probability and low-probability results are found in only a small fraction of patients suspected of having PE.

Comparable data do not exist for combining clinical suspicion with the results of noninvasive studies of the venous system of the lower extremities, yet the general bayesian principle applies: A high-probability venous study is more likely a true positive in the setting of high clinical suspicion, and a low-probability study is more likely a true negative when accompanied by low clinical suspicion than would be the case in either instance with no clinical information.

Confirming and Precluding the Diagnosis of Pulmonary Embolism or Deep Vein Thrombosis

Confirmation or preclusion of the diagnosis of PE or DVT requires the use of one or several imaging studies. Such studies are generally those used in nonpregnant individuals suspected of having venous thromboembolism. Of special interest in pregnant women is the radiation dose delivered to a fetus by traditional radiologic or nuclear medicine procedures. Initial concerns that noninvasive venous studies of the legs (impedance plethysmography and ultrasonography) might be rendered uninterpretable by the extrinsic pelvic mass of a gravid uterus have been shown to be largely unfounded when such procedures are performed with patients in the left lateral decubitus position; however, negative or equivocal findings in the legs must be interpreted in light of the increased tendency for DVT to begin in the pelvis in more than 10% of pregnant women with confirmed disease.

CONTRAST VENOGRAPHY. Ascending contrast venography remains the standard with which other modalities for the diagnosis of DVT are compared. Sensitivity and specificity are excellent, both approaching 100% with adequate studies, in the clinical setting of proximal or distal lower extremity disease. Unfortunately, venography takes 1 to 2 hours to perform and in as many as 10% of instances may be nondiagnostic or precluded by technical considerations, such as underfilling of the deep femoral system or inability to cannulate an appropriate foot vein in a massively swollen leg. Moreover, the increased propensity for DVT to originate in large-bore pelvic veins in pregnant women increases the likelihood of nondiagnostic or false negative results, whereas extrinsic compression by the uterine contents raises the possibility of false positive results if findings are not rigorously interpreted. Venography is invasive and associated with a substantial likelihood (up to 24%) of local discomfort and a small but measurable risk of systemic contrast reactions. Postvenography phlebitis may occur, but the risk of this complication may be minimized by the use of a heparinized saline flush. The risk to a fetus from the iodine in contrast media is low but unquantified. The estimated radiation dose to a fetus is 0.314 rad for complete unilateral venography in the mother, including fluoroscopy and spot films.[16] Venography limited to the leg, using an abdominal shield, is associated with a radiation exposure of less than 0.05 rad.[16]

PULMONARY ARTERIOGRAPHY. Pulmonary arteriography remains the gold standard for the diagnosis of PE. Indeed, experience from prospective trials has reinforced the importance of pulmonary arteriography in the 70% of instances in which ventilation-perfusion lung scans are nondiagnostic. The procedure is invasive, uncomfortable, and associated with a morbidity of 4 to 5%. The cited mortality of 0.2 to 0.3% reflects catheter complications and systemic contrast reactions, as well as the underlying comorbidity of many seriously ill patients undergoing this procedure. In general, pregnant women suspected of having PE have better physiologic reserve than most other categories of patients at risk for venous thromboembolism. The radiation exposure to the fetus of a maternal pulmonary arteriogram via the femoral route is 0.221 to 0.374 rad.[16] A pulmonary arteriogram via the brachial route in a patient with abdominal shielding delivers less than 0.05 rad to the fetus.[16]

VENTILATION-PERFUSION LUNG SCINTIGRAPHY. Ventilation-perfusion lung scans have been used for several decades in the diagnosis of PE. Perfusion lung scanning involves intravenous injection of technetium-labeled albumin microspheres or macroaggregates. Minimal immediate risk is generally posed by the injection other than in the rare patient with severe pulmonary hypertension. Technetium aerosols have largely supplanted the xenon gas previously used in ventilation scanning.

Among nonpregnant patients studied prospectively, a normal or nearly normal perfusion scan correctly precludes the diagnosis of PE in 91% of instances and if the pretest clinical suspicion is low, in 96% of cases.[15] Similarly, a high-probability ventilation-perfusion scan correctly establishes the diagnosis of PE in 88% of instances, and the likelihood rises to 96% if concurrent clinical suspicion is also high. Unfortunately, only 23% of patients with suspected PE fall into these diagnostic categories. The results of lung scanning in the majority of patients suspected of having PE have been categorized traditionally as low probability, intermediate probability, or indeterminate (abnormal in areas of abnormality on an accompanying chest radiograph). These are all nondiagnostic categories; PE has been shown to occur in 15 to 20% of low-probability scans and in as many as 32 to 40% of intermediate-probability or indeterminate scans. Although pregnant patients have been excluded from the prospective studies that generated these results, there is no reason to suspect that they would differ in any significant regard, other than the expectation that they, as young patients with low rates of chronic illness, might have fewer chest radiograph abnormalities and a higher likelihood of normal perfusion scans when PE was not present. The performance of ventilation-perfusion scintigraphy is generally safe, except for rare patients with severe pulmonary hypertension or severe obstructive lung disease. With reduced doses of radiolabeled aerosol and perfusate, the radiation dose to the fetus can be limited to less than 0.05 rad.[16]

RADIOLABELED FIBRINOGEN SCANNING. Much of the incidence data for DVT in various clinical settings is based on the findings of ^{125}I-fibrinogen scans. In prospective studies, this technique has been shown to be quite sensitive in identifying disease in the distal venous system. It is only 60 to 80% sensitive for proximal venous disease, and results are not immediately available, because measurable radiolabel uptake by propagating clot takes hours to occur and a final diagnosis may not be available for up to 3 days.[17] In any event, ^{125}I-fibrinogen scanning is contraindicated in pregnant or lactating women. The estimated radiation dose to the fetus of a pregnant woman undergoing such a procedure is 2 rad.[16] Moreover, concentration of unbound ^{125}I in the fetal or neonatal thyroid can produce goiter and hypothyroidism. Radiolabeled fibrinogen poses potential, albeit small, risks of hepatitis or human immunodeficiency virus transmission. Other thrombus-seeking radionuclides have been developed, but none have been studied in pregnant women. The sensitivity of most such studies is adversely affected by heparin therapy, which poses a management problem because imaging requires hours to days.

IMPEDANCE PLETHYSMOGRAPHY. Impedance plethysmography measures changes in electric resistance in response to changes in venous volume in an extremity. This technique is highly sensitive to obstructive common iliac, external iliac, or femoral vein thrombi in symptomatic patients but may fail to detect isolated nonobstructive proximal thrombi. Serial testing by impedance plethysmography has been shown to be an effective method for ruling out DVT in nonpregnant, symptomatic patients with repeatedly negative results. Early concern about its use in pregnancy-associated DVT centered on two issues: (1) technical problems related to extrinsic compression of pelvic veins by the gravid uterus and (2) the high frequency of thrombi originating in the pelvic veins in pregnant women with DVT. The first concern is obviated when impedance plethysmography is performed with a pregnant woman in the left lateral decubitus position. Moreover, convincing prospectively obtained data have shown that anticoagulant therapy may be safely withheld from symptomatic pregnant women who have negative results after impedance plethysmography.[11] Impedance plethysmography poses no known or expected risk to a fetus.

ULTRASONOGRAPHY. Real-time ultrasonography has been extensively evaluated to assess its accuracy in detecting lower extremity DVT. It is often coupled with a Doppler study in what is termed a duplex scan, although it is not clear that a duplex scan is significantly better than real-time ultrasonography in diagnosing proximal lower extremity DVT. Criteria used to diagnose venous thrombi include (1) failure of the vascular lumen to collapse fully under pressure from the transducer probe and (2) detection of intraluminal clot (manifested in increased intravascular echogenicity). For proximal lower extremity DVT, the sensitivity and specificity of real-time ultrasonography/duplex scan are 96% and 99%, respectively, in nonpregnant patients.[17] Both sensitivity and specificity are substantially lower in distal disease (i.e., below the popliteal vein), but serial studies allow the identification of proximally propagating clot. Color-flow Doppler ultrasonography is a newer variant that appears to have excellent sensitivity and specificity for proximal lower extremity DVT and is possibly more accurate than real-time ultrasonography in diagnosing calf DVT.

The published experience with ultrasonographic techniques for the diagnosis of DVT in pregnant women is limited to comparison with historic controls.[12] Nonetheless, these data appear promising, and one may reasonably assume good diagnostic accuracy from real-time ultrasonography/duplex scan/color-flow Doppler ultrasonography for most pregnant women with suspected DVT. An important caveat, once again, is the pregnant woman suspected of having isolated iliac or other pelvic DVT, in whom alternate diagnostic modalities are generally required to confirm or preclude the diagnosis of DVT.

Ultrasonography poses no known risk to either a pregnant woman or her fetus. Ultrasonography has an added benefit in that an alternate diagnosis—abscess, Baker's cyst, or lymphadenopathy—may be established in as many as 15% of instances when the test is performed for suspected DVT.

OTHER IMAGING MODALITIES. Both magnetic resonance imaging (MRI) and x-ray computed tomography (CT) have been used to establish the diagnosis of pelvic thrombophlebitis, including iliofemoral disease, in pregnant women.[18] Early reports suggested excellent sensitivity and specificity for MRI in the diagnosis of lower extremity DVT. A review has called these data into question, although MRI may have a real role in the diagnosis of calf DVT.[19] Both MRI and CT are expensive, somewhat time-consuming, not uniformly available, and not validated sufficiently in pregnant women to endorse their routine use. Risks to the fetus are unquantified.

Diagnostic Algorithm

DEEP VEIN THROMBOPHLEBITIS. The initial imaging procedure of choice in a pregnant woman suspected of having lower extremity DVT is either impedance plethysmography or real-time ultrasonography (with or without color-flow Doppler imaging) (Table 39–1). A positive study result from either modality is prima facie evidence of DVT and constitutes sufficient grounds to justify treatment. Empirical intravenous heparin therapy should be initiated before imaging if the clinical index of suspicion is high and a delay of more than several hours is anticipated before study. Choice of procedure, impedance plethysmography versus real-time ultrasonography, is generally dictated by availability and specific expertise in a given institution. Contrast venography, with pelvic shielding, should be obtained if neither noninvasive modality is readily available.

In the setting of a high clinical index of suspicion of distal DVT, with an equivocal or negative noninvasive study result, one should proceed to venography or pursue serial noninvasive studies on days 1, 3, and 7 after the initial negative result.

There is no proven alternative to contrast venography in diagnosing the vexing problem of isolated de novo iliac DVT. Impedance plethysmography generally yields positive results with fully obstructing iliac vein disease and is a reasonable first choice. Venography or serial impedance plethysmography should be pursued in the setting of neg-

---

TABLE 39–1. Diagnostic Algorithm: Deep Vein Thrombophlebitis

- For *suspected iliofemoral DVT*, the initial imaging procedure of choice is either RTU or IPG, performed on the suspected leg with the patient in a lateral decubitus position.
  - A positive result constitutes grounds for therapy.
  - Empirical therapy should be initiated if a delay of more than 4 hours in obtaining the study is anticipated.
  - Contrast venography with pelvic shielding should be obtained if RTU or IPG is unavailable.
- For *suspected distal (calf) DVT,* with equivocal or negative noninvasive study results, obtain a contrast venogram or pursue serial noninvasive studies on days 1, 3, and 7 after the initial study.
  - A positive result at any point constitutes grounds for therapy.
  - MRI may reveal a clot (but its use in pregnancy has not been validated).
- For *suspected isolated iliac DVT,* the initial imaging modality should be IPG.
  - A positive result constitutes grounds for therapy.
  - A negative or equivocal result mandates either immediate contrast venography or empirical heparinization and serial IPGs.
  - MRI or computed tomography may yield the diagnosis, but negative results may still obligate contrast venography until the specificity of these diagnostic modalities is better established.

DVT, Deep vein thrombophlebitis; RTU, real-time ultrasonography; IPG, impedance plethysmography; MRI, magnetic resonance imaging.

ative or equivocal initial noninvasive study results when one strongly suspects iliac DVT. Given the high risk of PE from such proximal disease, patients evaluated with serial impedance plethysmography should be maintained on therapeutic heparin until the diagnosis is confirmed or excluded. The diagnosis of pelvic DVT, including iliac disease, may also be made by MRI or contrast CT, although the sensitivity and specificity of either of these modalities has not been determined.

PULMONARY EMBOLISM. For the past several decades, the initial imaging study of choice in pregnant women and others suspected of having PE has been radionuclide perfusion or ventilation-perfusion scanning (Table 39–2). Prospective trials have shown that one can confirm or exclude the diagnosis of PE with perfusion-scanning or ventilation-perfusion-scanning alone in only one quarter of cases, with a high probability of normal or nearly normal scan, respectively. In three quarters of cases, radionuclide scans yield low-probability, intermediate-probability, or indeterminate scans, which are associated with PE in 15 to 60% of cases. Adequate interpretation of radionuclide scans requires a chest radiograph, which may also suggest alternative diagnoses (e.g., pneumonia, pneumothorax, lung abscess). Indeterminate radionuclide scans and those of low or intermediate probability all necessitate further evaluation.

Although concordance of chest (PE) and leg (DVT) findings is limited, positive findings on impedance plethysmography or real-time ultrasonography constitute sufficient grounds for anticoagulant therapy independent of the diagnosis of PE, and it is not unreasonable to pursue either such study after an equivocal perfusion scan or ventilation-perfusion scan.

Nonetheless, one must anticipate the need to pursue pulmonary arteriography in 50 to 75% of instances to adequately confirm or rule out the diagnosis of PE. Approach through the brachial vein with pelvic shielding minimizes fetal radiation exposure, but pulmonary arteriography via the femoral route should be performed if an upper extremity approach is not possible.

MANAGEMENT

Supportive Measures

Women with suspected DVT should be placed at bed rest and their leg elevated while the diagnosis is pursued. If DVT is confirmed, bed rest and leg elevation should be maintained for a minimum of 3 to 5 days or until pain and swelling subside. Gradient support hose should be fitted and worn at all times when the patient is out of bed, until 6 weeks after delivery.

Severe hypoxemia after PE in pregnant women is uncommon, but supplemental oxygen is appropriate. Hyperventilation engendered by PE shifts the hemoglobin-oxygen dissociation curve and may reduce fetal oxygenation. Fetal monitoring in the acute setting is indicated. Shock from massive PE is generally accompanied by evidence of high right-sided filling pressures and generally responds to expanding intravenous volume. Such patients should be monitored and treated in an intensive care unit.

TABLE 39–2. Diagnostic Algorithm: Pulmonary Embolus

- Initial imaging procedure of choice is either radionuclide V/Q scan or a noninvasive modality directed at concurrent lower extremity deep vein thrombophlebitis, either RTU or IPG.
  - With V/Q scan, treatment is warranted with a high-probability scan, and the diagnosis of pulmonary embolism is functionally precluded with a normal scan.
    - One may anticipate a high-probability or normal V/Q scan in only a quarter of cases.
  - With RTU or IPG, treatment is warranted with a positive study result.
- If the result of initial V/Q scan is anything other than high probability or normal, one should obtain RTU or IPG of the suspect leg(s).
- If results of V/Q scan and RTU/IFG are not determinative, one should obtain a contrast pulmonary angiogram using appropriate shielding and a brachial approach if feasible.

V/Q, Ventilation-perfusion; RTU, real-time ultrasonography; IPG, impedance plethysmography.

Treatment Options and Risks in Pregnant Patients

UNFRACTIONATED HEPARIN. Heparin is the agent of choice for nearly all variants of thromboembolic disease in pregnancy. Intravenous heparin by continuous infusion is the standard of care for acute DVT or PE. Aggressive early treatment to achieve a prompt rise in the activated partial thromboplastin time (aPTT) to greater than or equal to 1.5 times control has been shown to be necessary to preclude recurrent venous thromboembolism. Failure to achieve an adequate anticoagulant effect has been associated with a 25% risk of recurrent venous thromboembolism, which can be reduced to 5% with adequate early treatment.[20] A supratherapeutic aPTT (>2.5 times control) early in therapy has not been associated with a risk of clinically important bleeding complications. Accordingly, one should anticipate administering at least 35,000 to 40,000 U in the first 24 hours of therapy by one of the recently developed and validated infusion protocols, monitoring the aPTT and adjusting therapy every 4 hours until a therapeutic level is achieved. Pregnancy is a hypercoagulable state, and many pregnant women with venous thromboembolism require prodigious heparin doses to achieve an adequate anticoagulant effect.

Subcutaneous heparin is the standard of care for primary and secondary prophylaxis of venous thromboembolism in pregnancy. Different clinical situations in pregnancy determine whether standard-dose (nonadjusted) heparin or adjusted-dose subcutaneous heparin should be used (see the later discussion of treatment recommendations.)

Heparin does not cross the placenta. Neither fetal malformations nor fetal hemorrhage is associated with its administration to pregnant women. A major review (1980) of the complications of anticoagulant use during pregnancy concluded that both heparin and warfarin use are associated with an adverse fetal outcome in one third of cases.[21] Reanalysis of the data on which this study was based demonstrates an adverse fetal outcome in only one fifth of cases associated with maternal heparin use; a subsequent review strongly suggested that any such increase in spontaneous abortion or premature delivery with neonatal death associated with maternal heparin use can be explained by the underlying pathologic conditions associated with heparin use.[22] Data now available from a cohort study of 100 consecutive pregnancies associated with heparin use suggest a rate of adverse fetal/neonatal outcomes comparable to that of a normal population.[23]

Maternal complications of heparin use include hemorrhage, thrombocytopenia, hypersensitivity, and osteoporosis. Using current monitoring and administration techniques, the risk of significant hemorrhage associated with heparin use in pregnant women is only 2%.[23] It has been noted that the anticoagulant effect of heparin may persist for as long as 28 hours at term, and termination of therapy should occur 24 hours before anticipated delivery.[13]

Thrombocytopenia, associated with immune endothelial cell injury and heparin-dependent platelet antibodies, may occur in as many as 1% of patients treated with heparin. Of note, heparin-induced thrombocytopenia is associated with paradoxical thrombosis. Heparin-associated hypersensitivity is rare and is generally manifested by urticaria, although full anaphylaxis has been reported.

Heparin-induced osteoporosis occurs by an un-

known mechanism. It appears dose related, generally associated with administration of more than 20,000 U per day for more than 20 weeks, although lower doses for shorter periods have also been associated with bone demineralization.[9, 13] Most patients experience only subclinical bone density loss, but vertebral compression fractures have been described in as many as 3% of pregnant women treated with prophylactic heparin throughout pregnancy.[24] The demineralization appears reversible in most instances within 6 to 12 months of termination of heparin use. It is not known whether supplemental calcium or vitamin D administration can prevent or reduce heparin-induced osteopenia.

Heparin is not secreted into breast milk and can be safely administered to nursing mothers.

LOW-MOLECULAR-WEIGHT HEPARINS. Several different low-molecular-weight heparins have been developed, and enoxaparin has been approved and released for use in the United States for the prevention of thromboembolic complications among patients undergoing hip replacement surgery. These low-molecular-weight heparins have shown better physiologic specificity than that of unfractionated heparin for early stages of the coagulation cascade. Although no trials in pregnant patients have been conducted, low-molecular-weight heparins have been studied among other patient populations and have shown comparable or better efficacy than unfractionated heparin in both acute treatment of venous thromboembolism and prophylaxis, with fewer immediate adverse reactions, especially hemorrhagic complications. The complication profile of low-molecular-weight heparins with long-term use is not well established, but thrombocytopenia appears to occur less commonly than with unfractionated heparin. Dosing is generally based only on body weight, and they are administered subcutaneously. Although the pharmacologic agents themselves are likely to cost much more than unfractionated heparin, overall treatment costs may be competitive when the administration and monitoring costs of unfractionated heparin are factored in. Low-molecular-weight heparins may ultimately supplant traditional heparin therapy for most indications.

ORAL ANTICOAGULANTS. Warfarin is contraindicated in pregnancy. Its use is associated with an adverse fetal outcome in one third of cases.[21] Oral anticoagulants cross the placenta, and fetal anticoagulation may persist several weeks after maternal termination of therapy. Maternal warfarin use is often associated with fetal intracranial hemorrhage in utero or at term. Fetal exposure to warfarin in the first 6 to 12 weeks of gestation is associated with a striking embryopathy, manifested as nasal hypoplasia and epiphyseal stippling, which may occur in 13 to 28.5% of exposed infants. Retardation has been described in as many as 30% of children with warfarin embryopathy.

Fetal warfarin exposure is also associated with serious central nervous system abnormalities, including dorsal midline dysplasia with agenesis of the corpus callosum, Dandy-Walker malformations, and midline cerebellar atrophy, as well as ventral midline dysplasia manifested as optic atrophy. These abnormalities occur at a rate comparable to that of warfarin embryopathy but appear to be associated with warfarin exposure during any trimester of pregnancy.[21] It has been conjectured that they represent deformations following intracranial hemorrhage rather than true malformations.

Maternal complications of warfarin use include hemorrhage (reported in as many as 25% of patients treated using older, more intensive regimens than those now in use) and cutaneous necrosis in patients with underlying protein C or protein S deficiency begun on oral anticoagulant therapy without antecedent heparinization.

In sum, warfarin should not be administered to pregnant women other than in the rare instance of an absolute need for anticoagulation, as in a patient who has a mechanical heart valve and who is hypersensitive to heparin or who has developed thrombocytopenia while on heparin. Such women should be counseled, preferably before pregnancy, of the risks of such treatment. Warfarin does not appear to induce an anticoagulant effect in nursing infants whose mothers receive the drug.[13]

THROMBOLYTIC AGENTS. Thrombolytic agents are not approved for use in pregnant women. Concern centers primarily on the special risk of uteroplacental bleeding. Urokinase and streptokinase have been used rarely in managing both DVT and PE in pregnancy. In the few case reports that exist, the patients so treated appeared to benefit and suffered no major fetal or obstetric complications. There are no reports of the use of tissue thromboplastin activator for venous thromboembolism in pregnancy. Consideration of the use of thrombolytic therapy for venous thromboembolism in pregnancy should be confined to patients with life-threatening PE manifested by hemodynamic compromise or respiratory failure or in those with limb-threatening DVT. Subsequent heparinization is a necessary part of thrombolytic therapy.

ASPIRIN. Aspirin is teratogenic in animals, but debate persists about its teratogenicity in humans. Maternal aspirin use in any dose produces measurable hemostatic abnormalities in the mother, but maternal bleeding has been associated with ingestion of more than 1 gm per day. Neonatal hemorrhage may also occur with maternal ingestion of 1 to 4 tablets per day near term.

Aspirin in low doses, 60 to 150 mg per day, administered during the second and third trimesters of pregnancy to women at high risk for pregnancy-induced hypertension, reduces the incidence of pregnancy-induced hypertension and low-birthweight babies.[25] Aspirin at a dosage of 80 mg per day throughout pregnancy, coupled with a prednisone taper, administered to women with antiphospholipid antibodies and previous fetal loss appears to substantially improve the outcome of pregnancy.[26] At these low aspirin doses, neonatal adverse effects and developmental abnormalities have not been noted.

ANTITHROMBIN III CONCENTRATE. Antithrombin III concentrate has been administered to pregnant women known to have severe congenital antithrombin III deficiency. Clinical experience in this setting is extremely limited.

INFERIOR VENA CAVAL FILTER PLACEMENT. There is a modest experience with the use of Greenfield's inferior vena caval filter during pregnancy, generally placed via the jugular vein. Its use should be considered in pregnant women who have venous thromboembolism and who have failed to respond to appropriate anticoagulant therapy or who have a major contraindication to anticoagulant therapy, such as active hemorrhage or heparin-induced thrombocytopenia.

Treatment Recommendations

ACUTE DEEP VENOUS THROMBOSIS OR PULMONARY EMBOLISM DIAGNOSED DURING PREGNANCY. In women with acute DVT or PE diagnosed during pregnancy, heparin in therapeutic intravenous doses (as described earlier) should be administered for 5 to 10 days, followed by subcutaneous injection of heparin to prolong the 6-hour postinjection aPTT to 1.5 times control (Table 39–3). Heparin administration should be halted 24 hours before anticipated delivery. In the postpartum period, adjusted-dose subcutaneous heparin should be restarted and continued for at least 2 and possibly as long as 6 weeks, if DVT or PE occurred early in pregnancy. This recommendation is based on the presumption that the primary risks—the hypercoagulable state and anatomic derangements associated with pregnancy—resolve quickly in the postpartum period. Women with an independent risk factor, such as antiphospholipid antibody, and women who experienced DVT or PE in the third trimester should conclude a minimum of 3 months' and perhaps as long as 6 months' secondary prophylaxis.

Oral anticoagulants may be used as secondary prophylaxis in the postpartum period. Warfarin

TABLE 39–3. Treatment Recommendations for Thromboembolic Complications of Pregnancy

CLINICAL ENTITY	ACUTE MANAGEMENT	PRIMARY OR SECONDARY PROPHYLAXIS
Acute DVT or PE during pregnancy	Intravenous heparin* for 5–10 days Hold for 24 hours before anticipated delivery	Adjusted-dose heparin† SC to term Adjusted-dose heparin† SC or warfarin‡ PO 2–12 wk postpartum
Prior history of DVT or PE		Heparin, 5000 U SC every 12 hr throughout pregnancy and immediate postpartum period
Women requiring long-term anticoagulation who seek to become pregnant		Adjusted-dose heparin† SC *or* Frequent pregnancy tests on warfarin with switch to adjusted-dose heparin† SC when pregnancy achieved
Antiphospholipid antibodies Prior history of fetal loss		Prednisone and low-dose aspirin
Antiphospholipid antibodies Prior history of DVT or PE		Adjusted-dose heparin† SC to term and through puerperium
Antiphospholipid antibodies Pregnant for first time or without previous complications		DVT surveillance with RTU or IPG *or* Heparin, 5000 U SC every 12 hr through pregnancy and puerperium May also consider use of prednisone and low-dose aspirin
Ovarian vein thrombosis	Intravenous heparin* for 5–10 days	Consider warfarin‡ PO or adjusted-dose heparin† SC for 6–12 wk
Septic pelvic thrombophlebitis	Intravenous heparin* for 5–10 days Appropriate antibiotic coverage	Warfarin‡ PO (in postpartum period) or adjusted-dose heparin† SC to conclude 3–6 mo

*Heparin infusion sufficient to maintain aPTT 1.5–2.5 × control.
†Heparin dose every 8–12 hr sufficient to maintain aPTT 6 hr after dose at 1.5 × control.
‡Warfarin dose sufficient to achieve an international normalized ratio of 2.0–3.0
DVT, Deep vein thrombophlebitis; PE, pulmonary embolus; RTU, real-time ultrasonography; IPG, impedance plethysmography; SC, subcutaneously; PO, orally; aPTT, activated partial thromboplastin time.

can be started concurrently with heparin in the immediate postpartum setting, and heparin terminated when the protime (PT) becomes therapeutic (International Normalized Ration [INR] of 2.0–3.0). Warfarin should then be continued at a dose sufficient to maintain an INR of 2.0 to 3.0. Although prospective studies using warfarin in the postpartum period have not been conducted, the current standard of care for warfarin use in general uses a target INR of 2.0 to 3.0; a higher INR (3.0–5.0) should be routinely used only for patients who fail to respond to lower-dose therapy or who require anticoagulation in the setting of mechanical heart valves. Duration of therapy is as noted earlier.

PREGNANT WOMEN WITH PRIOR HISTORY OF DEEP VEIN THROMBOSIS OR PULMONARY EMBOLISM. In light of the 4 to 12% risk of recurrence in untreated patients, prophylaxis with heparin, 5000 U subcutaneously every 12 hours, throughout pregnancy and for 2 to 6 weeks postpartum is recommended. Low-intensity warfarin (INR 2.0–3.0) may be substituted in the postpartum period.

PATIENTS REQUIRING LONG-TERM ANTICOAGULATION, ESPECIALLY THOSE WITH MECHANICAL PROSTHETIC HEART VALVES, WHO PLAN TO BECOME PREGNANT. One may reasonably choose either (1) adjusted-dose heparin subcutaneously or (2) frequent pregnancy tests while on warfarin with substitution of adjusted-dose subcutaneous heparin when pregnancy is achieved.

PREGNANT WOMEN WITH ANTIPHOSPHOLIPID ANTIBODIES. Pregnant women with antiphospholipid antibodies and a prior history of fetal loss should receive prednisone and low-dose aspirin. Those with antiphospholipid antibodies and a prior history of venous thromboembolism should receive adjusted-dose heparin subcutaneously. Women with antiphospholipid antibodies who are either pregnant for the first time or who have not experienced thromboembolic complications during previous pregnancies should receive DVT surveillance, using impedance plethysmography or real-time ultrasonography, or nonadjusted-dose heparin prophylaxis throughout pregnancy. One might also reasonably consider the use of prednisone and low-dose aspirin.

SPECIAL TOPICS

Ovarian Vein Thrombosis

Acute ovarian vein thrombosis has been described as an early postpartum complication in approximately 1 of 4000 deliveries.[27] The clinical presentation generally involves severe lower abdominal or pelvic pain and striking adnexal tenderness, with onset 2 to 3 days postpartum. Most patients are febrile, and some may complain of flank pain. The differential diagnosis includes acute appendicitis, ureterolithiasis, pyelonephritis, and septic pelvic thrombophlebitis. Computed tomography and MRI have been shown to be effective in confirming the diagnosis of suspected acute ovarian vein thrombosis.[18] Consensus favors the view that isolated ovarian vein thrombosis in the early postpartum period after an otherwise uncomplicated delivery is a nonseptic problem, although culture and tissue confirmation are generally unavailable and many women are treated empirically with antibiotics. Pulmonary emboli have been reported in association with acute ovarian vein thrombosis. The mainstay of therapy is full therapeutic heparinization for 5 to 10 days. Such patients generally do not receive secondary prophylaxis with warfarin, although it may be reasonable to pursue such therapy when a persistent clot is noted on follow-up imaging studies or when PE is part of the initial presentation. Treatment failures may require ligation of the affected ovarian vein or positioning of vena caval filters, recognizing the fact that the left ovarian vein generally drains into the left renal vein, which drains above the usual site of caval filter placement.

Septic Pelvic Thrombophlebitis

Septic pelvic thrombophlebitis in the postpartum period generally occurs as a complication of puerperal endometritis. Thrombi associated with this problem have been identified in ovarian and iliofemoral veins and in the vena cava. Septic pulmonary emboli have been reported in as many as 39% of untreated patients.[28] Clinical features include severe pelvic pain, fever, shaking chills, and other signs of sepsis, including shock. Those experiencing septic PE may also demonstrate cough, dyspnea, pleuritic chest pain, hemoptysis, tachycardia, and hypoxemia; infiltrates on chest radiograph may cavitate. Computed tomography, MRI, and appropriately obtained cultures generally support the suspected diagnosis.[18] Although no controlled trials of therapy have been carried out, the available experience favors concurrent treatment with full therapeutic heparinization and multiple antibiotics. Full resolution of symptoms and signs is often quite delayed, although defervescence generally occurs within 12 to 36 hours after initiation of combined therapy unless a surgical problem exists; some patients require surgical drainage of identified pelvic abscesses or hysterectomy. Prospective studies addressing secondary DVT/PE prophylaxis after septic pelvic thrombophlebitis have not been performed, but it is known that a subset of cases involve iliofemoral veins.[18] It is reasonable to consider secondary prophylaxis of at least 3 months' duration with adjusted-dose subcutaneous heparin or warfarin (in the postpartum period) after acute septic pelvic thrombophlebitis.

Cerebral Vein/Sinus Thrombosis

Atraumatic cerebral vein/sinus thrombosis is an entity noted nearly exclusively in postpartum women, although occasional cases have been reported among oral contraceptive users. Clinical features include headache, focal and generalized seizures, pareses, papilledema, cortical blindness, cranial nerve findings, and obtundation. The hallmark is a rapidly changing clinical status. Onset of symptoms may occur from several days to several weeks postpartum. The differential diagnosis includes postpartum eclampsia and postpartum pituitary hemorrhage (pituitary apoplexy). Computed tomography generally reveals edema, enhancement, small ventricles, and low-density areas. Confirmation has traditionally required cerebral angiography, although MRI (or magnetic resonance angiography) may yield the diagnosis. Treatment involves administration of anticonvulsants, antiedema agents, and acute anticoagulation if there is no evidence of hemorrhage on CT and if propagation of thrombosis is suggested by clinical features. More than 70% of patients with this clinical entity recover with little or no residua, although another 10% of patients die.

REFERENCES

1. Koonin LM, Atrash HK, Lawson HW. Maternal mortality surveillance, United States, 1979–1986. MMWR 1991;40(SS-1):1.
2. Franks AL, Atrash HK, Lawson HW, Colberg KS. Obstetrical pulmonary embolism mortality, United States, 1970–1985. Am J Public Health 1990;80:720.
3. Rochat RW, Koonin LM, Atrash HK, et al. Maternal mortality in the United States: Report of the Maternal Mortality Collaborative. Obstet Gynecol 1988;72:91.
4. Coon WW, Willis PW, Keller JB. Venous thromboembolism and other venous disease in the Tecumseh community health study. Circulation 1973;48:839.

5. Villasanta U. Thromboembolic disease in pregnancy. Am J Obstet Gynecol 1965;93:142.

6. Aaro LA, Juergens JL. Thrombophlebitis associated with pregnancy. Am J Obstet Gynecol 1971;109:1128.

7. Ginsberg JS, Brill-Edwards P, Burrows RF, et al. Venous thrombosis during pregnancy: Leg and trimester of presentation. Thromb Haemost 1992;67:519.

8. Rutherford SE, Montoro M, McGehee W, et al. Thromboembolic disease associated with pregnancy: An 11-year review (abstract). Am J Obstet Gynecol 1991;164:286.

9. Rutherford SE, Phelan JP. Deep venous thrombosis and pulmonary embolism in pregnancy. Obstet Gynecol Clin North Am 1991;18:345.

10. Bergqvist A, Bergqvist D, Hallböök T. Acute deep vein thrombosis (DVT) after cesarean section. Acta Obstet Gynecol Scand 1983;62:473.

11. Hull RD, Raskob GE, Carter CJ. Serial impedance plethysmography in pregnant patients with clinically suspected deep-vein thrombosis. Ann Intern Med 1990;112:663.

12. Polak JF, Wilkinson DL. Ultrasonographic diagnosis of symptomatic deep venous thrombosis in pregnancy. Am J Obstet Gynecol 1991;165:625.

13. Ginsberg JS, Hirsh J. Use of antithrombotic agents during pregnancy. Chest 1992;102:385S.

14. Mosely P. Pregnancy and thrombophlebitis. Surg Gynecol Obstet 1980;150:593.

15. The PIOPED investigators. Value of the ventilation/perfusion scan in acute pulmonary embolism. JAMA 1990;263:2753.

16. Ginsberg JS, Hirsh J, Rainbow AJ, et al. Risks to the fetus of radiologic procedures used in the diagnosis of maternal thromboembolic disease. Thromb Haemost 1989;61:189.

17. Richlie DG. Noninvasive imaging of the lower extremity for deep venous thrombosis. J Gen Intern Med 1993;8:271.

18. Brown CE, Lowe TW. Puerperal pelvic thrombophlebitis: Impact on diagnosis and treatment using x-ray computed tomography and magnetic resonance imaging. Obstet Gynecol 1986;68:789.

19. Vukov LF, Berquist TH, King BF. Magnetic resonance imaging for calf deep venous thrombophlebitis. Ann Emerg Med 1991;20:497.

20. Hull R, Raskob G, Hirsh J, et al. Continuous intravenous heparin compared with intermittent subcutaneous heparin in the initial treatment of proximal-vein thrombosis. N Engl J Med 1986;315:1109.

21. Hall JG, Pauli RM, Wilson KM. Maternal and fetal sequelae of anticoagulation during pregnancy. Am J Med 1980;68:122.

22. Ginsberg JS, Hirsh J, Turner DC. Risks to the fetus of anticoagulant therapy during pregnancy. Thromb Haemost 1989;61:197.

23. Ginsberg JS, Kowalchuk G, Hirsh J, et al. Heparin therapy during pregnancy: Risks to the fetus and mother. Arch Intern Med 1989;149:2233.

24. Dahlman T, Lindvall N, Hellgren M. Osteopenia in pregnancy during long-term heparin treatment: A radiologic study postpartum. Br J Obstet Gynecol 1990;97:221.

25. Imperiale TF, Stollenwerk-Petrulis A. A meta-analysis of low-dose aspirin for the prevention of pregnancy-induced hypertension. JAMA 1991;266:260.

26. Silveira LH, Hubble CL, Jara LJ. Prevention of anticardiolipin antibody-related pregnancy losses with prednisone and aspirin. Am J Med 1992;93:403.

27. Rosenblum R, Derrick FC, Willis A. Postpartum ovarian vein thrombosis. Obstet Gynecol 1966;28:121.

28. Collins CG, MacCallum EA, Nelson EW, et al. Suppurative pelvic thrombophlebitis: Study of 70 patients treated by ligation of inferior vena cava and ovarian vessels. Surgery 1951;30:298.

Human Immunodeficiency Virus Infection in Pregnancy: Epidemiology, Management, and Vertical Transmission

Kathleen A. Steger, Cecelia Jarek, and Donald E. Craven

Current estimates are that 8 to 10 million persons are infected with human immunodeficiency virus (HIV) worldwide.[1] By the year 2000, more than 40 million persons may be infected worldwide; most of these will be women and children. Because children are infected through vertical transmission, women and children are primary targets for prevention and intervention during the second decade of acquired immunodeficiency syndrome (AIDS).

More than 1 million persons in the United States are infected with HIV type 1, and approximately 360,000 cases of AIDS were reported to the Centers for Disease Control and Prevention as of May 1994. An increasing proportion of cases are occurring in women, most of whom are of childbearing age.[2-5] Early recognition of HIV infection in pregnant women will increase the opportunity to make informed reproductive choices and to institute preventive measures that may decrease vertical transmission of HIV to fetuses and infants.

In this chapter, the epidemiology and management of HIV infection in pregnant women are reviewed. Particular emphasis is directed at education and counseling of women during pregnancy, as well as the use of zidovudine (ZDV) and other strategies to interrupt perinatal transmission of HIV.

EPIDEMIOLOGY OF HUMAN IMMUNODEFICIENCY VIRUS AND ACQUIRED IMMUNODEFICIENCY SYNDROME IN WOMEN

In the United States, women represent a steadily growing but cumulatively relatively small proportion (13%) of reported patients with AIDS.[2] This is largely because of the preponderance of cases in homosexual or bisexual males and intravenous drug users during the first decade of the epidemic in the United States. The epidemiology of the epidemic in the United States, however, has since the outset varied from that in developing countries, where heterosexual transmission accounts for the vast majority of cases.[1] These areas have a 1:1 ratio of male-to-female AIDS cases, and pediatric AIDS is commonly acquired perinatally.[1, 6]

Trends in the United States

The number and proportion of AIDS cases in women in the United States has increased steadily from 7% in 1984 to the current 13%.[2-5] Of all AIDS cases in women, 85% have occurred in women of childbearing age, with approximately one fourth of the cases in women 20 to 29 years of age, many of whom were most likely infected as adolescents.[5] This trend has serious implications in terms of HIV prevention strategies and will result in increases in pediatric cases of HIV infection and AIDS. In fact, 85% of the more than 3000 pediatric AIDS cases in the United States have been attributed to maternal HIV infection.[5]

In terms of associated mortality, between 1985 and 1988, the HIV-associated death rate in women quadrupled and by 1992 was the fifth leading cause of death in women of reproductive age.[7] In addition, HIV infection and AIDS has disproportionately affected women in racial and ethnic minority groups. In 1990, although black and Hispanic women constituted 19% of the total population of women in the United States, they accounted for 72% of women diagnosed with AIDS in this country.[7] The disproportionate impact of AIDS on minority groups has important implications for prevention efforts and effective health care delivery systems.

It is important to note that the epidemiologic trends described are based on cumulatively reported AIDS cases and are therefore dependent on the quality of the surveillance activities, the long period between HIV infection and the development of symptoms, the relevance of the AIDS case definition to specific populations, and the cumulative nature of the statistics. The revision of the Centers for Disease Control and Prevention case definition for AIDS, effective January 1, 1993, includes specific HIV manifestations in women as well as HIV-infected people with CD4 lymphocyte counts of less than or equal to 200 per mm[3]. These revisions should result in an increase in reported AIDS cases among women.[8]

Human Immunodeficiency Virus and Acquired Immunodeficiency Syndrome in Pregnancy

Worldwide, perinatal transmission is the most common cause of HIV infection in children. In the United States, approximately 7000 infants are born to HIV-infected mothers each year.[6]

A national population-based survey was initiated in 1988 to measure the prevalence of HIV infection in women who were birthing babies in the United States. In this study, blood specimens collected on filter paper for newborn metabolic screening were tested anonymously for maternal HIV antibody.[9] Despite the relatively low overall seroprevalence rates in women with live births, 0.8 per 1000, rates ranged from 0.2 per 1000 to 6.6 per 1000, with the highest rates found in New York, New Jersey, Florida, and Massachusetts.[5] Some metropolitan areas had notably higher rates than the states overall. For example, in Massachusetts, the HIV seroprevalence rate was 8 per 1000 among infants born to women at inner-city hospitals, compared with a 2 per 1000 rate statewide.[5] The rate of 22 per 1000 at Boston City Hospital was several times higher than the mean rate for inner-city hospitals.[10] During the same period, the HIV infection rates for women seeking abortions or family planning services were 18 per 1000 and 16 per 1000, respectively. Intravenous drug use and immigration from an HIV-endemic country were significantly associated with HIV infection.[10] Hospital-specific data have been useful for monitoring the epidemic and for allocating resources for education, counseling, testing, and prevention.

Vertical Transmission

Of the 7000 infants born to HIV-infected mothers in the United States each year, approximately 1000 to 2000 are HIV infected.[6] Rates of vertical transmission of HIV from mothers to their babies have varied widely among studies.[11–17] Determination of the precise rates of transmission has been compromised by the persistence of passively acquired maternal immunoglobulin G (IgG) antibody against HIV for as long as 18 months. Numerous prospective studies of HIV-infected pregnant women provide the best estimates of the actual transmission rate, but these studies are not consistent in terms of the populations studied and in the methods used to determine infection in infants.[12–16, 18] Transmission rates may vary as a result of the stage of maternal HIV disease, the virulence of the viral strain, the use of different cultural practices such as breast-feeding, and factors related to the delivery.[11–16, 19–24] Other important variables may include infection control practices during the birth process; genetic factors affecting immunologic responses; cofactors such as other sexually transmitted diseases, which may affect the integrity of the placental barrier; and behavioral factors such as continued illicit drug use or malnutrition. This partial list of possible cofactors implicated in vertical HIV transmission illustrates the difficulty in determining which factors actually are important in vertical transmission and the relative importance of each one.

Although we know that HIV transmission may occur early in pregnancy, as shown by the detection of HIV from aborted fetal tissue and during the perinatal and postnatal period,[25, 26] the overall rate of HIV transmission or the rates associated

TABLE 40–1.   Rates of Vertical Transmission of Human Immunodeficiency Virus (HIV)

STUDY	COUNTRY	YEAR	POPULATION	INFANT DIAGNOSIS	TRANSMISSION RATE	RISK FACTORS	COMMENTS
Selected Maternal/Infant Studies							
Blanche et al[28]	France	1992	Prospective cohort (n = 117)	HIV antibody + at 18 mo or AIDS-related death	27%	Breast-feeding, but in small numbers	No correlation with maternal factors or route of delivery
European Collaborative Study[17]	European countries	1992	Prospective cohort (n = 721)	HIV antibody + at 18 mo, + culture antigen 2, or HIV-related death	14%	Vaginal delivery with episiotomy and fetal monitoring; maternal p24; CD4 <700, <34 wk gestation	In centers where these procedures are not done routinely, trend of increased risk with breast-feeding, possibly increased risk with cesarean section
Goedert et al[12]	United States	1989	Prospective cohort (n = 55)	Clinical or serologic evidence of HIV at 15 mo	29%	Lack of maternal gp 120 band; <37 wk gestation	No correlation with maternal CD4 count or neutralizing antibody
Halsey et al[13]	Haiti	1990	Prospective case-control (n = 230)	HIV antibody + on filter paper samples at 12 mo	25%	Virtually all infants were breast-fed, so comparison was not possible	Maternal HIV infection resulted in 12% increase in infant mortality at 24 mo
Hira et al[14]	Africa	1990	Prospective case-control (n = 109)	HIV antibody + at 24 mo or AIDS diagnosis	39%	Younger maternal age and advanced HIV disease	Poor prognosis for HIV-infected infants; 44% died by 24 mo compared with 12% of uninfected controls
Ryder et al[15]	Africa	1989	Prospective case-control (n = 92)	Culture of randomly selected cord blood	39%	Matenal CD4 count <400/mm³	High mortality in HIV-infected mothers' offspring, 21% versus 3.8% (p <0.001) at 12 mo
ZDV Prophylaxis Studies							
ACTG 076[22]	United States, France	1994	Randomized trial (n = 364)	HIV culture	25.5% placebo group; 8.3% in ZDV group (p <0.0001)	CD4 count > 200/mm³	Trial stopped due to significant effect noted
Boyer[62]	United States	1994	Nonrandomized prospective cohort (n = 68)	HIV culture	29% in no-ZDV group; 4% in ZDV group (p <0.01)	Duration of labor, p24 antigen	Significant reduction in vertical transmission of HIV associated with ZDV treatment
Selected Twin Studies							
Goedert et al[20]	United States	1991	Retrospective (n = 66 sets)	HIV antibody at 15 mo or HIV-related disorder	32%	Birth order, vaginal delivery	22 discordant sets; 18 of 22 twin A infected; trend toward protective effect of cesarean section
de Martino et al[21]	Italy	1991	(n = 22 sets)	HIV antibody at 15 mo or clinical diagnosis	25%	Significant increase among breast-fed subjects (56% versus 4%, p = 0.002)	No difference in gestational age, route of delivery, birth weight; concordance in HIV infection in all but one twin pair

HIV, Human immunodeficiency virus; AIDS, acquired immunodeficiency syndrome.
Adapted from Craven DE, Steger KA, Jarek C. Human immunodeficiency virus infection in pregnancy: Epidemiology and prevention of vertical transmission. Infect Control Hosp Epidemiol 1994;15:36–47.

with pregnancy, labor, delivery, and the postnatal period have not been determined.

Early studies suggested that the rates of vertical transmission of HIV might be as high as 60%, but these results were biased in that the studies involved populations of women who had already borne a child who was HIV infected.[27] More recent prospective studies designed to determine the rate of vertical transmission have produced results ranging from 7 to 77% (Table 40–1).[12–15, 17, 22, 28, 29]

In the European collaborative study, 14.4% of 721 babies became infected with HIV, and maternal risk factors for vertical transmission were p24 antigenemia and CD4 counts less than 700 per mm³.[17] Factors related to the delivery that were found to increase the risk of HIV transmission included vaginal delivery in which episiotomy, scalp electrodes, forceps, or vacuum extractors were used. Of note is that infants born before 34 weeks' gestation had nearly a fourfold greater risk of infection than those born later. The hypothesis offered for this finding was that women who are more likely to be infectious, as determined by antigenemia or AIDS, may be more likely to deliver before 34 weeks' gestation. Infections of the genital tract may also increase the risk of premature delivery and of transmission of HIV infection. Furthermore, infants born before 34 weeks may be more susceptible to infection because of diminished immunocompetence and low levels of passively acquired antibodies. A twofold but not statistically significant increase in the risk of infection was noted in those infants who were breast-fed compared with those who were not.[17]

Other vertical transmission studies have reported relatively consistent rates between 21 and 29%; however, associated risk factors have differed.[12, 13, 28] Although two of these studies documented a correlation between maternal factors and vertical transmission, Blanche and colleagues found no such association. The French group found a statistically significant increased risk of HIV infection among a small number of breast-fed children.[28] In the study by Halsey and associates in Haiti, virtually all of the 230 infants studied were breast-fed and the estimated vertical transmission rate of HIV was 25%.[13] The major finding of this report, however, was that mortality during a 2-year period was increased by nearly 12% in infants of HIV-infected mothers compared with those born to uninfected mothers.

Two African studies demonstrated higher vertical transmission rates. In a prospective case-control study in Zaire, Ryder and co-workers reported an overall vertical HIV transmission rate of 39%. Infection with HIV was determined by positive HIV culture in 92 randomly selected cord blood samples or by clinical diagnosis.[15] The risk of vertical transmission was associated with maternal CD4 lymphocyte counts less than 400 per mm³.[15] Similar findings were reported by Hira and colleagues from Zambia, where 39% of the 109 infants monitored for 24 months were determined to be HIV infected on the basis of HIV antibody at 24 months or an AIDS diagnosis.[14] Maternal risk factors associated with increased HIV transmission included younger age and advanced HIV disease.

St. Louis and co-workers reported that rates of perinatal transmission varied between 7 and 71% for specific subsets of African women.[29] Several risk factors were identified by univariate analysis, but only low CD4 counts (<600/mm³), high CD8 counts (>1800/mm³), p24 antigenemia, placental membrane inflammation, prolonged fever (>30 days), and low hemoglobin levels (<8.5 gm/L) were independently associated with perinatal transmission. Of note is that both Ryder and Hira and their groups reported a higher mortality for HIV-infected children than for uninfected controls.

Two studies have focused on vertical transmission of HIV in twin pairs.[20, 21] Goedert and colleagues assessed rates of HIV transmission retrospectively in 66 sets of twins.[20] Unlike the Italian study, in which there was concordance in all 18 twin pairs except one, Goedert's group reported that although the HIV infection rate among the infants was 32% overall, 10 sets were concordantly infected and 34 sets were concordantly uninfected.[20, 21]

The most interesting finding, however, was the significantly increased rate of infection among first-born twins in the 22 discordant sets (82% versus 18%, p = 0.004). Goedert and co-workers also reported a higher HIV infection rate among first-born twins delivered by the vaginal route than by cesarean section (50% versus 38%). Data from these small studies, a meta-analysis, and the European Collaborative study suggest that a substantial proportion of HIV transmission occurs during the birth process and may be preventable by cleansing the birth canal or by performing a cesarean section.[23, 24]

Important data from the AIDS Clinical Trials Group (ACTG) study protocol 076 demonstrated that perinatal transmission of HIV was reduced 68% in women who received ZDV, 500 mg per day, versus placebo. Therapy was started after the fourteenth week of gestation, continued through the intrapartum period, and then was given to infants for 6 weeks after birth.[22]

HUMAN IMMUNODEFICIENCY VIRUS STRUCTURE AND FUNCTION

Since the discovery that AIDS was caused by a ribonucleic acid (RNA) retrovirus in 1983, a great deal has been learned about the viral genome, structure, replication, and effect on the host (Fig. 40–1).[19, 30, 31] The *gag* region of the HIV genome codes for the core proteins (p24), and the *env* gene produces the envelope glycoproteins (gp 160, gp 120, gp 41). Both the *gag* and *env* are important in the pathogenesis, diagnosis, and treatment of

HIV infection. Antibody to the p24 core protein is important for HIV diagnosis in adults, and the p24 antigen is a useful marker of viral replication.[32] Of the envelope glycoproteins, gp 120 is essential for the attachment to the CD4 (T helper) lymphocyte, contains neutralizing antibody domains, epitopes for cytotoxic T-cell activity, and is one of the candidates for an HIV vaccine.

Reverse transcriptase, produced by the *pol* region of the genome, permits the HIV RNA to be transcribed into proviral deoxyribonucleic acid (DNA) before integration into genomic DNA of the infected cell (Fig. 40–2). Zidovudine (ZDV, azidothymidine), dideoxyinosine, and other antiviral drugs inhibit reverse transcriptase activity.[30] In addition, new drugs designed to inhibit the *tat* gene, which up-regulates HIV, are currently undergoing clinical trials in patients with advanced HIV disease. Other parts of the HIV life cycle depicted in Figure 40–2 are also potential sites for antiviral therapy or immunotherapy.

HOST RESPONSE TO HUMAN IMMUNODEFICIENCY VIRUS

CD4 lymphocytes are the central component of the host immune system and are involved in the induction of cytotoxic T-cell activity, natural killer cell function, activation of macrophages, and induction of B cells.[19] Progressive HIV infection is characterized by an increase in viral load coupled with a depletion of host CD4 lymphocytes, although the exact mechanisms of T-cell destruction are not well understood.[19] As a result of these immune deficits, persons with advanced HIV infection are susceptible to various life-threatening infections caused by bacteria, fungi, protozoa, and other viruses. The risk for these opportunistic infections increases as the CD4 lymphocyte count decreases, and some such as cytomegalovirus (CMV) retinitis, *Cryptococcus neoformans* meningitis, and disseminated disease caused by *Mycobacterium avium* complex are invariably found only in advanced HIV disease when CD4 counts are less than 200 per mm³ (Fig. 40–3).[31]

DIAGNOSIS OF HUMAN IMMUNODEFICIENCY VIRUS IN ADULTS

Diagnosis in Pregnancy

Infection with HIV can be diagnosed by viral isolation, markers for the presence of HIV (p24 antigen), polymerase chain reaction (PCR), or anti-

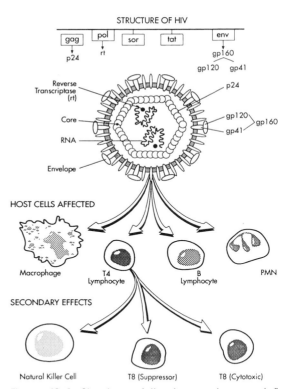

Figure 40–1. Structure of the human immunodeficiency virus (HIV) and genome and cells affected by the virus. PMN, Polymorphonuclear neutrophil. (From Craven DE, Steger KA, Jarek C. Human immunodeficiency virus infection in pregnancy: Epidemiology and prevention of vertical transmission. Infect Control Hosp Epidemiol 1994;15: 39.)

body responses detected by enzyme immunoassay, enzyme-linked immunosorbent assay (ELISA), Western blot, or immunofluorescence.[31, 32] Currently, enzyme immunoassay and Western blot antibody assays are most commonly used for diagnosis in adults and older children, whereas p24 antigen, PCR, and culture have been more useful for the diagnosis of HIV in newborns and children during the first year of life.[32, 33]

Antibody Tests

Enzyme-linked immunosorbent assay tests were introduced for screening blood before transfusion in April 1985.[32] Since then, ELISA tests have improved dramatically and now are highly sensitive, specific, inexpensive, and easy to perform. In the United States, a repeatedly positive ELISA test response is usually confirmed by the presence of specific protein bands present in the Western blot test, which is more expensive and specific than the ELISA.[31]

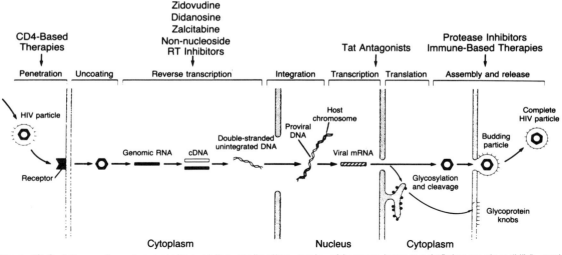

Figure 40-2. Schematic representation of the replication cycle of human immunodeficiency virus (HIV) and the sites of action of antiretroviral agents. (Reprinted from Johnson VA. New developments in antiretroviral drug therapy for HIV infection. In: Volberding P, Jacobson MA (eds). AIDS Clinical Review 1992. New York: Marcel Dekker, 1992, pp 69–104, by courtesy of Marcel Dekker, Inc.)

An indeterminate HIV test result is defined as a positive ELISA result with a Western blot that demonstrates antibody against one or more of the HIV proteins but does not meet the specific established criteria for a positive response.[32] Indeterminate test results may be encountered in women who have recently become infected or have end-stage HIV disease in which antibody is waning or with an antibody that cross-reacts with HIV. The chance that an indeterminate HIV test response will become positive is related to a woman's level of risk, but a woman with an indeterminate result should follow safe sexual practices, should be counseled about pregnancy planning, and should inform her sexual partner. Women with an indeterminate HIV test result should have the test re-

peated 1 to 3 months later or should have a p24 antigen test performed if the acute HIV syndrome is suspected.

p24 Antigen Test

The p24 antigen is commonly detected during the acute HIV infection and in women with advanced HIV disease.[32–34] A large amount of p24 antigen in blood has been associated with a poor prognosis, but levels may not correlate well with stage of HIV infection in some studies.

The use of an acid dissociation procedure that disrupts p24 antigen-antibody complexes has greatly increased the sensitivity of p24 antigen de-

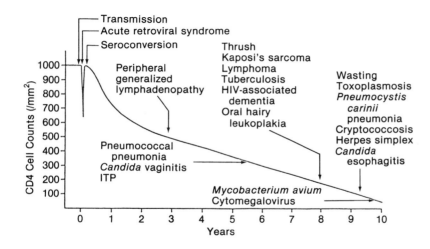

Figure 40-3. Summary of presentations of opportunistic infections by CD4 cell count/mm³. ITP, Idiopathic thrombocytopenia. (From Bartlett JG. The Johns Hopkins Hospital Guide to Medical Care of Patients with HIV Infection. 4th ed. Baltimore: Williams & Wilkins, 1994. Copyright John G. Bartlett, MD.)

tection assays. Using Coulter's assay for acid-dissociable p24 may increase mean levels two- to fivefold in adults, serving as a useful marker to monitor the efficacy of antiviral therapy.

DIAGNOSIS OF HUMAN IMMUNODEFICIENCY VIRUS IN NEWBORNS

Because IgG antibody crosses the placenta, all children born to an HIV-infected mother have maternal IgG antibodies against HIV, but 25% may also be infected with HIV.[12, 28, 35] Therefore, early diagnosis in children is often based on HIV culture, p24 antigen, or the presence of HIV DNA or RNA viral sequences detected by PCR.[33, 35–37]

Polymerase Chain Reaction

By comparison with HIV antigen and antibody tests, PCR uses a gene amplification technique that is rapid, automated, and highly sensitive and specific for detection of HIV DNA sequences.[37, 38] Polymerase chain reaction uses primers that anneal to the target sequences of HIV-1 DNA from the *gag* and *env* regions, which are subsequently amplified several thousandfold. Polymerase chain reaction is capable of detecting a single copy of a specific HIV gene segment. Thus, it is of value for the diagnosis of HIV in infants who have only a small amount of blood for HIV culture and passively acquired maternal antibodies. Rogers and co-workers identified five of seven neonates (<28 days of age) who developed AIDS a mean of 9.8 months after being identified as PCR, and no viral sequences were identified by PCR in nine neonates who remained well during the mean follow-up period of 16 months.[37]

Comeau and associates used PCR on newborn blood samples and identified 14 (67%) children who developed disease by 18 months and 9 (43%) of the 21 patients whose disease progressed more slowly.[35] Thus, more than 50% of the HIV-infected children could be identified by PCR at birth.[35] In the French multicenter study, PCR detected 22 (81%) of 27 positive infants versus 15 (56%) of the infants tested by HIV culture.[36]

Culture for Human Immunodeficiency Virus

Human immunodeficiency virus can be isolated from peripheral blood mononuclear cells and plasma throughout the course of HIV infection.[38] Quantitative levels of HIV in plasma and peripheral blood mononuclear cells appear to correlate with stage of HIV infection and prognosis.

HIV culture is a valuable tool for the diagnosis of HIV infection in infants born to HIV-infected mothers, but the procedures for culture are costly and laborious and may take several weeks. Burgard and co-workers used positive viral cultures at birth to identify 19 of 40 HIV-infected infants (48%, 95% confidence interval 32–63%); at 3 months of age, 30 (75%) were HIV-culture positive.[36] These data suggest that viral culture at birth can correctly identify about 50% of newborns infected with HIV and that the remaining 50% of infants may acquire HIV infection late in pregnancy, during delivery, or in the postpartum period.

p24 Antigen

Acid-dissociable p24 has been useful in the diagnosis of perinatally acquired HIV infection. In the French collaborative study, viral cultures were positive at birth in 19 (48%) of the 40 infants later found to be infected with HIV, whereas p24 antigen was present in only 18% of infants at birth. However, the presence of p24 antigen at birth was associated with severe, early HIV disease.[36] The presence of p24 antigenemia was detected in 16 (9%) of the 178 women tested at delivery, and a strong correlation was found between the presence of antigenemia in the mother and infant, 25% versus only a 7% rate of p24 antigenemia in the infants born to mothers who were p24 antigen negative.

SURROGATE MARKERS OF HUMAN IMMUNODEFICIENCY VIRUS DISEASE

CD4 Lymphocytes

By comparison, T-lymphocyte subset (CD4/CD8) analysis is a widely used test to assess the stage of HIV disease and eligibility for antiviral therapy and to assist in the diagnosis and prevention of opportunistic infection.[31] Both absolute number and percentage of CD4 cells are used: CD4 counts exceeding 500 per mm^3 are usually 29%, 200 to 500 per mm^3 correlate with 14 to 28%, and less than 200 per mm^3 corresponds to less than 14%. The use of percentage of CD4 cells reduces the variation noted with absolute CD4 counts, and better correlation is found with lower CD4 counts.

A large variation in absolute CD4 counts may be noted between laboratories and within the same laboratory. Limitations of the CD4 count include laboratory variation, differences in white blood cell count and lymphocyte percentage, and variations in the host diurnal rhythms, intercurrent illness, and the use of concurrent steroids. Despite limitations, absolute and percentage of CD4 lymphocyte count are helpful in guiding HIV therapy. Two CD4 determinations repeated at least 1 week apart are advised for initial evaluation. If the absolute T-helper number exceeds 500 per mm³, tests should be repeated every 4 to 6 months until the value is less than 500 per mm³. When the CD4 count is less than 200 per mm³, the risk of *Pneumocystis carinii* pneumonia (PCP) and prophylaxis against PCP should be initiated with trimethoprim-sulfamethoxazole, dapsone, or aerosolized pentamidine.[39]

The CD4 count is also useful for anticipating opportunistic infection caused by HIV infection. Tuberculosis, Kaposi's sarcoma, and oral thrush infection may be diagnosed when the CD4 counts are between 200 and 600 per mm³; PCP and toxoplasmosis usually appear at CD4 counts less than 200 per mm³; *M. avium complex,* CMV, and *C. neoformans* at CD4 counts less than 100 per mm³.

CD4 Lymphocytes in Pregnancy

Several studies have examined cellular immunity during pregnancy in non–HIV-infected patients. Most studies have reported that CD4 (T helper) cells and the CD4-to-CD8 (T suppressor) ratio are decreased and CD8 cells are increased during pregnancy and the postpartum period.[40–42]

Biggar and co-workers[40] compared changes in CD4/CD8 cells during pregnancy and the postpartum period in 37 HIV-infected women versus 65 seronegative women (Fig. 40–4). Both groups of women had declines in the percentage of CD4 cells in the early stages of pregnancy, but the seronegative women had increases in the percentage of cells during the 6 weeks before delivery and during the postpartum period, whereas the seropositives had a progressive decline in CD4 count during pregnancy and continuing into the postpartum period.

In a study of 20 pregnant HIV-infected women with a history of intravenous drug use compared with 24 seronegative controls, the former had significantly lower hematocrits, fewer lymphocytes per mm³, a lower CD4-to-CD8 ratio (0.90 ± 0.45 versus 1.59 ± 0.49), and lower CD4 counts (388 ± 200, range 117–753, versus 689 ± 316, range 240–1674).[43] Fifty-five percent of the 20 women

with asymptomatic HIV infection had CD4 counts less than 400 per mm³, compared with only 13% of the 24 seronegative pregnant patients with a history of injection drug use. Thus, seropositive pregnant women should have baseline CD4 counts. Women with lower CD4 counts (<500/mm³ or 29%) should have a repeat evaluation at least every trimester and perhaps more often if they are symptomatic or require prophylaxis against PCP.

PREGNANCY AND HUMAN IMMUNODEFICIENCY VIRUS DISEASE

The effect of pregnancy on the natural history of HIV infection is unknown and is the subject of great debate.[42–44] Some of the controversy is caused by differences in study populations, the stage of HIV disease, and the absence of matched control groups.

Natural History

Some small, uncontrolled studies and CD4 data have suggested that HIV infection progresses during pregnancy, whereas other small matched controlled studies of HIV-infected women have found no significant differences from controls.[43] In another study, rates of pregnancy among injection drug–using women enrolled in a methadone treatment program were 10 per 100 patient-years, and no significant differences were noted between HIV-seropositive and HIV-seronegative women.[43] Of note is that only 1 of 39 women who were asymptomatic and HIV infected developed symptomatic disease (oral candidiasis) during pregnancy, and none developed AIDS during the 13-month postpartum period.

High rates of bacterial pneumonia and severe vaginal candidiasis have been reported in HIV-infected women at all stages of disease.[45–48] In contrast to previous reports,[48] Selwyn and co-workers found no increase in the frequency of severe vaginal candidiasis in HIV-infected women, but higher rates of bacterial pneumonia were present in HIV-seropositive women than in seronegative controls (12% versus 0, p<0.05).[43] For these reasons, HIV-seropositive women should be carefully monitored during pregnancy for the presence of bacterial infections such as pneumonia.

Figure 40–4. Variation of mean CD4 lymphocyte percentages among HIV-negative and HIV-positive women during and after pregnancy. Note that the CD4 cell percentage in the HIV-negative women increased in the last 6 weeks of pregnancy and was significantly higher in the postpartum period than that in the HIV-positive women. (From Biggar RJ, Pahwa S, Minkoff H, et al. Immunosuppression in pregnant women infected with human immunodeficiency virus. Am J Obstet Gynecol 1989; 161:1239.)

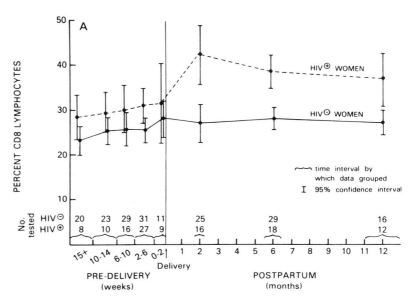

Obstetric Complications

Several investigators have studied obstetric complications and outcomes of HIV-infected women. In a retrospective study of pregnancy outcomes in 34 children who later developed HIV infection, Minkoff and co-workers found a greater number of women with premature rupture of the membranes, premature delivery, and babies with birth weights less than 2500 gm.[49] In the Edinburgh study, significantly increased rates of spontaneous abortion were reported, but no differences were observed in preterm delivery or low-birth-weight infants.[50]

In a large study from Zaire, Ryder and colleagues[15] reported that compared with seronegative controls, infants born to seropositive mothers were more likely to be premature and to have lower birth weight, a higher rate of chorioamnionitis, a higher fatality rate (p<0.001), but no difference in the rate of stillbirths. By comparison, asymptomatic HIV-infected women with intravenous drug use as a risk factor had no differences in the rate of spontaneous abortion, ectopic pregnancy, preterm delivery, stillbirth, or low-birth-weight neonates when compared with seronegative matched controls.[43]

Although obstetric complications occur in many women with HIV infection, it is difficult to assess the impact of confounding variables such as intravenous drug use, intercurrent sexually transmitted diseases, socioeconomic status, and access to medical care. Therefore, to assess correctly the impact of HIV infection on obstetric outcomes, HIV-infected women should be compared with matched seronegative controls.

MANAGEMENT OF HUMAN IMMUNODEFICIENCY VIRUS INFECTION IN PREGNANCY

Management of HIV infection in pregnancy has been the subject of several reviews.[34, 41, 51] The primary differences between pregnant women and other HIV-infected populations are the difficulty in differentiating symptoms of pregnancy from HIV infection, the potential effects of diagnostic tests, and the use of medications that may increase risk to a mother or cause damage to her fetus.

Counseling and Psychosocial Support

With the availability of ZDV and other early interventions for HIV infection, even during pregnancy, identification of HIV infection in pregnant women is crucial. Counseling should be sensitive and culturally appropriate, and testing should be voluntary but routinely offered and strongly endorsed or performed by the primary care provider. Human immunodeficiency virus infection should be discussed in the context of other sexually transmitted diseases, with risk reduction and prevention strategies included.

The AIDS epidemic has been superimposed on a number of societal issues including drug addiction, homelessness, violence, and poverty. The event of learning of one's HIV infection may have varying significance depending on one's level of social stability. For successful engagement in health care, attention must be given to stabilization of drug habits, housing, and abusive relationships. In addition, because women are most often the caretakers of dependent children, consideration for their immediate and long-term care must be addressed. A care plan that is specific to a woman and that integrates these social service needs is integral to successful medical management. Primary care providers should be cognizant of historical barriers to medical care among women. Approaches should be multidisciplinary and comprehensive and should involve the woman when possible.

It is important to realize that data suggest that women who are HIV infected often choose to continue pregnancies, even after having a child born with HIV infection.[11, 49, 52] A nondirective, nonjudgmental approach is recommended for reproductive counseling, but knowledge of HIV status as well as personal lifestyle characteristics is helpful. The presence of active, illicit drug use requires special attention because of its effect on compliance with health care, possible barriers to risk reduction, and the lack of appropriate drug treatment programs for women.[53, 54]

In terms of psychological impact of HIV on women, the issues are similar to those in the general HIV-infected population; however, additional issues may be related to the stresses of the pregnancy and possible infection of the child. An assessment of the support structure and family dynamics is particularly critical for HIV-infected pregnant women.

Medical Evaluation

Except for monitoring CD4 lymphocyte count and remaining alert for bacterial infections and opportunistic infections in patients with advanced HIV disease, the medical evaluation of the HIV-infected pregnant woman is similar to that for HIV-seronegative women.

A summary of the medical evaluation for HIV-infected patients is shown in Table 40–2. After a thorough obstetric and medical history, patients should have a physical examination to carefully evaluate skin lesions, the oropharynx, lymphadenopathy, and cardiopulmonary status. Laboratory tests depend in part on whether a patient has been previously assessed or treated for HIV infection. In addition to baseline blood screens, patients should have serologic tests, a urinalysis, and a tuberculin skin test with purified protein derivative

TABLE 40–2. Medical Evaluation of Pregnant Women Infected with Human Immunodeficiency Virus

Educational
　Risk reduction education
　Overall health promotion
Psychosocial
　Assessment, linkages, and support, including drug treatment
　Coordination of care and planning for family members
Medical
　Routine history and physical examination
　Baseline laboratory studies including:
　　Complete blood count, differential, platelets
　　Biochemistry screening profile
　　Urinalysis
　　Chest radiography if respiratory symptoms or disease present
　　Tuberculin skin test (purified protein derivative) with anergy panel
　　Serology test for syphilis
　　Toxoplasma serology
　　Hepatitis B surface antigen and antibody
　　Papanicolaou test
　　CD4 T-lymphocyte subsets each trimester and postpartum
　　　Consider zidovudine after first trimester as prophylaxis against perinatal HIV transmission
　　　If CD4 count is ≤200/mm³, give prophylaxis for *Pneumocystis carinii* pneumonia with Bactrim or aerosolized pentamidine if allergic to Bactrim

with an anergy panel. Chest radiographs should be performed only in the presence of respiratory symptoms or if results of the tuberculin test are positive.[55]

Except for syphilis, the frequency of other sexually transmitted diseases is not increased with HIV; however, all women should also be screened for gonorrhea and *Chlamydia*.[56] Genital *herpes simplex* may be more fulminant in presentation in HIV-infected women and more difficult to treat. Oral acyclovir can decrease the duration and severity of mucocutaneous disease, but its use in pregnancy should probably be limited to treatment of life-threatening or primary herpes simplex virus infection occurring in the third trimester. Current recommendations are that women with visible lesions or prodromal symptoms at the time of delivery should undergo cesarean section.

Physicians and other health care workers should be familiar with clinical manifestations of HIV disease in pregnant women. Monitoring the CD4 count during pregnancy may help prevent serious complications such as PCP. Because CD4 lymphocytes usually decrease during pregnancy, if the initial two tests performed at baseline are less than 750 per mm³, repeat counts should be performed at least every trimester, and if less than 300 per mm³, counts should be repeated monthly.

Figure 40–5. Summary of AIDS Clinical Trials Group (ACTG) study 076 indicating significantly decreased perinatal transmission of human immunodeficiency virus (HIV) for pregnant women treated with zidovudine (ZDV) versus placebo. (From Centers for Disease Control. Zidovudine for the prevention of HIV transmission from mother to infant. MMWR 1994;43:285.)

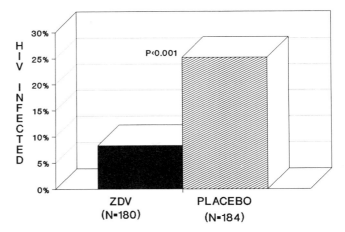

Antiretroviral Therapy

Studies of higher doses of ZDV during pregnancy demonstrate that the pharmacokinetics are similar to those in nonpregnant women, but information about the safety of ZDV during pregnancy is still scarce.[56–58] More information is needed about the effects of ZDV on the mother and the potential protective effect versus long-term risk to the fetus and newborn, most of whom will not become infected with HIV.

Data collected to date on small numbers of pregnant women suggest that ZDV is well tolerated and has not been associated with any serious acute side effects in the mother or child.[58, 59] As of December 31, 1991, the Burroughs Wellcome registry had enrolled 121 HIV-infected women who received ZDV during pregnancy.[59] Of the 31 outcomes reported after first-trimester exposure, only one birth defect was identified. During second-trimester exposure, one birth defect was identified in the 15 patients treated, and none of the 10 patients treated during the third trimester were found to have infants with birth defects. Five of the 58 total cases had induced abortions, and 2 patients were unavailable for follow-up.

Sperling and co-workers studied 43 pregnant women given doses of ZDV ranging from 300 to 1200 mg; 5 of the women had AIDS, 21 had HIV-related symptoms, and 14 were asymptomatic.[60] Seventeen of the patients had CD4 counts less than 200 per mm^3, 13 were between 200 and 500 per mm^3, and 7 had counts exceeding 500 per mm^3. Twelve women had ZDV prescribed during the first trimester, and 10 continued therapy throughout gestation. Only two minor toxic reactions were noted, and no pattern of adverse outcomes such as congenital malformation, premature birth, or fetal distress could be attributed to the drug. The use of

ZDV could have contributed to the oligohydramnios, anemia, or growth retardation observed in some of the patients, but other drugs were also used concomitantly with ZDV.

Zidovudine (200 mg orally three times daily) should be considered after the first trimester if the CD4 count is less than 500 per mm^3, and particularly if the patient is symptomatic. Because women have a lower mean body weight and mean lower hemoglobin values, they have a greater risk of anemia from ZDV therapy. Although dideoxyinosine and dideoxycytidine have significantly lower bone marrow toxicity, data on their efficacy and toxicity in women and during pregnancy are limited.[57, 58, 60, 61] Major side effects of these latter drugs are pancreatitis for patients receiving dideoxyinosine and peripheral neuropathy for patients treated with dideoxycytidine.

Data from the ACTG study protocol 076 suggest that the use of ZDV after the fourteenth week of gestation reduced perinatal transmission of HIV by 68%.[22] Of note is that all of the women had CD4 lymphocyte counts exceeding 200 per mm^3, and none had been receiving ZDV during their pregnancy (Table 40–3). The ZDV regimen of 500 mg per day was well tolerated and side effects were few, other than a reduction in hemoglobin of 1 gm per dl in the ZDV group versus the placebo group. Decreased HIV transmission to infants was also reported by Boyer and colleagues.[62]

Opportunistic Infection

In early pregnancy, women often experience fatigue, nausea, anorexia, and weight loss, which may be manifestations of HIV disease or HIV-related opportunistic infections.[51] Later in preg-

TABLE 40–3. Summary of the AIDS Clinical Trials Group (ACTG) Study Protocol 076 for Selection of Pregnant Women for Enrollment and Doses of Zidovudine Administered*

Patient Eligibility
• No prior antiretroviral treatment during current pregnancy or clinical indications for maternal antepartum antiretroviral therapy
• CD4 T-lymphocyte count >200/mm^3 at initial assessment

Zidovudine Regimen
• ZDV, 100 mg PO 5×/day, initiated at 14–34 wk gestation and continued for the remainder of the pregnancy
• Intravenous ZDV during labor; loading dose of 2 mg/kg body weight given over 1 hr, followed by continuous infusion of 1 mg/kg body weight/hr until delivery
• ZDV orally to the newborn (ZDV syrup at 2 mg/kg body weight every 6 hr) for the first 6 wk of life, beginning 8–12 hr after birth

Limitations of the Study
• Unknown efficacy of ZDV among women with CD4 T-lymphocyte counts ≤200 cells/mm^3 or among women who had previously used ZDV for extended periods and may be infected with ZDV-resistant strains of HIV
• Relative or independent contributions of the antepartum treatment, intrapartum treatment, or treatment of the infant not evaluable; the dose and duration of ZDV therapy not clear
• Risk or benefit of ZDV use in the first trimester not known
• No information about long-term side effects for infants and mothers treated with ZDV, including 75% of infants who did not become infected with HIV. However, long-term follow-up of infants and mothers is being conducted to monitor for possible late side effects

Current Recommendations
• Women of childbearing age should be informed of the results of ACTG protocol 076
• HIV-infected pregnant women meeting the protocol eligibility criteria should be informed of the potential benefits but unknown long-term risks of ZDV therapy as administered in ACTG protocol 076. The decision to use ZDV for prevention of perinatal transmission should be made by women in consultation with their health care providers
• Health care providers should inform their patients that this ZDV regimen substantially reduced but did not eliminate the risk of perinatal HIV transmission
• Until the potential risk for teratogenicity and other complications from ZDV therapy given in the first trimester can be assessed, ZDV therapy given only for the purpose of reducing the risk for perinatal transmission should not be instituted earlier than the 14th wk of gestation
• Public Health Service is developing further recommendations for the uses of ZDV for HIV-infected pregnant women whose clinical indications differ from the ACTG protocol 076 eligibility criteria and for counseling and HIV antibody testing for women of childbearing age

*Note the limitations of the study and current recommendations for the use of zidovudine to reduce perinatal transmission of HIV.
ZDV, Zidovudine; PO, orally; HIV, human immunodeficiency virus.
Data from Centers for Disease Control. Zidovudine for the prevention of HIV transmission from mother to infant. MMWR 1994;43:285.

nancy, women often note shortness of breath, pedal edema, rectal pain due to increased intra-abdominal pressure, dysphagia or heartburn, and sometimes headaches. Clinicians must be aware of the increased risk of common bacterial infections in HIV-infected pregnant women and the CD4 lymphocyte count at which opportunistic infections are likely to occur (see Fig. 40–3). Detailed information on the diagnosis and management of various opportunistic infections is available in several review articles.[31, 51, 56, 63]

Most of the serious opportunistic infections occur when the CD4 lymphocyte count is less than 300 per mm^3. In a study of the 56 HIV-infected pregnant women by Minkoff and co-workers, 16 patients had CD4 counts less than 300 per mm^3 and 7 (44%) developed opportunistic infection (6 PCP, 1 central nervous system toxoplasmosis), 1 developed pneumonia, and 1 patient had a postcesarean wound abscess.[64]

Pneumocystic pneumonia is the most common and serious opportunistic infection in pregnant women infected with HIV.[39, 56] It may present with subtle symptoms of mild dyspnea on exertion that may mimic pregnancy, and failure to diagnose the infection may result in severe maternal hypoxia with adverse sequelae for the fetus.[57] Initial episodes of PCP are associated with a maternal mortality of 5 to 10%, and the mortality rate increases with subsequent episodes.[56] Trimethoprim-sulfamethoxazole (Bactrim) is the treatment of choice for acute or subacute PCP during pregnancy.[51, 56, 65]

Prophylaxis against PCP should be considered if the CD4 count decreases to less than 200 per mm^3, with the understanding that CD4 counts usually decrease during pregnancy.[39, 40, 56] Possible drugs for prophylaxis include trimethoprim-sulfamethoxazole (1 double-strength tablet 3 times per week), aerosolized pentamidine (300 mg every 4 weeks via a Respirgard II jet nebulizer), or dapsone (50–100 mg/day). Although folic acid antagonists are usually considered to be contraindicated in pregnancy, trimethoprim-sulfamethoxazole has become the treatment of choice because its efficacy in nonpregnant patients has been superior to that of aerosolized pentamidine.[51, 65] In patients who cannot tolerate trimethoprim-sulfamethoxazole, aerosolized pentamidine should be considered. Because of the low concentrations of aerosolized pentamidine in the blood, most clinicians consider aerosolized pentamidine therapy acceptable for pregnant women, but it is more expensive and may be less effective than the other two regimens.[51, 56, 66]

Before aerosolized pentamidine therapy, patients should have a skin test for tuberculosis, a sputum culture for tuberculosis, and a chest radiograph if clinically indicated. Dapsone is a possible choice if glucose-6-phosphate dehydrogenase deficiency can be precluded. None of the drugs prescribed for PCP prophylaxis has a clear safety record or is recommended for use in pregnant women.[39, 56]

Although CMV infection is of concern for a mother and fetus, clinical disease usually occurs in patients with CD4 counts less than 100 per mm^3, and there are few data on CMV disease in pregnancy. Children infected with HIV and CMV disease, however, appear to have a more fulminant course of HIV infection.

Patients with AIDS have a higher than expected frequency of bacterial pneumonia overall, which is of particular concern during pregnancy.[43, 46] Pneumococcal vaccine, trivalent influenza vaccine, *Haemophilus influenzae,* type b conjugate vaccine, and tetanus-diphtheria boosters all are indicated at the first prenatal visit.

Unfortunately, very few drugs or vaccines have undergone controlled trials to evaluate pharmacokinetics and short- and long-term toxicity in pregnancy. Thus, clinicians must weigh the need to treat or prevent infection against the potential risk to a mother and fetus. In addition, the risks and benefits of all drugs used during pregnancy should be carefully explained to patients, informed consent should be considered, and each patient should be evaluated on an individual basis.

PREVENTION OF VERTICAL TRANSMISSION

Prevention of vertical transmission should be focused on HIV-infected women in pregnancy, at birth, and during the postpartum period. Intervention strategies, which are summarized in Table 40–4 and Figure 40–5, are discussed next.

Zidovudine Prophylaxis

Zidovudine may decrease vertical transmission to a fetus by reducing viremia and achieving high concentrations in the fetus.[36, 67–72] Perhaps the most effective and well-documented intervention strategy to prevent perinatal transmission of HIV has been the use of ZDV after the fourteenth week of pregnancy.[22] Eligibility criteria and the specific ZDV regimen used are summarized in Table 40–3. Transmission of HIV was reduced from 25.5% of the placebo group (95% confidence interval = 18.3–33.7%) versus 8.3% for the ZDV-treated group (95% confidence interval = 3.8–13.8%, p < 0.0001). The efficacy of ZDV in preventing perinatal transmission has been confirmed by Boyer and colleagues.[62] In their study, perinatal transmission of HIV occurred in 15 (33%) of the group without ZDV versus 1 (3%) of the women who received ZDV during pregnancy. Health care workers should be cognizant of the limitation of the ACTG study protocol 076 as well as the current public health recommendations, which are summarized in Table 40–4.[22, 38, 73–75]

General Intrapartum Strategies

Human immunodeficiency virus has been isolated from the blood, vaginal secretions, placenta, amniotic fluid, fetal tissue, and breast milk.[56, 76, 77] By definition, neonates who are culture positive for HIV within the first 48 hours of life have transplacental infection. Transplacental HIV infection appears to be less than 50%, with the majority of infants infected at birth.[12, 28, 56] Because bleeding from amniocentesis may result in fetal infection, the risks and benefits of amniocentesis should be carefully considered in HIV-infected patients.

Although controversial, several studies suggest that cesarean section is associated with reduced perinatal HIV transmission.[11, 15, 16, 20, 23, 24, 28] In the earlier study by the European Collaborative group, some instruments and procedures used in vaginal delivery were significantly associated with perinatal HIV transmission. The use of episiotomy, scalp electrodes for monitoring fetal heart rate, scalp blood sampling for pH evaluation, and instruments used for vaginal delivery should be avoided.[16, 17] Based on these data, care to maintain the skin barrier and to minimize exposure of the fetus to infected maternal secretions is advised.

Immune-Based Strategies

Immune-based therapies have also been investigated to prevent vertical transmission of HIV. However, because the routes, timing, and cellular mechanisms by which maternal-fetal transmission

TABLE 40–4. Strategies to Prevent Vertical Transmission of Human Immunodeficiency Virus

INTRAUTERINE TRANSMISSION	INTRAPARTUM TRANSMISSION	POSTPARTUM TRANSMISSION
Direct evidence: • HIV in placentas • In vitro infection of placenta-derived cells • Detection of HIV in fetal tissues at 8 wk of gestation • Case report describing HIV infection in premature infants • ZDV decreases perinatal transmission of HIV	Direct evidence: • Isolation of HIV from cervical and vaginal secretions of HIV-infected women • Intrapartum blood exposure • ZDV decreases perinatal transmission of HIV	Direct evidence: • Isolation of HIV from breast milk • Case reports of infants infected by "wet nurses" or newly infected mother • ZDV may decrease transmission
Indirect evidence: • Identification of 30% of infected newborns during neonatal period • Clinical observation of subset of infected infants whose disease progresses rapidly • Possible dysmorphic syndrome	Indirect evidence: • Some studies suggest decreased HIV transmission in women having cesarean section • Inability to detect HIV by current methods before 4 mo of age in up to 70% of infants • Observed bimodal distribution for expression of related symptoms (majority after 6 to 12 mo) • Discordant infection of HIV-exposed twins	Indirect evidence: • Data pooled from a number of studies to assess attributable risk of breast-feeding with HIV infection in the infant

Intervention:		Intervention:		Intervention:	
Maternal:	Fetal:	Maternal:	Newborn:	Maternal:	Infant:
Restrict viral replication Prevent and treat cofactors Administer ZDV after 14th wk of pregnancy Avoid amniocentesis	Increased functional immune competence Decreased fetal cell susceptibility	Decreased exposure to blood and body fluids Administer ZDV during delivery? Increased aseptic techniques/ Universal precautions	Maintain skin integrity Minimal invasive procedures/ increased asepsis Enhance immune competence (vaccine/ immunoglobulins)	Avoid breast-feeding if have safe alternatives Effective hand washing and asepsis	Infected— ZDV Uninfected— routine care

HIV, Human immunodeficiency virus; ZDV, zidovudine.
Adapted from Craven DE, Sleger KA, Jarek C. Human immunodeficiency virus infection in pregnancy: Epidemiology and prevention of vertical transmission. Infect Control Hosp Epidemiol 1994;15:41.

occurs are unclear, it is difficult to design appropriate interventions.[78] Clinical studies have suggested that the placental trophoblast and macrophages have an important role in the pathogenesis of fetal infection.[78] High titers of virus may be present in plasma and peripheral blood mononuclear cells during acute infection and with more advanced HIV disease.[38]

In many viral infections, the presence of neutralizing antibodies has been associated with clearance of infection and protection from reinfection. If neutralizing antibodies could decrease circulating titers of HIV, the use of hyperimmune globulin or active immunization of the mother could have a role in reducing prenatal and perinatal transmission of HIV.

Several investigators have suggested that neutralizing antibodies directed against different epitopes on the V3 loop of the gp 120 were associated

with reduced rates of HIV infection of the newborn,[2, 66, 79, 80] but others have not been able to reproduce these data.[13, 81–83] The discrepant results may be due in part to differences in the genetic sequence of the V3 loop region for the patient's strain versus the standard strains (MN or IIIb) used in the neutralizing antibody assay.

The goal for the next decade is to develop an active vaccine than can prevent infection, improve survival of patients already infected with the HIV virus, and decrease transmission to neonates. In addition, the use of HIV hyperimmune immunoglobulins should be evaluated as a means to reduce perinatal HIV transmission. Furthermore, immune therapy in combination with antiviral therapy to reduce vertical transmission may be effective. Data suggest that HIV infection could be prevented in animals vaccinated with an attenuated whole-cell vaccine.[84]

Breast-Feeding

Human immunodeficiency virus has been detected in breast milk by both culture and PCR.[76] Although little evidence suggests horizontal spread of HIV from mother to infant or among other household contacts,[77, 85] serious concerns have continued to be raised about the role of breast-feeding as a mechanism of HIV transmission.[86–90] Despite evidence from several case reports that implicates breast-feeding in HIV transmission, recommendations are complicated by the potential benefits associated with breast-feeding in terms of protection against infant deaths due to infectious diseases.[86–91] The risk-benefit assessment is particularly difficult to determine in areas where safe infant formulas are unavailable and HIV infection is common among women of childbearing age. In fact, the World Health Organization recommends that when safe and effective alternatives to breast-feeding are not available, breast-feeding by the biologic mother should be the method of choice.[92] However, the Centers for Disease Control and Prevention, the American College of Obstetrics and Gynecology, and the Academy of Pediatrics recommend that HIV-seropositive women living in the United States and other industrialized nations refrain from breast-feeding.[93–95]

Worldwide, more than 10 cases of apparent transmission of HIV via breast-feeding have been reported in mothers who were HIV infected postnatally.[96, 97] Although these reports have implicated breast-feeding as a mode of transmission of HIV from postnatally infected mothers, it has been argued that HIV transmission from mothers infected prenatally is rare.[98, 99] The relative importance of this mode of transmission in this setting is difficult to ascertain, because the majority of women in industrialized countries with known HIV infection do not breast-feed, and even when they do, horizontal transmission is more likely to be attributed to factors other than breast-feeding.

Although HIV transmission rates associated with breast-feeding in women infected postnatally vary, the overall risk of HIV transmission among the 42 children studied was 29%.[91] In an effort to quantitate the additional risk of transmission via breast-feeding, over and above transmission in utero or perinatally, Dunn and colleagues report an analysis of five studies in which mothers were infected prenatally.[91] The attributable risk of breast-feeding was 14% overall, although in two of the studies the rate was actually higher in the "never breast-fed" group. This overall rate was determined from grouped data, and other risk factors for HIV transmission may have been unevenly distributed across groups.[91]

At the very least, the finding that breast-feeding may be an important route of HIV transmission supports an advantage to routine screening of pregnant women for HIV infection, particularly in countries with available safe alternatives to breast-feeding.

SUMMARY

Women and children will become the most common groups of HIV-infected persons by the year 2000. The preponderance of HIV cases in women during their reproductive years demands attention to appropriate interventions to prevent perinatal transmission. Transmission of HIV may occur during pregnancy, intrapartum, or to a lesser extent postpartum. Data suggest that the use of ZDV can reduce perinatal transmission of HIV by 67% in women who have CD4 counts greater than 200 per mm^3. These striking findings will certainly result in greater use of ZDV after the first trimester of pregnancy. However, questions remain about how successful ZDV will be for women who have previously received ZDV, which may increase the risk of ZDV-resistant HIV isolates. Furthermore, the long-term risk of ZDV toxicity in children who were exposed to ZDV in utero but did not develop HIV infection needs further study. Finally, it is imperative to follow impeccable infection control practices during delivery, minimize mechanical trauma to neonates, and carefully counsel women on the potential risk of HIV transmission via breast-feeding.

REFERENCES

1. Chin J. Current and future dimensions of the HIV/AIDS pandemic in women and children. Lancet 1990;336:221.
2. AIDS Newsletter. MA Department of Public Health AIDS Surveillance Program, May 1994.
3. Centers for Disease Control. AIDS in women—United States. MMWR 1990;39:848.
4. Guinan ME, Hardy A. Epidemiology of AIDS in women in the United States: 1981 through 1986. JAMA 1987;257:2039.
5. Ellerbrock TV, Rogers M. Epidemiology of human immunodeficiency virus infection in women in the United States. Obstet Gynecol Clin North Am 1990;17:523.
6. Centers for Disease Control. National HIV Surveillance Summary, Results through 1991. Vol 3. Atlanta: US Department of Health and Human Services, Public Health Service, 1994.
7. Chu SY, Buehler JW, Berkelman RL. Impact of the human immunodeficiency virus epidemic on mortality in women of reproductive age, United States. JAMA 1990;264:225.
8. Centers for Disease Control. 1993 revised classification system for HIV infection and expanded surveillance case definition for AIDS among adolescents and adults. MMWR 1992;41 (RR-17):1.

9. Gwinn M, Pappaioanou M, George JR, et al. Prevalence of HIV infection in childbearing women in the United States: Surveillance using newborn blood samples. JAMA 1991;265:1704.

10. Donegan SP, Steger KA, Recla L, et al. Seroprevalence of human immunodeficiency virus in parturients at Boston City Hospital: Implications for public health and obstetric practice. Am J Obstet Gynecol 1992;167:622.

11. Scott GB, Fischl MA, Klimas N, et al. Mothers of infants with acquired immunodeficiency syndrome. JAMA 1985;253:363.

12. Goedert JJ, Mendez H, Drummond JE, et al. Mother to infant transmission of human immunodeficiency virus type 1: Association with prematurity or low anti-gp120. Lancet 1989;2:1015.

13. Halsey NA, Boulos R, Holt E, et al. Transmission of HIV-1 infection from mothers to infants in Haiti. Impact on childhood mortality and malnutrition. The CDS/JHU AIDS Project Team. JAMA 1990;264:2088.

14. Hira SK, Kamanga J, Bhat GJ, et al. Perinatal transmission of HIV-1 in Zambia. Br Med J 1989;299:1250.

15. Ryder RW, Nsa W, Hassig SE, et al. Perinatal transmission of the human immunodeficiency virus type 1 to infants of seropositive women in Zaire. N Engl J Med 1989;320:1637.

16. European Collaborative Study. Mother-to-child transmission of HIV infection. Lancet 1988;2:1039.

17. European Collaborative Study Group. Risk factors for mother-to-child transmission of HIV-1. Lancet 1992;339:1007.

18. Minkoff HL, Holman S, Beller E, et al. Routinely offered prenatal HIV testing (letter). N Engl J Med 1988;319:1018.

19. Pantaleo G, Graziosi C, Fauci AS. Immunopathogenesis in human immunodeficiency virus infection. N Engl J Med 1993;328:327.

20. Goedert JJ, Duliege AM, Amos CI, et al. The International Registry of HIV-Exposed Twins. High risk of HIV-1 infection for first-born twins. Lancet 1991;338:1471.

21. de Martino M, Tovo PA, Galli L, et al. HIV-1 infection in perinatally exposed siblings and twins. The Italian Register for HIV Infection in Children. Arch Dis Childhood 1991;66:1235.

22. Centers for Disease Control. Zidovudine for the prevention of HIV transmission from mother to infant. MMWR 1994;43:285.

23. Villari P, Chalmers TC, Lau J, Sacks HS. Cesarean section to reduce perinatal transmission of human immunodeficiency virus. Online J Curr Clin Trials. No. 2, 1993.

24. The European Collaborative Study. Caesarean section and risk of vertical transmission of HIV-1 infection. Lancet 1994;343:1464.

25. Courgnaud V, Laure F, Brossard A, et al. Frequent and early in utero HIV-1 infection. AIDS Res Hum Retroviruses 1991;7:337.

26. Jovaisas E, Koch MA, Schaeffer A, et al. LAV/HTLV-III in a 20-week fetus (letter). Lancet 1985;2:1129.

27. Scott GB, Mastrucci MT, Hutto SC, Parks WP. Mothers of infants with HIV infection: Outcome of subsequent pregnancies. Abstracts of the Third International Conference on AIDS. Washington, DC, 1987; THP.91.

28. Blanche SB, Rouzioux C, Guihard-Moscato ML, et al. A prospective study of infants born to women seropositive for human immunodeficiency virus type 1. N Engl J Med 1989;320:1643.

29. St Louis ME, Kamenga M, Brown C, et al. Risk factors for perinatal HIV-transmission according to maternal, immunologic, virologic and palcental factors. JAMA 1993;269:2853.

30. Johnson VA. New developments in antiretroviral drug therapy for HIV infection. In: Volberding P, Jacobson MA (eds). AIDS Clinical Review 1992. New York: Marcel Dekker, 1992, pp 69–104.

31. Gold JWM. HIV-1 infection: Diagnosis and management. Med Clin North Am. 1992;76(1):1.

32. Katzenstein DA, Holodnyi M. Quantitative virological measures of antiretroviral therapy. In: Volberding P, Jacobson MA (eds). AIDS Clinical Review 1992. New York: Marcel Dekker, 1992, pp 41–67.

33. Palomba E, Gay V, Barberis E, et al. Early diagnosis of human immunodeficiency virus infection in infants by detection of free and complexed p24 antigen. J Infect Dis 1992;165:394.

34. MacGregor SN. Human immunodeficiency virus infection in pregnancy. Clin Perinatol 1991;18:33.

35. Comeau AM, Hsu H-W, Schwerzler M, et al. Detection of HIV in specimens from newborn screening programs. N Engl J Med 1992;326:1703.

36. Burgard M, Mayaux M-J, Blanche S, et al. The use of viral culture and p24 antigen testing to diagnose human immunodeficiency virus infection in neonates. N Engl J Med 1992;327:1192.

37. Rogers MF, Ou C-Y, Kilbourne B, Schochetman G. Advances and problems in the diagnosis of human immunodeficiency virus infection in infants. Pediatr Infect Dis J 1991;10:523.

38. Ho DD, Moudgil T, Alam M. Quantitation of human immunodeficiency virus type 1 in the blood of infected persons. N Engl J Med 1989;321:1621.

39. Masur H. Prevention and treatment of *Pneumocystis* pneumonia. N Engl J Med 1992;327:1853.

40. Biggar RJ, Pahwa S, Minkoff H, et al. Immunosuppression in pregnant women infected with human immunodeficiency virus. Am J Obstet Gynecol 1989;161:1239.

41. Feinkind L, Minkoff HL. HIV in pregnancy. Clin Perinatol 1988;15:189.

42. Coyne BA, Landers DV. The immunology of HIV disease and pregnancy and possible interactions. Obstet Gynecol Clin North Am 1990;17:595.

43. Selwyn PA, Schoenbaum EE, Davenny K, et al. Prospective study of human immunodeficiency virus infection and pregnancy outcomes in intravenous drug users. JAMA 1989;261:1289.

44. Landesman SH. Human immunodeficiency virus infection in women: An overview. Semin Perinatol 1989;13:2.

45. Selwyn PA. Issues in the clinical management of intravenous drug users with HIV infection. AIDS 1989;3(Suppl 1):S201.

46. Witt DJ, Craven DE, McCabe WR. Bacterial infection in patients with acquired immunodeficiency syndrome and AIDS-related complex. Am J Med 1987;82:900.

47. Carpenter CCJ, Mayer KH, Fisher A, et al. Natural history of acquired immunodeficiency syndrome in women in Rhode Island. Am J Med 1989;86:771.

48. Rhoads JL, Wright C, Redfield RR, Burke DS. Chronic vaginal candidiasis in women with human immunodeficiency virus infection. JAMA 1987;257:3105.

49. Minkoff H, Nanda D, Menez R, et al. Pregnancies resulting in infants with acquired immunodeficiency syndrome or AIDS related complex: Follow up of mothers, children and subsequently born siblings. Obstet Gynecol 1987;69:288.

50. Johnstone FD, McCallum L, Brettle R, et al. Does HIV infection affect the outcome of pregnancy? Br Med J 1988;296:467.

51. Minkoff HL, DeHovitz JA. Care of women infected with the human immunodeficiency virus. JAMA 1991;266:2253.

52. Sunderland A, Minkoff H, Handte J, et al. The impact of human immunodeficiency virus serostatus on reproductive decisions of women. Obstet Gynecol 1992;79:1027.

53. Chavkin W. Mandatory treatment for drug use during pregnancy. JAMA 1991;266:1556.

54. Anastos K, Palleja S. Caring for women at risk of HIV infection. J Gen Intern Med 1991;6:S40.

55. Jacobs RF, Abernathy RS. Management of tuberculosis in pregnancy and the newborn. Clin Perinatol 1988;15:305.

56. Nanda D. Human immunodeficiency virus infection in pregnancy. Obstet Gynecol Clin North Am 1990;17:617.

57. Sperling RS, Stratton P. Treatment options for human immunodeficiency virus-infected pregnant women. Obstetric-Gynecologic Working Group of the AIDS Clinical Trials Group of the National Institute of Allergy and Infectious Diseases. Obstet Gynecol 1992;79:443.

58. Sperling RS, Stratton P, O'Sullivan MJ, et al. A survey of zidovudine use in pregnant women with human immunodeficiency virus infection. N Engl J Med 1992;326:857.

59. Zidovudine in Pregnancy Registry: International Interim Report January 1, 1989 through December 31, 1991. Research Triangle, NC: Burroughs Wellcome, 1992.

60. Sperling RS, Stratton P, O'Sullivan MJ, et al. A survey of zidovudine use in pregnant women with human immunodeficiency virus infection. N Engl J Med 1992;326:857.

61. Dancis J, Lee JD, Mendoza S, Liebes L. Transfer and metabolism of dideoxynosine by the perfused human placenta. J AIDS 1993;6:2.

62. Boyer PJ, Dillon M, Navale M, et al. Factors predictive of maternal-fetal transmission of HIV-1. Preliminary analysis of zidovudine given during pregnancy and/or delivery. JAMA 1994;271:1925.

63. Bartlett John G. The Johns Hopkins Hospital Guide to Medical Care of Patients with HIV Infection, 4th ed. Baltimore: Williams & Wilkins, 1994.

64. Minkoff HL, Henderson C, Mendez H, et al. Pregnancy outcomes among mothers infected with human immunodeficiency virus and uninfected control subjects. Am J Obstet Gynecol 1990;163:1598.

65. Minkoff HL, Moreno J. Drug prophylaxis for human immunodeficiency virus infected pregnant women: Ethical considerations. Am J Obstet Gynecol 1990;163:1111.

66. Ugen KE, Goedert JJ, Boyer J, et al. Vertical transmission of human immunodeficiency virus (HIV) infection. Reactivity of maternal sera with glycoprotein 120 and 41 peptides from HIV type 1. J Clin Invest 1992;89:1923.

67. Little BB, Bawdon RE, Christmas JT, et al. Pharmacokinetics of azidothymidine during late pregnancy in Long-Evans rats. Am J Obstet Gynecol 1989;161:732.

68. Lopez-Anaya A, Unadkat JD, Schumann LA, Smith AL. Pharmacokinetics of zidovudine (azidothymidine). I. Transplacental transfer. J AIDS 1990;3:959.

69. Liebes L, Mendoza S, Wilson D, Dancis J. Transfer of zidovudine (AZT) by human placenta. J Infect Dis 1990;161:203.

70. Lopez-Anaya A, Unadkat JD, Schumann LA, Smith AL. Pharmacokinetics of zidovudine (azidothymidine). III. Effect of pregnancy. J AIDS 1991;4:64.

71. Pons JC, Taburet AM, Singlas E, et al. Placental passage of azathiothymidine (AZT) during the second trimester of pregnancy: Study by direct fetal blood sampling under ultrasound. Eur J Obstet Gynecol Reprod Biol 1991; 40:229.

72. Toltzis P, Marx CM, Kleinman N, et al. Zidovudine-associated embryonic toxicity in mice. J Infect Dis 1991;163:1212.

73. Richman DD. Zidovudine resistance of human immunodeficiency virus. Rev Infect Dis 1990;12:S507.

74. Lyman WD, Tanaka KE, Kress Y, et al. Zidovudine concentrations in human fetal tissue: Implications for perinatal AIDS (letter). Lancet 1990;335:1280.

75. Barzilai A, Sperling RS, Hyatt AC, et al. Mother to child

76. Thiry L, Sprecher-Goldberger S, Jonckheer T, et al. Isolation of AIDS virus from cell free breast milk of three healthy virus carriers. Lancet 1985;2:891.

77. Friedland GH, Klein RS. Transmission of the human immunodeficiency virus. N Engl J Med 1987;317:1125.

78. Douglas GC, King BF. Maternal-fetal transmission of human immunodeficiency virus: A review of possible routes and cellular mechanisms of infection. Clin Infect Dis 1992;15:678.

79. Devash Y, Calvelli TA, Wood DG, et al. Vertical transmission of HIV is correlated with the absence of high affinity-avidity maternal antibodies to the gp 120 principal neutralizing domain. Proc Natl Acad Science U S A 1990;87:3445.

80. Rossi P, Moschese V, Lombardi V, et al. HIV-1 mother-to-child transmission. Lancet 1990;1:359.

81. Halsey NA, Markham R, Wahren B, et al. Lack of association between maternal antibodies to V3 peptides and maternal-infant HIV-1 transmission. J AIDS 1992;5:153.

82. Rubinstein A, Sicklick M, Gupta A, et al. Acquired immunodeficiency with reversed T4/T8 ratios in infants born to promiscuous and drug-addicted mothers. JAMA 1983;249:2350.

83. Parekh BS, Shaffer N, Pau CP, et al. Lack of correlation between maternal antibodies to V3 loop peptides of gp120 and perinatal HIV-1 transmission. The NYC Perinatal HIV Transmission Collaborative Study. AIDS 1991;5:1179.

84. Daniel MD, Kirchhoff F, Czajak SC, et al. Protective effects of a live attenuated SIV vaccine with a deletion in the nef gene. Science 1992;258:1938.

85. Friedland GH, Saltzman BR, Rogers MF, et al. Lack of transmission of HTLVIII/LAV infection to household contacts of patients with AIDS or ARC with oral candidiasis. N Engl J Med 1986;314:3444.

86. Van de Perre P, Simonon A, Msellati P, et al. Postnatal transmission of human immunodeficiency virus type 1 from mother to infant. A prospective cohort study in Kigali, Rwanda. N Engl J Med 1991;325:593.

87. Van de Perre P, Hitimana DG, Simonon A, et al. Postnatal transmission of HIV-1 associated with breast abscess. Lancet 1992;339:1490.

88. Hira SK, Mangrola UG, Mwale C, et al. Apparent vertical transmission of human immunodeficiency virus type 1 by breast-feeding in Zambia. J Pediatr 1990;117:421.

89. Palasanthiran P, Ziegler JB, Stewart GJ, et al. Breast feeding during primary maternal human immunodeficiency virus infection and the risk of transmission from mother-to-infant. J Infect Dis 1993;167:441.

90. Colebunders R, Kapita B, Nekwei W, et al. Breastfeeding and transmission of HIV. Lancet 1988;2:1487.

91. Dunn DT, Newell ML, Ades AE, Peckham CS. Risk of human immunodeficiency virus type 1 transmission through breast feeding. Lancet 1992;340:585.

92. Global programme on AIDS. Consensus statement from the WHO/UNICEF consultation on HIV transmission and breast-feeding. Wkly Epidemiol Rec 1992;67:177.

93. American College of Obstetricians and Gynecologists. Prevention of HIV Infection and AIDS. ACOG Committee Statement 1987. Washington, DC, 1987, pp 1–8.

94. Landesman S, Minkoff H, Holman S, et al. Serosurvey of human immunodeficiency virus infection in parturients: Implications for human immunodeficiency virus testing programs of pregnant women. JAMA 1987;258:2701.

95. American Academy of Pediatrics and American College of Obstetricians and Gynecologists. Guidelines for Perinatal Care. 2nd ed. Elk Grove Village, IL: The Academy, 1988.

96. Zeigler JB, Cooper DA, Johnson RO, et al. Postnatal transmission of AIDS-associated retrovirus from mother to infant. Lancet 1984;1:896.

97. Lederman SA. Estimating infant mortality from human immunodeficiency virus and other causes in breast-feeding and bottle-feeding populations. Pediatrics 1992;89:290.

98. Jelliffe DB, Jelliffe EFP. Postnatal transmission of HIV infection. N Engl J Med 1992;326:642.

99. Oxtoby MJ. Human immunodeficiency virus and other viruses in human milk: Placing the issue in broader perspective. Pediatr Infect Dis J 1988;7:825.

Infectious Disease in Pregnancy

Carol Sulis

Women of childbearing age are frequently exposed to (and care for) other adults, animals, and children suffering from a wide variety of contagious infectious diseases. Infections are common, and most infections are treated similarly whether or not a patient is pregnant. However, some infections that are mild in a mother may be teratogenic or fatal to her fetus; other infections that are mild in a nonpregnant host may be unusually severe in a pregnant woman (Table 41–1).

An increased frequency of complications associated with viral, parasitic, fungal, and certain bacterial pathogens is presumed to result from a depressed maternal cell-mediated immune response, which is most deficient late in pregnancy.[1] A mild elevation in basal temperature and circulating leukocytes during normal pregnancy and labor may confound evaluation and diagnosis. Concerns about pharmacokinetics and potential toxicity of antimicrobial agents complicate therapy (Table 41–2).[2–13]

Complications from congenital infections often occur early in the first trimester during fetal organogenesis, when a patient may not yet be aware of her pregnancy. It is prudent to determine pregnancy status before initiation of any diagnostic or therapeutic modality in all women of childbearing age. Pregnant patients should be instructed about the importance of preventing infectious diseases, with emphasis on good hygiene and scrupulous hand washing after exposure to potential pathogens.

This section focuses on common infectious complications caused by viruses, bacteria, and protozoa in pregnant women who are otherwise normal hosts. Special problems associated with human immunodeficiency virus infection are reviewed elsewhere (see Chapter 40).[14–16]

INFECTIONS ASSOCIATED WITH INCREASED MATERNAL MORBIDITY

Upper Respiratory Tract Infections

Historically important as the cause of devastating epidemics of puerperal sepsis, *Streptococcus pyogenes* (group A β-hemolytic streptococci) is a common cause of sore throat and upper respiratory tract infection. To prevent nosocomial spread, hospitalized patients with evidence of group A streptococcal colonization or infection should be placed in isolation until 24 hours of antibiotic therapy is completed.[17]

Pregnant women may be more susceptible to viral upper respiratory tract infections than nonpregnant women. Diseases due to the common cold viruses (rhinovirus, coronavirus) are usually trivial, self-limited, and characterized by rhinorrhea, sneezing, and congestion. Adenovirus infection is frequently associated with a dry cough and may evolve to pneumonia.

Pneumonia is uncommon (0.04–1% of pregnancies) but can be a cause of maternal mortality (0–4% case fatality rate). Pneumonia in the second and third trimesters of pregnancy has been associated with increased rates of premature labor and delivery and excess fetal loss. Symptoms of cough with pleuritic chest pain or fever should prompt an evaluation to rule out pneumonia, especially in a patient who smokes or has underlying lung disease or an antecedent upper respiratory tract infection.[18–20]

Community-Acquired Bacterial Pneumonia

Although precise rates are unavailable, it is presumed that the cause of bacterial pneumonia re-

TABLE 41–1. **Infections in Pregnancy**

INFECTIONS ASSOCIATED WITH INCREASED MATERNAL MORBIDITY	
Illness	**Comment***
Streptococcal infection	Localized infection with group A and group B β-hemolytic streptococci and pneumococcus more likely to disseminate during third trimester
Bacterial pneumonia	Increased risk of fetal loss, premature labor and delivery, and maternal death
Influenza	Increased attack rate and increased maternal death rate in 1918 and 1957 pandemics
Varicella	Increased rate of symptomatic pneumonitis; fetal embryopathy
Urinary tract infection	Pregnant women with asymptomatic bacteriuria have 20–40% chance of developing acute symptomatic urinary tract infection by third trimester; women with third-trimester pyelonephritis have 20–50% chance of premature labor
Viral hepatitis	Possible increased severity of disease when acute infection during thrid trimester, with potential for transmission to neonate during delivery

INFECTIONS ASSOCIATED WITH INCREASED FETAL MORBIDITY	
Etiology	**Comment†**
Cytomegalovirus	Congenital infection in 1% of all neonates; cytomegalic inclusion disease (hepatosplenomegaly, microcephaly, chorioretinitis); late sequelae (microcephaly, sensorineural hearing loss, mental or psychomotor retardation)
Group B streptococci	Severe infection in 1% of exposed neonates
Hepatitis B	Increased risk of congenital infection
Human immunodeficiency virus	Congenital infection in 30–60%
Listeria	Increased fetal wastage
Measles	Increased incidence of abortion
Mumps	Increased incidence of first-trimester abortion
Rubella	Increased incidence of abortion and in utero infection (congenital rubella syndrome)
Parvovirus B19	Increased fetal wastage; hydrops fetalis
Toxoplasmosis	Increased fetal wastage, congenital infection
Tuberculosis	Congenital infection rare; neonatal infection common unless infant isolated from mother postpartum
Varicella	Fetal varicella embryopathy (scarred atrophic limbs, eye anomalies, low birth weight, central nervous system involvement)
Chlamydia	Maternal infection associated with premature rupture of membrane and low birth weight. Neonatal transmission associated with conjunctivitis (20–50%) or pneumonia (10–20%)
Gonorrhea	Maternal infection associated with increased risk of spontaneous abortion, premature rupture of membranes, and perinatal infant mortality, but causal role has not been established. Proven sequelae (with unknown frequency) include ophthalmia neonatorum, neonatal sepsis or disseminated disease, and peripartum chorioamnionitis
Herpes simplex virus	30–50% risk of transmission during primary maternal infection; < 5% risk of transmission in recurrent maternal disease
Human papillomavirus	Laryngeal papillomatosis; mechanical obstruction to delivery
Syphilis	90–100% neonatal infection in primary maternal syphilis associated with congenital sequelae in 50% and stillbirth or abortion in remainder

OBSTETRIC INFECTIONS	
Etiology	**Comment‡**
Chorioamnionitis	Increased risk of premature labor, congenital infection, postpartum maternal morbidity
Necrotizing cellulitis	Increased postpartum maternal morbidity
Pelvic abscess	Increased postpartum maternal morbidity
Postpartum endometritis	Increased postpartum maternal morbidity
Septic thrombophlebitis	Increased postpartum maternal morbidity

*Complications that occur more frequently in pregnant than in nonpregnant women.

†Maternal disease usually no different from disease in nonpregnant women, but maternal infection is associated with significant fetal morbidity such as fetal malformation, growth retardation or prematurity, abortion or stillbirth, or congenital infection.

‡Obstetric disorders seen as complication of pregnancy, labor, or delivery.

flects that in the general population. *Streptococcus pneumoniae* is the most common community-acquired bacterial pneumonia in pregnant patients. Bacteremia with secondary meningitis may occur more frequently than in the general population.

Classic symptoms include sudden onset of shaking chills, which are followed by headache, fever, pleuritic chest pain, and production of purulent or rusty blood-tinged sputum. Lung examination may be unremarkable or may show evidence of consol-

TABLE 41–2.   Safety of Selected Antimicrobial Agents in Pregnancy

ANTIBIOTIC CLASS	COMMENT*†
Aminoglycoside	Use with discretion. Potential cranial nerve VIII toxicity, proved only after formal vestibular testing or audiogram in fetus exposed to streptomycin.
β-Lactam	
Cephalosporin	Considered safe; no human fetal toxicity reported.
Penicillin	Ticarcillin teratogenic in rats; use of all other penicillins considered safe in pregnancy.
Carbapenem	Insufficient human or animal data to assess toxicity in pregnancy.
Imipenem-cilastatin	Avoid use in pregnancy unless no alternative agent available.
Chloramphenicol	Use contraindicated near term because of association with gray baby syndrome.
Ethambutol	Use with discretion. Teratogenic in animals but no reported adverse reactions in human fetus.
Isoniazid	Use with discretion. Embryotoxic in some animals; increased incidence of psychomotor retardation, myoclonus, and seizures in small human series. Use may be associated with increased risk of hepatitis in pregnancy.
Macrolide	
Clindamycin	Category B; no known adverse effects on fetus.
Erythromycin	Estolate: absolutely contraindicated because of increased maternal risk of cholestatic hepatitis. Base: Category B; no known adverse effects on fetus. No data available on safety of azithromycin or clarithromycin.
Metronidazole	Use contraindicated. Conflicting data from animal models regarding teratogenic and carcinogenic potential. Unstable metabolites mutagenic in animals, but no confirmatory human data. Achieves high concentration in breast milk. Use in pregnancy generally contraindicated, especially during first trimester.
Monobactam	Probably safe. No mutagenesis or teratogenesis in extensive animal studies. No human fetal
Aztreonam	toxicity reported.
Nitrofurantoin	Use with discretion. Mutagenic; increased risk of hemolytic anemia in fetus or neonate with glucose-6-phosphate dehydrogenase deficiency.
Quinolone	Use contraindicated. Animal studies demonstrated irreversible degenerative changes in
Nalidixic acid	cartilage. No reports of mutagenesis or carcinogenesis.
Fluoroquinolone	
Rifampin	Use with discretion. Teratogenic in animals.
Sulfonamide	Category C; use with discretion. Use contraindicated at term because of increased risk of kernicterus in premature neonates.
Tetracycline	Category D; use contraindicated. May cause hypoplasia and discoloration of fetal teeth and inhibit long-bone growth. Mother at increased risk for acute fatty necrosis of the liver (which may be severe and cause death), pancreatitis, and renal damage (azotemia with high-dose intravenous use)
Trimethoprim	Category C; use with discretion. Teratogenic in rats. Folate antagonist.
Pyrazinamide	Use with discretion. Insufficient data to assess human fetal toxicity.
Vancomycin	Use with discretion. Theoretic auditory and renal toxicity in fetus.

ANTIVIRAL AGENT	COMMENT*†
Acyclovir	Use with discretion; not approved for use in pregnancy. No toxicity reported in small human series.
Amantadine	Use with extreme caution. Teratogenic and embryotoxic in rats.
Ribavarin	Use contraindicated. Mutagenic, teratogenic, embryocidal in animals.
Vidarabine	Use with extreme caution. Mutagenic and teratogenic in rodents. Use in pregnancy limited to treatment of severe systemic herpes simplex unresponsive to acyclovir.
Zidovudine	Mutagenic, embryotoxic in mice; no reported adverse reactions in human fetus. Use in pregnancy limited to treatment of patients infected with human immunodeficiency virus.

Table continued on following page

TABLE 41–2.   Safety of Selected Antimicrobial Agents in Pregnancy *Continued*

ANTIFUNGAL CLASS	COMMENT*†
Imidazole	
Ketoconazole	Use with extreme caution. Teratogenic and embryotoxic in rats. No reported adverse reactions in human fetus, but insufficient data to establish safety.
Miconazole	Use with caution. No reported adverse reactions in human fetus, but insufficient data to establish safety.
Flucytosine	Use with caution. Teratogenic in rats. No reported adverse reactions in human fetus, but insufficient data to establish safety.
Polyene	
Amphotericin B	Use with discretion. No reported adverse reactions in human fetus.
Nystatin	Topical agent. No reported adverse reactions in human fetus and considered safe for use during pregnancy.
Triazole	
Fluconazole	Use with extreme caution. Teratogenic in rats.
Itraconazole	No reported adverse reactions in human fetus, but insufficient data to establish safety.

*The following is a summary of the U.S. Food and Drug Administration classification for drugs used in pregnancy. Most antibiotics are category C agents and are assumed (though not proven) to be safe.
Category A: Controlled studies in pregnant women in the first trimester do not demonstrate risk to fetus.
Category B: Animal studies demonstrate no fetal risk, but there are no controlled studies in pregnant women.
Category C: Animal studies demonstrate adverse fetal effects, *and* there are no controlled studies in pregnant women *or* no data are available; drug should be used only when potential benefit outweighs potential risk to the fetus.
Category D: Human studies demonstrate fetal risk, but use may be acceptable when alternative therapies are unavailable.
Category X: Human and/or animal studies demonstrate fetal risk, and use is contraindicated in pregnancy.
   †Additional adverse reactions are well documented but not increased in pregnancy.

idation or pleural effusion. Diagnostic evaluation should include a complete blood count with differential white blood cell count, sputum Gram stain and culture, and blood cultures. A chest radiograph and arterial blood gas determination should be obtained if clinically warranted. Differential diagnosis includes pneumonia caused by *Haemophilus influenzae,* atypical organisms (*Legionella* species, *Mycoplasma pneumoniae, Chlamydia* species), and viruses. Primary influenza pneumonia or secondary bacterial pneumonia (*Staphylococcus aureus, S. pneumoniae, H. influenzae*) should be suspected when symptoms follow a flu-like illness. Empirical antibiotic therapy should be directed at suspected pathogens (Table 41–3). Early hospitalization, treatment with intravenous antibiotics, and supportive measures such as oxygen, antipyretics, and hydration may be warranted, especially when pneumonia occurs during the third trimester. Patients with persistent fever and pleural effusion should undergo diagnostic thoracentesis, with thoracostomy drainage if empyema is diagnosed.

Aspiration Pneumonia

Complications due to aspiration of respiratory secretions and gastric contents during labor and delivery continue to be an important cause of maternal mortality. Anesthesia and physiologic changes (delayed gastric emptying and decreased gastroesophageal sphincter tone) exacerbate the risk. Symptoms of chemical pneumonitis occur 6 to 8 hours after aspiration and may include cough, bronchospasm, or diffuse pulmonary edema. Evidence of bacterial infection is delayed and occurs 24 hours after aspiration. Physical findings may include tachypnea, fever, and evidence of pulmonary consolidation. Sputum Gram stain reveals sheets of polymorphonuclear leukocytes and mixed bacterial flora. Treatment should focus on mechanical removal of aspirated debris (suctioning) and maintenance of adequate oxygenation with bronchodilators and ventilatory support. Empirical antibiotics are begun once bacterial superinfection is confirmed (see Table 41–3).

Nosocomial Pneumonia

The etiology of other types of nosocomial pneumonia reflects the microbiologic environment of the specific institution. Colonization or infection with drug-resistant organisms (methicillin-resistant *S. aureus,* resistant gram-negative bacilli) or viruses are common and may be difficult to treat or may require use of relatively toxic agents. Benefits and risks of treatment should be assessed with the assistance of a pulmonary or infectious disease specialist on a case-by-case basis.

Influenza

Influenza A and B are caused by ribonucleic acid (RNA) orthomyxoviruses, which are subtyped

TABLE 41–3. Antimicrobial Agents in Pregnancy: Treatment of Respiratory Tract Infections

ORGANISM	SYMPTOMS	ANTIBIOTICS
Community-acquired bacterial pneumonia		Empirical therapy with ampicillin, cephalosporin, or erythromycin should be initiated pending identification of causative organism.
Streptococcus pneumoniae	Sudden onset of shaking chills, fever, rusty sputum with gram-positive diplococci; bacteremia common	Penicillin G, 400,000 U IV every 4 hr.
Haemophilus influenzae	More gradual onset; sputum with gram-negative coccobacilli	Ampicillin, 1–2 gm IV every 4–6 hr; cefuroxime, 1 gm IV every 8 hr, or ceftriaxone, 1–2 gm IV every 24 hr, if β-lactamase positive
Mycobacterium tuberculosis	Cough, night sweats, hemoptysis, weight loss	Empiric therapy with isoniazid, 300 mg/day PO *plus* rifampin, 600 mg/day PO, *plus* ethambutol, 2 gm/day PO *plus* pyridoxine, 50 mg/day PO pending sensitivity testing. Duration of therapy based on extent of disease.
Community-acquired atypical pneumonia		Empiric therapy with erythromycin, 500 mg PO or IV 4 times a day.
Legionella sp *Chlamydia* sp *Mycoplasma pneumoniae*	Variable onset. Dry cough, gastrointestinal complaints common in *Legionella*. Sputum Gram stain without organisms.	Erythromycin, 1 gm IV every 6 hr, is recommended for the treatment of *Legionella*.
Pneumonia following preceding URI *Staphylococcus aureus* *S. pneumoniae* *H. influenzae* *Streptococcus pyogenes*	Follows viral URI. CXR shows lobar infiltrate. Gram stain with PMN and bacteria.	Oxacillin, 1–2 gm IV every 4–6 hr *or* vancomycin, 1 gm IV every 12 hr, if methicillin resistance is suspected; addition of ceftriaxone, 1–2 gm IV every 24 hr, if *H. influenzae* or enteric gram-negative bacilli suspected.
Influenza A or Influenza B	Follows viral URI. Interstitial pneumonitis on CXR.	Amantadine, 100 mg PO every 12 hr, has been used in patients with severe underlying cardiac or pulmonary disease; safety and efficacy in pregnancy unknown, and extreme caution advised.
Aspiration pneumonia Mixed aerobes and anaerobes	Follows witnessed aspiration or period of depressed consciousness. Sputum with PMN and mixed bacterial flora.	Standard regimen: Penicillin 1–2 million units IV every 4 hr, *or* clindamycin, 600 mg IV every 8 hr. Use cefoxitin, 2 gm IV every 6–8 hr, *or* add third-generation cephalosporin to standard regimen if gram-negative bacilli are a concern.
Hospital-acquired pneumonia MRSA, resistant gram- negative bacilli, fungi	Follows colonization with hospital-specific pathogens, usually patient in intensive care unit or with serious underlying disease.	Vancomycin, 1 gm every 12 hr for MRSA; Third-generation cephalosporin *or* extended-spectrum penicillin (i.e., piperacillin) *plus* aminoglycoside *or* imipenem-cilastatin for resistant gram-negative enteric organism or *Pseudomonas aeruginosa*.
Varicella pneumonia	Follows chickenpox.	Acyclovir, 10–12.4 mg/kg every 8 hr used but not approved by Food and Drug Administration.

IV, Intravenously; PO, orally; URI, upper respiratory tract infection; CXR, chest radiograph; PMN, polymorphonuclear neutrophils; MRSA, methicillin resistant *Staphylococcus aureus*.

according to characteristics of their hemagglutinin (H) and neuraminidase (N) surface proteins. Protective antibody is subtype specific; however, frequent variation in the surface antigens results in large segments of the population being susceptible to reinfection (10–50% attack rate) and a potential for epidemic spread. Pregnancy was associated with an unusually high incidence of maternal in-

fection and death in the 1918 and 1957 influenza pandemic, but this association has not been observed subsequently. An incubation period of 1 to 2 days follows exposure to infectious virus in respiratory secretions. Disease begins abruptly with headache, high fever, chills, and myalgia. As these symptoms wane during the next 3 to 5 days, sore throat, rhinitis, and cough become more prominent, then slowly resolve over 1 to 2 weeks. Primary influenza pneumonia should be suspected when respiratory symptoms continue or worsen during the second week. Although some researchers describe an increased incidence of influenza pneumonia in pregnancy, most cases occur in patients with underlying cardiovascular disease. Hypoxia and progressive respiratory failure may require ventilatory support. Histologically, a diffuse hemorrhagic pneumonia is evident. The potential viral cause is strengthened when sputum Gram stain shows sheets of polymorphonuclear leukocytes with normal respiratory flora and chest radiography shows diffuse interstitial infiltrates. The diagnosis can be confirmed by the isolation of influenza from culture of respiratory secretions.

In contrast, a secondary bacterial pneumonia should be suspected when respiratory symptoms worsen after initial improvement. Common bacterial pathogens include *S. aureus, S. pneumoniae,* and *H. influenzae.* In addition to respiratory support, specific therapy is directed at the suspected pathogen. Primary influenza A pneumonia has been treated with oral amantadine (see Table 41–3).[13, 21, 22] Amantadine is not effective against influenza B, and its safety and efficacy in pregnancy have not been established. Antibiotic therapy should be considered unless bacterial superinfection is excluded. Although not routinely recommended in pregnancy, annual influenza vaccination should be given to those patients with chronic anemia, cardiovascular disease, diabetes mellitus, or immunodeficiency and to health care workers likely to be exposed to high-risk patients (Table 41–4). After exposures or during outbreaks of influenza A, the use of amantadine chemoprophylaxis in this selected group may decrease the incidence of both infection and mortality. Amantadine has numerous side effects, however, and is teratogenic in rats. Its safety has not been firmly established in pregnancy, and its use should be reserved for the high-risk patients described earlier (Table 41–5).

Varicella

Varicella (chickenpox) is a common childhood illness caused by a deoxyribonucleic acid (DNA) herpesvirus. Infection confers immunity, and fewer than 10% of adults are susceptible. An incubation period of 10 to 28 days follows exposure to virus in respiratory secretions or drainage from skin lesions. The virus replicates, then spreads hematogenously. Disease is characterized by fever, malaise, and a pruritic vesicular rash that begins on the face and trunk and spreads to the extremities. Lesions evolve over 2 to 4 days, then crust and resolve after 7 to 10 days. Virus remains latent in the dorsal root ganglia. Primary maternal varicella infection in the first trimester is associated with a 2 to 10% incidence of fetal varicella syndrome (scarred atrophic limb, eye anomalies, cerebral damage, low birth weight), but 25% of neonates have serologic evidence of infection. The risk of these severe sequelae associated with maternal zoster (shingles) or after primary maternal varicella in the second or third trimester is smaller, and 10 to 15% of neonates have serologic evidence of infection. When maternal symptoms develop in the perinatal period (5 days before through 2 days after delivery), neonates are at risk for perinatal varicella. A small number of neonates with perinatal varicella have developed unusually severe disseminated visceral and central nervous system disease, which was fatal in 30% of cases.

Adults with primary varicella are more prone to visceral complications than children, and 10 to 30% develop pneumonia. Patients may appear to have a mild case of varicella with scant lesions but 1 to 6 days into the illness abruptly develop cough and tachypnea with progression to respiratory failure. As many as 25% of adults with varicella pneumonia die, often as a result of complications from bacterial superinfection. Pregnant women with varicella pneumonia should be hospitalized and treated with oxygen and ventilatory support. High-dose intravenous acyclovir may shorten the duration of illness when given within 72 hours; however, there are insufficient data to determine whether acyclovir therapy improves maternal outcome or prevents congenital infection. Neonates at risk for perinatal varicella frequently are passively immunized with varicella-zoster immune globulin to abort or ameliorate infectious sequelae. The need for routine use of varicella-zoster immune globulin in these neonates is controversial, however, and there are insufficient data to establish efficacy (see Table 41–4).[13, 23–25]

Patients are most infectious for 1 to 3 days before the appearance of lesions and remain infectious until all lesions have crusted. Hospitalized patients (including neonates at risk for perinatal varicella) should be placed in strict respiratory isolation. Routine use of varicella-zoster immune globulin to prevent chickenpox in susceptible pregnant women after exposure is controversial. Varicella-zoster immune globulin may prevent maternal disease if given within 96 hours of exposure, but there are insufficient data to determine whether passive immunization protects the fetus.

TABLE 41–4. Immunization During Pregnancy

ACTIVE IMMUNIZATION

Vaccine	Reference	Comment
Tetanus toxoid Diphtheria toxoid	22, 28	Give at any time if patient lacks primary series or booster within past 10 yr.
Hepatitis B vaccine	22, 29–32	Can be used to prevent infection in susceptible women at high risk for exposure (household contact of carrier or active case, health care worker, intravenous drug abuse; may be used with HBIG).
Influenza vaccine Pneumococcal vaccine	21, 22 22, 33	Vaccine indicated only for high-risk patients with chronic underlying medical conditions. No known fetal anomalies.
Measles vaccine Mumps vaccine Rubella vaccine	22, 34 22, 34 22, 34–36	Live virus vaccines should be administered at least 3 mo before conception or immediately postpartum. No increase in congenital anomalies in women inadvertently given rubella vaccine during pregnancy.
Polio vaccine	22, 28	Primary series consists of three doses of enhanced potency inactive polio vaccine (IPV). If immediate protection is required (during an outbreak or because of foreign travel), one dose of oral polio vaccine (OPV) can be used to begin the primary series.

POSTEXPOSURE PROPHYLAXIS

Disease/Immune Globulin	Reference	Comment
Hepatitis A Immune serum globulin	22, 29	Immune globulin, 0.02 ml/kg IM (maximum 15 ml) in one dose given within 2 wk of exposure, may prevent maternal infection. No known adverse risk to fetus.
Hepatitis B Hepatitis B immune globulin (HBIG)	22, 29, 30	Use for maternal postexposure prophylaxis depends on type of exposure and maternal immune status. No known adverse risk to fetus. Give to neonate within 12 hr of delivery when mother is chronic carrier or had primary intrapartum infection.
Measles Immune serum globulin	22, 34	Immune globulin, 0.25 ml/kg IM (maximum 15 ml) in one dose given within 6 days of exposure, may prevent maternal disease. No known adverse risk to fetus, but efficacy in preventing abortion has not been established.
Varicella Varicella-zoster immune globulin (VZIG)	22, 23, 25	VZIG may prevent or abort complications of maternal disease if given within 96 hr of exposure. No known adverse risk to fetus. Immunization Practice Advisory Committee recommends administration of VZIG to neonate if mother develops chickenpox 5 days before or 2 days after delivery. No evidence that maternal administration prevents fetal infection.

IM, Intramuscularly.

Urinary Tract Infections

Symptomatic urinary tract infections occur in 1 to 2% of all pregnancies and are an important cause of maternal morbidity.[26, 27] The prevalence of asymptomatic bacteriuria is 4 to 7% in women of childbearing age. Increased prevalence is associated with lower socioeconomic status, older age, increased parity, and the presence of sickle cell disease. Extensive studies carried out before the availability of antibiotics established that 30 to 40% of bacteriuric pregnant women developed acute symptomatic pyelonephritis during the second or third trimester. In 1959, Kass showed that decreasing the prevalence of bacteriuria decreased the rate of prematurity and low birth weight. However, numerous subsequent studies have yielded conflicting results. Although their precise roles have not been established, several mechanisms are thought to contribute to the development of pyelonephritis in these women. Physiologic alterations of the urinary tract begin at about 7 weeks of gestation and include hormone-mediated dilation of the ureters and renal pelvis and decreased ureteral peristalsis. Incomplete bladder emptying and urinary stasis may result from a decrease in bladder tone or because of mechanical obstruction from the uterus. Changes progress throughout pregnancy and usually resolve within 2 months after delivery.

Symptoms of frequency, urgency, and dysuria with a positive urine culture are characteristic of cystitis. The presence of fever and chills with nausea and vomiting or flank pain suggests upper tract involvement. Older studies established that pyuria with isolation of more than 10^5 organisms from a midstream clean-catch urine sample was strongly correlated with infection. More recent studies have

TABLE 41–5. Prophylactic Antibiotics

CONDITION	REFERENCE	COMMENT
Asymptomatic bacteriuria	26, 27	See Table 41–6
Endocarditis		Same as for nonpregnant women
Group B streptococci (GBS)	41	Safety and efficacy of regimens for antenatal eradication of GBS carrier state have not been established. Ampicillin, 1–2 gm IV every 4 hr during labor and delivery in a pregnant woman with positive GBS culture *and* high-risk condition such as premature labor or >18 hr premature rupture of membranes may decrease the incidence of early-onset neonatal GBS infection and postpartum chorioamnionitis.
Haemophilus influenzae		Rifampin is usual prophylaxis after household or daycare contact with patient with invasive disease (meningitis) but is relatively contraindicated in pregnancy.
Neisseria meningitidis		Rifampin is usual prophylaxis after household or daycare contact with patient with invasive disease (meningitis, bacteremia) but is relatively contraindicated in pregnancy. Limited data suggest ceftriaxone, 250 mg IM, is effective.
Mycobacterium tuberculosis	22, 50–53	Patient with recent tuberculin skin test conversion within the past 1–2 yr and no active disease should begin prophylaxis with isoniazid, 300 mg/day PO, and pyridoxine, 50 mg/day PO.

IM, Intramuscularly; IV, intravenously; PO, orally.

demonstrated as few as 100 organisms per ml of urine in some symptomatic patients. The pathogens are the same as those found in nonpregnant women. *Escherichia coli* and other gram-negative bacilli are recovered from the urine of 60 to 85% of patients; enterococci and *Staphylococcus saprophyticus* are less common. Although their significance is unclear, several studies have found vaginal flora (lactobacilli, anaerobic streptococci, *Ureaplasma urealyticum, Gardnerella vaginalis*) in cultures of urine collected from as many as 25% of pregnant women.

Although screening is controversial because of cost and logistic difficulty, most authorities recommend that all pregnant women have an antenatal screening urine culture performed at 16 to 18 weeks of gestation to maximize yield. If the culture is negative at 16 weeks, the chance of developing a symptomatic urinary tract infection during pregnancy is very small, and additional screening is not generally recommended. If the culture is positive, most authorities recommend treatment to avoid the risk of progression to symptomatic urinary tract infection. The choice of antibiotic is guided by the expected sensitivity of the causative organisms (Table 41–6). Efficacy is greatest with a 7- to 10-day treatment course, although acceptable results from single-dose therapy have been noted in a small number of series. Urine should be recultured at the completion of therapy. Persistent

TABLE 41–6. Antimicrobial Agents in Pregnancy: Empirical Antibiotic Treatment of Urinary Tract Infections

ORGANISM	SYMPTOMS	ANTIBIOTICS
Asymptomatic bacteriuria in pregnancy		
E. coli (85%)	None	Ampicillin, 250 mg PO q.i.d. for 7–10 days *or* sulfisoxazole, 250–500 mg PO q.i.d. for 7–10 days (contraindicated near term), *or* nitrofurantoin, 100 mg PO q.i.d. for 7–10 days. Newer agents may be required if resistant organisms are suspected. Single-dose therapy less effective.
Enterococcus		
Staphylococcus saprophyticus		
Symptomatic bacteriuria in pregnancy		
Same as above	Cystitis	Same as above; consider suppressive therapy.*
	Pyelonephritis	Ampicillin, 1–2 gm IV every 4–6 hr, *plus* aminoglycoside or similar broad-spectrum coverage to start; consider suppressive therapy.*
Chronic suppression	Same as above	Nitrofurantoin, 50–100 mg PO at bedtime until delivery.*

*Use of nitrofurantoin is associated with a high frequency of side effects including fungal vulvovaginitis. Efficacy and safety of suppressive antibiotic therapy in pregnancy remains controversial. Patients who may benefit include those with persistent asymptomatic bacteriuria despite attempted eradication and those who have been treated for acute pyelonephritis. See text for full discussion.

IV, Intravenously; PO, orally; q.i.d., 4 times a day.

bacteriuria that occurs despite therapy with an effective antibiotic should prompt a second 7- to 10-day trial using a different antimicrobial agent. After successful treatment, most authorities recommend monthly screening urine cultures to verify absence of bacteriuria. The subset of patients with persistent bacteriuria are at particularly high risk for progression to pyelonephritis or may already have upper tract involvement. Treatment of these patients remains controversial; some authorities recommend use of oral suppressive antibiotics for the duration of the pregnancy, and others recommend treatment for presumed pyelonephritis (discussed later). Uncomplicated cystitis should be managed similarly.

In contrast, patients who progress to pyelonephritis have a 20 to 50% risk of premature labor, although the effect on prematurity remains controversial. Induction of labor may be caused by elaboration of bacterial products (phospholipase A_2) or host inflammatory mediators. Pregnant women with pyelonephritis should be hospitalized. Blood and urine cultures should be obtained before the initiation of intravenous antibiotics. Examination of a Gram-stained urine specimen may help guide empirical therapy, which should be revised once culture results become available (see Table 41–6). Fluid status and drug levels must be monitored closely to optimize therapy and avoid complications.

All patients have an increased risk of developing urinary tract colonization after bladder catheterization, which should be avoided during pregnancy if possible. Each institution has characteristic endemic pathogens that are frequently multidrug resistant. Treatment of nosocomial urinary tract infection often requires use of toxic antibiotics, and management should be individualized with the assistance of expert consultants.

Persistent bacteriuria or continued symptoms in the presence of appropriate antibiotic therapy warrants evaluation (ultrasonography or rarely intravenous pyelography) to exclude obstructive uropathy. Bacteremia and septic shock are potential complications but do not appear to occur with increased frequency during pregnancy. It is generally recommended that nonpregnant patients with uncomplicted pyelonephritis receive intravenous antibiotics for 48 hours after resolution of fever, followed by oral antibiotics to complete a 14-day course. Insufficient data are available to establish either the optimal duration of primary therapy or the efficacy or need for suppressive therapy in pregnant patients. Some authorities recommend continuing oral suppressive antibiotics for the duration of the pregnancy; others recommend frequent monitoring with re-treatment if infection recurs. Most agree that follow-up urine cultures immediately postpartum and a complete urologic evaluation 2 to 6 months after delivery are indicated.

INFECTIONS ASSOCIATED WITH INCREASED FETAL MORBIDITY

Many of the infections described next can be prevented by vaccination before conception (see Table 41–4).[15, 21, 22, 28–36] Sequelae of the remainder may be minimized by appropriate prenatal screening and management.

Cytomegalovirus

Cytomegalovirus (CMV) is a ubiquitous DNA herpesvirus. Fifty percent of adults have serologic evidence of past infection, and increased prevalence is associated with older age, parity, lower socioeconomic status, increased number of sex partners, and first pregnancy before age 15 years. In the United States, approximately 2% of susceptible women develop primary CMV during pregnancy, and 1% of all neonates are infected in utero.[37–39] Infection follows direct contact with virus in saliva, body secretions (including milk), and urine. Disease may be asymptomatic or may be characterized by a mild, mononucleosis-like syndrome with fever, malaise, myalgia, pharyngitis, and lymphadenopathy. Symptoms usually resolve in 3 to 5 weeks. The virus remains latent and periodically reactivates with accompanying viral shedding. No increased maternal morbidity is associated with CMV during pregnancy. However, CMV crosses the placenta, and congenital CMV occurs in 25 to 50% of primary maternal infections and 2 to 3% of recurrences. A severe congenital syndrome (cytomegalic inclusion disease) occurs in 5% of cases, and an infected fetus may be small for age and have various structural or functional organ impairments. Another 5 to 10% develop sensorineural hearing loss, chorioretinitis, or learning disabilities later in life. In contrast, most neonates exposed to CMV in the perinatal period (during delivery or nursing) remain asymptomatic. Viral culture confirms the presence of CMV but does not distinguish between primary or recurrent infection. The presence of CMV-specific immunoglobulin M suggests infection within the past 9 months, although elevation of immunoglobulin M levels may occur with reactivation. The antiviral agent ganciclovir may modulate the course of chronic CMV infection in immunodeficient patients but is contraindicated in pregnancy. In the absence of effective methods to prevent or treat congenital or perinatal CMV, routine screening during pregnancy is not recommended.

Because the virus is endemic, prevention of maternal exposure is probably not feasible, and a vaccine is not yet available. Pregnant women who anticipate exposure (health care workers, teachers) should follow infection control practices such as use of gloves and scrupulous hand washing.

Group B Streptococci

Streptococcus agalactiae (group B streptococcus) is a gram-positive coccus that causes about 12,000 cases of life-threatening perinatal infection in the United States each year.[17, 40, 41] Twenty percent to 40% of pregnant women are colonized with group B streptococci, and colonization is associated with premature rupture of membranes and premature delivery. Increased risk of colonization is associated with maternal age younger than 21 years, low parity, maternal diabetes, and use of an intrauterine contraceptive device. Group B streptococci may cause maternal chorioamnionitis, endomyometritis, and urinary tract infection. As many as 75% of women colonized with group B streptococci transmit the organism to the fetus. Transmission may occur in utero when the fetus aspirates infected amniotic fluid or during delivery through a colonized or infected vagina. A small number of colonized infants (1–2%) develop disease, and two neonatal syndromes are recognized. Early-onset disease occurs in the first 7 days of life and is characterized by bacteremia (98%), meningitis (10%), pneumonia, and a high mortality rate (20–50%). Increased risk of early-onset neonatal group B streptococcal disease is associated with prematurity and maternal factors such as amniotic fluid colonization, prolonged rupture of membranes, or a history of a previously infected delivery. Late-onset disease may be acquired intrapartum or postnatally. Infants present with meningitis in 30 to 60% of cases, and overall mortality is 10%.

Diagnosis of colonization or infection requires isolation of group B streptococci from samples of blood, body fluids, or secretions. Utility of more rapid tests is limited by low sensitivity and specificity.

Theoretically, most early-onset neonatal group B streptococcal disease could be prevented by identification and treatment of carriers before delivery, and routine screening at 26 to 32 weeks is recommended in high-risk populations.[41] Proponents of antepartum treatment have shown that

eradication of the carrier state may decrease the frequency of preterm labor but may not be practical because colonization may recur unless suppressive therapy is continued until delivery. Similarly, waiting until after delivery to treat neonates does not decrease the incidence of disease. To interrupt transmission of group B streptococci, most authorities now recommend intrapartum administration of intravenous ampicillin or penicillin to mothers with group B streptococcal colonization and the risk factors discussed earlier (preterm labor before 37 weeks, premature preterm rupture of membranes before 37 weeks, prolonged rupture of membranes greater than 18 hours, sibling born with group B streptococcal infection, or maternal fever during labor). Administration of systemic antibiotics to the mother treats incipient fetal infection, is associated with a greatly diminished incidence of neonatal disease, and may decrease the incidence of postcesarean endomyometritis. When these risk factors are present at delivery and the status of maternal group B streptococcal colonization is unknown, it may be reasonable to begin empirical antibiotics until culture results are available (see Table 41–5).

Hepatitis B

Hepatitis B virus is a DNA virus tropic for hepatocytes. Its prevalence is increased among certain high-risk populations (Asian, Eskimo, inhabitants of the tropics, intravenous drug abusers, prostitutes, health care workers), but pregnancy does not influence acquisition or severity of disease.[42] An incubation of 6 weeks to 6 months follows direct contact with virus in the body secretions or blood of patients with either acute infection or chronic carriage. Disease is frequently subclinical. Symptomatic infection begins with nausea, vomiting, low-grade fever, and fatigue and is followed by jaundice and liver tenderness. Viremia persists after 10% of acute infections, and about 50% of these hepatitis B surface antigen–positive chronic carriers develop liver disease (chronic hepatitis, cirrhosis, hepatocellular carcinoma). It is estimated that 0.1 to 0.5% of the U.S. population are hepatitis B carriers, and carriage rates as high as 70% have been reported in some high-risk groups. Congenital infection occurs in 95% of primary maternal infections and in 10 to 30% of pregnancies in chronic carriers. Subsequent disease may be prevented in 95% of congenitally infected neonates by prompt treatment with hepatitis B immune globulin and vaccine (see Table 41–4).[22, 29–32, 42] Although the prevalence of hepatitis B virus varies widely and universal screening may not be cost effective, most authorities recommend that pregnant women be tested for hepatitis B surface antigen before delivery. Women who are hepatitis B surface antigen positive should undergo routine evaluation and counseling according to Centers for Disease Control guidelines (safe sex, prophylaxis of sexual and household contact), and infants should receive hepatitis B vaccine and hepatitis B immune globulin within 12 hours of delivery. Women who are hepatitis B surface antigen negative but have a high risk of exposure (health care workers, household contacts of active cases or carriers) should be counseled about vaccination. In addition, routine hepatitis B vaccination of all neonates is now recommended.

Listeria

Listeria monocytogenes is a gram-positive bacillus that is widely distributed in the environment. Infections may occur sporadically or may be associated with food-borne epidemics. Several clinical syndromes have been described.[43] Pregnant women generally develop a mild flu-like illness after ingesting contaminated food. Symptoms include fever and chills, with a variable frequency of pharyngitis, myalgia, and gastrointestinal symptoms. Infection during pregnancy has been associated with septic abortion, chorioamnionitis, preterm labor, and congenital infection. Transplacental transmission may result in granulomatosis infantisepticum, a devastating neonatal infection characterized by disseminated microabscesses and extremely high mortality. Because of its nonspecific presentation, *Listeria* infection is often not suspected unless fetal distress is apparent. The optimal antibiotic regimen for the treatment of *Listeria* infection has not been established. Three weeks of intravenous penicillin or ampicillin appears to be effective for treatment of maternal infection and has been shown to improve fetal outcome in several small series. Because of the potential to improve fetal outcome when diagnosed early, *Listeria* infection should be considered in the differential diagnosis of febrile maternal illnesses.

Measles

Rubeola (measles) is caused by an RNA paramyxovirus. An incubation period of 10 to 14 days follows direct contact with the extremely infectious virus in either respiratory secretions or in aerosols. Disease begins with cough, coryza, and conjunctivitis, followed by the classic maculopap-

ular rash. Acute maternal infection is associated with 30 to 50% fetal mortality. Congenital anomalies have not been described in survivors. Data from the prevaccine era suggest that pregnant women with measles develop severe pneumonia with congestive heart failure and death more frequently than nonpregnant women. Although the incidence of measles has plummeted since the introduction of the live measles vaccine in 1969, recent outbreaks among previously immunized young adults have been reported. Susceptible adults should be vaccinated according to Immunization Practices Advisory Committee guidelines. The vaccine is contraindicated in pregnancy. Immune serum globulin may prevent disease in exposed, susceptible pregnant women, although its ability to protect the fetus has not been established (see Table 41–4).[22, 28, 34]

Mumps

Mumps is systemic disease caused by a paramyxovirus. Approximately 80 to 90% of adults are immune. An incubation period of 14 to 28 days follows direct contact with virus in respiratory secretions. A brief (1–2 days) prodrome of malaise, headache, low-grade fever, and anorexia is followed by tender, nonsuppurative swelling of the salivary glands. Maximal swelling occurs within 2 to 3 days and may be accompanied by high fever. The disease is subclinical in one third of patients and resolves in most within 1 week. Pregnancy does not appear to alter the course of the disease. In the prevaccine era, primary first-trimester maternal infection was associated with increased spontaneous abortion. No effective treatment for mumps has been found, and susceptible adults should be vaccinated according to Immunization Practices Advisory Committee guidelines (see Table 41–4).[22, 28, 34]

Rubella

Rubella (German measles) is caused by an RNA Rubivirus. An incubation period of 12 to 24 days follows exposure to infectious virus in respiratory secretions. The prodrome is characterized by malaise, fever, and anorexia. A maculopapular rash usually appears on the face, spreads to the body, and fades over 3 to 5 days. Adenopathy (especially posterior auricular, suboccipital, and posterior cervical) may persist for several weeks. Arthritis involving the fingers, wrists, and knees is more common in women, begins coincident with the rash, and usually resolves within 1 month. The disease course is not modified by pregnancy; however, primary maternal infection is associated with a 30 to 100% fetal infection rate. Sixty percent of first-trimester infections result in spontaneous abortion or a fetus with disordered organogenesis and multiple congenital defects. Classic congenital rubella syndrome is characterized by cardiac disease, cataracts or glaucoma, deafness, and mental retardation. No effective treatment is available, and emphasis is placed on prevention (see Table 41–4).[35, 36] Cases of congenital rubella syndrome have decreased since licensure of vaccine in 1969; however, it is estimated that 10 to 20% of women of childbearing age remain susceptible, and a recent upsurge has occurred in the number of cases of the syndrome among unvaccinated adults.[44] Neonates with congenital rubella syndrome may shed virus for as long as 1 year and should be strictly isolated to prevent nosocomial spread. Immune status should be ascertained in all pregnant women at the first prenatal visit. Termination of pregnancy should be considered when there is clear evidence of primary maternal infection during the first trimester. Single defects (such as unilateral hearing loss) are reported in 10% of infections occurring between the sixteenth and twentieth week of gestation, and termination is usually not considered. No cases of congenital rubella syndrome have been reported in maternal infection occurring after 22 weeks of gestation. Adults should be immunized according to Immunization Practice Advisory Committee guidelines. Vaccination is contraindicated during pregnancy. Although the vaccine virus crosses the placenta, no cases of congenital rubella syndrome have been attributed to inadvertent inoculation of pregnant women, and vaccination during pregnancy does not mandate termination of pregnancy.[44]

Parvovirus B19

Human parvovirus B19 (erythema infectiosum, fifth disease) is caused by a small DNA virus with worldwide distribution. Approximately 50% of adults in the United States are immune. Primary infection during the first half of pregnancy has been associated with an increased risk of hydrops fetalis and spontaneous abortion in several small series; however, the overall outcome of parvovirus B19 infection in pregnancy has not been established in prospective trials. Infection occurs primarily in the spring and summer and follows direct contact with the virus in respiratory secretions. Infection may be subclinical or followed in 6 to 8 days by low-grade fever, chills, malaise, and myalgia. These symptoms resolve during the next 1 to

4 days, although infectious virus can continue to be isolated from respiratory secretions. Children frequently develop a bright red macular rash on one or both cheeks (slapped cheek syndrome). The second phase of the illness begins 1 week later; children develop a lacy maculopapular rash on the extremities, and this may be evanescent or may persist for an additional week. Arthritis occurs and lasts 1 to 2 days in children and 2 to 4 weeks in adults. Infection in patients with preexisting blood dyscrasias has been associated with an aplastic crisis characterized by depletion of erythroid precursors from the bone marrow. Serologic diagnosis is useful, but tests are performed only at the Centers for Disease Control and Prevention and a few research laboratories. There is no treatment, and prevention strategies are generally not successful. Heightened surveillance for fetal hydrops may be warranted.[45–47]

Toxoplasmosis

Toxoplasmosis is caused by the intracellular parasite *Toxoplasma gondii*. A third of women in the United States have serologic evidence of past infection, and risk varies with age, geography, ethnicity, and history of exposure to cats. Infection occurs after exposure to oocysts in soil or tissue cysts in food. Eighty percent to 90% of infections are asymptomatic. Symptomatic adults may develop fever, night sweats, headache, malaise, pharyngitis, myalgia, lymphadenopathy, or rash as the trophozoites disseminate. Symptoms usually resolve over 4 to 6 weeks. Congenital infection may result when primary maternal infection occurs during pregnancy. Prospective studies have shown that the risk of infection ranges from 17% in the first trimester to 65% in the third trimester. Severe sequelae occur in 25% of fetuses infected during the first trimester and include spontaneous abortion, premature delivery, stillbirth, and a number of structural defects (microcephaly, intracerebral calcifications, chorioretinitis). Severe sequelae are observed in 11% of third-trimester infections and manifest as visual or hearing deficits, mental retardation, and seizures. Limited evidence suggests that treatment of an acute infection with spiramycin may reduce the risk of congenital infection. In the United States, it is estimated that acute toxoplasmosis occurs in 6 per 1000 pregnancies. Identification of infected mothers and neonates remains a problem. A number of serologic tests are available but are of limited use in establishing the onset of infection unless serial studies are performed. Isolation of trophozoites from cultures of blood, sterile body fluid, or placenta is consistent with acute infection; however, culture methods are limited by low sensitivity (tissue culture) or prolonged growth requirements (mouse culture). Furthermore, definitive diagnosis of fetal infection requires amniocentesis or percutaneous umbilical blood sampling with culture and serology.[48, 49] Because of the relatively low prevalence of toxoplasmosis in the United States, most authorities do not recommend routine screening.[45] If maternal infection does occur, management should be individualized with the assistance of an expert consultant. Most authorities do not recommend treating acute maternal infection. However, neonates at risk for developing congenital toxoplasmosis should be treated with antibiotics and monitored closely.

In an attempt to prevent infection, women should be instructed to eat well-cooked meats, wash hands carefully after digging in dry sandy soil, and avoid handling cat litter boxes.

Tuberculosis

Mycobacterium tuberculosis is an acid-fast bacillus that causes systemic disease. Infection follows inhalation of the organism in respiratory secretions or enviornmental aerosols. Approximately 10 million people in the United States have asymptomatic tuberculosis. Prevalence of infection is highest in immigrants from high-prevalence countries, health care workers, intravenous drug abusers, and people who are infected with human immunodeficiency virus, homeless, or of low socioeconomic status. During primary infection, the tubercle bacillus enters macrophages and disseminates throughout the body. One to 3 months after infection, a cell-mediated immune response develops and disease becomes latent, with formation of granulomas, fibrosis, and scarring. Without treatment, 5 to 10% of adults ultimately develop active disease. Active disease can be prevented by prophylactic treatment of those patients with asymptomatic infection. Infection status is most readily ascertained by tuberculin skin testing, which is interpreted according to Centers for Disease Control guidelines.[50, 51]

There is no clear evidence that pregnancy affects the course of asymptomatic tuberculosis infection or symptomatic disease. Congenital (in utero) infections are rare and are characterized by widespread dissemination of the tubercle bacilli, granuloma formation in the lungs and liver, and a high mortality rate. Postnatal acquisition occurs more frequently, and fulminant, disseminated disease is common.

Most authorities recommend routine prenatal tuberculin skin testing. Patients with positive tuberculin tests should be evaluated to preclude active disease. Evaluation should include a chest radiograph with abdominal shielding. Patients with active disease should submit three sputum samples for acid-fast bacillus smear and culture, then begin therapy with isoniazid, rifampin, and ethambutol (see Tables 41–2 and 41–5).[50–53] Hospitalized patients should be placed in respiratory isolation until infectiousness is determined. If multiple-drug-resistant tuberculosis is diagnosed, patients require treatment with a combination of agents that may be unsafe in pregnancy. In these cases, treatment must be individualized and expert guidance is advised.

Patients with no evidence of active disease but with documented skin test conversion within 1 to 2 years should begin prophylactic therapy with choice of drug (isoniazid, rifampin) based on local resistance patterns. Antituberculous drugs are relatively toxic to a mother and fetus, and close follow-up to monitor side effects is warranted. If resources permit, the source of infection should be sought, and household or close contacts should be tested for infection.

SEXUALLY TRANSMITTED DISEASES

Pelvic Inflammatory Disease

Pelvic inflammatory disease is an increasingly prevalent problem in the United States.[54] Affected women have a high incidence of ectopic pregnancy or infertility. Disease results from polymicrobial infection of endometrial or fallopian tube mucosa, which in many cases is damaged by prior sexually transmitted disease (STD) or use of an intrauterine contraceptive device. Pelvic inflammatory disease during pregnancy is uncommon after the first trimester, when the products of conception obliterate the uterine cavity. Diagnosis and management should conform to established guidelines (Table 41–7).[54–56] One component of prevention includes early recognition and treatment of STD.

Chlamydial Infection

Chlamydia trachomatis is a species of obligate intracellular bacteria thought to be the major cause of STD in the United States. An estimated 1 to 5% of U.S. women harbor *Chlamydia,* but rates as high as 75% occur among women in high-risk groups (age younger than 20 years, multiple sex partners, sex partner with nongonococcal urethritis, or prior history of STD). Clinical syndromes

TABLE 41–7. Antimicrobial Agents in Pregnancy: Empirical Antibiotic Treatment of Pelvic Infections

ORGANISM	SYMPTOMS	ANTIBIOTICS
Pelvic Inflammatory Disease		
Neisseria gonorrhoeae *Chlamydia trachomatis* Mixed aerobic and anaerobic bacteria, *Listeria monocytogenes*	Fever, abdominal pain	Cefoxitin, 2 gm IV every 6 hr, until patient is afebrile and asymptomatic for 48 hr. *Follow with* erythromycin, 500 mg PO q.i.d. for 10–14 days. *or* Clindamycin, 600 mg IV every 8 hr, *plus* gentamicin, 1.5 mg/kg IV every 8 hr until patient is afebrile and asymptomatic for 48 hr. Additional benefit derived from follow-up treatment with erythromycin, 500 mg PO q.i.d. for 10–14 days, has not been established in pregnancy.
Intra-amniotic Infection, Chorioamnionitis		
Mixed aerobic and anaerobic bacteria	Antenatal or peripartum fever without obvious source	Ampicillin, 1–2 gm IV every 4–6 hr, *plus* gentamicin, 1.5 mg/kg IV every 8 hr (or similar broad-spectrum coverage).
Postpartum Endometritis		
Same as above	Postpartum fever without obvious source, especially after cesarean section	Ampicillin, 1–2 gm IV every 4–6 hr, *plus* gentamicin, 1.5 mg/kg IV every 8 hr, *plus* clindamycin, 600 mg IV every 8 hr (or similar broad-spectrum coverage) *or* Cefoxitin, 2 gm IV every 6 hr until patient is afebrile and asymptomatic for 48 hr.

IV, Intravenously; PO, orally; q.i.d., 4 times a day.

include conjunctivitis, mucopurulent cervicitis, salpingitis, urethritis, and lymphogranuloma venereum. No distinctive in utero fetal infection has been described. However, maternal genital infection is associated with preterm rupture of membranes, premature labor and delivery, low birth weight, and an increased risk of postpartum endometritis. Neonatal transmission occurs as a fetus is bathed in infectious secretions during delivery. Conjunctivitis develops 3 to 20 days after birth in 20 to 50% of exposed neonates, and pneumonia occurs 5 days to 6 months after exposure in an additional 10 to 20%.

Diagnosis is made by microscopic inspection of exudate or tissue scrapings (stained with Giemsa's stain or fluorescein-conjugated monoclonal antibody) or by culture. Although an optimal regimen for treatment of chlamydial infection in pregnant women has not been established, maternal infection treated with 7 days of high-dose erythromycin (erythromycin base, 500-mg tablets four times a day for 7 days) appears to prevent perinatal infection.[57–60] Although the utility of routine screening remains controversial, most authorities recommend that high-risk women receive antenatal screening with treatment if indicated.

Patients infected with *Chlamydia* shed large numbers of organisms in secretions, and use of barrier precautions and scrupulous hand washing should be encouraged.

Gonorrhea

Neisseria gonorrhoeae, a gram-negative diplococcus, is the most commonly reported STD in the United States and occurs in 0.5 to 7% of pregnancies. Risk of acquisition is associated with age younger than 20 years, low socioeconomic status, and having a sex partner with gonorrhea. Infection may be limited to the lower urogenital tract (cervix, urethra) or may progress to involve the endometrium or fallopian tubes in as many as 20% of cases (pelvic inflammatory disease). Pregnant women appear to have an increased incidence of gonococcal pharyngitis and disseminated gonorrhea infection during the third trimester, although cases may reflect increased surveillance or reporting bias rather than a truly increased incidence. Diagnosis is made by isolation of the organism from culture of normally sterile body fluids (blood, joint fluid, cerebrospinal fluid) or secretions (vagina, rectum, pharynx). Although its role in causing perinatal complications has not been established, maternal gonococcal infection during pregnancy has been associated with a number of adverse fetal outcomes including increased risk of septic abortion, premature rupture of membranes, and perinatal mortality. Although PID is uncommon after the first trimester, patients with active gonorrhea at delivery are more likely to develop postpartum chorioamnionitis. Neonatal infection may cause purulent conjunctivitis (gonococcal ophthalmia neonatorum) 2 to 5 days after delivery or various less common local (wound abscess) or disseminated (bacteremia, arthritis, meningitis) infections.[61, 62]

Most authorities recommend that pregnant women have routine prenatal screening of endocervical cultures for gonorrhea. Treatment should follow established guidelines (one dose of ceftriaxone 250 mg intramuscularly for cervicitis, with follow-up test of cure cultures 4–7 days later.)[59] Pregnant women with PID or disseminated infection should be hospitalized for evaluation and intravenous antibiotics. The ability of antibiotics to reduce the adverse fetal outcomes noted earlier is controversial, and several studies have shown poor fetal outcome despite intrapartum therapy of maternal gonorrhea. Women with gonorrhea are at increased risk for other STDs and should also be screened for syphilis, *Chlamydia,* hepatitis B, and human immunodeficiency virus. In fact, because 30 to 50% of women with gonorrhea have coexisting chlamydial infection, most authorities recommend empirical addition of erythromycin (erythromycin base, 500 mg tablets four times a day for 7 days) unless *Chlamydia* culture is negative.

Herpes

Herpes simplex virus (HSV) is a DNA virus with worldwide distribution. Primary infection may be asymptomatic or may cause painful mucocutaneous ulcerations in oral (HSV 1) or anogenital (HSV 2) distribution. Lesions heal without scarring, and the virus becomes latent. Reactivation occurs with variable frequency and may be heralded by a prodrome of burning, itching, or tingling, followed by the appearance of vesicles. Insufficient data are available to estimate the prevalence, but in limited populations, primary HSV infection does not occur with increased frequency or severity during pregnancy.[63, 64] Neonatal HSV infection may occur in 30 to 50% of episodes of primary maternal HSV infection and in 1 to 4% of recurrent episodes. Death occurs in 50 to 60% of infected neonates, and severe sequelae (microcephaly, chorioretinitis, meningoencephalitis, seizures, mental retardation) develop in half of the survivors.

Diagnosis is made by obtaining a positive viral culture in an appropriate clinical setting. A number of serologic tests are available, but most cannot distinguish between primary and recurrent infection or determine the type of virus (HSV 1 or HSV 2). In nonpregnant patients, acyclovir has been used to treat disseminated HSV disease and may abort or suppress symptoms in patients with frequent recurrences. However, there are insufficient data about the safety of acyclovir in pregnancy or its efficacy in preventing neonatal transmission to formulate recommendations for prophylaxis.

Although antepartum cultures cannot be used to predict neonatal exposure because of the potential for reactivation shedding, some data show a decreased risk of neonatal infection when women with the typical prodrome or visible lesions during labor undergo cesarean delivery. Earlier protocols limited cesarean delivery to those women with membranes ruptured for less than 4 to 6 hours. However, because the mode of neonatal transmission remains unclear (direct inoculation from infectious cervical secretions or ascending infection after rupture of membranes), cesarean delivery should be strongly considered in women with imminent or active lesions regardless of the duration of membrane rupture.

Infected neonates may shed virus for prolonged periods, and caregivers should use barrier precautions and thorough hand washing to prevent nosocomial spread.

Papillomavirus

At least 60 types of human papillomavirus, a DNA virus in the papovavirus family, cause epithelial tumors of the skin and mucous membranes. Clinical manifestations include common warts, anogenital warts, and cervical carcinoma. The prevalence of uncomplicated genital warts (condylomata acuminata) in pregnancy is unknown. These warts may disseminate or grow dramatically during pregnancy. Involved tissues may bleed excessively and are easily lacerated during delivery. Rarely, exophytic lesions may grow so large that they obstruct the vagina and preclude vaginal delivery. Diagnosis is made clinically and confirmed by characteristic histology on biopsy samples of tissue from involved sites. There is no safe, effective therapy for human papillomavirus during pregnancy. Podophyllin, the standard therapy, is a mitotic poison, and its use is contraindicated in pregnant women. Variable success has been reported using topical trichloroacetic acid, cryotherapy, carbon dioxide laser cautery, and excision. The safety and efficacy of topical or intralesional interferon have not been established in pregnancy. Although a direct causal relationship has not been established, data from limited series suggest that maternal cervical human papillomavirus infection is associated with an increased incidence of neonatal laryngeal papillomatosis. However, insufficient data are available to recommend either routine screening or a strategy for the prevention of neonatal infection.[65]

Syphilis

Syphilis is caused by the spirochete *Treponema pallidum*.[66] The disease is divided into early (primary, secondary, early latent) and late (late latent, tertiary) stages. Congenital infection occurs in nearly all women who have primary infection during pregnancy and in 50% of women with latent syphilis and results in abortion or stillbirth in 50% of cases. The surviving neonates develop characteristic signs and symptoms including snuffles, rash, osteochondritis, cranial nerve VIII deafness, and interstitial keratitis. Rates of congenital syphilis in the United States have risen dramatically, with fewer than 100 cases per year reported in the late 1970s and nearly 4500 cases reported in 1991.[67] Diagnosis and management should follow standard guidelines.[59] A routine prenatal screen with a nontreponemal reagin test (Venereal Disease Research Laboratories, rapid plasma reagin) at the first prenatal visit is recommended. These nonspecific tests have low specificity, and all positive results must be confirmed by a specific treponemal test (microhemagglutination–*T. pallidum*, fluorescent treponemal antibody absorption). In most cases, treatment with penicillin has been shown to prevent the sequelae of congenital infection. The efficacy of other antibiotic regimens to prevent fetal infection is unknown, and neonates should be treated as if they have congenital syphilis.

OBSTETRIC INFECTIONS ASSOCIATED WITH INCREASED FETAL AND MATERNAL MORBIDITY

Chorioamnionitis

Chorioamnionitis is a histologic term used to describe inflammation of fetal membranes. Although its causal role has not been established, clinical chorioamnionitis (intra-amniotic infection) occurs in 5 to 28% of women with premature labor and in 1 to 2% of women who deliver at term. Specific risk factors in the development of intra-amniotic infection include prolonged rupture of membranes, multiple vaginal examinations, and prolonged labor. The frequency of intra-amniotic infection is also increased in young women with low parity, low socioeconomic status, and a history of bacterial vaginosis.[68–70] Most infections are

polymicrobial and are caused by a mixture of aerobes (gram-negative enteric bacilli [*E. coli, Klebsiella pneumoniae, Proteus* species], *Listeria*) and anaerobes (*Bacteroides* species, anaerobic streptococci, rarely *Clostridium* species). The contribution of coinfection with *Chlamydia, N. gonorrhoeae, Mycoplasma,* and *Ureaplasma* is uncertain. Intra-amniotic infection may result from hematogenous infection (*L. monocytogenes* and group A streptococci) or contiguous spread with ascending infection in the presence of ruptured membranes. Diagnosis should be suspected in a pregnant woman with fever and leukocytosis without a readily demonstrable source. Uterine tenderness and foul-smelling vaginal discharge are late signs. Isolation of organisms from aerobic and anaerobic culture of sterilely collected amniotic fluid is diagnostic, but infection can be suspected if neutrophils and bacteria are seen on smear. Bacteremia occurs in 3 to 12% of patients. Prenatal infection is associated with intrauterine growth retardation, fetal demise, premature delivery, and congenital infection. Infection late in pregnancy is associated with a lower rate of congenital infection but a higher risk of dysfunctional labor (up to 75%), often requiring oxytocin augmentation or cesarean delivery, and a higher rate of postpartum complications (wound infection in 4–7%, pelvic abscess or septic pelvic thrombophlebitis in 0–1%). Pneumonia has been reported in 2 to 25% of congenitally infected neonates; death occurs in 10% of premature births and 1 to 3% of term births. Once the diagnosis is suspected, antibiotics should be given to prevent fetal infection and suppress maternal disease (see Table 41–7).[68–71] In general, definitive treatment of polymicrobial infection requires evacuation of the infected uterine contents (i.e., delivery). An exception is made when *L. monocytogenes* is the sole pathogen. In this case, especially when prolongation of the pregnancy is desired, antibiotic therapy alone may eradicate infection. Broad antibiotic coverage is initiated empirically and continued until a patient has been afebrile and asymptomatic for 24 to 48 hours. Persistent fever should prompt a search for wound infection for pelvic abscess. No data support an extended course of antibiotic therapy unless a patient develops suppurative complications or is bacteremic. In complicated cases, the ultimate choice, dose, and duration of antibiotic are individualized, and surgical intervention may be required.

The prevalence of postpartum infections is increased in women who are obese, have frequent peripartum vaginal examinations, or undergo instrumentation (invasive fetal monitoring, cesarean delivery). These infections, which include postpartum endometritis, local wound infection, group A streptococcal puerperal sepsis, synergistic necrotizing gangrene, pelvic abscess, and septic pelvic thrombophlebitis are reviewed elsewhere.[72–74]

REFERENCES

1. Weinberg ED. Pregnancy-associated depression of cell-mediated immunity. Rev Infect Dis 1984;6:814.
2. Duff P. The aminoglycosides. Obstet Gynecol Clin North Am 1992;19:511.
3. Graham JM, Oshiro BT, Blanco JD. Limited-spectrum (first-generation) cephalosporins. Obstet Gynecol Clin North Am 1992;19:449.
4. Eriksen NL, Blanco JD. Extended-spectrum (second- and third-generation) cephalosporins. Obstet Gynecol Clin North Am 1992;19:461.
5. Campbell BA, Cox SM. The penicillins. Obstet Gynecol Clin North Am 1992;19:435.
6. Dinsmoor MJ. Imipenem-cilastatin. Obstet Gynecol Clin North Am 1992;19:475.
7. Sopor DE. Clindamycin. Obstet Gynecol Clin North Am 1992;19:483.
8. Graham EM. Erythromycin. Obstet Gynecol Clin North Am 1992;19:539.
9. Hager WD, Rapp RP. Metronidazole. Obstet Gynecol Clin North Am 1992;19:497.
10. Clark P. Aztreonam. Obstet Gynecol Clin North Am 1992;19:519.
11. Saravanos K, Duff P. The quinolone antibiotics. Obstet Gynecol Clin North Am 1992;19:529.
12. Egerman RS. The tetracyclines. Obstet Gynecol Clin North Am 1992;19:551.
13. Watts DH. Antiviral agents. Obstet Gynecol Clin North Am 1992;19:563.
14. Sperling RS, Stratton P, and the members of the Obstetric-Gynecologic Working Group of the AIDS Clinical Trials Group of the National Institute of Allergy and Infectious Diseases. Treatment options for human immunodeficiency virus-infected pregnant women. Obstet Gynecol 1992;79:443.
15. Ukwu HN, Graham BS, Lambert JS, Wright PF. Perinatal transmission of human immunodeficiency virus-1 infection and maternal immunization strategies for prevention. Obstet Gynecol 1992;80:458.
16. Human immunodeficiency virus infections. ACOG Technical Bulletin 1992;165:1.
17. Faro S. Streptococcal infections. In: Gleicher N (ed). Principles and Practice of Medical Therapy in Pregnancy. 2nd ed. Norwalk, CT: Appleton & Lange, 1992, pp 522–528.
18. Noble PW, Lavee AE, Jacobs MM. Respiratory diseases in pregnancy. Obstet Gynecol Clin North Am 1988;15:419.
19. Rodriques J, Niederman MS. Pneumonia complicating pregnancy. Clin Chest Med 1992;13:679.
20. McColgin SW, Glee L, Brian BA. Pulmonary disorders complicating pregnancy. Obstet Gynecol Clin North Am 1992;19:697.
21. Centers for Disease Control (CDC). Prevention and control of influenza: Recommendations of the Immunization Practices Advisory Committee (ACIP). MMWR 1992;41(RR-9):5.
22. Immunization during pregnancy. ACOG Technical Bulletin 1991;160:1.
23. Brunell PA. Varicella in pregnancy, the fetus, and the newborn: problems in management. J Infect Dis 1992;166(Suppl 1):S42.
24. Perinatal viral and parasitic infections. ACOG Technical Bulletin 1993;177:1.
25. Immunization Practices Advisory Committee. Varicella-zoster immune globulin for the prevention of chickenpox. MMWR 1984;33:84.
26. Andriole VT, Patterson TF. Epidemiology, natural history, and management of urinary tract infections in pregnancy. Med Clin North Am 1991;75(2):359.
27. Martens MG. Pyelonephritis. Obstet Gynecol Clin North Am 1989;16(2):305.
28. CDC. Update on adult immunization: Recommendations of the Immunization Practices Advisory Committee (ACIP). MMWR 1991;40(RR-12):1.
29. CDC. Protection against viral hepatitis: Recommendations of the Immunization Practices Advisory Committee (ACIP). MMWR 1990;39(RR-2):1.
30. CDC. Hepatitis B virus: A comprehensive strategy for eliminating transmission in the United States through universal childhood vaccination: Recommendations of the Immunization Practices Advisory Committee (ACIP). MMWR 1991;40(RR-13):1.
31. American Academy of Pediatrics. Universal hepatitis B immunization. Pediatrics 1992;89:795.
32. Guidelines for Hepatitis B virus screening and vaccination during pregnancy. ACOG Committee Opinion 1992;103:1.
33. Immunization Practices Advisory Committee. Pneumococcal polysaccharide vaccine. MMWR 1989;38:64.
34. CDC. Measles prevention: Recommendations of the Immunization Practices Advisory Committee (ACIP). MMWR 1989;38(9-S):1.
35. Rubella and pregnancy. ACOG Technical Bulletin 1992;171:1.
36. CDC. Rubella prevention: Recommendations of the Immunization Practices Advisory Committee (ACIP). MMWR 1990;39(RR-15):1.
37. Trofatter KF. Cytomegalovirus. In: Gleicher N (ed). Principles and Practice of Medical Therapy in Pregnancy. 2nd ed. Norwalk, CT: Appleton & Lange; 1992, pp 633–637.
38. Dobbins JG, Stewart JA, Demmler GJ. Surveillance of congenital cytomegalovirus disease, 1990–1991. MMWR 1992;41(SS-2):35.
39. Lamy ME, Mulongo KN, Gadisseux JF, et al. Prenatal diagnosis of fetal cytomegalovirus infection. Am J Obstet Gynecol 1992;166:91.
40. Zangwill KM, Schuchat A, Wenger JD. Group B streptococcal disease in the United States, 1990: Report from a multistate active surveillance system. MMWR 1992;41(SS-6):25.
41. Group B streptococcal infections in pregnancy. ACOG Technical Bulletin 1992;170:1.
42. Samuels P, Cohen AW. Pregnancies complicated by liver disease and liver dysfunction. Obstet Gynecol Clin North Am 1992;19:745.
43. Armstrong D. *Listeria monocytogenes*. In: Mandell GL, Douglas RG, Bennett JE (eds). Principles and Practice of Infectious Disease. 3rd ed. New York: Churchill Livingstone, 1990, pp 1587–1593.
44. CDC. Increase in rubella and congenital rubella syndrome—United States, 1988–1990. MMWR 1991;40:93.
45. Perinatal viral and parasitic infections. ACOG Technical Bulletin 1993;177:1.
46. Rodis JF, Quinn DL, Gary GW, et al. Management and outcomes of pregnancies complicated by human B19 parvovirus infection: A prospective study. Am J Obstet Gynecol 1990;163:1168.
47. Sheikh AU, Ernest JM, O'Shea M. Long term outcome in fetal hydrops from parvovirus B19 infection. Am J Obstet Gynecol 1992;167:337.
48. Remington JS, Desmonts G. Toxoplasmosis. In: Remington JS, Klein JO (eds). Infectious Diseases of the Fetus and Newborn Infant. 3rd ed. Philadelphia: WB Saunders, 1990, pp 89–195.

49. Lappalainen M, Koskela P, Koskiniemi M, et al. Toxoplasmosis acquired during pregnancy: Improved serodiagnosis based on avidity of IgG. J Infect Dis 1993;167:691.

50. American Thoracic Society: Diagnostic standards and classification of tuberculosis. Am Rev Respir Dis 1990;142:725.

51. American Thoracic Society: Treatment of tuberculosis and tuberculous infection in adults and children. Am Rev Respir Dis 1986;134:355.

52. Snider DE, Layde PM, Johnson MW, Lyle MA. Treatment of tuberculosis during pregnancy. Am Rev Respir Dis 1980;122:65.

53. Vallejo JG, Starke JR. Tuberculosis and pregnancy. Clin Chest Med 1992;13:693.

54. CDC. Pelvic inflammatory disease: Guidelines for prevention and management. MMWR 1991;40(RR-5):1.

55. Graham JM, Blanco JD. Pelvic inflammatory disease. In: Gleicher N (ed). Principles and Practice of Medical Therapy in Pregnancy. 2nd ed. Norwalk, CT: Appleton & Lange, 1992, pp 722–726.

56. Pastorek JG. Pelvic inflammatory disease and tubo-ovarian abscess. Obstet Gynecol Clin North Am 1989;16(2):347.

57. Livengood CH. *Chlamydia* infections. In: Gleicher N (ed). Principles and Practice of Medical Therapy in Pregnancy. 2nd ed. Norwalk, CT: Appleton & Lange; 1992, pp 617–626.

58. Bowie WR, Holmes KK. *Chlamydia trachomatis* (trachoma, perinatal infections, lymphogranuloma venereum, and other genital infections). In: Mandell GL, Douglas RG, Bennett JE (eds). Principles and Practice of Infectious Disease. 3rd ed. New York: Churchill Livingstone, 1990, pp 1426–1440.

59. CDC. 1989 Sexually transmitted disease treatment guidelines. MMWR 1989;38(S-8):1.

60. CDC. *Chlamydia trachomatis* infections: Policy guidelines for prevention and control. MMWR 1985;34(Suppl 3):53.

61. Handsfield HH. *Neisseria gonorrhoeae.* In: Mandell GL, Douglas RG, Bennett JE (eds). Principles and Practice of Infectious Disease. 3rd ed. New York: Churchill Livingstone, 1990, pp 1613–1629.

62. Gutman LT, Holmes KK. Gonococcal infection. In: Remington JS, Klein JO (eds). Infectious Diseases of the Fetus and Newborn Infant. 3rd ed. Philadelphia: WB Saunders, 1990, pp 848–865.

63. Prober CG, Corey L, Brown ZA, et al. The management of pregnancies complicated by genital infections with herpes simplex virus. Clin Infect Dis 1992;15:1031.

64. Perinatal herpes simplex virus. ACOG Technical Bulletin 1988;122:1.

65. Reichman RC, Bonnez W. Papillomaviruses. In: Mandell GL, Douglas RG, Bennett JE (eds). Principles and Practice of Infectious Disease. 3rd ed. New York: Churchill Livingstone, 1990, pp 1191–1200.

66. Tramont EC. *Treponema pallidum* (syphilis). In: Mandell GL, Douglas RG, Bennett JE (eds). Principles and Practice of Infectious Disease. 3rd ed. New York: Churchill Livingstone, 1990, pp 1794–1808.

67. CDC. Summary of notifiable diseases, United States, 1991. MMWR 1991;40:46.

68. Gilstrap LC, Cox SM. Acute chorioamnionitis. Obstet Gynecol Clin North Am 1989;16(2):373.

69. Blanco JD. Intra-amniotic infections. In: Gleicher N (ed). Principles and Practice of Medical Therapy in Pregnancy. 2nd ed. Norwalk, CT: Appleton & Lange; 1992, pp 712–716.

70. Gibbs RS, Romero R, Hillier SL, et al. A review of premature birth and subclinical infection. Am J Obstet Gynecol 1992;166:1515.

71. Kirschbaum T. Antibiotics in the treatment of preterm labor. Am J Obstet Gynecol 1993;168:1239.

72. Gibbs RS. Infection after cesarean section. Clin Obstet Gynecol 1985;28:697.

73. Duff P. Pathophysiology and management of postcesarean endomyometritis. Obstet Gynecol 1986;67:269.

74. Cox SM, Gilstrap LC. Postpartum endometritis. Obstet Gynecol Clin North Am 1989;16(2):363.

42

Lung Disease in Pregnancy

Anne Meneghetti and John Bernardo

The lungs and upper airways undergo well defined changes during pregnancy. Hormonal variations alter mucosal characteristics and ventilatory patterns. Mechanical changes within the abdomen caused by the enlarging uterus alter the shape of the thoracic cavity and affect lung mechanics. Compensatory mechanisms adjust for these changes to ensure adequate ventilation and oxygen delivery to a mother and her developing fetus, especially near term.

Although a healthy woman has little difficulty adjusting to the compromises imposed by pregnancy, the altered physiology modifies the expression of specific respiratory tract diseases in various ways. Furthermore, treatment of respiratory tract disease in pregnancy must take into consideration the effects of treatment on a developing fetus. This chapter examines the effects of pregnancy on the lungs and respiratory system and reviews the diagnosis and treatment of several specific respiratory disorders during pregnancy.

NORMAL PHYSIOLOGIC CHANGES IN THE LUNGS DURING PREGNANCY

Pregnancy induces significant changes in the shape of the thoracic cavity, substantial increases in tidal volume and minute ventilation, and consequent alterations in acid-base status. Mechanically, the gravid uterus exerts an upward force displacing the diaphragm cranially a maximum of 4 cm and expanding the transverse thoracic diameter by a maximum of 2.1 cm.[1] Although the result is a net decrease in resting lung volume, diaphragmatic and thoracic muscular range of motion is unimpaired[2] and vital capacity remains unchanged (Fig. 42–1).[3] One extensive study demonstrated no alterations in lung volumes in normal women until the second half of pregnancy. At this time, a decrease in both expiratory reserve volume and residual volume contributed to an 18% mean decrease in functional residual capacity. This decrease in functional residual capacity implies that airway closure may be more likely to occur with regular tidal breathing, especially when a patient is supine (Table 42–1).[4, 5] Both obesity and the recumbent position are associated with further reductions in functional residual capacity and expiratory reserve volume.[6] Despite these diminished lung volumes, tidal volume and inspiratory reserve volume increase, resulting in an unchanged vital capacity.[7]

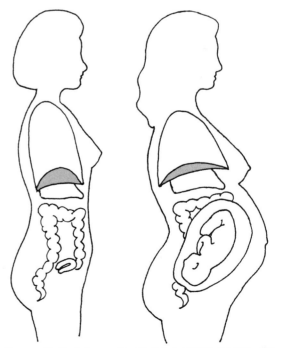

Figure 42–1. Schematic of the position of the diaphragm in the nonpregnant and pregnant woman.

TABLE 42–1. Lung Volumes in Pregnancy

	LUNG VOLUMES	CHANGE IN PREGNANCY
Tidal volume (TV)	Air moved in and out while breathing at rest	Increases by 50%
Functional residual capacity (FRC)	Volume at the end of a normal expiration, comprising RV + ERV	Decreases
Expiratory reserve volume (ERV)	Volume that could be expelled from FRC to reach RV	Decreases
Residual volume (RV)	Volume left after a forced maximal expiration	Decreases
Inspiratory capacity (IC)	Volume able to be forcibly inspired from the point of natural end-expiration	Increases
Vital capacity (VC)	Volume of air expired from maximal inspiration to maximal expiration = IRV + TV + ERV	Unchanged
Total lung capacity (TLC)	Maximal gas contained by the lungs	Minimally decreases

Countless studies of airway flows throughout pregnancy have confirmed no alterations in the forced expiratory volume in 1 second (FEV_1) or the ratio of FEV_1 to the forced vital capacity (FEV_1/FVC), suggesting that pregnancy does not hamper large airway function.[8] One study noted that the FEV_1 and peak expiratory flow rate during pregnancy are reduced when a patient is in the supine versus the seated position.[5] The diffusing capacity of the lung for carbon monoxide (DLCO) may increase in the first trimester then decrease in the latter half of pregnancy to a value near or slightly below the nonpregnant level, before rising again postpartum.[9] With exercise, the DLCO increases appropriately.[10]

The most consistent alteration of respiratory physiology during pregnancy is an increase in ventilation. This increase is present during the first trimester and by term is between 48 and 57% above the normal resting nonpregnant level.[7] Although both oxygen consumption and basal metabolic rate increase in pregnancy (by 21 and 14%, respectively), the increase in ventilation exceeds them (48%).[2] The increased minute ventilation (the product of tidal volume and respiratory rate) of pregnancy is due to a 50% increase in tidal volume while the respiratory rate remains unchanged (Fig. 42–2).[2] Circulating progesterone may increase respiratory center sensitivity to the partial pressure of carbon dioxide (Pco_2),[11] leading to increased tidal

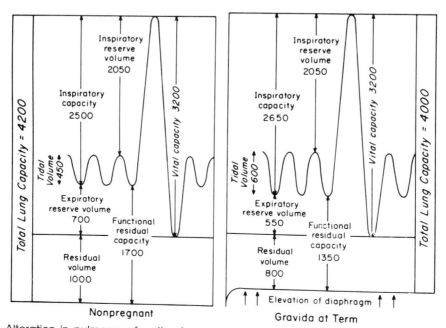

Figure 42–2. Alteration in pulmonary function in pregnancy. (From Leontic EA. Respiratory disease in pregnancy. Med Clin North Am 1977;61:111.)

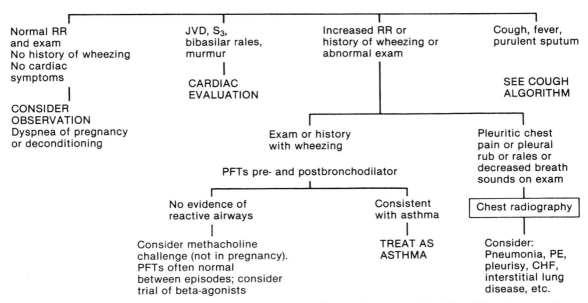

Figure 42–3. Dyspnea of pregnancy. RR, Respiratory rate; JVD, jugular venous distention; PFT, pulmonary function test; PE, pulmonary embolism; CHF, congestive heart failure.

volumes. The resulting increase in ventilation causes a decrease in P_{CO_2} to a plateau of 27 to 32 mm Hg (normal is 35–45).[8] The arterial pH is maintained between 7.4 and 7.45 by renal mechanisms that compensate for the respiratory alkalosis: the kidneys increase bicarbonate excretion to yield serum levels of 18 to 21 mEq per liter.[8]

Arterial partial pressure of oxygen (P_{O_2}) actually increases during pregnancy, as might be predicted by the lowered P_{CO_2}. Mean P_{O_2} ranges from 101 to 108 mm Hg.[12] Near term, the alveolar-arterial gradient* is noted to be slightly increased to a mean of 14 mm Hg in the seated position and to 20 mm Hg supine.[13] This increased alveolar-arterial gradient in later pregnancy partially offsets the predicted increase in arterial P_{O_2} expected from lowering the P_{CO_2}, but the P_{O_2} remains near 100 even at term.[12]

CHARACTERISTIC CHANGES IN THE AIRWAYS IN NORMAL PREGNANCY

Dyspnea of Pregnancy

As many as 60 to 70% of gravid women note dyspnea at some point during the course of pregnancy.[2] This symptom does not correlate with any measurable decrement in pulmonary function tests

(PFTs).[3] If dyspnea were related to mechanical factors, one would predict dyspnea to worsen as pregnancy progressed; however, this symptom is most frequently noted in the first two trimesters[3] and is often ameliorated near term. Many have supposed that this sensation is somehow related to the increase in resting ventilation, which is out of proportion to the body's demand. Although dyspnea may be physiologic in pregnancy, tachypnea is not, and a respiratory rate greater than 18 to 20 should be considered abnormal (Fig. 42–3).

NASOPHARYNGEAL COMPLICATIONS OF PREGNANCY

Vascular engorgement of the nasal turbinates to the point of obstruction can occur during menstruation.[14] Various hormonal influences acting in a sustained manner during gestation may result in persistent nasal mucosal congestion, often noted from the end of the first trimester until parturition.[14] Inhalation of allergens and noxious substances can further aggravate congestion. Preexisting structural abnormalities such as septal deviation or polyps are additional causes of obstruction in gravid women. In many pregnant women, the false vocal cords and larynx may appear swollen and red; this edema may cause changes in voice and difficulty in nasal breathing, especially near term. Epistaxis is more frequent, especially in the setting of respiratory tract infec-

---

*On room air at sea level, alveolar-arterial gradient is $[(760-47) \times 0.21 - (Pa_{CO_2}/0.8)] - Pa_{O_2}$ from arterial blood gas.

tions.[15] Chronic use of topical nasal decongestants may result in rebound engorgement of the nasal mucosa known as rhinitis medicamentosa.

Examination may reveal boggy, pale, edematous nasal mucosa with a clear discharge, consistent with allergic rhinitis. Erythematous mucosa is more likely associated with sinusitis or rhinitis medicamentosa. Without a history of purulent nasal discharge, facial pain, and fever, sinusitis can be notoriously difficult to confirm without sinus radiographs or computed tomography.

If symptoms are tolerable, ideally no pharmacologic therapy should be instituted in the absence of acute infection. Treatment of rhinitis in pregnancy depends on the suspected cause (Table 42–2). Rhinitis medicamentosa may resolve after a week of complete abstention from nasal vasoconstrictors, but patients may require inhaled corticosteroids to reverse the rebound edema. Allergic rhinitis may respond to antihistamines/decongestants or topical nasal steroids.[16] Extensive studies of pregnant and lactating women are not available, but inhaled beclomethasone, two puffs per nostril twice daily, has been used with success. Although some patients may experience relief in a few days, others require up to several weeks before maximal effects are noted. Aqueous versions of nasal steroids may be better tolerated than pressurized aerosol preparations. The drug should be discontinued if a significant nosebleed occurs. In addition to or instead of these medications, nasal topical saline spray, available without a prescription, often provides considerable relief.

Nasal polyps may be treated with inhaled steroids. Oral steroids should be reserved for severe nasal polyposis or symptomatic eosinophilic rhinitis unresponsive to other therapy.[17] Vasomotor rhinitis is nonallergic chronic congestion, usually without significant rhinorrhea but with prominent postnasal drip and sore throat, precipitated by strong odors, irritants, and other factors. Treatment for this form of rhinitis is empirical.

The antihistamines brompheniramine and diphenhydramine should be avoided because of increased risk of fetal malformations.[18] If an antihistamine is absolutely necessary, tripelennamine (pyribenzamine)[12] in doses of 25 to 50 mg every 6 hours as needed, or 100 mg of the sustained-release formulation twice daily to a maximum of 200 mg daily,[17] or chlorpheniramine 4 mg orally up to four times a day or 8 to 12 mg of the sustained release formulation twice daily[19] is recommended. Note that antihistamines themselves do not directly relieve nasal congestion. Therefore, a decongestant is often given concomitantly. The decongestant pseudoephedrine (30–60 mg every 6 hours or 120 mg of the timed-release capsule every 12 hours)[17] is considered safe in pregnancy, but phenylephrine and phenylpropanolamine should be avoided.[18]

COMMON RESPIRATORY DISORDERS IN PREGNANCY

Asthma in Pregnancy

Asthma is an inflammatory disorder in which variable airflow obstruction is at least partially reversible spontaneously or with treatment. Asthma is characterized by increased airway responsiveness to various stimuli. Wheezing and dyspnea are common symptoms, resulting from pathologic contraction of airway smooth muscle and secretion of abnormal mucus, which obstructs airways. Various types of asthma have been identified. It is imperative that clinicians recognize that not all patients with asthma wheeze; in some patients, airway hyperresponsiveness is manifested solely by episodic dyspnea or cough.

Extrinsic asthma refers to an immunoglobulin E–mediated bronchospastic response within minutes of inhaling an allergen or a delayed response 6 to 12 hours later. Common allergens include pollens, animal antigens, molds, and dust mites. This disease may appear seasonal, episodic, or chronic, depending on a patient's exposure to the offending antigen and her response. Some patients may also have allergic rhinoconjunctivitis or a history of atopic dermatitis. *Intrinsic asthma* is not immunoglobulin E mediated, despite the occasional presence of increased eosinophils in the sputum and peripheral blood. Patients may be able to identify various triggers such as cold air, noxious odors, smoke, stress, gastroesophageal reflux,

TABLE 42–2. Treatment of Rhinitis in Pregnancy

CAUSE	TREATMENT
Allergic rhinitis	Avoid allergen if possible Pseudoephedrine, tripelennamine, intranasal cromolyn or beclomethasone, intranasal saline spray
Bacterial rhinosinusitis	Saline nasal spray/irrigation Oral amoxicillin, cefaclor, erythromycin for 2–3 wk Pseudoephedrine
Rhinitis medicamentosa	Discontinue topical vasoconstrictors Intranasal beclomethasone
Vasomotor rhinitis	Pseudoephedrine

Modified from Incaudo G. Diagnosis and treatment of rhinitis during pregnancy and lactation. Clin Rev Allergy 1987; 5:325. Modified and printed with permission.

sinusitis, or upper respiratory tract infections. In some cases, the attacks may have no identifiable cause. Some patients may have mixed types of asthma, in which both allergic and nonimmunologic triggers are identified. *Variant or cough asthma* manifests as a nonproductive cough, often episodic, and may be associated with an antecedent upper respiratory tract illness. Bronchial hyperreactivity may persist for weeks after an otherwise resolved upper respiratory tract infection.

Aspirin-induced asthma is noted in sensitive patients minutes to hours after ingestion of nonsteroidal anti-inflammatory drugs. The resulting bronchospasm can be life threatening, and patients may continue to experience chronic symptoms long after ingestion of aspirin. These patients should be provided with a list of over-the-counter aspirin- and nonsteroidal anti-inflammatory drug–containing medications to avoid. Nasal polyposis is occasionally associated with aspirin sensitivity. *Exercise-induced asthma* is wheezing noted shortly after discontinuance of exercise. Although mild bronchospasm may be noted during exercise as well, patients who wheeze markedly at the onset of exercise may simply have poorly controlled ordinary asthma. The temperature and humidity of the air may affect symptoms: cold, dry air tends to induce more wheezing for a given minute ventilation than does warm, moist air.[20]

About 1% of pregnant women have asthma.[21] The course for each individual patient is unpredictable, although the course of asthma for a given woman may be consistent with successive pregnancies.[22] Those with the most severe disease are not surprisingly at greatest risk for deterioration during pregnancy.[23] Upper respiratory tract infections are perhaps the most common cause of asthma exacerbation during pregnancy. Uncontrolled wheezing is associated with increased mortality of pregnant women and their fetuses.[24] Low birth weight,[23] hyperemesis, vaginal hemorrhage, toxemia, complicated labor, and increased neonatal mortality are reportedly more common in asthmatic mothers,[25] but the incidence of congenital malformations is not increased. Pregnancy outcome even in women with steroid-dependent asthma approximates that of the population at large when asthma is well controlled.[26] At the time of labor and delivery, 90% of asthmatic women in one large study were completely asymptomatic.[22]

Diagnosis

Although a patient with active expiratory wheezing occasionally comes to a physician's office, the diagnosis of reactive airways disease is often made by history. Physical examination during an acute attack may show tachypnea (respiratory rate >20), tachycardia, pulsus paradoxus, nasal flaring, use of accessory neck and shoulder muscles, rib retractions, and inability to complete a sentence. Lung examination reveals wheezing, especially on expiration, and a long forced expiratory time. Some wheezes may be heard only when a patient is asked to inhale deeply and then exhale quite forcibly. Stridor, a high-pitched inspiratory sound often heard best by auscultation over the anterior neck, should be distinguished from wheezing. Stridor may be noted with life-threatening upper airways obstruction due to foreign body aspiration, epiglottitis, anaphylaxis, or goiter, and it should be evaluated immediately.

Because symptoms of asthma may be fleeting or noted only in response to specific stimuli such as allergens, cold air, upper respiratory tract infections, or exercise, the findings on examination and results of PFTs may be normal between episodes. In some patients, subtle clues such as reduced small airways flow manifest as a low forced expiratory flow rate (FEF_{25-75}; also called maximum midexpiratory flow rate) on spirometry (Fig. 42–4). In those with normal PFT results, the study may be repeated with measurements before and after a cold air challenge.

Alternatively, a methacholine challenge test may be used to provoke bronchoconstriction in persons with presumed latent reactive airways. However, the effects of methacholine on developing fetuses are not known; therefore, the test should not be performed during pregnancy. In fact, the manufacturer recommends performing a methacholine challenge test within 10 days of onset of menses or within 2 weeks after a negative pregnancy test. It is also not known whether inhaled methacholine is excreted in breast milk. Inhalational challenge is also not recommended for patients taking β-blockers, because response to methacholine can be prolonged in these patients.[27]

Clinical history may suggest certain allergic triggers (dust mites, animals, pollens, molds) to be avoided, but initial skin testing may be deferred until postpartum to avoid potentially severe systemic reactions.[28] Chest radiographs are seldom indicated in routine evaluation of a pregnant asthmatic woman. Radiographic findings are usually normal for pregnancy, although hyperinflation may be seen in some asthma sufferers. Baseline PFTs, when a patient is least symptomatic, should be measured in all asthmatic patients for future reference. Tuberculin skin testing (purified protein derivative, by the Mantoux technique) should be performed in all patients. If the reaction is significant, a chest radiograph is indicated immediately for those with any symptom of active tuberculosis;

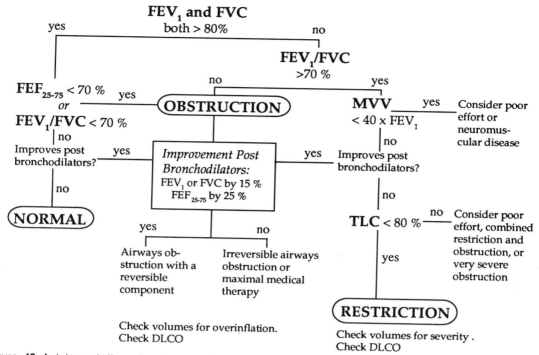

Figure 42-4. Interpretation of pulmonary function testing. (From Meneghetti A. Pulmonary Fellows Guide. Unpublished, 1991.)

otherwise, it may be deferred until the second or third trimester. All patients with new onset of asthma should have their thyroid-stimulating hormone measured, because hypothyroidism may clinically present as wheezing.

Treatment

Treatment of a gravid asthmatic patient differs little from that of a nonpregnant woman, except that a practitioner must also consider the pharmacologic effect of each medication upon the developing fetus. One begins with identifying and controlling any recognizable exacerbants such as allergens. Physical activity should not be limited. Medications should be kept to the minimum required to control symptoms, and if a patient improves during the course of pregnancy, tapering or discontinuing the medication is appropriate.

Smoking should be discontinued. Behavioral modification approaches to smoking cessation are encouraged; no controlled trials have investigated nicotine patch use during pregnancy. Patients should be counseled about the risks that uncontrolled asthma pose to a fetus and should be advised that well-controlled studies of most medications in pregnant asthmatic women are lacking.

Gastroesophageal reflux disease may exacerbate bronchial hyperreactivity via an incompletely understood mechanism. Women with gastroesophageal reflux may complain of a sour taste or dyspepsia, more pronounced on recumbency, which may be alleviated by antacids. Asthmatic women who note this association should avoid substances that reduce lower esophageal sphincter tone, such as caffeine, theophylline, oral β_2-agonists, chocolate, alcohol, fatty foods, and mint. Pregnancy itself may reduce lower esophageal sphincter tone in response to various stimuli.[28] Patients suffering from this exacerbant should avoid the supine position postprandially for several hours if possible and should raise the head of their bed by several inches to minimize the effects of reflux at night.

Bacterial sinusitis and respiratory tract infections should be treated promptly with antibiotics such as amoxicillin, erythromycin, or cefaclor,[29] based on sputum Gram stain if obtainable. All chronically asthmatic patients should receive an annual influenza vaccination during the fall/winter season; however, it is recommended that it be given during the second or third trimester of pregnancy.[30]

Inhalant allergen immunotherapy for those with extrinsic asthma carries the potential risk of severe systemic reactions and therefore should be closely monitored during pregnancy. It is recommended that those patients who are already showing benefit from an immunotherapy program and who are not prone to systemic reactions continue treatment, perhaps with a reduction in dose.[29] Immunotherapy should not be initiated during pregnancy because of the unknown potential for systemic reactions. Those who are known or are suspected to be sensitive to inhalant allergens should take avoidance measures. For example, it may be helpful to keep animals out of the house, especially out of the bedroom. Patients with dust mite sensitivity should encase their mattress and pillows in airtight plastic covers, use air conditioning to maintain a low humidity level, wash bedding weekly in 130°F water, and avoid dusting and vacuuming or wear a mask during and immediately after these activities. When pollen counts are high, the outdoors should be avoided by patients with hayfever.

For all asthmatic patients, β-blockers, especially those that are not β-1 selective, may exacerbate asthma and are best avoided if possible. Cough preparations containing iodides should also be avoided, because these compounds are concentrated in the fetal thyroid, resulting in fetal goiter and hypothyroidism, and are also teratogenic.[31] Iodine may also contaminate breast milk.[32] Tetracyclines should be avoided because of their effects on fetal bones and teeth. Sedatives and narcotics are respiratory depressants and should be avoided if possible in those at risk for respiratory decompensation. During lactation, the same medications used to treat gestational asthma may be continued, because levels of drugs reaching a breast-fed baby are usually less than that received by a fetus through the placenta. Both theophylline and corticosteroids are secreted in small amounts into breast milk.

One may initially prescribe an inhaled β₂-agonist as needed. Once β-agonist use exceeds four times a day, an anti-inflammatory medication should be started, and the β-agonist is continued as needed. Inhaled steroids are the anti-inflammatory agent of choice, using up to four puffs of beclomethasone four times daily or cromolyn sodium two puffs four times daily. If necessary, both anti-inflammatory agents may be used simultaneously. Several weeks of therapy are required before maximal effects are achieved. If a patient has seasonal asthma, treatment with anti-inflammatory agents should begin several weeks before the anticipated season. For exercise-induced asthma, cromolyn sodium or an inhaled β-agonist may be used 15 to 30 minutes before activity. β-Agonists and anti-inflammatory inhalers are often helpful in variant asthma as well. Only when anti-inflammatory therapy is unsuccessful is theophylline or an oral corticosteroid used.

There is generally no reason to use home nebulizers instead of metered-dose inhalers unless a patient is physically unable to use an inhaler effectively. To optimize delivery, the use of a spacer device that attaches to the mouthpiece of the inhaler is encouraged. Cylinder or accordian-type spacers allow a patient to actuate an inhaler directly into the spacer before slow inhalation of the drug, thus eliminating the need to coordinate inhalation and activation of the metered-dose inhaler. Patients should demonstrate use of the inhaler to ensure proper technique (Table 42–3).

A peak flow meter for home assessment should be considered for women with severe or labile disease. Predicted peak expiratory flows for women are in the range of 380 to 550 liters per minute and are not altered in pregnancy.[19] Flows in excess of 200 liters per minute suggest mild to moderate severity, and those of 50 to 100 suggest marked decompensation. More important than the absolute number is the pattern for a particular individual: a 20 to 25% decrease from a patient's usual best baseline flow rate on repeated good efforts may be an early sign of an exacerbation. For patients using this tool, a daily log of each morning's best reading should be kept. If a patient is regularly using inhaled bronchodilators, measurements should be taken consistently either before or after the morning dose.

Medications

Drug treatment of asthma is summarized in Table 42–4.

BETA₂-AGONISTS. This class of drug binds to β₂-receptors in bronchial smooth muscle and secretory cells to promote bronchodilation and diminish mucus secretion. Metaproterenol, albuterol,

---

TABLE 42–3.   Directions for Use of a Metered-Dose Inhaler

Remove cap from mouthpiece.
Shake the inhaler.
Exhale completely.
Position the mouthpiece approximately 4–6 inches away from a widely opened mouth. (Some patients prefer the use of a spacer.)
Simultaneously actuate the device while *slowly* inhaling to total lung capacity.
Hold breath for 10 sec or as long as feasible.
Repeat the above steps 2–3 min later for the next puff.
The drug canister should be removed from the plastic case daily and the case washed in soapy water.
Before going on a trip, it may be helpful to estimate the amount of the drug remaining in a canister by removing it from the plastic case and placing it in a bowl of water. If it sinks below the surface, there is a significant amount of the drug left. If it floats on the surface, the canister may be nearly empty.

TABLE 42–4. **Drug Treatment of Asthma**

Inhaled β-agonist, 2 puffs as needed*
|
Once β-agonist use exceeds q.i.d.,
begin an anti-inflammatory drug:
inhaled beclomethasone, 2–4 puffs b.i.d.–q.i.d.
or
Cromolyn sodium, 2 puffs q.i.d.
and taper β-agonist use if possible
|
Add theophylline, 200–300 mg orally b.i.d.†
|
Add oral steroids,
a short tapered course over weeks
or chronic dosing
(≤ 10 mg prednisone every other day if possible)

---

*Cromolyn sodium may be used either prophylactically or continuously as an initial choice, especially in those with extrinsic or exercise-induced asthma. It may also be used concomitantly with inhaled steroids.
†Monitor serum levels to achieve 5–12 μg/ml.
q.i.d., 4 times a day; b.i.d., 2 times a day.

---

terbutaline, and pirbuterol are commonly available in metered-dose inhalers. Inhaled, they rapidly relieve bronchospasm, and very little reaches the systemic or placental circulation.[18] Duration of action is generally 3 to 6 hours. Because terbutaline may inhibit labor and preserve or even increase uteroplacental blood flow in pregnant women,[33] it may be an ideal choice for pregnant asthmatic women. Although there are no well-controlled studies of pregnant asthmatic women, oral β₂-agonists at bedtime may occasionally be necessary in women who have nocturnal exacerbations of asthma. Although human experience with inhaled and systemic use has not shown evidence of fetal injury,[19] use of a metered-dose inhaler nightly is considered preferable, because inhaled agents are assumed to have a greater margin of safety than oral agents. Salmeterol is a new β₂-agonist with a longer duration of action. However, if patients experience symptoms in between the every 12-hour dosing, they must use a short-acting β₂-agonist to control these breakthrough symptoms. Because studies in pregnant women are lacking, it is pref-

erable to use short-acting agents, as there has been more clinical experience with them.

CROMOLYN SODIUM. This anti-inflammatory drug inhibits the degranulation of mast cells. When administered before exposure to a trigger, it may inhibit both the early and late phases of wheezing, which can occur up to 6 to 12 hours after an initial attack. As many as 2 puffs four times a day may be required for 4 to 6 weeks to optimize its prophylactic effect.[34] It has no role in an acute attack already in progress. Human anecdotal experience[35] and animal studies suggest its safety, and this drug has been used with success in pregnant asthmatic women. Nedocromil sodium is a newer inhaled anti-inflammatory agent. Although animal studies have shown no harm to fetuses, there are no adequate studies in pregnant women, and there has been less clinical experience with this agent than with cromolyn.

INHALED STEROIDS. These agents inhibit inflammation of the airways (Table 42–5). Patients should be cautioned that results may not be noticeable in some cases for days to weeks of regular use. To achieve a prophylactic effect, regular daily use should be emphasized even for asymptomatic patients. Patients should be warned not to reach for these agents (or cromolyn) to abort acute bronchospasm. Based on animal studies and human experience in pregnancy, inhaled beclomethasone dipropionate may be the best choice for gestational asthma.[29] The lack of systemic absorption averts adrenal insufficiency. One prospective study of 45 pregnant women showed no increase in fetal malformations when less than 16 inhalations per day (800 μg) were used.[26] To avoid oral candidiasis, the mouth should be rinsed with water after the prescribed number of inhalations.

ORAL STEROIDS. Glucocorticoids relieve bronchospasm and mucosal edema and inhibit inflammation. A short course such as 40 to 60 mg of prednisone daily to start, then tapered off over 1 to 2 weeks, might be used to alleviate an exacerbation. If steroids are needed continuously to control wheezing, an alternate-day regimen of less

---

TABLE 42–5. **Comparable Dosing of Inhaled Steroid Preparations**

MEDICATION	STARTING DOSE	USUAL DOSE	MAXIMUM DOSE
Beclomethasone (Beclovent, Vanceril) 42 μg per puff	12–16 puffs daily, then taper	2 puffs (84 μg) t.i.d.–q.i.d. or 4 puffs (168 μg) b.i.d.	20 puffs daily (840 μg)
Flunisolide (AeroBid) 0.5 mg per puff	2 puffs b.i.d. (1 mg)	2 puffs b.i.d. (1 mg)	4 puffs b.i.d. (2 mg)
Triamcinolone (Azmacort) 100 μg per puff	12–16 puffs daily (b.i.d. dosing may be effective), then taper	2 puffs (200 μg) t.i.d.–q.i.d.	16 puffs daily (1600 μg)

b.i.d., 2 times a day; t.i.d., 3 times a day; q.i.d., 4 times a day.

than 10 mg of prednisone daily is preferable. While patients are receiving oral steroids, it is not clear that inhaled steroids offer further benefit; however, inhaled steroids may be used after an oral steroid taper. For an effective transition, patients should begin inhaled steroids during the final week(s) of an oral steroid taper.

Although steroids have been shown to be teratogenic (mainly cleft palate) in some animal species, human evidence has failed to suggest any birth defects,[36] and they should not be withheld from pregnant women whose symptoms are not controlled by other agents. One study showed no increased risk of abortion, stillbirth, uterine hemorrhage, toxemia, or neonatal death when mothers received an average daily dose of 8.2 mg of prednisone.[37] No evidence of adrenal insufficiency was noted in the infants of these women; however, because maternal adrenal function may be suppressed, supplemental steroids are usually given to a woman at the time of labor, such as 100 mg of hydrocortisone intravenously every 8 hours at least until the stress of labor and delivery is over. In general, any patient who has received high-dose steroids for 2 or more weeks may be at risk for adrenal suppression for as long as 1 year. However, in pregnant patients, adrenal insufficiency due to remote steroid use is not common; hydrocortisone is recommended routinely during labor only for those pregnant patients who have received systemic steroids within the last 4 weeks preceding delivery.[19] Such patients should also be given stress doses of hydrocortisone during periods of severe infection, trauma, surgery, or other stress.

Well-known side effects of oral steroids include salt and water retention, hypokalemic alkalosis, and hypertension. Patients should be monitored for glucose intolerance and questioned for symptoms of peptic ulcer disease. Prolonged use may lead to myopathy, osteoporosis, skin fragility, cutaneous anergy, cataracts, immunosuppression, and cushingoid habitus.

ANTICHOLINERGICS. These agents may relieve bronchospasm by inhibiting vagal mechanisms. Atropine crosses the placenta and may induce fetal tachycardia, which may not in itself be harmful.[21] It should be administered with caution to patients with tachydysrhythmias. Inhaled ipratropium may be even safer than atropine, but human data in pregnancy and lactation are insufficient to warrant use in pregnancy unless other measures are ineffective.

XANTHINE BRONCHODILATORS. The precise mechanism of bronchodilation for aminophylline and theophylline is unknown. These agents appear to be generally safe for a developing fetus.[38] However, in both pregnant and nonpregnant asthmatic patients, these drugs demonstrate greater toxicity and less efficacy than inhaled bronchodilators[26] and are therefore considered third-line therapy. In nonpregnant women, aminophylline has been shown to inhibit uterine activity[39] and theoretically might have a similar effect in pregnant women by increasing cyclic adenosine monophosphate in uterine smooth muscle.

Drug levels should be monitored in all patients receiving theophylline preparations. Some studies have observed an increased proportion of free drug for any given theophylline level during pregnancy,[40] and a more prudent goal for drug levels in a gravid patient might be 5 to 12 μg per ml instead of the 10 to 20 μg per ml used for nonpregnant patients.[29] Furthermore, theophylline clearance may be reduced in the third trimester, so levels should be closely monitored during this time.[40] Theophylline half-life is reduced in smokers, for whom dosing requirements may be higher. Moreover, if a patient discontinues smoking, a reduction in dose may be required to avoid toxicity. Erythromycin, caffeine, ciprofloxacin, and oral contraceptives may raise serum theophylline levels by decreasing clearance. Those with chronic heart or liver disease may also need reduced theophylline dosing. Side effects of methylxanthines include nausea, vomiting, heartburn, diarrhea, headache, insomnia, tremor, dysrhythmias, and seizures, which can occur even at therapeutic levels. Long-acting preparations are convenient. For patients with prominent nocturnal symptoms, sustained-release theophylline may be taken at bedtime.

STATUS ASTHMATICUS

Respiratory distress that does not resolve with a few doses of a nebulized β-agonist deserves aggressive treatment. The absence of wheezing on examination may be misleading; very severe bronchospasm may decrease breath sounds so that the entire chest sounds quiet. As such a patient improves, wheezing may become more evident than before. Pulsus paradoxus is the decrease of systolic blood pressure during inspiration. A decrease of greater than 18 to 20 mm Hg suggests a more severe attack. The upper chest and clavicular area should be palpated in any severely asthmatic patient to detect subcutaneous emphysema. A shielded chest radiograph is indicated in patients whose physical examination findings suggest pneumonia, in those with subcutaneous emphysema, and in patients with pleuritic chest pain. Serum electrolyte levels should be monitored, because dehydration is not uncommon during asthma exacerbations. An increased white blood cell count

TABLE 42–6. Management of Status Asthmaticus

PHARMACOLOGIC	SUPPORTIVE
Nebulized β-agonist such as terbutaline (2–4 mg in 2 ml saline) repeated every 15–20 min until distress is relieved*	Humidified oxygen by nasal cannula to achieve $Po_2 > 70$ or oxygen saturation > 95%
IV Solu-Medrol, 125 mg every 6 hr until improvement, followed by taper over several days	IV fluid
Consider IV aminophylline, 5 mg/kg bolus† over 30 min followed by 0.5 mg/kg/hr	Chest radiograph
Consider nebulized atropine sulfate, 1 mg	Antibiotics if bacterial infection is suspected
If no response, consider subcutaneous terbutaline,‡ 0.25 mg (may be repeated once, 30 min later)	

*Heart rate should be monitored; however, initial rate may be high due to respiratory distress, and this should not necessarily preclude cautious use of β-agonists.

†If a patient is already on oral theophylline, a stat level should be obtained. If <5 μg/ml, load 2.5 mg/kg over 30 min; if >5 μg/ml, no loading dose is needed—begin maintenance dose. Maintenance dose should be reduced by 1/3 to 1/2 in those with chronic liver or heart disease. In all cases, follow levels, beginning 12 hr after initial dose, to achieve levels between 5 to 12 μg/ml. Switch to oral theophylline once the patient is stable.

‡Preferable to epinephrine, 0.3 ml of 1:1000 subcutaneously.

IV, Intravenous.

may be due to infection or stress. An elevated total eosinophil count often correlates with steroid-reversible asthma.

The first intervention should be repeated nebulized β-agonists, which are preferable to subcutaneous injections of epinephrine or terbutaline (Table 42–6). Supplemental oxygen per nasal cannula to achieve a Po_2 of 70 or an oxygen saturation by oximeter of 95% should be given. Jeopardy to a fetus exists when the maternal Po_2 is less than 60 mm Hg.[41] In all but the mildest of exacerbations, arterial blood gas determinations are usually indicated and are helpful in gauging the severity of an attack. Note that blood gas values in pregnant women should be interpreted with the awareness of the expected compensated respiratory alkalosis of pregnancy. Hence, a normal pH near 7.4 and a carbon dioxide near 40 may be a sign of impending respiratory failure in an acutely dyspneic pregnant woman. Certainly, a pH less than 7.35 and any hypercarbia should prompt consideration of monitoring in an intensive care unit. Intravenous fluids are usually warranted and should contain glucose if a patient is not glucose intolerant.

The second pharmacologic intervention is intravenous glucocorticoids. Because the onset of action may be several hours after the initial dose, they should be administered early if a patient has not responded within the first half-hour or so of other therapy. In patients responding poorly to other treatment, intravenous aminophylline may also be considered.

It should be borne in mind that wheezing can be a symptom of several conditions in addition to asthma (Table 42–7).

SINUSITIS

Bacterial sinusitis may be as much as six times more common in pregnant than in nonpregnant women,[42] and occult sinus disease may exacerbate asthma. A history of purulent nasal discharge; frontal, retro-orbital, or malar headache; and fever may be noted. Nasal polyposis and other forms of nasal obstruction are predisposing factors. Despite a classic presentation, definitive diagnosis may be difficult without sinus radiographs or computed tomography scan. Empirical treatment with penicillins or cephalosporins for 2 to 3 weeks should be effective: amoxicillin, 500 mg three times daily, is a typical regimen for non–penicillin-allergic patients with sinusitis. Tetracyclines, ciprofloxacin (and other fluoroquinolones), and sulfonamides should be avoided in pregnancy. Simultaneous decongestants and topical nasal saline spray may speed recovery.

ACUTE BRONCHITIS

The incidence of bronchitis during pregnancy is similar to that in nonpregnant women.[43] Approxi-

TABLE 42–7. All That Wheezes Is Not Asthma

Bronchiolitis
Allergic reactions
Congestive heart failure
Mitral stenosis
Hypersensitivity pneumonitis
Pulmonary embolus
Hypothyroidism

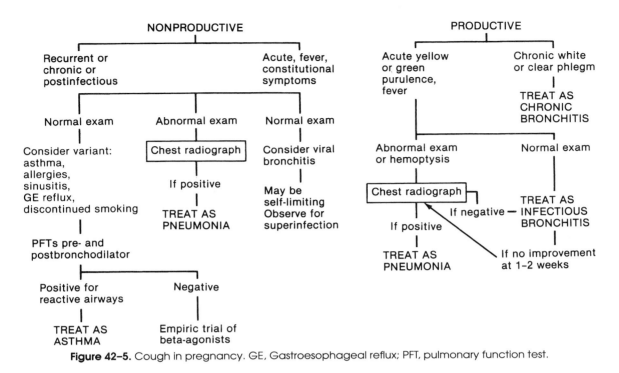

Figure 42–5. Cough in pregnancy. GE, Gastroesophageal reflux; PFT, pulmonary function test.

mately half the cases encountered are due to viral infections.[7] Patients with viral illnesses should be alerted for signs of complicating bacterial superinfection presenting as otitis, sinusitis, purulent bronchitis, or pneumonia. Although acute bronchitis is usually self-limited, hyperemia of airways mucosa due to gestational hormones may extend the course of illness. Treatment includes bed rest, oral hydration, and antibiotics such as penicillins, cephalosporins, or erythromycin if thick yellow or green secretions persist. Expectorants containing iodide should be avoided in pregnancy, but guaifenesin or dextromethorphan (2 tsp four times daily as needed) is acceptable.[19] Narcotic analgesia is a respiratory depressant and should not be administered during an asthma exacerbation or to any patient at risk for sudden respiratory decline. Additionally, some narcotics such as codeine cause histamine release and thus may precipitate bronchospasm in some sensitive individuals; therefore, they should be used only as a last resort for intolerable coughing. A chest radiograph to preclude pneumonia is seldom indicated in the presence of normal findings on physical examination; however, if a patient does not show improvement within several days to a week, a shielded chest radiograph may be indicated.

CHRONIC BRONCHITIS

Unlike variant asthma, which manifests as a nonproductive cough, a diagnosis of chronic bron-

chitis requires a productive cough for at least 3 months out of the year for at least 2 years (Fig. 42–5). Inhaled β-agonists or inhaled corticosteroids may ameliorate symptoms in some patients. Expectorants containing iodide should be avoided in pregnancy. Guaifenesin or dextromethorphan, 2 tsp orally up to four times a day,[19] is recommended if medicine is necessary. When smoking is suspected to be the cause, discontinuance is strongly encouraged.

PNEUMONIA

Pneumonia occurs in fewer than 1% of all deliveries but is responsible for a significant percentage of nonobstetric maternal deaths.[44] The risk for premature delivery is higher if pneumonia is contracted between the twentieth and thirty-sixth week of pregnancy.[45] Etiologic agents are similar to those found in nonpregnant patients, including pneumococcus and *Mycoplasma,* as well as viruses. In smokers, β-lactamase–resistant *Haemophilus influenzae* and *Moraxella catarrhalis* are also common pathogens. Management includes sputum Gram stain, sputum cultures and sensitivity tests, blood cultures, monitoring of electrolytes, antibiotics, bed rest, and hydration. A chest radiograph is usually indicated in the setting of abnormal findings on a chest examination but need not be repeated during pregnancy if a patient demonstrates clinical improvement. Supplemental humidified oxygen by nasal cannula or face mask should ensure a Po_2 of at least 70 or a corresponding oxygen saturation by oximeter of 95%. Sedatives and narcotics depress respiratory function and should be avoided. Hospitalization, supplemental oxygen, and intravenous hydration should be considered for patients at 32 to 40 weeks of gestation.[7]

Antibiotics such as penicillin, cephalosporins, and erythromycin should be considered as first choices for community-acquired pneumonia in pregnant or lactating women.[46] Tetracyclines, ciprofloxacin, and sulfonamides should be avoided. Antibacterials should be continued for at least 5 days after a patient is afebrile.[7] Although breast-feeding during pneumonia has been contraindicated by some, passive immunity may be conferred to a fetus via immunoglobulins in the mother's milk.[7]

Although influenza pneumonia is not a common cause of maternal death, one should remain alert for acute decompensation due to bacterial superinfection, especially by pneumococci and staphylococci. Amantadine hydrochloride is effective if given within 48 hours of the onset of symptoms and can be an effective prophylactic agent in those exposed to influenza A. However, because of insufficient studies in pregnancy, it is not recommended for uncomplicated cases of influenza pneumonia in all pregnant women but should be considered in those with severe infection or preexisting lung disease.[47] Although no strong evidence specifically contraindicates vaccination with the available killed viral vaccines for pregnant patients, pregnant women should be considered to have the same balance of benefits and risks associated with the influenza vaccine as do nonpregnant women.[7] Influenza vaccination is customarily delayed until after the first trimester.

Varicella pneumonia is also uncommon during pregnancy, but fatal cases have been reported. Pneumonia usually becomes apparent on days 4 to 6 of the illness and is correlated with the severity of the exanthem and fever.[48] Because of the potential for devastating illness, pregnant women seronegative to varicella should be considered for prophylaxis with varicella-zoster immune globulin within 4 days of close exposure to chickenpox.[48] Although prophylaxis with acyclovir for such exposures is controversial, this drug should not be withheld from pregnant women with life-threatening varicella pneumonia. Some authorities recommend intravenous acyclovir beginning on day 3 or 4 for pregnant women with an extensive exanthem and fever[47] in hopes of averting pneumonic complications.

Pneumocystis carinii pneumonia often appears subacutely over several weeks with fever, cough, and dyspnea. The findings on chest radiography may be normal or may show bilateral interstitial infiltrates. Diagnosis is made by demonstration of cysts in sputum or bronchial secretions. *P. carinii* pneumonia should be suspected in patients known to be human immunodeficiency virus positive, patients with hemophilia, injection drug abusers, and those having received blood transfusions before 1985. The few reports on the outcome of *P. carinii* pneumonia in pregnant women have been discouraging.[49]

OTHER LUNG DISEASES IN PREGNANCY

Tuberculosis

The course of pregnancy is not altered by tuberculosis,[7] but at least 15% of patients who remain untreated will deteriorate after delivery.[55] The tuberculin (purified protein derivative) skin test response probably remains normal throughout the course of pregnancy.[51] In two large series, a positive history or physical examination usually suggested the need for a radiographic examination in patients who were later found to have a roentgenographic abnormality.[52] In asymptomatic skin test–positive patients, chest radiography may be deferred until the second or third trimester; however, a positive skin test reaction should prompt an immediate chest radiograph if such symptoms as cough, fever, weight loss, or night sweats are present. Patients with abnormal findings on a chest radiograph consistent with active tuberculosis should collect three morning sputum samples for acid-fast bacilli smear and culture.

Because of the emergence of multidrug-resistant strains of tuberculosis and the complex nature of treatment from both individual and public health perspectives, further evaluation and pharmacologic therapy may be best handled by prompt referral to those expert in the management of tuberculosis. The provider should be reminded that the use of rifampin may render some oral contraceptives ineffective, and patients taking these drugs simultaneously should be advised to use effective barrier methods if avoidance of pregnancy is desired.

No increased risk appears to be associated with having a chest radiograph during pregnancy.[53] The amount of radioactivity delivered to a fetus during a standard posteroanterior chest film is equivalent to that of a cross-country plane flight (36 mrad) and can be diminished by lead shielding.[54] However, a semielective chest radiograph should be delayed until after the first trimester to avoid even this small amount of exposure to rapidly dividing fetal cells.

Bronchiectasis

Bronchiectasis is a sequela of chronic suppurative infection or inflammatory bronchitis. Patients present with chronic purulent sputum and often have characteristic radiographic findings. Patients may benefit from inhaled bronchodilators and percussion with postural drainage. Rotating oral antibiotics may control chronic purulent secretions. Although data are scant, patients appear to tolerate pregnancy well.[7]

Sarcoidosis

Sarcoidosis is a systemic granulomatous disease of uncertain cause. It is noted to have an incidence in pregnancy of 0.02 to 0.05%.[55] Bilateral hilar lymphadenopathy or interstitial infiltrates may be seen on a chest radiograph, and diagnosis is suggested by noncaseating granulomas on biopsy of affected tissues. Infectious causes of granulomatous disease, such as tuberculosis, must be ruled out. Indications for steroids in gravid or nongravid patients include worsening pulmonary function and treatment for various nonpulmonary manifestations such as active uveitis. Exacerbations are rare during pregnancy, but patients with active disease during pregnancy may suffer an exacerbation 3 to 6 months postpartum.[56]

Histoplasmosis

Histoplasmosis should be suspected in patients who give an appropriate travel or residential history for the Mississippi River/Ohio River/St. Lawrence River valleys, the Caribbean, or Central and South America. Those exposed to building demolition may also be at risk. Patients may be asymptomatic or may be acutely symptomatic with fever, chills, and cough 1 to 3 weeks after exposure. They may suffer a rapidly fatal course or may only have a chronic productive cough. A chest radiograph may show cavities, hilar and mediastinal lymphadenopathy with calcification, or parenchymal granulomas, which also may be calcified. Diagnosis is established by sputum culture of *Histoplasma capsulatum*. A positive precipitin test result may occur within days after infection, and rising complement-fixation antibodies support the diagnosis. Positive skin tests suggest exposure but cannot distinguish current from previous disease.

Although most cases are self-limited and benign, the provider must weigh the risks and toxicity from antifungal therapy to a woman and her fetus in cases severe enough to warrant therapy.

Coccidioidomycosis

Coccidioidomycosis is endemic to the southwestern United States, Mexico, and South America. An incubation period of 1 to 3 weeks follows the inhalation of spores; then fever, chills, cough, fatigue, arthralgia, and upper respiratory tract symptoms ensue. A chest radiograph may show parenchymal infiltrates or mediastinal or hilar lymphadenopathy. As with histoplasmosis, sputum smear, culture, and serologic titers are indicated. Skin testing cannot distinguish current from previous disease. Although most infections resolve spontaneously without treatment, coccidioidomycosis has a tendency to disseminate during pregnancy.

In 33 cases of this disease in pregnancy, increased spontaneous abortion in the first trimester and premature labor in the third trimester were noted. Seven of 11 women who contracted this disease in the third trimester died.[57] The appropriateness of surgery or antifungal therapy should be guided by an expert in the management of fungal diseases.

Pulmonary Embolism

Pulmonary embolism is second only to abortion as a cause of maternal death;[58] however, the increased risk of a pulmonary embolism appears to be associated primarily with the postpartum period.[59] One series noted superficial and deep venous thrombophlebitis in 12 and 2 per 1000 pregnancies, respectively.[60] More than 75% (10 of 13) occurred in the first month postpartum (especially within the first 3 days after delivery). Definite pulmonary embolism was diagnosed in 13 of 32,337 pregnancies (0.4 per 1000). Only rarely do patients have a classic presentation with pleuritic chest pain, hemoptysis, tachypnea, oxygen desaturation, tachycardia, classic electrocardiographic findings, a wedge-shaped pulmonary infiltrate, and a swollen leg (see Chapter 39).

Restrictive Lung Disease

Restrictive lung diseases include decreased lung volumes due to previous surgery, kyphoscoliosis, interstitial lung diseases, and abnormalities in chest wall musculature. In general, these diseases are well tolerated in pregnancy. A vital capacity of 1 liter has often been considered the minimal vital capacity requirement necessary to sustain a successful pregnancy, yet successful pregnancies have been reported with a vital capacity of only 800 ml.[61] Treatment includes supportive measures and oxygen supplementation if necessary.

Emphysema

Emphysema is unlikely to occur in women of childbearing age in the absence of an inherited α_1-antitrypsin deficiency. Pulmonary function tests demonstrate airways obstruction without response to bronchodilators, and a low DLCO.

Primary Pulmonary Hypertension

Primary pulmonary hypertension is a disease of unknown cause. Women present with gradually worsening dyspnea on exertion. Maternal mortality has been reported to exceed 50%.[62] Pulmonary hypertension resulting from underlying chronic pulmonary disease (secondary pulmonary hypertension) is generally considerably much less severe than primary pulmonary hypertension and does not carry this high mortality rate. No effective treatment for this disorder has been found, other than supportive measures and supplemental oxygen.

Catamenial Pneumothorax

Catamenial pneumothorax is characterized by typically right-sided chest pain, temporally related to menstruation, in women in their third or fourth decade of life. Endometriosis near pleural surfaces may have a role in the development of pneumothoraces in this disorder. Most pneumothoraces are small and self-resolving; thoracotomy tube drainage may be required for larger, symptomatic lesions.

Pleuritic Chest Pain

In the setting of a dry cough, fever, and a pleural friction rub on examination, sharp pleuritic chest pain may represent viral pleurisy, which should resolve without specific treatment. Vigorous coughing due to any cause may result in a sprain of the intercostal muscles or a rib fracture, causing pleuritic chest pain and splinting. Pneumonia with a pleural reaction and pulmonary embolus with infarction may also cause pleuritic chest pain. Although most pulmonary emboli associated with pregnancy occur postpartum,[59] a previous history of pulmonary embolism or evidence of peripheral thrombophlebitis on examination should raise suspicion. A chest radiograph and noninvasive studies of the lower extremities may be considered for diagnostic purposes.

Narcotics, sedatives, and iodine-containing products should be avoided during pregnancy. Nonsteroidal anti-inflammatory drugs should be avoided in those patients who are aspirin sensitive, and large doses of aspirin should be avoided near term because of increased bleeding and the risk of premature closure of the fetal ductus arteriosus.

REFERENCES

1. Thomson KJ, Cohen ME. Studies on the circulation in pregnancy. II. Vital capacity observations in normal pregnant women. Surg Gynecol Obstet 1938;66:591.
2. Prowse CM, Gaensler EA. Respiratory and acid-base changes during pregnancy. Anesthesiology 1965;26:381.
3. Cugell DW, Frank NR, Gaensler EA, Badger TL. Pulmonary function in pregnancy. I. Serial observations in normal women. Am Rev Tuberc 1953;67:568.
4. Russell IR, Chambers WA. Closing volume in normal pregnancy. Br J Anesth 1981;53:1043.
5. Norregaard O, Schultz P, Ostergaard A, et al. Lung function and postular changes during pregnancy. Respir Med 1989;83:467.
6. Comroe JH, Forster RE, DuBois AB, et al. In: The Lung: Clinical Physiology and Pulmonary Function Tests. Chicago: Year Book Medical Publishers, 1962.
7. Leontic EA. Respiratory disease in pregnancy. Med Clin North Am 1977;61:111.
8. Weinberger SE, Weiss ST, Cohen WR, et al. Pregnancy and the lung. Am Rev Respir Dis 1980;121:559.
9. Milne JA, Mills RJ, Coutts JRT, MacNaughton MC, et al. The effect of human pregnancy on the pulmonary transfer factor for carbon. Clinical Science and Molecular Medicine 1977; 53:271.
10. Bedell GN, Adams RW. Pulmonary diffusing capacity during rest and exercise. A study of normal persons with atrial septal defect, pregnancy, and pulmonary disease. J Clin Invest 1962;41:1908.
11. Lyons HA, Antonio R. The sensitivity of the respiratory center in pregnancy and after the administration of progesterone. Trans Assoc Am Physicians 1959;72:173.
12. Templeton A, Kelman GR. Maternal blood gases, ($P_{A}O_2$-PaO_2), physiological shunt and V_D/V_T in normal pregnancy. Br J Anaesth 1976;48:1001.
13. Awe RJ, Nicotra MB, Newson TD, Viles R. Arterial oxygenation and alveolar-arterial gradients in term pregnancy. Obstet Gynecol 1979;53;182.
14. Holmes TH, Goodell H, Wolf S, et al. Quoted in Baker DC and Strauss RB: The physiologic treatment of nasal obstruction. Clin Plast Surg 1977;4:123.
15. Bonica JJ. In: Principles and Practice of Obstetric Analgesia and Anesthesia. Philadelphia: FA Davis, 1967, pp 27–39.
16. Marbry RL. Intranasal steroid injection during pregnancy. South Med J 1980;73:1176.
17. Incaudo GA. Diagnosis and treatment of rhinitis during pregnancy and location. Clin Rev Allergy 1987;5:325.

18. Stablein JJ, Lockey RF. Managing asthma during pregnancy. Compr Ther 1984;10(3):45.

19. Executive Summary: Management of Asthma During Pregnancy. Report of the Working Group on Asthma and Pregnancy, NIH Publication No. 93-3279A. Bethesda, Md: National Institutes of Health, National Heart, Lung and Blood Institute, March 1993.

20. Greenberger PA. Asthma in pregnancy. Symposium on medical disorders during pregnancy. Clin Perinatol 1985;12(3):571.

21. Weinstein AM, Dubin BD, Podleski WK, et al. Asthma and pregnancy. JAMA 1979;241:1161.

22. Schatz M, Harden K, Forsythe A, et al. The course of asthma during pregnancy, post-partum, and with successive pregnancies: A prospective analysis. J Allergy Clin Immunol 1988;81:509.

23. Gluck JC, Gluck PA. The effects of pregnancy on asthma: A prospective study. Ann Allergy 1976;37:164.

24. Gordon M, Niswander KR, Berendes H, et al. Fetal morbidity following potentially anoxigenic obstetric conditions. VII. Bronchial asthma. Am J Obstet Gynecol 1970;106:421.

25. Bahna SL, Bjerkedal T. The course and outcome of pregnancy in women with bronchial asthma. Acta Allergol 1972;27:397.

26. Greenberger PA, Patterson R. Beclomethasone diproprionate for severe asthma during pregnancy. Ann Intern Med 1983;98:478.

27. Physicians' Desk Reference, 47th ed. Montvale, NJ: Medical Economics, 1993.

28. Robert SF, Gerald SR, Carol J, et al. Altered lower esophageal sphincter function during early pregnancy. Gastroenterology 1978;74:1233.

29. Schatz M. Asthma during pregnancy: Interrelationships and management. Ann Allergy 1992;68:123.

30. Centers for Disease Control. Prevention and control of influenza. MMWR 1984;33:253.

31. Romero R, Lockwood C. In: Niebyl JR (ed). Drug Use in Pregnancy. 2nd ed. Philadelphia: Lea & Febiger, 1988, pp 67–82.

32. Varheer H. Drug excretion in breast milk. Postgrad Med 1974;56:97.

33. Schatz M, Hoffman CP, Zeiger RS, et al. The course and management of asthma and allergic disease during pregnancy. In: Middleton E, Reed CE, Ellis CF, et al (eds). Allergy: Principles and Practice. 3rd ed. St Louis: CV Mosby, 1988, pp 1093–1155.

34. D'Alonzo GE. The pregnant asthmatic patient. Semin Perinatol 1990;14(2):119.

35. Wilson J. Use of Cromoglycate during pregnancy. J Pharmacol Med 1982;8:45.

36. Briggs GG, Freeman RK, Yaffe SJ. Drugs in Pregnancy and Lactation. 3rd ed. Baltimore: Williams & Wilkins, 1990, pp 237–238, 520–521.

37. Schatz M, Patterson R, Zeitz S, et al. Corticosteroid therapy for the pregnant asthmatic patient. JAMA 1975; 233:804.

38. Greenberger P, Patterson R. Safety of therapy for allergic symptoms during pregnancy. Ann Intern Med 1978; 89:234.

39. Coutinho EM, Vieria Lopes AC. Inhibition of uterine motility by aminophylline. Am J Obstet Gynecol 1971; 110:726.

40. Gardener MJ, Schatz M, Cousius L, et al. Longitudinal effects of pregnancy on the pharmacokinetics of theophylline. Eur J Clin Pharmacol 1987;31:289.

41. Hernandez E, Angell CS, Johnson JWC. Asthma in pregnancy: Current concepts. Obstet Gynecol 1980;55:739.

42. Sorri M, Bortikanen-Sorri AL, Karja J. Rhinitis during pregnancy. Rhinology 1980;18:83.

43. Horstman DM. Viral infections. In: Barrow GN, Ferris TF (eds). Medical Complications During Pregnancy. Philadelphia: WB Saunders, 1975, pp 416–437.

44. Spector SL. Reciprocal relationship between pregnancy and pulmonary disease. Chest 1984;86(3):1S.

45. Barnes CG. Disorders of the respiratory system I. In: Barnes CG (ed.). Medical Disorders in Obstetric Practice. 4th ed. Oxford, England: Blackwell Scientific, 1974.

46. Philipson A. Pharmacokinetics of antibiotics in pregnancy and labor. Clin Pharmacol 1979;4:297.

47. Centers for Disease Control. Influenza—United States. MMWR 1984;33:252.

48. Prober CG, Gershon AA, Grose C. Consensus: Varicella-zoster infections in pregnancy and the perinatal period. Pediatr Infect Dis J 1990;9:865.

49. Minkoff H, deRagt RH, Landesman S, et al. *Pneumocystis carinii* pneumonia associated with adult immunodeficiency syndrome in pregnancy: A report of three maternal deaths. Obstet Gynecol 1986;67:284.

50. Selikoff IJ, Dorgman HL. Management of tuberculosis. In: Rovinsky JJ, Guttmacher AF (eds). Medical, Surgical, and Gynecologic Complications of Pregnancy. 2nd ed. Baltimore: Williams & Wilkins, 1965.

51. Present PA, Comstock GW. Tuberculin sensitivity in pregnancy. Am Rev Respir Dis 1975;112:413.

52. Mattox JH. The value of routine prenatal chest x-ray. Obstet Gynecol 1973;41:243.

53. Swartz HM, Reichling BA. Hazards of radiation exposure for pregnant women. JAMA 1978;239:1907.

54. Bonebreak CR, Noller DK, Loehener CP, et al. Routine chest roentgenography in pregnancy. JAMA 1978; 240:2747.

55. O'Leary JA. Ten year study of sarcoidosis and pregnancy. Am J Obstet Gynecol 1962;84:462.

56. Mayock RL, Sullivan RD, Greening RR, et al. Sarcoidosis and pregnancy. JAMA 1957;164:158.

57. Vaughn JE, Ramirez H. Coccidioidomycosis as a complication of pregnancy. Calif Med J 1951;74:121.

58. Henderson SR, Lund CJ, Creasman WT. Antepartum pulmonary embolism. Am J Obstet Gynecol 1972;112:476.

59. Handin RI. Thromboembolitic complications of pregnancy and oral contraceptives. Prog Cardiovasc Dis 1974;16:395.

60. Aaro LA, Juergens JL. Thrombophlebitis associated with pregnancy. Am J Obstet Gynecol 1971;109:1128.

61. Hung CT, Pelosi M, Lunger A, et al. Blood gas measurements in the kyphoscoliotic gravida and her fetus: Report of a case. Am J Obstet Gynecol 1975;121:287.

62. McCaffrey RM, Dunn LJ. Primary pulmonary hypertension in pregnancy. Obstet Gynecol Surv 1964;19:567.

43

Neurologic Problems in Pregnancy

Nagagopal Venna

A variety of neurologic disorders are encountered in pregnancy and the puerperium. A few conditions such as eclampsia are unique to the pregnant state. Some entities that are rare in the general population such as cerebral venous thrombosis have a particular predilection for women in the postpartum period. Many common conditions such as migraine, epilepsy, multiple sclerosis, and cerebral aneurysms can complicate pregnancy. The evaluation and treatment of these problems should consider the complex interaction of pregnancy with the disorders as well as the impact of laboratory tests and treatment methods on both the mother and the fetus.

SEIZURES IN PREGNANCY

Epilepsy

Epilepsy is one of the most common neurologic conditions that occur in pregnancy. There are approximately 400,000 women of childbearing age in the United States who have epilepsy, and an increasing number of them are choosing to become pregnant because of improved seizure control and more enlightened attitudes toward epilepsy in society. Women with epilepsy now regularly seek advice regarding the risks posed by epilepsy to the pregnancy and its effects on the offspring. Over the last 3 decades, the interrelationships of pregnancy and epilepsy have been studied in retrospective and in prospective systematic studies in Europe, Japan, and the United States. A body of knowledge has accumulated on which to base sound advice to the patient and to provide optimal care to the pregnant woman.

Effects of Antiepileptic Drugs

CONGENITAL MALFORMATIONS. For women with epilepsy who plan to become preg-

nant or who find themselves pregnant, one of the major concerns is the risk of harm to the fetus from the antiepileptic drugs, in particular the risk of malformations. Many studies since the 1960s have confirmed the small but definite increase in the risk of congenital malformations in the children born to mothers with epilepsy.[1-3] Malformations occur at a rate of about 2% in the general population; the risk is increased to approximately 4% in the offspring of epileptic mothers who do not take antiepileptic drugs and further enhanced to 6% among the mothers taking antiepileptic drugs during pregnancy. A few reports indicate a slight increase in the risk of malformation even in the children of fathers with epilepsy. Viewing this in a different perspective, 90% of the patients who have epilepsy have a normally developed child, emphasizing the relatively small magnitude of the risk. The risk should also be considered in the context of other factors such as concurrent malnutrition, alcoholism, drug abuse, and epilepsy in the father and malformations in the family. The risk of malformation is present with all the first-line drugs currently used, namely, phenytoin, carbamazepine, valproic acid, phenobarbital, and primidone. The risk is about the same degree, although there are some qualitative differences in the type of malformations so that no one drug is devoid of this teratogenic potential. The exception is the drug trimethadione, which is still occasionally used for petit mal epilepsy.[4] This drug has a high incidence of major and multiple malformations and should not be used in pregnancy or in women of reproductive age. The risk of malformations is higher when more drugs are used in polypharmacy than when a single drug for epilepsy is used. Evidence also suggests that higher maternal blood levels of the drug increase the risk further. No malformations have been described that are found to be unique to a particular antiepileptic drug.

The malformations have been classified as major, minor, and dysmorphic features. Major malformations are defects of neural tube closure that result in spina bifida aperta, often associated with hydrocephalus but not anencephaly, and congenital heart disease such as ventricular septal defect, cleft lip, and cleft palate. Normal development of these structures takes place in the first trimester of pregnancy, with neural tube closing by 4 weeks, lip formation by 8 weeks, and palate formation by 10 weeks. Minor malformations described with antiepileptic drugs are in the form of hypospadias (the urethra opens on the underside of the penis or the perineum), club feet, and equinovarus deformity of the legs (the heel is turned inward from the midline of the leg and the foot is plantar stressed). Minor dysmorphic features are of no serious medical significance and consist of changes such as epicanthal folds, broad and flat nasal bridge, upturned nasal tip, long philtrum, rotated ears, and hypoplasia of the nails and of the distal phalanges of the hands. Hypertelorism (an abnormal increase in the distance between the eyes) has also been frequently described. With the exception of hypertelorism, many of the dysmorphic features become markedly less noticeable when these children are followed to the age of about 4 years.

Phenytoin, a widely used antiepileptic drug, was initially linked to the so-called fetal hydantoin syndrome of craniofacial defects and a constellation of minor malformations and dysmorphic features described earlier, but it is now clear that a similar syndrome occurs with the use of all of the usual antiepileptic drugs.

Carbamazepine is also widely used and for a time was advocated as the drug of choice with the least teratogenic potential in pregnant women. However, with more systematic accumulation of data, this conclusion has proved to be incorrect.[5] The usual major and minor malformations have all been described with carbamazepine. This drug has been associated with a neural tube defect in an estimated 0.9% of fetuses exposed to it. Carbamazepine, however, when used during gestation has fewer negative effects on subsequent childhood cognitive development than phenytoin and may be preferred for use during pregnancy for this reason.[6]

Phenobarbital and primidone are generally used less nowadays than in the past but have been associated with the whole spectrum of malformations that occur with the use of other drugs. Much attention was focused on valproate, the most recent drug on the scene and now widely used for both petit mal, grand mal, and partial seizures. Of particular concern has been the occurrence of spina bifida with meningomyelocele and hydrocephalus.[7] This association has now been confirmed, and

it is estimated that 1 to 2% of fetuses exposed to valproate develop this malformation. It has been seen in patients whose only drug is valproic acid, and the evidence suggests that the risk is higher with doses higher than 1000 mg per day. Other malformations that were described are bilateral radial hypoplasia and urogenital malformations.

The mechanisms by which antiepileptic drugs induce malformations are only now being delineated. This research has been aided by studies of embryogenesis in experimental animals that are exposed to controlled levels of antiepileptic drugs. All antiepileptic drugs cross the placenta freely and enter the fetal circulation. A common pathophysiologic mechanism appears to be interference with folate metabolism of the embryo and the fetus. This is especially notable with valproate, phenytoin, and barbiturates, which are known to alter folate metabolism. A recent study has shown that nutritional supplementation of folate in pregnancy has a significant protective effect against neural tube defects in women who previously had a child with a neural tube defect. A targeted study has not yet been done in pregnant epileptic patients.[8]

The role of reactive epoxide metabolites of antiepileptic drugs has also been explored in experimental animals. Metabolites such as epoxides, catechol, quinone, and semiquinone are known to be reactive substances capable of binding to embryonic nucleic acids and can disrupt normal development. In experimental animal studies, the coadministration of drugs that decreased these reactive metabolites has led to a decrease in malformations.

BLEEDING TENDENCIES IN THE NEWBORN. A rare disorder in the newborn that is related to the use of antiepileptic drugs is the occurrence of bleeding induced by suppression of vitamin K–dependent clotting factors. The clotting mechanisms of the mother are unaffected, however. This can lead to serious internal bleeding in infants born to mothers taking phenobarbital, primidone, and phenytoin, as well as carbamazepine, diazepam, and ethosuximide. This generally occurs in the immediate period after delivery with intracranial or abdominal bleeding. The diagnosis may be difficult because of the presentation with shock. Mortality has been as high as 30% because of delayed recognition of this complication.[9]

DRUG RESIDUES. Phenytoin, carbamazepine, and valproic acid are excreted in breast milk in low concentrations but have no clinically evident effects on the baby. However, phenobarbital, primidone, clonazepam, and lorazepam can achieve milk levels of up to 60% of the maternal blood levels.[10] Breast-fed infants may thus become drowsy and irritable and may experience difficulties in feeding. Even when not breast-fed, the infants exposed to phenobarbital in utero may have slow clearance of the drug because of its long half-life in infants—up to 300 hours and longer in premature infants. Some infants may develop withdrawal symptoms several days after delivery with jitteriness and, rarely, withdrawal seizures.

NEONATAL GROWTH RETARDATION. Whether intrauterine exposure to antiepileptic drugs causes pre- or postnatal growth retardation has not been determined definitively. There is, however, no strong evidence that the use of antiepileptic drugs is related to the incidence of microcephaly.

POSTNATAL COGNITIVE DEVELOPMENT. Antiepileptic drugs have been implicated in neonatal psychomotor developmental delay. One study indicates a 40% increase in cognitive dysfunction in babies born to mothers taking antiepileptic drugs during pregnancy.[11] This most closely correlated with the number of seizures occurring during pregnancy, especially partial seizures, and with lower educational level of the parents. It appears that most children born to mothers with epilepsy who are on antiepileptic drugs during pregnancy have normal psychomotor development.

Epilepsy during Pregnancy

A common concern for the patient with epilepsy who becomes pregnant is the effect of pregnancy on seizures. Studies of large numbers of patients have shown that in approximately 50% of patients, seizures are unchanged and occasionally are actually better controlled during pregnancy.[1] In the other half, seizures, whether generalized or partial, become more frequent in pregnancy and return to prepregnant level within 6 weeks after delivery. The most consistent predictor of seizure control is the degree of seizure control in the 2 years preceding the pregnancy: if the woman has more than one seizure a month, the chances are high that seizure control will be worse during pregnancy. If seizures are rare or occur at a rate of fewer than one in 9 months, the rate tends to remain stable. The behavior of seizures in a previous pregnancy does not predict the course of seizures in a current pregnancy. Status epilepticus is rare, with an incidence of approximately 1% in patients with epilepsy. In about 1 to 2% of their pregnancies, epileptic seizures may occur during and in the immediate 24 hours after labor and delivery.

The mechanism for worsening of seizures during pregnancy is complex, but decreased levels of antiepileptic drugs seem to be important. Notable drops in the total drug blood levels, usually maximal in the first trimester, have been documented for phenytoin, carbamazepine, valproic acid, and phenobarbital, in descending order of magnitude.[12] The levels rapidly swing back to baseline in the first few weeks of the postpartum period. Recent pharmacodynamic studies have shown, however, that the physiologically active fraction of the free drug, not bound to serum proteins, is much less depressed than the total drug levels for phenytoin and carbamazepine. Free valproate levels may actually increase, whereas phenobarbital and primidone free fractions decrease the most. This is consistent with the observation that many patients have subtherapeutic or low therapeutic levels of antiepileptic drugs during pregnancy without loss of seizure control.

Many factors contribute to the decrease in blood concentrations of antiepileptic drugs including the fact that pregnant women decrease their intake of the drugs because of fear of injuring the fetus. They may also be unable to ingest full doses because of hyperemesis and nausea. In some, absorption of the drugs from the gastrointestinal tract is markedly decreased. Increased total blood volume, distribution of the drug in the fetal circulation, and enhanced maternal clearance of antiepileptic drugs by the liver and the kidney contribute to the low levels.

The altered hormonal environment of pregnancy may lower the seizure threshold also. Estrogens are known to have such an effect in experimental animals, whereas progesterone seems to have an antiseizure effect. The role of the hormonal environment is suggested by the rare phenomenon of women who experience seizures exclusively during pregnancy (gestational epilepsy).

Seizures in pregnancy can have obvious adverse effects. Partial complex seizures with alteration of consciousness and generalized tonic-clonic seizures with loss of consciousness and falls can lead to accidental injury to the mother and the fetus, including abruptio placentae. Although there is no documented evidence that the occasional, single, generalized tonic-clonic seizure is harmful to the fetus, frequent seizures can be harmful through the mechanism of prolonged periods of hypoxemia. Status epilepticus is clearly detrimental to the fetus as well as to the mother and should be promptly arrested.[13]

The risk of spontaneous abortion does not appear to be higher in women with epilepsy. However, therapeutic abortions induced by prostaglandin may cause convulsions in these women.[14] As a result, these agents should not be used in women with epilepsy.

Antiepileptic Drugs, Labor, Delivery, and Puerperium

A generalized tonic-clonic seizure may occur during labor or within 24 hours after delivery in 1 to 2% of patients with epilepsy. This may be related in part to the stress of labor; more frequently, it is caused by missing a dose of the antiepileptic drug.

Guidelines for the Management of Epilepsy in Pregnancy

Preconception and prenatal counseling is important when a patient with epilepsy plans to become pregnant or seeks advice during pregnancy. A reasonable amount of knowledge has been accumulated on which to base the guidelines as depicted in Table 43–1.[15] Many aspects of the counseling and management of seizures are best done by collaboration among the primary care physician, obstetrician, and neurologist. This coordinated effort is particularly important in women who have severe seizure disorders.

A principal aim of the treatment plan is the optimal use of antiepileptic drugs, balancing the risks of uncontrolled seizures against the teratogenic effects of the medications. For each patient, the possibility of withdrawal of antiepileptic medication should be contemplated, especially during the first trimester, which is the most critical period for organogenesis. This is possible in patients with self-limited seizure disorders. For example, it is not rare to see patients who have had seizures related to specific provoking factors, such as alcohol or drug withdrawal, or to metabolic derangements due to intercurrent illness who were given antiepileptic drugs and continued to take them indefinitely. Some patients have simple partial seizures and may experience only olfactory hallucinations, simple sensory symptoms, or focal motor twitches without generalization or alteration of consciousness. Rarely, adults may have only petit mal seizures. When follow-up and compliance are assured and seizures have been infrequent, it is possible to withhold antiepileptic drugs for at least the first trimester of pregnancy. Drug withdrawal is also feasible in a patient who has not had seizures in the preceding 2 to 3 years on medications and who has no significant underlying neurologic disease. All of these decisions are best made in consultation with a neurologist on an individual basis.

In most instances, however, antiepileptic drugs are needed but can be modified. No one drug is completely free of teratogenic risks or clearly superior to another in this regard. Trimethadione, however, which is used for petit mal epilepsy, should be prohibited because of its high risk of malformations. In most instances, whatever antiepileptic drug was most appropriate and efficacious for the patient before conception should be continued in pregnancy as well.

If possible, only one drug should be used for management of seizures. Polypharmacy enhances teratogenic risk. In current practice, increasing numbers of patients are given effective monotherapy. The minimum effective dose should be given, aiming at a low therapeutic blood level of antiepileptic drug. In this regard, it is important to adjust the dose according to clinical seizure control and not simply to follow blood levels. Many patients have low therapeutic or even subtherapeutic levels of phenobarbital, carbamazepine, phenytoin, and valproate, and yet seizure control is adequate because the free fractions of these drugs are higher. Blood levels of these drugs should be monitored on a monthly basis. If seizures are not well controlled, free plasma levels should be obtained wherever possible to provide a more accurate guide for the adjustment of dose. For valproate, the drug should be given in divided doses, three to four times a day to avoid high peak levels and to keep the total daily dose of the drug to less than 1000 mg whenever possible. Based on studies showing the protective effect of folate against neural tube defects, it is recommended that all patients on antiepileptic drugs receive supplements of folate, 4.0 mg per day, beginning 3 months before conception through the first trimester.

TABLE 43–1.   Preconception and Prenatal Counseling for Women with Epilepsy

Topics for discussion with the patient:
1. Teratogenic potential of antiepileptic drugs
2. Teratogenic time window of the first trimester of pregnancy
3. Dangers of seizures in pregnancy
4. Risk of increased frequency of seizures in pregnancy
5. Methods of optimal use of antiepileptic drugs
6. Monitoring seizure control by clinical and blood levels of antiepileptic drugs monthly
7. Methods of monitoring fetal health by ultrasound and alpha-fetoprotein measurements
8. Question of withdrawal of antiepileptic drugs for the first trimester of pregnancy
9. Inadvisability of switching antiepileptic drugs
10. History of major malformation in previous pregnancies and in the family
11. Folate supplementation before conception and in the first trimester
12. Postpartum monitoring of levels of antiepileptic drugs

Monitoring of Fetal Health

A family history of malformations, especially neural tube defects, is important to obtain. In patients taking valproate or carbamazepine or a combination of drugs, serum alpha-fetoprotein should be obtained at 16 weeks (Table 43–2). It is estimated that this assay identifies approximately 75% of pregnancies associated with neural tube defects. High-resolution ultrasonography performed by an experienced laboratory should be obtained at about 18 weeks. Ultrasonography identifies about 94% of cases.[16] When the results of these two tests are inconclusive, amniocentesis for alpha-fetoprotein is recommended, taking into consideration that the risk of miscarriage is 1% with this procedure. Ultrasonography at 24 weeks is sensitive to the detection of craniofacial as well as serious congenital heart disease.

Management of Labor and Delivery

It is important to ensure that the mother is given her usual antiepileptic drugs before and during delivery because of the risk of seizures occurring during this time. Otherwise, the method of delivery is guided by obstetric indications alone.

Management in the Postpartum Period

All infants born to mothers taking antiepileptic drugs should be given vitamin K, 20 mg intramuscularly at birth, to avoid internal bleeding. Some advise administration of vitamin K to the mother during the last month of pregnancy as well.

Follow-up evaluation of the mother at 2 weeks and 6 weeks after delivery is important to monitor blood levels of the antiepileptic drugs. Rebound of drug levels to above the therapeutic range with resultant toxicity is a frequent occurrence.

Breast-feeding the Infant

Valproate, carbamazepine, and phenytoin do not cross into the breast milk in significant amounts.

TABLE 43–2. Monitoring of Fetal Health

1. Serum–amniotic fluid alpha-fetoprotein at 16 weeks of pregnancy for detection of neural tube defects.
2. Ultrasound of fetus at 18 weeks to detect neural tube defects.
3. Ultrasound of fetus at 24 weeks to detect cleft palate, cleft lip, and heart malformation.
4. Precautions about breast-feeding if mother is taking barbiturates or benzodiazepines.

However, it is best to avoid breast-feeding when the mother is taking phenobarbital or primidone; 60% of maternal blood concentrations are found in the neonatal circulation and their long half-life in newborns is also of concern.

Oral Contraceptive Drugs in Epilepsy

The effectiveness of oral contraceptive drugs may be diminished by the concomitant use of antiepileptic drugs.[17] Phenobarbital, primidone, phenytoin, and carbamazepine are powerful inducers of the liver's microsomal enzyme systems, and they accelerate the metabolism of the estrogens and progesterone of the contraceptive pill. Such an acceleration can promote a decrease in blood levels of these hormones of approximately 50% or more. This had lead to an occasional contraception failure in women on long-term therapy with antiepileptic drugs, at a rate that is estimated to be 25 times higher than that in women who are not on these drugs. However, failure of oral contraceptives is unpredictable in the individual patient. Breakthrough bleeding while taking the pill suggests a lower concentration of sex hormones and a consequent failure to prevent ovulation, but this is not completely reliable. It is generally recommended that women taking phenytoin, barbiturates, or carbamazepine be given a combined pill with an ethinyl estradiol content of at least 50 μg of estradiol. If the patient experiences breakthrough bleeding while taking the pill with a lower dose of estradiol, it is another indication to increase to 50 μg of estradiol. In some cases, it may be necessary to increase it further.[18] It seems that subcutaneous contraceptive steroid implants may be more effective in this context because of less rapid clearance by the liver compared with that of the orally administered drug.

Valproic acid, clonazepam, and the new GABA-mimetic drug vigabatrin do not have such interactions with the oral contraceptive pill and may be preferable to the enzyme-inducing antiepileptic drugs in selected cases.

NEW ONSET SEIZURES

Seizures may occur for the first time during pregnancy and the puerperium. A systematic approach is needed to identify the cause of seizures, the possibility of recurrence, and the appropriateness of therapy (Table 43–3).

Seizures Related to Syncope

Syncope is common in pregnancy. When it is sufficiently prolonged, it is not uncommonly asso-

---

TABLE 43–3. New Onset Seizures in Pregnancy and the Puerperium

---

Related to the Pregnant State:
1. Toxemia of pregnancy
2. Cerebral cortical venous thrombosis of puerperium
3. Prolonged vasopressin infusion
4. Syncopal seizures
5. Gestational epilepsy

Unrelated to Pregnancy:
1. Epilepsy. First seizures of idiopathic epilepsy
2. Drug or alcohol withdrawal

---

ciated with brief myoclonic jerks of the limbs and trunk, which are often misconstrued as a primary seizure disorder. Occasionally when the patient is unable to obtain a recumbent position, the myoclonic jerks may progress to a generalized tonic-clonic convulsive seizure. A careful history is the clue to the diagnosis. Patients describe light-headedness, dizziness, blurring of vision, and perspiration for minutes before loss of consciousness, which occurs while the patient is sitting or standing. The patient falls limply to the ground. Observers may note pallor and describe myoclonic jerks, going on to generalized convulsions. Interval neurologic examination is normal. A normal electroencephalogram is further supportive evidence, but the critical factor is a careful history accompanied by a normal neurologic examination.

Seizures due to toxemia of pregnancy are discussed in Chapter 36. Seizures due to cortical vein thrombosis are discussed later in this chapter.

Seizures Due to Intravenous Vasopressin Infusion

Rarely, generalized tonic-clonic seizures may appear in a woman after prolonged induction of labor by intravenous vasopressin (Pitressin) infusion. The infusion results in hyponatremia due to water retention, with clouding of consciousness, confusion, and seizures. The infusion should be stopped. Generally, no other treatment is required.

Gestational Epilepsy

Gestational epilepsy is rare but has been documented.[1] Patients may experience generalized tonic-clonic or partial complex seizures. By definition, these occur only during the pregnancy and remit spontaneously between pregnancies, suggesting a special role of the hormonal environment

of pregnancy in inducing the seizures. They tend to occur in the sixth and seventh months of pregnancy. Neurologic examinations are typically normal, but an electroencephalogram may show a temporal epileptic focus. The diagnosis is to a large extent one of exclusion and long-term follow-up, which shows that seizures recur for brief periods only during the pregnancies.

New onset seizures may also be due to withdrawal from alcohol or drugs. More often, they may herald the onset of idiopathic epilepsy because this syndrome occurs most often in young adults up to the age of 25 years. Thus, there is a large overlap between the age groups prone to develop idiopathic epilepsy and the reproductive years.[1]

A new onset seizure in a pregnant woman is an indication for neurologic consultation. A detailed history is critical, focusing on symptoms of syncope preceding the seizure as well as other factors such as a drug or alcohol use or settings for electrolyte imbalance such as vasopressin infusion. A thorough neurologic and a general physical examination are necessary. A computed tomography (CT) scan can be obtained as clinically indicated. In occasional cases when cortical vein thrombosis is suspected, a magnetic resonance imaging (MRI) scan of the brain is helpful. Cerebrospinal fluid examination may also be appropriate.

SEIZURES IN THE PUERPERIUM

Cortical Vein Thrombosis

Cerebral cortical vein and cerebral venous sinus thromboses are rare but have a specific predilection for women in the puerperium.[19] Most cases occur in the first 2 to 3 weeks after childbirth, but rare cases have been described in pregnancy as early as the first trimester. The exact mechanism for the development of venous thrombosis is not known but is in keeping with the hypercoagulable state of this period and the tendency for venous thrombosis in the limbs and pelvis. In the nonpregnant women, oral contraceptive use also increases the risk of this rare disorder.[20]

Cortical vein thrombosis leads to hemorrhagic infarction of the brain, often beginning in the occipital lobes and in the parasagittal areas of the frontal and parietal lobes. Arterial blood flow is present, but venous drainage is blocked, resulting in hemorrhages into the cortex and the subcortical structures. The lesions can be small or large, causing progressive massive swelling of the brain with bilateral parasagittal infarctions and consequent brain herniation syndromes. This is especially likely to occur when the venous thrombosis spreads from the cortical veins into the superior sagittal and other sinuses with consequent marked elevations of intracranial pressure. Other patients develop only large venous sinus thrombosis without involvement of the cortical veins.

Patients develop a subacute illness with severe and persistent headaches, often associated with blurring and impairment of vision, sometimes to the point of bilateral cortical blindness. Generalized or focal and secondary generalized seizures are common and can be intractable because of the hemorrhagic cortical infarctions. Patients may develop focal neurologic symptoms, especially unilateral or bilateral leg weakness and cortical blindness. Elevated intracranial pressure is manifested by papilledema. The clinical picture ranges from mild cases with headache and mild visual disturbances to progressive obtundation, status epilepticus, and brain herniation syndromes resulting in death.

A high degree of suspicion is needed for the diagnosis of early and mild cases. The combination of headaches and visual disturbances often leads to an incorrect diagnosis of migraine. Cortical blindness is often misconstrued as hysterical blindness until seizures occur. An MRI scan of the brain is the test of choice for cortical vein thrombosis. Infarctions in the brain in the parasagittal locations on both sides of the superior sagittal sinus in the frontal and parietal regions are frequent.[21] The parasagittal location and the spread across the arterial territories are characteristic of venous infarctions. Bilateral occipital lobe infarctions are also common. Varying degrees of edema and a hemorrhagic component are readily identified. The MRI scan in most cases also detects the presence of thrombus as a high signal in the superior sagittal, straight, and transverse sinuses in various combinations. Magnetic resonance venography increases the chances of detecting cortical vein thrombosis. When these facilities are not available, an angiogram with an examination of the venous phase can also help in the diagnosis. A CT scan of the brain can show similar abnormalities but is less sensitive in detecting clot in the venous sinuses. A contrast-enhanced study may show a clot at the confluence of the superior sagittal and straight sinuses as a filling defect (the empty triangle sign).

There is a wide clinical spectrum of severity and progression of the disease: some patients have minor symptoms that do not progress further, and they gradually get better. In others, the neurologic deterioration is progressive. Whenever there are indications of clinical deterioration, intravenous heparin therapy is generally recommended, although this therapy is still controversial. Increasing numbers of cases have been treated successfully despite the presence of small cortical hemorrhages seen on CT or MRI scans of the brain.[22] Case reports documenting dramatic clinical improvement in previously moribund patients treated with heparin have been reported. There have also been case reports of patients treated with thrombolytic agents in the form of streptokinase, or heparin and urokinase in combination.[23] However, there have been no controlled studies.

Supportive therapy consists of anticonvulsant drugs and treatment of brain edema with dexamethasone sodium phosphate (Decadron) and mannitol. The mortality rate for this condition is approximately 25%. However, survivors often make excellent clinical recovery, largely because the arterial supply to the brain is retained and veins recanalize.

Back Pain in Pregnancy

Low back pain is common in pregnancy, occurring in nearly half of pregnant women, and is often due to mechanical stresses on the facet joints and on the posterior spinous ligaments.[24] The stretching on the lumbar spine due to the exaggerated lordosis and the stretching of the abdominal muscles and shortening of the paraspinal muscles also contribute to the back pain syndrome. This is further aided by the relaxation of the pelvic girdle and sacroiliac joints. In this syndrome, pain is located over the lumbar spine and spreads to the thighs. It is not associated with neurologic symptoms of paresthesias or with bladder or bowel control difficulties. Back pain is increased by physical activity and is improved with rest, although many patients experience worsening of the pain at night. Results of a neurologic examination are normal, without indication of nerve root injury. A compression test of the pelvis and the sacroiliac joint may reproduce the symptoms, whereas results of the straight leg raising test are normal. Restriction of physical activity, local application of heat, and wearing a maternity belt tend to alleviate the back pain. In most instances, conservative therapy is the treatment of choice; the pain syndrome gradually resolves within several months after childbirth.

Soft intervertebral disk herniation is not rare in pregnancy.[25] Its features are similar to those occurring in nonpregnant patients, and it most frequently occurs at the L4–5 and L5–S1 levels with radicular syndromes of L5 and S1 nerve roots. The diagnosis is made on the basis of the history and physical examination. A CT or an MRI scan of the lumbar spine is not necessary in the vast majority of the cases unless there is a progressive neurologic deficit of cauda equina syndrome with caudal anesthesia or bladder or bowel involvement, or both, from central disk herniation. Conservative therapy of rest and mild analgesic medications is sufficient for most patients. The syndrome tends to resolve gradually after delivery but may occur again in subsequent pregnancies.

PERIPHERAL NERVE PROBLEMS IN PREGNANCY

Carpal Tunnel Syndrome

Carpal tunnel syndrome is the most common mononeuropathy of pregnancy[26] and is related to fluid accumulation and swelling of soft tissues within the carpal tunnel and relaxation of the transverse carpal ligament with consequent entrapment of the median nerves. Symptoms are prominent and usually begin in the second and third trimesters with painful numbness in the hand and fingers, aggravated by use of the hand. Nocturnal awakening because of pain in the hand is a characteristic feature. Although paresthesias affect the thumb, index, and middle fingers, many patients relate symptoms that affect the entire hand, which manifest as dropping objects, decreased grip strength, and pain radiating proximally to the elbow or shoulder. Physical examination reveals a positive Tinel's sign of tingling on tapping the median nerve at the wrist. Phalen's sign of forced passive palmar flexion of the hand may also reproduce the symptoms.

The carpal tunnel syndrome of pregnancy is self-limited and gets better promptly after delivery in the vast majority of the cases. Thus, conservative treatment is the best approach in most cases. Night-time wearing of splints to the wrist often brings remarkable relief along with the reassurance of its benign natural course. Analgesics in the form of nonsteroidal anti-inflammatory medications may be helpful if splints are not adequate. However, this benefit should be evaluated carefully (see Chapter 34). When symptoms are severe, injection of methylprednisolone into the carpal tunnel may bring relief. Surgical treatment of carpal tunnel syndrome is rarely necessary. In most patients, symptoms resolve within 3 months; but in approximately 20% of patients, the syndrome may recur in subsequent pregnancies.

Foot Drop after Labor

This is not an uncommon complication of labor and is due to compression of the peroneal nerve behind the knee as it winds around the neck of the fibula. It is caused by improper positioning of the legs during prolonged labor. It can also result from a proximal lesion of the lumbosacral plexus at the pelvic brim from compression of the L4–5 roots by the fetal head. This is especially likely to happen when the mother is small and the baby is big or in a transverse lie and labor is prolonged. It is also likely to happen with a midforceps delivery. Clinical differentiation of a lumbar plexus radiculopathy and a distal peroneal nerve palsy may be difficult. However, an electromyographic examination 2 to 3 weeks after the onset of the problem indicates denervation in the hamstring as well as in the gluteal muscles supplied by the L5 root, pointing to a proximal localization. Most patients recover spontaneously over a period of 6 weeks to 3 months.

Multiple Sclerosis in Pregnancy

Multiple sclerosis is the most common chronic neurologic disorder of young adults in the United States. Of the estimated 200,000 Americans with this disease, two thirds are women. Thus, the clinical scenario of a woman with multiple sclerosis who plans to become pregnant is somewhat common. Many questions of interactions between the pregnancy and the multiple sclerosis often arise in clinical practice. Several studies examining these issues with particular reference to the effects of pregnancy on central nervous system demyelination and the effects of repeated pregnancies on the long-term course of the disease and disability have been completed.[27] These studies have demonstrated that multiple sclerosis does not adversely affect fertility, conception, pregnancy, labor, delivery, or fetal health. There is also no good evidence that pregnancy triggers the first episodes of multiple sclerosis. Longitudinal studies have demonstrated consistently that multiple sclerosis is ameliorated during pregnancy, especially during the second and third trimesters. It is postulated that the complex hormonal and immunologic changes that occur during pregnancy have a modulatory effect on the immunopathogenic mechanism of multiple sclerosis. This has also been shown with other autoimmune diseases during pregnancy. In contrast, studies have also consistently shown that the risk of exacerbation of multiple sclerosis is increased during the first 6 months of the puerperium to about two to three times the risk in nonpregnant patients. It is estimated that approximately 20 to 40% of women with multiple sclerosis will experience an exacerbation in the first 3 months after delivery. A few studies have looked at the long-term outcome in terms of total disability in multiple sclerosis in relation to single or multiple pregnancies. It appears that there is no significant effect. Spinal anesthesia has traditionally been avoided in multiple sclerosis patients during delivery because of the possibility of exacerbation, although a causal link has not been established. There are a few instances in which epidural spinal anesthesia has been used successfully and safely, although no large studies are available.[28]

Guidelines for Advice to Patients Regarding Pregnancy and Multiple Sclerosis

From a medical perspective, the decision to have children should be based primarily on the severity of the existing neurologic disability, the person's mental and physical capacity to nurture the baby, and the availability of support systems, rather than on the effects of pregnancy on multiple sclerosis. Patients are advised that the outcome of pregnancy is not affected adversely by multiple sclerosis and that pregnancy ameliorates multiple sclerosis temporarily. They should also be appraised of the increased risk of flare-up of the disease during the first 6 months following the delivery, but that the long-term outcome of the disease is not significantly altered by single or multiple pregnancies. The patient should be counseled to plan for additional help and support in the care of the baby.

Patients with multiple sclerosis often are concerned about the risk of the disease in their offspring. It is clear that there is a genetic predisposition to develop multiple sclerosis, although this is a complex polygenic susceptibility: there is a 40% chance of an identical twin of a person with multiple sclerosis developing multiple sclerosis. The risk of multiple sclerosis in a child whose mother has multiple sclerosis is about 3% compared with an incidence of 0.1% in the general population.[29] The overall risk of multiple sclerosis in a child born to a mother with the disease is low.

The various immunomodulatory and immunosuppressive therapies that are commonly used for exacerbations of multiple sclerosis are best avoided during pregnancy because of the potential toxic effects on the fetus. Corticosteroids are best avoided, especially during the first trimester of pregnancy because of adrenal suppression in the fetus as well as virilization in the female fetus. Cytotoxic and other immunosuppressive drugs should also be avoided because they provide only temporary symptomatic benefit. Interferon-β, approved for use in multiple sclerosis, has been shown to decrease the number of exacerbations over the first 2 years of its treatment. Use of interferon-β is also best avoided during pregnancy because the effects on the fetus are not yet known. There are no neurologic reasons that preclude breast-feeding.

HEADACHE SYNDROMES IN PREGNANCY

Severe headache occurring during pregnancy is a common problem. It is a matter of concern because the headache may be the presenting symptom of a serious underlying cause, such as rupture of an arteriovenous malformation, or of a cerebral aneurysm, eclampsia, and, rarely, brain tumor or cerebral venous thrombosis. Fortunately in most cases, headaches are due to tension headaches, migraines, or a combination of the two. Evaluation of new onset headache in pregnancy should always include a careful history; thorough general physical and neurologic examinations; and, whenever appropriate, neuroimaging and spinal fluid examinations.

Migraine

The clinical features and diagnosis of migraine are detailed in Chapter 58. As migraine is most common in women in their reproductive years, it is frequently encountered in the context of pregnancy.[30] The migraine syndrome in women who have had migraine is markedly ameliorated or remits during pregnancy in two thirds of cases. The mechanism of this protective effect of pregnancy is not known, but the estrogen-mediated decreased response of the cranial blood vessels to adrenergic stimulation as well as the increase in endorphins may have a role. In approximately one third of patients with preexisting migraine, headaches may become more frequent, more severe, or both. Occasionally, migraine may appear for the first time during pregnancy, or a patient with common migraine may for the first time develop complicated migraine, with visual or other neurologic symptoms. It is not uncommon for headaches to become more frequent. Sleep deprivation, decreased or irregular food intake, and physical and psychological stresses are common triggering factors. The relationship of migraine to the incidence of eclampsia is not established. There is no excessive risk caused by migraine to the offspring of mothers with migraine compared with that to those without migraine.

The diagnosis of migraine is reliably made on

the basis of a careful history or clinical examination. The criteria are the same for pregnant as for nonpregnant patients. However, when neurologic symptoms appear for the first time in pregnancy, the possibility of an underlying arteriovenous malformation should be evaluated by appropriate investigations. The combination of headaches and visual symptoms are also seen with eclampsia and cortical venous thrombosis and can be misdiagnosed as classic migraine. A subarachnoid hemorrhage from a ruptured aneurysm or arteriovenous malformation should be ruled out in the patient who presents with a new-onset ''thunderclap'' type of headache before designating this as a migraine headache.

Headaches should be treated using nonpharmacologic methods whenever possible. Provocative factors such as hunger and sleep deprivation should be avoided. Only simple analgesics should be used along with reassurance about the benign nature of the underlying headache syndrome. Acetaminophen is the most widely used and appears to be safe. Aspirin is probably best avoided because of its inhibition of prostaglandin synthesis, which can delay the onset of labor, prolong the course of labor, and possibly increase blood loss during labor and can affect hemostasis in the newborn as well as lead to premature closure of the ductus arteriosus. There is no documented evidence of the teratogenecity of aspirin. Occasional severe headaches can be treated with codeine. Ergot alkaloids are to be avoided, although there is no good evidence that the commonly used ergotamine has any effect on the uterus. Nonsteroidal anti-inflammatory medications can be used, but they should be avoided in the last weeks of pregnancy so that they do not bring on premature closure of the ductus arteriosus.

In most situations, reassurance and symptomatic therapy for the occasional headaches and preventive nonpharmacologic methods help the patient to cope with the headaches quite well. Occasionally, one encounters a patient who has frequent recurrences of severe headaches during pregnancy for whom prophylactic therapy may be appropriate. Propranolol has been used successfully and safely for this purpose as well as for the control of hypertension in pregnancy. It is used in the lowest possible dose, ranging from 40 to 160 mg in divided doses. It is best avoided during the last phases of pregnancy because it crosses the placenta and may cause bradycardia, hypoglycemia, and decreased fetal response to hypoxemia in the newborn.[31] Tricyclic antidepressants should be used with caution and in the smallest possible dose, beginning at 10 mg at night time, and can be increased up to 75 to 100 mg per day. These are also best avoided in the first trimester and at term because the tricyclics cross the placenta and may cause tachycardia, myoclonic jerks, and urinary retention in the newborn.[32] These medications do not enter into the breast milk in any significant amount so that breast-feeding need not be avoided.

Tension Vascular Headaches

The characteristics of this syndrome are described in Chapter 58. Tension headaches are one of the most common, recurrent type of headache during pregnancy, and their characteristics are the same as those in nonpregnant patients. They are often precipitated by the psychological and physical stresses of pregnancy and are worsened by sleep deprivation and poor nutrition. The diagnosis is established by a characteristic clinical picture combined with a normal general physical and neurologic examination and by careful follow-up when the diagnosis is made for the first time in pregnancy.[33] In most patients, therapy consists of nonpharmacologic methods, with reassurance and avoidance of triggering factors, and if necessary simple analgesics in the form of acetaminophen. On rare occasions, prophylactic therapy is needed.

Subarachnoid Hemorrhage Due to Rupture of Cerebral Aneurysms

When a new-onset severe headache develops in a pregnant patient, subarachnoid hemorrhage is a major concern. Aneurysmal or subarachnoid hemorrhage continues to be a leading cause of obstetric morbidity and mortality in modern clinical practice.[34, 35] Rupture of aneurysms is three times higher in pregnant women than in nonpregnant women and is estimated to occur in about 1 in 10,000 pregnancies. The older the pregnant patient, the more likely the subarachnoid hemorrhage is due to an aneurysm rather than a cerebral arteriovenous malformation. Aneurysms may rupture during any part of the pregnancy, but the risk of bleeding increases with advancing phases of gestation. However, contrary to expectation, first bleeding of an aneurysm is rare during labor, although rebleeding is not uncommon. The heightened risk of rupture of the aneurysm continues in the first weeks after delivery. The mechanism by which pregnancy and the puerperium predispose to the rupture of brain aneurysms has not been defined but appears to be related to hormonal and hemodynamic factors that weaken the wall of the aneurysm.

Clinical features of subarachnoid hemorrhage are well known and are identical to those seen in nonpregnant patients. Abrupt, razor-sharp onset of severe, persistent headache accompanied by photophobia, neck pain, and neck stiffness are usual. Depending on the amount of subarachnoid hemorrhage, patients also demonstrate various levels of decreased consciousness, confusion, ocular motor nerve palsies, hemiparesis, paraparesis, and subhyaloid hemorrhages. Uncommonly, focal or generalized seizures can occur.

In addition to the typical picture of moderate to severe subarachnoid hemorrhage that is easy to recognize, some patients experience mild sentinel bleeding from an aneurysm. This is important to recognize so that devastating recurrent bleeding can be prevented and the prognosis for the mother and baby improved. Thus, any sudden headache that is persistent and whose clinical characteristics do not fit into well-defined syndromes such as migraine or tension headache and for which no alternative explanations are available in the form of eclampsia should raise the possibility of a subarachnoid hemorrhage even though the headache may not qualify as the ''worst headache of the patient's life.''

Brain CT scan without contrast material is the test of choice to detect an acute subarachnoid hemorrhage. It should be scrutinized to detect small amounts of blood around the brain stem, in the suprasellar cisterns, and in interhemispheric and sylvian fissures. Brain CT scan reveals subarachnoid hemorrhage in more than 90% of cases. It provides valuable information about the amount of subarachnoid hemorrhage and the presence of intracerebral clot, hydrocephalus, and infarction, which helps in making decisions about the management of the patient.

Brain MRI scanning is not sensitive to acute subarachnoid blood. When a brain CT scan is negative and when the clinical suspicion of subarachnoid hemorrhage is strong, a spinal tap should be done without hesitation. Spinal fluid should be spun immediately and compared with water to detect mild or early xanthochromia, an invaluable sign of bleeding into the subarachnoid space as opposed to a traumatic tap. A cerebral arteriogram is the definitive test for confirmation of the aneurysm and for detecting the presence of multiple aneurysms.

Subarachnoid hemorrhage from a bleeding cerebral aneurysm has a high morbidity and mortality rate, both from the initial bleeding and from recurrent bleeding. Aneurysms have a 50% incidence of rebleeding in the first 3 weeks after the initial rupture. Patients are also at risk for cerebral infarction resulting from vasospasm, which is maximal in the second week after the initial bleed. They may develop further complications from the mass effect of an intracerebral hematoma, hydrocephalus, or, occasionally, seizures.

Treatment of the aneurysm takes priority and should be guided by general principles applicable to the nonpregnant patient. This treatment is best done in the intensive care unit in conjunction with experienced neurosurgeons and neurologists. The main medical therapies are moderate control of blood pressure, usually with nimodipine (a calcium channel blocker); controlled intravascular volume expansion, which decreases the ischemic complications; sedation; and antiseizure medications. Neurosurgical intervention is needed for evacuation of hematomas or for treatment of hydrocephalus. The definitive treatment of the aneurysm is clipping, and the timing of this procedure is similar to that used with nonpregnant patients. In general, if aneurysmal rupture occurs in the later stages of pregnancy, it is recommended that the delivery be performed at 38 weeks of gestation by elective cesarean section. No specific therapy is available to decrease the risk of recurrent bleeding during the puerperium. Depending on the clinical situation, when the aneurysm ruptures in the early stages of pregnancy, it may be clipped successfully and the pregnancy continued to term without adverse effects on the fetus. There have been unusual instances of severe subarachnoid hemorrhage with brain death, when the mother was maintained on artificial support until term when the fetus could be delivered safely.

Subarachnoid Hemorrhage Due to Arteriovenous Malformations

Rupture of cerebral arteriovenous malformation is another important cause of subarachnoid hemorrhage in the pregnant patient.[34, 36] Pregnancy poses a serious threat to the patients who harbor cerebral arteriovenous malformations as well as the rare patients with spinal cord arteriovenous malformations. It is estimated that the risk of known cerebral arteriovenous malformation rupture during pregnancy is as high as 80%. Arteriovenous malformations are more common causes of subarachnoid hemorrhage in younger patients between the ages of 15 and 25 years and in primigravidas compared with aneurysmal subarachnoid hemorrhages, which are more common in older and multiparous women. The mechanism for vulnerability during this phase of pregnancy is not known. In contrast to aneurysmal subarachnoid hemorrhage, arteriovenous malformations may bleed for the first time during labor.

The clinical manifestations of subarachnoid hemorrhage from arteriovenous malformations are similar to those caused by aneurysmal subarachnoid hemorrhage. However, in many cases, the clinical picture, including the neurologic impairment, is milder. The patients are more likely to have seizures as a complication of arteriovenous malformation rupture. The spectrum of neurologic impairments is also variable, from headache with neck stiffness to catastrophic intracerebral and intraventricular hemorrhage. The patient may have a history suggesting subarachnoid hemorrhage during previous pregnancies more often than would a patient with an aneurysm, probably indicating the less catastrophic natural course of arteriovenous malformations and in keeping with the fact that arteriovenous malformations may bleed several times over a period of years. The neurologic examination is significant for neck stiffness and various neurologic focal deficits depending on the location and extent of the intracerebral hemorrhage. The CT scan of the brain is valuable in detecting both acute subarachnoid and intracerebral bleeding. A CT scan with intravenous contrast infusion reveals the characteristic serpiginous tangle of blood vessels. An MRI scan of the brain is a sensitive test and shows the extent of the malformation much more precisely than the CT scan. It has also been known to be positive in angiographically occult arteriovenous malformations. The cerebral angiogram is, however, very useful in defining the exact arterial feeders and the type and extent of the venous drainage.

Treatment of cerebral arteriovenous malformations that have ruptured is best done in collaboration with a neurologist and neurosurgeon in an intensive care setting. Cerebral ischemic complications are rare with hemorrhage due to arteriovenous malformations, in contrast to the complication rate with aneurysmal subarachnoid hemorrhage, and the medical management of the condition is less complex. In most patients with a stable neurologic status, with arteriovenous malformations that are inoperable because of the deep location within the cerebral hemispheres or brain stem, or with malformations that are massive, the pregnancy is allowed to proceed to 38 weeks. At this time, the infant is delivered by elective cesarean section to avoid the increased intracranial pressure from the Valsalva maneuver, which is known to increase the incidence of recurrent bleeding during parturition. Safe delivery of the baby also has been done by the vaginal route, but the use of epidural anesthesia and forceps is recommended. The usual indication for emergency neurosurgery during pregnancy is the presence of an enlarging intracerebral hematoma with progressive clinical neurologic deterioration. In such cases, evacuation of the hematoma may be function-saving as well as lifesaving. Definitive treatment of the arteriovenous malformation is planned after completion of the pregnancy. Patients who survive the rupture of an arteriovenous malformation should avoid future pregnancies unless the arteriovenous malformation is completely resected. Subsequent pregnancies pose a threat of recurrent bleeding and a higher morbidity and mortality. Definitive treatment of arteriovenous malformations is still evolving: complete surgical resection is feasible for smaller, more accessible malformations. Others have been treated with a combination of embolization and surgery. Proton beam therapy has been used increasingly for large or deep malformations that are not accessible for surgical removal. Proton beam therapy is quite effective but takes 1 to 2 years before a significant decrease in the size of the malformation is achieved. The patient should be advised against pregnancies during this interval.

NEUROLOGIC LABORATORY INVESTIGATIONS IN PREGNANT WOMEN

Lumbar Puncture

There are no specific contraindications to the use of a lumbar puncture during pregnancy. Its indications are the same as those in nonpregnant patients. The issue usually arises in suspected cases of subarachnoid hemorrhage and, rarely, meningitis. Technically, lumbar puncture is not more difficult in the pregnant woman, although it may be more uncomfortable to the patient.

Computed Tomography Scan of the Brain

In general, any neuroradiologic test should be done only for specific, urgent, and well-considered indications during pregnancy. These tests should be avoided in the first trimester of pregnancy when radiation is most likely to interfere with normal organogenesis. However, brain CT scanning can be done safely for proper indications and with good technique and protection of the fetus and ovaries by using an abdominal lead shield. The usual indication for an urgent CT scan during pregnancy is the suspicion of intracranial hemorrhage; less commonly it is done for other headache modalities and new-onset seizures. With the proper technique, the potential fetal radiation exposure is usually less than 5 rad, and it is unlikely to cause any dysfunction.

Magnetic Resonance Imaging Scan of the Brain and Spine

Both these tests are extremely sensitive imaging techniques for the brain and the contents of the spine. They are only rarely needed in the commonly encountered neurologic problems of pregnancy but are very helpful in imaging arteriovenous malformations of the brain and detecting cerebral venous thrombosis. In the vast majority of cases of low back pain and sciatica, diagnosis and treatment can be provided on the basis of the clinical examination. In the rare cases when central disk herniation causes progressing cauda equina syndrome, an MRI scan of the spine may be needed. The safety or hazards of MRI to the fetus have not been established. Thus, it is best avoided, especially in the first trimester of pregnancy. It may be used, however, when clearly needed, and this is a matter of clinical judgment.

REFERENCES

1. Knight AH, Rhind EG. Epilepsy and pregnancy. A study of 163 pregnancies in 59 patients. Epilepsia 1975;16:99.
2. Dravet C, Julian C, Legras C, et al. Epilepsy, antiepileptic drugs and malformations in children of women with epilepsy. Neurology 1992;42(suppl 5):75.
3. Tanganelli P, Regesta G. Epilepsy, pregnancy and major birth anomalies. Neurology 1992;42(suppl 5):89.
4. Feldman GL, Weaver DD, Lovrien EW. The fetal trimethadione syndrome: A report of an additional family and further delineation of this syndrome. Am J Dis Child 1977;131:89.
5. Rosa FW. Spina bifida in infants of women treated with carbamazepine during pregnancy. N Engl J Med 1991;324:674.
6. Scolnik D, Nulman I, Rovet J, et al. Neurodevelopment of children exposed in utero to phenytoin and carbamezepine monotherapy. JAMA 1994;271:767.
7. Lindhout D, Schmidt D. In-utero exposure to valproate and neural-tube defects. Lancet 1986;2:1392.
8. MRC Vitamin Study Research Group (Nicolas Wald). Prevention of neural-tube defects: Results of Medical Research Council vitamin study. Lancet 1991;338:131.
9. Gimowsky ML, Petrie R. Maternal anticonvulsants and fetal hemorrhage. J Reprod Med 1986;31:61.
10. Kuhnz W, Koch S, Helge H, et al. Primidone and phenobarbital during lactation period in epileptic women: Total and free drug serum levels in nursed infants and their effects on neonatal behavior. Dev Pharmacol Ther 1988;11:147.
11. Granstrom ML, Gaily E. Psychomotor development in children of mothers with epilepsy. Neurology 1992;42(suppl 5):144.
12. Yerby MS, Frid PN, McCormick K. Antiepileptic drug disposition during pregnancy. Neurology 1992;42(suppl 5):12.
13. Mendez-Quijada J, Mores AF, Juavinao N. Status epilepticus in pregnancy, a case report. J Reprod Med 1990;35:289.
14. Brandenburg H, Jahoda MGJ, Wladimiroff JW, et al. Convulsion in epileptic woman after administration of prostaglandin E2 derivative. Lancet 1990;2:1138.
15. Delgado-Escueta AV, Janz D. Consensus guideline: Preconception counseling, management and care of the pregnant woman with epilepsy. Neurology 1992;42(suppl 5):149.
16. Hobbins JC. Prognosis and management of neural-tube defects today. N Engl J Med 1991;324:690.
17. Orme MLE. The clinical pharmacology of oral contraceptive steroids. Br J Clin Pharmacol 1982;16:31.
18. Mattson RH, Cramer JA, Darney PD, et al. Use of oral contraceptives by women with epilepsy. JAMA 1986;256:238.
19. Ameri A, Bowsser MG. Cerebral venous thrombosis in cerebral ischemia: Treatment and prevention. Neurol Clin 1992;10:87.
20. Buchanan DS, Brazinsky JH. Dural sinus and cerebral venous thrombosis and incidence in young women receiving oral contraceptives. Arch Neurol 1970;22:440.
21. McMurdo SK, Brant-Zawadski M, Bradley WG, et al. Dural sinus thrombosis study using intermediate field strength MR imaging. Radiology 1986;161:83.
22. Einhaupl KM, Villringer A, Meister W, et al. Heparin treatment in sinus venous thrombosis. Lancet 1991;338:597.
23. DiRocco C, Ianelli A, Leone G, et al. Heparin-urokinase treatment in aseptic dural sinus thrombosis. Arch Neurol 1981;38:431.
24. Berg G, Hammar M, Moller-Nielsen J, et al. Low-back pain during pregnancy. Obstet Gynecol 1988;72:71.
25. LeBan MM, Perrin JCS, Latimer FR. Pregnancy and herniated lumbar disc. Arch Phys Med Rehab 1983;64:319.
26. Voitk AJ, Mueller J, Farlinger DE, et al. Carpal tunnel syndrome in pregnancy. Can Med Assoc J 1983;128:277.
27. Birk K, Ford C, Smeltzer S, et al. The clinical course of multiple sclerosis during pregnancy and puerperium. Arch Neurol 1990;47:738.
28. Warren TM, Dattas, Ostheimer GW. Lumbar epidural anesthesia in a patient with multiple sclerosis. Anesth Analg 1982;61(12):1022.
29. Sadovnic AD, Baird PA, Ward RH. Multiple sclerosis; updated risks for relatives. Am J Med Genet 1988;29(3):533.
30. Somerville BW. A study of migraine in pregnancy. Neurology 1972;22:824.
31. Finnstrom O, Ezitis J, Ryden G, et al. Neonatal effects of beta-blocking drugs in pregnancy. Acta Obstet Gynecol Scand 1984;118:91.
32. Webster PA. Withdrawal symptoms in neonates associated with maternal antidepressant therapy. Lancet 1973;2:318.
33. Weinberger J, Lsauersen NH. Vascular headache in pregnancy. Am J Obstet Gynecol 1982;143:842.
34. Dias MS, Sekhar LN. Intracranial hemorrhage from aneurysms and arteriovenous malformations during pregnancy and puerperium. Neurosurgery 1990;27:855.
35. Wiebers DO. Subarachnoid hemorrhage in pregnancy. Semin Neurol 1988;8:226.
36. Sadasivah B, Malik GM, Lee C, et al. Vascular malformations and pregnancy. Surg Neurol 1990;30:305.

INFECTIOUS DISEASE IN WOMEN

Gynecologic Infections

44

Vaginitis

Phyllis L. Carr

EPIDEMIOLOGY

Vaginitis is one of the most common medical problems of women presenting to a physician's office. Despite the frequency of this complaint, the pathophysiology of this process is not thoroughly understood. The interaction of normal host defense mechanisms, pathogenic organisms, and changes in substrate that allow an alteration in the balance of organisms all contribute to vaginal infection. An understanding of the normal vaginal ecology and the effects of the cyclic changes of the menstrual cycle on the vaginal microbiology is necessary to appropriately evaluate vaginal complaints.

NORMAL VAGINAL ECOLOGY AND CYCLIC CHANGES

The physiologic secretion of the vagina includes substances from the vulvar, sebaceous, sweat, Bartholin's and Skene's glands, as well as exfoliated cells, cervical mucus, and secretions of the endometrial cavity and fallopian tubes. Normal secretions pool in the posterior fornix and do not adhere to the vaginal walls. The average pH of the secretions is between 3.8 and 4.5. Normal vaginal flora, composed predominantly of lactobacilli, contribute to the inhibition of pathogens by maintaining this acidic environment. Other organisms present in low concentrations include small numbers of *Staphylococcus epidermidis,* diphtheroids, streptococci, *Gardnerella vaginalis, Escherichia coli,* and anaerobic bacteria. A higher pH is maintained during menstruation, and along with the change in pH, there is a slight alteration in the flora. Aerobes decrease premenstrually, and *Staphylococcus aureus* organisms increase at the time of menstruation.

HORMONAL CHANGES

In the prepubertal female, low estrogen levels result in few lactobacilli, a thin vaginal mucosa, minimal glycogen production, and an alkaline pH. There is little protection against vaginal infection; poor hygiene can result in vaginal infection. Higher estrogen levels at puberty cause a thickening of the vaginal epithelium and an attendent increase in glycogen. Lactobacilli split the glycogen produced by the epithelial cells into glucose and maltose. The increase in glycogen results in greater numbers of lactobacilli and, consequently, in relative protection against vaginal infections. The very high levels of estrogen during pregnancy result in the thickest vaginal epithelium, high levels of glycogen and lactobacilli, and the most acidic pH. In the postmenopausal woman, estrogen levels again fall, resulting in atrophic vaginal epithelium, low glycogen levels, decreased lactobacilli, a more alkaline pH, and a greater susceptibility to vaginal infection.

PATHOPHYSIOLOGY OF INFECTION AND SUSCEPTIBILITY

The high estrogen levels in pregnancy and in women on high-dose oral contraceptives are felt to predispose women to yeast infections by providing more glycogen. The glycogen provides the increased growth medium for yeast to proliferate. Pregnancy is also associated with decreased levels of cell-mediated immunity, which contribute to the occurrence of yeast infections. Antibiotics, especially the broad-spectrum antibiotics, reduce the normal protective resident bacterial population and predispose to increased yeast infections. Tight-fitting garments and occlusive materials are also associated with higher rates of vaginal yeast infection.

Factors that predispose women to *Trichomonas vaginalis* and bacterial vaginosis are less well understood. In bacterial vaginosis there is again a relative decrease in lactobacillus and an overgrowth of anaerobic bacteria, including *Bacteroides* and *Peptostreptococcus,* and a concomitant increase in *G. vaginalis.* Total organism counts increase to 10^7 to 10^{11}, from normal levels of 10^5 to 10^7, and the pH increases to greater than 4.5. Both trichomonads and bacterial vaginosis have been associated with sexual transmission, although both infections can occur in the absence of sexual activity. For reasons not well understood, use of the oral contraceptive pill has been associated with a lower rate of *Trichomonas* infection and bacterial vaginosis. Chemicals including douches, chlorinated pools, and perfumed toilet paper can cause vaginitis, generally in the form of an allergic or a contact dermatitis.

CLINICAL PRESENTATION AND SYMPTOMS

Typically, women present with a complaint of vaginal discharge, pruritus, irritation, odor, or, less commonly, urinary symptoms of frequency or dysuria in the absence of urinary infection (25%). The discharge is variably described as thick and white to yellow—the classic ''cottage cheese'' appearance of yeast vaginitis; profuse, watery, and green as in *Trichomonas* infection; or a thin, homogeneous, gray, malodorous discharge characteristic of bacterial vaginosis. Despite the classic descriptions of discharge in each of the various infections, there

is considerable overlap in the clinical presentation of each entity. Accurate diagnosis requires the performance of additional office procedures and the appropriate use and interpretation of laboratory results.

The evaluation of a patient with suspected vaginitis should include a careful abdominal examination that checks for pelvic tenderness that might indicate pelvic inflammatory disease and for costovertebral angle tenderness that indicates urinary tract infection. The speculum examination should first evaluate the cervix to determine whether the source of discharge is cervical or vaginal. If the discharge appears to be cervical, chlamydial and gonococcal cultures should be obtained. A vaginal discharge should be cultured for yeast and trichomonads if cultures are available. Next, the pH should be determined, and normal saline and potassium hydroxide wet mounts obtained. If the wet preparations are clearly diagnostic, cultures may not be required. They are useful, however, in the patient without a clear diagnosis at the time of the visit (Fig. 44–1).

INFECTIOUS CAUSES

Candidal Vulvovaginitis

Most adult women have at least one episode of candidal vaginitis, and for some women, these infections are a recurring problem. The majority of candidal infections (80%) are due to *Candida albicans.* Other *Candida* species, including *glabrata* and *tropicalis* account for the remainder. Asymptomatic colonization is reported to occur in up to 15 to 20% of women. The strain types recovered from symptomatic and asymptomatic women are similar. It is unclear whether damage to the vaginal mucosa is required to produce infection. Both filamentous and budding forms of yeast are found in vaginal infections, although filamentous forms appear more likely to be associated with invasion. There is normally a balance between lactobacilli and *Candida* with each providing factors necessary for the other's growth.

Predisposing Factors

An increase in glycogen production is felt to predispose to yeast infections. Diabetes and nondiabetic glycosuria are associated with such an increase, as are increased levels of estrogen, such as occur in pregnancy and in women on high-dose formulations of the oral contraceptive. Estrogens enhance the ability of *Candida* to adhere to vaginal epithelial cells. *Candida* has been shown to

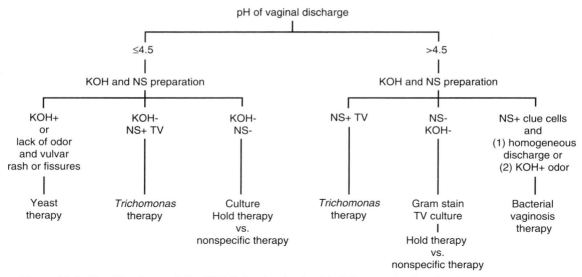

Figure 44–1. Algorithm for vaginitis. KOH, Potassium hydroxide; NS, normal saline; TV, *Trichomonas* vaginitis.

have a receptor for female reproductive hormones, which facilitate yeast mycelial formation and thus virulence. Decreased T-cell immunity during pregnancy also increases the likelihood of yeast vaginitis, especially in the last trimester. T cells normally inhibit *Candida* proliferation and germination. Newer, low-dose estrogen oral contraceptives have not always been shown to increase the occurrence of yeast vaginitis. Corticosteroids predispose to yeast infections through their effects on T-cell immunity.

Broad-spectrum antibiotics, particularly ampicillin, tetracyclines, metronidazole, and the cephalosporins predispose to vaginal yeast infections by eradicating normal flora and perhaps by a direct stimulatory effect on *Candida* growth kinetics. Normal flora, particularly the lactobacillus, elaborate bacteriocins that inhibit yeast proliferation and germination. The daily intake of 8 ounces of lactobacillus acidophilus–containing yogurt has been shown to decrease *Candida* colonization and vaginitis.

Recurrent Disease

Some women who have chronic and recurrent yeast vaginitis do not have any of these predisposing factors. A number of theories have been postulated to account for their infections. An acquired *Candida* antigen-specific cutaneous anergy has been described in which there is reduced T-lymphocyte reactivity to *Candida* antigen, which permits *Candida* proliferation and germination. This is thought to account for 40 to 70% of recurrent candidal vaginitis.

Many women report a stress-induced vaginitis. This susceptibility in ovulating women has been postulated to result from the binding of β-endorphin to macrophages, increasing production of prostaglandin E_2, which stimulates *Candida* germination. *Candida* has been found to have "opiate-like" receptors as well as the receptors that react with steroid hormones.

It has long been noted that many women acquire yeast infections just before menstruation. The late luteal phase just before menstruation has been shown to have the lowest levels of cell-mediated immunity to *C. albicans* and to subsequently permit germination of yeast. This is mediated by progesterone; estrogen has no effect. Women with higher progesterone levels or whose macrophages are highly sensitive to progesterone-induced immunosuppression are felt to have increased susceptibility.

It is also unclear how much of "recurrent" infection is actual relapse as opposed to reinfection. Although the results of vaginal cultures at the completion of therapy are generally negative, repeat cultures at 30 days have been found to produce positive results with identical strains to the prior positive culture. This seems to result from a failure to eradicate all yeast from the vagina and implies that small numbers of yeast persist that are able to reestablish infection at a later time. Trends toward shorter courses of therapy may result in inadequate eradication of the organism.

Dietary features have been postulated as an etiology of recurrent yeast vaginitis, particularly those with high dietary sucrose and artificial sweeteners that lead to high levels of urine sugars.

There is no conclusive evidence that diet plays a role in promoting recurrent vaginal yeast infections.

A persistent intestinal reservoir of *Candida* has been postulated in which the perianal area provides a source of vaginal reinfection. Simultaneously positive vaginal and rectal cultures with identical strains have been found in some studies. However, long-term oral nystatin therapy has not been shown to decrease vaginal reinfection. The overall importance of an intestinal reservoir in recurrent yeast vaginitis is probably slight.

A shift in pathogens has also been postulated. Some studies have shown an increase in the number of non–*C. albicans* pathogens, especially *C. glabrata* and *C. tropicalis,* from roughly 10% of infections in the 1970s to 20% in the 1980s. Shortened courses of therapy are felt to have selected for fungi that are not as sensitive to the imidazoles, including *C. glabrata* and *C. tropicalis.* However, other studies have not confirmed this observation.

Sexual transmission of yeast has also been an area of controversy. Asymptomatic penile yeast carriage has been described in 5 to 25% of male partners of symptomatic women with vaginal yeast infection. Identical strains have been found in the majority of sexual partners. Clearly, yeast vaginitis occurs in women who are not sexually active, and the contribution of sexual transmission is probably not substantial.

Factors that influence the virulence of candidal infections are not well understood. Adherence to vaginal epithelial cells is greater for *C. albicans* than for *C. tropicalis,* and this may explain why more clinical infection is seen with the former organism. Adherence to epithelial cells is also increased in germinating cells that are more virulent. Although the symptoms of vaginal yeast infection are not strictly related to the number of organisms, the majority of women with symptomatic yeast infection have large numbers of yeast present, as well as evidence of germination.

Not all symptoms of candidal vaginitis are necessarily due to infection. An irritative or hypersensitivity phenomenon may also be important. The candidal vaginitis with prominent secretions may be more of a hypersensitivity reaction, whereas the vulvitis may be an invasive form of the infection. Anti-*Candida* IgE has been found in the vaginal washes of 18 to 20% of patients with recurrent vaginitis, suggesting an immediate hypersensitivity response localized to the vagina. Exposure to *Candida* results in increased production of prostaglandin E_2, which transiently inhibits cell-mediated immunity, increasing the susceptibility to candidal vaginitis. An allergic reaction to components of the partner's semen has also been de-

scribed for coitus-related recurrent vaginitis. This reaction has been reported to lessen with the use of condoms.

As recurrent yeast vaginitis can be a marker for immune deficiency, any woman with recurring or difficult to treat vaginitis must be evaluated for human immunodeficiency virus infection. Recurrent candidal vaginitis has been recognized as an early feature of acquired immunodeficiency syndrome in women, often appearing before other diagnoses that define this syndrome.

Diagnosis

Elements of the history and physical examination can be helpful in reaching a diagnosis. Of particular interest is the recent use of broad-spectrum antibiotics, pregnancy, or the use of oral contraceptives, especially if they contain high levels of estrogen. The presence of pruritus or a vulvar rash, fissures, and a lack of odor to the discharge are all suggestive of a diagnosis of yeast vaginitis, particularly in the presence of a pH less that 4.5. The potassium hydroxide wet preparation should be obtained with a large amount of discharge to facilitate the finding of hyphae (Fig. 44–2). Presumptive hyphae on wet mount, particularly in the setting of clinical features suggestive of yeast, is highly predictive of yeast. The lack of hyphae in the presence of budding yeast can suggest *C. glabrata.* Culture can be helpful if the wet mount is not diagnostic of yeast, which occurs in 20 to 30% of cases.

Treatment

For initial treatment of women with occasional yeast vaginitis, there are many options. Over-the-

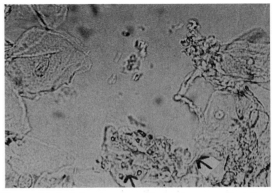

Figure 44–2. Fully developed, acute mycotic infection. Note the many buds *(arrow)* and white blood cells and the occasional mycelia *(arrow)*. (From Jovanovic R, Congema E, Nguyen HT. Antifungal agents vs. boric acid for treating chronic mycotic vulvovaginitis. J Reprod Med 1991; 36:595.)

counter treatments include miconazole (Monistat) and clotrimazole (Gyne-Lotrimin). These agents should generally be used as initial therapy in a patient with an uncomplicated yeast infection. Patients should not treat themselves without medical guidance unless they have had a prior documented yeast infection with exact replication of symptoms.

The location of infection may be helpful in determining the mode of therapy. For patients with more of a vulvitis, the topical cream forms may be more effective, whereas for patients with more of a discharge and vaginitis, the tablets may be more acceptable and have a higher cure rate. Boric acid vaginal suppositories are also effective when used twice a day for 14 days. Gentian violet can be effective, but many patients find this treatment unacceptable. There is also a considerable rate of severe allergic reaction. Terconazole (Terazol) has had a higher cure rate in some studies, probably because of increased occurrence of *C. glabrata.* One-dose oral regimens have been described, including fluconazole, 150 mg.

For chronic or recurrent candidal infection, it is important to consider predisposing factors that may contribute to infection. Although many diabetic patients have recurring yeast vaginitis, oral glucose tolerance tests are seldom helpful in explaining frequent vaginitis in women who are not clearly diabetic and should not be ordered routinely. Discontinuation of oral contraceptives is effective for many women in decreasing the frequency of yeast vaginitis. Evaluation of clothing, eliminating nylon and tight-fitting garments, can also be helpful. Encouraging daily intake of lactobacillus acidophilus–containing yogurt can decrease the colonization of *Candida* and the incidence of candidal vaginitis. For women with a history of yeast infections recurrently complicating a course of antibiotic therapy, prophylactic yeast therapy should be advised. This is generally an over-the-counter agent used nightly on days 1 and 3, or longer, depending on the time course of antibiotic treatment.

When these initial measures are ineffective, longer treatment regimens are probably necessary, usually for 10 to 14 days. For women who have monthly recurrences before their menstrual period, an intravaginal candicide nightly for several days before this may be effective, such as 600 mg of boric acid, or an agent such as Aci-Jel once a month. Ketoconazole, 200 mg orally twice a day for 5 to 7 days each month, is also effective but more toxic. Persons on a regimen of ketoconazole, 100 mg orally every day for 6 months, have been shown to have only a 5% recurrence rate. This low dose is felt to have a fungistatic effect by inhibiting germination of yeast. For women who have an allergic vaginitis from *Candida,* hyposensitization with *Candida* antigen has been reported to be effective.

Bacterial Vaginosis

The pathophysiology of bacterial vaginosis is not well understood, despite the fact that this is the second most common cause of vaginitis in women and in some series the most common. Symptoms are thought to result from increased numbers of anaerobic bacteria, concomitant with a decrease in the number of lactobacilli and normal flora. A number of other organisms are also recovered including *G. vaginalis, Mycoplasma hominis,* and *Mobiluncus.* The bacteriology is complex, and the precise role of these other organisms is unclear. *G. vaginalis,* a pleomorphic gram-variable bacillus, is present in many women who have no symptoms of vaginal infection, and the presence of this organism on culture does not imply infection. Carrier rates of *Gardnerella* in some series are as high as 10 to 40% of normal women. Only in the setting of decreased numbers of lactobacilli and increased anaerobic organisms such as *Peptostreptococcus* and *Bacteroides* does the presence of *Gardnerella* signify infection.

The role of sexual transmission of bacterial vaginosis is unclear. Many studies have revealed higher rates of this infection in clinics that deal with sexually transmitted diseases. *Gardnerella,* however, has been cultured from adolescents who are not sexually active. Similar organisms have been cultured from male sexual contacts of women with bacterial vaginosis. It has also been observed that women with intrauterine devices have a higher rate of bacterial vaginosis (20% vs. 6%).

A number of complications appear to be associated with bacterial vaginosis, including pelvic inflammatory disease. Tubo-ovarian abscesses with facultative and anaerobic bacteria have been found in women with bacterial vaginosis. Women with bacterial vaginosis have higher rates of abdominal pain and adnexal tenderness on clinical examination, even when frank pelvic inflammatory disease is not present. Premature rupture of membranes, chorioamnionitis, and preterm delivery are also described with bacterial vaginosis. Women with *Bacteroides* cultured from the vagina were found to be more likely to give birth before 37 weeks of gestation and to have infants weighing less than 2500 gm. Postpartum endometritis occurs at five times the rate in women with vaginosis following cesarian section. Sixty percent of women with postpartum endometritis had organisms associated with bacterial vaginosis recovered from the endometrial cavity. Wound infection, including episiotomy, is also more common in women with bacterial vaginosis. These complications increase the importance of accurate diagnosis of bacterial vaginosis in certain clinical circumstances, including the third trimester of pregnancy and before pelvic surgery.

Diagnosis

The gold standard of diagnosis is a clinical one, requiring three of four criteria: (1) a thin homogeneous discharge, (2) a pH of 4.5 or higher, (3) an amine or fishy odor with the addition of potassium hydroxide, and (4) the presence of clue cells on microscopy. The normal saline wet mount should utilize a small amount of discharge with a large amount of saline to disperse the epithelial cells and facilitate the finding of clue cells. A clue cell is a squamous epithelial cell whose border is obscured by adherent *Gardnerella* organisms (Fig. 44–3). Because *Gardnerella* can normally be part of the

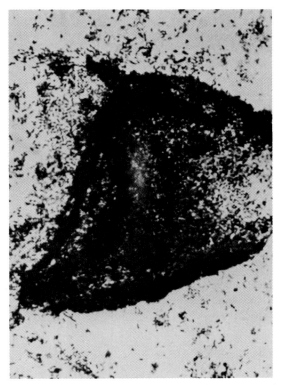

Figure 44–3. Vaginal epithelial cell with a clue cell appearance in which attachment of bacteria to the cell wall produces a loss of the cell border. (From Eschenbach DA. Bacterial vaginosis: Emphasis on upper genital tract complications. Obstet Gynecol Clin North Am 1989, 16:600. Courtesy of Sharon Hillier, PhD.)

indigenous vaginal flora, the presence of clue cells indicates greater numbers of *Gardnerella,* which is thought to be indicative of infection. The proliferation of anaerobic bacteria results in the increased production of amines, which causes the fishy odor characteristic of this discharge. This odor is intensified when 10% potassium hydroxide is added to vaginal secretions, converting the amines to a more volatile state. This is also the basis of gas-liquid chromatography of vaginal secretions to diagnose bacterial vaginosis. The discharge generally contains few white blood cells, although this is not always the case and cannot be used to exclude the diagnosis. A pH of less than 4.5, however, does virtually exclude bacterial vaginosis.

Other methods of diagnosis are currently being evaluated largely because of the clinician variability in diagnosis and the association of bacterial vaginosis with upper reproductive tract complications that makes accurate diagnosis and treatment vital. The Gram stain has been shown to have a high predictive value in identifying women with bacterial vaginosis. This appears to be better than gas-liquid chromatography, the proline aminopeptidase test or vaginal cultures in predicting infection.

The Spiegel criteria is one system that utilizes the Gram stain to diagnose bacterial vaginosis. Fewer than five lactobacillus morphotypes per high power field and five or more *Gardnerella* morphotypes with five or more other morphotypes (gram-positive cocci, small gram-negative rods, curved gram-variable rods, or fusiforms) per high power field are diagnostic of bacterial vaginosis (Fig. 44–4).

The vaginal infection and prematurity study group has developed a scoring system from 0 to 10 that allows for gradations in the severity of bacterial vaginosis, utilizing the most reliable of bacterial morphotypes to create a summary score of the alteration in vaginal flora (Table 44–1). A score of 0 to 3 represents normal flora, 4 to 6 is indeterminate, and 7 to 10 indicates bacterial vaginosis.

In summary, a diagnosis of bacterial vaginosis can be made by the presence of three of four of the criteria previously noted or by Gram stain utilizing the Spiegel criteria. The vaginal infection and premature study group scoring system may also be helpful in making more standardized diagnostic criteria. Gas-liquid chromatography, the proline aminopeptidase test, and vaginal cultures are less helpful in making a diagnosis.

Treatment

Treatment consists of metronidazole, 500 mg orally twice a day for 7 days. More recent regi-

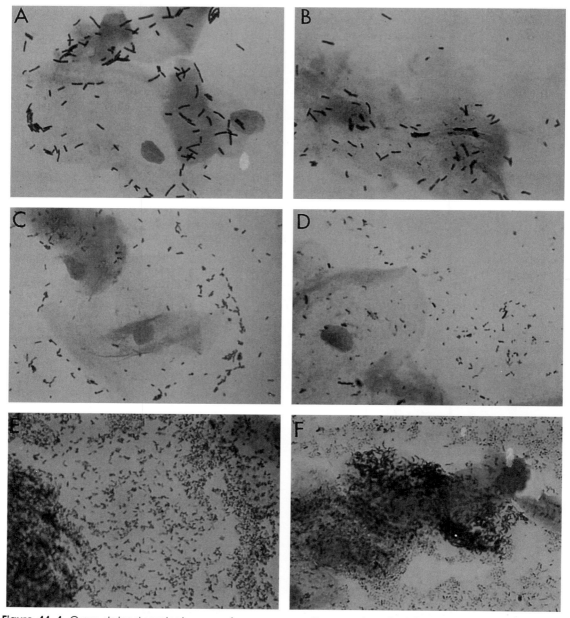

Figure 44–4. Gram-stained vaginal smears from women with normal vaginal flora (*A* and *B*), intermediate vaginal flora (*C* and *D*), or bacterial vaginosis (*E* and *F*). *A*, The 4+ lactobacillus morphotypes, no small gram-negative or gram-variable rods (score = 0); *B*, 3+ lactobacillus morphotypes, 1+ *Gardnerella* spp. morphotypes (score = 2); *C*, 3+ lactobacillus morphotypes and 3+ small gram-variable rods (score = 6); *D*, 2+ lactobacillus morphotypes and 4+ small gram-negative and -variable rods (score = 6); *E*, no lactobacilli and 4+ gram-negative and -variable rods (score = 8); note the margin of clue cells on the left; *F*, no lactobacilli and 4+ gram-negative rods and curved rods (score = 10); note the *Mobiluncus* spp. morphotypes on the clue cell (center of field). (From Nugent RP, Krohn MA, Hillier SL. Reliability of diagnosing bacterial vaginosis is improved by a standardized method of Gram stain interpretation. J Clin Microbiol 1991; 29:299.)

mens have consisted of 2 gm orally on days 1 and 3, which results in lower rates of secondary yeast infection, with cure rates of 80 to 90%. Metronidazole vaginal gel 0.75% twice a day for 5 days is also available and has the advantage of fewer systemic reactions, although the efficacy is not as well established. Other regimens include clindamycin, 300 mg orally twice a day for 7 days, and clinda-

TABLE 44–1. Scoring System (0 to 10) for Gram-Stained Vaginal Smears*

SCORE†	LACTOBACILLUS MORPHOTYPES	*GARDNERELLA* AND *BACTEROIDES* SPP. MORPHOTYPES	CURVED GRAM-VARIABLE RODS
0	4+	0	0
1	3+	1+	1+ or 2+
2	2+	2+	3+ or 4+
3	1+	3+	
4	0	4+	

*Morphotypes are scored as the average number seen per oil immersion field. Note that less weight is given to curved gram-variable rods. Total score = lactobacilli + *G. vaginalis* and *Bacteroides* spp. + curved rods.

†0, No morphotypes present; 1, <1 morphotype present; 2, 1 to 4 morphotypes present; 3, 5 to 30 morphotypes present; 4, 30 or more morphotypes present.

From Nugent RP, Krohn MA, Hillier SL. Reliability of diagnosing bacterial vaginosis is improved by a standardized method of Gram stain interpretation. J Clin Microbiol 1991; 29:297.

mycin cream, 2% vaginally nightly for 7 nights. Although these may be safer regimens in women of childbearing age than metronidazole, their efficacy is not as well established. Ampicillin (500 mg four times a day for 7 days, cure rate 40–60%), doxycycline, and sulfonamide creams are not as effective in treating bacterial vaginosis. Ofloxacin, 300 mg twice a day for 7 days, has also been used for bacterial vaginosis. If women are sexually active, the partner may also be treated, although two randomized, double-blind trials have not shown a benefit from treating the sexual partner.

Trichomonas Vaginitis

Trichomonas accounts for 10 to 25% of vaginal infections, depending on the population studied, although the incidence has been declining for the past 20 years. This infection is found in higher numbers in sexually transmitted disease clinics, and risk factors for infection include cigarette smoking, lower socioeconomic status, and having a greater number of sexual partners.

The organism can be recovered from most male sexual contacts of women with the infection; however, less than 20% of men are symptomatic. The organism is a motile protozoan with four flagella, slightly larger than a leukocyte (Fig. 44–5). It is felt to be cytotoxic by the vigorous mechanical motions, which cause a variable amount of erythema of the vaginal mucosa. The characteristic ''strawberry cervix'' or intraepithelial microabscesses are infrequently seen, usually in less than 5 to 10% of patients. Virulence varies widely among the different strains. Twenty-five to 50% of

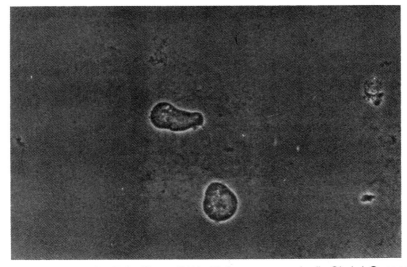

Figure 44–5. *Trichomonas vaginalis.* (From Hammill HA. *Trichomonas vaginalis.* Obstet Gynecol Clin North Am 1989; 16:532.)

women positive for *T. vaginalis* are asymptomatic. Many of these women relate symptoms, however, when asked specific questions.

Sexual infection is not the only mode of transmission. The organism can survive in tap water, chlorinated swimming pools, and hot tubs. When recurrent infection is a problem, these modes of spread should be considered.

This organism is also associated with complications, including pelvic inflammatory disease. The motility of the organism is felt to facilitate the movement of microorganisms from the vagina to the fallopian tubes, acting as a vector for pelvic infection. It has also been associated with premature rupture of membranes in pregnancy and neonatal respiratory tract infection. Because of the association of *Trichomonas* infection with smoking and low socioeconomic status, it is difficult to determine the impact of *T. vaginalis* infection in adverse pregnancy outcome, including preterm labor and low birth weight infants.

Diagnosis

The symptomatic patient usually describes a copious amount of discharge, which on nitrous paper has a very alkaline pH, usually 6 to 7, and many white blood cells. The diagnosis can be made by viewing the organism on a normal saline wet mount 65 to 75% of the time and is the most cost-effective mode of diagnosis. Although a Papanicolaou smear can suggest *Trichomonas* infection, the diagnosis should be confirmed by wet mount or culture before treatment because of the high false positive rate. Culture is still the most sensitive diagnostic modality and is relatively inexpensive. Many laboratories, however, do not offer *Trichomonas* cultures. With the increasing incidence of metronidazole resistance, cultures may become more standard. A polymerase chain reaction–based test is also being evaluated for the diagnosis of *Trichomonas* infection, as well as a direct fluorescent antibody test and enzyme immunoassay. The organism has been found to coexist with a number of other infections, including gonococcal infection and bacterial vaginosis. It has not been found with concurrent yeast infection.

Treatment

Treatment consists of metronidazole, 500 mg orally twice a day for 7 days or 2 gm orally in a single dose. This results in a cure rate of 86 to 97%. The Centers for Disease Control and Prevention recommends treating the sexual partner at the time of diagnosis. Metronidazole can be given in

pregnancy after 20 weeks of gestation in a 500 mg dose twice daily for 3 to 5 days.

Although there are resistant strains, it is generally a relative resistance, and higher doses of metronidazole are associated with cure, such as 750 mg four times a day for 6 to 10 days. Highly resistant infection with *Trichomonas* has been reported. A combination of vaginal metronidazole, 250 mg a day for 5 days, given concurrently with oral metronidazole therapy has been effective. Intravenous metronidazole regimens have also been used. Hypertonic saline (20%) can relieve symptoms, but this should not be used in pregnancy because of the danger of premature rupture of membranes. Intravaginal nonoxynol 9 has also relieved symptoms but seldom results in cure. Although treatment in pregnancy is somewhat controversial, invasive technologies such as chorionic villus sampling, in vitro fertilization, and cerclage placement may require preprocedure therapy to avoid procedure-related infection and complications.

Group B Streptococcus

Group B streptococci are found more frequently in women with intrauterine devices and during the first half of the menstrual cycle. The organism was isolated from 18% of college women and from 23% of pregnant women screened in an inner city population. Generally this organism is not felt to cause symptoms and does not require therapy except in pregnancy. Eradication of the organism in pregnancy, however, has been difficult. It is best treated at the time of delivery. This results in adequate neonatal prevention of complications associated with group B streptococcus.

Staphylococcus aureus

S. aureus is also found more frequently during menstruation in women and has been implicated in toxic shock (see Chapter 47). The organism does not cause symptoms of vaginitis, and does not require treatment for this purpose.

Gram-Negative Rods

Not infrequently vaginal cultures yield a gram-negative rod. This most commonly occurs in the setting of barrier contraceptives and in postmenopausal women as an overgrowth phenomena. Treatment consists of a povidone-iodine (Betadine) douche, which is available without a prescription, given nightly on days 1 and 3.

NONINFECTIOUS CAUSES

Atrophic Vaginitis

In postmenopausal women, atrophic vaginitis can be a frequently overlooked cause of discomfort. Women complain of either a dry sensation or a watery discharge and occasionally of slight spotting or bleeding. Other frequent symptoms include pruritus, burning, irritation, a feeling of pressure and dyspareunia. The vaginal mucosa appears thinned, smooth, and light pink to almost white. The diagnosis can also be made from routine Papanicolaou smears. Atrophic vaginitis is easily treated with either oral or topical estrogen therapy, such as Premarin cream, 1 gm vaginally at night one or two times a week. If estrogen therapy is contraindicated, a vaginal acidifier or lubricant such as Aci-Jel or Replens may be helpful.

A milder form of this problem occurs after delivery and during lactation and results from the relative estrogen deficiency. This can also be seen in patients with eating disorders or athletic amenorrhea and in women on low-dose oral contraceptives. Medications that can also cause similar symptoms include tamoxifen, danazol, leuprolide, and nafarelin.

Other Causes

Other causes of vaginal complaints can include the neurodermatitis of diabetes, the presence of a foreign body such as a tampon, or chemical causes such as perfumed toilet paper and deodorants. Cervicitis should also be considered in the work-up of these patients. Careful attention should be given to the appearance of the cervix and the presence of any discharge near the os to determine the site of origin. Studies of vaginitis and vaginal discharge report a 6 to 12% incidence of *Chlamydia* infection. Other important considerations include the timing in the menstrual cycle, stress, and recent sexual activity. Many women mistake normal changes in the cervical fluid during the menstrual cycle for vaginal infection. Stress can also increase the rate of vaginal desquamation, which can be mistaken for a pathologic discharge when it actually has a physiologic cause. The presence of sperm in the vagina results in an alkaline pH, which can be misleading, suggesting *Trichomonas* vaginitis or bacterial vaginosis. An improvement in symptoms followed by a recurrence of symptoms in the middle of therapy can result from an allergic response to the therapy or from destabilization of the normal vaginal flora from therapy, including a secondary yeast infection from antibiotic therapy for bacterial vaginosis. Studies of patients with clinically unconfirmed chronic vulvovaginitis have revealed a high incidence of psychiatric problems, including depression and a history of prior early traumatic sexual experiences including abuse. These issues should be explored in any patient with unconfirmed recurrent vulvovaginitis.

RECOMMENDED READING

Amsel R, Totten PA, Spiegel CA, et al. Nonspecific vaginitis: Diagnostic criteria and microbial and epidemiological associations. Am J Med 1983;74:14.

Aubaert J, Hee JS. Treatment of vaginal trichomonas: Single 2 gram compared to 7 day course. J Reprod Med 1982;27:743.

Bard DS. Trichomonas vaginalis (urogenital trichomoniasis). In: Monif GRG (ed). Infectious Diseases in Obstetrics and Gynecology. 2nd ed. Philadelphia: Harper & Row, 1982, pp 286–300.

Beard MK. Atrophic vaginitis: Can it be prevented as well as treated? Postgrad Med 1992;91:257.

Berg AO, Heidrich FE, Fihn SD, et al. Establishing the cause of genitourinary symptoms in women in a family practice. JAMA 1984;251:620.

Bleker OP, Folkertsma K, Dirks-Go SIS. Diagnostic procedures in vaginitis. Eur J Obstet Gynecol Reprod Biol 1989;31:179.

Boyer KM, Gadzala CA, Kelly PD, et al. Selective intrapartum chemoprophylaxis of neonatal group B streptococcal early onset disease: 2. Predictive value of prenatal cultures. J Infect Dis 1983;148:802.

Bump RC, Zuspan FP, Buesching WJ, et al. The prevalence, six-month persistence, and predictive values of laboratory indicators of bacterial vaginosis (nonspecific vaginitis) in asymptomatic women. Am J Obstet Gynecol 1984;150:918.

Carr PL, Thabault P, Levenson S, Friedman RH. Vaginitis in a community based practice. Society for General Internal Medicine. April, 1992. Clin Res 1992;40:554A.

Cotch MF, Pastorek JG, Nugent RP, et al. for the Vaginal Infections and Prematurity Study Group. Demographic and behavioral predictors of *Trichomonas vaginalis* infection among pregnant women. Obstet Gynecol 1991;78:1087.

Dombrowski MP, Sokol RJ, Brown WJ, et al. Intravenous therapy of metronidazole-resistant *Trichomonas vaginalis*. Obstet Gynecol 1987;69:524.

Drutz DJ. Lactobacillus prophylaxis for *Candida* vaginitis. Ann Intern Med 1992;116:419.

Elvik SL. Vaginal discharge in the prepubertal girl. J Pediatr Health Care 1990;4:181.

Eschenbach DA. Bacterial vaginosis: Emphasis on upper genital tract complications. Obstet Gynecol Clin North Am 1989;16:593.

Eschenbach DA, Hillier SL. Advances in diagnostic testing for vaginitis and cervicitis. J Reprod Med 1989;34:555.

Eschenbach DA, Hillier SL, Critchlow C, et al. Diagnosis and clinical manifestations of bacterial vaginosis. Am J Obstet Gynecol 1988;158:819.

Faro S. Bacterial vaginitis. Clin Obstet Gynecol 1991;34:582.

Friedrich EG. Vaginitis. Am J Obstet Gynecol 1985;152:247.

Hagar WD, Brown ST, Kraus SJ, et al. Metronidazole for vaginal trichomonas. JAMA 1980;1219:244.

Hammill HA. Normal vaginal flora in relation to vaginitis. Obstet Gynecol Clin North Am 1989;16:329.

Hammill HA. *Trichomonas vaginalis.* Obstet Gynecol Clin North Am 1989;16:531.

Hill LVH, Embil JA. Vaginitis: Current microbiologic and clinical concepts. Can Med Assoc J 1986;134:321.

Hilton E, Isenberg HD, Alperstein P, et al. Ingestion of yogurt containing lactobacillus acidophilus as prophylaxis for candidal vaginitis. Ann Intern Med 1992;116:353.

Horowitz BJ, Giaquinta D, Ito S. Evolving pathogens in vulvovaginal candidiasis: Implications for patient care. J Clin Pharmacol 1992;32:248.

Hurley R. Recurrent *Candida* infection. Clin Obstet Gynaecol 1981;8:209.

Jerve F, Berdal TB, Bohman P, et al. Metronidazole in the treatment of non-specific vaginitis (NSV). Br J Vener Dis 1984;60:171.

Jovanovich R, Congema E, Nguyen HT. Antifungal agents vs. boric acid for treating chronic mycotic vulvovaginitis. J Reprod Med 1991;36:593.

Kalo-Klein A, Witkin SS. *Candida albicans* and cellular immune system interactions during different stages of the menstrual cycle. Am J Obstet Gynecol 1989;161:1132.

Kent HL. Epidemiology of vaginitis. Am J Obstet Gynecol 1991;165:1168.

Krohn MA, Hillier SL, Eschenbach DA. Comparison of methods for diagnosing bacterial vaginosis among pregnant women. J Clin Microbiol 1992;27:1266.

Livengood CH, Lossick JG. Resolution of resistant vaginal trichomoniasis associated with the use of intravaginal nonoxynol 9. Obstet Gynecol 1991;78:954.

Losick JG, Kent HL. Trichomoniasis: Trends in diagnosis and management. Am J Obstet Gynecol 1991;165:1217.

Monif GRG. Classification and pathogenesis of vulvovaginal candidiasis. Am J Obstet Gynecol 1985;152:935.

Nugent RP, Krohn MA, Hillier SL. Reliability of diagnosing bacterial vaginosis is improved by a standardized method of Gram stain interpretation. J Clin Microbiol 1991;29:297.

O'Connor MI, Sobel JD. Epidemiology of recurrent vulvovaginal candidiasis: Identification and strain differentiation of *Candida albicans.* J Infect Dis 1986;154:358.

Rhoads JL, Wright C, Redfield RR, Burke DS. Chronic vaginal

candidiasis in women with human immunodeficiency virus infection. JAMA 1987;257:3105.

Rigg D, Miller MM, Metzger WJ. Recurrent allergic vulvovaginitis: Treatment with *Candida albicans* allergen immunotherapy. Am J Obstet Gynecol 1990;162:332.

Riley DE, Roberts MC, Takayama T, Krieger JN. Development of a polymerase chain reaction-based diagnosis of *Trichomonas vaginalis.* J Clin Microbiol 1992;30:465.

Roy S. Nonbarrier contraceptives and vaginitis and vaginosis. Am J Obstet Gynecol 1991;165:1240.

Schaaf VM, Perez-Stable EJ, Borchardt K. The limited value of symptoms and signs in the diagnosis of vaginal infections. Arch Intern Med 1990;150:1929.

Sobel JD. Recurrent vulvovaginal candidosis. What we know and what we don't. Ann Intern Med 1984;101:390.

Sobel JD. Epidemiology and pathogenesis of recurrent vulvovaginal candidiasis. Am J Obstet Gynecol 1985;152:924.

Sobel JD. Recurrent vulvovaginal candidiasis. A prospective study of the efficacy of maintenance ketoconazole therapy. N Engl J Med 1986;315:1455.

Sobel JD. Pathophysiology of vulvovaginal candidiasis. J Reprod Med 1989;34(8 Suppl):S572.

Sobel JD. Pathogenesis and treatment of recurrent vulvovaginal candidiasis. Clin Infect Dis 1992;14(suppl 1):S148.

Spiegel CA, Amsel R, Eschenbach D, et al. Anaerobic bacteria in nonspecific vaginitis. N Engl J Med 1980;303:601.

Spiegel CA, Amsel R, Holmes KK. Diagnosis of bacterial vaginosis by direct Gram stain of vaginal fluid. J Clin Microbiol 1983;18:170.

Stewart DE, Whelan CI, Fong IW, Tessler KM. Psychological aspects of chronic, clinically unconfirmed vulvovaginitis. Obstet Gynecol 1990;76:852.

Svedberg JA, Petravage JB. Vulvovaginitis: Diagnosis and management. Compr Ther 1991;17:17.

Sweet RL. Importance of differential diagnosis in acute vaginitis. Am J Obstet Gynecol 1985;152:921.

Underhill RA, Peck J. Causes of therapy failure after treatment of *T. vaginalis.* Br J Clin Pract 1974;28:134.

Witkin SS. Imunologic factors influencing susceptibility to recurrent candidal vaginitis. Clin Obstet Gynecol 1991;34:662.

Woodcock KR. Treatment of *T. vaginalis* with a single oral dose of metronidazole. Br J Vener Dis 1972;48:65.

Sexually Transmitted Diseases

Howard Libman

Women are affected by a wide variety of sexually transmitted diseases (STDs) (Table 45–1). Gonorrhea and chlamydial infections produce urethritis, cervicitis, and pelvic inflammatory disease (PID). Human papillomavirus (HPV) is the cause of genital warts and squamous intraepithelial neoplasia of the cervix. Syphilis is responsible for myriad systemic and mucocutaneous abnormalities. Herpes simplex virus (HSV) infection is associated with a recurrent vesicular skin eruption and molluscum contagiosum with clustered papules. Infestations with scabies and pediculosis are characterized by a pruritic dermatitis. Less common STDs, including lymphogranuloma venereum, chancroid, and donovanosis, manifest with papular or ulcerative genital lesions.

SEXUALLY TRANSMITTED DISEASES IN PRIMARY CARE

A careful and complete sexual history should be performed on all patients as part of primary care practice. An appearance of openness to discussion and sensitivity about STDs by the health care provider are generally sufficient to prompt even the reluctant patient to discuss her concerns. Questions should be asked using terminology that is understandable to the patient, and assumptions should not be made regarding sexual orientation or types of sexual activity in which the patient participates. All women who engage in or have a partner or partners who engage in unprotected sexual relationships with one or more persons should be considered at risk for STDs.

Patients diagnosed with one STD should be screened for other common sexually transmitted conditions. Regular laboratory evaluation for gonorrhea, chlamydial infection, syphilis, and human immunodeficiency virus (HIV) is recommended for women at high risk, and routine screening for these diseases should also be considered as part of prenatal care. Appropriate management of an STD includes identification, screening, and treatment of the patient and her current sexual partner or partners. Women should be cautioned about unprotected sexual relations with new partners, and the use of condoms or other appropriate barrier methods should be advocated to control the spread of STDs.[1]

GONORRHEA

Gonorrhea is caused by *Neisseria gonorrhoeae,* a gram-negative, kidney-shaped, diplococcal bacterium. The clinical spectrum of gonococcal disease in women includes asymptomatic carriage, urethritis, cervicitis, salpingitis, proctitis, pharyngitis, and disseminated infection. In 1991, there were 620,478 cases of gonorrhea reported in the United States, approximately 40% of which occurred in women.[2] The risk of male-to-female transmission during a single sexual contact has been estimated to be as high as 50%.[3]

Symptoms and Signs

The incubation period of gonococcal infection averages 3 to 5 days, with a range of 1 to 14 days. Although the majority of women with gonorrhea present with symptoms, asymptomatic or minimally symptomatic disease is also common.[4] Urethritis in women manifests as dysuria and frequency. Purulent discharge is sometimes elicited on palpation of the urethra or Bartholin's glands. Cervicitis may be asymptomatic or associated with vaginal spotting or increased vaginal discharge. On physical examination, purulent drainage is often visible from the cervical os.

Abdominal pain, which occurs in 10 to 20% of

463

TABLE 45–1.   Sexually Transmitted Diseases in Women

INFECTION	CLINICAL SYNDROME
Gonorrhea	Urethritis, cervicitis, pelvic inflammatory disease
Chlamydia or *Ureaplasma*	Urethritis, cervicitis, pelvic inflammatory disease
Human papillomavirus	Condylomata acuminata, cervical dysplasia
Syphilis	Primary: chancre; secondary: mucocutaneous disease; tertiary: neurologic and cardiovascular disease; latent
Herpes simplex virus	Recurrent vesicular → ulcerative skin eruption
Chancroid	Ulcerative skin eruption
Lymphogranuloma venereum	Papular → ulcerative skin eruption
Donovanosis	Papular → ulcerative skin eruption
Molluscum contagiosum	Papular skin eruption
Scabies	Infestation of genital region
Pediculosis	Infestation of genital region
Trichomoniasis*	Urethritis, vaginitis, cervicitis
Human immunodeficiency virus (HIV)*	Increased risk of opportunistic infections or neoplasia with advancing immunodeficiency
Hepatitis B and C viruses	Jaundice, nausea or vomiting, abdominal pain
Cytomegalovirus	Infectious mononucleosis syndrome

*Discussed elsewhere in text. See Chapter 44 for trichomoniasis and Chapters 40, 48, and 49 for HIV.

women with gonorrhea, is generally indicative of endometritis, salpingitis, or tubo-ovarian abscess formation.[5] Gonococcal PID generally develops a few days following the onset of menses.[6] The patient may appear acutely ill, and physical examination may reveal fever, uterine and adnexal tenderness, and pain on manipulation of the cervix. An adnexal mass generally indicates the presence of a tubo-ovarian abscess. Infertility resulting from fallopian tube obstruction is the most important long-term complication of PID, occurring in up to 20% of women following a single episode and in more than 50% with multiple episodes.[7] Other potential sequelae include an increased risk of recurrent PID, ectopic pregnancy, and chronic abdominal pain secondary to adhesions.[5]

Acute perihepatitis (Fitz-Hugh–Curtis syndrome), manifesting as right upper quadrant pain, may occur through spread of infection from the fallopian tube to the liver capsule.[8] Pharyngeal and anorectal infections, affecting 40% and 10 to 20%, respectively, of women with gonorrhea, are only sometimes symptomatic. Gonococcal pharyngitis is usually exudative but cannot be distinguished clinically from streptococcal or viral infection. Gonococcal proctitis may manifest with tenesmus and mucopurulent rectal discharge. Disseminated gonococcal infection most often appears as migratory polyarthralgias-tenosynovitis associated with a hemorrhagic pustular eruption on the peripheral extremities.[9] If the condition is not promptly diagnosed and treated, an oligoarticular or monoarticular arthritis involving the knees, elbows, or more distal joints may evolve over several days.

Gonorrhea may be transmitted to neonates by infected mothers during pregnancy or at the time of delivery.[10] Increased risks of spontaneous abortion, premature labor, early rupture of the fetal membranes, and perinatal infant mortality have been described.[11] The most common manifestation of gonorrhea in newborns—conjunctivitis—is now largely prevented in the United States by routine topical administration of silver nitrate solution. Systemic neonatal gonococcal diseases, such as pneumonia, bacteremia, meningitis, and arthritis, are generally seen only in premature infants.[12]

Laboratory Findings

Endocervical and rectal cultures are recommended in all women with suspected gonorrhea; cultures from other sites should be obtained as indicated by the history of exposure and nature of the presenting clinical syndrome. In patients with localized gonococcal disease, Gram stain of the appropriate site may reveal polymorphonuclear leukocytes and intracellular gram-negative diplococci. A single endocervical culture has a sensitivity of 90% in women with gonococcal cervicitis.[13] Approximately 50% of patients with disseminated gonococcal infection have positive results on blood or synovial fluid cultures.[8, 9] Cultures for *N. gonorrhoeae* should be obtained on a selective medium (Thayer-Martin plate), which is placed in an enhanced carbon dioxide atmosphere (e.g., candle jar) and promptly incubated at 35 to 37°C. Results are generally available within 24 to 48 hours.

TABLE 45–2. Treatment of Common Sexually Transmitted Diseases

INFECTION	TREATMENT	ALTERNATIVE TREATMENT
Gonorrhea, localized	Ceftriaxone 125–250 mg IM × 1	Ciprofloxacin, ofloxacin, spectinomycin,* cefotaxime
Gonorrhea, disseminated	Ceftriaxone 1 gm IV q.d. × 7–10 days	Cefotaxime, ceftizoxime
Chlamydia or *Ureaplasma*	Doxycycline 100 mg p.o. b.i.d. × 7 days	Tetracycline, erythromycin, ofloxacin, azithromycin
Human papillomavirus	Topical podophyllin, trichloroacetic acid, or 5-fluorouracil, or cryotherapy	Electrocauterization, laser therapy, conventional surgery, intralesional interferon-α
Syphilis	Primary, secondary, and early latent stages: benzathine penicillin 2.4 mU IM × 1 Late latent and tertiary stages: benzathine penicillin 2.4 mU IM weekly × 3 Neurosyphilis: penicillin G 12–24 mU IV daily × 15 days	Doxycycline or tetracycline
Herpes simplex virus	Primary infection: acyclovir 400 mg p.o. t.i.d. × 7–10 days Recurrent infection: no therapy Prevention of frequent recurrences: acyclovir 400 mg p.o. b.i.d.	
Molluscum contagiosum	Curettage	Trichloroacetic acid, cryotherapy
Scabies	5% Permethrin	Lindane
Pediculosis	5% Permethrin	Lindane, pyrethrins with piperonyl butoxide

*Not effective for the treatment of pharyngitis.
IM, Intramuscularly; IV, intravenously; q.d., every day, p.o., orally; t.i.d., three times a day; b.i.d., twice a day.

Diagnosis

Gonococcal urethritis and cervicitis may be suspected on the basis of Gram stain results but should be confirmed by culture. Differential diagnosis includes infection with *Chlamydia trachomatis* or *Ureaplasma urealyticum.* Gonococcal pharyngitis and proctitis may be suspected from the history but should always be verified by culture. Pelvic inflammatory disease and disseminated gonococcal infection are generally clinical diagnoses, although in some cases *N. gonorrhoeae* may grow from cultures of the cervix, blood, or synovial fluid.

Treatment

Because of the increasing prevalence of strains of *N. gonorrhoeae* that are resistant to penicillin and tetracycline, ceftriaxone is now considered the treatment of choice for both localized and disseminated gonococcal infection (Table 45–2).[14] Patients with gonorrhea should be treated concurrently for chlamydial infection with a tetracycline or erythromycin derivative (see later discussion). Pelvic inflammatory disease, which may be gonococcal, chlamydial, or polymicrobial in origin, should be managed with either ceftriaxone or cefoxitin, or doxycycline, or clindamycin, and an aminoglycoside.

For patients who are allergic to cephalosporins, ciprofloxacin or spectinomycin are acceptable alternatives. Treatment of gonococcal infection during pregnancy consists of ceftriaxone or spectinomycin; ciprofloxacin and other fluoroquinolones are contraindicated because of teratogenic effects in laboratory animals. Sexual contacts of persons with documented gonorrhea should be empirically treated for active disease.

Follow-up Care

Patients diagnosed with gonococcal infection should have cultures performed from the involved site or sites following completion of the treatment regimen to document eradication of the pathogen. Because the rectum is a common source of relapsing infection in women, routine culture of this site has been recommended after therapy.

CHLAMYDIAL INFECTION

C. trachomatis and *U. urealyticum,* formerly known as the T strain mycoplasma, are common causes of urethritis, mucopurulent cervicitis, and PID in women. In addition, *C. trachomatis* has been implicated in the dysuria-pyuria syndrome.[15] Chlamydial proctitis and Fitz-Hugh–Curtis syndrome have also been described in women.

Because chlamydial disease is not reportable to state and federal agencies, its true incidence is unknown. However, nongonococcal urethritis has been estimated to be twice as common as gonococcal infection. Gonococcal and nongonococcal urethritis affect similar patient populations and often occur concurrently; *C. trachomatis* has been isolated from the cervix in up to 60% of women diagnosed with gonorrhea.[16] Oral contraceptive use may predispose to chlamydial infection in women.[17]

Symptoms and Signs

The incubation period for nongonococcal urethritis ranges from 7 to 21 days. As many as 70% of women with chlamydial infection are asymptomatic and have normal results on pelvic examination. Symptomatic chlamydial urethritis and cervicitis are often clinically indistinguishable from gonococcal disease. Patients present with dysuria, frequency, vaginal spotting or increased discharge, or a combination of these. On physical examination, the cervix may be inflamed and friable, and mucopurulent discharge is frequently visible emanating from the os.[18] Chlamydial proctitis manifests as rectal pain associated with mucopurulent discharge.

Pelvic inflammatory disease has been estimated to occur in more than 10% of women with chlamydial infection. The syndrome manifests in a manner similar to that of gonococcal PID, but some women with endometrial and tubal involvement may be asymptomatic or have mild symptoms.[19] Infertility, ectopic pregnancy, and chronic pelvic pain have been described as sequelae of chlamydial PID.

C. trachomatis infection in pregnancy has been correlated with premature delivery and early rupture of the membranes, although these findings have not been demonstrated in all studies.[20] Other potential complications include neonatal infection, manifested by conjunctivitis or pneumonitis, and late postpartum endometritis.[12]

Laboratory Findings

Gram stain of urethral or cervical discharge reveals polymorphonuclear leukocytes (generally $\geq$ 30/1000-power field) without intracellular bacteria. Chlamydial antigens from clinical specimens can be detected using enzyme-linked immunosorbent assay and direct immunofluorescent techniques, with results generally reported within 48 hours.[16, 21] Chlamydial cell culture, which is avail-

able in some clinical laboratories, appears more sensitive than antigen detection but is more expensive. The test is performed by staining inoculated cell cultures with iodine, Giemsa, or fluorescent antibody.

Diagnosis

A presumptive diagnosis of nongonococcal urethritis or cervicitis is made clinically in the absence of Gram stain evidence of *N. gonorrhoeae* from affected sites. Positive chlamydial antigen or culture results provide confirmation. The diagnosis of PID is made clinically; *C. trachomatis* is sometimes identified from antigen detection or culture of cervical discharge.

Treatment

The treatment of choice for nongonococcal urethritis or cervicitis is doxycycline or tetracycline (see Table 45–2).[22] Ofloxacin and azithromycin may be used as alternatives, but they are much more expensive.[23, 24] Erythromycin base should be used as alternative therapy during pregnancy, although it may be poorly tolerated; the estolate form is to be avoided because of its association with abnormal liver function tests. Tetracycline derivatives and fluoroquinolones are teratogenic and are contraindicated in pregnant women. The management of PID (see earlier discussion) should generally include an agent effective against *C. trachomatis*. Because of the high infectivity rate of chlamydial disease, sexual contacts of patients with the infection should be empirically treated.

Follow-up Care

Repeat chlamydial antigen detection or culture from the infected site should be performed in patients following completion of their course of treatment.

HUMAN PAPILLOMAVIRUS

Human papillomavirus is the cause of genital warts (condylomata acuminata). In addition, certain strains of the virus, especially types 16 and 18, have been associated with squamous intraepithelial neoplasia, a precancerous lesion of the cervix.[25]

Symptoms and Signs

The incubation period for HPV infection averages 1 to 2 months, with a range from 1 to 20 months. Genital warts are commonly asymptomatic in women. They manifest most often as single or multiple skin-colored papular lesions on the posterior introitus or labia; on pelvic examination, similar lesions may be visible on the cervix or in the vagina or perirectal region.[26, 27] Local symptoms, such as itching, burning, or pain, occur in some cases. Warts greater than 1 cm in diameter may take on a "cauliflower-like" or pedunculated appearance. Lesions may stay the same size over time, become larger, or show evidence of spontaneous remission.

There is significant evidence associating HPV infection with cervical cancer. Women with a history of genital warts are four times as likely to develop in situ carcinoma of the cervix than those without such a history.[28] Furthermore, more than 90% of cervical cancers contain deoxyribonucleic acid from HPV.[29] HIV-infected women with HPV disease appear to be at particularly high risk for the development of neoplastic lesions of the cervix.[25]

The presence of large genital warts during pregnancy may interfere with normal vaginal delivery and, if traumatized, be a source of significant bleeding.[30] Some cases of laryngeal papillomatosis in the newborn may be related to vaginal delivery in HPV-infected women.[31]

Laboratory Findings

There is no generally available serologic test for HPV infection, and the virus is not routinely cultured from affected sites. Cytology (Papanicolaou smear) results may show evidence of HPV infection in the demonstration of condylomata or cervical intraepithelial neoplasia, but the test is of relatively low sensitivity.[32] Histologic examination reveals the characteristic findings of acanthosis, koilocytosis, parakeratosis, and hyperkeratosis. Antigens to HPV can be detected in cytologic or histologic specimens using an immunoperoxidase staining technique.

Diagnosis

Diagnosis is based on the clinical appearance of lesions. The application of 3 to 5% acetic acid solution, which renders warts white in color, may be useful before pelvic examination to facilitate recognition of vaginal and cervical lesions. Differential diagnosis of genital warts includes condylomata lata, which are flat, moist, gray-appearing lesions associated with secondary syphilis. A syphilis serology test should be performed on all patients with suspected HPV infection.

Treatment

Initial treatment of genital warts consists of the application of topical agents or cryotherapy. Depending on the size and number of warts, several successive treatments may be necessary. Unfortunately, there are few controlled studies comparing the efficacy of different therapeutic methods. No matter what treatment is used, recurrences are common, but their frequency is variable over time.

Weekly administration of a 25% or 50% solution of podophyllin applied directly to the warts on the external genitalia is often effective.[33] Patients should be instructed to wash the compound off within 4 hours of application. Podofilox, which is a 0.5% solution of podophyllotoxin, is available by prescription for home use. The recommended treatment regimen is twice daily application for three consecutive days each week. Other topical agents employed in the management of condylomata include trichloroacetic acid (80–90% solution applied weekly) and 5-fluorouracil (5% cream applied daily), the latter of which appears particularly useful for the treatment of vaginal lesions.

Cryotherapy with liquid nitrogen, electrocauterization, laser therapy, or conventional surgery can also be used to treat genital warts.[34] Intralesional interferon-α has also been employed with some success but is expensive.[35] Because small amounts of podophyllin and 5-fluorouracil may be absorbed systemically, these agents should not be used during pregnancy; trichloroacetic acid, cryotherapy, and laser therapy appear to be safe treatment methods.

Follow-up Care

Infection with HPV is a chronic condition, and the relapse rate of genital warts exceeds 75%. Patients should be reexamined regularly for response to therapy and evidence of recurrence. Women with HPV infection on cervical cytologic examination should be referred for gynecologic evaluation and colposcopy. Because HPV infection is a risk factor for cervical dysplasia, women with an HPV-infected sexual partner should have a pelvic examination and a Papanicolaou smear performed at least twice per year.

SYPHILIS

In 1991, 128,569 cases of syphilis were reported in the United States.[2] Of the cases of primary and secondary syphilis, approximately 45% were diagnosed in women.

Symptoms and Signs

The incubation period ranges from 9 to 90 days, with a mean of 21 days. Syphilis is categorized as primary, secondary, latent, or tertiary. Primary syphilis manifests as single or multiple, nontender genital ulcerations with indurated borders. Lesions are most often located on the labia or in the vagina but may also be identified in the mouth or perirectal region. Nontender regional lymphadenopathy is generally present. If left untreated, primary syphilis resolves within 6 weeks.

Secondary syphilis occurs 3 to 6 weeks after the appearance of the chancre and is associated with a wide variety of clinical manifestations.[36] A generalized erythematous, maculopapular skin rash beginning on the trunk and proximal extremities and extending to involve the palms and soles is most characteristic (Fig. 45–1). Constitutional symptoms and generalized lymphadenopathy are also common. Mouth ulcerations (''mucous patches''), condylomata lata, and alopecia may occur as well. Less often, there is clinical evidence of meningitis or polyarthritis. Without treatment, the syndrome of secondary syphilis improves within several weeks but may relapse one or more times over the course of the subsequent year.

Only one third of patients infected with *Treponema pallidum* ever develop tertiary syphilis. In the immunocompetent host, a latency period follows for 10 or more years before manifestations of tertiary syphilis become evident. However, some patients with HIV infection may have more rapidly advancing disease.[37] Neurologic complications of syphilis include aseptic meningitis, posterior column disease, and dementia. Cardiovascular syphilis is manifested by aortitis or saccular aneurysm of the ascending aorta.

Congenital syphilis is the result of maternal spirochetemia associated with the early stages of the infection during pregnancy. Neonatal complications include abortion, neonatal death, congenital abnormalities, and latent infection.[12] Osteochondritis, snuffles, hepatosplenomegaly, lymphadenopathy, rash, and anemia constitute the early clinical signs of congenital syphilis.

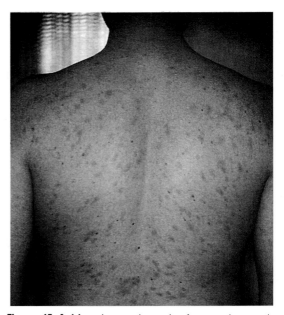

Figure 45–1. Maculopapular rash of secondary syphilis (see color section). (From Callen JP, Greer KE, Hood AF, et al. Color Atlas of Dermatology. Philadelphia: WB Saunders, 1993, p 122.)

Laboratory Findings

Serologic tests for syphilis are categorized as nontreponemal (VDRL [Venereal Disease Research Laboratories], RPR [rapid plasma reagin]) or treponemal (MHA–TP [microhemagglutination assay–*T. pallidum*], FTA-ABS [fluorescent treponemal antibody absorption]). Nontreponemal tests are sensitive but nonspecific and are used primarily for screening purposes. Positive results are reported as a titer. Treponemal tests are more specific but also more costly to perform and are used to confirm positive results on screening tests. False-positive nontreponemal test results, usually of low titer ($\leq 1:8$), occur during pregnancy and in a wide variety of acute and chronic infectious and inflammatory diseases. False-positive treponemal test results are less common. The percentage positivity of serologic tests for each of the stages of syphilis is shown in Table 45–3.

Diagnosis

The diagnosis of syphilis is suspected clinically and confirmed by serologic test results or, less commonly, by darkfield microscopy of a chancre during the primary stage. Lumbar puncture with cerebrospinal fluid analysis should be performed

TABLE 45–3. Syphilis Serologies and Stage of Disease

	STAGE OF DISEASE		
TYPE OF SEROLOGY	Primary	Secondary	Latent or Tertiary
Nontreponemal (VDRL, RPR)	70–80%	99%*	<30%†
Treponemal (MHA–TP, FTA-ABS)	65–85%	100%	95–98%

*If there is a strong clinical suspicion of secondary syphilis and nontreponemal test is nonreactive, laboratory should be requested to dilute specimen further to rule out prozone reaction.
†Includes patients who have received treatment of syphilis.
VDRL, Venereal Disease Research Laboratories; RPR, rapid plasma reagin; MHA–TP, microhemagglutination assay–*Treponema pallidum*; FTA-ABS, fluorescent treponemal antibody absorption.

in any patient who has neurologic symptoms or signs and is recommended in all individuals with late latent syphilis.[34] Differential diagnosis of genital ulcerations includes primary syphilis, HSV infection, chancroid, lymphogranuloma venereum, and donovanosis (Table 45–4). Differences in the clinical appearance and evolution of the lesions are generally sufficient to distinguish among these conditions.

Treatment

Treatment regimens for syphilis are outlined in Table 45–2. Therapy for primary, secondary, and early latent syphilis consists of benzathine penicillin, 2.4 million units intramuscularly. Therapy for late latent syphilis (>1 year duration) consists of a total of 7.2 million units of benzathine penicillin given over 3 weeks. Neurosyphilis is treated with a 2-week course of high-dose intravenous penicil-

lin G. A tetracycline derivative should be used as alternative therapy in the patient who is allergic to penicillin with primary, secondary, or latent syphilis. Recent sexual contacts of patients with active syphilitic lesions should be treated empirically for early disease.

The management of syphilis during pregnancy is essentially the same as that just described, although tetracyclines are contraindicated because of their teratogenic effects. It is recommended that patients with neurosyphilis and pregnant women with any stage of syphilis who have a history of penicillin allergy be desensitized to the drug in a hospital setting.

Follow-up Care

Patients with syphilis should be monitored monthly for clinical and serologic response to ther-

TABLE 45–4. Differential Diagnosis of Genital Ulcerations

DISEASE	CLINICAL MANIFESTATIONS	DIAGNOSTIC EVALUATION
Primary syphilis	Painless, clean-appearing ulcer with indurated border; nontender regional adenopathy	Darkfield examination; VDRL/RPR (screening) and MHA–TP, FTA-ABS (confirmatory) serologies
Herpes simplex virus infection	Painful clustered vesicles on erythematous base that evolve into shallow ulcers; tender regional adenopathy and constitutional symptoms with primary infection	Tzanck smear; culture of vesicular fluid
Chancroid	Painful ulceration with ragged edges; tender regional adenopathy	Culture
Lymphogranuloma venereum	Painless papule progressing to ulcer that heals quickly; fluctuant or necrotic regional adenopathy; constitutional symptoms present	Complement fixation or indirect fluorescence antibody titer
Donovanosis	Painless papule that progresses to granulomatous ulcer; may be associated with pseudobubos	Histology

VDRL, Venereal Disease Research Laboratories; RPR, rapid plasma reagin; MHA–TP, microhemagglutination assay–*Treponema pallidum*; FTA-ABS, fluorescent treponemal antibody absorption.

apy. Nontreponemal test results decrease in titer with effective treatment, whereas treponemal test results remain positive indefinitely. A fourfold drop in nontreponemal serologic titer, indicative of adequate therapy, should occur within 3 months in early syphilis and within 6 months in latent disease.[38] Most patients with primary, secondary, and early latent syphilis convert to a negative titer within 2 years. Some patients with late latent and tertiary syphilis may remain serofast over time at a low titer.

HERPES SIMPLEX VIRUS

Herpes simplex virus infection is a common STD manifesting as a self-limited, recurrent genital skin eruption. Herpes simplex virus type II (HSV II) is responsible for 70 to 90% of cases of herpes genitalis.

Symptoms and Signs

The incubation period for HSV infection ranges from 2 to 10 days. Up to 60% of patients with primary HSV infection are asymptomatic.[39] Symptomatic primary infection with HSV is generally associated with both constitutional and localized symptoms. There may be fever and fatigue, and physical examination reveals painful clustered vesicular lesions on an erythematous base located on the vulva or labia or in the vagina (Fig. 45–2). Less frequently, the cervix, buttocks, or perineal region may be involved. Tender regional lymphadenopathy is often present. The skin lesions usually ulcerate over a few days and then gradually crust over and heal within 3 weeks.

Recurrences can be precipitated by trauma, menstruation, or emotional or physical stress. A

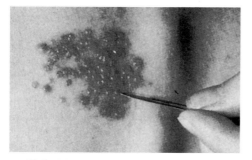

Figure 45–2. Primary herpes simplex virus (see color section). (From Lookingbill DP, Marks JG Jr. Principles of clinical diagnosis. In: Moschella SL, Hurley HJ. Dermatology. 3rd ed. Vol. 1. Philadelphia: WB Saunders, 1992, p 219.)

prodrome of local burning, itching, or tingling is common. Recurrent HSV infection manifests similarly to the primary infection, although it is less often associated with constitutional symptoms, and healing generally occurs within 10 days.[40] The frequency of recurrent disease varies from once per month to less than once per year.[41] Patients infected with HIV and other immunocompromised hosts may experience severe local recurrences or disseminated disease.

Infection with HSV II can be transmitted during pregnancy or at the time of delivery. Primary infection in a pregnant woman may result in abortion, prematurity, and disseminated neonatal disease.[42] The risk of neonatal transmission from women with asymptomatic or recurrent HSV infection appears to be significantly lower than that from women with primary infection.[43] However, the presence of active genital lesions associated with either primary or recurrent infection is considered an indication for caesarean section.[12]

Laboratory Findings

A Tzanck smear is prepared by aspirating a vesicular lesion, letting the specimen air dry, and staining it with Wright or Giemsa stain (Fig. 45–3). On microscopic examination under high power, multinucleated giant cells are diagnostic. Herpes simplex virus culture of vesicular fluid is also available in some clinical laboratories, with results available within 7 days. There is no clinically useful serologic test for HSV infection.

Diagnosis

Diagnosis of HSV infection is often made clinically. Primary infection may be confirmed by either a Tzanck smear or an HSV culture. The differential diagnosis of genital ulcer disease is described in Table 45–4.

Treatment

Oral acyclovir has been shown to increase the rate of healing and decrease the duration of viral shedding and is the treatment of choice for primary herpes genitalis (see Table 45–2).[44] The drug is given in the dose of 400 mg three times per day for 7 to 10 days. Topical acyclovir ointment is of little, if any, clinical utility. Severe cases of HSV infection in the immunocompromised host should be treated with intravenous acyclovir.

The effect of any preparation of acyclovir in the

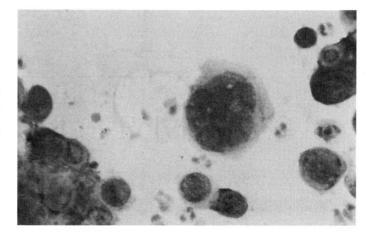

Figure 45-3. A positive Tzanck smear from herpes simplex blister (see color section). (From Callen JP, Greer KE, Hood AF, et al. Color Atlas of Dermatology. Philadelphia: WB Saunders, 1993, p 169.)

treatment of recurrent disease is less convincing. However, oral acyclovir given in reduced dosage has been shown to be effective in decreasing the frequency of recurrent disease in patients with six or more recurrences per year.[45] The drug is well tolerated, and the emergence of resistant viral strains does not appear to be a problem.[46]

Acyclovir has not been demonstrated to have any teratogenic effects. However, experience with the drug during pregnancy is limited, and it should be used in this circumstance only if there is a compelling clinical indication.

Follow-up Care

Patients should be informed that HSV infection is a chronic and recurrent condition and that the risk of transmitting the infection, although diminished when skin lesions are absent, persists in asymptomatic individuals and never disappears completely. Infrequent recurrences can be managed by the patient alone using analgesics; frequent or severe exacerbations should be brought to the attention of the health care provider.

CHANCROID

Chancroid, an ulcerative skin disease caused by the bacterium *Haemophilus ducreyi,* has increased in frequency in the United States over the past decade, with outbreaks reported in many urban areas.[47] Following an incubation period of 4 to 7 days, a painful erythematous papule becomes evident. It evolves into a pustule and subsequently ruptures to form a tender ulceration with ragged edges. Multiple ulcerations are common in

women, with lesions most often occurring on the labia and cervix and in the perianal region; autoinoculation may occur. The diagnosis of chancroid is made clinically. Gram stain is not useful, and culture is not very sensitive. Serologic studies should always be performed to rule out syphilis. Treatment consists of ceftriaxone (1 dose of 250 mg intramuscularly) or erythromycin (500 mg orally four times per day for 7 days).

LYMPHOGRANULOMA VENEREUM

Lymphogranuloma venereum is a manifestation of infection caused by a limited number of serotypes of *C. trachomatis.* The primary lesion consists of a painless papule, vesicle, or erosion that heals after a few days. This is followed by unilateral or bilateral regional lymphadenopathy that may drain cutaneously over time. An anorectal syndrome has also been described in women. The diagnosis of lymphogranuloma venereum is made clinically and is supported by a specific complement fixation test ($\geq$1:80 or fourfold rise in titer over 1 week). Treatment consists of a 2-week course of doxycycline or tetracycline. Erythromycin base should be used as an alternative during pregnancy.

DONOVANOSIS

Donovanosis, also known as granuloma inguinale, is caused by the gram-negative bacterium *Calymmatobacterium granulomatis.* It is rarely described in the United States. The primary lesion is a papule on the external genitalia that enlarges and subsequently ulcerates.[48] The diagnosis of dono-

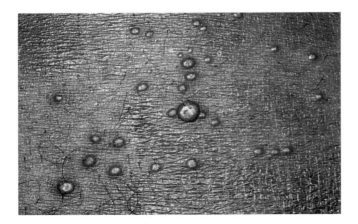

Figure 45–4. Multiple molluscum contagiosum (see color section). (From Callen JP, Greer KE, Hood AF, et al. Color Atlas of Dermatology. Philadelphia: WB Saunders, 1993, p 286.)

vanosis is made by examination of skin scrapings demonstrating histiocytes, plasma cells, and the causative organism; differential diagnosis includes primary syphilis and chancroid. Treatment consists of at least a 2-week course of tetracycline derivative or trimethoprim-sulfamethoxazole.

MOLLUSCUM CONTAGIOSUM

Molluscum contagiosum is a viral infection of the skin caused by a DNA poxvirus that is transmitted by direct body contact. The condition appears, following an incubation period of 2 to 7 weeks, as grouped 1- to 5-mm nodules with central umbilication; lesions are most often found on the genitals, thighs, and buttocks (Fig. 45–4). Diagnosis is made clinically.[49] Left untreated, skin lesions may persist from weeks to years and may spread through autoinoculation. Treatment, consisting of curettage, liquid nitrogen, or trichloroacetic acid, speeds resolution of the condition.

SCABIES

Scabies, caused by a highly contagious mite, *Sarcoptes scabiei,* manifests as an intensely pruritic dermatitis that is thought to represent a cell-mediated hypersensitivity response to the mite or its products.[50] Following an incubation period of 4 weeks, the infestation appears with intense itching, which usually increases in severity at night. Physical examination shows excoriations and small linear crusts. Common sites of involvement include the interdigital webbing of hands, wrists, axillae, waist, lower buttocks, umbilicus, feet, and ankles. Frequent washing of the affected areas or use of

topical corticosteroids may alter the clinical appearance of lesions.

Diagnosis is often presumptive; definitive diagnosis requires demonstration of burrows through the use of mineral oil or ink, or demonstration of the mite by epidermal shave biopsy. Treatment consists of topical 5% permethrin (Elimite) or 1% lindane (Kwell). Both permethrin and lindane are available as a cream, and lindane is available as a lotion. They should be applied from the neck to the toes, left on for 8 hours, and washed off thoroughly. Lindane is potentially neurotoxic and is contraindicated in pregnant and nursing women.

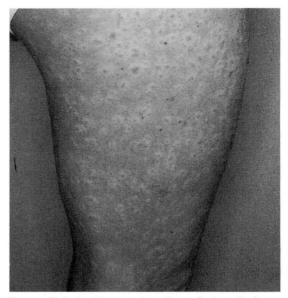

Figure 45–5. Pruritic papules. (From Callen JP, Greer KE, Hood AF, et al. Color Atlas of Dermatology. Philadelphia: WB Saunders, 1993, p 85.)

Clothes and bed linens of infected individuals should be washed in hot water, and all close personal contacts should be treated concurrently.

PEDICULOSIS

Pediculosis pubis is caused by *Phthirus pubis,* also known as the crab louse. It is transmitted principally by intimate body contact, inhabiting the genital region. Clinical manifestations include intense pruritus; excoriations from scratching; and visible adult lice, eggs (nits), or both attached to pubic hair.[50] Diagnosis is made by identification of the parasite or its eggs. Treatment consists of 1% permethrin (Nix) applied to the pubic area and left on for 10 minutes, followed by combing to remove nits. Alternative treatments include lindane (Kwell) or pyrethrins with piperonyl butoxide (RID). As with scabies, bed linens and clothing should be washed in hot water, and recent sexual contacts should be treated at the same time as the patient.

REFERENCES

1. Cates W Jr. Epidemiology and control of sexually transmitted diseases: Strategic evolution. Infect Dis Clin North Am 1987;1:1.
2. Centers for Disease Control. Summary of notifiable diseases, United States, 1991. MMWR 1992;40(53):1.
3. Thin RNT, Williams IA, Nicol CS. Direct and delayed methods of immunofluorescent diagnosis of gonorrhea in women. Br J Vener Dis 1971;47:27.
4. McCormack WM, Stumacker RJ, Johnson K, et al. Clinical spectrum of gonococcal infections in women. Lancet 1977;1:1182.
5. Holmes KK, Eschenbach DA, Knapp JS. Salpingitis: Overview of etiology and epidemiology. Am J Obstet Gynecol 1980;138:893.
6. Platt R, Rice PA, McCormack WM. Risk of acquiring gonorrhea and prevalence of abnormal adnexal findings among women recently exposed to gonorrhea. JAMA 1983;250:3205.
7. Sweet RL. Pelvic inflammatory disease and infertility in women. Infect Dis Clin North Am 1987;1:199.
8. Lopez-Zeno JA, Keith LG, Berger GS. The Fitz-Hugh–Curtis syndrome revisited: Changing perspectives after half a century. J Reprod Med 1985;30:567.
9. Holmes KK, Counts GW, Beaty HN. Disseminated gonococcal infection. Ann Intern Med 1971;74:979.
10. Gutman LT, Wilfert KM. Gonococcal disease in infants and children. Sex Transm Dis 1984;52:384.
11. Edwards LE, Barrada MI, Hamann AA, et al. Gonorrhea in pregnancy. Am J Obstet Gynecol 1978;132:637.
12. Watts DH, Eschenbach DA. Sexually transmitted diseases in pregnancy. Infect Dis Clin North Am 1987;1:253.
13. Barlow D, Phillips I. Gonorrhoea in women: Diagnostic, clinical and laboratory aspects. Lancet 1978;1:761.
14. Schwarcz SK, et al. National surveillance of antimicrobial resistance in *Neisseria gonorrhoeae:* The gonococcal isolate surveillance project. JAMA 1990;264:1413.
15. Stamm W, et al. Causes of the acute urethral syndrome in women. N Engl J Med 1980;303:409.
16. Centers for Disease Control. *Chlamydia trachomatis* infections: Policy guidelines for prevention and control. MMWR 1985;34(suppl):53.
17. Washington AE, et al. Oral contraceptives, *Chlamydia trachomatis* infection, and pelvic inflammatory disease: A word of caution. JAMA 1985;253:2246.
18. Brunham RC, et al. Mucopurulent cervicitis: The ignored counterpart of urethritis in men. N Engl J Med 1984;311:1.
19. Mardh PA, et al. *Chlamydia trachomatis* infection in patients with acute salpingitis. N Engl J Med 1977;296:1377.
20. Hillier SL, et al. A case-control study of chorioamnionic infection and chorioamnionitis in prematurity. N Engl J Med 1988;319:972.
21. Batteiger BE, Jones RB. Chlamydial infections. Infect Dis Clin North Am 1987;1:55.
22. Toomey KE, Barnes RC. Treatment of *Chlamydia trachomatis* genital infection. Rev Infect Dis 1990;12:S645.
23. Batteiger BE, Jones RB, White A. Efficacy and safety of ofloxacin in the treatment of nongonococcal sexually transmitted disease. Am J Med 1989;87(suppl 6C):75S.
24. Stamm W. Azithromycin in the treatment of uncomplicated genital chlamydial infections. Am J Med 1991;91(suppl 3A):19S.
25. Syrjanen KJ. Current concepts of human papillomavirus infections of the genital tract and their relationship to intraepithelial neoplasia and squamous cell carcinoma. Obstet Gynecol Surv 1984;39:252.
26. Chuang TY, Perry HO, Kurland LT, et al. Condyloma acuminatum in Rochester, Minnesota, 1950–78: Epidemiology and clinical features. Arch Dermatol 1984;120:469.
27. Oriel JD. Natural history of genital warts. Br J Vener Dis 1971;47:1.
28. Franchesci S, Doll R, Gallwey J, et al. Genital warts and cervical neoplasm: An epidemiological study. Br J Cancer 1983;48:621.
29. zur Hausen H. Genital papillomavirus infections. Prog Med Virol 1985;32:15.
30. Young RL, Acosta AA, Kaufman RH. The treatment of large condylomata acuminata complicating pregnancy. Obstet Gynecol 1973;41:65.
31. Mounts P, Kashima H. Association of human papillomavirus subtype and clinical course in respiratory papillomatosis. Laryngoscope 1984;94:28.
32. Lorincz AT, Temple GF, Patterson JA, et al. Correlation of cellular atypia and human papillomavirus DNA in exfoliated cells from the uterine cervix. Obstet Gynecol 1986;68:508.
33. Miller RA. Podophyllin. Int J Dermatol 1985;24:491.
34. Centers for Disease Control. 1989 Sexually transmitted disease treatment guidelines. MMWR 1989;38(suppl 8)1.
35. Eron LJ, Judson F, Tucker S, et al. Interferon therapy for condyloma acuminata. N Engl J Med 1986;315:1059.
36. Chapel TA. The signs and symptoms of secondary syphilis. Sex Trans Dis 1980;7:161.
37. Johns DR, Tierney M, Felsenstein D. Alteration in the natural history of neurosyphilis by concurrent infection with human immunodeficiency virus. N Engl J Med 1987;316:1569.
38. Brown ST, Zaidi A, Larsen SA. Serological response to syphilis treatment: A new analysis of old data. JAMA 1985;253:1296.
39. Guinan M, Wolinsky SM, Reichman RC. Epidemiology of genital herpes simplex virus infections. Epidemiol Rev 1985;7:127.
40. Guinan M, MacCalman J, Kern ER, et al. The course of untreated recurrent genital herpes simplex infections in 27 women. N Engl J Med 1981;304:759.

41. Corey L, Adams HG, Brown ZA, et al. Genital herpes simplex virus infections: Clinical manifestations, course, and complications. Ann Intern Med 1983;98:958.

42. Hutto C, Arvin A, Jacobs R, et al. Intrauterine herpes simplex virus infections. J Pediatr 1987;110:97.

43. Prober CG, Sullender WM, Yakusama LL, et al. Low risk of herpes simplex virus infections in neonates exposed to the virus at the time of vaginal delivery to mothers with recurrent genital herpes simplex virus infections. N Engl J Med 1987;316:240.

44. Bryson YJ, Dillon M, Lovett M, et al. Treatment of the first episodes of genital herpes simplex virus infection with oral acyclovir: A randomized double-blind controlled trial in normal subjects. N Engl J Med 1983;308:916.

45. Douglas JM, Critchlow C, Benedetti J, et al. A double-blind study of oral acyclovir for suppression of recurrences of genital herpes simplex virus infection. N Engl J Med 1984;310:1551.

46. Kaplowitz LG, Baker D, Gelb L, et al. Prolonged continuous acyclovir treatment of normal adults with frequently recurring genital herpes simplex virus infection: The acyclovir study group. JAMA 1991;265:747.

47. Schmid GP, Sanders LL Jr, Blount JH, et al. Chancroid in the United States; reestablishment of an old disease. JAMA 1987;258:3265.

48. Sehgal VN, Shyam-Prasad AL. Donovanosis: Current concepts. Int J Dermatol 1986;25:8.

49. Brown ST, Nalley JF, Kraus SJ. Molluscum contagiosum. Sex Transm Dis 1981;8:227.

50. Orkin M, Maibach HI. Current views of scabies and pediculosis pubis. Cutis 1984;33:85.

Pelvic Inflammatory Disease

Judith L. Steinberg and Peter A. Rice

Pelvic inflammatory disease (PID) is a cause of significant morbidity for women of childbearing years. Each year, approximately 1 million women experience an episode of symptomatic PID, costing nearly $3 billion for direct expenditure of medical services.[1] PID denotes infection of the upper genital tract including, either singly or in combination, endometritis, salpingitis, tubo-ovarian abscess, and pelvic peritonitis. Although a percentage of women are acutely symptomatic and may require hospitalization, it is the sequelae of PID that are most devastating—tubal infertility, ectopic pregnancy, chronic abdominal pain, and recurrent PID. It has become evident that what manifests as symptomatic PID is simply the tip of the iceberg and that the residua of subclinical infection detected only years later during an infertility evaluation may be especially prevalent. Therefore, it is of utmost importance to have a low threshold for the diagnosis of PID and to emphasize prevention efforts.

EPIDEMIOLOGY

Incidence and Prevalence Estimates

Pelvic inflammatory disease is not a reportable disease in the United States, and for this reason estimates of its incidence and prevalence are approximate.[2] In the 1980s, an annual mean of approximately one quarter of a million women in the United States were hospitalized for PID, with approximately two thirds of these hospitalizations attributed to acute PID and the remainder to chronic PID.[3] During the same period, women with acute PID made approximately 1.2 million visits to private physicians' offices annually; approximately a third of these represented a woman's initial visit for PID. Comparable data on the number of women treated in public clinics, emer-

gency rooms, and hospital outpatient departments in this 10-year period are not available.

Sexually active women in younger age groups have higher rates of hospitalization for acute PID but lower rates of hospitalization for chronic pelvic pain that results from acute or recurrent PID. Data regarding office visits for PID show the age distribution to be similar to that of hospitalizations for acute PID. Nonwhite women have higher average annual hospitalization rates than white women for both acute and chronic PID. Similarly, rates of office visits for PID are slightly higher for nonwhite women.[3] For acute PID, hospitalization rates are higher for women who are single, separated, or divorced than for women who are married or widowed. For both acute and chronic PID in the United States, average annual hospitalization rates are highest in the South and lowest in the Northeast, with intermediate rates in the Midwest and West.

Although office visit rates for PID appear to have remained unchanged in the decade of the 1980s compared with the previous decade,[3] hospitalization rates decreased 36%, from 3.5 to 2.2 hospitalizations per 1000 women (Fig. 46–1). A relatively smaller decrease in hospitalization rates was observed among 15 to 19 year olds (10%) compared with a 40% decrease for the 20- to 24-year-old age group, resulting in the younger age group's having the highest hospitalization rate in the late 1980s, even without adjusting for the proportion of sexually active women.[3]

Demographic and Social Indicators of Risk

Age, socioeconomic status, marital status, and rural or urban residence have been correlated with the risk of acquiring sexually transmitted diseases (STDs) (Table 46–1).[4] Age is inversely related to

475

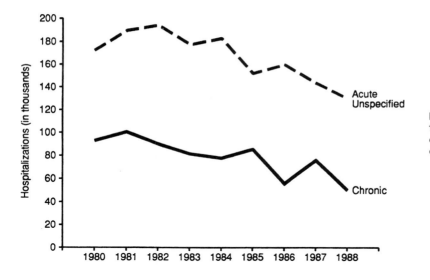

Figure 46–1. Pelvic inflammatory disease. Hospitalization among women 15–44 years of age, United States, 1980–1988.

PID rates and directly correlated with PID sequelae (e.g., tubal damage and infertility).[5] Sexually experienced teenagers are three times more likely to be diagnosed as having PID than are 25- to 29-year-old women.[6] Both biologic and behavioral characteristics of adolescents may account for these differences.[7]

Low levels of education, unemployment, and low income as measures of socioeconomic status have been associated with an increased risk of

TABLE 46–1. Specific Risk Variables Affecting Acquisition of Sexually Transmitted Diseases and Development of Pelvic Inflammatory Disease and Its Sequelae

| | PROGRESSION OF DISEASE | | |
RISK VARIABLE	Acquisition of STD	Development of PID	Development of PID Sequelae
Demographic and social indicators			
Younger age	+	+	−
Lower socioeconomic status	+	+	•
Single marital status	+	+	•
Residence, urban or rural	+	•	•
Individual behavior and practices			
Sexual behavior			
Age at first sexual intercourse	+	•	•
Number of partners	+	•	•
Frequency of sexual intercourse	+	•	•
Rate of acquiring new partners	+	•	•
Contraceptive practice			
Barrier	−	−	−
Hormonal	+	−	•
Intrauterine device	•	+	+
Health care behavior			
Evaluation of symptoms	−	−	−
Compliance with treatment instructions	−	−	−
Partner notification	−	−	−
Others			
Douching	•	+	•
Menstrual cycle (chlamydial/gonococcal infection)	+	+	•
Smoking	+	+	•
Substance abuse	+	+	•

STD, Sexually transmitted disease; PID, pelvic inflammatory disease; +, increased risk; −, decreased risk; •, no association reported. From Centers for Disease Control and Prevention. Pelvic inflammatory disease: Guidelines for prevention and management. MMWR 1991;40(RR-5):1.

developing PID.[4] Data on marital status show that women who have never married and women who are divorced or separated are at increased risk of developing PID.[4] In addition, urban residence is often suggested to be associated with an increased risk of developing PID, but no studies have compared PID rates among urban and rural populations.

Individual Behavior Practices

Sexual Behavior

Although STD-related PID results from having intercourse with an individual harboring an STD, the precise behavior, if any, in the development of PID remains unclear. Several aspects of sexual behavior, however, have been associated with an increased risk of PID. These include young age at first sexual intercourse, multiple sex partners,[8] greater frequency of sexual intercourse,[9] and increased rates of acquiring new partners within the previous 30 days.[10]

Contraceptive Practice

Contraceptive choice affects the risk of PID as well as the risk of an STD and tubal infertility (see Table 46–1). Because of complex interrelationships, precise etiologic associations are difficult to ascertain.

BARRIER METHODS. When properly used, mechanical and chemical barriers decrease the risk of STD, PID, and tubal infertility. Condoms, when used consistently and correctly throughout sexual activity, appear highly effective for reducing the risk of acquisition and transmission of STDs that cause PID,[11, 12] leading to a decreased risk of hospitalization for PID,[13] tubal pregnancy,[14] and tubal infertility.[15] Latex condoms offer greater protection against agents that cause STDs, particularly viruses, than natural membrane condoms.[16]

Vaginal spermicides also appear to decrease a woman's risk of acquiring bacterial STDs, particularly cervical infection with *Chlamydia trachomatis* and *Neisseria gonorrhoeae*.[17, 18] Use of a diaphragm appears to decrease a woman's risk of developing PID[13] and tubal infertility,[15] although its precise mechanical protective effect against PID has not been determined because most women use a spermicide with a diaphragm. Finally, the combination of a spermicide and diaphragm, as well as other combinations of barrier methods, may further decrease the risk of acquiring an STD and developing PID.[19]

ORAL CONTRACEPTIVES. Current data on the use of oral contraception and the risk of lower and upper genital tract infection and sequelae are inconsistent. Women who use oral contraceptives have an increased risk of *C. trachomatis* infection of the cervix[20] but a lower risk of developing symptomatic, clinically overt PID.[21, 22] No substantial increase or decrease in the risk of tubal infertility is noted among women using oral contraceptives.[15] Because of the questions raised by these findings, the risk of developing PID and its sequelae attributable to *C. trachomatis* among women using oral contraceptives is undetermined. Oral contraception may reduce the risk of PID that is not attributable to *C. trachomatis*.

INTRAUTERINE DEVICES. Women who use intrauterine devices are probably at increased risk of developing PID that may not be STD related.[23] Most of this increased risk occurs in the first months after insertion of an intrauterine device. Lower risks of PID have been reported with the current generation of intrauterine devices than with types used in earlier years.[24]

Health Care–Seeking Behavior

Early detection and appropriate treatment of lower genital tract disease in both women and men may reduce the incidence and severity of PID. Prompt evaluation, compliance with management instructions, and referral of sex partners are likely to decrease the risk of developing PID.[25]

Other Risk Variables

Vaginal douching, menses, cigarette smoking, and substance abuse have also been suggested as variables influencing the risk of developing PID. Data from several reports suggest that women with acute PID are more likely to have a history of douching than women without PID.[10, 26] Current data, however, do not provide sufficient information to determine whether positive associations are attributable to characteristics of the women who douche or to douching itself. Consequently, no conclusion can be reached about the precise relationship between douching and PID.

Women with chlamydial or gonococcal salpingitis have experienced onset of symptoms substantially more often within 7 days of onset of menses than at other times in the menstrual cycle.[27] For nonchlamydial, nongonococcal salpingitis, the reverse relationship has been found.[27]

In two studies examining the effect of cigarette smoking on relative risk of having PID, women who were current smokers had a twofold increased relative risk of PID.[8, 28] A dose-response relationship was observed in one study[28] but not in the other.[8] Also, alcohol and illicit drug use, particularly use of cocaine, have been associated with gonorrhea and PID.[10, 29]

PATHOPHYSIOLOGY

Microbiology

Pelvic inflammatory disease is caused by microorganisms that ascend from the lower (cervix and vagina) to the upper genital tract (uterus and fallopian tubes). These organisms can be divided into two main groups: those organisms that are transmitted during sexual intercourse, such as *C. trachomatis* and *N. gonorrhoeae* (the STD organisms), and bacterial species indigenous to the flora of the lower genital tract (endogenous organisms).[30] In young women, the majority (up to 60%) of cases of PID are caused by *C. trachomatis* and *N. gonorrhoeae.*[31] In cases of PID in which no STD organisms can be identified, microbiologic studies of specimens from the upper genital tract have resulted in isolation of a number of other bacterial species (most frequently *Streptococcus* species, *Escherichia coli,* and *Haemophilus influenzae*) and anaerobes (most frequently *Prevotella, Bacteroides* species, *Peptostreptococcus,* and *Peptococcus*).[30, 32] This observation has led to the concept of a polymicrobial etiology of PID.[32] Most often, the species distribution of non-STD isolates from the upper genital tract has been similar to that found in bacterial vaginosis. In STD-associated cases of salpingitis, a number of microbial species in addition to *C. trachomatis* or *N. gonorrhoeae* are often isolated from the fallopian tubes.

Theories of Pathogenesis

A prerequisite for ascending infection may be an infection of the columnar epithelium of the cervix by *C. trachomatis* or *N. gonorrhoeae.* However, the precise factors that determine the spread of these microorganisms or (other) vaginal flora from the lower to the upper genital tract are poorly understood. The ascent of microorganisms in most cases of PID is canalicular—that is, through the internal cervical orifice, into the endometrial cavity, through the uterotubal junction, into the fallopian tubes, and into the pelvic cavity.[30] Interruption of this route of spread, for example by ligation of the fallopian tubes, prevents salpingitis[33]; this disease is also rare in surgically sterilized women.[34] Furthermore, a continuum of infection that includes the bacterial species isolated and histopathologic evidence of infection has been demonstrated, beginning at the cervix and moving to the endometrium and finally up into the fallopian tubes in cases of salpingitis.[30]

Major barriers that protect the endometrium and the rest of the upper genital tract from *C. trachomatis* and *N. gonorrhoeae* and the vaginal flora include the endocervical canal itself and the mucous plug within the endocervix.[35] *C. trachomatis* and *N. gonorrhoeae* cause mucopurulent endocervicitis that damages the endocervical canal and results in breakdown of these barriers, permitting ascending infection.[36–39] Ascendance may also occur because of loss of the clearance mechanism normally provided by healthy ciliary epithelial cells in the cervix. Although the chlamydiae and gonococci are primary pathogens of the cervix and may cause ascending infection by themselves, the changes they cause within the endocervical canal may also allow other flora to breach this barrier and ascend to infect the endometrium and then the fallopian tubes, both of which are usually thought to be sterile. Two additional anatomic sphincter-like structures may protect the more distal upper genital tract beyond the endometrium. The uterotubal junction and the ampullo-isthmic junction may provide additional natural barriers against the movement of infectious agents from the endometrium into the fallopian tubes.

In healthy sexually active women, representative species of endogenous bacterial vaginal flora have been demonstrated in the pelvic cavity, often without evidence of ongoing infection.[40–43] Experimental observations also suggest that microorganisms may be transported upward through the genital tract, often without causing infection.[44] In an analogous fashion, passive transport of particulate matters and dyes from the vagina and cervix upward into the genital tract has been repeatedly demonstrated in healthy women at the time of ovulation and postcoitally.[45] Thus, a physiologic postcoital upward flushing of microorganisms through the genital tract may bring bacteria into the fallopian tubes.

Sexual activity is a prerequisite for the acquisition of PID. This disease is rare in celibate women.[30, 46, 47] This observation has raised questions of vector-directed mechanisms in causing upper tract infection—that is, that causative organisms could be transported upward into the genital tract by coitus-related factors such as spermatozoa or orgasmic uterine myometrial activity.[30, 45] Bacteriospermia has frequently been documented in males, and adherence of bacteria to spermatozoa has been characterized experimentally.[45] Spermatozoa with adhered microorganisms have also been shown capable of migrating through cervical secretions.[45] Another vector often discussed in this context is *Trichomonas vaginalis*. This flagellate has been demonstrated in the upper genital tract both in cases of PID and in women with no signs of salpingitis.[45] Bacteria have been shown to adhere to this organism.[45]

The anatomy and physiology of women may combine to facilitate ascendance of *C. trachomatis* and *N. gonorrhoeae* (and vaginal flora) and therefore increase the susceptibility to PID. Age is an important risk factor for the development of PID.[48, 49] Extension of the endocervical columnar epithelium outward beyond the endocervix (cervical ectopy) occurs commonly in adolescents, in whom the prevalence of PID is highest. A larger area is thus covered by columnar and squamocolumnar epithelium, and this area may be more susceptible to infection, for example infection caused by *C. trachomatis*.[50, 51] It is possible that other specific age-related changes in cervical mucus or defense mechanisms within the endocervical canal determine whether lower genital infections persist, ascend, or are cleared. During the normal menstrual cycle, changes that occur in cervical mucus may permit passage of organisms, particularly at midcycle, when estrogen levels are high and progesterone levels are relatively lower. Increased levels of progesterone, occurring after ovulation, result in more viscous and less abundant cervical mucus that may be less penetrable to bacteria (as it is to spermatozoa). In addition, the more viscous mucus acts as a plug to seal off the uterine cavity, and organisms may gain access to the uterine cavity during menses after the mucous plug has been expelled.[52] Most cases of clinically apparent chlamydial or gonococcal PID have their onset during or shortly after menstrual bleeding.[5, 53] Retrograde menstrual bleeding, which has been documented in the majority of menstruating women, may also facilitate movement of organisms into the fallopian tubes.[54] This observation, together with evidence that amenorrheic women rarely acquire salpingitis, suggests that chlamydial or gonococcal infection in the endometrium might spread via retrograde menstrual bleeding into the fallopian tubes.[5]

None of these hypotheses is unanimously agreed on, and more evidence is required before these or other proposed mechanisms of ascent of salpingitis-causing organisms are proved.

Vaginal and cervical microorganisms can be introduced above the internal cervical orifice by dilation and curettage, insertion of an intrauterine device, hysterosalpingography, intrauterine insemination, or any other procedure in which materials are passed through the cervical orifice into the uterine cavity. Acute salpingitis has developed within 6 weeks of such procedures in as many as 12% of cases.[30]

ASSESSMENT OF PATIENTS WITH SUSPECTED PELVIC INFLAMMATORY DISEASE

Clinical and Routine Laboratory Features

It is difficult to diagnose PID because its manifestation may range from asymptomatic to a surgical emergency. In recent years, silent PID, or asymptomatic disease, has become evident as infertility workups show adherent fallopian tubes in women who have no prior history of PID.[55, 56] In addition, upper genital tract disease (i.e., endometritis) frequently accompanies mucopurulent cervicitis but remains undetected for lack of signs and symptoms of classic PID.[57, 58] Laparoscopic evaluations have shown similar degrees of tubal inflammation and ultimate damage in both silent and symptomatic PID.[55] Therefore, it is essential that diagnostic schemas for PID be inclusive of a broad range of presentations, using a low threshold for the diagnosis of mild disease. Moreover, these findings underscore the need for prevention, early diagnosis, and appropriate treatment of lower genital tract infection.

Patients with PID classically present with lower abdominal or pelvic pain. Associated symptoms may include fever, abnormal vaginal discharge, menstrual irregularity, dysuria, vomiting, and proctitis symptoms. Physical examination may reveal a documented temperature exceeding 38.3°C; evidence of cervicitis; cervical, uterine, or adnexal tenderness; and a palpable adnexal mass. Laboratory analysis may show elevations in peripheral white blood cell count, erythrocyte sedimentation rate, and acute-phase reactants, such as C-reactive protein. *N. gonorrhoeae* or *C. trachomatis* or both may be detected in cervical discharge. However, individually, none of these signs and symptoms is sufficiently sensitive nor specific to establish a diagnosis of PID.[59]

Combinations of signs and symptoms are generally used to make a clinical diagnosis of PID. When such combinations have been examined, however, none has been found to be at once highly sensitive and specific.[59] For example, if the clinical criteria of lower abdominal pain, evidence of lower genital tract infection, and motion tenderness on pelvic examination (Table 46–2) are used to make a diagnosis of PID, laparoscopy confirms salpingitis in approximately 60% of patients and

TABLE 46–2. Criteria for Establishing a Clinical Diagnosis of Pelvic Inflammatory Disease

Minimal Criteria
- Lower abdominal pain*
- Adnexal tenderness
- Cervical motion tenderness

Additional Useful Criteria

Routine
- Oral temperature >38.3° C
- Abnormal cervical or vaginal discharge
- Elevated erythrocyte sedimentation rate and/or C-reactive protein
- Cervical infection with *N. gonorrhoeae* or *C. trachomatis*

Elaborate
- Histopathologic evidence on endometrial biopsy
- Tubo-ovarian abscess on sonography
- Laparoscopic abnormalities consistent with pelvic inflammatory disease

*May be absent in atypical pelvic inflammatory disease.
From Centers for Disease Control and Prevention. Pelvic inflammatory disease: Guidelines for prevention and management. MMWR 1991;40(RR-5):1.

other pelvic pathology or no other upper tract findings in the remaining 40%.[35] Other pelvic pathology might include ectopic pregnancy, appendicitis, endometriosis, hemorrhagic ovarian cyst, ovarian tumor or torsion, and mesenteric lymphadenitis. In the presence of normal findings on laparoscopic examination, PID may be limited to involvement of the endometrium only. When one or more other features are added to the diagnostic criteria—elevated erythrocyte sedimentation rate, temperature exceeding 38.3°C, and palpable adnexal mass—the specificity of a diagnosis of PID improves with a resultant loss in sensitivity (Table 46–2).[59] In fact, the sensitivity and specificity of the complete criteria are 17% and 99%, respectively.[59]

Isolation or detection of pathogens from genital tract sites can aid in the diagnosis of PID as well as reveal the microbial etiology. For example, when *N. gonorrhoeae* or *C. trachomatis* is detected at the cervix, the positive predictive value of clinical criteria increases to approximately 90%.[60]

Additional Testing

To help improve diagnostic accuracy, more elaborate testing has been suggested, including such procedures as endometrial biopsy, laparoscopy, and ultrasonography. Because identification of bacteria at the cervical level does not necessarily predict which ones will be pathogenic in the upper genital tract, potential pathogens may be more accurately identified with cultures of endometrial aspirates or biopsy samples, peritoneal fluids, and fallopian tube exudates. Of note, correlation of culture results at different sites is often variable.[61]

The criteria for diagnosis of endometritis on endometrial biopsy are based on the finding of a plasma cell infiltrate. In one study,[62] endometrial biopsy had a sensitivity and specificity of 70% and 92%, respectively, in predicting laparoscopically confirmed salpingitis. In a second study,[63] endometrial biopsy confirmed the presence of endometritis in 89% of patients given a clinical diagnosis of PID. Thus, endometrial biopsy may be a more sensitive indicator of PID than laparoscopy. These observations are in keeping with the presumed pathogenesis of the disease; laparoscopy may not identify pelvic infection that has not yet reached the fallopian tubes. The relative ease of endometrial biopsy in relation to laparoscopy is one argument for its use. It may prove particularly useful early in the course of PID, when diffuse involvement of the endometrium is more likely and sampling of the endometrium is less likely to miss an involved area.

Laparoscopy is often considered the gold standard for the diagnosis of PID. Its use increases the sensitivity and specificity of the diagnosis.[64] On laparoscopy, the tubes appear erythematous and edematous and may exude purulent or seropurulent material from the ostia. The tubes may be fixed to pelvic structures to a variable extent. In severe PID, the entire pelvis may be filled with an inflammatory mass; a tubo-ovarian abscess may be present.[30, 65] Limitations of laparoscopy as a diagnostic tool are its lack of utility in diagnosing earlier stages of PID, such as endometritis; its possible insensitivity in detecting more subtle early changes of the tubes, which are found in mild salpingitis[61, 66]; and the costs and risks of the procedure.

Pelvic ultrasonography has a role in the diagnosis and follow-up of pelvic abscesses. However, its utility in the diagnosis of PID is limited. Intravaginal ultrasonography has been examined as a noninvasive alternative to laparoscopy, sometimes in combination with endometrial biopsy.[61] The sensitivity and specificity of intravaginal ultrasonography alone or in combination have not yet been adequately determined; therefore, this technique is not recommended for routine use.

Recommendations for Diagnosis

No simple and standard algorithm can be accurately applied to the diagnosis of PID. Rather, criteria for the diagnosis of PID must be flexible so that mild disease can be detected and severe disease diagnosed accurately. First, one must consider PID in the differential diagnosis of not only lower abdominal pain but also other symptoms such as vaginal discharge and menstrual irregularity. An assessment of the severity of the illness must then be made. If the presentation is mild, then few indicators would be required to make a diagnosis of PID. The Centers for Disease Control and Prevention (CDC) recommends instituting therapy for PID when all three of the following minimal criteria for pelvic infection are met: (1) lower abdominal tenderness, (2) adnexal tenderness, and (3) cervical motion tenderness.[67] A competing diagnosis, such as ectopic pregnancy or appendicitis, should be excluded. In all cases of suspected PID, cervical specimens should be analyzed for the presence of *N. gonorrhoeae* and *C. trachomatis* (see Table 46–2).

Mild or Asymptomatic Pelvic Inflammatory Disease

In the setting of a mild presentation, PID should be diagnosed in women who have an abnormal cervical discharge and any upper tract sign, such as lower abdominal pain, cervical motion, or uterine or adnexal tenderness. The isolation of *C. trachomatis* or *N. gonorrhoeae* from the cervix would argue in favor of the diagnosis, but these results are often not known at the time of presentation. In addition, although more data are needed, a diagnosis of asymptomatic PID should be considered in women who present with an abnormal cervical discharge and menstrual irregularity in the absence of signs or symptoms, because menstrual irregularity may be suggestive of endometritis. Endometrial biopsy is not currently recommended for women with mild or asymptomatic presentations, although the utility of this procedure in diagnosis and determination of microbial cause suggests a future role.

Severe Pelvic Inflammatory Disease

In the case of a severe presentation, diagnostic criteria must be highly specific. Competing diagnoses must be accurately excluded so that appropriate management can be rapidly instituted. A diagnosis of PID would require the fulfillment of a higher number of criteria. The CDC's additional routine criteria for diagnosing PID are (1) oral temperature greater than 38.3°C, (2) abnormal cervical or vaginal discharge, (3) elevated erythrocyte sedimentation rate, (4) elevated C-reactive protein, and (5) laboratory documentation of cervical infection with *N. gonorrhoeae* or *C. trachomatis*. In addition, more elaborate and expensive tests may be required, such as endometrial biopsy, laparoscopy, or ultrasonography (Table 46–3).[67] The combination of endometrial biopsy and laparoscopy would offer the greatest sensitivity and specificity. Ultrasonography would be indicated in the evaluation and follow-up of suspected pelvic masses.

Some have argued that laparoscopy should be routine in the diagnosis of PID. In addition to its diagnostic accuracy, preliminary studies have suggested its therapeutic utility in managing complications of PID and possibly shortening hospital stays.[68–70] Others have argued that routine use of laparoscopy for patients hospitalized with presumed PID is cost effective.[71] However, the use of an invasive and expensive test in patients who are only mildly ill generally has not been advocated. Although diagnostic accuracy may be poor with clinical criteria, the risk of delayed management of a competing diagnosis is small in the setting of a mild presentation.

TREATMENT

Four principles form the basis for recommendations regarding the treatment of PID. First, the goals of treatment are both short term and long term: resolution of the acute signs and symptoms of the disease and preservation of fertility. That treatment affects fertility outcome is suggested by comparisons of post-PID fertility rates from the pre- and postantibiotic eras.[30] Swedish studies[72] have also suggested the importance of early diagnosis and treatment for improving tubal pathology. In experimental infection, tubal pathology may be adversely affected by treatment delay.[73]

Second, treatment requires broad-spectrum antibiotic therapy. As noted previously, PID is often polymicrobial in etiology; antibiotics must be directed toward not only *N. gonorrhoeae* and *C. trachomatis* but also Enterobacteriaceae, streptococci, anaerobes, and possibly *Mycoplasma*. Third, treatment is usually empirical. Therapy must be initiated before culture data are available. Moreover, culture data may not accurately or completely reflect the involved pathogens. Finally, the

TABLE 46–3. Treatment of Pelvic Inflammatory Disease: Guidelines Proposed by the Centers for Disease Control

INPATIENT TREATMENT

Regimen A

Cefoxitin, 2 gm IV every 6 hr, or cefotetan, 2 gm IV every 12 hr   *plus*   Doxycycline, 100 mg IV or PO every 12 hr

Regimen B

Clindamycin, 900 mg IV every 8 hr   *plus*   Gentamycin, loading dose IV or IM (2 mg/kg body weight) followed by a maintenance dose (1.5 mg/kg) every 8 hr

OUTPATIENT TREATMENT

Regimen A

Cefoxitin, 2 gm IM plus probenecid, 1 gm PO, in a single dose concurrently; or ceftriaxone, 250 mg IM, or other parenteral third-generation cephalosporin (e.g., ceftizoxime or cefotaxime)   *plus*   Doxycycline, 100 mg PO 2 times a day for 14 days

Regimen B

Ofloxacin, 400 mg PO 2 times a day for 14 days   *plus*   Either clindamycin, 450 mg PO 4 times a day, or metronidazole, 500 mg PO 2 times a day for 14 days

IV, Intravenously; IM, intramuscularly; PO, orally. Adapted from Centers for Disease Control and Prevention. Sexually transmitted diseases treatment guidelines. MMWR 1993;42(RR-14):75.

choice of therapy for PID must be flexible. Given its polymicrobial etiology, PID is not one disease. For example, more severe presentations and complicated PID may involve more endogenous organisms; the emphasis of therapy must then shift to target these pathogens more adequately.

The CDC's recommendations for treatment of PID[67] are provided in Table 46–3. Recommended inpatient regimens include cefoxitin or cefotetan plus doxycycline or high-dose clindamycin plus gentamycin. The former is preferred if either *C. trachomatis* or *N. gonorrhoeae* is isolated. These regimens are continued until at least 48 hours after a patient has improved; a 14-day course of therapy is completed with oral doxycycline or clindamycin. Doxycycline is preferred if *Chlamydia* is isolated. A clindamycin-containing regiman is preferable for the treatment of tubo-ovarian abscesses. The recommended outpatient regimens are (A) a single dose of cefoxitin and probenecid or ceftriaxone plus doxycycline for 14 days or (B) ofloxacin plus either clindamycin or metronidazole for 14 days.

Enterobacteriaceae and anaerobes are targeted to a greater extent by the inpatient regimen, particularly regimen B. Although not first-line therapy, gentamycin and clindamycin treat *N. gonorrhoeae* and *C. trachomatis,* respectively. The outpatient regimens place their emphasis on STD-related pathogens primarily, including penicillinase-producing and tetracycline-resistant *N. gonorrhoeae* and *C. trachomatis.* Outpatient regimen B also includes excellent treatment for endogenous anaerobic flora.

The data that support these recommendations are deficient in several respects. Although many studies have investigated PID treatment,[74–79] no study has adequately addressed efficacy of therapy in relation to the long-term goal of preservation of fertility. Studies have been limited by small sample sizes, incomplete culture data (upper tract specimens were inconsistently obtained), inadequate follow-up, and lack of precision and standardization of the diagnosis of PID and the definition of cure. Few studies systematically required laparoscopy or endometrial biopsy for diagnosis or determination of cure. Finally, minimal data on outpatient regimens are available.

According to the available studies, the two recommended inpatient regimens produce clinical and microbiologic evidence of cure in more than 90% of cases. Data are insufficient to discern the relative efficacy of the regimens. Of note, *N. gonorrhoeae* and *C. trachomatis* were adequately eradicated from the cervix by clindamycin-aminoglycoside regimens in short-term follow-up.

Outpatient regimen A was studied in 24 women with probable PID; 92% were clinically cured or improved.[80] One concern about this regimen is its questionable efficacy in the eradication of endogenous flora that produce PID. Doxycycline has poor *in vitro* activity against coliforms, *Gardnerella,* viridans streptococci, and anaerobes.[81] Furthermore, it is unlikely that a single dose of a cephalosporin would be sufficient to eradicate these organisms. Not known, however, is the clinical significance of the persistence of endogenous flora in pathologic lesions. To address this issue, the CDC added outpatient regimen B as an alternative in its 1993 treatment guidelines. Ofloxacin provides activity against *N. gonorrhoeae, C. trachomatis, Mycoplasma,* Enterobacteriaceae, and some gram-positive organisms. The addition of metronidazole or clindamycin treats the anaerobic flora. Clindamycin also adds to the gram-positive (aerobic) spectrum of the regimen. However, this regimen is significantly more expensive (three- to fivefold higher) than outpatient regimen A (ceftriaxone and doxycycline) and has not been studied in clinical trials, particularly with respect to the possibility of side effects.

Other alternative regimens that have been suggested include ampicillin or amoxicillin and a β-lactamase inhibitor, such as sulbactam or clavulanic acid. These have activity against endogenous organisms as well as penicillinase-producing *N. gonorrhoeae.* Their efficacy against *Chlamydia,* however, is questionable.[75, 82, 83] Studies of ampicillin-sulbactam or amoxicillin-clavulanic acid often in combination with doxycycline reveal clinical cure rates of greater than 90%.[75] One small study[84] suggested improved posttreatment tubal pathology with parenterally administered ampicillin-sulbactam as compared with cefoxitin (plus doxycycline if *Chlamydia* was isolated). However, this was not confirmed in a second study of ambulatory therapy.[82] In fact, this study documented a poor clinical response with both ampicillin-sulbactam and cefoxitin-doxycycline.

Other alternative regimens include metronidazole plus doxycycline, which has had variable results in clinical trials.[75, 85] This regimen fails to treat tetracycline-resistant *N. gonorrhoeae* and provides poor treatment for Enterobacteriaceae, streptococci, and *Gardnerella.* Ciprofloxacin as a single agent for the treatment of PID has resulted in high clinical cure rates in several small studies.[75, 85-87] Although ciprofloxacin provides effective treatment for *N. gonorrhoeae* and other gram-negative aerobes, it is relatively inactive against *Chlamydia* and anaerobes. Thus, as a single agent, it is unlikely to be an effective treatment of PID. A new orally administered third-generation cephalosporin, cefpodoxime, in combination with doxycyline may also prove to be an effective outpatient regimen.[81]

A controversial issue in the treatment of PID is the indication for hospitalization. Because of the potential inadequacy of an outpatient regimen and the risk of serious sequelae, some experts argue that all patients with PID require inpatient therapy. However, no data document the relative efficacy of treatment regimens on preservation of fertility, nor are dose-response data available. Based on the opinions of a panel of STD expert advisors, the CDC[67] recommends hospitalization when (1) the diagnosis is uncertain, (2) surgical emergencies

such as appendicitis or ectopic pregnancy cannot be excluded, (3) a pelvic abscess is suspected, (4) the patient is pregnant, (5) the patient is an adolescent (because compliance with therapy may be unpredictable and long-term sequelae may be particularly severe for adolescents), (6) severe illness or nausea and vomiting precludes outpatient management, (7) the patient is unable to follow or tolerate an outpatient regimen, (8) the patient has failed to respond to outpatient therapy, and (9) clinical follow-up within 72 hours of starting antibiotic treatment cannot be arranged. If outpatient therapy is chosen, careful observation is mandatory. Patients should be re-evaluated by 72 hours after the start of therapy.

An important aspect of therapy is prevention of reinfection. Thus, sex partners of women with PID should be evaluated and treated empirically for infection with *N. gonorrhoeae* and *C. trachomatis.*[67] Partners should abstain from sex until after re-evaluation at the completion of therapy. The CDC recommends a microbiologic re-examination of the lower genital tract 7 to 10 days after the completion of therapy.[67] To further evaluate for the presence of persistent infection, some STD experts recommend a second screening for *N. gonorrhoeae* and *C. trachomatis* 4 to 6 weeks after therapy.[67]

SEQUELAE

The long-term sequelae of PID are significant; these include infertility, ectopic pregnancy, chronic abdominal pain, and recurrent PID. In a large cohort study from Sweden,[88] of women who were laparoscopically diagnosed with PID, tubal infertility occurred in 11.4% after one episode. Increased age adversely affected reproductive outcome; the tubal infertility rate after one episode of PID was 19% in women age 25 to 34 years and 9% in those age 15 to 24 years (Table 46–4). Another important factor affecting fertility outcome was the laparoscopic grade of PID. For example, after one episode of PID, the tubal infertility rates were 6%, 13%, and 30% for mild, moderate, and severe disease, respectively. Other smaller studies[89-92] have found an adverse fertility outcome with complicated PID, including tubo-ovarian abscess.

The relationship between microbial cause of PID and fertility outcome has been examined in several studies. In the Swedish cohort study[88, 93] and in a smaller Canadian study,[90] better fertility outcomes were noted with gonococcal as opposed to nongonococcal PID. Data from the latter study suggested that a chlamydial cause adversely af-

TABLE 46–4.   Tubal Infertility after Laparoscopically Verified Acute Salpingitis

NUMBER OF EPISODES OF PELVIC INFLAMMATORY DISEASE	NUMBER OF WOMEN	% INFERTILE DUE TO TUBAL OCCLUSION BY AGE GROUP		
		15–24 yr*	25–34 yr*	Total 15–34 yr*
None (control subjects)	150	0	0	0
One, total	484	9.4	19.2	11.4
Mild disease		3.5†	7.8†	6.1†
Moderately severe disease		10.8†	22.0†	13.4†
Severe disease		27.3†	40.0†	30.0†
Two	163	20.9	31.0	23.1
Three or more	61	51.6	60.0	54.3

*Age at time of first episode of pelvic inflammatory disease
†Percent of those in subgroup.
From Weström L. Impact of sexually transmitted diseases on human reproduction: Swedish studies of infertility and ectopic pregnancy. In: Holmes KK, Mardha P-A, Sparling PF, et al (eds): Sexually Transmitted Diseases. 2nd ed. New York: McGraw-Hill, 1990, pp 593–614. Reproduced with permission from McGraw-Hill, Inc.

fected fertility outcome. In a small retrospective cohort study,[94] infection with *C. trachomatis* was significantly associated with involuntary infertility in women with one PID episode but not those with prior histories of PID. However, a third study[95] did not confirm differences in infertility rates based on microbial causes. Of note, many seroepidemiologic studies have implicated chlamydial infection as a factor in tubal infertility.[96–99] Prior gonococcal and mycoplasmal infections have also been implicated but may be less strongly associated with tubal occlusion than chlamydial disease.[99–101]

The kind of contraceptive used may be another factor affecting post-PID fertility outcome. In the Swedish study,[72, 95] oral contraceptive users were more likely to have mild disease and therefore improved fertility rates.

In the Swedish cohort study,[72] ectopic pregnancy occurred in 1 of 24 (4.1%) subsequent pregnancies of women with PID and 1 of 129 pregnancies of control women. Thus, a history of PID confers a seven- to tenfold increased risk of ectopic pregnancy. In addition, as with tubal infertility, seroepidemiologic studies have implicated chlamydial and gonococcal infections as risk factors for tubal pregnancies.

Chronic abdominal pain (duration >6 months) was noted in 18% of women in the Swedish cohort study and was related to the number of PID episodes.[30, 93] When women with post-PID chronic abdominal pain are evaluated laparoscopically, pelvic adhesions are usually found.

Recurrence of PID was noted in 23% of women who were monitored in the early Swedish studies.[72] However, the rate decreased to 12% after 1977 and 4% after 1980, coincident with the institution of partner notification and epidemiologic

treatment. In a small retrospective cohort study,[94] recurrent PID occurred in 43% of women. Using multivarate analysis, significant predictors of recurrent PID were initiation of sexual intercourse at a young age and longer duration of abdominal pain during the index episode of PID.

PREVENTION

Several facts argue in favor of prevention as a critical tool for the management of PID. First, even with treatment, the long-term sequelae of PID are significant. Second, the diagnosis of mild or subclinical disease is often missed and symptoms do not correlate with the degree of tubal damage. Last, the optimal treatment regimen for the preservation of fertility is not known.

Given the pathogenesis of PID, primary prevention requires prevention of lower genital tract infection. This may be accomplished by (1) abstaining from sex, (2) postponing initiation of sexual activity, (3) limiting the number of sexual partners, and (4) avoiding sex with partners who show physical signs of STDs or who are from high-risk groups.[102] In addition, barrier contraception—condoms, diaphragms, and spermicides, such as nonoxynol 9—is protective when used consistently and appropriately against the acquisition of genital tract pathogens. As mentioned earlier, the data on oral contraceptives are unclear, and precise etiologic associations are difficult to ascertain. Oral contraceptives may increase the risk for acquisition of chlamydial infection[20] yet reduce the risk of PID and the severity of tubal damage.[72, 103]

The goal of secondary prevention of PID is to prevent acscension of lower genital tract pathogens to the upper tract. This is accomplished by early detection and appropriate treatment of lower genital tract disease. In addition to improving access to care and the health care–seeking behaviors of individuals, early detection requires targeted screening of high-risk individuals because lower genital tract disease is so often asymptomatic. Screening for gonococcal and chlamydial infection is suggested for (1) women with multiple sexual partners or a new sexual partner, (2) prostitutes, (3) illicit drug users, and (4) pregnant women. In addition, screening should be routine in high-prevalence settings, such as STD clinics, adolescent or family planning clinics that serve a high proportion of adolescents, jails, and emergency rooms.[2, 102, 104]

In performing screening, it is important to know the sensitivity and specificity of the screening tests that are being used. Because of their convenience and cost, direct antigen tests are often used to screen for chlamydial infection. Although these tests are specific, they are often insensitive indicators of disease as compared with culture, because their sensitivities are limited by the numbers of organisms present in the sample obtained. This is particularly relevant in asymptomatic women being screened; because they often have low levels of infection, they may have no symptoms.[105] Unfortunately, chlamydial culture is also an imperfect gold standard with a sensitivity of approximately 65%.[106] In addition, culture is expensive, is not widely available, and may also be insensitive in asymptomatic populations or those infected with small numbers of organisms. Insensitivity of culture in these populations is a particular problem when specimens collected must be frozen or held on ice until they can be processed for culture, because these holding conditions reduce the number of viable chlamydiae.[105] Newer *Chlamydia* detection methods that use ligase or polymerase chain reaction to amplify low copy numbers of chlamydial deoxyribonucleic acid[106–108] hold great promise and should replace antigen detection and culture as these tests become more widely available commercially and diagnostic laboratories adapt and streamline this new technology.

Several issues are notable in the appropriate treatment of lower genital tract infection. First, it is impossible to distinguish gonococcal from chlamydial cervicitis by clinical findings alone. Therefore, rather than waiting for culture results, patients found to have cervicitis should be treated for both infections. Second, given the high rate of endometritis in women with cervicitis,[57, 58] some experts have advocated treating cervicitis as if it were PID, with a longer course of doxycycline.[109] Third, because bacterial vaginosis may be a risk factor for PID,[110] early recognition and treatment of this disease may be an important secondary preventive measure.

Secondary prevention also involves notification, evaluation, and treatment of sex partners of patients with STDs to prevent secondary spread of disease in the community. Female partners of patients with gonorrhea or chlamydial infection are a high-risk group; epidemiologic treatment (even before signs or symptoms of disease may be evident) provides for early treatment of presumptive lower genital tract disease. Moreover, epidemiologic treatment of sex partners of women with cervicitis or PID protects against reinfection.

Tertiary prevention involves early detection and treatment of PID to prevent long-term sequelae. As noted previously, some animal and human studies have suggested the importance of early treatment of PID in limiting tubal damage.[72, 73] However, there are no data on the effect of the recommended treatment regimens on preservation of fertility. Strategies for tertiary prevention include lowering the threshold for the diagnosis of PID so that mild or early disease will be detected and treated. In addition, patients should be informed of warning signs and symptoms so that they will seek health care at the earliest time.

REFERENCES

1. Washington AE, Katz P. Cost and payment source for pelvic inflammatory disease: Trends and projections, 1983 through 2000. JAMA 1991;266(18):2565.
2. Centers for Disease Control and Prevention (CDC). Pelvic inflammatory disease: Guidelines for prevention and management. MMWR 1991;40:(RR-5):1.
3. Rolfs RT, Galaid EL, Zaidi AA. Epidemiology of pelvic inflammatory disease: Trends in hospitalizations and office visits, 1979–1988. Joint Meeting of the Centers for Disease Control and National Institutes of Health about Pelvic Inflammatory Disease Prevention, Management, and Research in the 1990s. Bethesda, MD, September 4–5, 1990.
4. Washington AE, Aral SO, Wolner-Hanssen P, et al. Assessing risk for pelvic inflammatory disease and its sequelae. Joint Meeting of the Centers for Disease Control and National Institutes of Health about Pelvic Inflammatory Disease Prevention, Management, and Research in the 1990s. Bethesda, MD, September 4–5, 1990.
5. Cates W. Rolfs RT, Aral SO. Sexually transmitted disease, pelvic inflammatory disease, and infertility: An epidemiologic update. Epidemiol Rev 1990;12:199.
6. Bell TA, Holmes KK. Age-specific risks of syphilis, gonorrhea, and hospitalized pelvic inflammatory disease in sexually experienced U.S. women. Sex Transm Dis 1984;11:291.
7. Cates W Jr. The epidemiology and control of STD in adolescents. In: Schydlower M, Shafer M-A (eds). AIDS and the Other Sexually Transmitted Diseases. Adolescent Medicine: State of the Art Reviews. Vol 1. Philadelphia: Hanley & Belfus, 1990, pp 409–427.
8. Marchbanks PA, Lee NC, Peterson HB. Cigarette smoking as a risk factor for pelvic inflammatory disease. Am J Obstet Gynecol 1990;162:639.
9. Lee NC, Rubin GL, Borucki R. The intrauterine device and pelvic inflammatory disease revisited: New results

from the Women's Health Study. Obstet Gynecol 1988;72:1.

10. Wolner-Hanssen P, Eschenbach DA, Paavonen J, et al. Association between vaginal douching and acute pelvic inflammatory disease. JAMA 1990;263:1936.

11. Austin H, Louv WC, Alexander WJ. A case-control study of spermicides and gonorrhea. JAMA 1984;251:2822.

12. Grimes DA, Cates W. Family planning and sexually transmitted diseases. In: Holmes KK, Mardh P-A, Sparling PF, Wiesner PJ (eds). Sexually Transmitted Diseases. 2nd ed. New York: McGraw-Hill Information Services, 1990, pp 1087–1094.

13. Kelaghan J, Rubin GL, Ory HW, et al. Barrier-method contraceptives and pelvic inflammatory disease. JAMA 1982;248:184.

14. Li D-K, Daling JR, Stergachis AS, et al. Prior condom use and the risk of tubal pregnancy. Am J Public Health 1990;80:964.

15. Cramer DW, Goldman MB, Schiff I, et al. The relationship of tubal infertility to barrier method and oral contraceptive use. JAMA 1987;257:2446.

16. CDC. Condoms for prevention of sexually transmitted diseases. MMWR 1988;37:133.

17. Louv WC, Austin H, Alexander WJ, et al. A clinical trial of nonoxynol-9 for preventing gonococcal and chlamydial infections. J Infect Dis 1988;158:518.

18. Rosenberg MJ, Rojanapithayakorn W, Feldblum PJ, Higgins JE. Effect of the contraceptive sponge on chlamydial infection, gonorrhea, and candidiasis: A comparative clinical trial. JAMA 1987;257:2308.

19. Judson FN, Ehret JM, Bolin GF, et al. In vitro evaluations of condoms with and without nonoxynol-9 as physical and chemical barriers *Chlamydia trachomatis,* herpes simplex virus type 2, and human immunodeficiency virus. Sex Transm Dis 1989;16:51.

20. Washington AE, Gove S, Schachter J, Sweet RL. Oral contraceptives, *Chlamydia trachomatis* infection, and pelvic inflammatory disease: A word of caution about protection. JAMA 1985;253:2246.

21. Senanayake P, Kramer DG. Contraception and the etiology of pelvic inflammatory disease: New perspectives. Am J Obstet Gynecol 1980;138:852.

22. Wolner-Hanssen P, Eschenbach DA, Paavonen J, et al. Decreased risk of symptomatic chlamydial pelvic inflammatory disease associated with oral contraceptive use. JAMA 1990;263:54.

23. World Health Organization, Mechanisms of Action of Safety and Efficacy of Intrauterine Devices. Technical Report Series 753. Geneva, Switzerland: World Health Organization, 1987.

24. Lee NC, Rubin GL, Oreg HW, Burkman RJ. Type of intrauterine device and the risk of pelvic inflammatory disease. Obstet Gynecol 1983;62:1.

25. CDC. Study of epidemiologic methods for control of gonorrhea reinfections, Louisville, Kentucky, 1976–1981. Atlanta: U.S. Department of Health and Human Services, Public Health Service, CDC.

26. Forrest KA, Washington AE, Daling JR, Sweet RL. Vaginal douching as a possible risk factor for pelvic inflammatory disease. J Natl Med Assoc 1989;81:159.

27. Sweet RL, Blankfort-Doyle M, Robbie MO, Schachter J. The occurrence of chlamydial and gonococcal salpingitis during the menstrual cycle. JAMA 1986;255:2062.

28. Scholes D, Daling JR, Stergachis AS. Cigarette smoking and risk of pelvic inflammatory disease. Am J Epidemiol 1990;132:759.

29. Fullilove RE, Fullilove MT, Bowser BP, Gross SA. Risk of sexually transmitted disease among black adolescent crack users in Oakland and San Francisco, Calif. JAMA 1990;263:851.

30. Westrom L, Mardh P-A. Acute pelvic inflammatory disease (PID). In: Holmes KK, Mardh P-A, Sparling PF, et al. (eds). Sexually Transmitted Diseases. 2nd ed. New York: McGraw-Hill, 1990, pp 593–614.

31. Mardh P-A. An overview of infectious agents of salpingitis, their biology, and recent advances in methods of detection. Am J Obstet Gynecol 1980;138:933.

32. Eschenbach DA, Buchanan TM, Pollock HM, et al. Polymicrobial etiology of acute pelvic inflammatory disease. N Engl J Med 1975;293:166.

33. Falk HC. Interpretation of the pathogenesis of pelvic infections as determined by cornual resection. Am J Obstet Gynecol 1946;52:66.

34. Vessey M, Huggins G, Lawles M, et al. Tubal sterilization: Findings in a large prospective study. Br J Obstet Gynecol 1983;90:203.

35. Odeblad E. The functional structure of human cervical mucus. Acta Obstet Gynecol Scand 1968;47(Suppl 1):57.

36. Rees E, Tait A, Hobson D, et al. *Chlamydia* in relation to cervical infection and pelvic inflammatory disease. In: Hobson D, Holmes KK (eds). Nongonococcal urethritis and related infections. Washington, DC: American Society for Microbiology, 1977, pp 67–76.

37. Brunham RC, Paavonen J, Stevens CE, et al. Mucopurulent cervicitis: The ignored counter-part of urethritis in the male. N Engl J Med 1984;311:1.

38. Swinker ML, Young SA, Cleavenger RL, et al. Prevalence of *Chlamydia trachomatis* cervical infection in a college gynecology clinic: Relationship to other infections and clinical features. Sex Transm Dis 1988;15:133.

39. Paavonen J, Critchlow CW, DeRouen T, et al. Etiology of cervical inflammation. Am J Obstet Gynecol 1986;154:556.

40. Heinonnen PK, Teisala K, Punnonen R, et al. Anatomic sites of upper genital tract infection. Obstet Gynecol 1985;66:384.

41. Paavonen J, Teisala K, Heinonnen PK, et al. Microbiological and histopathological findings in acute pelvic inflammatory disease. Br J Obstet Gynecol 1987;94:454.

42. Weisner D, Sonntag H-G, Semm K. Bakteriologische Untersuchungen von Douglasflussigkeit. Geburtshilfe Frauenheilkd 1980;40:1118.

43. Spence MK, Branco LJ, Patel J, et al. A comparative evaluation of vaginal, cervical, and peritoneal flora in normal, healthy females. Sex Transm Dis 1982;9:37.

44. Rank RG, Sanders MM. Ascending genital tract infection as a common consequence of vaginal inoculation with the guinea pig inclusion conjunctivitis agent in normal guinea pigs. In: Bowie WR, Caldwell HD, Jones RP, et al (eds). Chlamydial Infection. Proceedings of the Seventh International Symposium in Human Chlamydial Infections. Cambridge: Cambridge University Press, 1990, pp 249–252.

45. Keith LG, Berger GS, Lopez-Zeno J. New concepts on the causation of pelvic inflammatory disease. Curr Probl Obstet Gynecol Fertil 1986;9:3.

46. Stemmer W. Ober die Ursachen von Eileiterentzundungen. Zentralbl Gynakol 1941;63:1062.

47. Falk V. Treatment of acute-tuberculous salpingitis with antibiotics alone and in combination with glucocorticoids. Acta Obstet Gynecol Scand 1965;44(Suppl 1 &6):1.

48. Westrom L, Svensson L, Wolner-Hanssen P, et al. Chlamydial and gonococcal infection in a defined population of women. Scand J Infect Dis 1982;S32:157.

49. Fredricksson B, Hagstrom B, Evaldson G, et al. *Gardnerella*-associated vaginitis and anaerobic bacteria. Gynecol Obstet Invest 1984;17:236.

50. Svensson L, Westrom L, Mardh P-A. *Chlamydia trachomatis* in women attending a gynecological outpatient

clinic with lower genital tract infection. Br J Vener Dis 1981;57:259.

51. Harrison HR, Phil D, Costin M, et al. Cervical *Chlamydia trachomatis* infection in university women: Relationship to history of contraception, ectopy and cervicitis. Am J Obstet Gynecol 1985;153:244.

52. Graney DO, Vontver LA. Anatomy and physical examination of the female genital tract. In: Holmes KK, Mardh P-A, Sparling PF, et al. (eds). Sexually Transmitted Diseases. 2nd ed. New York: McGraw-Hill, 1990, pp 105–115.

53. Westrom L. Diagnosis, etiology, and prognosis of acute salpingitis. Lund, Sweden: Studentlitteratur AB, 1976.

54. Halme J, Hammond MG, Hulka J, et al. Retrograde menstruation in healthy women and in patients with endometriosis. Obstet Gynecol 1984;64:151.

55. Patton DL, Moore DE, Spadoni LR, et al. A comparison of the fallopian tube's response to overt and silent salpingitis. Obstet Gynecol 1989;73:622.

56. Wolner-Hanssen P, Kiviat NB, Holmes KK. Atypical pelvic inflammatory disease: Subacute, chronic, or subclinical upper genital tract infection in women. In: Holmes KK, Mardh PA, Sparling PF, et al. (eds). Sexually Transmitted Diseases. 2nd ed. New York: McGraw-Hill, 1990, pp 615–616.

57. Paavonen J, Kiviat N, Brunham TC, et al. Prevalence and manifestations of endometritis among women with cervicitis. Am J Obstet Gynecol 1985;152:280.

58. Donegan SP, Page D, Greenberg M, et al. Asymptomatic acute endometritis as a complication of male to female transmission of *Neisseria gonorrhoeae* and *Chlamydia trachomatis* (Abstract 32). Eighth International Society for Sexually Transmitted Diseases Research. Copenhagen, Denmark, September 1989.

59. Kahn JG, Walker CK, Washington E, et al. Diagnosing pelvic inflammatory disease. A comprehensive analysis and considerations for developing a new model. JAMA 1991;214(18):2594.

60. Stamm WE. Measures to control *Chlamydia trachomatis* infections: An assessment of new national policy guidelines. JAMA 1986;256 (9):1178.

61. Expert Committee on Pelvic Inflammatory Disease, National Institutes of Health. Pelvic inflammatory disease. Research directions in the 1990s. Sex Transm Dis 1991;18(1):46.

62. Wasserheit JN, Bell TA, Kiviat NB, et al. Microbial causes of proven pelvic inflammatory disease and efficacy of clindamycin and tobramycin. Ann Intern Med 1986;104:187.

63. Paavonen J, Aine R, Teisala K, et al. Comparison of endometrial biopsy and peritoneal fluid cytologic testing with laparoscopy in the diagnosis of acute pelvic inflammatory disease. Am J Obstet Gynecol 1985;151:645.

64. Hadgu A, Westrom L, Brooks CA, et al. Predicting acute pelvic inflammatory disease: A multivariate analysis. Am J Obstet Gynecol 1986;155:954.

65. Hager WD, Eschenbach DA, Spence MR, Sweet RL. Criteria for diagnosis and grading of salpingitis. Obstet Gynecol 1983;61(1):113.

66. Sellors J, Mahony J, Goldsmith C, et al. The accuracy of clinical findings and laparoscopy in pelvic inflammatory disease. Am J Obstet Gynecol 1991;164:113.

67. CDC. 1993 Sexually transmitted diseases treatment guidelines. MMWR 1993;42(RR-14):75.

68. Reich H, McGlynn F. Laparoscopic treatment of tuboovarian and pelvic abscess. J Reprod Med 1987;32:747.

69. Adducci JE. Laparoscopy in the diagnosis and treatment of pelvic inflammatory disease with abscess formation. Int Surg 1981;66:359.

70. Henry-Suchet J, Soler A, Loffredo V. Laparoscopic treatment of tuboovarian abscess. J Reprod Med 1984;29:579.

71. Method MW, Urnes PD, Neahring R, et al. Economic considerations in the use of laparoscopy for diagnosing pelvic inflammatory disease. J Reprod Med 1987;32(10):759.

72. Westrom L. Pelvic inflammatory disease: Bacteriology and sequelae. Contraception 1987;36:111.

73. Swensen CE, Sung ML, Schacter J. The effect of tetracycline treatment on chlamydial salpingitis and subsequent fertility in the mouse. Sex Transm Dis 1986;13:40.

74. Brunham RC. Therapy for acute pelvic inflammatory disease (PID): A critique of recent treatment trials. Am J Obstet Gynecol 1984;148:235.

75. Peterson HB, Walker CK, Kahn JG, et al. Pelvic inflammatory disease. Key treatment issues and options. JAMA 1991;266(18):2605.

76. Peterson HB, Galaid EI, Zenilman JM. Pelvic inflammatory disease: Review of treatment options. Rev Infect Dis 1990;12(Suppl 6):S656.

77. Walters MD, Gibbs RS. A randomized comparison of gentamicin-clindamycin and cefoxitin-doxycycline in the treatment of acute pelvic inflammatory disease. Obstet Gynecol 1990;75:867.

78. Landers DV, Wolner-Hanssen P, Paavonen J, et al. Combination antimicrobial therapy in the treatment of acute pelvic inflammatory disease. Am J Obstet Gynecol 1991;164:849.

79. Soper DE, Despres B. A comparison of two antibiotic regimens for treatment of pelvic inflammatory disease. Obstet Gynecol 1988;72:7.

80. Wolner-Hanssen P, Paavonen J, Kiviat N, et al. Outpatient treatment of pelvic inflammatory disease with cefoxitin and doxycycline. Obstet Gynecol 1988;71:595.

81. Hasselquist MB, Hillier S. Susceptibility of upper-genital tract isolates from women with pelvic inflammatory disease to ampicillin, cefpodoxime, metronidazole, and doxycycline. Sex Transm Dis 1991;18(3):146.

82. Kosseim M, Ronald A, Plummer FA, et al. Treatment of acute pelvic inflammatory disease in the ambulatory setting: Trial of cefoxitin and doxycycline versus ampicillin-sulbactam. Antimicrob Agents Chemother 1991;55(8):1651.

83. Crombleholme WR, Schachter J, Grossman M, et al. Amoxicillin therapy for *Chlamydia trachomatis* in pregnancy. Obstet Gynecol 1990;75:752.

84. Bruhat MA, Le Bouedec G, Pouly JL, et al. Treatment of acute salpingitis with sulbactam/ampicillin. Int J Gynecol Obstet 1989;2(Suppl):41.

85. Heinonen PK, Teisala K, Aine R, Miettinen A. Brief report: Intravenous and oral ciprofloxacin in the treatment of proven pelvic inflammatory disease. A comparison with doxycycline and metronidazole. Am J Med 1989;87(Suppl 5A):152S.

86. Crombleholme WR, Schachter J, Ohm-Smith M, et al. Efficacy of single-agent therapy for the treatment of acute pelvic inflammatory disease with ciprofloxacin. Am J Med 1989;87(Suppl 5A):142S.

87. Thadepalli H, Mathai D, Scotti R, et al. Ciprofloxacin monotherapy for acute pelvic infections: A comparison with clindamycin plus gentamicin. Obstet Gynecol 1991;78:696.

88. Westrom L. Impact of sexually transmitted diseases on human reproduction: Swedish studies of infertility and ectopic pregnancy. In: Sexually Transmitted Diseases Status Report, NIAID Study Group, No 81-2213. Washington, DC, NIH Publications, 1980, p 43.

89. Rivlin ME. Clinical outcome following vaginal drainage of pelvic abscess. Obstet Gynecol 1983;61:169.

90. Brunham RC, Binns B, Guijon F, et al. Etiology and outcome of acute pelvic inflammatory disease. J Infect Dis 1988;158(3):510.

91. Brumsted JR, Clifford PM, Nakajima ST, Gibson M. Reproductive outcome after medical management of complicated pelvic inflammatory disease. Fertil Steril 1988;50(4):667.

92. Landers DV, Sweet RL. Tubo-ovarian abscess: Contemporary approach to management. Rev Infect Dis 1983;5:876.

93. Westrom L. Effect of acute pelvic inflammatory disease on fertility. Am J Obstet Gynecol 1975;121:707.

94. Safrin S, Schachter J, Dahrouge D, Sweet RL. Long-term sequelae of acute pelvic inflammatory disease. A retrospective cohort study. Am J Obstet Gynecol 1992;166:1300.

95. Svensson L, Mardh P-A, Westrom L. Infertility after acute salpingitis with special reference to *Chlamydia trachomatis* associated infection. Fertil Steril 1983;40:322.

96. Moore DE, Foy HM, Daling JR. Increased frequency of serum antibodies to *Chlamydia trachomatis* in infertility due to distal tubal disease. Lancet 1982;2:574.

97. Brunham RC, Maclean IW, Binns B, Peeling RW. *Chlamydia trachomatis*: Its role in tubal infertility. J Infect Dis 1985;152:127.

98. De Muylder X, Laga M, Tennstedt C, et al. The role of *Neisseria gonorrhoeae* and *Chlamydia trachomatis* in pelvic inflammatory disease and its sequelae in Zimbabwe. J Infect Dis 1990;162:501.

99. Moore DE, Cates W Jr. Sexually transmitted disease and infertility. In: Holmes KK, Mardh PA, Sparling PF, et al. (eds). Sexually Transmitted Diseases. 2nd ed. New York: McGraw-Hill, 1990, pp 763–769.

100. Moller BR, Taylor-Robinson D, Furr PM, et al. Serological evidence that chlamydiae and mycoplasmas are involved in infertility in women. J Reprod Fertil 1985;73:237.

101. Robertson JN, Ward ME, Connway D, Caul EO. Chlamydial and gonococcal antibodies in sera of infertile women with tubal obstruction. J Clin Pathol 1987;40:377.

102. Washingon AE, Cates W, Wasserheit JN. Preventing pelvic inflammatory disease. JAMA 1991;266(18):2574.

103. Wolner-Hansson P, Svensson L, Mardh P-A, Westrom L. Laparoscopic findings and contraceptive use in women with signs and symptoms suggestive of acute salpingitis. Obstet Gynecol 1988;66:233.

104. CDC. Recommendations for the Prevention and Management of *Chlamydia trachomatis* Infections, 1993. MMWR 1993;42(RR-12):22.

105. Lin JS L, Jones WE, Yan L, et al. Underdiagnosis of *Chlamydia trachomatis* infection. Diagnostic limitations in patients with low-level infection. Sex Transm Dis 1992;19(5):259.

106. Schachter J, Stamm WE, Quinn TC, et al. Ligase chain reaction to detect *Chlamydia trachomatis* infection of the uterus. J Clin Microbiol 1994; 32:2540.

107. Loeffelholz MJ, Lewinski CA, Silver SR, et al. Detection of *Chlamydia trachomatis* in endocervical specimens by polymerase chain reaction. J Clin Microbiol 1992;30: 2847.

108. Bass CA, Jungkind DL, Silverman NS, Bondi JM. Clinical evaluation of a new polymerase chain reaction assay for detection of *Chlamydia trachomatis* in endocervical specimens. J Clin Microbiol 1993;30:2648.

109. Mardh P-A. Pelvic inflammatory disease and related disorders; novel observations. Scand J Infect Dis 1990;69(Suppl):83.

110. Eschenbach DA, Hillier S, Critchlow C, et al. Diagnosis and clinical manifestations of bacterial vaginosis. Am J Obstet Gynecol 1988;158:819.

111. Handsfield H. Recent developments in STDs: II. Viral and other syndromes. Hosp Prac 1991;27(1):175.

Toxic Shock Syndrome

M. Anita Barry

Toxic shock syndrome (TSS) is an acute multisystem disorder associated with specific strains of *Staphylococcus aureus.* A similar syndrome has been described with certain streptococcal strains.[1] An association between staphylococcal TSS and menstruation has been well documented, with the majority of cases occurring in young women.

EPIDEMIOLOGY

Most reported cases of TSS in the United States have occurred in females; 93% of cases reported to the national passive surveillance system have been in women, with a peak incidence in those 15 to 19 years of age.[2] Data from an enhanced active surveillance system established in 1986 in selected geographic areas confirmed this finding; of the 116 definite and 63 probable cases identified, 85% occurred in females. Of these cases, 55% were associated with menstruation.[3] Specific risk factors for menstrual TSS identified to date include the use of tampons, particularly tampons of high absorbency.[4] The reported incidence of TSS in the United States increased in 1977 after the introduction of superabsorbency tampons and peaked in 1980. Case rates have steadily declined since, a trend believed to be at least partially related to the removal of superabsorbency tampons from the market.

Incomplete reporting of cases makes the incidence of disease difficult to determine. However, data from women members of a large prepaid health plan in California showed rates of 0.4 per 100,000 woman-years, 2.2 per 100,000 woman-years, and 1.5 per 100,000 woman-years in time periods before the introduction of superabsorbency tampons, during the period of superabsorbency product availability, and after the withdrawal of these products, respectively.[5]

The low incidence of nonmenstrual cases makes temporal trends difficult to determine.[2] In a study by Petitti and Reingold, the case rate in men remained stable at 0.1 per 100,000 despite fluctuations observed among women.[5] Nonmenstrual cases have been associated with surgical and nonsurgical wounds, with the postpartum state, and in conjunction with influenza outbreaks.[2, 6] Cases have also been reported in users of contraceptive sponges and diaphragms, but few data are available to assess risk in these groups.[3]

Recurrence of disease in untreated, menstrual TSS cases has been clearly documented. These recurrences may occur after asymptomatic menses. As many as 12 episodes in an individual have been documented.[7, 8]

PATHOGENESIS

More than 90% of menstrual TSS cases have been associated with a staphylococcal strain that produces a protein, TSS toxin 1 (TSST-1). Although TSST-1 may produce clinical findings through a direct toxic effect, a major role for endogenous mediators such as interleukin-1 seems more likely.[9] The protective effect of antibodies against TSST-1 is not clearly defined, although TSST-1 antibody was protective in one reported study of nongenital TSS.[10]

In nonmenstrual cases, TSST-1 can be isolated in only about 60% of reported cases.[11] Other enterotoxins (A through E) are likely to be playing a major part in these cases.

CLINICAL PRESENTATION

Although much of the available information on TSS is derived from severe cases, particularly those requiring hospitalization, milder forms of the syndrome are likely to occur. Diffuse multisystem involvement, often with a rapid onset, is the rule. Table 47–1 lists criteria for the Centers for Disease Control and Prevention surveillance definition.[12] Fever, hypotension, and a diffuse erythroderma are common presenting symptoms.[8, 12, 13] Multiple der-

TABLE 47–1. Centers for Disease Control and Prevention Criteria for the Diagnosis of Toxic Shock Syndrome

Fever: temperature $\geq 38.9°$ C
Hypotension: systolic blood pressure <90 mm Hg for adults, or orthostatic drop in diastolic blood pressure ≥ 15 mm Hg from lying to sitting, or orthostatic syncope
Rash: diffuse macular erythema
Desquamation of palms and soles 1 to 2 wk after onset of illness
Involvement of three or more of the following organ systems:
   Gastrointestinal: vomiting or diarrhea at onset of illness
   Muscular: severe myalgia or creatine phosphokinase $\geq 2\times$
   Lymph nodes: enlargement
   Mucous membrane hyperemia: vaginal, conjunctival, or oropharyngeal
   Renal: Blood urea nitrogen or creatinine $\geq 2\times$ ULN, or pyuria in the absence of urinary tract infection
   Hepatic: bilirubin, serum levels of glutamic-oxalacetic or -pyruvic transaminase $\geq 2\times$ ULN
   Hematologic: platelets $<100,000/mm^3$
   Central nervous system: disorientation without alterations in consciousness or focal neurologic signs
Negative results of serologic tests if obtained to Rocky Mountain spotted fever, leptospirosis, or rubeola

ULN, Unilateral lymphadenopathy.

matologic changes have been described, including a diffuse sunburn-like rash with erythema of the palms and soles early in the course of illness. A generalized erythematous, urticarial, maculopapular, pruritic rash occurring at 7 to 14 days has also been reported in more than 50% of patients.[14] Localized desquamation involving the fingers, toes, palms, and soles and generalized desquamation occur at 10 to 21 days. Mucous membrane changes include erythema and injection of the conjunctivae and mouth, tongue, pharynx, vagina, and tympanic membranes. Clinical findings in a large case series, with their respective reported frequencies, included temperature $38.9°C$ or greater (100%), rash or desquamation (100%), hypotension (100%), vomiting (89%), diarrhea (84%), mucous membrane hyperemia (91%), myalgias (94%), and disorientation (69%).[8] Common laboratory abnormalities in the same series were abnormal findings on urinalysis (88%), elevated levels of blood urea nitrogen or creatinine (52%), elevated bilirubin values (54%), thrombocytopenia (42%), and hypocalcemia (43%). In addition, the electrocardiogram may show diffuse loss of voltage, flattened T waves, and diffuse nonspecific ST-T wave changes. Metabolic acidosis, acute renal failure, hepatic failure, pulmonary edema, the adult respiratory distress syndrome, and disseminated intravascular coagulation may also occur.

Long-term sequelae have been reported to follow TSS. In a case-control study, women with TSS were matched with women hospitalized for acute appendicitis and appendectomy. Women with TSS were significantly more likely than controls to have fatigue, hair loss, nail changes, problems with concentration, reading difficulty, memory loss, emotional changes, and conditions involving joint, cardiac, muscle, and genitourinary systems.[15]

Clinical characteristics in nonmenstrual cases may differ from those in menstrual cases. In one series, nonmenstrual cases were more likely to be nosocomially acquired, to have prior antimicrobial therapy, and to have an earlier onset of fever and rash in relation to the initial symptoms. By stepwise analysis, four factors were noted to be more common among nonmenstrual cases than menstrual cases: delayed onset of TSS symptoms after precipitating injury or event, more frequent central nervous system manifestations, less frequent musculoskeletal involvement, and a higher degree of anemia. Overall mortality did not differ significantly between the two groups, with a 12.5% mortality in nonmenstrual cases compared with 4.8% in menstrual cases.[16]

DIAGNOSIS

Diagnosis of TSS is based on clinical and laboratory findings. Isolation of a TSST-1–producing *Staphylococcus* from a patient with compatible signs and symptoms supports the diagnosis. However, because normal persons may carry TSST-1–producing *Staphylococcus,* a single laboratory test does not confirm the diagnosis. For retrospective diagnosis, an increase in serum antibody to TSST-1 provides supporting evidence, but this test is not widely available.

THERAPY

Removal of potentially infected foreign bodies with drainage of infected sites is crucial. Anti-staphylococcal β-lactamase-resistant antimicrobial agents should be administered in maximal doses. Supportive therapy with administration of fluids and pressors as needed is a cornerstone of therapy. The use of steroids has been suggested, but data to support their efficacy are not available. Immune globulin preparations have also been suggested and appear to be protective in a rabbit model of TSS if given in a timely fashion.[7] However, additional data are needed.

PREVENTION

Women who develop TSS should be advised to discontinue tampon use. Little information is available on therapy for recurrent cases. Use of intravenous immune globulin for patients lacking antibody to TSST-1 and empirical use of rifampin have been suggested, but additional data are needed.[7]

REFERENCES

1. Stevens DL, Tanner MH, Winship J, et al. Severe group A streptococcal infections associated with a toxic shock-like syndrome and scarlet fever toxin A. N Engl J Med 1989;321:1.
2. Broome CV. Epidemiology of toxic shock syndrome in the United States: Overview. Rev Infect Dis 1989;11(Suppl 1):S14.
3. Gaventa S, Reingold AL, Hightower AW, et al. Active surveillance for toxic shock syndrome in the United States, 1986. Rev Infect Dis 1989;11(Suppl 1):S28.
4. Reingold AL, Broome CV, Gaventa S, et al. Risk factors for menstrual toxic shock syndrome: Results of a multi-state case-control study. Rev Infect Dis 1989;11(Suppl 1):S35.
5. Petitti DB, Reingold AL. Recent trends in the incidence of toxic shock syndrome in Northern California. Am J Public Health 1991;81:1209.
6. Centers for Disease Control and Prevention. Toxic shock syndrome following influenza—Oregon; Update on influenza activity—United States. MMWR 1987;36:64.
7. Chesney PJ. Clinical aspects and spectrum of illness of toxic shock syndrome: Overview. Rev Infect Dis 1989;11(Suppl 1):S1.
8. Davis JP, Osterholm MT, Helms CM, et al. Tristate toxic shock syndrome study. II. Clinical and laboratory findings. J Infect Dis 1982;145:441.
9. Parsonnet J. Mediators in the pathogenesis of toxic shock syndrome: Overview. Rev Infect Dis 1989;11(Suppl 1):S263.
10. Jacobson JA, Kasworm E, Daly JA. Risk of developing toxic shock syndrome associated with toxic shock syndrome toxin-1 following non-genital staphylococcal infection. Rev Infect Dis 1989;11(Suppl 1):S8.
11. Garbe PL, Arko RJ, Reingold AL, et al. *Staphylococcus aureus* isolates from patients with nonmenstrual toxic shock syndrome. JAMA 1985;253:2538.
12. Shands KN, Schmid GP, Dan BB, et al. Toxic shock syndrome in menstruating women: Association with tampon use and *Staphylococcus aureus* and clinical features in 52 cases. N Engl J Med 1980;303:1436.
13. Tofte RW, Williams DN. Clinical and laboratory manifestations of toxic shock syndrome. Ann Intern Med 1982;96(Suppl part 2):843.
14. Chesney PJ, Crass BA, Polyak MB, et al. Toxic shock syndrome: Management and long term sequelae. Ann Intern Med 1982;96:847.
15. Davis JP, Vergeront JM, Amsterdam LE, et al. Long-term effects of toxic shock syndrome in women: Sequelae, subsequent pregnancy, menstrual history, and long-term trends in catamenial product use. Rev Infect Dis 1989;11(Suppl 1):S50.
16. Kain KC, Schulzer M, Chow AW. Clinical spectrum of nonmenstrual toxic shock syndrome (TSS): Comparison with menstrual TSS by multivariate discriminant analyses. Clin Infect Dis 1993;16:100.

Acquired Immunodeficiency Syndrome in Women

48

Human Immunodeficiency Virus Infection: Epidemiology, Risk Assessment, and Testing

Elcinda L. McCrone

Since the beginning of the acquired immunodeficiency syndrome (AIDS) pandemic, more than 4 million women worldwide have been infected with the human immunodeficiency virus (HIV); 600,000 women worldwide[1] and 46,000 women in the United States[2] have AIDS. In most large central African cities and some large cities in the United States, such as New York City, AIDS has become the leading cause of death for women age 25 to 44 years.[1] Overall in the United States in 1993, AIDS became the fourth leading cause of death for women in this age group.[3] This chapter reviews the current trends in the epidemiology of HIV infection to provide a foundation on which primary care practitioners may assist efforts to improve HIV case detection, education, and prevention. An approach to HIV counseling and testing is discussed.

EPIDEMIOLOGY

Global Epidemiology

According to the World Health Organization's mid-1990s estimates, more than 10 million people worldwide are infected with HIV, approximately 6 million men and 4 million women.[4] At least 6 million of those with HIV infection are in Africa. At least 1 million persons in each of North America, South America, and Asia and 500,000 in Europe are infected. Worldwide, only about 10% of the HIV infections are acquired by injection drug

use, 10% are perinatally transmitted, and 5% are transmitted through blood products. About 75% of the HIV infections worldwide are acquired through sexual intercourse, and 80% of these are heterosexually transmitted.[4]

The global patterns of HIV infection are determined by the frequency of each mode of transmission and the time at which the HIV epidemic entered each area. These patterns are more easily conceptualized by outlining the three distinct epidemiologic patterns described by the World Health Organization in the mid-1980s.[5] Pattern I describes the epidemic in North America and Western Europe, where infection began in the late 1970s to early 1980s and affected primarily homosexual men and intravenous drug users. These areas bear only about 10 to 15% of the world's HIV burden. Pattern II areas include sub-Saharan Africa and parts of the Caribbean. Infection began in the mid-to-late 1970s and occurs predominantly in heterosexual men and women. Latin America is evolving from a pattern I area into a pattern II area and is designated as pattern I/II. In the late 1980s, infection emerged in the pattern III areas of Asia, the Middle East, Eastern Europe, and North Africa. No specific mode of transmission predominates in these pattern III areas, but some researchers have noted an increase in prevalence of infection in prostitutes and intravenous drug users. The greatest rate of rise in new HIV infections in the 1990s is occurring in Southeast Asia, particularly Thailand, which experienced a 500% increase in HIV infections in 1992, much of it associated with rapid growth of the sex trade and heroin use. Likewise, India is experiencing an expansion of HIV infection, which is already greater in magnitude than that of Thailand.

Epidemiology in the United States

As with the global AIDS epidemic, the epidemic in the United States represents a composite of many smaller epidemics in different subgroups and in different regions of the country. An increasing number of cases are being diagnosed in smaller cities and rural areas, especially in the South and Midwest. Minority women are disproportionately affected with AIDS; 72% of the women with AIDS are African American and Hispanic.

From 1981 through 1993, 360,000 adults and adolescents with AIDS have been reported to the Centers for Disease Control and Prevention (CDC).[2] A 3.5% increase in new cases was reported in 1992.[6] Nationally, transmission among homosexual and bisexual men still remains the most common means of acquisition of HIV infection (Table 48–1); however, since 1991, the number of newly diagnosed cases of AIDS in this risk category has declined. The largest proportionate increase in the number of new AIDS cases has occurred in the heterosexual transmission exposure category; this increase in heterosexual transmission has been larger in women than in men (9.8 versus 2.5%, respectively, in 1992).[6]

TABLE 48–1. Cases of Acquired Immunodeficiency Syndrome in the United States, by Exposure Category*

	% OF TOTAL CASES
Mode of Transmission	
Male sex with male	54%
Injection drug use	24%
Male/male sex and injection drug use	7%
Hemophilia	1%
Heterosexual	6%
Blood transfusion recipient	2%
Undetermined	6%
Gender	
Male	87%
Women	13%
Race/ethnicity	
White	50%
Black	32%
Hispanic	17%
Other	1%

*Total cases reported as January 1, 1994.
From Massachusetts Department of Public Health. AIDS surveillance summary. AIDS Newsletter 1994;10:1.

More than 46,000 women with AIDS have been reported to the CDC through 1993, accounting for 13% of the total AIDS cases.[2] Although in the 4-year period of 1988 to 1991 the acquisition of HIV infection by women through their own injection drug use rose steadily, by 1992, heterosexual transmission accounted for more HIV infection in women than did their own injection drug use,[6] particularly in the South, the Midwest, and the West. Regional differences are noted, however, and injection drug use still remains the predominant mode of transmission in the Northeast.

HETEROSEXUAL TRANSMISSION

In Africa, heterosexual transmission is overwhelmingly the most common source of HIV infection for both women and men. The major groups at risk for HIV infection are prostitutes, men who frequent prostitutes, and men and women with multiple sex partners.[7, 8] In contrast, heterosexual transmission accounts for only 7% of AIDS cases in the United States,[2] with more than half of the heterosexual transmission to women involved in sex with an injection drug user. The risk group of the index case does not appear to be associated with the facility of transmission between men and women.[9, 10] It has been suggested that male-to-female heterosexual transmission may occur with greater facility, perhaps enhanced by specific cofactors.

Many studies have attempted to identify potential cofactors that may facilitate heterosexual transmission. Some studies have postulated the following as potential cofactors: sex during menses,[9] cervical ectopy,[11] advanced disease in the infected partner,[9, 12, 13] and receptive anal intercourse.[9, 10, 12, 13] Sexually transmitted diseases (STDs) have inconsistently been identified as potential cofactors for transmission of HIV infection. A large European multicenter group found an increased male-to-female transmission rate with a history of *Chlamydia* infection or syphilis in either partner but no association with gonorrhea, genital warts, or genital herpes.[9] The reverse associations were found by an Italian multicenter study group in which the presence of genital warts but not syphilis correlated with an increased rate of transmission; this Italian study also did not show any correlation with genital herpes.[13] After controlling for sexual exposure, an African study found the presence of gonorrhea, *Chlamydia* infection, and *Trichomonas* infection to correlate with HIV transmission but found a much lower correlation with genital ulcers.[14]

In the United States and Western Europe, the

TABLE 48–2. Education about Human Immunodeficiency Virus Transmission and Infection

TOPICS FOR DISCUSSION	POINTS OF EMPHASIS
Clinical staging of HIV infection	Viral etiology of HIV infection
	HIV is incurable
	No preventive vaccine
	Difference between HIV infection and acquired immunodeficiency syndrome
	Average 10-year latent period
Transmission of HIV infection	Most HIV-infected people do not look ill
	Any HIV-infected person can transmit the disease
	HIV is transmitted by sexual contact: vaginal intercourse, anal intercourse, and oral sex
	HIV is transmitted by sharing needles with an infected person
	HIV may be transmitted through contact with blood or semen of an infected individual
	HIV may be transmitted to the fetus during pregnancy by an infected mother
Common misconceptions about HIV transmission	Currently, the risk of HIV transmitted by blood transfusions or blood products is remote
	HIV is *not* transmitted by casual or household contact, sharing dishes or bathrooms
	HIV infection is *not* transmitted by coughing, sneezing, kissing, or touching
	HIV is *not* transmitted by donating blood
	HIV is *not* transmitted by mosquito bites

HIV, Human immunodeficiency virus.

overall prevalence of HIV infection in female partners of infected men has been shown to be 20 to 25,[10] whereas studies of the prevalence of HIV infection in male partners of HIV-infected women have demonstrated transmission rates of 1 to 12%.[9, 15] This difference in the pattern of transmission between men and women has not been documented in Africa and other pattern II countries, where more than 50% of those with HIV infection are women. When the transmission rates are stratified according to the number of potential cofactors present, a somewhat linear pattern of transmission can be noted. The transmission rate from male to female in the presence of none of the previously mentioned cofactors has been shown to be 7 to 10%,[9, 12] with one risk factor about 30%,[9] and with two or more cofactors 50 to 70%.[9, 12] A similar linear correlation has been demonstrated with female-to-male transmission, in which the transmission rate was 1% with no cofactors, 16% with one cofactor, and 57% with two.[9]

It has not been determined if the pathophysiology of certain STDs enables then to serve as cofactors, thereby facilitating HIV transmission, or if a history of STDs is simply a marker for unsafe sexual practices. The associations of various STDs with HIV infection may merely reflect the geographic prevalence of different STDs superimposed on the HIV epidemic rather than a causal relationship.

RISK ASSESSMENT AND PREVENTION

The rapid expansion of the HIV epidemic in women emphasizes the need for effective education and prevention strategies to forestall further heterosexual and perinatal spread of infection. The trusting relationship established by the primary care physician should afford a comfortable environment through which to ascertain an individual patient's risk of having or acquiring HIV infection; however, only 11% of primary care physicians question their patients about high-risk behaviors.[16] With the growing importance of heterosexual transmission in the United States, any sexually active individual must be considered to be at risk and should receive education on disease transmission and prevention (Table 48–2). Safe sex practices should be discussed and proper condom use demonstrated (Table 48–3).

A detailed history and physical examination should be performed to ascertain whether a woman may be at high risk for having or acquiring HIV infection (Table 48–4). An accurate drug use and sexual history is important to assess the degree of risk and to target areas for risk reduction. A drug use history should begin with asking about prescribed medications, then over-the-counter medications, followed by injection or noninjection illicit drug use. This discussion offers an opportunity to provide education about drugs and

TABLE 48–3. Education about Safer Sex Practices

TOPIC FOR DISCUSSION	POINTS TO EMPHASIZE
Risky sexual behaviors	Vaginal or anal intercourse without a condom
	Use of oil-based lubricants: Vaseline, Crisco, butter
	Sharing sex toys not protected by condoms
	Use of lambskin or natural condoms
	Unrolling condom before use (increases potential for breaking)
Safer sexual behaviors	Massaging, caressing, kissing, masturbating
	Using a latex condom with nonoxynol-9 spermicide
	Using a condom for fellatio
	Using a dental dam (or plastic food wrap) for cunnilingus
	Avoiding contact of mucous membranes or cuts with menstrual blood
Proper condom use[33]	Use a new condom with each act of intercourse
	Use the correct size condom
	Use a latex condom with nonoxynol-9 spermicide in the tip
	Use water-based lubricants only: K-Y jelly, diaphragm jelly
	Apply condom to erect penis before genital contact
	Hold base of condom when withdrawing penis
	Immediately remove condom
	Immediately wash ejaculate off skin, penis, and hands
Misconceptions about sexual practices	Withdrawal of the penis before ejaculation offers no protection against HIV infection
	Birth control pills, diaphragms, and intrauterine devices offer no protection against HIV infection
	Douching does not protect against HIV infection
	Having sex with only one partner does not ensure protection against HIV infection

HIV, Human immunodeficiency virus.

alcohol, which interfere with judgment and impulse control, leading to unsafe sexual practices (Table 48–5).

An accurate sexual history is often difficult to obtain and may be uncomfortable for both the patient and the physician. It may provide a patient with support and put her more at ease to acknowledge that the questions may be uncomfortable but are necessary to assess the risk for HIV infection and other diseases. The questions must be phrased

TABLE 48–4. Women at Highest Risk for Human Immunodeficiency Virus Infection

CATEGORY	INDICATORS OF POTENTIAL HIV INFECTION
Historical indicators	Women from countries with a high rate of heterosexual transmission
	Women with multiple sexual partners (especially prostitutes)
	Injection drug users
	Transfusion recipients between 1978 and 1985
	Sexual partners of HIV-infected persons, injection drug users, bisexuals, or hemophiliacs
	Women delivering HIV-infected children
	Women with a history of a sexually transmitted disease
Clinical indicators	Unexplained chronic constitutional symptoms
	Unexplained chronic generalized adenopathy
	Unexplained diarrhea or wasting
	Unexplained encephalopathy
	Unexplained thrombocytopenia
	Unexplained thrush or chronic vaginal candidiasis
	Genital ulcer or other active sexually transmitted disease
	Pelvic inflammatory disease
	Recurrent bacterial pneumonias
	Tuberculosis
	Chronic skin or nail infections
	Recurrent herpes zoster

HIV, Human immunodeficiency virus.

TABLE 48–5. Relative Risk of Sexual Behaviors

DEGREE OF RISK	SEXUAL BEHAVIOR
Highest risk	Unprotected anal intercourse
	Unprotected vaginal intercourse
	Oral-anal sex (''rimming'')
Moderate risk	Anal intercourse with condom
	Vaginal intercourse with condom
	Unprotected oral-genital sex
Lower risk	Oral sex with condom or barrier
	Deep kissing (''French,'' ''wet'')
Lowest risk	Dry kissing
	Hugging
	Holding hands
	Massage

From Carr R, Wald A, Shanahan C, Hein D. HIV education and prevention. In: Libman H, Witzburg RA (eds). HIV Infection—A Clinical Manual. 2nd ed. Boston: Little, Brown & Co, 1993, pp 423–431.

in a nonjudgmental fashion with sensitivity to a woman's cultural and educational background, avoiding references to stereotypes and using ordinary language. Initial open-ended questions can be followed by more specific lines of questioning. For example, a woman should not be asked if she is promiscuous, but she should be asked how many sexual partners she has had; she should not be asked if she is a lesbian or heterosexual but should be asked if she has sex with men, women, or both. Women who have sex only with other women may still be at risk for having or acquiring HIV infection. Although woman-to-woman transmission is rare, lesbian women have acquired HIV infection through injection drug use and sexual relationships with infected men.[17, 18]

The number of sexual partners since 1975 and the presence of sexual contact with drug-injecting partners should be determined. Eighty percent of male injection drug users have partners who do not inject drugs.[19] However, a woman may not know or may have inaccurate information about her sex partner's risk factors, even if she has a steady partner.[20] She should be asked if she has regularly or intermittently used condoms and if she has engaged in anal intercourse. Many individuals, especially prostitutes and injection drug users, may practice safe sex with their casual partners but not with their regular partners. A history of pelvic inflammatory disease or STD is an indicator of unsafe sexual practices. Counseling on and testing for HIV infection should be encouraged in women who have been determined to be at increased risk.

Risk reduction methods should be discussed with women who are engaging in risky behaviors. If appropriate, intervention should include referral to a drug treatment program and education about safer substance use. Such education includes em-

phasizing using sterile needles or participating in needle exchange programs, if available, and not sharing needles. If needles and syringes are being reused, the patient should be instructed to rinse the syringe and needle twice with bleach and then twice with water. Success is more likely to be achieved in modifying high-risk sexual or drug behavior than in eliminating these behaviors.[21] Focusing on the personal adverse consequences of drug use is not likely to be effective, because those who abuse drugs have already accepted the risk to themselves; but they may be persuaded to change their behavior for the benefit of their partner and children. Behavior modification will more likely succeed if advice is heard repeatedly and from multiple sources; recovering addicts and community-based outreach services are very effective sources of information.[22]

Successful drug abuse intervention does not, however, guarantee that safe sex practices will also be implemented. Asking steady sexual partners to use condoms may be interpreted as an admission of infidelity or may imply mistrust. Because no method of protection is safe, effective, and controllable by a woman, women must rely on their sexual partner's willingness to participate in safe sexual practices. Other than celibacy, the male condom is currently the primary method of preventing sexual transmission of HIV. A contraceptive sponge impregnated with nonoxynol-9 has been approved as a female contraceptive and has been shown to be viricidal for HIV in vitro.[23, 24] When this contraceptive device was evaluated in prostitutes, HIV transmission was actually enhanced,[25] perhaps because of mucosal abrasions from frequent sexual activity. However, in another study of women with less frequent sexual contact, consistent use of a nonoxynol-9 spermicide was effective in reducing the incidence of HIV infection.[26] Larger studies are needed to evaluate the effectiveness of this device in preventing the transmission of HIV infection.

When developing a specific risk-reduction plan with each patient, a physician must be aware of the social and cultural misconceptions about HIV infection and the barriers to successful implementation of behavioral change, particularly among minority populations. Some African Americans feel that they are blamed for the disease because of scientific evidence suggesting that the disease originated in Africa. Another prevalent misconception is that the purpose of needle exchange programs is to promote drug use among minority populations. Minority groups may feel that HIV was introduced into their population to control their population growth and that condom use is promoted for the same reasons. Despite extensive

AIDS education efforts, many minority women believe that AIDS can be acquired by sneezing, using toilet seats, or eating foods prepared by a person with AIDS.[27]

Prevention efforts must address these misconceptions. Minority individuals may be unwilling to participate in prevention programs because of previous negative experiences with public health groups. Education is most effective if it is delivered orally and by a member of the minority group; this is particularly true for injection drug users.[21] Any written information must be linguistically and educationally appropriate. Providing educational programs for impoverished African American and Hispanic women may be particularly difficult.[27]

HUMAN IMMUNODEFICIENCY VIRUS TESTING

The initial screening test for detection of antibodies to HIV is an enzyme-linked immunoassay. It was designed to have a high degree of sensitivity to reduce the occurrence of false negatives at the expense of false positives. Most commercially available tests have a sensitivity of at least 99.5% and a specificity of greater than 99.8% in high-risk populations.[28] In low-risk populations, the incidence of false positives is higher. A positive result of an enzyme-linked immunoassay is repeated on the same serum sample. If it is again positive, a confirmatory Western blot test is performed.

The Western blot confirms the presence of antibodies to HIV-1 by identifying antibodies to specific viral proteins encoded by the *gag* (group-specific antigen/core), *env* (envelope), and *pol* (polymerase) gene products (see Chapter 49). The specific pattern and intensity of banding are dependent on the sensitivity of the commercial test kit and which antibodies were circulating at the time the sample was obtained. Most commercial test kits are quite sensitive to anti-p24 antibody (*gag* gene product), and it is often the first antibody to appear during seroconversion. Antibodies to the *pol* (p31, p51, p66), *env* (gp 41, gp 120, gp 160), and other *gag* (p18, p55) gene products may appear somewhat later. Interpretive criteria for a positive test result have not been standardized. Some disagreement is expressed about whether antibodies from all three gene products must be present for a test to be considered positive. The CDC has recommended that the Western blot be considered positive when any two of the three most diagnostically significant bands—anti p-24, anti-gp 41, and anti-gp 160/120—are present.[29] The absence of any band correlating with a viral gene product is considered a negative test result.

A Western blot that cannot be interpreted as positive or negative is classified as indeterminant; 10 to 20% of sera reactive by enzyme-linked immunoassay are indeterminant by Western blot.[30] An indeterminant result may represent early production of antibody against viral core antigens, loss of core antibody late in HIV disease, cross-reactive antibody to HIV-2, or cross-reactivity to nonviral proteins. The presence of a solitary anti-p24 band in a high-risk individual may represent early seroconversion; repeat enzyme-linked immunoassay and Western blot should be performed in 1 month and repeated in 3 to 6 months if results of the latter are persistently indeterminant and the patient is still engaging in high-risk behavior.[31] An indeterminant Western blot test result in a low-risk patient should be repeated in 3 to 6 months.[30] More specific assays, such as HIV-1 culture, polymerase chain reaction, and a recombinant envelope assay, may be used to evaluate for early seroconversion or clarification of a persistently indeterminant result.[31]

HUMAN IMMUNODEFICIENCY VIRUS PRETEST AND POSTTEST COUNSELING

Although health care providers need to be aware of the regulations pertaining to HIV testing in their own state, it is strongly recommended that all patients who are being HIV tested receive complete pretest and posttest counseling (Tables 48–6 and 48–7).[32] Providers must also be aware of their state's HIV reporting requirements and the limitations on confidentiality of the HIV test results. Before testing, the physician and patient should discuss the ethical and legal responsibilities for partner notification and the duty to warn partners who may be at risk for transmission of infection.[33] All state health departments have professional partner notification services available to maintain the anonymity of the index case. Women may be fearful of notifying their partners because of the threat of domestic violence.[34] High-risk women who refuse HIV testing because of the fear of partner notification or discrimination should be strongly encouraged to seek testing at an anonymous testing center.

Testing and counseling for HIV should be carried out in a supportive environment by adequately trained individuals. Sufficient time must be allotted in both pre- and posttest counseling to ensure a complete exchange of information and to be sure that a patient completely understands the testing process and the implications of the test results, as

TABLE 48–6. Human Immunodeficiency Virus Pretest Counseling

TOPICS FOR DISCUSSION	POINTS TO EMPHASIZE
Description of HIV testing	HIV testing is voluntary
	Anonymous HIV testing may be available
	HIV test results are confidential
	Testing is performed on blood
	Antibody testing not antigen, window period 3–6 months
	A positive result represents infection with the virus, not acquired immunodeficiency syndrome
	A negative result probably means no infection wth HIV unless potential exposure has occurred within 6 months
	An indeterminant test may be measuring antibody other than HIV, repeat in 3–6 months
Benefits of HIV testing	Modify high-risk behavior to prevent primary infection if result is negative
	Modify high-risk behavior to prevent transmission if test is positive
	Receive early treatment services
	Consider infection status in family planning
Risks of HIV testing	False positive or false negative test results
	Fear of disclosure
	Discrimination in employment, housing, medical care
	Psychological distress
Psychosocial assessment	Ask patient's motives for wanting testing
	Assess personal support systems
	Ask what a negative or positive test result would mean for patient
	Formulate a plan for patient if result positive
	Suggest that patient bring support person along for test results
	Schedule follow-up appointment for test results
Contraindication to testing	Pre- and posttest counseling unavailable
	Inability to provide informed consent
	Lack of personal support systems
	Suicidality

HIV, Human immunodeficiency virus.

well as to allow time to assess medical and psychosocial needs. Written material that is linguistically and educationally appropriate should be provided; however, written material should not replace oral communication.

Counseling has been shown to affect behavior positively by encouraging risk-reducing sexual and drug use behaviors that prevent primary infection by those at risk and prevent transmission to others by those who are already infected.[35, 36] However, such counseling may also provoke anxiety in patients. A patient may feel that safe sex guidelines interfere with her lifestyle and place limitations on social behavior and relationships with sexual partners. By adopting risk-reducing behaviors, a patient may feel stigmatized and may be perceived by her peer group as being infected.

Counselors should anticipate various emotional responses to a patient's learning of a positive test result. Common reactions include silence, sadness, crying, fear, anger, and concern for family and partner. A patient should be assessed for the possibility of suicide (ideation, threat, or gesture) and asked whether she has a plausible suicide plan. A

plan for crisis intervention should be developed, particularly if she has a past history of suicide ideation, psychiatric illness, substance abuse, and poor impulse control. The diagnosis of HIV infection may carry with it the disclosure of belonging to a certain risk group, and a patient may feel societal and family discrimination. She may harbor feelings of rejection and fear of loss of job, housing, and children. Single mothers from impoverished communities are particularly vulnerable to feelings of helplessness. A patient's ability to understand the test results may be impaired by concurrent substance abuse or impaired cognition secondary to advanced HIV disease. Emotional distress and anxiety may also interfere with a patient's ability to absorb the information presented at a counseling session. An additional follow-up posttest counseling session may be necessary.

A social service assessment is an important component of a posttest evaluation, particularly if the test result is positive. A basic needs assessment should include an evaluation of living arrangements, both housing and personal supports, finances, transportation, food, and medical needs. A

TABLE 48–7. Human Immunodeficiency Virus Posttest Counseling

TEST RESULT	POINTS TO EMPHASIZE
Negative	Ask what test result patient expects
	Assess reaction to test result
	Assess for survival guilt
	Remind patient of window period
	Retest in 3–6 months if patient concerned about false negative
	Reinforce risk reduction behaviors
Positive	Ask what test result patient expects
	Discuss meaning of test result, infection versus acquired immunodeficiency syndrome
	Prepare for strong emotions, allow time for discussion
	Discuss patient's plan for next 24 hours
	Anticipate suicidal behavior
	Assess support systems
	Refer to support group
	Assess social services needs
	Discuss precautions to prevent transmission
	Discuss risks of pregnancy, contraception
	Discuss partner attitudes about safe sex
	Discuss partner notification, potential for violence
	Discuss natural history of HIV infection
	Reiterate benefits of early care
	Encourage healthy lifestyle
	Provide information on treatment and access to research protocols
	Consider staging evaluation for HIV disease
	Schedule follow-up medical care

HIV, Human immunodeficiency virus.

woman should be asked to prioritize her needs. Referrals should be made for appropriate entitlements and women's support groups. Community support systems might include religion, meditation, spiritual healing, and acupuncture.

REFERENCES

1. Chin J. Current and future dimensions of the HIV/AIDS pandemic in women and children. Lancet 1990;336:221.
2. Massachusetts Department of Public Health. AIDS surveillance summary. AIDS Newsletter 1994;10:1.
3. Centers for Disease Control and Prevention (CDC). Update: Mortality attributable to HIV infection among persons aged 25–44 years—United States, 1991 and 1992. MMWR 1993;42(45):869.
4. World Health Organization. Current and Future Dimensions of the HIV/AIDS Pandemic—A Capsule Summary (Publication no. WHO/GPA/RES/SFI/91.4). Geneva: World Health Organization, 1991.
5. Mann J, Chin J, Quinn T. The international epidemiology of AIDS. Sci Am 1988;259:82.
6. CDC. Update: Acquired immunodeficiency syndrome—United States, 1992. MMWR 1993;42:547.
7. Quinn TC, Mann JM, Curran JW, Piot P. AIDS in Africa: An epidemiologic paradigm. Science 1986;234:955.
8. Plummer FA, Simonsen JN, Cameron DW, et al. Cofactors in male-female sexual transmission of human immunodeficiency virus type 1. J Infect Dis 1991;163:233.
9. European Study Group on Heterosexual Transmission of HIV. Comparison of female to male and male to female transmission of HIV in 563 stable couples. Br Med J 1992;304:809.
10. Padian N, Marquis L, Francis D, et al. Male-to-female transmission of human immunodeficiency virus. JAMA 1987;258:788.
11. Moss GB, Clemetson D, D'Costa L, et al. Association of cervical ectopy with heterosexual transmission of human immunodeficiency virus: Results of a study of couples in Nairobi, Kenya. J Infect Dis 1991;164:588.
12. European Study Group. Risk factors for male to female transmission of HIV. Br Med J 1989;298:411.
13. Lazzarin A, Scarcco A, Musicco M, et al. Man-to-woman sexual transmission of the human immunodeficiency virus: Risk factors related to sexual behavior, man's infectiousness, and woman's susceptibility. Arch Intern Med 1991;151:2411.
14. Laga M, Manoka A, Kivuvu M, et al. Non-ulcerative sexually transmitted diseases as risk factors for HIV-1 transmission in women: Results from a cohort study. AIDS 1993;7:95.
15. Padian NS, Shiboski SC, Jewell NP. Female-to-male transmission of human immunodeficiency virus. JAMA 1991;266:1664.
16. Ferguson K, Stapleton J, Helms CM. Physician's effectiveness in assessing risk for human immunodeficiency virus infection. Arch Intern Med 1991;151:561.
17. Chu SY, Buehler JW, Fleming PL, Berkelman RL. Epidemiology of reported cases of AIDS in lesbians, United States 1980–89. Am J Public Health 1990;80:1380.
18. Chu S, Hammett T, Buehler J. Update: Epidemiology of reported cases of AIDS in women who report sex only with other women, United States, 1980–1991. AIDS 1992;6:518.
19. DesJarlais DC, Friedman SR. The psychology of preventing AIDS among intravenous drug users: A social learning conceptualization. Am Psychol 1988;43:865.
20. Shayne V, Kaplan B. Double victims: Poor women and AIDS. Women Health 1991;17:21.

21. Becker MH, Joseph JG. AIDS and behavioral change to reduce risk: A review. Am J Public Health 1988;78:394.
22. CDC. Assessment of street outreach for HIV prevention—selected sites, 1991–1993. MMWR 1993;42:873.
23. Hicks DR, Martin LS, Getchell JP. Inactivation of HTLV-III/LAV-infected cultures of normal human lymphocytes by nonoxynol-9 in vitro. Lancet 1985;2:1422.
24. Polsky B, Baron PA, Gold JWM, et al. In vitro inactivation of HIV-1 by contraceptive sponge containing nonoxynol-9. Lancet 1988;1:1456.
25. Kreiss J, Ngugi E, Holmes K, et al. Efficacy of nonoxynol 9 contraceptive sponge use in preventing heterosexual acquisition of HIV in Nairobi prostitutes. JAMA 1992;268:477.
26. Zekeng L, Feldblum PJ, Oliver RM, Kaptue L. Barrier contraceptive use and HIV infection among high-risk women in Cameroon. AIDS 1993;7:725.
27. Nyamathi A, Bennett C, Leake B, et al. AIDS-related knowledge, perceptions, and behaviors among impoverished minority women. Am J Public Health 1993;83:65.
28. CDC. Update: Serologic testing for antibody to human immunodeficiency virus. MMWR 1988;36:833.
29. CDC. Interpretive criteria used to report Western blot results for HIV-1-antibody testing—United States. MMWR 1991;40:692.
30. CDC. Interpretation and use of the Western blot assay for serodiagnosis of human immunodeficiency virus type 1 infections. MMWR 1989;38(S-7).
31. Celum CL, Coombs RW, Lafferty W, et al. Indeterminate human immunodeficiency virus type 1 Western blots: Seroconversion risk, specificity of supplemental tests, and an algorithm for evaluation. J Infect Dis 1991;164:656.
32. CDC. Recommendations for HIV testing services for inpatients and outpatients in acute-care hospital settings and technical guidance on HIV counseling. MMWR 1993;42(RR-2):1.
33. CDC. 1993 Sexually transmitted diseases treatment guidelines. MMWR 1993;42(RR-14):1.
34. North RL, Rothenberg KH. Partner notification and the threat of domestic violence against women with HIV infection. N Engl J Med 1993;329:1194.
35. Higgins DL, Galavotti C, O'Reilly KR, et al. Evidence for the effects of HIV antibody counseling and testing on risk behaviors. JAMA 1991;266:2419.
36. Ross MW, Wodak A, Gold J. The association of needle cleaning with reduced seroprevalence among intravenous drug users sharing injection equipment. J Acquir Immune Defic Syndr 1992;5:849.

Human Immunodeficiency Virus Infection: Pathogenesis, Natural History, and Management

Elcinda L. McCrone and Lisa R. Hirschhorn

Comprehensive health care for women must focus on the early recognition of human immunodeficiency virus (HIV) infection in women, eliminating the barriers to care, and providing access to treatment and prophylactic therapies both in the primary care setting and through access to clinical trials. Biologically, other than gynecologic manifestations and the incidence of certain opportunistic infections, the course of HIV infection in women appears to be no different from that in men,[1, 2] but the psychosocial aspects may differ, resulting in different choices for medical care. Women with HIV infection are more likely than men to be poor and nonwhite[3] and may be less likely to seek health care for themselves because of their responsibility for and competing health needs of their partner and children, who also may be HIV infected. They are also more likely to seek care at hospitals with less experience in treating HIV-related disease, correlating with increased mortality.[4, 5] Primary care providers must understand the pathogenesis of the disease and the barriers to care in order to provide optimal service to these women. This chapter reviews the pathophysiology of HIV infection and its clinical sequelae. In addition, guidelines for the primary care management of women with HIV infection are discussed.

PATHOGENESIS OF HUMAN IMMUNODEFICIENCY VIRUS INFECTION

Human immunodeficiency virus belongs to the retrovirus family, named for their ability to transfer viral genomic ribonucleic acid (RNA) into pro-

viral deoxyribonucleic acid (DNA) by a reverse transcriptase enzyme. This DNA provirus incorporates into the host chromosome, establishing a chronic, slowly progressive infection that is unable to be eradicated by the host's immune system. Human immunodeficiency virus has three structural genes: *env, gag,* and *pol.*[6] The *env* gene codes for a single polypeptide, glycopeptide (gp) 160, which is posttranscriptionally cleaved into two structural components, gp 120 and gp 41 (Fig. 40–1). Some HIV vaccines currently in therapeutic trials use these outer structural components. The gp 120 binds to the CD4 receptor of target cells, whereas the gp 41 is involved in syncytia formation (attachment of infected to uninfected cells). The *gag* gene codes for the structural components of the inner shell of the virus, including the p24 protein, which can be used clinically as a surrogate marker for viral replication. The *pol* gene codes for the reverse transcriptase and endonuclease enzymes, essential for viral replication and targets for antiretroviral therapy. Other HIV genes code for regulatory functions, such as inducing viral latency (*nef*), enhancing viral replication (*tat*), converting the production of regulatory to structural proteins during viral replication (*rev*), facilitating assembly and export of virions during viral budding (*vpu*), and increasing infectivity of the virus (*vif*).[6–8]

Human immunodeficiency virus preferentially infects T-helper (CD4) lymphocytes, monocytes, macrophages, eosinophils, natural killer cells, and antigen-presenting dendritic cells.[7] After attachment of the viral gp 120 protein to the CD4 surface receptor of the target cell, HIV enters the cell by fusion of the cell and viral membranes. The

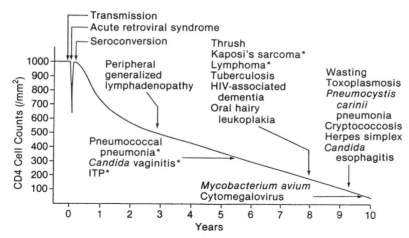

Figure 49–1. Occurrence of complications related to infection with the human immunodeficiency virus (HIV) based on CD4 lymphocyte count. Decline in CD4 cell count based on sequential tests in 318 seroconverters in the MAC study (J Infect Dis 1992;165:352). Approximate time of complications relative to CD4 cell count is based on experience of MACS with 888 diagnoses that defined the acquired immunodeficiency syndrome (A. Munoz, personal communication) and multiple published reports. Asterisks indicate conditions that are observed over a broad range of CD4 cell counts. ITP, Idiopathic thrombocytopenic purpura; PCP, *Pneumocystis carinii* pneumonia; CMV, cytomegalovirus. (From Bartlett JG. The Johns Hopkins Hospital Guide to Medical Care of Patients with HIV Infection. 4th ed. Baltimore: Williams & Wilkins, 1994. Copyright John G. Bartlett, MD.)

viral reverse transcriptase transcribes the viral RNA to proviral DNA, which accumulates in the cytoplasm or becomes incorporated into the DNA of the host's chromosome. A cellular latent phase may occur, followed by viral expression, replication, assembly, and budding. These steps in the viral life cycle can serve as potential targets for the development of pharmacologic and immunologic therapies to prevent and treat HIV infection.

After the initial infection, the disease appears to be clinically asymptomatic. However, during this prolonged latent period, which lasts from months to 10 years or more, active viral replication occurs in the lymphoid tissue.[9] The mechanisms that determine the rate of the progression from HIV infection to acquired immunodeficiency syndrome (AIDS) are not completely understood but probably involve complex interactions between cytokines produced by two subsets of CD4 lymphocytes, TH-1 and TH-2, and CD8 suppressor lymphocytes.[10, 11] Under the influence of cytokines produced by a subset of CD4 helper cells (TH-1), the CD8 lymphocytes may have a role in controlling the initial HIV infection,[12] but as a slow, programmed cell death (apoptosis) induced by viral activation depletes the number of CD4 cells, the CD8 lymphocytes are no longer able to limit viral replication. As viral replication increases, genomic mutations occur, resulting in the emergence of more virulent, cytopathic strains.[13] The emergence of these cytopathic, syncytia-inducing viral strains

has been correlated with a more rapid progression to AIDS.[14, 15] Elucidation of these immunopathogenic mechanisms may lead to more effective immunotherapies to inhibit or slow the progression of HIV disease.

CLASSIFICATION OF HUMAN IMMUNODEFICIENCY VIRUS INFECTION

In January 1993, the Centers for Disease Control and Prevention (CDC) revised their case definition for AIDS and proposed a clinical staging system incorporating CD4 lymphocyte counts (Table 49–1).[16] Clinical category A includes the acute HIV syndrome and progressive generalized lymphadenopathy (previous CDC classification group 2). Category B includes symptomatic conditions that are attributable to HIV infection, or are indicative of a defect in cell-mediated immunity, or have a course that is complicated by HIV infection (Table 49–2). The new AIDS definition (Table 49–3) includes all previous AIDS-defining conditions plus CD4 counts less than 200 cells per mm^3 (or CD4 percentage less than 14), pulmonary tuberculosis (TB), recurrent bacterial pneumonias (two episodes or more in 12 months), and the first gender-specific AIDS-defining condition, invasive cervical carcinoma.

TABLE 49–1.   Centers for Disease Control and Prevention 1993 Revised Classification System for Human Immunodeficiency Virus Infection

CD4 + T-CELL CATEGORIES	CLINICAL CATEGORIES		
	(A) Asymptomatic, Acute (Primary) HIV or PGL*	**(B)** Symptomatic, Not (A) or (C) Conditions†	**(C)** AIDS-Indicator Conditions‡
>500 cells/mm³	A1	B1	C1
200–499 cells/mm³	A2	B2	C2
<200 cells/mm³ AIDS-indicator T-cell count	A3	B3	C3

*Clinical category A includes acute (primary) HIV infection.
†Includes symptomatic conditions not included in category C (see Table 49–2).
‡See Table 49–3.
HIV, Human immunodeficiency virus; PGL, persistent generalized lymphadenopathy; AIDS, acquired immunodeficiency syndrome.
From Centers for Disease Control and Prevention. 1993 revised classification system for HIV infection and expanded surveillance case definition for AIDS among adolescents and adults. MMWR 1993;41(RR-17):1.

NATURAL HISTORY AND INCIDENCE OF HUMAN IMMUNODEFICIENCY VIRUS–RELATED COMPLICATIONS

Information on the natural history of HIV infection in women has been limited. Early reports suggested a more fulminant course in women.[17] This shorter survival in women may have been related to delayed diagnosis due to underrecognition of HIV infection in women and limited access to health care. Studies demonstrate that with comparable access to health care, antiretroviral therapy,

TABLE 49–2.   Centers for Disease Control and Prevention Clinical Classification Category B, Symptomatic Human Immunodeficiency Virus Infection*

Bacillary angiomatosis
Candidiasis, oropharyngeal (thrush)
Candidiasis, vulvovaginal; persistent, frequent, or poorly responsive to therapy
Cervical dysplasia (moderate or severe)/cervical carcinoma in situ
Constitutional symptoms, such as fever (38.5°C) or diarrhea lasting >1 month
Hairy leukoplakia, oral
Herpes zoster (shingles), involving at least two distinct episodes or more than one dermatome
Idiopathic thrombocytopenic purpura
Listeriosis
Pelvic inflammatory disease, particularly if complicated by tubo-ovarian abscess
Peripheral neuropathy

*Includes but is not limited to these conditions.
From Centers for Disease Control and Prevention. 1993 revised classification system for HIV infection and expanded surveillance case definition for AIDS among adolescents and adults. MMWR 1993;41(RR-17):1.

and prophylaxis for opportunistic infections, the course of HIV infection in women is no more rapid and may even be less fulminant than that in men.[2, 18, 19]

Other than gynecologic manifestations and the incidence of a few opportunistic infections, the natural history of HIV infection in women is probably similar to that in men.[1, 2] *Pneumocystis carinii* pneumonia (PCP) is the most common AIDS-defining diagnosis in both women and men.[1, 20] A few differences in the incidence of several other AIDS-indicator diagnoses have been reported, with an increased incidence of *Candida* esophagitis, herpesvirus infections, and extrapulmonary TB and a lower incidence of Kaposi's sarcoma in women than in men.[1]

A high prevalence of the new AIDS-defining infections, recurrent bacterial pneumonias and pulmonary TB, have been reported in women and intravenous drug users of both sexes.[19, 20] Although cervical carcinoma and its precursor, human papillomavirus (HPV)–related cervical squamous intraepithelial lesion (SIL, or cervical intraepithelial neoplasia) occur with increased frequency in HIV-infected women,[21, 22] the reported number of AIDS-defining cases of cervical carcinoma has been relatively small.[23] Fifty-four percent of the total number of new AIDS cases reported to the CDC in 1993 met the AIDS definition by the new criteria. Of these 55,432 AIDS cases that met the new definition, 91% met the new criteria by having a CD4 count less than 200 cells per mm³. A proportionately larger number of women, injection drug users, and blacks accounted for the remaining 9% who met the revised case definition with a new AIDS-defining opportunistic infection, epidemiologically reflecting the populations infected with TB.[23]

TABLE 49–3.   Centers for Disease Control and Prevention 1993 Revised Acquired Immunodeficiency Syndrome Case-Defining Conditions

Candidiasis of bronchi, trachea, or lungs
Candidiasis, esophageal
Cervical cancer, invasive*†
Coccidioidomycosis, disseminated or extrapulmonary†
Cryptococcosis, extrapulmonary
Cryptosporidiosis, chronic intestinal (>1 month's duration)
Cytomegalovirus disease (other than liver, spleen, or nodes)
Cytomegalovirus retinitis (with loss of vision)
Encephalopathy, HIV-related dementia†
Herpes simplex: chronic ulcer(s) (>1 month's duration); or bronchitis, pneumonitis, or esophagitis
Histoplasmosis, disseminated or extrapulmonary†
Isosporiasis, chronic intestinal (>1 month's duration)†
Kaposi's sarcoma†
Lymphoma, Burkitt's (or equivalent term)
Lymphoma, immunoblastic (or equivalent term)
Lymphoma, primary, of brain†
Mycobacterium avium complex or *Mycobacterium kansasii,* disseminated or extrapulmonary
Mycobacterium tuberculosis, any site (pulmonary* or extrapulmonary)†
Mycobacterium, other species or unidentified species, disseminated or extrapulmonary
Pneumocystis carinii pneumonia
Pneumonia, recurrent*†
Progressive multifocal leukoencephalopathy
Salmonella septicemia (nontyphoidal), recurrent†
Toxoplasmosis of brain
Wasting syndrome due to HIV†

*Added to the revised case definition in 1993.
†Requires positive HIV serology.
HIV, Human immunodeficiency virus.
From Centers for Disease Control and Prevention. 1993 revised classfication system for HIV infection and expanded surveillance case definition for AIDS among adolescents and adults. MMWR 1993;41 (RR-17):1.

CLINICAL SPECTRUM AND MANIFESTATIONS OF HUMAN IMMUNODEFICIENCY VIRUS DISEASE IN WOMEN

The mean time from HIV seroconversion to AIDS is 8 to 10 years[24]; however, a small number of individuals, long-term survivors, have remained asymptomatic for 20 years or more.[25] Longitudinal studies on cohorts of women have demonstrated a decline in mean CD4 cell count of 50 to 70 cells per mm^3 per year,[18, 26] similar to the rate of decline described in men. The mean time for CD4 lymphocyte counts to drop to less than 500 and 200 cells per mm^3 after seroconversion has been 5.1 years and 9.6 years, respectively.[26]

The insidious decline in CD4 lymphocyte numbers during the course of HIV infection is accompanied by functional abnormalities of CD4 lymphocytes, polymorphonuclear leukocytes, and macrophages, which result in dysfunction of both cell-mediated and humoral immunity. The infectious and neoplastic complications of HIV infection are a result of these immunologic abnormalities and are related to the degree of immunosuppression. The occurrence of some common

manifestations of HIV infection at various stages of CD4 lymphocyte depletion is depicted in Figure 49–1, and the frequency of these complications is shown in Table 49–4. Treatment options for the management of many common infectious complications of HIV infection in women are summarized in Table 49–5. Many recommendations change rapidly as newer and more effective therapeutic options are introduced; therefore, this table should be used to help guide rather than dictate treatment options. A number of references are cited to provide more information about the efficacy, toxicity, and choice of treatments for these conditions.

Acute Retroviral Syndrome

The acute retroviral syndrome typically occurs 1 to 3 weeks after HIV exposure. Although this primary infection may be asymptomatic,[9, 27] symptoms ranging from a mild mononucleosis-like illness with fever, headache, pharyngitis, morbilliform rash, adenopathy, myalgias, and arthralgias to aseptic meningitis or meningoencephalitis occur in 50 to 70% of individuals.[27] Laboratory abnor-

TABLE 49–4. Frequency of Acquired Immunodeficiency Syndrome–Defining Complications

COMPLICATION	INITIAL AIDS-DEFINING DIAGNOSIS IN WOMEN*	INITIAL AIDS-DEFINING DIAGNOSIS IN MEN*	OVERALL FREQUENCY OF OCCURRENCE†
Pneumocystis carinii pneumonia	52%	53%	75–85%
Candida esophagitis	20%	13%	20–30%
HIV wasting syndrome	19%	17%	70–90%
HIV-associated encephalopathy	7%	7%	40–70%
Toxoplasmosis encephalitis	6%	5%	5–15%
Cytomegalovirus	6%	9%	80–90%
Disseminated *Mycobacterium avium* infection	6%	6%	30–40%
Cryptococcal meningitis	5%	8%	8–12%
Chronic mucocutaneous herpes simplex	4%	4%	10–25%
Extrapulmonary tuberculosis	2%	3%	
Cryptosporidiosis	2%	2%	5–10%
Lymphoma	2%	4%	3–5%
Kaposi's sarcoma	2%	13%	15–25%

AIDS, Acquired immunodeficiency syndrome; HIV, human immunodeficiency virus.

*Adapted from Fleming PL, Ciesielski CA, Byers RH, et al. Gender differences in reported AIDS-indicative diagnoses. J Infect Dis 1993;168:61. Used with permission of the University of Chicago Press.

†Adapted from Bartlett JG. The Johns Hopkins Hospital Guide to Medical Care of Patients with HIV Infection. 4th ed. Baltimore: Williams & Wilkins, 1994. Copyright John G. Bartlett, MD.

malities are nonspecific, including leukopenia followed by lymphocytosis, thrombocytopenia, and elevated serum levels of transaminases. A transient decline in the number of CD4 lymphocytes associated with a p24 antigenemia and a marked viremia may be noted.[7, 9, 27] Diagnosis can be attempted early in the syndrome by p24 antigen testing, HIV culture, or polymerase chain reaction (in a research setting). Most symptoms remit within 2 weeks, but a diffuse lymphadenopathy may persist in one third of patients. Seroconversion usually occurs 1 to 4 weeks after acute infection, with nearly all individuals demonstrating antibodies within 3 months.[7] However, isolated case reports have described seroconversion being delayed for as long as 42 months,[28] and rare instances of seroreversion have also been noted[29] (see HIV testing in Chapter 48.)

CD4 Lymphocyte Count as a Surrogate Marker

The total CD4 count or percentage is currently the best, most practical surrogate marker for monitoring the clinical course of progression of HIV infection.[30–33] It is widely used to guide patient management, particularly with regard to initiating and monitoring the response to antiretroviral therapy and initiating prophylactic medications (Table 49–6). However, CD4 counts do not always correlate with a patient's clinical course, particularly in those on antiretroviral therapy.[33] The p24 anti-

gen is not widely used in directing the management of an individual case but may be useful to herald the more rapid progression of disease in patients with clinical deterioration but stable CD4 counts.[31]

CD4 lymphocyte measurements are affected by biologic and procedural variability and therefore must be interpreted cautiously. In addition to laboratory variation,[34] CD4 cell numbers are affected by a seasonal and diurnal fluctuation,[35, 36] corticosteroid use, and intercurrent illnesses such as cytomegalovirus, TB, and hepatitis B.[37] Because of the great variability in CD4 counts, values affecting therapeutic decision-making should be repeated in 1 week for verification. Because of the potential for great variability in the CD4 count, some physicians prefer to use the CD4 percentage to monitor the course of HIV infection. CD4 cell counts of greater than 500 per mm^3, 200 to 500 per mm^3, and less than 200 per mm^3 correspond to CD4 percents of greater than 29%, 14 to 28%, and less than 14%, respectively.

Manifestations of Disease with CD4 Count Greater than 500 Cells per mm^3

Most individuals with CD4 counts greater than 500 cells per mm^3 are asymptomatic, but a few experience mild cutaneous and mucosal manifestations, such as seborrheic dermatitis, bacterial folliculitis, aphthous ulcers, herpes labialis, and cervical SIL; the risk of developing an AIDS-defining condition or dying during the subsequent 18 to 24 months is less than 5%.[31]

TABLE 49–5. Management of Common Human Immunodeficiency Virus–Related Infectious Complications

CONDITION	THERAPY	ALTERNATIVE THERAPY	ADDITIONAL REFERENCES
Skin			
Bacillary angiomatosis	Erythromycin (250–500 mg PO q.i.d. × 2–8 wk)	Doxycycline (100 mg PO b.i.d. × 2–8 wk)	120
Eosinophilic folliculitis	Itraconazole (200 mg PO once or twice daily)	High-potency topical steroid	121
Molluscum contagiosum	Freeze, surgical removal	Retin-A cream used by some dermatologists for severe cases	122
Seborrheic dermatitis	Topical ketoconazole or 1% hydrocortisone cream		122
Herpes zoster	Acyclovir (800 mg PO 5 ×/day or 10 mg/kg IV every 8 hr) × 7–10 days until lesions crust	IV acyclovir for disseminated, ophthalmic nerve, or visceral involvement Foscarnet (40 mg/kg IV every 8 hr) for resistant virus	122
Eye			
Cytomegalovirus retinitis	Ganciclovir (GCV, 5 mg/kg IV every 12 hr × 14–21 days, then 5 mg/kg IV daily 5–7 days/wk) or Foscarnet (60 mg/kg every 8 hr × 14–21 days then 90–120 mg/kg IV daily)	Oral GCV and GCV retinal implants currently in clinical trials	123, 124
HIV retinopathy	No treatment necessary		
Oral Cavity			
Aphthous ulcers	Mouth rinses with 0.12% chlorhexidine gluconate (Peridex), 2% viscous lidocaine, or Miles solution‡	For severe cases: prednisone (40 mg PO/day × 1–2 wk, then taper) Thalidomide (100 mg PO daily) (investigational)	125
Candidiasis (thrush)	Clotrimazole troches (10 mg PO 5 ×/day) or Nystatin (500,000 U swish and swallow 5 ×/day) until symptoms resolve, then suppressive therapy 2–4 ×/day	Ketoconazole (200 PO mg daily) or Fluconazole (50–100 mg PO daily) or Itraconazole (200 mg PO daily) For refractory cases, amphotericin B (0.3–0.5 mg/kg IV daily)	126
Herpes simplex virus	Acyclovir (200 mg PO 5 ×/day × 10 days) Maintenance therapy may be required: acyclovir (200 mg PO t.i.d. or 400 mg b.i.d.)	Acyclovir (5 mg/kg IV every 8 hr × minimum 7 days) or Foscarnet (40 mg/kg IV every 8 hr or 60 mg/kg IV every 12 hr)	127
Oral hairy leukoplakia	Most lesions asymptomatic, no treatment required	Acyclovir (800 mg PO 5 ×/day × 2–3 wk)	
Periodontitis/gingivitis	Mouth rinses with 0.12% chlorhexidine gluconate (Peridex) b.i.d., and rigorous dental hygiene	For more severe cases: add metronidazole (250 mg PO t.i.d. × 7–14 days)	
Respiratory			
Bacterial pneumonia	Standard therapy usually adequate, noting increased risk of *S. pneumoniae* and *H. influenzae*	May see increased risk of gram-negative pneumonias in patients with more advanced diseases	
Pneumocystis carinii pneumonia			
Mild to moderate disease	Trimethoprim (15–20 mg/kg/day) plus sulfamethoxazole (75 mg/kg/day PO divided t.i.d.–q.i.d. × 21 days), then prophylaxis (see Table 49–7)	Pentamidine (4 mg/kg daily IV × 21 days) or Trimethoprim (15–20 mg/kg/d divided t.i.d.–q.i.d.) plus dapsone* (100 mg/day × 21 days), then prophylaxis Other alternatives: Atovaquone (750 mg PO t.i.d.) or Clindamycin (600 mg IV every 6–8 hr or 300–450 mg PO every 6 hr) plus primaquine* (15 mg base PO daily)	128, 129

TABLE 49–5.   Management of Common Human Immunodeficiency Virus–Related Infectious Complications *Continued*

CONDITION	THERAPY	ALTERNATIVE THERAPY	ADDITIONAL REFERENCES
Moderate to severe disease (Po_2 <70 mm Hg or alveolar-arterial gradient >35)	Trimethoprim (15 mg/kg/day) plus sulfamethoxazole (75 mg/kg/day IV × 21 days divided t.i.d.–q.i.d.) plus Prednisone (40 mg PO b.i.d. × 5 days then 40 mg daily × 5 days then 20 mg daily to end of therapy)	Pentamidine (4 mg/kg IV daily × 21 days) Salvage for refractory disease: Trimetrexate (45 mg/m^2 IV/day) plus 5 mg folinic acid PO	128, 129
Tuberculosis			
MDR not suspected	INH (300 mg) plus pyridoxine (50 mg) plus rifampin (600 mg) plus pyrazinamide (15–30 mg/kg) plus ethambutol (or streptomycin) (15–25 mg/kg) PO daily × 2 mo, then INH plus rifampin for total 9–12 mo if no drug resistance identified	Directly observed intermittent therapy an option if coordinated with local public health officials In areas with <4% INH resistance, some clinicians use INH plus rifampin plus pyrazinamide as initial therapy	79, 130, 131
MDR suspected	Consult medical expert experienced in treatment of MDR-tuberculosis and the local health department		132
Sinusitis	Standard therapy usually adequate, but longer duration may be required		133, 134
Gastrointestinal			
Candida esophagitis	Fluconazole (100–200 mg PO daily × 14–21 days or until resolution of symptoms)	Ketoconazole (200–400 mg PO b.i.d.) Itraconazole (100–200 mg PO daily) For refractory cases, amphotericin B (0.3–0.5 mg/kg IV daily)	135
Herpes simplex virus esophagitis	Acyclovir (200–800 mg PO 5 ×/day or 5 mg/kg IV every 8 hr × 7–10 days)	Foscarnet (40 mg/kg IV every 8 hr or 60 mg IV every 12 hr × 10–14 days or until resolved)	
Cytomegalovirus colitis or esophagitis	Ganciclovir (5 mg/kg IV b.i.d. × 14–21 days) Foscarnet (60 mg/kg every 8 hr or 90 mg/kg every 12 hr IV × 14–21 days)		
Cryptosporidium	Symptomatic treatment with antidiarrheal agents (Lomotil, loperamide, denatured tincture of opium) and nutritional supplements No therapy proven effective	Following therapies possibly effective: Paromomycin (500–750 mg PO q.i.d. × 14–28 days then 500 mg PO b.i.d.); Hyperimmune bovine colostrum; Azithromycin and atovaquone also in clinical trials	136, 137
Isospora belli	Trimethoprim plus sulfamethoxazole (2 DS b.i.d. or 1 DS t.i.d. × 2–4 wk, then 1–2 DS PO daily suppressive therapy)	Pyrimethamine (50–75 mg PO daily plus 5 mg folinic acid daily) × 1 mo, then pyrimethamine (25 mg PO daily) plus folinic acid suppressive therapy	
Salmonella	Amoxicillin (500–1000 mg PO t.i.d. × 2–4 wk)† Ciprofloxacin (500–750 mg PO b.i.d. × 2–4 wk) Consider IV therapy initially if systemically ill or malabsorption present Suppressive therapy may be required to prevent relapse	Trimethoprim (5–10 mg/kg/day PO) plus sulfamethoxazole Third-generation cephalosporins also effective	136
Wasting	Nutritional supplements (Ensure, Sustecal, Advera, others) Elemental diet for severe malabsorption (e.g., Vionex TEN)	Megace (40–80 mg PO b.i.d.–q.i.d.) Dronabinol (Marinol) (2.5 mg PO b.i.d.) Parenteral hyperalimentation used by some clinicians in severe cases	
Gynecologic			
Bacterial vaginosis	Standard treatment usually adequate: metronidazole (500 mg b.i.d. PO × 7 days)	Metronidazole (2 gm PO × 1 day) or Metronidazole gel (5 gm intravaginally b.i.d. × 5 day) or Clindamycin cream (5 gm intravaginally at bedtime × 7 days)	49

Table continued on following page

TABLE 49–5. **Management of Common Human Immunodeficiency Virus–Related Infectious Complications**
Continued

CONDITION	THERAPY	ALTERNATIVE THERAPY	ADDITIONAL REFERENCES
Candida vaginitis	Intravaginal miconazole suppository or cream (× 7 days) Clotrimazole troche or cream (× 7 days)	Ketoconazole (200 mg PO daily or b.i.d. × 5–7 days) Fluconazole (150 mg × 1 or 100 mg PO daily × 5–7 days)	49
Herpes simplex labialis	Acyclovir (200 mg PO 5 ×/day × 10 days) Maintenance therapy may be required: acyclovir (200 mg t.i.d. or 400 mg b.i.d.) PO	Acyclovir (5 mg/kg IV every 8 hr × at least 7 days) Foscarnet (40 mg/kg IV every 8 hr or 60 mg/kg IV every 12 hr)	49
Pelvic inflammatory disease	Outpatient: ceftriaxone (250 mg IM) plus doxycycline (100 mg PO b.i.d. × 14 days) Inpatient: cefoxitin (2 gm every 6 hr IV) plus doxycycline (100 mg PO or IV b.i.d.)	Outpatient: ofloxacin (400 mg PO b.i.d.) plus clindamycin (450 mg PO q.i.d.) or metronidazole (500 mg PO b.i.d.) × 14 days Inpatient: clindamycin (900 mg every 8 hr IV) plus gentamicin IV or IM	49
Syphilis	Standard treatment recommended by Centers for Disease Control and Prevention: 1° and 2°: benzathine penicillin G 2.4 mU IM every wk × 1–2 Latent: Cerebrospinal fluid evaluation recommended. Treat according to results	In early syphilis, some recommended exam of cerebrospinal fluid before treatment plus additional doses of penicillin	49, 62
Nervous System			
Toxoplasma gondii	Pyrimethamine (100–200 mg PO loading dose, then 50–100 mg/day PO) plus folinic acid (10 mg/day PO) plus sulfadiazine (4–8 gm/day PO) × 6 wk, then pyrimethamine (25–50 mg/day PO) plus folinic acid (5 mg/day PO) plus sulfadiazine (2–4 gm/day PO) for suppression	Pyrimethamine + folinic acid + clindamycin (600 mg IV or 300–450 mg PO every 6 hr) × 6 wk, then pyrimethamine (25–50 mg/day PO) plus folinic acid (5 mg/day PO) plus clindamycin (300 mg PO q.i.d.) for suppression	
Cryptococcus neoformans	Amphotericin B (0.5–1.0 mg/kg IV daily for 2–4 wk induction) then Fluconazole (200–400 mg PO daily) for suppression In severe cases, some clinicians add 5-flucytosine (75–100 mg/kg/day PO) to initial regimen	For milder cases, fluconazole, 400 mg daily × 2–4 wk, then Fluconazole, 200–400 mg daily PO for suppression Itraconazole 200 mg PO b.i.d. in clinical trials	138
Progressive multifocal leukoencephalopathy	No proven treatment	Clinical trials of systemic or intrathecal ara-C in progress High-dose ZDV (200 mg PO every 4 hr) may have benefit	
HIV dementia	Unknown ZDV (1000–1200 mg/day PO) may have some benefit	Nimodipine in clinical trials	
Peripheral neuropathy	Tricyclics at low dosages (e.g., amitriptyline, 25–50 mg PO at bedtime; nortriptyline, 10–50 mg PO at bedtime) Topical capsaicin-containing ointments (e.g., Zostrix)	Tegretol, mexiletine (not approved for this use and in clinical trials)	
Systemic			
Coccidioidomycosis	Amphotericin B (0.5–1.0 mg/kg IV daily × 8 wk, minimum 2–2.5 gm total dose), then Fluconazole (400 mg PO daily) or amphotericin B (1 mg/kg/wk IV) maintenance	Itraconazole (200 mg PO b.i.d.) Fluconazole (400–800 mg PO b.i.d.)	

TABLE 49–5. **Management of Common Human Immunodeficiency Virus–Related Infectious Complications**
Continued

CONDITION	THERAPY	ALTERNATIVE THERAPY	ADDITIONAL REFERENCES
Histoplasmosis	Amphotericin B (0.5–1.0 mg/kg/day IV × 8 wk) minimum 1–2.5 gm total dose), then Itraconazole (300 mg PO b.i.d. × 3 days, then 200 mg PO b.i.d. maintenance)	Itraconazole (200 mg PO b.i.d.) as initial therapy in milder cases	
Mycobacterium avium complex	Newer macrolides (clarithromycin, 500 mg PO b.i.d., or azithromycin, 500 mg PO daily) plus ethambutol (15 mg/kg PO) with or without clofazamine (100 mg PO daily)	Additional agents for patients with severe disease or who are intolerant or failing initial therapy include: Rifabutin (450–600 mg PO daily)§ Ciprofloxacin (750 mg PO b.i.d.) Amikacin (7.5 mg/kg IV/IM daily)	139
Tuberculosis MDR not suspected	Same regimen as for pulmonary disease. Central nervous system and skeletal disease may require longer duration of treatment		79, 131, 132
MDR not suspected	Consult medical expert experienced in treatment of MDR tuberculosis and the local health department		132

*Test for glucose-6-phosphate dehydrogenase deficiency before initiating therapy.
†Because of increasing rates of ampicillin-resistant *Salmonella,* many clinicians use quinolones or third-generation cephalosporins initially.
‡Miles solution: 60 mg hydrocortisone, 20 ml mycostatin, 2 gm tetracycline, and 120 ml viscous lidocaine.
§Uveitis reported in patients treated concurrently with clarithromycin and rifabutin, this combination should be used with caution.
b.i.d., 2 times a day; t.i.d., 3 times a day; q.i.d., 4 times a day; IV, intravenously; IM, intramuscularly; PO, orally; HIV, human immunodeficiency virus; ZDV, zidovudine; INH, isoniazid; MDR, multidrug resistance; DS, double strength; TEN, total enteral nutrition.
Adapted with permission from Bartlett JG. The Johns Hopkins Guide to Medical Care of Patients with HIV Infection. 4th ed. Baltimore: Williams & Wilkins, 1994; and from Lane HC, Laughon BE, Fallon J, et al. Recent advances in the management of AIDS-related opportunistic infections. Ann Intern Med 1994;120:945. For more information on specific medications and associated toxicities, consult The Medical Letter.[140]

Manifestations of Disease with CD4 Count 200 to 500 Cells per mm³

As CD4 lymphocyte counts fall to 200 to 500 cells per mm³, HIV-related dermatologic and mucosal complications increase in frequency and severity. Conditions such as pulmonary TB, herpes zoster, oropharyngeal and vaginal candidiasis, oral hairy leukoplakia, eosinophilic folliculitis, idiopathic thrombocytopenic purpura, salmonellosis, and Hodgkin's disease occur with increased frequency. Recurrent bacterial sinopulmonary infections with *Streptococcus pneumoniae, Haemophilus influenzae,* and *Moraxella catarrhalis* are common. Patients may suffer from intermittent fevers, diarrhea, weight loss, and other constitutional symptoms. The risk of developing an AIDS-defining condition or dying during the subsequent 18 to 24 months is 20 to 30%.[31]

Manifestations of Disease with CD4 Count Less than 200 cells per mm³

Although individuals with CD4 lymphocyte counts less than 200 cells per mm³ may remain asymptomatic for a period of time, the marked suppression of cell-mediated immunity predisposes to various opportunistic infections. The frequency of the more common AIDS-defining complications is summarized in Table 49–4. Manifestations of HIV disease that are seen noted this stage of illness include PCP, cerebral toxoplasmosis, cryptococcosis, histoplasmosis, coccidioidomycosis, cryptosporidiosis, isosporiasis, microsporidiosis, esophageal candidiasis, HIV dementia, B-cell lymphomas, and cervical cancer. The median survival during this stage of illness is 18 to 24 months.[31]

As the CD4 lymphocyte counts drop below 100 cells per mm³, complications include cytomegalovirus retinitis, *Mycobacterium avium* complex, and progressive multifocal leukoencephalopathy. Careful clinical evaluation and prophylactic therapy for many of these opportunistic infections may be recommended (Table 49–7). CD4 counts less than 50 cells per mm³ are associated with a median survival of 12 months,[38] with the majority of deaths occurring after the CD4 count falls below 50 cells per mm³.[39] Bacterial pneumonias due to *Staphylo-*

TABLE 49–6. CD4-Specific Recommendations for the Care of Human Immunodeficiency Virus-Infected Women*

CD4 COUNT	RECOMMENDED CARE
CD4 >500 cells/mm^3	CD4 counts every 3–6 months depending on level and state of health
CD4 ≤500 cells/mm^3	CD4 counts every 2–3 months Discuss antiviral therapy (see Table 49–9), encourage if symptomatic (e.g., thrush, fevers, weight loss) Consider referral for discussion of research protocols if client is interested in treatment
CD4 ≤300 cells/mm^3	CD4 counts every 2–3 months Discuss antiviral therapy, encourage if symptomatic from HIV infection PCP prophylaxis if symptomatic from HIV infection (see Table 49–7)
CD4 ≤200 cells/mm^3	CD4 counts every 2–3 months until <50 Encourage antiviral therapy (see Table 49–9) PCP prophylaxis (see Table 49–7) Routine funduscopic exam every 3–6 months Consider toxoplasmosis prophylaxis if positive serology (see Table 49–7)[143]
CD4 <100 cells/mm^3	CD4 counts every 2–3 months until <50, then only to monitor response to changes in treatment or as clinically indicated Encourage antiretroviral therapy (see Table 49–9) PCP prophylaxis (see Table 49–7) Consider MAC prophylaxis (see Table 49–7) Consider toxoplasmosis prophylaxis if positive serology (see Table 49–7)[143] Routine funduscopic exam every 3–6 months

*These recommendations are based on CD4 counts but should be interpreted with respect to an individual patient's clinical status, competing health issues, other medications, and personal preferences. The recommendations supplement health maintenance evaluation (see Table 49–8). More frequent CD4 count measurements are suggested if the disease is clinically progressing or if CD4 cell counts are approaching a level where a change in therapy is recommended. See Table 49–9 for specific guidelines for the choice of antiretroviral therapy and Table 49–7 for recommendations for prophylactic therapy.

PCP, *Pneumocystis carinii* pneumonia; MAC, *Mycobacterium avium complex*; HIV, human immunodeficiency virus.

coccus aureus, H. influenzae, and *S. pneumoniae* are common causes of death in this population.[40]

Gynecologic Manifestations

Candida vaginitis, genital ulcer diseases (such as herpes and syphilis), pelvic inflammatory disease (PID), HPV diseases (condylomata, SIL, and carcinoma), and menstrual irregularities occur at all stages of HIV infection and are often the earliest manifestations of HIV disease in women. The frequency and severity of these gynecologic conditions increase with the degree of immunosuppression. Atypical manifestations and suboptimal responses to standard therapy are common.[41]

Vaginal Candidiasis

The most common gynecologic disorder in HIV-infected women is chronic vaginal candidiasis.[17, 18] Persistent or recurrent disease can occur at higher mean CD4 counts than in oral candidiasis.[42] Recurrent vaginal candidiasis may imply progressive immunosuppression and herald the onset of other opportunistic infections.[43] Vulvovaginal candidiasis generally responds well to topical therapy; however, systemic therapy with an imidazole is sometimes required in refractory cases (see Table 49–5). Maintenance or suppressive therapy may be necessary, especially in women with moderate to severe immunosuppression.[44]

Genital Tract Infections and Pelvic Inflammatory Disease

Little is known about the clinical course and management of PID in HIV-infected women. High rates of HIV infection (4–16.7%) have been found in women hospitalized for PID,[45–47] and a number of studies have suggested that women with HIV may have an inadequate response to standard treatment. Compared with HIV-negative women, HIV-infected women presented with less abdominal tenderness and lower leukocyte counts and, despite similar regimens, had a higher risk of requiring surgical treatment for their disease.[47, 48] In recognition that the natural history and management of PID may be altered by HIV infection, PID was added to the CDC classification system for symptomatic HIV infection (see Table 49–2).[16] However, current recommendations for the initial management of PID in this population do not differ from those for women not known to be HIV infected (see Table 49–5).[49]

Despite the wide prevalence of lower genital tract infections in women in general, very little information is available on the prevalence of bacterial vaginosis or trichomoniasis in HIV-infected women. The Multicenter PID-HIV Study Group found similar rates of cervical gonorrhea and *Chlamydia* (approximately 25%), bacterial vaginosis (50%), *Trichomonas* (20%), and vaginal candidiasis (20%) in both HIV-infected and -uninfected women.[50] However, a Baltimore group

TABLE 49–7.   Prophylaxis of Human Immunodeficiency Virus–Related Infectious Complications

CONDITION	FIRST CHOICE	ALTERNATIVES	INDICATIONS
Pneumocystis carinii pneumonia	TMP-SMX (1 DS tablet daily PO or 3 ×/wk), or TMP-SMX (1 SS tablet daily PO)	Aerosolized pentamidine (300 mg monthly via Respigard II nebulizer) Dapsone* (25 mg/day or 100 mg PO 2–3 ×/wk) Pentamidine (4 mg/kg IM/IV every 2–4 wk)	History of prior PCP, or CD4 cell count <200/mm³, or CD4 cell count >200/mm³ with persistent HIV-related symptoms: fever, thrush, weight loss
Tuberculosis			
INH sensitive	INH (300 mg PO daily) plus pyridoxine (50 mg PO daily × 12 mo)	Rifampin (600 mg PO daily × 12 mo)	History or presence of positive result of purified protein derivative test with > 5 mm induration in the absence of prior adequate treatment for latent or active TB, or Anergy and high risk for prior exposure to TB[141]
Drug resistant	If only INH resistance, rifampin (600 mg PO daily × 12 mo) Otherwise contact expert in treatment of drug-resistant TB	Potential regimens include pyrazinamide plus ethambutol, with or without ciprofloxacin	
Mycobacterium avium complex (MAC)	Rifabutin (300 mg PO daily)	Clarithromycin (500 mg PO b.i.d.) or Azithromycin (500 mg PO 3 ×/wk)	CD4 cell counts < 100/mm³ and no MAC infection
Toxoplasma gondii	TMP-SMX (1 DS tablet PO daily or 3 ×/wk), or TMP-SMX (1 SS tablet PO daily)	Dapsone (as for PCP prophylaxis) plus pyrimethamine (50 mg PO) and folinic acid (5 mg PO 2–3 ×/wk)	CD4 cell count < 100–200/mm³ and positive *Toxoplasma* IgG
Cryptococcus neoformans	None recommended	Some clinicians use fluconazole (50–100 mg PO daily)[142]	CD4 cell count <1 100/mm³

TMP-SMX, Trimethoprim plus sulfamethoxazole; DS, double strength (160 mg trimethoprim plus 800 mg sulfamethoxazole); SS, single strength (80 mg trimethoprim plus 400 mg sulfamethoxazole); INH, isoniazid; PCP, *Pneumocystis carinii* pneumonia.

*Test for glucose-6-phosphate dehydrogenase deficiency before initiating therapy.

Adapted from Gallant JE, Moore R, Chaisson RE. Prophylaxis for opportunistic infections in patients with HIV infection. Ann Intern Med 1994; 120:932; Bartlett JG. The Johns Hopkins Hospital Guide to Medical Care of Patients with HIV Infection. 4th ed. Baltimore: Williams & Wilkins, 1994.

found that HIV-infected women were more likely to have syphilis (15 versus 5%), gonorrhea (20 versus 13%), and *Trichomonas* (28 versus 16%).[51]

The genital ulcer diseases (herpes simplex virus, syphilis, and chancroid) occur with greater frequency and severity in HIV-infected women[18] and may be more refractory to therapy. The diagnosis of herpetic lesions may be more difficult owing to atypical manifestations, such as severely ulcerating perineal disease,[52] and bacterial superinfection. Herpetic ulcers may respond more slowly to therapy, and because frequent recurrences are common, suppressive oral therapy may be necessary.[53, 54]

The incidence of primary and secondary syphilis has increased to its highest level in 40 years.[55] The current epidemic of syphilis overlaps epidemiologically with the HIV epidemic, particularly among black heterosexuals in urban areas.[56] In recent years, the syphilitic epidemic has shifted from the urban areas of the East, West, and Gulf coastal areas to the Midwest, paralleling that of the HIV epidemic.[55] In women, the epidemics of both syphilis and HIV infection are strongly linked to the use of crack cocaine and low socioeconomic status.[55] Concurrent HIV infection does not appear to alter the Venereal Disease Research Laboratories

positivity rate in the diagnosis of syphilis[57, 58] or the usual serologic response to treatment.[59, 60]

The incidence of early neurosyphilis has risen dramatically in the HIV era. Individuals infected with HIV and early primary or secondary syphilis have been shown to have a high incidence of asymptomatic and clinically apparent neurosyphilis.[61] A high relapse rate after treatment of primary infection has been described, especially when conventional doses of penicillin have been used.[62] Because the magnitude of these increased risks has not been adequately quantified, the CDC has not altered its treatment recommendations for HIV-infected individuals with early syphilis from those without concurrent HIV infection (see Table 49–5), although careful evaluation (1, 2, 3, 6, 9, and 12 months) after therapy is recommended; cerebrospinal fluid examination before therapy is recommended in all HIV-infected individuals presenting with latent syphilis.[49] Some clinicians recommend a more aggressive approach to both diagnosis and therapy, suggesting a cerebrospinal fluid examination on all HIV-infected patients with syphilis regardless of neurologic symptoms and stage of disease.[62, 63]

Some literature suggests that the presence of

certain sexually transmitted diseases may serve as cofactors and facilitate the transmission of HIV between sexual partners[64, 65] (see Heterosexual Transmission in Chapter 48). The strong correlation between the incidence of sexually transmitted diseases and the prevalence of HIV infection demonstrates the need for prevention efforts against these concurrent epidemics.

Cervical Disease

Infection with HPV, the etiologic agent of venereal warts, is associated with the development of cervical SIL and cervical cancer. A number of studies have shown a three- to twelvefold increased risk of SIL and cervical cancer in HIV-infected women.[21, 22, 66–69] This increased risk appears to be related to a synergistic effect between HIV-induced immunosuppression and HPV cervical infection, with increased rates of SIL reported in women who are coinfected with HIV and HPV compared with women infected with only one of these viruses.[21] As a result of this increased risk of cervical neoplasia, invasive cervical cancer was added to the CDC AIDS case definition in 1993.[16] Women with HIV infection and SIL or cervical cancer appear to have higher rates of multicentric disease, a more advanced stage of disease at the time of diagnosis, and a poorer response to treatment than their seronegative counterparts.[70, 71] A number of studies have also reported that the relative risk of these conditions is related to the degree of HIV-induced immunosuppression (as measured by decreasing CD4 cell counts),[67, 72] as is a poorer response to treatment. Maiman and colleagues reported that in HIV-positive women with SIL treated with a standard protocol, recurrence rates were 18% in women with CD4 cell counts greater than 500 cells per mm^3 and 45% in women with CD4 counts less than 500 cells per mm^3.[70]

Because of the increased incidence of SIL and of more aggressive disease, particularly in women with more advanced HIV infection, the optimal screening technique and schedule is unknown. One study comparing Papanicolaou (PAP) smears with colposcopic biopsies as a routine screening procedure found that PAP smears were significantly less sensitive in detecting SIL (3 versus 41%).[73] Another study has not confirmed this finding.[74] The role of colposcopy in the routine care of HIV-positive women remains controversial, and a clinical trial is ongoing to resolve the issue. Recommendations from the Agency for Health Care Policy and research are for semiannual PAP smears, with colposcopic follow-up for abnormal cytologic findings. The expert panel specifically did not recommend the use of colposcopy as a routine screening tool.[75]

The appropriate management of SIL and cervical cancer in HIV-infected women is also unknown because of increased rates of recurrent disease and decreased response to standard treatment modalities.[70] More information on the natural history and management of these conditions is needed; a study evaluating the role of local chemotherapy (intravaginal 5-fluorouracil) after standard ablative treatment of SIL to prevent recurrent disease is in progress.

APPROACH TO THE PRIMARY CARE MANAGEMENT OF WOMEN INFECTED WITH HUMAN IMMUNODEFICIENCY VIRUS

The evaluation and primary medical care of a woman infected with HIV must recognize the need for a comprehensive and multidisciplinary spectrum of services to address the medical, social, and psychological effects of her infection. A guideline for the initial and subsequent evaluation of a woman with HIV infection is summarized in Table 49–8. The assessment begins with a complete history, including previous medical problems (especially opportunistic infections), sexual and drug history, contraceptive use, and family and support systems. A comprehensive physical examination, with particular attention to the skin, oral cavity, neurologic findings, and lymph nodes, should be performed at each evaluation. A baseline indirect and direct funduscopic examination should be performed, although many physicians defer the initial indirect funduscopy until the CD4 counts are less than 200 to 500 cells per mm^3. As the CD4 cell counts fall below 100 cells per mm^3, the indirect funduscopy should be repeated at least every 6 months. A complete pelvic examination with PAP smear and cultures for *Chlamydia* and *N. gonorrhoeae* should be included. The PAP smear should be repeated every 6 months, with aggressive follow-up for abnormal results. Dental examination and prophylaxis should be performed every 3 to 6 months.

Routine laboratory work including hematology, chemistries (including liver function tests), CD4 cell count and percent, toxoplasmosis titer, hepatitis B serology, and Venereal Disease Research Laboratories should be performed at the initial evaluation. Because of daily variability, the CD4 cell count should be repeated at the next visit to obtain a more stable baseline measure before initiating antiretroviral therapy or prophylaxis for opportunistic infections.[76] The role of other prognos-

TABLE 49–8. Primary Care Health Maintenance Schedule

ASSESSMENT	FREQUENCY
Physical examination	Every 3–6 months, more often if clinically indicated
Papanicolaou smear	Every 6 months, more often if abnormal
Weight and nutritional assessment	Every 3–6 months, more often if clinically indicated
CD4 cell count	Every 3–6 months, more often as counts approach targets for interventional therapy (see Table 49–6)
Complete blood count	Every 6 months if asymptomatic, every 3–6 months if symptomatic, more often if on myelotoxic medications
Chemistry panel	Yearly if asymptomatic, every 2–4 months if on toxic medications
Purified protein derivative and anergy panel	Yearly, omit if anergic for 2 consecutive years
Toxoplasma titer	Baseline, yearly if negative
Venereal Disease Research Laboratories (VDRL)	Yearly
Hepatitis B serologies	Baseline
Hepatitis C serology	Baseline
Immunizations	
Pneumovax	Initially
Haemophilus B vaccine	Initially
Hepatitis B vaccine	Initially if serology negative and patient at risk
Influenza vaccine	Every November
Diphtheria/tetanus	Every 10 years
Counseling	Initially, then as needed
Psychosocial assessment	
Safer sex education	
Drug use education	
Living will, do-not-resuscitate orders	Yearly

From El-sadr W, Oleske JM, Agins BD, et al. Evaluation and Management of Early HIV Infection. U.S. Department of Health and Human Services, Public Health Service, Agency for Health Care Policy and Research, 1994 (U.S. Department of Health and Human Services PHS Agency for Health Care Policy and Research, ed. Clinical Practice Guideline; Vol 7, AHCPR Publication No. 94-0572); Soloway B, Hecht F. Primary care: Charting materials. AIDS Clin Care 1991; 3(6):44.

tic markers of HIV progression, such as p24 antigen and β_2-microglobulin, in general practice is unknown, although some clinicians order these tests to help guide treatment choices.[32] Once the clinical stage of HIV infection has been determined from history, examination, and CD4 cell counts, options for prophylaxis for opportunistic infections (see Table 49–7) and antiretroviral therapy (Table 49–9) should be discussed.

A skin test for TB, using the standard Mantoux method (5 U intermediate-strength purified protein derivative [PPD] injected intradermally) along with two delayed-type hypersensitivity controls (two of the following: mumps, *Candida albicans,* or tetanus toxoid)[77] should be performed yearly or until anergic for 2 consecutive years. Because of increased risks of reactivation of TB,[78, 79] women who have a positive PPD skin test (>5 mm of induration) or who are anergic and at high risk for past exposure to TB should be evaluated with a chest radiograph to preclude the possibility of active disease; if active TB is not present, prophylactic therapy, usually with isoniazid for 1 year, should be initiated unless otherwise contraindicated.[77, 80] Women with a negative PPD skin test should receive skin testing every 6 to 12 months,

depending on the risk of ongoing exposure to TB.[80]

Because of increased rates of bacterial infections and potential for morbidity due to viral illnesses, vaccines are an important part of the preventive care of women with HIV infection.[81–83] Because immunologic response correlates with the stage of disease, pneumococcal vaccine and possibly *H. influenzae* type B vaccines should be given as early as possible to women who have not received them in the past[83–85]; influenza vaccine should be administered when seasonally appropriate.[83, 84] Other vaccines such as tetanus and measles should be kept up to date. If a patient does not have evidence of prior hepatitis B infection and is at continuing risk for exposure through sexual activity or injection drug use, the hepatitis B vaccine should be given using the standard dose regimen.[84]

Education and counseling are a crucial component of the care of HIV-infected women. Information about HIV and its sequelae should be reviewed, and safe sexual practices discussed. Dietary counseling should be given to encourage adequate nutrition and decrease the risk of exposure to pathogens that may result in significant

TABLE 49–9. Antiretroviral Treatment Recommendations from the 1993 National Institute of Allergy and Infectious Diseases State-of-the-Art Panel on Antiretroviral Therapy in Human Immunodeficiency Virus-Infected Patients

CLINICAL STATUS	CD4 + CELL COUNT (cells/mm³)	RECOMMENDATION
No Previous Antiretroviral Therapy		
Asymptomatic	>500	No therapy
Asymptomatic	200–500	ZDV or no therapy
Symptomatic	200–500	ZDV
Asymptomatic	<200	ZDV
Symptomatic	<200	ZDV
Previous Antiretroviral Therapy		
Stable	≥300	Continue ZDV
Stable	<300	Continue ZDV or change to ddI
Progressing	50–500	Change to ddI or ddC
Progressing	<50	Change to ddI or ddC
Intolerant to ZDV		
Stable or progressing	<500	Change to ddI or ddC

ZDV, Zidovudine; ddI, didanosine; ddC, zalcitabine.
From Sande MA, Carpenter CCJ, Cobbs CG, et al. Antiretroviral therapy for adult HIV-infected patients: Recommendations from a state-of-the-art conference. JAMA 1993; 270:2583.

morbidity or mortality.[86] Restrictions should include avoiding raw eggs and undercooked chicken (for *Salmonella* and *Campylobacter* species), undercooked meat (for *Toxoplasma gondii* in patients with negative serologies), and unpasteurized milk (for *Listeria monocytogenes*). Finally, when appropriate, issues of disclosure, health care proxies, living wills, and guardianship of children should be discussed. This discussion requires time, education, and sensitivity on the part of health care providers and may be facilitated by the involvement of individuals with experience in these areas.

PROPHYLAXIS OF INFECTIOUS COMPLICATIONS

Some of the major advances in the care of HIV-infected individuals have been in the area of prevention of infections such as PCP and TB.[87–89] Current recommendations for prophylactic regimens in HIV-infected individuals are summarized in Table 49–7. The benefits of each prophylactic therapy must be weighed against its efficacy, cost, and drug toxicity. The potential for adverse drug interactions with multiple concurrent medications must also be considered. Prophylactic interventions such as immunizations and evaluation for TB prophylaxis should be performed on entering the health care system (see Table 49–8). The timing of other interventions, including prophylaxis for PCP and *M. avium* complex, is determined primarily by the CD4 cell count (see Table 49–7).

ANTIRETROVIRAL THERAPY

Therapeutic choices and decisions surrounding the treatment of HIV infection must integrate continually changing information from clinical trials, ongoing laboratory research, clinical experience, and patients' preferences. As more treatment options and information from clinical investigations become available, these decisions become more complex. In addition to conflicting data from clinical trials, the efficacy of available treatments has been limited by toxicity, the development of drug resistance, and the inability to reverse HIV-mediated immunosuppression. In this setting, there may not be an ideal choice, and the best treatment option should be decided individually for each patient.

Four drugs with anti-HIV activity have currently been approved by the Food and Drug Administration for treatment of HIV-infected individuals; zidovudine (3'-azido-3'-deoxythymidine [AZT, ZDV]), didanosine (dideoxyinosine [ddI]), zalcitabine (dideoxycytidine [ddC]), and stavudine (2',3'-didehydro-3'-cleoxythymidine [d4T]).[90–94] All four agents are nucleoside analogues that inhibit HIV reverse transcriptase. Initial studies found that ZDV prolonged survival in patients with advanced HIV infection and delayed clinical progression for at least 1 year in individuals with less advanced disease.[90, 91, 95] Studies comparing these drugs found that ZDV was superior to either ddI or ddC as initial antiretroviral therapy,[96, 97] whereas ddI and ddC appeared to be equally effective second-line therapy in individuals with prior ZDV treatment.[98] The spectrum of toxicity is different for these agents (Table 49–10). Major toxicities of ZDV include neutropenia, anemia, nausea, and myopathy. Dideoxyinosine can cause pancreatitis (which may be fatal), painful neuropathy, and diarrhea, and ddC is associated with stomatitis, neuropathy (more frequently than ddI), and pancreatitis (less commonly than ddI).

Unfortunately, treatment with ZDV has been shown to be limited by toxicity and the development of drug resistance, with little impact on survival or quality of life.[95, 99, 100] The Veteran Affairs Cooperative Study found that ZDV treatment had no impact on survival after 2 years of follow-up, although some delay in progression to AIDS was observed.[101] More recently, the Concorde Study reported no benefit in either clinical progression or survival in individuals treated with ZDV for 3 years.[99, 102] Laboratory investigations have confirmed that drug resistance develops in individuals treated with ZDV, with an increased risk of resistance associated with more advanced disease or longer duration of treatment.[103, 104] The development of this resistance is associated with an increased risk of disease progression in ZDV-treated patients that is independent of other prognostic factors.[14, 105, 106] Clinical trials have shown that although ZDV remains the choice for initial treatment, individuals with prior ZDV therapy (as little as 2–4 months) may benefit from changing antiretroviral therapy to ddI, a drug that is active against ZDV-resistant HIV.[96, 107, 108]

ZDV has also been shown to decrease vertical transmission in a large study performed by the AIDS Clinical Trial Group (ACTG 076).[109] Pregnant women with CD4 cell counts greater than 200 per mm^3 with no prior ZDV treatment were given ZDV or placebo after the first trimester and intravenous ZDV or placebo during labor; the infants received the same medication for the first 6 weeks of life. Transmission was found to be reduced by 68% from 25.5% in the placebo group to 8.3% in the ZDV group.[23] Based on the results of this study, it is recommended that ZDV be offered to pregnant women with HIV infection, although the efficacy of this regimen in women with prior ZDV treatment or lower CD4 cell counts remains unknown.

Based on clinical and laboratory observations, increasing interest is expressed about earlier use of combination treatment using agents that target the same or different steps in HIV replication in order to delay the onset of drug resistance.[109a] One study compared ddC with ZDV monotherapy and ZDV-ddC combination therapy in patients with prior ZDV therapy and CD4 cell counts less than 300 per mm^3. Overall, combination treatment did not offer any clinical advantage[110]; however, in a subanalysis, the combination regimen delayed clinical progression in individuals with CD4 cell counts between 150 and 300 cells per mm^3. Finally, some studies have suggested that the combination of ZDV plus acyclovir (800 mg two to four times a day) may offer a survival advantage to individuals with advanced HIV infection.[111] A

TABLE 49–10. Recommended Regimens and Potential Toxicities of Selected Antiretroviral Drugs

DRUG	DOSAGE	TOXICITY	COMMENTS
ZDV	100 mg PO 5 ×/day, or 200 mg t.i.d.	Anemia, leukopenia, nausea, skin and nail discoloration, hepatitis	Higher rates of toxicity in patients with more advanced human immunodeficiency virus infection Some studies have suggested lower doses (300 mg daily) be effective with reduced toxicity[145]
ddI	200 mg PO b.i.d.; 125 mg PO b.i.d. for <60 kg	Pancreatitis (rarely fatal), diarrhea, painful neuropathy	Buffer reduces absorption of rifabutin, dapsone, ketoconazole. Must take 2 tablets with each dose
ddC	0.75 mg PO t.i.d.	Painful neuropathy, stomatitis, pancreatitis	Stomatitis resolves without stopping medication
D4T	40 mg PO b.i.d. 30 mg PO b.i.d. for <60 kg	Neuropathy, pancreatitis	
3TC	150–300 mg PO b.i.d. in clinical trials	Neutropenia (rare), neuropathy (rare), macrocytosis	Used in combination therapy in clinical trials
Nevirapine	400 mg PO daily in clinical trials	Rash (rarely Stevens-Johnson syndrome), hepatitis	Decreased incidence of rash in patients started on 200 mg daily

b.i.d., Twice a day; t.i.d., 3 times a day.

From Sande MA, Carpenter CCJ, Cobbs CG, et al. Antiretroviral therapy for adult HIV-infected patients: Recommendations from a state-of-the-art conference. JAMA 1993; 270:2583. Copyright 1993, American Medical Association.

number of other trials addressing the role of combination therapy as initial or secondary treatment are currently in progress.

Because of the limited efficacy of current antiretrovirals, the development of drug resistance, and treatment-limiting toxicities, a number of other agents and therapeutic strategies are also in clinical use or trials. Another nucleoside reverse transcriptase inhibitor, 3TC,[112] has been shown to have anti-HIV activity and is currently in clinical trials and is also available through a compassionate use program. Nonnucleoside reverse transcriptase inhibitors such as nevirapine are also being studied, and although these agents have been shown to have specific anti-HIV-1 activity, the rapid development of resistance has limited their potential use to combination therapies.[103] Research is continuing on agents that block other steps of the HIV life cycle, including *tat* inhibitors (which did not show activity in early clinical trials) and protease inhibitors.[108] Efforts to affect the immune system are also being studied. Vaccines derived from envelope glycoproteins (gp 160 and gp 120) and designed to induce neutralization antibodies and enhance cell-mediated immunity are in clinical trials[113, 114]; immunotherapy with interferon has shown promising results but dose-limiting toxicity.[115] Finally, patients and providers express growing interest about alternative therapies such as acupuncture and herbal therapies.[116] Such therapies that show promising antiretroviral activity in the laboratory or clinical benefit should be considered for evaluation in clinical trials, recognizing their potential for efficacy and for toxicity.

In the setting of often conflicting results of clinical trials, the National Institute of Allergy and Infectious Diseases convened an expert panel to make recommendations to guide the use of antiretrovirals. These guidelines are summarized in Table 49–9.[117] This panel emphasized that each treatment decision should be individualized, using the recommendations as guidelines, and that the ultimate decision rested with the patient. The guidelines suggest consideration of ZDV (600 mg daily in three divided doses) or observation alone in asymptomatic individuals with CD4 cell counts greater than 200 per mm^3 and strongly recommend treatment for patients with lower CD4 cell counts or symptoms. In individuals with evidence of clinical progression on ZDV or ZDV intolerance, the panel recommended switching to either ddI or ddC. Many of the studies from which these recommendations derive did not enroll adequate numbers of women to determine if gender-specific differences in efficacy or toxicity exist.[118] It is essential that efforts be made to overcome women's real and perceived barriers to enrollment in

clinical trials so that these important questions can be studied.

REFERENCES

1. Fleming PL, Ciesielski CA, Byers RH, et al. Gender differences in reported AIDS-indicative diagnoses. J Infect Dis 1993;168:61.
2. Lemp GF, Hirozawa AM, Cohen JB, et al. Survival for women and men with AIDS. J Infect Dis 1992;166:74.
3. Hellinger FJ. The use of health services by women with HIV infection. Health Serv Res 1993;28:543.
4. Bastian L, Bennett CL, Adams J, et al. Differences between men and women with HIV-related *Pneumocystis carinii* pneumonia: Experience from 3,070 cases in New York City in 1987. J Acquir Immune Defic Syndr 1993;6:617.
5. Stone VE, Seage GR, Hertz T, Epstein AM. The relation between hospital experience and mortality for patients with AIDS. JAMA 1992;268:2655.
6. Greene WC. The molecular biology of human immunodeficiency virus type 1 infection. N Engl J Med 1991;324:308.
7. Levy JA. Pathogenesis of human immunodeficiency virus infection. Microbiol Rev 1993;57:183.
8. Steffy K, Wong-Staal F. Genetic regulation of human immunodeficiency virus. Microbiol Rev 1991;55:193.
9. Pantaleo G, Graziosi C, Fauci AS. The immunopathogenesis of human immunodeficiency virus infection. N Engl J Med 1993;328:327.
10. Clerici M, Shearer GN. A TH1 to TH2 switch is a critical step in the etiology of HIV infection. Immunol Today 1993;14:107.
11. Collaborative DHPG Treatment Study Group. Treatment of serious cytomegalovirus infections with 9-(1,3-dihydroxy-2-propoxymethyl)guanine in patients with AIDS and other immunodeficiencies. N Engl J Med 1986;1986:801.
12. Mackewicz CE, Ortega HW, Levy JA. CD8 + cell anti-HIV activity correlates with the clinical state of the infected individual. J Clin Invest 1991;87:1462.
13. Levy JA. HIV pathogenesis and long term survival. AIDS 1990;7:1401.
14. St. Clair M, Hartigan P, Andrews J, et al. Zidovudine resistance, syncytium-inducing phenotype, and HIV disease progression in a case-control study. J Acquir Immune Defic Syndr 1993;6:891–897.
15. Koot M, Keet IPM, Vos AHV, et al. Prognostic value of HIV-1 syncytium-inducing phenotype for rate of CD4 + cell depletion and progression to AIDS. Ann Intern Med 1993;118:681.
16. Centers for Disease Control and Prevention (CDC). 1993 revised classification system for HIV infection and expanded surveillance case definition for AIDS among adolescents and adults. MMWR 1993;41(RR-17):1.
17. Rothenberg R, Woelfel M, Stoneburner R, et al. Survival with the acquired immunodeficiency syndrome. N Engl J Med 1987;317:1297.
18. Carpenter CCJ, Mayer KH, Stein MD, et al. Human immunodeficiency virus infection in North American women: Experience with 200 cases and a review of the literature. Medicine 1991;70:307.
19. Selwyn PA, Alcabes P, Hartel D, et al. Clinical manifestations and predictors of disease progression in drug users with human immunodeficiency virus infection. N Engl J Med 1992;327:1697.
20. Farizo KM, Buehler JW, Chamberland ME, et al. Spectrum of disease in persons with human immunode-

ficiency virus infection in the United States. JAMA 1992;267:1798.

21. Vermund S, Kelly K, Klein R, et al. High risk of human papillomavirus infection and cervical squamous intraepithelial lesions among women with symptomatic human immunodeficiency virus infection. Am J Obstet Gynecol 1991;165:392.

22. Mandelblatt JS, Fahs M, Garibaldi K, et al. Association between HIV infection and cervical neoplasia: Implications for clinical care of women at risk for both conditions. AIDS 1993;6:173.

23. CDC. Update: Impact of the expanded AIDS surveillance case definition for adolescents and adults on case reporting—United States, 1993. MMWR 1994;43(9):160.

24. Buchbinder S, Heessol N, O'Malley P, et al. HIV disease progression and the impact of prophylactic therapies in the San Francisco City Clinic Cohort (SFCCC): A 13 year follow-up (abstract WC42). Seventh International World Conference on AIDS, Florence, Italy, June 16–21, 1991.

25. Learmont J, Tindall B, Evans L, et al. Long-term symptomless HIV-1 infection in recipients of blood products from a single donor. Lancet 1992;340:863.

26. Flanigan TP, Imam N, Lange N, et al. Decline of CD4 lymphocyte counts from the time of seroconversion in HIV-positive women. J Womens Health 1992;1:231.

27. Tindall B, Cooper DA, Donovan B, Penny R. Primary human immunodeficiency virus infection: Clinical and serologic aspects. Infect Dis Clin North Am 1988;2:329.

28. Wolinsky SM, Rinaldo CR, Kwok S, et al. Human immunodeficiency virus type 1 (HIV-1) infection a median of 18 months before a diagnostic western blot. Ann Intern Med 1989;111:961.

29. Farzadegan H, Polis MA, Wolinsky SM, et al. Loss of human immunodeficiency virus type 1 (HIV-1) antibodies with evidence of viral infection in asymptomatic homosexual men: A report from the multicenter AIDS cohort study. Ann Intern Med 1988;108:785.

30. Stein DS, Korvick JA, Vermund SH. CD4 + lymphocyte cell enumeration for prediction of clinical course of human immunodeficiency virus disease: A review. J Infect Dis 1992;165:352.

31. MacDonell KB, Chimiel JS, Poggensee L, et al. Predicting progression to AIDS: Combined usefulness of CD4 lymphocyte counts and p24 antigenemia. Am J Med 1990;89:706.

32. Fahey JL, Taylor JMG, Detels R, et al. The prognostic value of cellular and serologic markers in infection with human immunodeficiency virus type 1. N Engl J Med 1990;322:166.

33. Choi S, Lagakos SW, Schooley RT, Volberding PA. CD4 + lymphocytes are an incomplete surrogate marker for clinical progression in persons with asymptomatic HIV infection taking zidovudine. Ann Intern Med 1993;118:674.

34. CDC. Guidelines for the performance of CD4 T-cell determinations in persons with human immunodeficiency virus infection. MMWR 1992;41(RR-8):1.

35. Van Rood Y, Goulmy E, Blokland E, et al. Month-related variability in immunological test results; implications for immunological follow-up studies. Clin Exp Immunol 1991;86:349.

36. Malone JL, Simms TE, Gray GC, et al. Sources of variability in repeated T-helper lymphocyte counts from HIV-1-infected patients: Total lymphocyte count fluctuations and diurnal cycle are important. J Acquir Immune Defic Syndr 1990;3:144.

37. Laurence J. T-cell subsets in health, infectious disease, and idiopathic CD4 + T lymphocytopenia. Ann Intern Med 1993;119:55.

38. Yarchoan R, Venzon DJ, Pluda JM, et al. CD4 count and the risk for death in patients infected with HIV receiving antiretroviral therapy. Ann Intern Med 1991;115:184.

39. Phillips AN, Elford J, Sabin C, et al. Immunodeficiency and the risk of death in HIV infection. JAMA 1992;268:2662.

40. Stein M, O'Sullivan P, Wachtel T, et al. Causes of death in persons with human immunodeficiency virus infection. Am J Med 1992;93:387.

41. Minkoff HL, DeHovitz JA. Care of women infected with the human immunodeficiency virus. JAMA 1991;266:2253.

42. Imam N, Carpenter CCJ, Mayer KH, et al. Hierarchical pattern of mucosal candida infections in HIV-seropositive women. Am J Med 1990;89:142.

43. Rhoads JL, Wright C, Redfield RR, Burke DS. Chronic vaginal candidiasis in women with human immunodeficiency virus infection. JAMA 1987;257:3105.

44. Sobel JD. Candidal vulvovaginitis. Clin Obstet Gynecol 1993;36:153.

45. Safrin S, Rush J, Mills J. Influenza in patients with human immunodeficiency virus infection. Chest 1990;98:33.

46. Sperling RS, Friedman FJ, Joyner M, et al. Seroprevalence of human immunodeficiency virus in women admitted to the hospital with pelvic inflammatory disease. J Reprod Med 1991;36:122.

47. Hoegsberg B, Abulafia O, Sedlis A, et al. Sexually transmitted diseases and human immunodeficiency virus infection among women with pelvic inflammatory disease. Am J Obstet Gynecol 1990;163:1135.

48. Korn AP, Landers DV, Green JR, Sweet RL. Pelvic inflammatory disease in human immunodeficiency virus–infected women. Obstet Gynecol 1993;82:765.

49. CDC. 1993 sexually transmitted disease treatment guidelines. MMWR 1993;42(RR-14):1.

50. Irwin K, O'Sullivan M, Sperling R, et al. The microbiologic etiology of pelvic inflammatory disease (PID) in HIV + and HIV − women; preliminary findings of a multicenter study. (Abstract PO-B23-1937). Ninth International Conference on AIDS, Berlin, Germany, June 6–11, 1993.

51. Zenilman JM, Erickson B, Fox R, et al. Effect of HIV posttest counseling on STD incidence. JAMA 1992;267:843.

52. Quinnan GV, Masur H, Rook AH, et al. Herpes virus infections in the acquired immune deficiency syndrome. JAMA 1984;252:72.

53. Strauss SE, Siedlin M, Takiff H, et al. Oral acyclovir to suppress recurring herpes simplex virus infections in immunodeficient patients. Ann Intern Med 1984;100:522.

54. Conant MA. Prophylactic and suppressive treatment with acyclovir and the management of herpes in patients with acquired immunodeficiency syndrome. J Am Acad Dermatol 1988;18:186.

55. CDC. Primary and secondary syphilis—United States, 1982–1990. MMWR 1991;40:314.

56. Rolfs R, Nakashima A. Epidemiology of primary and secondary syphilis in the United States, 1981–1989. JAMA 1990;264:1432.

57. Rompalo AM, Cannon RO, Quinn TC, Hook EWI. Association of biologic false-positive reactions for syphilis with human immunodeficiency virus infection. J Infect Dis 1992;165:1124.

58. Matlow AG, Rachlis AR. Syphilis serology in human immunodeficiency virus-infected patients with symptomatic neurosyphilis: Case report and review. Rev Infect Dis 1990;12:703.

59. Gourevitch MN, Selwyn PA, Davenny K, et al. Effects of HIV infection on the serologic manifestations and response to treatment of syphilis in intravenous drug users. Ann Intern Med 1993;118:350.

60. Romanowski B, Sutherland R, Fick GH, et al. Serologic response to treatment of infectious syphilis. Ann Intern Med 1991;114:1005.

61. Johns DR, Tierney M, Felsenstein D. Alteration in the natural history of neurosyphilis by concurrent infection with the human immunodeficiency virus. N Engl J Med 1987;316:1569.

62. Musher DM, Hamill RJ, Baughn RE. Effect of human immunodeficiency virus (HIV) infection on the course of syphilis and on the response to treatment. Ann Intern Med 1990;113:872.

63. Lukehart SA, Hook EW, Baker-Zander SA, et al. Invasion of the central nervous system by *Treponema pallidum*: Implications for diagnosis and treatment. Ann Intern Med 1988;109:855.

64. Laga M, Manoka A, Kivuvu M, et al. Non-ulcerative sexually transmitted diseases as risk factors for HIV-1 transmission in women: Results from a cohort study. AIDS 1993;7:95.

65. Plummer FA, Simonsen JN, Cameron DW, et al. Cofactors in male-female sexual transmission of human immunodeficiency virus type 1. J Infect Dis 1991;163:233.

66. Feingold AR, Vermund SH, Burk RD, et al. Cervical cytologic abnormalities and papillomavirus in women infected with human immunodeficiency virus. J Acquir Immune Defic Syndr 1990;3:896.

67. Marte C, Kelly P, Cohen M, et al. Papanicolaou smear abnormalities in ambulatory care sites for women infected with the human immunodeficiency virus. Am J Obstet Gynecol 1992;166:1232.

68. Conti M, Agarossi A, Parazzini F, et al. HPV, HIV infection, and risk of cervical intraepithelial neoplasia in former intravenous drug abusers. Gynecol Oncol 1993;49:344.

69. Ellerbrock T, Wright TC, Chaisson MA, et al. Strong independent association between HIV infection and cervical intraepithelial neoplasia (CIN) (Abstract WS-B07-5). Ninth International Conference on AIDS, Berlin, Germany, June 6–11, 1993.

70. Maiman M, Fruchter R, Serur E, et al. Recurrent cervical intraepithelial neoplasia in human immunodeficiency virus-seropositive women. Obstet Gynecol 1993;82:1170.

71. Adachi A, Fleming I, Burk R, et al. Women with human immunodeficiency virus infection and abnormal Papanicolaou smears: A prospective study of colposcopy and clinical outcome. Obstet Gynecol 1993;81:372.

72. Shafer A, Friedmann W, Mielke M, et al. The increased frequency of cervical dysplasia-neoplasia in women infected with the human immunodeficiency virus is related to the degree of immunosuppression. Am J Obstet Gynecol 1991;164:593.

73. Maiman M, Tarricone N, Viera J, et al. Colposcopic evaluation of human immunodeficiency virus-seropositive women. Obstet Gynecol 1991;78:84.

74. Wright T. Personal communication (submitted for publication).

75. El-sadr W, Oleske JM, Agins BD, et al. Evaluation and Management of Early HIV Infection. Rockville, MD: U.S. Department of Health and Human Services, Public Health Service, Agency for Health Care Policy and Research, 1994 (U.S. Department of Health and Human Services PHS Agency for Health Care Policy and Research, ed. Clinical Practice Guideline; Vol 7, AHCPR Publication No. 94-0572).

76. National Institute of Allergy and Infectious Diseases. State-of-the-art conference on azidothymidine therapy for early HIV infection. Am J Med 1990;89:335.

77. CDC. Purified protein derivative (PPD)-tuberculin anergy and HIV infection: Guidelines for anergy testing and management of anergic persons at risk of tuberculosis. MMWR 1991;40(RR-5):27.

78. Selwyn PA, Hartel D, Lewis V, et al. A prospective study of the risk of tuberculosis among intravenous drug users with human immunodeficiency virus infection. N Engl J Med 1989;320:545.

79. Barnes PF, Bloch AB, Davidson PT, Snyder DJ. Tuberculosis in patients with human immunodeficiency virus infection. N Engl J Med 1991;324:1644.

80. CDC. Screening for tuberculosis and tuberculosis infection in high-risk populations and the use of preventative therapy for tuberculous infection in the United States: Recommendations of the advisory committee for elimination of tuberculosis. MMWR 1990;39(RR-8):1.

81. Janoff E, Breiman R, Daley C, Hopewell P. Pneumococcal disease during HIV infection: Epidemiologic, clinical, and immunologic perspectives. Ann Intern Med 1992;117:314.

82. Witt D, Craven D, McCabe W. Bacterial infection in patients with acquired immunodeficiency syndrome (AIDS) and AIDS-related complex. Am J Med 1987;82:900.

83. CDC. Recommendations of the advisory committee on immunization practices (ACIP): Use of vaccines and immune globulins in persons with altered immunocompetence. MMWR 1993;42(RR-4):1.

84. Craven D, Fuller J, Barber T, Pelton S. Immunization of adults and children infected with human immunodeficiency virus. Infect Dis Clin Prac 1992;1:411.

85. Steinhoff M, Auerbach B, Nelson K, et al. Antibody responses to *Haemophilus influenza* type B vaccines in men with human immunodeficiency virus infection. N Engl J Med 1991;325:1837.

86. Kales C, Holzman R. Listeriosis in patients with HIV infection: Clinical manifestations and response to therapy. J Acquir Immune Defic Syndr 1990;3:139.

87. Graham N, Zeger S, Park L, et al. The effects on survival of early treatment of human immunodeficiency virus infection. N Engl J Med 1992;326:1037.

88. Pape JW, Jean SS, Ho JL, et al. Effect of isoniazid prophylaxis on incidence of active tuberculosis and progression of HIV infection. Lancet 1993;342:268.

89. Gallant JE, Moore R, Chaisson RE. Prophylaxis for opportunistic infections in patients with HIV infection. Ann Intern Med 1994;120:932.

90. Fischl M, Richman D, Grieco M, et al. The efficacy of azidothymidine (AZT) in the treatment of patients with AIDS and AIDS-related complex. N Engl J Med 1987;317:185.

91. Volberding PA, Lagakos SW, Koch MA, et al. Zidovudine in asymptomatic human immunodeficiency virus infection: A controlled trial in persons with fewer than 500 CD4-positive cells per cubic millimeter. N Engl J Med 1990;322:941.

92. Cooley T, Kunches L, Saunders C, et al. Once-daily administration of 2,3-dideoxyinosine (ddI) in patients with the acquired immunodeficiency syndrome or AIDS-related complex: Results of a phase I trial. N Engl J Med 1990;322:1340.

93. Yarchoan R, Thomas RV, Allain J-P, et al. Phase I studies of 2′,3′-dideoxycytidine in severe human immunodeficiency virus infection as a single agent and alternating with zidovudine (AZT). Lancet 1988;1:76.

94. Browne M, Mayer K, Chafee S, et al. 2,3-Didehydro-3-deoxythymidine (d4T) in patients with AIDS or AIDS related complex: A phase I trial. J Infect Dis 1993;167:21.

95. Cooper D, Gateli J, Kroon S, et al. Zidovudine in persons with asymptomatic HIV infection and CD4 + cell counts greater than 400 per cubic millimeter. N Engl J Med 1993;329:297.

96. Dolin R, Amato D, Fischl M, et al. Efficacy of didanosine (ddI) versus zidovudine (ZDV) in patients with 0 or less than or equal to 16 weeks of prior ZDV therapy: The ACTG of the NIAID (Abstract WS-B24-1). Ninth International Conference on AIDS, Berlin, Germany, 1993.

97. Follansbee S, Drew L, Olson R, et al. The efficacy of zalcitabine (ddC, HIVID) versus zidovudine (ZDV) as monotherapy in ZDV naive patients with advanced HIV disease: A randomized, double-blind, comparative trial (ACTG 114; N3300) (Abstract PO-B26-2113). Ninth International Conference on AIDS, Berlin, Germany, June 6–11, 1993.

98. Abrams D, Goldman A, Launer C, et al. A comparative trial of didanosine or zalcitabine after treatment with zidovudine in patients with human immunodeficiency virus infection: The Terry Beirn Community Programs for Clinical Research on AIDS. N Engl J Med 1994;330:657.

99. Concorde Coordinating Committee. Concorde: MRC/ANRS randomised double-blind controlled trial of immediate and deferred zidovudine in symptom-free HIV infection. Lancet 1994;343:871.

100. Lenderking W, Gelber R, Cotton D, et al. Evaluation of the quality of life associated with zidovudine treatment in asymptomatic human immunodeficiency virus infection: The AIDS Clinical Trials Group. N Engl J Med 1994;330:738.

101. Hamilton J, Hartigan P, Simberkoff M, et al. A controlled trial of early versus late treatment with zidovudine in symptomatic human immunodeficiency virus infection. N Engl J Med 1992;326:437.

102. Lipsky J. Concorde lands (commentary). Lancet 1994;343:866.

103. Larder B, Darby G, Richman D. HIV with reduced sensitivity to zidovudine (AZT) isolated during prolonged therapy. Science 1989;243:1731.

104. Richman D, Havlir D, Corbeil J, et al. Nevirapine resistance mutations of human immunodeficiency virus type 1 selected during therapy. J Virol 1994;68:1660.

105. D'Aquila R, Johnson V, Kuritzakes D, et al. HIV-1 drug resistance and syncytium-inducing phenotype: Associations with disease progression among ACTG 116B/117 subjects: The NIH AIDS Clinical Trials Group (ACTG) Virology Committee Resistance Working Group and the ACTG Protocol 116B/117 Team (Abstract PO-B26-2046:476). Ninth International Conference on AIDS, Berlin, Germany, June 6–11, 1993.

106. Montaner J, Singer J, Schecher M, et al. Clinical correlates of in vitro HIV-1 resistance to zidovudine: Results of the multicentre Canadian AZT trial. AIDS 1993;7:186.

107. Kahn JO, Lagakos SW, Richman DD, et al. A controlled trial comparing continued zidovudine with didanosine in human immunodeficiency virus infection. N Engl J Med 1992;327:581.

108. Spruance S, Pavia A, Peterson D, et al. Didanosine compared with continuation of zidovudine in HIV-infected patients with signs of clinical deterioration while receiving zidovudine. Ann Intern Med 1994;120:360.

109. Connor EM, Sperling RS, Gelber R, et al. Reduction of maternal-infant transmission of human immunodeficiency virus type 1 with zidovudine treatment. N Engl J Med 1994;331:1173.

109a. Hirsch MS, D'Acquila RT. Therapy for human immunodeficiency virus infection. N Engl J Med 1993;328:1686.

110. Fischl M, Collier A, Stanley K, et al. The safety and efficacy of zidovudine (ADV) and zalcitabine (ddC) or ddC alone versus ZDV. (Abstract WS-B25-1). Ninth International Conference on AIDS, Berlin, Germany, June 6–11, 1993.

111. Cooper D, Pehrson P, Pedersen C, et al. The efficacy and safety of zidovudine alone or as cotherapy with acyclovir for the treatment of patients with AIDS and AIDS-related complex: A double-blind randomized trial. European-Australian Collaborative Group. AIDS 1993;7:197.

112. Pluda J, Cooley T, Montaner J, et al. Phase I/II study of 3TC (GR 109714X) in adults with ARC or AIDS. (Abstract WS-B26-2). Ninth International Conference on AIDS, Berlin, Germany, June 6–11, 1993.

113. Redfield R, Birx D, Vahey M, et al. HIV vaccine therapy: Phase 1 safety and immunogenicity using gp160. (Abstract Tu39-TuB 0563). Eighth International Conference on AIDS, Amsterdam, The Netherlands, 1992.

114. Allan JD, Conanat M, Lavelle J, et al. Safety, and immunogenicity of MN and IIIB rgp 120/HIV-1 vaccines in HIV-1 infected subjects with CD4 counts >500 cells/mm³ (Abstract PO-B27-2137). Ninth International Conference on AIDS, Berlin, Germany, June 6–11, 1993.

115. Lane H, Davey V, Kovacs J, et al. Interferon-alpha in patients with asymptomatic immunodeficiency virus (HIV) infection. A randomized, placebo-controlled trial. Ann Intern Med 1990;112:805.

116. Abrams DI. Alternative therapies in HIV infection. AIDS 1990;4:1179.

117. Sande MA, Carpenter CCJ, Cobbs CG, et al. Antiretroviral therapy for adult HIV-infected patients: Recommendations from a state-of-the-art conference. JAMA 1993;270:2583.

118. Cotton DJ, Finkelstein DM, He W, et al. Determinants of accrual of women to a large, multicenter clinical trials program of human immunodeficiency virus infection. J Acquir Immune Defic Syndr 1993;6:1322.

119. Bartlett JG. The Johns Hopkins Hospital Guide to Medical Care of Patients with HIV Infection. 4th ed. Baltimore: Williams & Wilkins, 1994.

120. Koehler JE, Tappero JW. Bacillary angiomatosis and bacillary peliosis in patients infected with human immunodeficiency virus. Clin Infect Dis 1993;17:612.

121. King C, Heon V, Berger T, Conant M. Itraconazole for the treatment of HIV-associated eosinophilic folliculitis. (Abstract PO-B20-1887). Ninth International Conference on AIDS, Berlin, Germany, June 6–11, 1993.

122. Cockerell C. Human immunodeficiency virus infection and the skin, a crucial interface. Arch Intern Med 1991;151:1295.

123. Studies of Ocular Complications of AIDS Research Group in Collaboration with the AIDS Clinical Trials Group. Mortality in patients with the acquired immunodeficiency syndrome treated with either foscarnet or ganciclovir for cytomegalovirus retinitis. N Engl J Med 1992;326:213.

124. Palestine AG, Polis MA, DeSmet MD, et al. A randomized, controlled trial of foscarnet in the treatment of cytomegalovirus retinitis in patients with AIDS. Ann Intern Med 1991;115:665.

125. Bach M, Howell D, Valenti A, et al. Apthous ulceration of the gastrointestinal tract in patients with the acquired immunodeficiency syndrome (AIDS). Ann Intern Med 1990;112:465.

126. Daar E, Meyer R. Bacterial and fungal infections in medical management of AIDS patients. Infect Dis Clin North Am 1992;76:2173.

127. Erlich KS, Jacobson MA, Koehler JE, et al. Foscarnet therapy for severe acyclovir-resistant herpes simplex virus type-2 infections in patients with the acquired immunodeficiency syndrome (AIDS). Ann Intern Med 1989;110:710.

128. Lane HC, Laughon BE, Fallon J, et al. Recent advances in the management of AIDS-related opportunistic infections. Ann Intern Med 1994;120:945.

129. Sattler FR, Feinberg J. New developments in the treatment of *Pneumocystis carinii* pneumonia. Chest 1992;101:451.

130. Iseman MD, Cohn DL, Sbarbaro JA. Directly observed treatment of tuberculosis: We can't afford not to try. N Engl J Med 1993;324:576.

131. CDC. Initial therapy for tuberculosis in the era of multidrug resistance: Recommendations of the advisory council for the elimination of tuberculosis. MMWR 1993;42(RR-7):1.

132. Iseman MD. Treatment of multidrug-resistant tuberculosis. N Engl J Med 1993;329:784.

133. Small C, Kaufman A, Armenaka M, Rosenstreich D. Sinusitis and atopy in human immunodeficiency virus infection. J Infect Dis 1993;167:283.

134. Zurlo J, Feuerstien I, Lebovics R, Lane H. Sinusitis in HIV-1 infection. Am J Med 1992;93:157.

135. Laine L, Dretler RH, Conteas CN, et al. Fluconazole compared with ketoconazole for the treatment of *Candida* esophagitis in AIDS: A randomized trial. Ann Intern Med 1992;117:655.

136. Smith P, Quinn T, Strober W, et al. Gastrointestinal infections in AIDS. Ann Intern Med 1992;116:63.

137. Peterson C. Cryptosporidiosis in patients infected with the human immunodeficiency virus. Clin Infect Dis 1992;15:903.

138. Britton C. Progressive multifocal leukoencephalopathy: Disease progression, stabilization and response to intrathecal ARA-C in 26 patients (Abstract ThB1512). Eighth International Conference on AIDS, Amsterdam, The Netherlands, July 19–24, 1992.

139. Benson C. Treatment of disseminated disease due to the *Mycobacterium avium* complex in patients with AIDS. Clin Infect Dis 1994;18(Suppl 3):S237.

140. The Medical Letter. Drugs for AIDS and associated infections. Med Lett Drugs Ther 1993;35:79.

141. CDC. Purified protein derivative (PPD)-tuberculin anergy and HIV infection: Guidelines for anergy testing and management of anergic persons at risk for tuberculosis. MMWR 1991;40(RR-5):27.

142. Wheat LJ, Goldman M. Antifungal prophylaxis in AIDS: Should it be the standard of care. AIDS Clin Care 1994;6(4):27.

143. Carr A, Tindall B, Brew BJ, et al. Low-dose trimethoprim-sulfamethoxazole prophylaxis for toxoplasmic encephalitis in patients with AIDS. Ann Intern Med 1992;117:106.

144. Soloway B, Hecht F. Primary care: Charting materials. AIDS Clin Care 1991;3(6):44.

145. Collier A, Bozzette S, Coombs R, et al. A pilot study of low-dose zidovudine in human immunodeficiency virus infection. N Engl J Med 1990;323:1015.

CARDIOVASCULAR DISEASE IN WOMEN

50

Hypertension

Ellen Cohen, Mary E. Wheat, Deborah M. Swiderski, and Pamela Charney

Hypertension is the most common chronic medical condition and the most common reason for office visits in the United States. Depending on one's definition of hypertension (160/95 versus 140/90), hypertension affects between 35 and 50 million persons nationwide. It confers progressively greater risk for cerebrovascular and cardiovascular morbidity and mortality as blood pressure rises. In 1981, approximately 2 million years of life and 500,000 years of productive life were lost in the United States as a result of hypertension. Hypertension is also the most common indication for the use of prescription drugs.

Blood pressure must be measured accurately to diagnose hypertension in individual patients. Using an appropriate cuff size, at least two different measurements taken in a relaxed state during a single visit are averaged. Patients should not have used tobacco or caffeine within 30 minutes of measurement. Furthermore, hypertension should never be diagnosed from a single visit's measurement alone.

Given that risk of cardiovascular complications increases as blood pressure rises, the cutoff for defining elevated blood pressure has been gradually lowered. The most recent national recommendations define the spectrum of hypertension as beginning at 140/90.[1] Other groups, particularly in Europe, have used a definition of 160/95. When comparing different clinical studies regarding epidemiology and therapy of hypertension, it is important to be aware of differences between studies both in techniques used to measure blood pressure and in its definition.

EPIDEMIOLOGY: THE MAGNITUDE OF THE PROBLEM

Several large population-based surveys have examined the epidemiology of hypertension in the United States according to race and gender. The most reliable data pertain to blacks and whites. Some information is available about hypertension in Latinos, but no population-based data have been reported for Asian Americans. Blacks have much higher prevalence rates of hypertension than whites (Fig. 50–1). Black women have a higher overall prevalence of hypertension than black men. White women and men have closely comparable rates. However, in both black and white hypertensive individuals, women have a much greater likelihood of having their blood pressure effectively controlled at the time of screening.[2] These studies also show that women have a much greater likelihood than men of knowing that they have high blood pressure and of taking antihypertensive medications at the time of screening.

Information about the prevalence of hypertension in Latina American women is based on several population surveys, all of which are somewhat problematic in terms of their ability to be generalized to the diverse Latino population in the United States.[3–6] The only survey that used a probability sample to investigate hypertension prevalence in different Latino subgroups in the United States[5] found prevalence rates of hypertension in both women and men that were considerably less than those found in either blacks or whites. Interpretation of these results must, however, be viewed

521

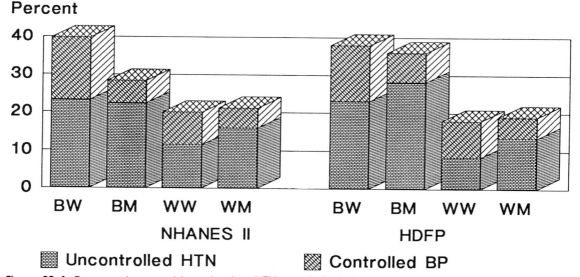

Figure 50-1. Race and sex and hypertension (HTN): controlled plus uncontrolled HTN. NHANES II, National Health and Nutrition Examination Survey II; HDFP, Hypertension Detection and Follow-up Program; BP, blood pressure; BW, black women; BM, black men; WW, white women; WM, white men.

cautiously because of problems in how the blood pressure determinations were performed.[6] Latina women, like black and white women, are also more likely than men to be aware of their high blood pressure and to have controlled hypertension.

Another method of analyzing gender differences in hypertension is to examine relative incidence rates as the population ages. Among blacks and whites, women and men develop hypertension at similar rates in all age groups, with steadily increasing incidence rates at each 10-year age interval. At all ages, black women and men consistently have incidence rates at least twice those of their white counterparts. As the population ages, women and men develop hypertension at similarly increasing rates, while at the same time men are dying at younger ages than women. Thus, in older age groups, hypertensive women actually outnumber hypertensive men in the overall population.

The potential sequelae of hypertension include stroke, myocardial infarction, congestive heart failure, and renal insufficiency. Treatment of hypertension is justified by the well-documented reduction of such endpoints when blood pressure is reduced. Because cardiovascular disease is the major cause of morbidity and mortality in women and men older than 60 years in the United States, the most clinically relevant way to look at the relative risk of hypertension in women and men is in terms of its contribution to cardiovascular events. Hypertensive men have a higher incidence of total cardiovascular endpoints than do hypertensive

women at all ages, as demonstrated by 20-year follow-up data from the Framingham study. However, the attributable risk percent—that is, the proportion of such events that could theoretically be prevented by removing hypertension as a risk factor—is actually similar or higher in women than in men at all ages. Extrapolating Framingham data to the entire white U.S. population shows that the absolute number of cardiovascular events attributable to hypertension may be somewhat greater in women than in men by age 65 to 74 years (Fig. 50–2).

These epidemiologic data make it clear that hypertension is common in women, that many women are treated for hypertension, and that such treatment, if effective in reducing related adverse outcomes, has major public health implications.

TARGET ORGAN ASSESSMENT

Preventing damage to target organs is the ultimate goal of reducing elevated blood pressure. As discussed earlier, men have a higher incidence rate of total cardiovascular endpoints than women at all ages. However, when one looks at a specific endpoint such as stroke, which has the closest association with hypertension as a risk factor, hypertensive men and women have a similarly increased relative risk of stroke over time (2.3 for women, 2.7 for men at 18 years' follow-up in the Framingham study).[7]

The significance of left ventricular hypertrophy

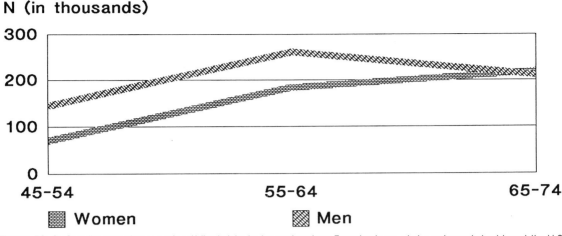

Figure 50-2. Cardiovascular events attributable to hypertension: Framingham data extrapolated to white U.S. population.

as a sequela of hypertension has been elucidated by the Framingham study. Echocardiographically proven left ventricular hypertrophy was independently associated with an increased risk of all measured endpoints.[8] For most endpoints, women had a somewhat higher relative risk than men (for risk of cardiovascular disease, women 1.49 and men 1.57; for cardiovascular death, women 2.12 and men 1.73; for death from all causes, women 2.01 and men 1.49). Several studies have shown that treatment with certain antihypertensive agents can reverse left ventricular hypertrophy.[9] At present, however, there are insufficient data to show that reversing left ventricular hypertrophy will decrease the number of adverse events.

Several studies have examined the contribution of hypertension to the development of renal disease, using serum creatinine determinations in population-based studies. Women on average have lower serum creatinine values than men, a difference that is not taken into account in some data analyses, making the validity of their gender-specific findings questionable. The one study that did correct for normal gender differences in serum creatinine values found that both women and men with higher blood pressure levels in 1974 had an increased risk of hypercreatininemia 15 years later[10] (relative odds 1.56 in women, 2.08 in men).

Overall, it appears that women and men suffer similar consequences of hypertension at fairly comparable rates. Hypertensive women should thus be monitored for the development of cerebrovascular disease and renal insufficiency. Whether or not hypertensive women or men should routinely be evaluated echocardiographically for the

presence of left ventricular hypertrophy remains controversial.

MANAGEMENT OF HYPERTENSION

Evaluation for Secondary Causes

Elevated blood pressure in women has multiple secondary causes. The most common of these, alcohol use (discussed later), oral contraceptives, and noncompliance with treatment, are often overlooked by clinicians.

Oral contraceptives are cited as the most frequent reversible cause of secondary hypertension. Cohort studies of women taking estrogen-progestogen pills show an average 5- to 7-mm Hg increase in systolic blood pressure, with a smaller 1- to 2-mm Hg rise in diastolic blood pressure. This increase is more likely to occur in women in their mid-30s and older. The risk of developing hypertension is increased two- to sixfold and affects about 5% of women.[11] Some data suggest that these changes differ among races.[12, 13] Increases in blood pressure seem to be attributable to both the estrogenic and progestogenic content. Few data are available on the risks of hypertension associated with progesterone-only methods (e.g., progestin only oral contraceptives, depo-medroxyprogesterone, or subcutaneous progestin implants). Unlike oral contraceptives, postmenopausal estrogen therapy is associated with a decrease in blood pressure and is not contraindicated in hypertension.

Women using oral contraceptives need periodic monitoring of their blood pressure. If overt hyper-

TABLE 50–1. A Quarter Century of Hypertension Treatment Studies

STUDY	NUMBER OF SUBJECTS	PERCENTAGE OF WOMEN	ANALYSIS BY GENDER
Hypertension Detection and Follow-up Program	10,940	46	Decreased mortality in black women and all men Possible increased mortality in white women (Reduced strokes in all groups)
The Australian Therapeutic Trial	3427	37	36% decrease in adverse outcome in women (p = N.S.) 26% decrease in adverse outcome in men (p < 0.05)
Medical Research Council Trial	17,354	48	26% increased mortality in women (p = N.S.) 15% decreased mortality in men (p = < 0.05) Reduced total cardiovascular events in women and men
European Working Party on Hypertension in the Elderly	840	70	18% reduction in cardiovascular mortality in women (p = N.S.)
Systolic Hypertension in the Elderly Program	4736	57	Decreased strokes in black and white women and white men: Reductions in other cardiovascular events in total population
Medical Research Council Trial in Older Adults	4396	58	Decreased strokes in women and men
Multiple Risk Factor Intervention Trial	12,866	0	Not applicable
The Oslo Study	785	0	Not applicable
Veterans Administration Cooperative Study	523	0	Not applicable

tension occurs, the medication should be discontinued, and in most cases blood pressure normalizes within 3 months. For women whose pressure increases to the high normal range and who have high cardiovascular risk profiles, other contraceptive options should be explored and the risks of an unwanted pregnancy weighed against the risks of an increase in blood pressure.

Renovascular disease, the cause of elevated blood pressure in about 0.5% of all hypertensive individuals, is important to diagnose because its treatment may enable cessation of antihypertensive therapy. Atherosclerosis is responsible for about two thirds of all renovascular hypertension and occurs twice as frequently in younger men than women, with the sex distribution equalizing in the elderly. Fibromuscular dysplasia, on the other hand, is the most common cause of renovascular hypertension before age 40 years and occurs predominantly in women.[14, 15] Findings suggestive of renovascular hypertension include abdominal bruits and lack of response to intensive pharmacotherapy.

Pheochromocytoma is an exceedingly rare cause of hypertension (0.1%) but should be suspected in women because it may first appear during pregnancy and, if not identified, can be associated with adverse outcomes. Orthostatic hypotension, sweating, pallor, and tachycardia should alert a clinician to the possibility of pheochromocytoma.[16] Thyroid disease occurs 10 times more frequently in women than men; however, its role as a cause of hypertension remains unclear.[17]

Effects of Treatment on Hypertensive Complications

The efficacy of treatment of hypertension can be evaluated in terms of several clinical endpoints. The major clinical trials have examined and combined different endpoints, making comparisons between studies somewhat confusing[2] (Table 50–1). Furthermore, trials have enrolled variable proportions of women subjects and may or may not analyze data for women separately. None of the major treatment trials set out to examine effects of hypertension therapy in gender and race subgroups; thus, the post hoc analyses must be viewed with caution.

The clinical endpoint with the strongest evidence of benefit from blood pressure reduction in both black and white women and men is the incidence of stroke. This finding has now been demonstrated clearly in several treatment trials, including black and white women of all ages.[18, 19] Furthermore, it has also been shown that reduction of isolated systolic hypertension in older adults reduces stroke rates.[20]

When looking at effects of antihypertensive therapy on other cardiovascular endpoints in women, studies have shown conflicting results.

Given the inadequate numbers of women enrolled and their relatively low rates of cardiovascular events, it is difficult to draw conclusions about the effects of antihypertensive therapy on nonstroke cardiovascular outcomes in women.

Another way to assess the effect of antihypertensive therapy is to look at overall mortality rates. Here again, gender analysis yields conflicting results, particularly among white women. In post hoc analyses of the three major treatment studies including women, one suggested benefit, one showed no effect, and one suggested increased risk in treated white women.

Overall, these data demonstrate the efficacy of antihypertensive therapy in reducing stroke rates in both women and men, black and white. However, given the small numbers of women studied and differences in data reported, conclusions about effects on other cardiovascular events and mortality cannot be drawn.

Blood Pressure Response to Pharmacotherapy

Innumerable small and large trials have compared blood pressure response to various drugs, which include variable proportions of women subjects. However, exceedingly few of these studies include gender analysis or offer meaningful information about differences or similarities between women and men in terms of blood pressure response to drugs.[18–22] Two small studies suggested that diltiazem might be particularly effective in women.[23, 24] A small study in middle-aged, obese black women found a thiazide to be more effective than clonidine.[25] Interestingly, hypertensive women have been observed to have lower renin levels than men,[26] possibly providing a physiologic explanation for these findings.

Nonpharmacologic Therapy

Because all antihypertensive drug therapies have at least some adverse effects, whether biomedical or financial, nonpharmacologic therapy should be used as primary or adjunctive therapy in all hypertensive individuals. Fewer well-designed studies have explored the role of nonpharmacologic than drug therapy in reducing blood pressure, but women have been included in most trials. Thus, although gender-specific analyses of different lifestyle modifications have been infrequently performed, the recommendations reasonably apply to women. Physical activity is the least well-studied nonpharmacologic antihypertensive therapy in women[27]; however, because isotonic exercise has other well-documented benefits in women, including reducing the risk of osteoporosis, facilitation of weight control, improvement in lipid profile and glucose tolerance, and decreased overall mortality, its inclusion in the primary or adjunctive treatment of elevated blood pressure is justified.

Among the nonpharmacologic therapies, the best evidence supports the use of weight reduction and sodium restriction. Well-designed randomized controlled trials including women have examined these interventions either alone[28–32] or in conjunction with drug therapy.[21, 31, 33] A nutritional program including both weight management and sodium reduction significantly slowed the return of hypertension (defined as >140/90).[34] Relatively small amounts of weight loss (e.g., 5–10 lb) have produced significant reductions in both systolic and diastolic blood pressure. Sodium restriction in these studies is generally defined as a no-added-salt diet, allowing about 2 gm (88 mmol) of sodium daily.

Other dietary manipulations include potassium supplementation, magnesium and calcium supplementation, and reduction of saturated fat.[35] Well-designed trials of dietary changes demonstrate conflicting results. Prudent recommendations would indicate assessing these parameters and supplementing potassium, calcium, and magnesium if deficiencies exist. Of note, one study demonstrated that a 10-mmol increase in daily potassium intake was significantly protective against stroke mortality in women, independent of various risk factors including blood pressure.[36] Health considerations other than hypertension may support reducing fat intake; however, neither reduction of saturated fat nor an increase of polyunsaturated fats has been shown to have a consistent antihypertensive effect in either women or men.

Alcohol intake has been associated with increased blood pressure in several large cross-sectional and cohort studies that included both substantial numbers of women and gender analyses.[37–39] The risk of hypertension appears to follow a J-shaped curve, being lowest in those reporting one to seven drinks per week. The risk of increased blood pressure increases significantly at intakes greater than two to three drinks per day. Clinicians should also remember that elevated blood pressure can occur in the context of alcohol withdrawal. Hence, assessment of alcohol intake in those at risk for hypertension and recommendations that consumption be limited to not more than one drink per day are reasonable.

Women who smoke should be advised to stop. Although they cannot be told that this will reduce their blood pressure, they can be told that it will reduce their risk of cardiovascular events such as stroke.[40] Caffeine is associated with a transient increase in blood pressure in infrequent users; however, cessation of caffeine intake has not been shown to have any effect on reducing blood pressure.

Relaxation techniques have been shown to reduce blood pressure in women and men in some studies[41] but not in others.[31, 42] A trial of relaxation techniques is reasonable in women who are interested in this approach.

The advantages of nonpharmacologic therapy include the avoidance of adverse drug effects and medication costs. Furthermore, because questions remain about optimal drug therapy in women, particularly those who are white and younger, nonpharmacologic therapy may be particularly advantageous in this group.

SIDE EFFECTS OF ANTIHYPERTENSIVE DRUGS

The side effects of antihypertensive drugs are legion. They include serious adverse effects such as metabolic disturbances, high financial cost, and negative quality-of-life issues. Proper selection of indicated antihypertensive drugs minimizes such risk and may even confer benefit.[43, 44]

Serum Lipids

Levels of serum lipids, including total, high-density, and low-density lipoprotein cholesterol, have been shown to be related to cardiovascular endpoints in women and men. The protective effects of high-density lipoprotein have been shown to be particularly important in women. The potential benefits of antihypertensive drug therapy in reducing cardiovascular risk may be compromised by adverse alterations in lipid levels caused by these medications.

Although lipid physiology is known to differ by gender, few studies of antihypertensive therapy have included gender analysis of effects on lipids.[2] Such analysis must include menopausal status as a critical confounding variable. The Medical Research Council Trial did show an increase in total cholesterol in both women and men treated with bendrofluazide, propranolol, or methyldopa; however, neither specific lipoprotein levels nor menopausal status were reported. Boehringer and colleagues[45] found an increase in low-density lipoprotein and total cholesterol in postmenopausal

but not premenopausal women treated with chlorthalidone. Unfortunately, menopausal status was defined by age alone. In a study of both pharmacologic and nonpharmacologic therapy of hypertension,[21] chlorthalidone raised total cholesterol whereas nutritional therapy lowered it. In a multiple regression analysis for change in total cholesterol level, gender was not a significant predictor.

Because lipid effects of antihypertensive drugs currently receive much attention, it is essential that future research on antihypertensive therapies include analysis of lipid effects by gender. In addition, menopausal status must be defined by clinical and laboratory markers.

Sexual Side Effects

Because sexual side effects are a common reason for patients' dissatisfaction or noncompliance with antihypertensive therapy, it is important to document their effect on women. The sexual response cycle has similar physiologic mechanisms in women and men. It would therefore seem reasonable to hypothesize that medications that cause sexual dysfunction in men may have similar effects in women. Although few of the earlier treatment trials examined sexual side effects in women,[46] studies are now reporting these data.

One study showed no statistically significant sexual impairment in women treated with low-dose chlorthalidone or atenolol as compared with placebo.[47] Interestingly, sexual function improved in women and men treated with weight loss regardless of concurrent assignment to drug therapy or placebo. Although the Systolic Hypertension in the Elderly Program did not include a separate gender analysis of sexual side effects, 57% of subjects were women, and no statistically significant increase in sexual side effects was noted in the drug-treated participants.[20] Croog and colleagues provided a more detailed analysis of sexual side effects among black men and women on atenolol, verapamil, and captopril.[48] In men taking captopril, sexual function improved significantly. Women demonstrated a numerically larger improvement on the sexual function scale used, but this trend failed to reach statistical significance because fewer women were randomized to captopril. The Treatment of Mild Hypertension Study[22] reported a 3% incidence of problems related to sexual activity in women, as compared with a 10% incidence in men. However, no statistically significant differences were found between any of the six drug and placebo treatment groups in women or men. A large postmarketing study of captopril reported a statistically significant improvement in sexual quality of life among both women and men.[49] Importantly, no placebo control was used.

Assessment of sexual side effects has been further confounded by study methods. Many studies have framed their questions about sexual function in terms of male physiology (e.g., erection, ejaculation). One study evaluated the utility of a self-recorded diary for assessing sexual function in women.[50] Future treatment trials must continue to include such survey instruments.

The preliminary data suggest that women experience sexual dysfunction with antihypertensives analogous to that previously reported in men. More detailed information is needed about gender-specific sexual side effects of various pharmacologic agents as determined by studies that include adequate numbers of women and that stratify subjects by gender at randomization.

THERAPY FOR THE INDIVIDUAL WOMAN

Because the goal of antihypertensive therapy is to reduce risk, treatment of blood pressure is warranted when benefits of therapy outweigh the adverse effects of treatment. The exact level of blood pressure at which pharmacologic therapy should begin remains an area of controversy, particularly for white women. Some would institute drug therapy at blood pressure levels greater than 140/90; others would pursue nonpharmacologic therapies until diastolic blood pressure rose above 95 or a woman showed evidence of target organ damage. Because of its lower risk profile, nonpharmacologic therapy (Table 50–2) must always be considered the cornerstone of blood pressure treatment. Its benefit has been demonstrated not only in those labeled hypertensive but also in those with high-normal blood pressure (systolic 130–139 or diastolic 85–89) who are at high risk of developing frank hypertension.

When a woman has been labeled as having mild (140–159/90–99) or moderate (160–179/100–109) hypertension, a vigorous 3- to 6-month trial of

TABLE 50–2. Nonpharmacologic Therapy to Reduce Blood Pressure

Weight reduction if overweight
Sodium restriction
Potassium, magnesium, and calcium repletion if depleted
No more than one alcoholic drink daily
Moderate physical activity
Relaxation technique training

indicated nonpharmacologic therapy should be pursued. If hypertension persists or if she shows evidence of target organ damage or of other cardiovascular risk factors, then addition of pharmacologic treatment is appropriate. Because epidemiologic data suggest more dramatic benefit from pharmacologic therapy in black women than white, the treatment threshold may be lower in blacks. Nonpharmacologic therapy should continue to be used, particularly in view of its favorable impact on side effects such as sexual dysfunction.

Women who have mild or moderate hypertension and who have not responded to nonpharmacologic therapy should be begun on monotherapy. In older women, particular attention should be paid to standing as well as sitting blood pressure to avoid exacerbation of possible orthostatic hypotension. Various agents are available, and selection is influenced by consideration of cost, potential side effects, and comorbid conditions in an individual woman. Medications should be initiated at low doses to minimize side effects.[51, 52]

Estrogen therapy is not contraindicated in women with hypertension; indeed, some regimens appear to reduce blood pressure.[53] Furthermore, because estrogen therapy reduces cardiovascular risk, it may be of particular benefit in women with hypertension. Women beginning estrogen therapy should have their blood pressure monitored, however, because a small proportion may experience an increase in blood pressure. No data are available on the effect of route of administration (e.g., transdermal versus oral) on blood pressure levels and outcome.

β-Blockers and diuretics are the only antihypertensive medications for which documentation shows that use reduces mortality as well as blood pressure.[54] Consequently, the Fifth Report of the Joint National Committee on Detection, Evaluation, and Treatment of Blood Pressure recommends use of these drug classes as initial pharmacotherapy of hypertension unless specific contraindications exist.[1]

Other authorities contest this recommendation, noting that the relative failure of antihypertensive therapy to decrease rates of myocardial infarction, as compared with stroke, may be a result of unfavorable effects of these agents on lipid and glucose metabolism.[55] Noting that calcium channel antagonists, angiotensin-converting enzyme inhibitors, and selective α_1-adrenergic blockers all are effective monotherapies for blood pressure reduction, they cite evidence of favorable metabolic and vascular actions of these drugs that could augment their effectiveness in reducing cardiovascular complications of hypertension.

TABLE 50–3. Individualizing Antihypertensive Therapy

DRUG CLASS	ADVANTAGES WITH COMORBID CONDITIONS	CONTRAINDICATIONS OR SPECIAL MONITORING REQUIRED
Initial Agents		
Thiazide diuretics	Osteoporosis; CHF; cost	Glucose intolerance; hypercholesterolemia; preeclampsia; IHSS; gout
Loop diuretics	Renal insufficiency; diabetes; gout	
Potassium-sparing diuretics		Renal insufficiency; use of angiotensin-converting enzyme inhibitors
β-Blockers	Angina; IHSS; vascular headaches; post-MI	CHF; type I diabetes; bronchospasm; bradycardia or heart block; peripheral vascular disease
Angiotensin-converting enzyme inhibitors	CHF; diabetes; hypercholesterolemia	Pregnancy or planning pregnancy; IHSS; renal artery stenosis or severe bilateral renal arterial disease
Calcium antagonists	Angina; diabetes; IHSS*; hypercholesterolemia; vascular headaches	CHF; bradycardia or heart block*
α₁-Antagonists	Hypercholesterolemia	IHSS
Supplemental Agents		
α₂-Agonists	Pregnancy or planning pregnancy (methyldopa)	Depression; liver disease (methyldopa)
Direct vasodilators	Pregnancy or planning pregnancy (hydralazine)	Angina; IHSS; post-MI
Reserpine	Cost	Depression; peptic ulcer disease

*Diltiazem, verapamil.
IHSS, Idiopathic hypertrophic subaortic stenosis; CHF, congestive heart failure; MI, myocardial infarction.

This controversy certainly is even more speculative as it relates to women than to men. Fewer data are available in every area; certain assumptions, such as the effect of lipid alterations on outcome, are far more uncertain in women because these effects are related to hormonal status, and women have not been included in any outcome-oriented lipid treatment trials. Other gender-related effects—for example, the potentially beneficial effect of thiazide diuretics on calcium metabolism and osteoporosis—have not yet been quantified. The cost of pharmacotherapy also increases with the newer agents, a fact that may more adversely affect women, who are more likely to be poor or to lack insurance.[56]

Diuretics and β-blockers can be initial therapy in women unless contraindications exist. Lower doses of diuretics in particular have been shown to be equally efficacious in higher doses while minimizing side effects.[52] Adverse metabolic effects should be monitored when these agents are used; particularly for women with other cardiovascular risk factors, an unfavorable change in lipid or glucose metabolism supports use of another agent. Furthermore, as indicated in Table 50–3, choice of an antihypertensive agent should always be individualized, with consideration of both indications and contraindications for each woman. Most antihypertensive agents are effective in reducing blood pressure in older women[57]; however, concern for orthostatic hypotension may dictate therapy. Black women, who may have lower renin levels than whites, may fare better with a diuretic or calcium channel blocker.[58]

Comorbid conditions should always be considered in the selection of antihypertensives. For example, although β-blockers should be avoided in women with asthma, they may represent an excellent choice in a woman with angina or frequent migraines. Thiazide diuretics may be particularly desirable in women at risk for osteoporosis[43, 44] (e.g., thin, white women); they would be contraindicated in a woman with renal calculi. Angiotensin-converting enzyme inhibitors or calcium channel blockers may be of theoretic benefit in diabetic women.[59] Figure 50–3 outlines a treatment algorithm for hypertensive women.

Hypertension is one of the risks for cardiovascular disease. Other modifiable risk factors should also be addressed. Some of these are part of the nonpharmacologic treatment of hypertension itself—for example, encouragement of moderate physical activity and weight reduction. Diabetes should be appropriately treated, smoking cessation strongly encouraged, and any lipid abnormalities addressed. Foremost, a collaborative working relationship between a woman and her physician should be emphasized to facilitate adherence and

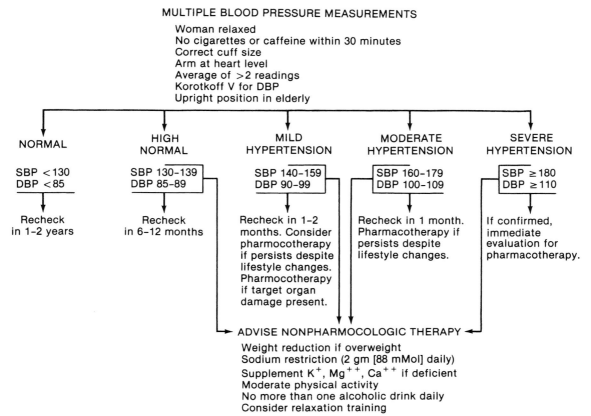

MULTIPLE BLOOD PRESSURE MEASUREMENTS
Woman relaxed
No cigarettes or caffeine within 30 minutes
Correct cuff size
Arm at heart level
Average of >2 readings
Korotkoff V for DBP
Upright position in elderly

NORMAL	HIGH NORMAL	MILD HYPERTENSION	MODERATE HYPERTENSION	SEVERE HYPERTENSION
SBP <130 DBP <85	SBP 130–139 DBP 85–89	SBP 140–159 DBP 90–99	SBP 160–179 DBP 100–109	SBP ≥180 DBP ≥110
Recheck in 1–2 years	Recheck in 6–12 months	Recheck in 1–2 months. Consider pharmocotherapy if persists despite lifestyle changes. Pharmocotherapy if target organ damage present.	Recheck in 1 month. Pharmacotherapy if persists despite lifestyle changes.	If confirmed, immediate evaluation for pharmacotherapy.

ADVISE NONPHARMOCOLOGIC THERAPY
Weight reduction if overweight
Sodium restriction (2 gm [88 mMol] daily)
Supplement K^+, Mg^{++}, Ca^{++} if deficient
Moderate physical activity
No more than one alcoholic drink daily
Consider relaxation training

Figure 50–3. Treatment algorithm for hypertension. SBP, Systolic blood pressure; DBP, diastolic blood pressure.

accurate reporting of side effects during prolonged treatment of a chronic condition.

REFERENCES

1. The Fifth Report of the Joint National Committee on Detection, Evaluation and Treatment of High Blood Pressure. JAMA 1993;153:154.
2. Anastos K, Charney C, Charon R, et al. Hypertension in women: What is really known? Ann Intern Med 1991;115:287.
3. Stern MP, Gaskill SP, Allen CR, et al. Cardiovascular risk factors in Mexican Americans in Laredo, Texas. II. Prevalence and control of hypertension. Am J Epidemiol 1981;113:556.
4. Franco LJ, Stern MP, Rosenthal M, et al. Prevalence, detection, and control of hypertension in a biethnic community: The San Antonio Heart Study. Am J Epidemiol 1985;121:684.
5. Pappas G, Gergen PJ, Carroll M. Hypertension prevalence and the status of awareness, treatment, and control in the Hispanic Health and Nutrition Examination Survey (HHANES), 1982–84. Am J Public Health 1990;80:1431.
6. Geronimus AT, Neidert LJ, Bound J. A note on measurement of hypertension in HHANES. Am J Public Health 1990;80:1437.
7. Kannel WB, Wolf PA, Verter J, McNamara PM. Epidemiologic assessment of the role of blood pressure in stroke. The Framingham Study. JAMA 1970;214:301.
8. Levy D, Garrison R, Savage D, et al. Prognostic implications of echocardiographically determined left ventricular mass in the Framingham Heart Study. N Engl J Med 1990;322:1561.
9. Schulman S, Weiss J, Becker L, et al. The effects of antihypertensive therapy on left ventricular mass in elderly patients. N Engl J Med 1990;322:1350.
10. Perneger TV, Nieto J, Whelton PK, et al. A prospective study of blood pressure and serum creatinine. Results from the ''Clue'' Study and the ARIC Study. JAMA 1993;269:488.
11. Woods JW. Oral contraceptives and hypertension. Hypertension 1988;11(Suppl II):II-11.
12. Khaw K, Peart WS. Blood pressure and contraceptive use. Br Med J 1982;285:402.
13. Layde PM, Beral V, Kay CR. Further analyses of mortality in oral contraceptive users. Royal College of General Practitioners Oral Contraception Study. Lancet 1981;1:541.
14. Mann SJ, Pickering TC. Detection of renovascular hypertension, state of the art. Ann Intern Med 1992;117:845.
15. Ram C, Venkata S. Renovascular hypertension. Cardiol Clin 1988;6:483.
16. Manger WM, Gifford RW. Pheochromocytoma. In: Laragh JH, Brenner BM (eds): Hypertension: Pathophysiology, Diagnosis, and Management. Vol II. New York: Raven Press, 1990, p 1639.
17. Klein I. Thyroid hormone and blood pressure regulation. In: Laragh JH, Brenner BM (eds): Hypertension: Pathophysiology, Diagnosis, and Management. Vol II. New York: Raven Press, 1990, p 1661.

18. Five-year findings of the hypertension detection and follow-up program (HDFP). III. Reduction in stroke incidence among persons with high blood pressure. HDFP Cooperative Group. JAMA 1982;247:633.
19. MRC trial of treatment of hypertension in older adults: Principal results. MRC Working Party. Br Med J 1992;304:405.
20. Prevention of stroke by antihypertensive drug treatment in older persons with isolated systolic hypertension. Final results of the Systolic Hypertension in the Elderly Program. SHEP Cooperative Research Group. JAMA 1991;265:3255.
21. Oberman A, Wassertheil-Smoller S, Langford HG, et al. Pharmacologic and nutritional treatment of mild hypertension: Changes in cardiovascular risk status. Ann Intern Med 1992;112:89.
22. The Treatment of Mild Hypertension Study. The Treatment of Mild Hypertension Research Group. Arch Intern Med 1991;151:1413.
23. Applegate W, Phillips H, Schnaper H, et al. A randomized controlled trial of the effects of three antihypertensive agents on blood pressure control and quality of life in older women. Arch Intern Med 1991;151:1817.
24. Massie B, MacCarthy E, Ramanathan K, et al. Diltiazem and propranolol in mild to moderate essential hypertension as monotherapy or with hydrochlorothiazide. Ann Intern Med 1987;107:150.
25. Reisin E, Weed SG. The treatment of obese hypertensive black: A comparative study of chlorthalidone versus clonidine. J Hypertens 1992;10:489.
26. Meade T, Imeson J, Gordon D, Peart W. The epidemiology of plasma renin. Clin Sci 1983;64:273.
27. Aroll B, Beaglehole R. Does physical activity lower blood pressure: A critical review of the clinical trials. J Clin Epidemiol 1992;45:439.
28. Trials of Hypertension Collaborative Research Group. The effects of nonpharmacologic interventions on blood pressure of persons with high normal levels. JAMA 1992;267:1213.
29. Hypertension Prevention Trial Research Group. The hypertension prevention trial: Three-year effects of dietary changes on blood pressure. Arch Intern Med 1990;150:153.
30. Stamler R, Stamler J, Gosch F, et al. Primary prevention of hypertension by nutritional-hygienic means: Final results of a randomized, controlled trial. JAMA 1989;262:1801.
31. Reisin E, Abel R, Modan M, et al. Effect of weight loss on the reduction of blood pressure in overweight hypertensive patients. N Engl J Med 1978;298:1.
32. Cutler J, Follman D, Elliott P, Suh I. An overview of randomized trials of sodium restriction and blood pressure. Hypertension 1991;17(SI):27.
33. Erwteman T, Nagelkerke N, Lubsen J, et al. β-blockade, diuretics and salt restriction for the management of mild hypertension: A randomized double blind trial. Br Med J 1984;289:406.
34. Stamler R, Stamler J, Grimm R, et al. Nutritional therapy for high blood pressure: Final report of a four-year randomized controlled trial—the hypertension control program. JAMA 1987;257:1484.
35. Kaplan N. Long-term effectiveness of nonpharmacological treatment of hypertension. Hypertension 1991;18(SI):153.
36. Khaw K, Barrett-Connor E. Dietary potassium and stroke-associated mortality. N Engl J Med 1987;316:235.
37. Klatsky A, Friedman G, Armstrong M. The relationships between alcoholic beverage use and other traits to blood pressure: A new Kaiser Permanente study. Circulation 1986;73:628.
38. Witteman J, Willett W, Stampfer M, et al. Relation of moderate alcohol consumption and risk of systemic hypertension in women. Am J Cardiol 1990;65:633.
39. Ueshima H, Ozawa H, Baba S, et al. Alcohol drinking and high blood pressure: Data from a 1980 national cardiovascular survey of Japan. J Clin Epidemiol 1992;45:667.
40. Kawachi I, Colditz F, Stampfer M, et al. Smoking cessation and decreased risk of stroke in women. JAMA 1993;269:232.
41. Patel C, Marmot M, Terry D, et al. Trial of relaxation in reducing coronary risk: Four year follow up. Br Med J 1985;290:1103.
42. van Montfrans G, Karemaker J, Wieling W, et al. Relaxation therapy and continuous ambulatory blood pressure in mild hypertension: A controlled study. Br Med J 1990;300:1368.
43. Felson D, Sloutskis D, Anderson J, et al. Thiazide diuretics and the risk of hip fracture. Results from the Framingham Study. JAMA 1991;265:370.
44. LaCroix A, Wienpahl J, White L, et al. Thiazide diuretic agents and the incidence of hip fracture. N Engl J Med 1990;322:286.
45. Boehringer K, Weidmann P, Mordasini R, et al. Menopause-dependent plasma lipoprotein alterations in diuretic-treated women. Ann Intern Med 1982;97:206.
46. Drugs that cause sexual dysfunction: An update. Med Lett Drugs Ther 1992;34:73.
47. Wassertheil-Smoller S, Blaufox M, Oberman A, et al. Effect of antihypertensives on sexual function and quality of life: The TAIM study. Ann Intern Med 1991;114:613.
48. Croog S, Kong W, Levine S, et al. Hypertensive black men and women: Quality of life and effects of antihypertensive medications. Arch Intern Med 1990;150:1733.
49. Schoenberger J, Tests M, Ross A, et al. Efficacy, safety and quality-of-life assessment of captopril antihypertensive therapy in clinical practice. Arch Intern Med 1990;150:301.
50. Hodge R, Harward M, West M, et al. Sexual function of women taking antihypertensive agents: A comparative study. J Gen Intern Med 1991;6:290.
51. Kaplan N. The appropriate goals of antihypertensive therapy: Neither too much nor too little. Ann Intern Med 1992;116:686.
52. Kaplan N. The case for low dose diuretic therapy. Am J Hypertens 1991;4:970.
53. Wren B, Routledge D. Blood pressure changes: Oestrogens in climacteric women. Med J Aust 1981;2:528.
54. Alderman M. Which antihypertensive drugs first—and why! JAMA 1992;267:2786.
55. Weber MA, Laragh JH. Hypertension: Steps forward and steps backward. Arch Intern Med 1993;153:149.
56. Horton JA. The Women's Health Data Book: A profile of women's health in the United States. The Jacobs Institute of Women's Health. Washington, DC: Elsevier, 1992.
57. Tjoa H, Kaplan N. Treatment of hypertension in the elderly. JAMA 1990;264:1015.
58. Moser M. Hypertension treatment results in minority patients. Am J Med 1990;88(Suppl 3B):24S.
59. Kasiske B, Kalil R, Ma J, et al. Effect of antihypertensive therapy on the kidney in patients with diabetes: A meta-regression analysis. Ann Intern Med 1993;118:129.

Cholesterol Screening and Management

Joanne Murabito

Heart disease is the leading cause of death among American women. Coronary artery disease (CAD) risk in women is associated with elevated total cholesterol levels, elevated low-density lipoprotein (LDL) cholesterol levels, and possibly elevated triglyceride levels. High-density lipoprotein (HDL) cholesterol is inversely related to coronary risk and is an especially powerful predictor of coronary events in women. Cholesterol and its lipoproteins, as well as the risk of CAD, may be modified by menopause, estrogen therapy, and oral contraceptive use.

CORONARY DISEASE RISK IN WOMEN

Cholesterol, cigarette smoking, and hypertension all are significant risk factors for CAD in women, and the relationship of these risk factors to CAD is as strong in women as it is in men.[1] Diabetes mellitus is not only associated with greater risk of CAD than the other risk factors in women but essentially cancels any advantage women have over men in terms of the risk of CAD.

Cholesterol

Coronary artery disease incidence rises continuously with increasing cholesterol level.[2-4] Prospective studies of women have shown elevations in risk of CAD to occur at higher total cholesterol levels than those observed in men. Increased risk of CAD in women has been reported with cholesterol levels above the range of 235 to 265 mg per dl.[4, 5] As women age, mean cholesterol level rises, and about the time of menopause, the average cholesterol level in women exceeds the average level in men. More than 23% of adult women in the

United States have a total cholesterol value greater than 260 mg per dl.[1]

The risk of CAD associated with an elevated cholesterol level is markedly enhanced in the presence of other known CAD risk factors, resulting in a multiplicative rather than an additive increase in risk.[6] For each 1% reduction in total cholesterol level, a 2% reduction in risk for CAD has been observed.[7] Lower cholesterol levels have also been associated with lower overall mortality.[8]

Low-Density Lipoprotein Cholesterol

Most cholesterol is contained in LDL. Elevated levels of LDL cholesterol have been associated with an increased risk for coronary events in both women and men. A 1% increase in LDL cholesterol corresponds to slightly more than a 2% increase in CAD risk.[9]

High-Density Lipoprotein Cholesterol

High-density lipoprotein is inversely related to coronary incidence and is the most powerful lipid predictor of CAD risk in women. An increase of 1 mg per dl in HDL cholesterol level is associated with a 3% decrease in CAD risk and a nearly 5% decrease in cardiovascular disease mortality in women.[10] This potent association between CAD incidence and HDL cholesterol level exists throughout all levels of total cholesterol.[11] Even in the presence of a desirable total cholesterol level (<200 mg/dl), a low HDL cholesterol level confers increased risk for CAD in both women and men. Framingham Study women with the lowest cholesterol levels (<211 mg/dl) and coexistent low levels of HDL cholesterol (<46 mg/dl) were observed to have an increased incidence of myocardial infarction.[12] In the presence of an elevated HDL cholesterol level, a minimal increment is noted in the incidence of coronary events in individuals with desirable cholesterol levels compared with those with elevated cholesterol levels.[11]

Ratio of High-Density Lipoprotein to Total Cholesterol

The ratio of total cholesterol to HDL cholesterol level is strongly associated with CAD and may be more useful in predicting CAD risk than total cholesterol or HDL cholesterol level alone. A ratio of less than or equal to 4.5 represents an average risk for CAD, whereas a ratio less than 3.5 is associated with half the average risk for a coronary event.[13] Current management guidelines, however, do not incorporate this ratio for women but continue to use the same absolute LDL cutoff points for both women and men.

Triglyceride

Elevated triglyceride levels are associated with CAD risk in univariate analysis but lose their predictive value with adjustment for other lipid risk factors. Two different mechanisms have been proposed to explain the adverse consequences of hypertriglyceridemia on CAD risk. Triglyceride-rich lipoproteins may be atherogenic, or the metabolic derangements associated with elevated triglyceride levels, such as the lowering of HDL cholesterol level and possibly the induction of a procoagulant state, may explain the connection between triglycerides and CAD.[14] The Framingham Study has shown that in women but not in men, triglycerides were significantly associated with CAD incidence even after adjustment for age and pertinent risk factors including total cholesterol.[15] Women,[15] men with high ratios of total cholesterol to HDL cholesterol,[16, 17] and diabetic patients[18] appear to be particularly prone to the effects of elevated triglyceride values.

REDUCTION IN CORONARY RISK WITH CHOLESTEROL-LOWERING TREATMENT

Both primary and secondary intervention trials have demonstrated the efficacy of cholesterol-lowering diet and medication in reducing CAD incidence.[7, 19, 20] This benefit can only be extrapolated to women because the major randomized placebo-controlled trials have been conducted in middle-aged men, either excluding women or including women in small numbers precluding sex-specific analyses of treatment outcomes.

More recently, angiographic trials have been able to demonstrate stabilization and regression of coronary atherosclerotic lesions with the reduction of LDL cholesterol. The Cholesterol-Lowering Atherosclerosis Study demonstrated stabilization and regression of coronary artery lesions in both native coronary arteries and coronary artery bypass vessels more frequently in the cholesterol-lowering treatment group.[21] The first report of the effect of therapy in women[22] demonstrates that women as well as men in the cholesterol-lowering treatment group achieved regression of coronary lesions whereas those in the control group were observed to have coronary lesion progression. The Program on the Surgical Control of Hyperlipidemia was the first trial to demonstrate not only stabilization of atherosclerotic coronary lesions with cholesterol lowering but, in turn, a true reduction in clinical coronary events.[23]

MENOPAUSE AND ESTROGEN EFFECTS ON LIPIDS AND CORONARY RISK

Menopause

Unfavorable changes in lipid profiles have been noted to occur at the time of menopause. After a natural menopause, women have increases in total cholesterol, LDL cholesterol, and triglyceride levels and a decline in HDL cholesterol level when compared with premenopausal women, even after adjusting for age.[24] These lipid changes may partly explain the rise in CAD incidence after menopause. Investigators in the Framingham Heart Study did not observe myocardial infarction or death due to CAD in premenopausal participants; however, these events occurred after either a natural or a surgical menopause.[25] In contrast, the Nurses Health Study reported no association between natural menopause and increased CAD risk; excess risk was confined to those women who had undergone hysterectomy and bilateral oophorectomy without the benefit of estrogen therapy.[26]

Estrogen Therapy

Epidemiologic studies consistently report that postmenopausal women receiving estrogen therapy have half the risk for coronary events as nonusers. This reduction in risk is present for the clinical outcomes of myocardial infarction, cardiovascular death, and all-cause mortality, as well as the anatomic outcome of severe CAD documented at cardiac catheterization.[27–31] Furthermore, the beneficial effect of estrogen persists even when adjusting for age and other CAD risk factors. The effects of estrogen on CAD risk are believed to be mediated partly through favorable changes in HDL and LDL cholesterol levels. Of note, these data are derived from observations of women almost exclusively on unopposed estrogen therapy. Concurrent administration of progestins may negate many of the favorable lipid modifications of estrogen and in turn diminish the estrogen-associated reduction in CAD risk. Although unlikely, given the congruent findings of many case-control, prospective, and angiographic investigations, the beneficial impact of estrogen may be related to confounding factors or prevention bias.

Unopposed oral estrogen therapy has been definitely shown to positively alter cholesterol and lipoproteins in a dose-dependent manner. Conjugated equine estrogen at 0.625 mg daily has been found to increase HDL cholesterol levels 10% and triglyceride levels 11% and decrease LDL cholesterol levels by 4%. A daily dose of 1.25 mg increased HDL cholesterol and triglyceride levels 14% and 17%, respectively, and decreased LDL cholesterol level 8%.[32] Estradiol valerate (2 mg/day) appears to have even more favorable lipid effects, increasing HDL cholesterol 15% and decreasing LDL cholesterol levels 16%.[32] Transdermal estradiol does not produce the same positive effect on lipids.[33]

The effects of estrogen-progestin combination therapy on cholesterol and lipoproteins are difficult to assess owing to small sample sizes, different estrogen-progestin combinations, and short duration of follow-up in most studies. Progestins, even the less androgenic medroxyprogesterone acetate, administered in a cyclic fashion attenuate the estrogen-induced rise in HDL cholesterol levels.[32, 34–36] Continuous estrogen-progestin therapy has also been shown to diminish the HDL-raising effects of estrogen. Conjugated estrogen, 0.625 mg, used continuously with medroxyprogesterone acetate (either 2.5 mg/day or 5 mg/day) resulted in a 4.5% rise in HDL cholesterol levels rather the expected 10% rise with unopposed therapy.[37] Further trials are needed not only to evaluate the lipid alterations of combined estrogen-progestin therapy but also the associated impact on coronary events and mortality.

Oral Contraceptives

Cardiovascular disease risk is increased in current users of oral contraceptives, especially in older women, cigarette smokers, and women with other cardiovascular risk factors.[38] Past users of oral contraceptives appear to have a risk of cardiovascular disease similar to that of never users. The Nurses Health Study investigators could not document any increase in cardiovascular risk with increased duration of oral contraceptive use nor any risk trends with time since discontinuation of use.[39] Most risk assessment studies were performed when women were prescribed relatively high hormone doses; risk data are lacking for the newer low-dose preparations, which it is hoped will be associated with less marked cardiovascular effects. Several mechanisms are believed to contribute to the increased cardiovascular risk associated with the oral contraceptives, including unfavorable changes in lipid profiles, glucose tolerance, blood pressure, and platelet function and coagulation.

Comparison of the lipid changes associated with various oral contraceptives is difficult because of content differences, sample size limitations, and short follow-up in most reports. Additionally, biphasic and triphasic preparations are in use as well as new third-generation gonane progestins. Users of estrogen-dominant oral contraceptives have significantly higher HDL cholesterol and triglyceride levels than nonusers.[40] The progestin-dominant oral contraceptives produce the greatest detrimental impact on lipids, lowering HDL cholesterol and raising LDL cholesterol levels.[35, 40] The adverse lipid alterations induced by progestins are directly related to their degree of androgenic potency. Norgestrel and levonorgestrel are associated with the greatest androgenic effects, and norethindrone and ethynodiol diacetate produce less androgenic effect. Oral contraceptives containing third-generation gonane progestins have become available in the United States and are reportedly associated with favorable lipid effects, providing an attractive option.[41]

CHOLESTEROL SCREENING GUIDELINES

Adults Free of Coronary Disease

All adults age 20 years or older without known CAD should have nonfasting total and HDL cholesterol levels measured at least once every 5 years, along with an assessment of other CAD risk factors (Fig. 51–1).[42] Total cholesterol levels are classified identically in women and men as follows: less than 200 mg per dl, desirable level; 200 to 239 mg per dl, borderline-high level; and greater than 240 mg per dl, high level. An HDL cholesterol level less than 35 mg per dl is considered low and is recognized as an independent risk factor for CAD. A second confirmatory measurement is required if the total cholesterol level is elevated or if HDL cholesterol level is low. The average of the two cholesterol measurements

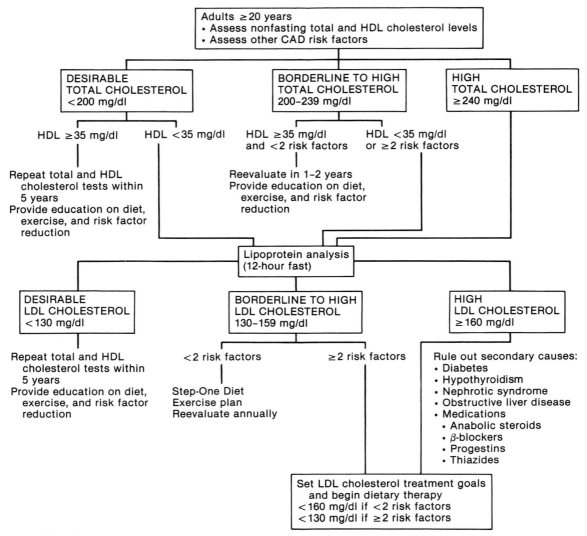

Figure 51-1. Screening for high blood cholesterol in adults without coronary artery disease (CAD). In adults with coronary disease, perform a lipoprotein analysis. When the low-density lipoprotein (LDL) cholesterol is optimal (≤100 ml/dl), educate on diet, exercise, and risk factor reduction and repeat the lipoprotein analysis. When the LDL cholesterol is >100 mg/dl, initiate therapy. HDL, High-density lipoprotein. (Modified from Summary of the second report of the National Cholesterol Education Program (NCEP) expert panel on detection, evaluation, and treatment of high blood cholesterol in adults (Adult Treatment Panel II). JAMA 1993;269:3015–3023.)

should be used to determine further screening strategy.

In patients with a desirable total cholesterol level, the HDL cholesterol level determines further screening. When the HDL cholesterol level is 35 mg per dl or greater, screening cholesterol measurements should be repeated within 5 years and general dietary, exercise, and risk factor education provided. For patients with a borderline-high cholesterol level with an HDL cholesterol level equal to or greater than 35 mg per dl and fewer than two CAD risk factors, re-evaluation in 1 to 2 years and education on dietary modifications, exercise, and risk factor reduction is required. Further evaluation with a fasting lipoprotein analysis is recommended for all other patients, including (1) patients with desirable total cholesterol and HDL cholesterol levels less than 35 mg per dl, (2) patients with borderline-high cholesterol and HDL cholesterol levels less than 35 mg per dl or two or more CAD risk factors, and (3) all patients with high cholesterol levels.[42] Lipoprotein analysis necessitates a

TABLE 51–1. The Step-One Diet

	CHOOSE	DECREASE
Fish, chicken, turkey, and lean meats	Fish, poultry without skin, shellfish, lean cuts of beef, lamb, pork, or veal	Fatty cuts of beef, lamb, pork; spare ribs, organ meats, regular cold cuts, sausage, hot dogs, bacon, sardines, roe
Skim and low-fat milk, cheese, yogurt, and dairy substitutes	Skim or 1% milk (liquid, powdered, evaporated) Buttermilk	Whole milk (4% fat): regular, evaporated, condensed; cream, half and half, 2% milk, imitation milk products, most nondairy creamers, whipped toppings
	Nonfat (0% fat) or low-fat yogurt	Whole-milk yogurt
	Low-fat cottage cheese (1% or 2% fat)	Whole-milk cottage cheese (4% fat)
	Low-fat cheeses, farmer, or pot cheeses (all of these should be labeled no more than 2–6 gm fat/ounce)	All natural cheeses (e.g., blue, Roquefort, Camembert, cheddar, Swiss)
		Low-fat or ''light'' cream cheese Low-fat or ''light'' sour cream Cream cheeses, sour cream
	Sherbet Sorbet	Ice Cream
Eggs	Egg whites (2 whites = 1 white egg in recipes), cholesterol-free egg substitutes	Egg yolks
Fruits and vegetables	Fresh, frozen, canned, or dried fruits and vegetables	Vegetables prepared in butter, cream, or other sauces
Breads and cereals	Homemade baked goods using unsaturated fats sparingly, angel food cake, low-fat crackers, low-fat cookies	Commercial baked goods: pies, cakes, doughnuts, croissants, pastries, muffins, biscuits, high-fat crackers, high-fat cookies
	Rice, pasta	Egg noodles
	Whole-grain breads and cereals (oatmeal, whole wheat, rye, bran, multigrain, etc.)	Breads in which eggs are major ingredient
Fats and oils	Baking cocoa	Chocolate
	Unsaturated vegetable oils: corn, olive, rapeseed (canola oil), safflower, sesame, soybean, sunflower	Butter, coconut oil, palm oil, palm kernel oil, lard, bacon fat
	Margarine or shortening made from one of the unsaturated fats listed above Diet margarine	
	Mayonnaise, salad dressings made with unsaturated oils listed above	Dressings made with egg yolk
	Low-fat dressings	
	Seeds and nuts	Coconut

From The Expert Panel. Report of the National Cholesterol Education Program Expert Panel on Detection, Evaluation, and Treatment of High Blood Cholesterol in Adults. Arch Intern Med 1988;148:36.

12-hour fast and includes measurement of total cholesterol, HDL cholesterol, and triglyceride levels. LDL cholesterol is calculated from these measurements using Friedewald's equation as follows:

LDL cholesterol =
  (total cholesterol − HDL cholesterol) − (triglycerides/5).

Low-density lipoprotein cholesterol level cutoff points have been defined to identify desirable (<130 mg/dl), borderline-high-risk (130–159 mg/dl), or high-risk (160 mg/dl or greater) levels. For patients with a desirable LDL cholesterol level, general dietary, physical activity, and risk factor education should be provided and retesting performed within 5 years. Patients with borderline-high-risk LDL cholesterol level and less than two CAD risk factors need re-evaluation annually as well as education on the step-one diet (Table 51–1) and physical activity. A cholesterol-lowering treatment program is reserved for patients with a borderline-high-risk LDL cholesterol level and at least two CAD risk factors and for all patients with a high-risk LDL cholesterol level. Familial lipoprotein disorders and secondary causes including diabetes, hypothyroidism, nephrotic syndrome, chronic renal failure, obstructive liver disease, and drugs need consideration in patients with high

TABLE 51–2. Coronary Disease Risk Factors to Consider in Screening for and Management of High Blood Cholesterol

RISK FACTORS ASSOCIATED WITH INCREASED RISK OF CORONARY ARTERY DISEASE
Age: men ≥ 45 years, women ≥ 55 years or premature menopause without estrogen therapy
Family history of premature coronary artery disease (age < 55 years in a father or male first-degree relative or age < 65 years in a mother or female first-degree relative)
Cigarette smoking
Hypertension
High-density lipoprotein cholesterol level < 35 mg/dl
Diabetes mellitus
RISK FACTOR ASSOCIATED WITH DECREASED RISK OF CORONARY ARTERY DISEASE*
High-density lipoprotein cholesterol level ≥ 60 mg/dl

*Subtract one risk factor.
Modified from Summary of the Second Report of the National Cholesterol Education Program (NCEP) Expert Panel on Detection, Evaluation, and Treatment of High Blood Cholesterol in Adults (Adult Treatment Panel II). JAMA 1993;269:3015.

LDL cholesterol levels. Laboratory evaluation to preclude secondary causes should include, when clinically appropriate, glucose, thyroid-stimulating hormone, creatinine, albumin, and liver function tests.

Screening and management recommendations incorporate the presence of known CAD and pertinent CAD risk factors in order to identify those patients at highest risk for a new coronary event and thus those most likely to benefit from cholesterol-lowering interventions. Risk factors to consider in the evaluation of elevated cholesterol levels are listed in Table 51–2. The risk of CAD in women lags behind that of men by approximately 10 years and rises progressively after menopause. Therefore, age and premature menopause (without estrogen therapy) have been included as risk factors in addition to family history of premature CAD, cigarette smoking, hypertension, low HDL

cholesterol level, and diabetes. Concern has been raised about the use of identical HDL cholesterol level cutoff points for women and men. An HDL cholesterol level of 35 mg per dl represents the twenty-fifth percentile for men and just below the tenth percentile for women and therefore may be too low for women.[43] Because of the powerful inverse association between HDL cholesterol and CAD risk, one risk factor may be subtracted if the HDL cholesterol level is 60 mg per dl or greater.

Adults with Coronary Disease or Other Atherosclerotic Disease

All adults with evidence of CAD, peripheral arterial disease, or symptomatic carotid artery disease require a fasting lipoprotein analysis. The average of two LDL cholesterol measurements taken 1 to 8 weeks apart should be used to determine appropriate treatment. An optimal LDL cholesterol level for patients with existing disease is less than 100 mg per dl. For those who meet this level, individualized dietary and exercise education is provided and lipoprotein analysis repeated annually. When the LDL cholesterol level exceeds 100 mg per dl, the patient requires a clinical evaluation including assessment for secondary causes and familial disorders as well as initiation of cholesterol-lowering therapy.

CHOLESTEROL-LOWERING TREATMENT

Dietary Therapy

Cholesterol-lowering intervention begins with dietary modification. Low-density lipoprotein cholesterol level cutoff points for initiation of dietary treatment and minimum LDL cholesterol level treatment goals depend on a patient's personal history of CAD and CAD risk factors (Table 51–3). For patients with CAD, dietary therapy is begun

TABLE 51–3. Cholesterol-Lowering Treatment Guidelines Based on LDL Cholesterol Level

| PATIENT CATEGORY | LDL CHOLESTEROL TREATMENT INITIATION LEVEL | | MINIMUM LDL CHOLESTEROL GOAL |
	Diet	Drug	
No CAD and < 2 risk factors	≥ 160 mg/dl	≥ 190 mg/dl*	< 160 mg/dl
No CAD and ≥ 2 risk factors	≥ 130 mg/dl	≥ 160 mg/dl	< 130 mg/dl
CAD	> 100 mg/dl	≥ 130 mg/dl	≤ 100 mg/dl

* > 220 mg/dl if premenopausal woman or man < 35 years.
CAD, Coronary artery disease; LDL, low-density lipoprotein.
Modified from Summary of the Second Report of the National Cholesterol Education Program (NCEP) Expert Panel on Detection, Evaluation, and Treatment of High Blood Cholesterol in Adults (Adult Treatment Panel II). JAMA 1993;269:3015.

when the LDL cholesterol level exceeds 100 mg per dl. In patients who do not have CAD but who are at high risk because of their CAD risk factors, dietary treatment is instituted when the LDL cholesterol level is 130 mg per dl or greater. For those with fewer than two CAD risk factors, dietary treatment is initiated when the LDL cholesterol level is 160 mg per dl or greater.

Dietary intervention is carried out in two steps: the step-one diet (see Table 51–1), in which total fat intake is restricted to less than 30% of calories, saturated fat to less than 10% of calories, and cholesterol to less than 300 mg per day; and the step-two diet, which further restricts saturated fat to less than 7% of caloric intake and cholesterol to less than 200 mg per day. The step-two diet is used as the initial dietary treatment in patients with CAD. Weight reduction and regular exercise need to be used in conjunction with dietary modifications. The average expected reduction in cholesterol is 30 to 40 mg per dl on the step-one diet, with an additional decline of 15 mg per dl on the step-two diet.[43]

After initiation of the step-one diet, cholesterol measurement and dietary adherence should be assessed at 4 to 6 weeks and 3 months. If the goal LDL cholesterol level has not been reached after 3 months of dietary therapy, referral to a registered dietitian is often necessary for progression to the step-two diet or a second trial of the step-one diet. Once LDL cholesterol goals are met, cholesterol measurement and dietary counseling need to be repeated quarterly in the first year and biannually thereafter.

Drug Therapy

Drug therapy is added to dietary treatment when at least 6 months of dietary modifications have failed to meet LDL cholesterol level goals. In adults free of CAD, drug treatment is begun with an LDL cholesterol level exceeding 190 mg per dl in the absence of risk factors and 160 mg per dl or greater if two or more risk factors are present (see Table 51–3). Because premenopausal women without other risk factors are at low risk for a coronary event, drug therapy can be delayed unless their LDL cholesterol is greater than 220 mg per dl. In patients with known CAD or other atherosclerotic disease, drug treatment is indicated for an LDL cholesterol level of 130 mg per dl or greater. Drug treatment goals are the same as those for dietary therapy (see Table 51–3).

The major classes of drugs effective in lowering cholesterol are listed in Table 51–4. The drugs of first choice for the treatment of hypercholesterol-

emia have traditionally been the bile acid sequestrants and nicotinic acid because of the documented reduction in CAD risk observed in clinical trials of these medications as well as their long-term safety records.[7, 19] Although both types of medications effectively lower LDL cholesterol levels, nicotinic acid has a more favorable effect on raising HDL cholesterol and additionally lowers triglyceride values. The Food and Drug Administration–approved hydroxymethylglutaryl coenzyme A (HMG-CoA) reductase inhibitors (lovastatin, pravastatin, simvastatin, fluvastatin) have powerful effects on lowering cholesterol, appear to be safe in short-term drug trials (long-term safety has not yet been proved), and have the added advantage of greater ease of patients' adherence.[45–48] Therefore, many clinicians are opting to use hydroxymethylglutaryl coenzyme A reductase inhibitors as first-line agents to lower cholesterol levels. In postmenopausal women, estrogen therapy can be considered because it lowers LDL cholesterol and raises HDL cholesterol levels. Gemfibrozil effectively lowers triglycerides and in some patients modestly reduces LDL cholesterol and raises HDL cholesterol levels.

Bile Acid Sequestrants

The primary action of the bile acid sequestrants is to bind bile acids in the intestine. Interruption of the enterohepatic circulation depletes hepatic cholesterol stores and increases hepatic LDL cholesterol receptor activity, which promotes removal of LDL cholesterol from plasma. Sequestrant therapy may also increase HDL cholesterol and triglyceride levels. Initial doses of the bile acid sequestrants effectively reduce LDL cholesterol level 10 to 15%, and maximal doses reduce LDL cholesterol level 15 to 30%.[43]

The cholesterol-lowering effects of 4 gm of cholestyramine are equivalent to that of 5 gm of colestipol. Cholestyramine is available in standard formulation, a reduced-calorie formulation, and a flavored bar. The usual starting dose of cholestyramine is 4 gm once or twice daily, with a maximal dose of 24 gm per day. Colestipol is available in standard powder formulation, and the usual starting dose is 5 gm twice daily and maximal daily dose is 30 gm.

Bile acid sequestrants are not absorbed from the gastrointestinal tract, limiting systemic toxicity. Side effects are mainly gastrointestinal and include constipation, bloating, epigastric fullness, nausea, and gas. Constipation can often be overcome with a high-fiber diet. The sequestrants interfere with the absorption of a number of medications and should therefore be administered 1 hour before or

TABLE 51–4. Drugs Effective in Lowering LDL Cholesterol*

DRUG	REDUCE RISK OF CORONARY ARTERY DISEASE	LONG-TERM SAFETY	LDL LOWERING	HDL	TRIGLY-CERIDES	STARTING DOSE	MAXIMUM DOSE	SIDE EFFECTS	MONITORING
Cholestyramine Colestipol	Yes	Yes	15–30%	↑	↑	4 gm twice daily 5 gm twice daily	24 gm/day 30 gm/day	Dose-dependent upper and lower gastrointestinal	Dosing schedules of coadministered drugs
Nicotinic acid	Yes	Yes	15–30%	↑	↓	100–250 mg as single dose or 3 divided doses with meals	3 gm/day Rarely, doses up to 6 gm are used	Flushing, upper gastrointestinal, and hepatic	Uric acid, liver function, glucose
Lovastatin	Not proven	Preliminary evidence	25–45%	↑	↓	20 mg once daily with evening meal	80 mg/day	Gastrointestinal and hepatic, miscellaneous including muscle pain	Liver function, creatine phosphokinase, lens
Simvastatin Pravastatin Flurastatin						5–10 mg 10–20 mg 20 mg	40 mg 40 mg 40 mg		
Gemfibrozil	Yes	Yes	5–15%†	↑	↓	600 mg twice daily 30 minutes before meals	600 mg twice daily	Gastrointestinal, occasional hepatic, rare hematologic	Should not be given to patients with gallbladder disease

*Estrogen therapy may be considered in postmenopausal women.
†May increase LDL cholesterol in hypertriglyceridemic patients.
LDL, Low-density lipoprotein cholesterol; HDL, high-density lipoprotein cholesterol.
Modified from The Expert Panel. Report of the National Cholesterol Education Program Expert Panel on Detection, Evaluation, and Treatment of High Blood Cholesterol in Adults. Arch Intern Med 1988;148:36.

3 to 4 hours after other medications. The medications affected include antibiotics, β-blockers, digoxin, phenobarbital, thiazide diuretics, thyroid hormone, and warfarin anticoagulants. The potential increase in triglyceride levels necessitates avoidance of these drugs in patients with moderate to severe hypertriglyceridemia. In addition, occasional and usually transient elevations in liver transaminases and alkaline phosphatase levels have been noted. Long-term use may be associated with fat-soluble vitamin (A, D, K) deficiencies.

Nicotinic Acid

The exact mechanism of action of nicotinic acid on lipoproteins has not been fully established. Nicotinic acid lowers both total and LDL cholesterol and triglyceride and raises HDL cholesterol levels. Reductions of LDL cholesterol levels by 15 to 30% can be achieved with this drug. Nicotinic acid is available in 100-mg and 500-mg tablets as well as sustained-release formulations. The initial starting dose is 100 to 250 mg per day, with a gradual increase in the total daily dose until 1.5 gm per day is achieved. The maximal daily dose of nicotinic acid is 6 gm per day.

A number of significant side effects associated with nicotinic acid often limit patients' adherence. In addition, this medication is contraindicated in patients with active peptic ulcer disease, liver disease, and gout and must be used carefully in those with diabetes or asymptomatic hyperuricemia. Flushing and itching are common side effects on initiation of therapy and appear to be prostaglandin mediated. Flushing can be minimized by pretreatment with aspirin or nonsteroidal anti-inflammatory medications, by administering the drug with meals, or by treatment with a sustained-release preparation, which is more costly. Tolerance to the flushing generally develops during the first several weeks of therapy. Dry skin can often be treated with moisturizers, and gastrointestinal side effects can be minimized by administering the medication with meals. Metabolic effects include abnormalities of liver function, hyperglycemia, and hyperuricemia. Liver function, uric acid, and glucose should be measured before treatment and once the therapeutic dose has been reached or increased. Drug interactions are few and include postural hypotension when administered concurrently with antihypertensive medications and myopathy when administered in combination with lovastatin.

Hydroxymethylglutaryl Coenzyme A Reductase Inhibitors

The hydroxymethylglutaryl coenzyme A reductase inhibitors block the rate-limiting enzyme in cholesterol biosynthesis, resulting in an increase in LDL receptor activity in the liver and receptor-mediated removal of LDL cholesterol from plasma. In women, lovastatin produces sustained dose-related reductions in LDL cholesterol of 24 to 40% as well as increases in HDL cholesterol (7–9%) and modest reductions in triglyceride levels (9–18%).[48] Among women without CAD or two CAD risk factors, 82 to 95% achieved a goal LDL cholesterol level less than 160 mg per dl while on lovastatin.[48] For women with CAD or CAD risk factors, 40 to 87% (depending on lovastatin dose) achieved their goal LDL cholesterol level.[48] The usual starting dose of lovastatin is 20 mg administered with the evening meal, with adjustment to a maximal dose of 80 mg per day. Pravastatin and simvastatin were approved for use in 1991. The usual starting dose of pravastatin is 10 to 20 mg in the evening, with a maximal daily dose of 40 mg. The corresponding starting dose of simvastatin is 5 to 10 mg, with a maximal daily dose of 40 mg. Most recently approved is flurastatin, with a starting dose of 20 mg in the evening and a maximal dose of 40 mg.

Lovastatin is generally well tolerated; most side effects have been mild and transient.[45–48] Upper and lower gastrointestinal side effects, myalgia, fatigue, insomnia, headache, and rash all have been reported. Metabolic abnormalities include increases in liver transaminases and creatine phosphokinase levels. In a large multicenter trial, transaminase elevations above three times the upper limit of normal occurred in only 0.1% of women and were dependent on a lovastatin dose greater than 20 mg.[48] Additionally in that trial, myopathy (muscle symptoms and creatine phosphokinase level greater than 10 times normal) was rare and associated with the 80 mg per day dose.[48] Concern has also been raised about the possibility that this drug may induce or have an effect on the progression of lens opacities (cataracts); this effect has not been verified to date. Rare hypersensitivity syndromes have been noted. Although endocrine dysfunction has not been observed, a theoretical blunting of the pituitary-gonadal axis could occur in premenopausal women. Drug interactions are few; however, severe myositis (including rhabdomyolysis) has occurred when lovastatin was given concurrently with cyclosporine, gemfibrozil, nicotinic acid, and erythromycin. Estrogen therapy appears to have no significant effects on the efficacy or safety of lovastatin.[48]

Gemfibrozil

The primary mechanisms of action of gemfibrozil, a fibric acid derivative, have not been completely established. It is highly effective in reducing elevated triglyceride levels and has the associated effect of raising HDL cholesterol levels. Gemfibrozil has variable effects on LDL cholesterol and may increase LDL cholesterol level in patients with hypertriglyceridemia. In patients without elevated triglyceride levels, a reduction in LDL cholesterol level of 10 to 15% has been noted. Gemfibrozil is available in 300-mg capsules or 600-mg tablets. The recommended therapeutic dose is 600 mg twice daily one-half hour before meals.

Gemfibrozil is generally well tolerated. The most common side effects are upper gastrointestinal complaints and increased lithogenicity of bile. Therefore, preexisting gallbladder disease is a contraindication to use, as is liver or kidney dysfunction. Occasional abnormalities of liver function test results as well as rare changes in hematologic parameters have been observed. Drug interactions are few and include potentiation of oral anticoagulants and myositis (with possible rhabdomyolysis) when given concurrently with lovastatin.

Probucol

Probucol increases LDL cholesterol catabolism by an unclear mechanism, resulting in reduction of LDL cholesterol level of 8 to 15%. Unfortunately, this drug also reduces HDL cholesterol level by as much as 25%. Clinical usefulness is limited to patients who require treatment and are unable to tolerate other drugs. Probucol is available in 250-mg and 500-mg tablets. The usual dose is 500 mg twice per day. Side effects are mainly gastrointestinal and include diarrhea and gas. A prolongation of the Q-T interval has been observed, necessitating avoidance of this drug in patients with ventricular irritability or in patients taking other medications associated with prolongation of the Q-T interval.

Combination Drug Therapy

When single-drug therapy fails to meet LDL cholesterol treatment goals, a combination of two drugs can produce further reductions in LDL cholesterol levels. The combination of a bile acid sequestrant with either nicotinic acid or lovastatin has the potential of lowering LDL cholesterol levels by 40 to 50% or more, raising HDL cholesterol levels, and limiting the sequestrant-induced elevation in triglycerides.[43] The combination of nicotinic acid and lovastatin may be useful for severe hypercholesterolemia or in cases of coexistent hypertriglyceridemia; however, the risk of myositis

is increased. The addition of gemfibrozil to any of the other agents has the advantage of lowering triglyceride values, but further LDL cholesterol reduction is variable. Severe myopathies have been noted with the combination of lovastatin and gemfibrozil.

Drug Therapy Recommendations

Many factors need to be considered in selecting a medication once it becomes evident that drug treatment is indicated, including a patient's lipoprotein profile and medical history, the medication side effects, and cost. Importantly, patients need to be actively involved in establishing an acceptable treatment plan to aid with long-term adherence. Although bile acid sequestrants and nicotinic acid have traditionally been the agents of first choice because of both their documented efficacy in reducing coronary events and their safety profiles, these drugs are also associated with unpleasant side effects that limit patients' adherence. The hydroxymethylglutaryl coenzyme A reductase inhibitors are generally better tolerated and easier to use, thus providing an attractive treatment option. In postmenopausal women, estrogen therapy can be considered.

Bile acid sequestrants are the drugs of choice in patients with moderately elevated LDL cholesterol and normal triglyceride levels, especially in cases of primary prevention and when drug therapy is needed in premenopausal women. Niacin is the first-line agent in patients with elevated LDL cholesterol and low HDL cholesterol levels or coexistent hypertriglyceridemia. Furthermore, when medication cost is an issue, niacin is far cheaper than any other cholesterol-lowering drug. Adherence with niacin requires considerable patient education and may be difficult to achieve owing to the associated flushing that accompanies drug initiation. For patients who cannot tolerate niacin and require reduction in both LDL cholesterol and triglycerides, lovastatin or a sequestrant with gemfibrozil can be used. Lovastatin, with its powerful effects on LDL cholesterol and its ease of administration compared with the sequestrants and niacin, can also be used as first-line therapy. Lovastatin, however, does not raise HDL cholesterol and lower triglyceride levels to the same degree as niacin. Gemfibrozil is most beneficial in patients with high triglyceride levels and in diabetic patients with elevated triglyceride levels. Estrogen therapy can be considered in postmenopausal women with elevated LDL cholesterol levels.

After initiation of drug therapy, LDL cholesterol needs to be measured at 4 to 6 weeks and again at

3 months. If LDL cholesterol goals are met, patients can be evaluated every 4 months or sooner if medication side effects need to be assessed. If LDL cholesterol goals are not reached, patients can be switched to a different medication or to a combination of two medications.

Low Levels of High-Density Lipoprotein Cholesterol

No controlled clinical trials designed to determine the benefit of raising HDL cholesterol levels have been published. Nevertheless, given the powerful inverse association of HDL cholesterol levels with risk for CAD, efforts to raise HDL cholesterol levels by lifestyle modifications can be supported. Because cigarette smoking, obesity, and lack of physical activity all are associated with reduced HDL cholesterol levels, smoking cessation, weight loss, and regular exercise all can be advocated. In addition, avoidance of drugs known to reduce HDL cholesterol levels is prudent, including androgens, anabolic steroids, β-blocking agents, and progestational agents. When drug therapy is needed to lower LDL cholesterol levels in a patient who also has a low HDL cholesterol level, drugs that raise HDL cholesterol levels (such as niacin) should be used.

Elevated Triglycerides

Triglyceride levels are classified as normal (<200 mg/dl), borderline-high (200–400 mg/dl), high (400–1000 mg/dl), and very high (>1000 mg/dl).[42] Patients with borderline-high and high triglyceride levels may be at increased risk for CAD. Patients with very high triglyceride levels are at increased risk for pancreatitis. Nonpharmacologic measures including weight reduction and diet, exercise, and restriction of alcohol intake should be emphasized for all those with an elevated triglyceride level. In patients with very high triglyceride levels, drug treatment (gemfibrozil or nicotinic acid) is generally needed to reduce the risk of pancreatitis. No consensus has been reached about the use of drug treatment for borderline-high triglyceride values. Controlled clinical trials to establish efficacy of treatment in patients with high triglycerides, low HDL cholesterol, and desirable LDL cholesterol levels are not available. However, some authorities would consider drug treatment in this situation in cases in which lifestyle modifications have failed and CAD or CAD risk factors are present.

Pregnant Women

Elevations in cholesterol and triglyceride levels that occur during pregnancy are generally not clinically significant. Elevations in triglyceride levels usually return to prepregnancy levels by 6 weeks postpartum, whereas LDL cholesterol levels may remain elevated for 6 to 9 months postpartum.[43] Dietary modifications can be continued during pregnancy for women with preexisting lipid abnormalities, with avoidance of drug therapy, because fetal effects have been inadequately studied. For women with preexisting hypertriglyceridemia, triglyceride levels should be carefully monitored to assess the risk of pancreatitis.

REFERENCES

1. Eaker ED, Packard B, Thom TJ. Epidemiology and risk factors for coronary heart disease in women. Cardiovasc Clin 1989;19:129.
2. Kannel WB, Castelli WP, Gordon T, McNamara PM: Serum cholesterol, lipoproteins, and the risk of coronary heart disease. The Framingham Study. Ann Intern Med 1971;74:1.
3. Multiple Risk Factor Intervention Trial Research Group: Multiple risk factor intervention trial: Risk factor changes and mortality results. JAMA 1982;248:1465.
4. Task Force on Cholesterol Issues, American Heart Association. The cholesterol facts: A summary of the evidence relating dietary fats, serum cholesterol, and coronary heart disease. A joint statement by the American Heart Association and the National Heart, Lung, and Blood Institute. Circulation 1990;81:1721.
5. Bush TL, Fried LP, Barrett-Connor E. Cholesterol, lipoproteins, and coronary heart disease in women. Clin Chem 1988;34:B60.
6. Anderson KM, Wilson PWF, Odell PM, Kannel WB. An updated coronary risk profile: A statement for health professionals. Circulation 1991;83:356.
7. The Lipids Research Clinics Program: The Lipid Research Clinics Coronary Primary Prevention Trial results. I. Reduction in incidence of coronary heart disease. JAMA 1984;251:351.
8. Anderson KM, Castelli WP, Levy D. Cholesterol and mortality: 30 years of follow-up from the Framingham Study. JAMA 1987;257:2176.
9. Wilson PWF. High-density lipoprotein, low-density lipoprotein and coronary artery disease. Am J Cardiol 1990;66:7A.
10. Gordon DJ, Probstfield JL, Garrison RJ, et al. High-density lipoprotein cholesterol and cardiovascular disease. Four prospective American studies. Circulation 1989;79:8.
11. Castelli WP, Garrison RJ, Wilson PWF, et al. Incidence of coronary heart disease and lipoprotein cholesterol levels: The Framingham Study. JAMA 1986;256:2835.
12. Abbott RD, Wilson PWF, Kannel WB, Castelli WP. High density lipoprotein cholesterol, total cholesterol screening, and myocardial infarction. The Framingham Study. Arteriosclerosis 1988;8:207.
13. Castelli WP. Cardiovascular disease in women. Am J Obstet Gynecol 1988;158:1553.
14. Grundy SM, Vega GL. Two different views of the relationship of hypertriglyceridemia to coronary heart disease implications for treatment. Arch Intern Med 1992;152:28.

15. Wilson PWF, Anderson KM, Castelli WP. The impact of triglycerides on coronary heart disease: The Framingham Study. Atheroscler Rev 1991;22:59.

16. Manninen V, Tenkanen L, Koskinen P, et al. Joint effects of serum triglyceride and LDL cholesterol and HDL cholesterol concentrations on coronary heart disease risk in the Helsinki Heart Study: Implications for treatment. Circulation 1992;85:37.

17. Assmann G, Schulte H. Triglycerides and atherosclerosis results from the Prospective Cardiovascular Munster Study. Atheroscler Rev 1991;22:51.

18. Austin MA. Plasma triglyceride and coronary heart disease. Arterioscler Thromb 1991;11:2.

19. Coronary Drug Project Research Group. Clofibrate and niacin in coronary heart disease. JAMA 1975;231:360.

20. Canner PL, Berge KG, Wenger N, et al. Fifteen year mortality in Coronary Drug Project patients: Long-term benefit with niacin. J Am Coll Cardiol 1986;8:1245.

21. Blankenhorn DH, Nessim SA, Johnson RL, et al. Beneficial effects of combined colestipol-niacin therapy on coronary atherosclerosis and coronary venous bypass grafts. JAMA 1987;257:3233.

22. Kane JP, Malloy MJ, Ports TA, et al. Regression of coronary atherosclerosis during treatment of familial hypercholesterolemia with combined drug regimens. JAMA 1990;264:3007.

23. Buchwald H, Varco RL, Matts JP, et al. Effect of partial ileal bypass surgery on mortality and morbidity from coronary heart disease in patients with hypercholesterolemia: Report of the program on surgical control of the hyperlipidemias (POSCH). N Engl J Med 1990;323:946.

24. Matthews KA, Meilahn E, Kuller LH, et al. Menopause and risk factors for coronary heart disease. N Engl J Med 1989;321:641.

25. Gordon T, Kannel WB, Hjortland MC, McNamara PM. Menopause and coronary heart disease: The Framingham Study. Ann Intern Med 1978;89:157.

26. Colditz GA, Willett WC, Stampfer MJ, et al. Menopause and the risk of coronary heart disease in women. N Engl J Med 1987;316:1105.

27. Stampfer MJ, Willett WC, Colditz GA, et al. A prospective study of postmenopausal estrogen therapy and coronary heart disease. N Engl J Med 1985;313:1044.

28. Bush TL, Barrett-Connor E, Cowan LD, et al. Cardiovascular mortality and noncontraceptive use of estrogen in women: Results from the Lipid Research Clinics Program Follow-up Study. Circulation 1987;75:1102.

29. Bush TL, Cowan LD, Barrett-Connor E, et al. Estrogen use and all-cause mortality preliminary results from the Lipid Research Clinics Program Follow-up Study. JAMA 1983;249:903.

30. Sullivan JM, Zwaag RV, Lemp GF, et al. Postmenopausal estrogen use and coronary atherosclerosis. Ann Intern Med 1988;108:358.

31. Stampfer MJ, Colditz GA. Estrogen replacement therapy and coronary heart disease: A quantitative assessment of the epidemiologic evidence. Prev Med 1991;20:1.

32. Bush TL, Miller VT. Effects of pharmacologic agents used during menopause. Impact on lipids and lipoproteins. In: Mishell D (ed). Menopause: Physiology and Pharmacology. Chicago: Year Book Medical Publishers, 1986, pp 187–208.

33. Judd H. Efficacy of transdermal estradiol. Am J Obstet Gynecol 1987;156:1326.

34. Knopp RH. Estrogen replacement therapy for reduction of cardiovascular risk in women. Curr Opin Lipidol 1991;2:240.

35. Knopp RH. Cardiovascular effects of endogenous and exogenous sex hormones over a woman's lifetime. Am J Obstet Gynecol 1988;158:1630.

36. Rijpkema AHM, van der Sanden AA, Ruijs AHC. Effects of post-menopausal oestrogen-progestogen replacement therapy on serum lipids and lipoproteins: A review. Maturitas 1990;12:259.

37. Weinstein L, Bewtra C, Gallagher JC. Evaluation of a continuous combined low-dose regimen of estrogen-progestin for treatment of the menopausal patient. Am J Obstet Gynecol 1990;162:1534.

38. Stadel BV. Oral contraceptives and cardiovascular disease. N Engl J Med 1981;305:612.

39. Stampfer MJ, Willett WC, Colditz GA, et al. A prospective study of past use of oral contraceptive agents and risk of cardiovascular diseases. N Engl J Med 1988;319:1313.

40. Wahl P, Walden C, Knopp R, et al. Effect of estrogen/progestin potency on lipid/lipoprotein cholesterol. N Engl J Med 1983;308:862.

41. Harvengt C, Desager JP, Gaspard U, et al. Changes in lipoprotein composition in women receiving two low-dose oral contraceptives containing ethinyl estradiol and gonane progestins. Contraception 1988;37:565.

42. Summary of the second report of the National Cholesterol Education Program (NCEP) Expert Panel on detection, evaluation, and treatment of high blood cholesterol in adults (Adult Treatment Panel II). JAMA 1993;269:3015.

43. Gotto AM Jr. Primary and secondary prevention of coronary artery disease. Curr Opin Cardiol 1992;7:553.

44. The Expert Panel. Report of the National Cholesterol Education Program Expert Panel on detection, evaluation, and treatment of high blood cholesterol in adults. Arch Intern Med 1988;148:36.

45. Bradford RH, Shear CL, Chremos AN, et al. Expanded Clinical Evaluation of Lovastatin (EXCEL) Study results I. Efficacy in modifying plasma lipoproteins and adverse event profile in 8245 patients with moderate hypercholesterolemia. Arch Intern Med 1991;151:43.

46. Bradford RH, Shear CL, Chremos AN, et al. Expanded Clinical Evaluation of Lovastatin (EXCEL) Study results III. Efficacy in modifying lipoproteins and implications for managing patients with moderate hypercholesterolemia. Am J Med 1991;91(Suppl 1B):18S.

47. Dujovne CA, Chremos AN, Poll JL, et al. Expanded Clinical Evaluation of Lovastatin (EXCEL) Study results: IV. Additional perspectives on tolerability of lovastatin. Am J Med 1991;91(Suppl 1B):25S.

48. Bradford RH, Downtown M, Chremos AN, et al. Efficacy and tolerability of lovastatin in 3390 women with moderate hypercholesterolemia. Ann Intern Med 1993;118:850.

Coronary Artery Disease

Nanette K. Wenger

Although coronary artery disease (CAD) has traditionally been viewed as a problem of men, it is also the major cause of death in women in the United States, accounting for a quarter of a million deaths annually. Further, CAD is a major contributor to illness, disability, and an unfavorable quality of life for women. As was evident in data from the Framingham Heart Study, CAD affects predominantly older women, in that any initial manifestation of CAD occurred about a decade later in women than in men, and myocardial infarction (MI) occurred an average of 20 years later.[1] The reasons for this gender–age disparity are poorly understood. Thus, although CAD occurs less commonly in women than in men at middle age, the gender difference decreases with increasing age. Despite the lower prevalence of CAD in women than in men, deaths due to CAD in women equal those in men, attesting to the more adverse outcomes among women. Because women constitute the majority of the elderly population, the age group in which cardiovascular and coronary diseases are more prevalent among women, cardiovascular deaths in elderly women now exceed those among elderly men in the United States.

With aging of the population and with a life expectancy of women that is 6 to 7 years greater than for men, we can anticipate an escalating occurrence of morbidity and mortality from CAD among women as the size of the population of elderly women increases, unless major improvements occur in the preventive, diagnostic, and management strategies for CAD in women. The challenge is to reduce the risk for cardiovascular disease in women by encouraging their adoption of healthy lifestyles and by instituting other preventive interventions and to educate women and their health care providers to vigorously evaluate and manage CAD in women to reduce their morbidity and mortality.[2]

CORONARY RISK FACTORS: PREVENTION OF CORONARY ARTERY DISEASE

Traditional CAD risk factors, common to both genders, are highly prevalent in women in the United States, with obesity and diabetes mellitus encountered more frequently among women than men. Further, the risk of death due to both coronary and cardiovascular disease is greatest among women who are educationally and socioeconomically disadvantaged. Risk factors for CAD, particularly hypertension, obesity, and cigarette smoking, as well as physical inactivity, tend to cluster among black, Hispanic, and Native American women. Diabetes mellitus appears to impart greater CAD risk for women than for men, and elevated triglyceride levels appear to engender risk only for women. Although hypertension is more prevalent in men than women at younger age, hypertension is more common in women after age 45 to 50 years.

Oral contraceptive use,[3] pregnancy, oophorectomy, hysterectomy, and premature menopause are CAD risk factors unique to women. The preventive role of postmenopausal hormone therapy warrants urgent investigation.[4] Case-control and cohort studies of estrogen therapy suggest a 35 to 50% lowering of CAD risk, even among otherwise high-risk postmenopausal women; however, randomized trials have not been undertaken, and question has been raised about the component of this apparent benefit that may be a healthy cohort or adherent patient effect. Further, in women with an intact uterus, unopposed estrogen therapy increases endometrial hyperplasia and the risk of uterine cancer; estrogen-progestin combinations, which limit endometrial hyperplasia, can decrease the risk of uterine cancer, but the efficacy of combined estrogen-progestin administration in favorably altering CAD risk has not yet been assessed. Estrogen use has several biologically plausible explanations for benefit: It reduces circulating lipid levels, as well as lipid uptake into the vascular wall. However, only about one third of the postulated estrogen benefit can be attributed to favorable lipid alterations. In nonhuman primates, estrogen administration has restored normal vascular reactivity to atherosclerotic coronary vessels; whether comparable effects occur with estrogen-progestin compounds is not yet known.

ANGINA PECTORIS

Information about angina pectoris, derived from the Framingham Heart Study, was based solely on the clinical history, before the availability of coronary arteriographic confirmation. Angina was described as the major initial manifestation of CAD in women, occurring in 56% of Framingham women compared with 43% of men. Within 5 years of the diagnosis of angina, 25% of Framingham men developed MI, whereas 86% of Framingham women considered to have angina never suffered MI;[5] the misinterpretation of angina as entailing a favorable prognosis among women, based on these data, likely had an adverse impact on the preventive approach to and the clinical care for CAD in women in subsequent years. A challenge to the benignity of angina pectoris in women came only with publication of data from the Coronary Artery Surgery Study Registry,[6, 7] which documented the results of coronary arteriography among men and women referred to participating hospitals by their treating physicians for chest pain symptoms considered severe enough to merit evaluation for coronary artery bypass graft (CABG). Fifty percent of women in this Registry population had little or no evidence of coronary artery atherosclerotic obstruction, as compared with 17% of the men. If such was the case in Framingham, perhaps the lack of progression from angina to MI in women reflected the sizable portion of Framingham women whose chest pain syndromes were due to causes other than coronary atherosclerotic obstruction. Indeed, a retrospective review of the Framingham data showed that among women age 60 to 69 years described to have angina, their angina entailed the same adverse prognosis as it did for Framingham men.

Thus, a pivotal approach to women with chest pain syndromes is to differentiate those due to coronary atherosclerotic heart disease (and to identify its risk or severity characteristics) from that due to other causes (see the later section on diagnostic testing). The clinical history alone is inadequate to do so, and objective confirmation is required. To date, the optimal timing and use of noninvasive and invasive diagnostic procedures remain obscure.

CHEST PAIN WITH NORMAL CORONARY ARTERIES

Chest pain syndromes, at times with evidence of myocardial ischemia at exercise electrocardiography (ECG) or exercise radionuclide testing but with normal coronary arteries at coronary arteriography, occur frequently in women, particularly younger women, and generally have a favorable prognosis.

The so-called variant[8, 9] or Prinzmetal's angina, due to coronary artery spasm in the absence of atherosclerotic obstructive lesions, typically has a benign course[10]; pain often occurs cyclically, is rarely activity precipitated, and responds well to vasodilator therapies.

A decrease in coronary vasodilator reserve has been postulated as yet another cause of chest pain in women,[11] with the pain having both typical and atypical characteristics of myocardial ischemia. Coexisting hypertension is frequent, often with left ventricular hypertrophy and ventricular diastolic dysfunction; most patients have a good symptomatic response to calcium channel–blocking drugs, although chest pain syndromes may persist in some. The relationship between left ventricular hypertrophy or diastolic dysfunction and loss of coronary vasodilator reserve, if any, remains enigmatic. Because women with this presentation often have abnormalities on their resting ECG, as well as evidence of myocardial perfusion abnormalities at exercise radionuclide scintigraphy, coronary arteriography is warranted to preclude significant obstructive atherosclerotic coronary lesions.

Attention is being directed toward syndrome X,[12] a chest pain syndrome associated with insulin resistance; microvascular endothelial dysfunction, decreased coronary vasodilator reserve, abnormalities of coronary vascular resistance, and complicating neurohormonal and possibly other endothelial abnormalities have been described as contributory. Some patients with this syndrome also appear to have abnormal patterns of pain perception. Although the outcome is generally favorable, with frequent satisfactory symptomatic response to coronary vasodilator drugs, a subset of women with syndrome X develop ventricular dysfunction and cardiomyopathy.

MYOCARDIAL INFARCTION

Myocardial infarction was less often the initial presentation of CAD in Framingham women, occurring in 35% of women as compared with 50% of men. However, women had a greater mortality with an initial MI, 39% as compared with 31% for men.[13] In the Multicenter Postinfarction Study, diabetes imparted an adverse prognosis for women, independent of ejection fraction.[14] Cardiac rupture complicating MI is also more frequent among women.[15, 16] Even with the contemporary lessening of mortality from MI, the excess MI mortality among women persists; the hospital mortality for women in the Myocardial Infarction Triage and Intervention Registry was 16%, as compared with 11% for men.[17]

Framingham women also had an excess of unrecognized MI, which occurred in 35% of women as compared with 27% of men.[18] Further, about half of these unrecognized infarctions were characterized as silent. It is currently well recognized that both older age and concomitant diabetes and hypertension increase the likelihood of silent or unrecognized MI; these predisposing features characterized women with MI in Framingham as well as contemporary populations of women with MI. Despite these findings, gender differences, if any, in the occurrence of silent ischemia are not known.

Equally important and also currently evident is the excess late morbidity and mortality of women who survive MI. One year mortality in the Framingham Heart Study was 45% for women as compared with 10% for men,[18] and 40% of women versus 13% of men sustained reinfarction within the first year. Contemporary data confirm both the excess of deaths for women after MI and the greater risk of recurrent infarction and of heart failure among surviving women than for their male counterparts;[19, 20] women and particularly black women had more postinfarction angina as well.[19] After MI, reinfarction was more prevalent in women, occurring in 32% versus 23% of men, with a comparably greater occurrence of stroke or transient ischemic attack. The prognosis was unfavorable despite better preservation of left ventricular function both at hospital admission and postinfarction, an attribute associated with favorable MI outcomes in men.[19, 21] The explanations for gender disparity in the left ventricular function-MI prognosis relationship are conjectural. The increased occurrence of non–Q-wave infarction among women, reported in several series,[19, 22, 23] likely renders them more susceptible to reinfarction; this occurrence leads to greater morbidity and mortality. To what extent the gender differences in outcomes can be ascribed to older age and to comorbid illness remains obscure.

Psychosocial complications following MI are also described as more common in women[24, 25]: anxiety, depression, sexual dysfunction, and guilt feelings about their illness. Return to work was less frequent and more delayed for women than men, despite early resumption of high-intensity household tasks among women.[25] The complex relationships of these observations in women to their older age at infarction, increased severity or complications of MI, lesser social support, and increased poverty rate compared with men should be elucidated.

SUDDEN DEATH

Sudden death occurred less often in Framingham women than men, 37% versus 46%.[1] It also was encountered at an older age in women, typically after 65 to 74 years, about 20 years later than in men. After MI, women are also less likely than men to die suddenly.[26]

In the Multicenter Postinfarction Trial,[27] ventricular arrhythmias independently predicted an adverse outcome for men but not for women, despite a comparable gender occurrence of these arrhythmias. Although not yet confirmed in other cohorts, the relationship of this observation to the lesser occurrence of sudden death in women requires attention. Probable concordant evidence is offered by the less frequent inducibility of ventricular tachycardia or ventricular fibrillation in women at electrophysiologic study of patients who were known to have CAD and who survived a cardiac arrest.[28]

DIAGNOSTIC TESTING: STATE OF THE ART

Exercise testing provides the cornerstone for noninvasive evaluation of myocardial ischemia; exercise-based tests are designed to increase myocardial oxygen demand serially, such that the test result will be abnormal when myocardial ischemia occurs (Table 52–1).

The combination of a carefully taken clinical history, assessment of CAD risk factors, and appropriate choice of an exercise-based test can determine the need for invasive testing (i.e., coronary arteriography).

As with any noninvasive diagnostic procedure, the pretest likelihood of disease limits the value of the information derived. It is important, however, to realize that exercise testing is not a purely bayesian phenomenon in that interpretation of the results is also dependent on the intensity of the exercise performed and the severity of the

TABLE 52–1. Diagnostic and Therapeutic Strategies in Women

DIAGNOSTIC TEST	DATA ON USE FOR WOMEN
Exercise electrocardiogram	Low pretest probability in young women limits likelihood of abnormal test results
	In older women, limited by patient's ability to perform exercise
Exercise radionuclide (thallium) tests	Use of gender-based criteria necessary to prevent false positive test results from breast tissue artifact
Technetium-99m scanning	No gender-specific data available
Pharmacologic radionuclide perfusion (dipyridamole) tests	No gender-specific data available
Gated blood-pool scanning	Criteria using increase in ventricular ejection fraction not applicable in women
Exercise echocardiography	High sensitivity and specificity in women
Therapeutic Strategies	
Aspirin	Similar benefits in secondary prevention in women
Antianginals	Theoretic advantage of vasodilators, no gender-specific data
Thrombolytic therapy	Similar benefits in women
Exercise rehabilitation	Similar benefits for women
Percutaneous transluminal coronary angioplasty	Increased mortality, possibly because women are older; greater comorbidity; more severe disease
Coronary artery bypass graft	Increased mortality, may be due to other risk factors (age, diabetes) or to technical difficulties and increased reocclusion with smaller coronary arteries

abnormalities induced and that abnormal test data are dependent on the severity and extent of the underlying CAD.[29] However, when the pretest likelihood of CAD, particularly that of multivessel CAD, is very low, there is little possibility that an abnormal test result can provide evidence for myocardial ischemia. A significant problem is thus posed in evaluating chest pain in young and middle-aged women who have few CAD risk factors and who have a very low pretest likelihood of CAD. On the other hand, in populations of older women (often with multiple CAD risk factors) being evaluated for chest pain, problems of older age, of comorbidity, or of a sedentary lifestyle may limit the ability to exercise adequately and thus curtail the information available from an exercise test. Further, preexisting ECG abnormalities related to hypertension, mitral valve prolapse, and the like may limit the diagnostic accuracy of the exercise ECG.[30, 31] Women appear more likely than men to have ST-T abnormalities on the resting ECG.

Nevertheless, for older women with a history typical of angina and a normal resting ECG, a simple exercise ECG test, with evaluation of ST-segment depression, is reasonable. Also, because of the low probability of CAD in younger women with chest pain syndromes, an adequate intensity negative (normal) exercise ECG provides substantial power to preclude myocardial ischemia as etiologic[30, 31]; this high negative predictive value,

comparable to that for men, has been inadequately appreciated and applied. In women whose resting ECG is abnormal, exercise radionuclide myocardial perfusion studies, typically using thallium-201 imaging, provide the best predictive accuracy,[29, 32–34] significantly better than that of exercise ECG.[35] Because of the relatively poor imaging characteristics of the thallium-201 isotope, interposition of breast tissue between the heart and the imaging camera may provide false positive results; gender-based criteria for interpretation, considering breast tissue imaging artifacts, have improved the accuracy of exercise thallium test results for women.[34]

Thallium exercise testing is also recommended for women with some features of chest pain typical of angina and others atypical of angina, in that the clinical description of the chest pain helps define the most appropriate diagnostic procedures.[29, 30, 36, 37] In several reports, when chest pain was typical of angina, 60 to 75% of women had evidence of significant CAD,[38] with one quarter to one half having multivessel CAD. Chest pain characterized as probable angina was associated with a 30 to 40% prevalence of significant CAD in women and 4 to 22% occurrence of multivessel CAD.[36] Only about 5% of women with nonspecific chest pain symptoms had evidence of CAD, and virtually none had multivessel CAD,[38] suggesting that exercise testing provides little diagnostic value in this population.[36]

Gender-specific data are not yet available for technetium-99m sestamibi imaging.

Pharmacologic radionuclide perfusion testing, using thallium-201 to identify areas of myocardial malperfusion, is applicable to evaluate women who have chest pain and who are unable to exercise, but its use is based on data validated for men. Gender-specific information is lacking.

Exercise radionuclide ventriculographic (gated blood pool) studies often fail to provide adequate diagnostic accuracy for women.[39–41] The traditional male model for diagnosis, in which failure to increase the ventricular ejection fraction with exercise suggests CAD, does not apply to women. Women have a smaller ventricular end-diastolic volume at rest and increase their exercise stroke volume predominantly by increasing the end-diastolic volume[42] (i.e., using Starling's mechanism); this contrasts with men who increase their exercise stroke volume from a larger initial end-diastolic volume primarily by increasing the ventricular ejection fraction. In one study, more than one third of women, as compared with fewer than 10% of men (with normal coronary arteries at arteriography), failed to increase their ejection fraction with exercise.[40, 41] Peak exercise ejection fraction may be a better diagnostic indicator in women.[43, 44]

Exercise echocardiography, as well as dipyridamole echocardiography, performed in small numbers of women with a high prevalence of CAD, has been described to have high sensitivity and specificity (about 86% each) for the diagnosis of CAD.[45, 46] The development of new wall-motion abnormalities as indicators of myocardial ischemia is suggested to retain its predictive accuracy with single-vessel disease, a common finding in women.

The role of cardiac fluoroscopic detection of coronary arterial calcification is under evaluation; older age and multivessel CAD appear associated with an improved predictive accuracy.[29, 47–49] The simplicity and widespread availability of this inexpensive procedure warrant elucidation of its value.

The optimal algorithm for identification of women with chest pain at high risk of a coronary event or of early death due to CAD remains to be developed.

Substantial documentation in recent years has shown that women with chest pain syndromes receive more delayed and less intensive diagnostic evaluation than do men, with fewer invasive diagnostic and therapeutic procedures, even after abnormal noninvasive test results.[50] Despite the almost doubled performance of coronary arteriography and a threefold increase in CABG and percutaneous transluminal coronary angioplasty

(PTCA) in women in recent years, myocardial revascularization procedures are still undertaken less frequently than for men. Whether this difference represents a gender bias, denying women equal access to care; an inappropriately aggressive pattern of evaluation for men; or suitable procedure use for both genders cannot be ascertained in the absence of outcome data. Nevertheless, information from several studies suggests that the performance of coronary arteriography may be the predominant determinant of access to myocardial revascularization.[51] In one such study, no gender difference was apparent in the referral for myocardial revascularization of patients with high-mortality-risk characteristics after coronary arteriography; that more men than women with non–high-risk coronary arteriographic and clinical characteristics were referred for revascularization was considered by some to suggest more appropriate care for women,[52, 53] in that surgery was undertaken predominantly when survival benefit was likely. Although this conclusion may be valid when only mortality endpoints are considered, data from the postinfarction Survival and Ventricular Enlargement trial suggest that other aspects are also relevant. Before the index infarction that determined eligibility for the Survival and Ventricular Enlargement trial, infarction that resulted in an ejection fraction less than 40%, men were almost twice as likely as women to have been referred for coronary arteriography and subsequent CABG. This occurred despite the fact that women reported significantly greater physical activity limitation due to anginal symptoms, 50% versus 31% in men.[54] Clearly, the burden of functional impairment due to anginal symptoms warrants consideration, in addition to survival data[54–56]; and clearly, in the cohort of the Survival and Ventricular Enlargement trial, medical management had been unable to prevent preinfarction functional disability in half of the women.

THERAPEUTIC STRATEGIES

Medical Management

Virtually none of the antianginal (anti-ischemic) drugs used daily in clinical practice has been studied for gender comparison. Only timolol, a β-blocking drug, was shown to have comparable gender benefit in limiting reinfarction.[57] Aspirin, in the ISIS-2 study, showed comparable gender protection against reinfarction.[58]

On a theoretic basis, the smaller coronary artery size in women and the greater predisposition of women to vasospastic problems such as Prinzmetal's angina and Raynaud's phenomenon suggest that drugs causing coronary vasodilation might be anticipated to provide preferential benefit. Studies are needed to validate this plausible but untested concept.

Thrombolytic therapy, administered in the early hours of acute MI, has occasioned major improvement in survival in patients eligible for its use. With inclusion of elderly patients in clinical trials, women with acute MI were reasonably represented in some studies of coronary thrombolysis, and equal gender benefit was demonstrated.[59] This equal gender benefit occurred despite an excess of bleeding complications in women, particularly serious intracranial bleeding. Thrombolytic therapy is typically administered in a fixed-dose regimen, raising concern about whether the lesser body mass of women fosters a relatively higher thrombolytic dose; in several studies of thrombolytic therapy, lowering of drug dose resulted in fewer bleeding complications. Clearly, dose-ranging studies are needed in women, particularly because the benefit of thrombolytic therapy appears even greater in elderly than in younger patients, reflecting the higher risk status of MI at elderly age.

Also of concern is that women are less eligible for thrombolytic therapy owing to their late arrival at the hospital after symptom onset. Whether this situation reflects the misperception that CAD is not a serious problem for women remains uncertain. Comorbidity and possibly older age further contribute to lack of eligibility of women for thrombolytic therapy, as does the increased frequency of non–Q-wave infarction in an elderly population, such that ECG criteria for initiating thrombolysis may not be met. However, even among women who have acute MI and who are eligible for thrombolytic therapy by standard criteria, physicians tend to use less coronary thrombolysis,[60] possibly for fear of bleeding complications. This practice raises concern, given the higher case fatality rate for women than for men.

Despite the reduced MI mortality among both men and women after thrombolytic therapy,[59] the in-hospital and 1-year gender ratio of MI deaths was not altered by coronary thrombolysis. One-year mortality rates for women were twice those for men, 29.8% versus 15.2%.[61]

After MI, fewer women than men are referred for exercise rehabilitation by their treating physicians,[62] despite documentation of an equal percentage increase in functional capacity in men and women so treated. Additionally, even when referred, women are less likely to have good attendance records and are more prone to cease participating.[25] The contribution of the design, scheduling, and site of many exercise rehabilita-

tion programs, structured to meet the needs of the predominant population (middle-aged and working men) and their relative lack of applicability to elderly women, warrant examination.

Myocardial Revascularization Procedures

Because randomized clinical trial data on myocardial revascularization procedures both for men and for women are lacking, outcome information is based on observational studies. However, in all reported clinical and registry series of CABG and PTCA, women are older, have an excess of hypertension and diabetes, and have more severe and unstable angina with a resultant greater likelihood of requiring urgent or emergency procedures. These characteristics are likely to impart an adverse prognosis. The smaller coronary artery size of women may engender technical procedural difficulties that may increase operative mortality, limit the completeness of myocardial revascularization, and adversely affect CABG patency. In most reported series, however, women also less frequently have multivessel CAD, prior MI, and abnormal ventricular systolic function; based on the male model of CAD, these features should suggest favorable revascularization outcomes.

In virtually all surgical case series, female gender was the major characteristic predicting an adverse procedural outcome, both an excess death rate and an excess of surgical complications among CABG survivors.[63–65] The risk of perioperative mortality for women after CABG is almost twice that of men. This was the case in the Coronary Artery Surgery Study, in which the perioperative mortality rate was 4.5% in women versus 1.9% in men[24, 66]; perioperative heart failure was also more common in women. Contemporary data from the Myocardial Infarction Triage and Intervention Registry show an overall higher surgical mortality related to more elderly, medically complex, and seriously ill patients undergoing CABG; 13% of women as compared with 6.5% of men died during the hospital stay for CABG.[17, 67] As noted earlier, women have a greater perioperative occurrence of heart failure symptoms; given their preserved ventricular systolic function, these symptoms likely represent ventricular diastolic dysfunction.[68] Inappropriate recognition of the mechanism for heart failure and thus inappropriate treatment for its symptoms may compromise outcome.

The most treacherous period for women seems to be the operative and perioperative phase of CABG, and temporal features of this high-risk status warrant more detailed examination. The contribution of severe or unstable angina, mandating urgent or emergency CABG, should also be addressed.[69, 70] A disproportionate number of women with unstable angina are enrolled in several CABG series,[63–65] as well as in the NHLBI PTCA Registry.[71] It remains controversial whether women indeed have an excess of unstable angina or whether this preponderance reflects gender-related differing indications for CABG and PTCA or delayed referral. Internal thoracic artery grafting, the current vessel of choice owing to its superior long-term patency rates, is a more laborious procedure that is less likely to be performed when surgery is undertaken on an urgent or emergency basis; saphenous vein grafts provide less satisfactory long-term conduits. Even with elective CABG, only one internal thoracic artery is likely to be used in diabetic patients to avert problems in wound healing; some surgeons consider internal thoracic artery grafting unwise at advanced age. Thus, elderly diabetic women appear likely to receive less optimal vascular conduits. Among women who undergo CABG and who survive to be discharged from the hospital, their 5- and 10-year survival rates, including relative symptom-free survival, are either comparable to or better than those for men, possibly related to the women's lack of prior MI and preserved ventricular systolic function.[63]

Women are more likely to have adverse psychosocial outcomes than are men after CABG[72]; a lesser and later return to work, more frequent depression, and decreased resumption of preoperative activities. The potential contributions to their psychosocial impairment of older age, greater comorbidity, lesser social support, widowhood, limited financial resources, and the like have yet to be evaluated.

Although the early PTCA Registry and case series reports described a lesser success rate and an excess of procedural and hospital mortality rates among women,[71] PTCA procedural success has serially improved with refinements in angioplasty equipment and techniques and increased experience of the operators.[73] Nevertheless, despite a comparable PTCA procedural risk for both genders in contemporary series, the hospital mortality after PTCA remains higher in women, with most of this hospital mortality, as well as the excess late mortality, attributable to coexisting medical problems and older age.[74] Again, these data are derived only from observational series.

Data compiled at the Emory University School of Medicine,[75–77] encompassing the years 1974 to 1991, showed that 6903 of the 30,089 coronary arteriographic procedures were performed in women. During the same time period, 13,368 patients underwent CABG, of whom 2648 were women. Based on coronary arteriographic criteria, no bias was evident in the referral of women for CABG; however, information is lacking about the population from which the women referred for coronary arteriography were derived.[75]

From earlier to recent years, the population undergoing CABG at Emory has become progressively older, with a concomitant increase in surgical mortality; however, mortality for women increased to a greater extent than for men because women were relatively older and had more frequent emergency CABG and more prevalent diabetes; in very recent years, an excess of triple-vessel and left main CAD was present in women undergoing CABG, further increasing mortality.[76]

Examination of data regarding a first elective PTCA during the years 1980 to 1990 showed that 2667 of the 10,286 total PTCA procedures at Emory were performed in women. As in other series, gender success was comparable; however, women had a higher hospital death rate, only partially attributable to older age. The lesser 5-year survival of women after PTCA appeared entirely related to comorbid medical problems, principally older age.[77]

SUMMARY

We know that the female heart is vulnerable to coronary atherosclerotic heart disease and that the disease becomes clinically manifest at an older age in women than in men. Thus, CAD is likely to engender greater morbidity and mortality in women as the U.S. population ages and with female gender predominance at elderly age. Women with symptomatic CAD appear to sustain greater morbidity, more functional limitations, and consequently a substantially greater impairment of quality of life than do men.[54] The effect of postmenopausal hormone therapy, a potential preventive approach unique to women, must be examined, as well as other preventive strategies designed to retard or minimize CAD in women.[78]

Once women develop clinically overt CAD, their prognosis is less favorable than that for men. Women are more likely than men to die during or after MI, as well as after PTCA and CABG; reasons for this striking gender difference in prognosis remain poorly understood. The contributors to these features of older age and comorbidity, as compared with less frequent and possibly more delayed diagnostic procedures and surgical interventions, remain to be ascertained. Contemporary prognosis of CAD is influenced both by access to diagnostic procedures and by the therapies selected; these, in turn, may be influenced by physicians' decisions, by patients' decisions, by reimbursement issues, and by societal perceptions of the importance of CAD as a problem for U.S. women.

Prospectively derived, contemporary, gender-specific information must be obtained to determine which components of the traditional male model of CAD are applicable to both genders and at elderly age. The impact of earlier diagnosis and therapy of CAD in women must be examined to ascertain whether therapies initiated at earlier age, with less advanced and unstable CAD and with less severe comorbidity but particularly with less urgency or emergency of the surgical procedures undertaken for severe or unstable angina pectoris, will offer improved outcomes. Importantly, as for other diseases in elderly populations, mortality rates must be viewed as only a partial assessment of outcome; the impact of therapies on morbidity, on functional status, and on other aspects of life quality must equally be assessed.[2]

REFERENCES

1. Lerner DJ, Kannel WB. Patterns of coronary heart disease morbidity and mortality in the sexes: A 26-year follow-up of the Framingham population. Am Heart J 1986;111:383.
2. Wenger NK. Coronary heart disease in women: An overview (myths, misperceptions, and missed opportunities). In: Wenger NK, Speroff L, Packard B (eds). Cardiovascular Health and Disease in Women. Greenwich, CT, Le Jacq Communications, 1993, pp 21–29.
3. Engel HJ, Engel E, Lichtlen PR. Angiographic findings after myocardial infarction in women aged ≤ 50 years—role of oral contraceptives. In: Oliver MF, Vedin A, Wilhelmsson C (eds). Myocardial Infarction in Women. New York: Churchill Livingstone, 1986, pp 173–185.
4. Tepper R, Goldberger S, May JY, et al. Hormonal replacement therapy in postmenopausal women and cardiovascular disease: An overview. Obstet Gynecol Surv 1992;47:426.
5. Kannel WB, Feinleib M. Natural history of angina pectoris in the Framingham Study. Prognosis and survival. Am J Cardiol 1972;29:154.
6. The Principal Investigators of CASS and their Associates. The National Heart, Lung, and Blood Institute Coronary Artery Surgery Study (CASS). Circulation 1981;63(Suppl I):I-1.
7. Kennedy JW, Killip T, Fisher LD, et al. The clinical spectrum of coronary artery disease and its surgical and medical management, 1974–1979. Coronary Artery Surgery Study. Circulation 1982;66(Suppl III):III-16.
8. Selzer A, Langston M, Ruggeroli C, Cohn K. Clinical syndrome of variant angina with normal coronary arteriogram. N Engl J Med 1976;295:1343.
9. Pasternak RC, Hutter AM Jr, DeSanctis RW, et al. Variant angina. Clinical spectrum and results of medical and surgical therapy. J Thorac Cardiovasc Surg 1979;78:614.
10. Scholl J-M, Veau P, Benacerraf A, et al. Long-term prognosis of medically treated patients with vasospastic angina and no fixed significant coronary atherosclerosis. Am Heart J 1988;115:559.
11. Cannon RO III, Watson RM, Rosing DR, Epstein SE. Angina caused by reduced vasodilator reserve of the small coronary arteries. J Am Coll Cardiol 1983;1:1359.
12. Cannon RO III, Camici PG, Epstein SE. Pathophysiological dilemma of syndrome X. Circulation 1992;85:883.
13. Kannel WB, Abbott RD. Incidence and prognosis of myocardial infarction in women: The Framingham Study. In: Eaker ED, Packard B, Wenger NK, et al (eds). Coronary Heart Disease in Women. New York: Haymarket Doyma, 1987, pp 208–214.
14. Smith JW, Marcus FI, Serokman R, with the Multicenter Postinfarction Research Group. Prognosis of patients with diabetes mellitus after acute myocardial infarction. Am J Cardiol 1984;54:718.
15. Vlodaver Z, Edwards JE. Rupture of ventricular septum or papillary muscle complicating myocardial infarction. Circulation 1977;55:815.
16. Radford MJ, Johnson RA, Daggett WM Jr, et al. Ventricular septal rupture: A review of clinical and physiologic features and an analysis of survival. Circulation 1981;64:545.
17. Maynard C, Litwin PE, Martin JS, Weaver D. Gender differences in the treatment and outcome of acute myocardial infarction. Results from the Myocardial Infarction Triage and Intervention Registry. Arch Intern Med 1992;152:972.
18. Kannel WB, Sorlie P, McNamara PM. Prognosis after initial myocardial infarction. The Framingham Study. Am J Cardiol 1979;44:53.
19. Tofler GH, Stone PH, Muller JE, et al. Effects of gender and race on prognosis after myocardial infarction: Adverse prognosis for women, particularly black women. J Am Coll Cardiol 1987;9:473.
20. Greenland P, Reicher-Reiss H, Goldbourt U, et al. In-hospital and 1-year mortality in 1,524 women after myocardial infarction. Comparison with 4,315 men. Circulation 1991;83:484.
21. Tofler GH, Stone PH, Muller JE, Braunwald E. Clinical manifestations of coronary heart disease in women. In: Eaker ED, Packard B, Wenger NK, et al (eds). Coronary Heart Disease in Women. New York: Haymarket Doyma, 1987, pp 215–221.
22. Johansson S, Bergstrand R, Schlossman D, et al. Sex differences in cardioangiographic findings after myocardial infarction. Eur Heart J 1984;5:374.
23. Pohjola S, Siltanen P, Romo M. Five-year survival of 728 patients after myocardial infarction. A community study. Br Heart J 1980;43:176.
24. Fisher LD, Kennedy JW, Davis KB, et al. Association of sex, physical size, and operative mortality after coronary artery bypass in the Coronary Artery Surgery Study (CASS). J Thorac Cardiovasc Surg 1982;84:334.
25. Boogaard MAK, Briody ME. Comparison of the rehabilitation of men and women postmyocardial infarction. J Cardiopulmonary Rehabil 1985;5:379.
26. Waters DD. General discussion of session III. In: Eaker ED, Packard B, Wenger NK, et al (eds). Coronary Heart Disease in Women. New York: Haymarket Doyma, 1987, pp 264–266.
27. Moss AJ, Carleen E, and the Multicenter Postinfarction Research Group. Gender differences in the mortality risk associated with ventricular arrhythmias after myocardial infarction. In: Eaker ED, Packard B, Wenger NK, et al (eds). Coronary Heart Disease in Women. New York: Haymarket Doyma, 1987, pp 204–207.

28. Vaitkus PT, Kindwall KE, Miller JM, et al. Influence of gender on inducibility of ventricular arrhythmias in survivors of cardiac arrest with coronary artery disease. Am J Cardiol 1991;67:537.

29. Hung J, Chaitman BR, Lam J, et al. Noninvasive diagnostic test choices for the evaluation of coronary artery disease in women: A multivariate comparison of cardiac fluoroscopy, exercise electrocardiography and exercise thallium myocardial perfusion scintigraphy. J Am Coll Cardiol 1984;4:8.

30. Weiner DA, Ryan TJ, McCabe CH, et al. Exercise stress testing. Correlations among history of angina, ST-segment response and prevalence of coronary-artery disease in the Coronary Artery Surgery Study (CASS). N Engl J Med 1979;301:230.

31. Hlatky MA, Pryor DB, Harrell FE Jr, et al. Factors affecting sensitivity and specificity of exercise electrocardiography. Multivariable analysis. Am J Med 1984;77:64.

32. Melin JA, Wijns W, Vanbutsele RJ, et al. Alternative diagnostic strategies for coronary artery disease in women: Demonstration of the usefulness and efficiency of probability analysis. Circulation 1985;71:535.

33. Sternby NH. Sex differences in atherosclerosis. In: Oliver MF, Vedin A, Wilhelmsson C (eds). Myocardial Infarction in Women. New York: Churchill Livingstone, 1986, pp 166–169.

34. Goodgold HM, Rehder JG, Samuels LD, Chaitman BR. Improved interpretation of exercise T1-201 myocardial perfusion scintigraphy in women: Characterization of breast attenuation artifacts. Radiology 1987;165:361.

35. Friedman TD, Greene AC, Iskandrian AS, et al. Exercise thallium-201 myocardial scintigraphy in women: Correlation with coronary arteriography. Am J Cardiol 1982;49:1632.

36. Chaitman BR, Bourassa MG, Davis K, et al. Angiographic prevalence of high-risk coronary artery disease in patient subsets (CASS). Circulation 1981;64:360.

37. Guiteras Val P, Chaitman BR, Waters DD, et al. Diagnostic accuracy of exercise ECG lead systems in clinical subsets of women. Circulation 1982;65:1465.

38. Chaitman BR, Bourassa MG, Lam J, Hung J. Noninvasive diagnosis of coronary heart disease in women. In: Eaker ED, Packard B, Wenger NK, et al (eds). Coronary Heart Disease in Women. New York: Haymarket Doyma, 1987, pp 222–228.

39. Greenberg PS, Berge RD, Johnson KD, et al. The value and limitation of radionuclide angiocardiography with stress in women. Clin Cardiol 1983;6:312.

40. Higginbotham MB, Morris KG, Coleman RE, Cobb FR. Sex-related differences in the normal cardiac response to upright exercise. Circulation 1984;70:357.

41. Gibbons RJ, Lee KL, Cobb F, Jones RH. Ejection fraction response to exercise in patients with chest pain and normal coronary arteriograms. Circulation 1981;64:952.

42. Hanley PC, Zinsmeister AR, Clements IP, et al. Gender-related differences in cardiac response to supine exercise assessed by radionuclide angiography. J Am Coll Cardiol 1989;13:624.

43. Gibbons RJ, Lee KL, Pryor D, et al. The use of radionuclide angiography in the diagnosis of coronary artery disease—a logistic regression analysis. Circulation 1983;68:740.

44. Gibbons RJ, Fyke FE III, Clements IP, et al. Noninvasive identification of severe coronary artery disease using exercise radionuclide angiography. J Am Coll Cardiol 1988;11:28.

45. Sawada SG, Ryan T, Fineberg NS, et al. Exercise echocardiographic detection of coronary artery disease in women. J Am Coll Cardiol 1989;14:1440.

46. Masini M, Picano E, Lattanzi F, et al. High dose dipyridamole-echocardiography test in women: Correlation with exercise-electrocardiography test and coronary arteriography. J Am Coll Cardiol 1988;12:682.

47. Rifkin RD, Parisi AF, Folland E. Coronary calcification in the diagnosis of coronary artery disease. Am J Cardiol 1979;44:141.

48. Hamby RI, Tabrah F, Wisoff BG, Hartstein ML. Coronary artery calcification: Clinical implications and angiographic correlates. Am Heart J 1974;87:565.

49. Ghazzal ZMB, Weintraub WS, Renwick G, et al. Calcification of the coronary arteries and the diagnosis of coronary heart disease in women. Emory J Med 1991;5:9.

50. Ayanian JZ, Epstein AM. Differences in the use of procedures between women and men hospitalized for coronary heart disease. N Engl J Med 1991;325:221.

51. Krumholz HM, Douglas PS, Lauer MS, Pasternak PC. Selection of patients for coronary angiography and coronary revascularization early after myocardial infarction: Is there evidence for a gender bias? Ann Intern Med 1992;116:785.

52. Bickell NA, Pieper KS, Lee KL, et al. Referral patterns for coronary artery disease treatment: Gender bias or good clinical judgment? Ann Intern Med 1992;116:791.

53. Laskey WK. Gender differences in the management of coronary artery disease: Bias or good clinical judgement? Ann Intern Med 1992;116:869.

54. Steingart RM, Packer M, Hamm P, et al. Sex differences in the management of coronary artery disease. N Engl J Med 1991;325:226.

55. Wenger NK. Exclusion of the elderly and women from coronary trials. Is their quality of care compromised? JAMA 1992;268:1460.

56. Gurwitz JH, Col NF, Avorn J. The exclusion of the elderly and women from clinical trials in acute myocardial infarction. JAMA 1992;268:1417.

57. Pedersen TR, for the Norwegian Multicenter Study Group. Six-year follow-up of the Norwegian Multicenter Study on timolol after acute myocardial infarction. N Engl J Med 1985;313:1055.

58. ISIS-2 (Second International Study of Infarct Survival) Collaborative Group. Randomised trial of intravenous streptokinase, oral aspirin, both, or neither among 17,187 cases of suspected acute myocardial infarction: ISIS-2. Lancet 1988;2:349.

59. Gruppo Italiano per lo Studio della Streptochinasi nell'Infarto Miocardico (GISSI). Effectiveness of intravenous thrombolytic treatment in acute myocardial infarction. Lancet 1986;i:397.

60. Maynard C, Althouse R, Cerqueira M, et al. Underutilization of thrombolytic therapy in eligible women with acute myocardial infarction. Am J Cardiol 1991;68:529.

61. Gruppo Italiano per lo Studio della Streptochinasi nell'Infarto Miocardico (GISSI). Long-term effects of intravenous thrombolysis in acute myocardial infarction: Final report of the GISSI study. Lancet 1987;ii:871.

62. Oldridge NB, LaSalle D, Jones NL. Exercise rehabilitation of female patients with coronary artery disease. Am Heart J 1980;100:755.

63. Loop FD, Golding LR, MacMillan JP, et al. Coronary artery surgery in women compared with men: Analyses of risks and long-term results. J Am Coll Cardiol 1983;1:383.

64. Kahn SS, Nessim S, Gray R, et al. Increased mortality of women in coronary artery bypass surgery: Evidence for referral bias. Ann Intern Med 1990;112:561.

65. Gardner TJ, Horneffer PJ, Gott VL, et al. Coronary artery bypass grafting in women. A ten-year perspective. Ann Surg 1985;201:780.

66. Kennedy JW, Kaiser GC, Fisher LD, et al. Clinical and

angiographic predictors of operative mortality from the collaborative study in coronary artery surgery (CASS). Circulation 1981;63:793.

67. Maynard C, Weaver WD. Treatment of women with acute MI. New findings from the MITI Registry. J Myocardial Ischemia 1992;4:27.

68. Judge KW, Pawitan Y, Caldwell J, et al. Congestive heart failure symptoms in patients with preserved left ventricular systolic function: Analysis of the CASS Registry. J Am Coll Cardiol 1991;18:377.

69. Wenger NK. Gender, coronary artery disease, and coronary bypass surgery. Ann Intern Med 1990;112:557.

70. Tobin JN, Wassertheil-Smoller S, Wexler JP, et al. Sex bias in considering coronary bypass surgery. Ann Intern Med 1987;107:19.

71. Cowley MJ, Mullin SM, Kelsey SF, et al. Sex differences in early and long-term results of coronary angioplasty in the NHLBI PTCA Registry. Circulation 1985;71:90.

72. Stanton BA, Jenkins CD, Denlinger P, et al. Predictors of employment status after cardiac surgery. JAMA 1983;249:907.

73. Holmes DR Jr, Holubkov R, Vlietstra RE, et al. Comparison of complications during percutaneous transluminal coronary angioplasty from 1977 to 1981 and from 1985 to 1986: The National Heart Lung, and Blood Institute Percutaneous Transluminal Angioplasty Registry. J Am Coll Cardiol 1988;12:1149.

74. Savage MP, Goldberg S, Hirshfeld JW, et al. Clinical and angiographic determinants of primary coronary angioplasty success. J Am Coll Cardiol 1991;17:22.

75. Weintraub WS, Cohen CL, Wenger NK. Is there a bias against performing coronary revascularization in women (Abstract)? Circulation 1992;86(Suppl I):I.

76. Weintraub WS, Wenger NK, Jones EJ, et al. Changing demography of coronary surgery patients: Differences between men and women (abstract). Circulation 1992:86(Suppl I):I.

77. Weintraub WS, Wenger NK, Delafontaine P, et al. PTCA in women compared to men: Is there a difference in risk (abstract)? Circulation 1992;86(Suppl I):I.

78. Grady D, Rubin SM, Petitti DB, et al. Hormone therapy to prevent disease and prolong life in postmenopausal women. Ann Intern Med 1992;117:1016.

RHEUMATOLOGIC DISORDERS IN WOMEN

53

Inflammatory and Noninflammatory Arthropathies

Richard Polisson and Margaret Seton

The inflammatory and noninflammatory arthropathies are common in women, beginning in adolescence and extending well into the postmenopausal years. Although few of these disorders present as life-threatening emergencies, many of the arthropathies, such as rheumatoid arthritis (RA), are associated with profound morbidity and early mortality. In this chapter, the rheumatic diseases that affect diarthrodial joints are outlined and the issues of diagnosis and management addressed.

THE INFLAMMATORY ARTHRITIDES

Rheumatoid Arthritis

Pathogenesis and Epidemiology

Rheumatoid arthritis is a chronic systemic inflammatory disorder manifested by symmetric small and large joint synovitis with a variable spectrum of extra-articular manifestations. The cause of RA is unknown. Thought to be mediated by T-cell responses to ''arthritogenic'' peptides, the cytokines produced by these activated T cells and other cellular and humoral events cause an intense inflammatory response, usually localized to the joint space. Stimulated by growth factors, blood vessels grow into the synovium, drawing activated mononuclear cells to the site. These produce biologically active cytokines that drive pannus formation, bone erosion, and cartilage destruction. In contrast to the intense mononuclear cell response observed in the synovium, an influx of phagocytic polymorphonuclear cells is observed in the synovial fluid. Here local production of rheumatoid factor, activation of complement, and elaboration of proteolytic enzymes are thought to have an additional role in the pathogenesis of the disease.

Rheumatoid arthritis is more common in women than in men, with a prevalence estimated to be 1 to 2% worldwide. The disease may have an acute or stuttering onset, may remit only to return years later, or may progress inexorably to disability or early death. Although certain prognostic indicators, such as late or early age of onset, male sex, and positive rheumatoid factor, may auger a more severe course, clinical observation over time is more important for establishing the diagnosis, predicting disease outcome, or deciding on treatment options. Rheumatoid arthritis is a lifelong disease for which there is no cure, and for that reason, a compassionate and lifelong view of therapies must

553

be undertaken. Early referral to a rheumatologist is indicated to facilitate appropriate therapeutic decisions about the use of second-line drugs.

Clinical Features and Differential Diagnosis

Patients with RA present with fatigue and pain, describing prolonged morning stiffness usually lasting longer than 30 minutes and loss of ability to perform activities of daily living. The history and physical examination frequently reveal certain signs and symptoms that are characteristic of the disease (Table 53–1). In RA, the biochemical processes described earlier are manifested principally in the joints, which may be boggy, tender, and sometimes warm. A profound loss of strength and decreased range of motion of the affected joints are evident. Although other extra-articular manifestations of rheumatic disease may be present at the onset of disease, these manifestations often occur later in the disease process (Table 53–2). It is important to note the texture of the skin, the presence or absence of rashes, any associated ulcers of the mucous membranes, evidence of adenopathy, and signs of a thyroid mass. The salivary glands should be examined for evidence of dry eyes or dry mouth. The heart, lungs, and

TABLE 53–1. 1987 American College of Rheumatology Criteria for the Classification of Rheumatoid Arthritis*

1. Morning stiffness in and around the joints, lasting at least 1 hour before maximal improvement.
2. At least 3 joint areas simultaneously have had soft tissue swelling or fluid (not bony overgrowth alone) observed by a physician. The 14 possible areas are right or left PIP, MCP, wrist, elbow, knee, ankle, and MTP joints.
3. At least one area swollen (as defined above) in a wrist, MCP, or PIP joint.
4. Simultaneous involvement of the same joint areas (defined in 2) on both sides of the body (bilateral involvement of PIPs, MCPs, or MTPs is acceptable without absolute symmetry).
5. Subcutaneous nodules over bony prominences or extensor surfaces or in juxta-articular regions, observed by a physician.
6. Demonstration of abnormal amounts of serum rheumatoid factor by any method for which the result has been positive in fewer than 5% of normal control subjects.
7. Radiographic changes typical of rheumatoid arthritis on posteroanterior hand and wrist radiographs, which must include erosions or unequivocal bony decalcification localized in or most marked adjacent to the involved joints (osteoarthritis changes alone do not qualify).

*For the diagnosis of rheumatoid arthritis, four of the seven criteria are required.
PIP, Proximal interphalangeal; MCP, metacarpophalangeal; MTP, metatarsophalangeal.

TABLE 53–2. Extra-articular Features of Rheumatoid Arthritis

1. Subcutaneous nodules—associated with seropositivity and more aggressive arthritis
2. Serositis with pleuropericarditis—usually asymptomatic; tamponade is rare (pericardial fluid may have a profoundly low glucose concentration)
3. Pulmonary disease—diffuse interstitial fibrosis with restrictive results on pulmonary function tests; multiple pulmonary function tests; multiple pulmonary nodules
4. Neuropathy from entrapment or vasculitis (mononeuritis multiplex)
5. Inflammatory eye disease—episcleritis, scleritis, corneal stromal loss occasionally vision threatening
6. Felty's syndrome—splenomegaly, anemia, thrombocytopenia, neutropenia, recurrent infections, leg ulcers
7. Sjögren's syndrome—keratoconjunctivitis sicca, serologic abnormalities
8. Systemic necrotizing vasculitis—severe, potentially life-threatening extra-articular feature with manifestations similar to periarthritis nodosa

abdomen need to be assessed carefully, and the size of the spleen noted. Peripheral pulses, nail bed changes, and detailed neurologic findings should also be recorded.

The differential diagnosis for early-onset RA is extensive and depends somewhat on whether the process described is acute or chronic, whether the pattern of joint involvement is migratory or additive, and whether the process observed is monarticular, oligoarticular, or polyarticular. Many of the rheumatic diseases may mimic the early presentation of RA, including systemic lupus, Sjögren's syndrome, mixed connective tissue disease, overlap syndromes, and seronegative spondyloarthropathies. Also included in the differential diagnosis are endocrinopathies, most commonly thyroid dysfunction; regional musculoskeletal complaints such as fibromyalgia; bacterial infections including rheumatic fever or disseminated gonococcal infection; viral syndromes such as human immunodeficiency virus, parvovirus, or hepatitis virus; and crystal-induced arthropathies.

The initial laboratory evaluation includes a routine urinalysis, complete blood count with differential, Westergren's sedimentation rate, and chemistry analysis including liver function tests and determinations of creatinine, calcium, phosphorus, albumin, and alkaline phosphatase. Antinuclear antibody and rheumatoid factor should also be determined, although these tests lack sufficient sensitivity or specificity to be pathognomonic in the absence of the typical clinical stigmata. A chest radiograph, electrocardiogram, and aldolase or creatine phosphokinase determination may also be required, depending on the physical findings, but these are not mandatory in all patients. If unusual skin lesions are present, a dermatologic consultation with biopsy should be arranged. In early RA, radiographs of the joints involved show soft tissue changes and perhaps periarticular osteopenia. For this reason, in the absence of other atypical findings, radiographic studies of all the involved joints early in the disease are unnecessary. However, in patients with aggressive or more advanced RA, the marginal joint erosion as defined on plain radiographs is the harbinger of a destructive, deforming process (Fig. 53–1) and suggests that disease-modifying antirheumatic drug therapy may be appropriate.

Treatment

The standard treatment pyramid for RA, beginning initially with salicylates and nonsteroidal anti-inflammatory drugs (NSAIDs), is being challenged as being too conservative. A more aggressive approach in which second-line or disease-modifying antirheumatic agents are used earlier in the disease is recommended. The initial treatment continues to involve patient education, encouragement, and full-dose salicylate or NSAID therapy.

Follow-up should be attentive, and early referral to a rheumatologist should be made when patients show evidence of progressive disease or do not respond promptly to initial therapy. Although low doses of glucocorticoids (5–10 mg/day of prednisone or equivalent) may provide some comfort initially, they offer no solutions in terms of long-term outcome. For that reason, glucocorticoids should be avoided unless they are part of a long-term treatment strategy that incorporates other medications. Second-line therapies, such as gold salts, methotrexate, hydroxychloroquine, or sulfasalazine, are effective in short-term studies of RA; however, their potential for toxicity should not be ignored. The decision to initiate these agents should be made with the assistance of a rheumatologist familiar with the indications for and potential complications of the drugs.

Studies of experimental therapy are now under way with antibodies that block specific adhesion molecules found in vessel walls and with toxins that target the CD4 receptor, which is up-regulated in activated T cells. Anticytokines, induction of tolerance through oral antigens (type II chicken collagen), modification of diet with noninflammatory fatty acids (fish oils and γ-linolenic acid), and the use of tetracyclines in the treatment of RA are options also under active investigation. These medical insights, coupled with advances in the field of reconstructive surgery, provide significant benefit to the patient with progressive disease.

Seronegative Spondyloarthropathies

Pathogenesis and Epidemiology

The term spondyloarthropathy is derived from the Greek words spondylos (vertebra), arthron (joint), and pathos (suffering). These seronegative spondyloarthropathies form a heterogeneous group

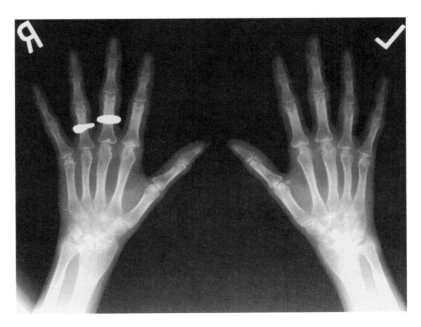

Figure 53–1. Radiographic features of rheumatoid arthritis (RA). Erosive, seropositive RA—hands. Note the marginal erosions, particularly the metacarpophalangeal joints, diffuse loss of carpal joint space with fusion and destruction of wrist joint articulation, and ulnar styloid erosion. These are the hands of a young woman on methotrexate, hydroxychloroquine sulfate (Plaquenil Sulfate), and nonsteroidal anti-inflammatory drugs.

of disorders, some characterized by axial entheso-pathies, sacroiliitis, and the presence of the HLA-B27 serologic markers. Others are characterized more by an asymmetric oligoarthritis of large joints in the context of gastrointestinal or other mucosal inflammation or infection. The classification of spondyloarthropathy as psoriatic arthritis, ankylosing spondylitis, the arthropathy of inflammatory bowel disease, or Reiter's syndrome serves to describe the major features of the disease present, but clinically, these seronegative spondyloarthropathies exist as a continuum (Table 53–3).

As the word seronegative suggests, patients test negative for rheumatoid factors and antinuclear antibody and manifest extra-articular features of rheumatic disease that are descriptive of the spondyloarthropathies. These extra-articular manifestations include uveitis (especially in HLA-B27–positive individuals), mucosal ulcers (including oral, urogenital, and gastrointestinal ulcerations), cervicitis, psoriasis (including the pustular dermatitis in the form of keratoderma blennorrhagicum), aortitis, and apical lung disease.

The pathogenesis of these arthritides is unknown. The recognition that HLA-B27, a class I major histocompatibility antigen, was present in more than 90% of white patients with ankylosing spondylitis (despite a 6% prevalence in the white population at large) led to epidemiologic studies and basic immunologic research in an effort to elucidate the scientific basis for this observation. Further, it was noted that enteric or urogenital infections with such organisms as *Klebsiella, Salmonella, Campylobacter, Yersinia, Shigella,* or *Chlamydia* were associated with the development of a reactive arthritis in susceptible individuals, many of whom were HLA-B27 positive. These findings led to the concept of a shared immunogenic region or epitope between the infecting organism and the HLA-B27 molecule that resulted in specific autoimmunity directed against the articular structures or periarticular ligament insertions. The implication here is that the infectious agent stimulates an immune response, with antibodies cross-reacting with a homologous structure on the host HLA-B27 molecule, forming the basis for the molecular mimicry theory. This theory implies the perpetuation of the infection at a subclinical level to drive the chronic inflammatory response or some other intrinsic pertubation of the immune system to account for the persistence of articular and periarticular inflammation.

The other theory proposed to explain the pathogenesis of the seronegative spondyloarthropathies

TABLE 53–3. **Comparison of Seronegative Spondyloarthropathies**

	ANKYLOSING SPONDYLITIS	REITER'S SYNDROME	PSORIATIC ARTHROPATHY	INTESTINAL ARTHROPATHY
Sex distribution	Male ≥ female	Male ≥ female	Male ≥ female	Female = male
Age at onset (yr)	≥ 20	≥ 20	Any age	Any age
Uveitis	+	+ +	+	+
Peripheral joints	Lower limb, often	Lower limb, often	Upper > lower limb	Lower > upper limb
Sacroiliitis	Always	Often	Often	Often
Plantar spurs	Common	Common	Common	Common
HLA-B27 positive	90%	90%	20% (50% with sacroiliitis)	5% (50% with sacroiliitis)
Enthesopathy	+	+	+	? +
Aortic regurgitation	+	+	? +	?
Response to therapy (indomethacin, phenylbutazone)	+ + +	+	+ +	+
Onset	Gradual	Sudden	Variable	Peripherally: sudden; axial: gradual
Urethritis	−	+	−	−
Conjunctivitis	+	+ + +	+	+
Skin involvement	−	+	+ + +	−
Mucous membrane involvement	−	+ +	−	+
Spine involvement	+ + +	+	+	+
Symmetry	+	−	−	+

From Schumacher HR Jr. Primer on Rheumatic Diseases. 9th ed. Atlanta: Arthritis Foundation, 1988, p 143 (Table 29–2). Modified from Calin A. Spondylarthritis. Scientific American Medicine. Vol. 3. 1982, p 16.

is that an arthritogenic peptide of bacterial origin is presented to the immune system by the HLA-B27 molecule. This theory implies that the disease is mediated not by cross-reactive antibodies but by cytotoxic T lymphocytes with specificity for this HLA-B27-peptide complex. The exact mechanism by which an infectious agent might trigger this cell-mediated immune response is not intuitively evident, because the processing of bacterial antigens tends to rely on an exogenous pathway of peptide presentation in the context of class II molecules, to use larger peptide fragments, and to depend on CD4-positive helper T lymphocytes. One proposal is that an empty class I HLA-B27 molecule binds this exogenous peptide, priming the cytotoxic T lymphocyte for subsequent cross-reactivity with the HLA-B27 arthritogenic-peptide complex.

A third theory of the pathogenetic significance of the HLA-B27 molecule is that this is simply a genetic marker that may be closely linked to an immune response gene that determines susceptibility to spondyloarthropathy. However, not all HLA-B27–positive individuals develop ankylosing spondylitis, and 5 to 10% of white and as many as 50% of African American patients are HLA-B27 negative.

Finally, in any discussion of pathogenesis in which infectious organisms are implicated, the observation of *Chlamydia* (or its antigen) persisting in the synovium of patients with Reiter's syndrome suggests that the latter disorder is not a postinfectious reactive arthritis but a persistent infection. These observations raise the issue of adequate antibiotic therapy in some individuals.

The prevalence of ankylosing spondylitis in the general population approaches 2%, with estimates that 10 to 20% of HLA-B27–positive individuals with first-degree relatives with spondylitis will also develop clinically apparent disease. Although ankylosing spondylitis may be as common in women as in men, women seem to present or be identified less commonly with back pain attributed to sacroiliitis than men. The frequency of HLA-B27 in the white population affected by ankylosing spondylitis is 90 to 95%. It is slightly less in Reiter's syndrome and *Salmonella*-reactive arthropathy and is near 60% for those patients who have psoriasis and inflammatory bowel disease and who exhibit concomitant sacroiliitis. However, the absence of this genetic marker in the presence of spondylitis and sacroiliitis does not preclude a diagnosis of a seronegative spondyloarthropathy. This is particularly true in nonwhites, in whom the frequency of the HLA-B27 marker may be less than 1%.

Clinical Features

Patients with seronegative spondyloarthropathies generally present with an oligoarticular arthritis, asymmetric in distribution, primarily in large rather than small joints and usually involving the lower extremities. Patients with ankylosing spondylitis may present with low back pain or stiffness that does not resolve with rest and that is sustained for months. Exercise and NSAIDs may be described as easing the pain. Associated signs or symptoms may include iritis, hip pain (less commonly other peripheral joints are involved), cervical, or thoracic pain. An associated enthesopathy (inflammation at the site of tendon insertion), such Achilles tendinitis or plantar fasciitis, is common, as are constitutional symptoms of malaise, low-grade fever, and weight loss. Other accompanying symptoms such as iritis, mucocutaneous lesions, low back pain, bloody diarrhea, psoriasis, or a family history positive for seronegative spondyloarthropathy help define the diagnostic category of the disease. Considerable morbidity is associated with these diseases. The rheumatologic manifestations of psoriasis bear an inconstant relationship to flares in the skin, whereas the peripheral arthropathy of inflammatory bowel disease (but not axial enthesitis) tends to wax and wane with the gastrointestinal disease activity. Some evidence supports the increased expression of these diseases in patients with human immunodeficiency virus infection.

Physical examination should include an assessment of cervical extension, respiratory excursion, and lumbar flexion. Evidence for iritis and aortic insufficiency should be sought, and peripheral joints as well as the spine and sacroiliac joints should be examined. The skin should be evaluated for psoriatic lesions, oral ulcers, keratoderma blennorrhagicum, Achilles tendinitis, dactylitis, nail bed pitting, or onycholysis. Abdominal, genital, and rectal examinations with stool Hemoccult testing are indicated. A detailed neurologic examination yields generally normal findings early in disease. Features favoring the diagnosis of one seronegative spondlyoarthropathy over another are outlined in Table 53–3.

Initial laboratory evaluation should include a complete blood count with differential, erythrocyte sedimentation rate, chemistry and electrolyte determinations, urinalysis, and urethral or stool cultures when appropriate. Ferguson's views of the sacroiliac joints may be obtained; however, the radiographic findings do not affect the initial treatment. Therefore, an argument could be made to avoid x-rays in women of childbearing potential, unless the diagnosis remains unclear over time.

HLA-B27 markers are not necessary, although the finding of a positive HLA-B27 result is interesting and sometimes supports the diagnosis.

Treatment

Therapy should include full doses of NSAIDs (discussed later). Anecdote suggests that indomethacin may be the "best" NSAID for this disease continuum; however, this has not been validated by controlled clinical trials. Caution should be used in patients with inflammatory bowel disease, because these drugs have been reported to exacerbate their underlying bowel disease. Sulfasalazine may be the treatment of choice for these patients. Systemic glucocorticoids should be avoided in the spondyloarthropathies; they may not be effective, and for patients with psoriatic arthritis, tapering glucocorticoids may induce a flare in cutaneous disease. If peripheral joint complaints become refractory to treatment, second-line therapy with low doses of methotrexate may be indicated. Early referral to a rheumatologist is appropriate.

THE NONINFLAMMATORY ARTHRITIDES

Osteoarthritis

Pathogenesis and Epidemiology

Survey studies confirm radiographically that osteoarthritis is present in most individuals by 65 years of age; however, only a small percentage have symptomatic disease (Table 53–4). Osteoar-

thritis is a common joint disorder, more common in women than men and more common with advancing age in both genders. Although obesity, antecedent trauma, and advancing age are identified risk factors for osteoarthritis of the knee in women, the predisposing causes of generalized osteoarthritis and osteoarthritis of the hips are less clear.

Osteoarthritis may often be present as a simple clinical observation or radiographic finding. Its presence alone does not indicate treatment. The disease process tends to be a noninflammatory condition, wear and tear of the joint space with fraying cartilage, subchondral bone thickening, and reactive bone formation along the weight-bearing aspect of the joint (Fig. 53–2). When the mechanics of the joint become compromised by the process, then osteoarthritis can lead to considerable pain and disability.

Clinical Features and Differential Diagnosis

Clinically, osteoarthritis may be described by the pattern of joint involvement and the duration of symptoms. It is a progressive, monarticular or polyarticular arthrosis, usually without clinical signs of systemic inflammation or local pannus formation. The disease typically affects the small distal joints of the hands, the axial joints of the cervical and lumbar spine, and large weight-bearing joints of the lower extremities. Osteoarthritis is classically defined radiographically by joint space narrowing, reactive bony sclerosis, and osteophyte formation. It is usual for a woman to present with symptoms of progressive pain in one

TABLE 53–4. Prevalence of Radiographic Osteoarthritis in Three Major Joint Sites

		JOINT SITE		
AGE	SEX	Hip	Knee	Distal Interphalangeal Joint
< 55	Men	1%	2%	10%
	Women	1%	5%	20%
55–65	Men	3%	10%	45%
	Women	2%	20%	60%
> 65	Men	6%	25%	50%
	Women	4%	40%	80%
Approximate overall prevalence of symptomatic osteoarthritis in adults in the United States		0.7%	1.6%	3.0%
Approximate % of those with advanced radiographic changes with symptoms		80–90% (M = F)	30–40% (F > M)	10–20% (F > M)

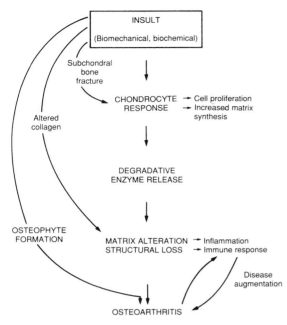

Figure 53-2. Pathogenesis of osteoarthritis. (From Schumacher HR Jr. Primer on Rheumatic Diseases. 9th ed. Atlanta, Ga: The Arthritis Foundation, 1988, p 173. Copyright 1988. Used by permission of the Arthritis Foundation.)

or more joints, often the knees, with onset 2 to 3 years earlier. Patients often describe a stiffness or pain that occurs on the first five to six steps of weight bearing after rest and then subsides. This gelling phenomenon is quite characteristic of osteoarthritis; however, the duration of the stiffness is considerably less than that observed in patients with RA. The most consistent finding by history is the relationship of pain to activity or weight bearing and the easing of pain by rest and recumbency. Therefore, pain tends to worsen toward the end of the day, in contradistinction to the prolonged morning stiffness of the inflammatory arthritides. Night pain is a feature of end-stage osteoarthritis.

Osteoarthritis has a predilection for involvement of the distal interphalangeal and proximal interphalangeal joints in the hand. The evident bony enlargements of these joints are named Heberden's and Bouchard's nodes, respectively. The carpometacarpal joint of the thumb is also frequently affected, but in contrast to RA the metacarpophalangeal joints are relatively spared. Osteoarthritis of the other joints of the upper extremities (i.e., the wrist, elbow, and shoulder) is extremely uncommon. Complaints related to these areas should raise the question of another underlying disease, antecedent trauma, nonarticular disease, or referred pain (i.e., from the cervical spine). Both the cervi-

cal and lumbar spine may be involved in osteoarthritis, and the predominant complaint may be secondary to the nerve root impingement caused by osteophyte formation or degenerative disk disease. In the lower extremity, the hips and knees are most commonly involved, followed by the metatarsophalangeal joint of the first toe. Symptomatic problems with the ankle or presenting complaints in the midfoot or small joints of the toe are unusual.

On physical examination, obesity is often a concomitant finding. An antalgic gait may be present, but patients do not appear systemically ill. Decreased cervical rotation and Heberden's and Bouchard's nodes are common. Stiffness of the lumbar spine, pain radiating into the buttock, or radicular irritation may be apparent. The hip may show early loss of internal or external rotation. Joint effusions may or may not be present on examination of the knees. If present, these are usually cool but may occasionally be warm to the touch and may be found in association with findings suggestive of internal derangement of the knee or ligamentous laxity. Varus or valgus deformities or patellofemoral crepitation should be sought. The ankle joint and small joints of the feet tend to be asymptomatic.

Radiographs confirm the physical findings of irregular bony overgrowth, varus or valgus deformities, and occasionally joint ankylosis and fusion. The radiographic hallmark of osteoarthritis is the osteophyte, in contrast to the marginal erosion or periarticular osteopenia seen in the inflammatory arthritides. Radiographs of the cervical spine may show an impingement of neural foramina in the C5 to C7 area by osteophytes, along with disk space narrowing. In diffuse idiopathic skeletal hyperostosis, an osteoarthritis-related syndrome, the anterior longitudinal ligament may show flowing calcification across several disk spaces. In osteoarthritis of the lumbar spine, disk space narrowing, vacuum phenomenon, facet sclerosis, and osteophyte formation are features of the disease process. In the hips and knees, the findings of asymmetric joint space narrowing along the weight-bearing axis, reactive bony sclerosis, bone cysts, and osteophyte formation are common.

Treatment

The management of osteoarthritis is an outpatient practice that can be undertaken in the office of the primary care provider. The principles of therapy are weight loss, strengthening of periarticular muscles, and unloading the diseased joint. A walking program is typically begun, along with physical therapy with attention to quadriceps strengthening or low back exercises and the judicious use of cervical collars, braces, or canes. Very often NSAIDs are useful for the relief of pain, although acetaminophen may be equally efficacious when the process is noninflammatory. Aspiration and intra-articular injection of glucocorticoids are occasionally useful adjunctive therapy for symptomatic osteoarthritis of the knee when warm synovial effusions can be documented.

When these measures do not prove effective, consultation with a rheumatologist is indicated to rule out causes contributing to the disease process or unusual associated diseases and to initiate a long-term strategy for treatment. If a patient presents with evident internal derangement of a joint, then direct referral to an orthopedic surgeon is indicated. Total joint replacements, however, are not a panacea and should in fact be avoided in young and obese patients, in whom complications and failure rates are high.

THE INFECTIOUS ARTHRITIDES

Nongonococcal Bacterial Arthritis

Pathogenesis and Epidemiology

In adults, nongonococcal bacterial arthritis tends to present in a monarticular fashion, with predilection for the knee. It is this presentation that mandates an emergency evaluation for any patient presenting with monarticular arthritis, because outcome is dependent on early recognition and appropriate treatment. This approach has not changed since early studies on bacterial invasion of the joint space were reported. The only caveat to add here is that in patients with a history of intravenous drug abuse, the presentation of septic arthritis may be more complex, often preferentially involving axial joints such as the sternoclavicular or sacroiliac joints.

Nongonococcal bacterial arthritis is a true infection of the joint space and reflects penetration of bacteria through the synovial lining. However, as noted in Table 53–5, other events are also important in the pathogenesis of joint destruction. Bacterial arthritis tends to occur as a result of hematogenous dissemination of bacteria, although direct trauma and contiguous bony infection are other causes. A significant predisposing factor appears to be preexisting arthropathy. This is important to note, because included here are patients with longstanding erosive RA, crystal arthropathies, severe osteoarthritis, and Charcot's joints. In this setting, where preexisting joint discomfort and joint effusions may be present, the index for suspicion of a superimposed bacterial process must be high or

TABLE 53–5. Septic Arthritis: Pathogenic Mechanisms

CAUSE	EFFECTS
Bacteria	Direct toxic effects on chondrocytes
	Synovial necrosis and abscess formation
Phagocytes	Metalloproteinase-induced cartilage degradation
	Loss of chondroitin sulfate and glycosaminoglycan
Synovium	Granulation tissue erosion of articular cartilage

From Medical Knowledge Self-Assessment Program (MKSAP). Rheumatology 1993, Table 38, p 152. Used by permission of S Karger AG, Basel.

the infection will be missed and the joint destroyed. Other predisposing factors include the presence of a prosthesis and underlying poor health of the patient. Chronic liver disease, systemic lupus, complement deficiencies, diabetes, cancer, acquired immunodeficiency syndrome, and intravenous drug use all constitute risk factors for septic arthritis because they are associated with impaired host defenses. Direct inoculation by arthrocentesis or arthroscopic procedures is distinctly unusual.

Clinical Features and Differential Diagnosis

In 80 to 90% of patients, the clinical presentation is of an acutely ill patient with a single painful, swollen joint. Fever may or may not be present. Physical examination demonstrates erythema, effusion, and loss of range of motion at the joint. Any potential source of bacterial invasion including skin sources should be sought. Evidence of endocarditis including changes in murmurs is also important.

The differential diagnosis of monarticular arthritis is extensive and includes the systemic inflammatory rheumatic diseases, acute trauma or internal derangement of the joint, hemorrhage into a joint, or a crystal-induced arthropathy. The diagnostic approach is straightforward. The joint must be tapped, and the synovial fluid examined under the microscope and sent for appropriate cultures. In the presence of a high suspicion for septic arthritis, there is no contraindication to joint aspiration. Any medical issues that place a patient at an increased risk for arthrocentesis, such as a recognized bleeding disorder, use of anticoagulants, or an overlying soft tissue wound, should prompt the internist to consult with specialists in orthopedics or rheumatology. Aspiration of a prosthetic joint should be performed by an orthopedist under sterile conditions in the operating room. The diagnostic yield from synovial fluid properly collected and processed is high. Routine laboratory studies should be performed, including blood cultures and radiographs of the affected joint. The synovial fluid should be Gram stained and examined under a polarized microscope. The presence of urate crystals or calcium pyrophosphate crystals does not preclude infection. A search for the source of the infection in each patient is indicated. If endocarditis is suspected, two-dimensional echocardiography should be performed to look for valvular vegetations.

In adults, the predominant organism is *Staphylococcus aureus*, although reports increasingly describe gram-negative organisms particularly *Pseudomonas aeruginosa*, especially among intravenous drug abusers. Streptococci, pneumococci, *Escherichia coli,* and polymicrobial infections are encountered in decreasing frequency. *Candida* and other fungal infections, tuberculosis, and other mycobacterial infections, Lyme disease, and the gonococcal arthritides must be considered and ruled out.

Treatment

Initial antibiotics should include coverage for methicillin-resistant staphylococci and gram-negative coverage, depending on the patient and the laboratory findings reported. The pending cultures and sensitivities allow more selective use of antibiotics. The usual length of treatment is 4 weeks, with oral antibiotics being used during the last 2 weeks. It is imperative that the joint be drained either by repeat aspirations at the bedside or by arthroscopic surgery. Early mobilization is indicated, and frequent reassessment of patients is necessary to reduce the morbidity and mortality of this disease. The outcome rests largely on the virulence of the infecting organism, as well as the delay in the diagnosis and the institution of treatment.

Gonococcal Arthritis

Pathogenesis and Epidemiology

Septic arthritis from disseminated gonococcal infection is a common infectious arthropathy encountered in younger sexually active women. The pathogenesis of gonococcal arthritis is probably different from joint space infections caused by other pyogenic organisms. For example, the host's susceptibility may be affected by inherited deficiencies of complement or by the local genitourinary environment (i.e., menses or pregnancy). Most importantly, the clinical expression of the disorder implicates an immune response to bacterial antigens similar to that observed with acute rheumatic fever following streptococcal infection.

Gonococcal arthritis, although previously a disorder of men, is now encountered with increasing frequency in women, especially those living in urban areas. It is the most commonly encountered cause of septic arthritis in that setting. However, it develops in only a small fraction of those individuals who are actually infected with *Neisseria gonorrhoeae*, lending credence to the notion that both organism and host factors are important features that determine the prevalence and virulence of the syndrome.

Clinical Features

In contrast to patients with nongonococcal septic arthritis, typical patients with disseminated gonococcal infection are relatively healthy but with prominent joint pain and fever. Dysuria or vaginal discharge may be apparent in only a minority of infected patients, and the arthropathy is distinctly different from that with joint space infections due to other causes. The arthritis is typically oligoarticular or occasionally polyarticular, migratory, or additive and frequently involves tenosynovial structures, often with prominent involvement of tendons and tendon sheaths of the hands and feet. The vesicular and pustular dermatitis with an erythematous base that is so characteristic of disseminated gonococcal infection is actually noted in only 40 to 50% of patients. In contrast to septic arthritis caused by *S. aureus, N. gonorrhoeae* is often difficult to grow in culture, especially if the organism is not plated at the bedside and placed immediately in an appropriate culture environment. The diagnosis is usually based on isolation of the gonococcus in culture; however, because of the relatively high frequency of negative synovial fluid cultures, newer diagnostic modalities are now being investigated. Polymerase chain reaction has been used to detect gene sequences that are responsible for expression of gonococcal proteins in culture-negative synovial fluids. It is hoped that further studies of this promising technique will determine its utility for detecting disseminated gonococcal infection.

Treatment

Historically, penicillin was highly successful in the treatment of disseminated gonococcal infection. However, the emergence of penicillinase-producing organisms has resulted in a significant change in the suggested therapeutic regimen. Third-generation cephalosporins or quinolones are now the initial drugs of choice pending the results of final culture and sensitivity tests. The suggested treatment protocol for disseminated gonococcal infection is shown in Table 53–6.

Lyme Disease

Pathogenesis and Epidemiology

Lyme disease was first recognized as a distinct clinical entity in the 1970s, when individuals with a febrile illness associated with erythema migrans and an oligoarticular inflammatory arthropathy were observed in clusters along the Connecticut shoreline. Some of those patients eventually improved with antibiotic therapy, and thus an infectious cause was assumed. *Borrelia burgdorferi*, an elusive spirochete, was defined as the cause of the syndrome in 1982. The epidemiology of Lyme disease is complex. *B. burgdorferi* is spread by the saliva of the nymphal *Ixodes dammini* tick, which prefers the white-footed mouse as its host.

Clinical Features and Treatment

The clinical features of Lyme disease are protean; therefore, misdiagnosis (both overdiagnosis and underdiagnosis) is common. The infection has been implicated as the cause of many inflammatory and noninflammatory conditions, including fibromyalgia and chronic fatigue syndrome. However, true Lyme disease has discrete clinical stages that in some ways resemble syphilis. In the early stage of infection, a patient may observe the development of erythema migrans after a tick bite; however, only 60 to 80% of patients with Lyme disease actually observe this characteristic rash. Regional adenopathy and constitutional symptoms may also be present. Within days to weeks, the spirochete disseminates to produce an entirely different set of signs, symptoms, and syndromes. In-

fected patients may experience a different skin rash, characterized by multiple smaller versions of erythema migrans with annular borders, episodic polyarthralgias and polyarthritis, and fatigue. After dissemination, the cardiac, neurologic, and musculoskeletal systems may also be involved to various degrees. Although heart involvement is rare, conduction system abnormalities such as atrioventricular block and myopericarditis have been reported. Both the central and peripheral nervous systems can be affected. Meningoencephalitis, cranial neuropathies (especially unilateral or bilateral Bell's palsy), and painful radiculoneuropathies are the usual manifestations. Finally, in the later stages of the disease, an inflammatory oligoarticular arthritis of the large weight-bearing joints is frequently noted. Contrary to popular belief, this arthropathy only rarely causes serious disability.

Because of the vague clinical features, the illness is frequently difficult to diagnose. The serologic tests are imperfect, and results must be interpreted along with other criteria. True Lyme disease may be diagnosed when the appropriate clinical features (i.e., erythema migrans, central nervous system or cardiac disorders, arthritis) are observed in association with results of an enzyme-linked immunosorbent assay. One must recognize that false negative results may be observed early in the course of the illness; likewise, false positive results may occur in patients with other spirochetal or autoimmune diseases. The treatment usually involves the use of doxycycline (for early limited infections) or parenteral ceftriaxone (for disseminated or refractory infections). Specific treatment regimens are noted in Table 53–7.

TABLE 53–6. Treatment of Disseminated Gonococcal Infection

1. Ceftriaxone, 1 gm IV daily for 7–10 days
2. Ceftizoxime or cefotaxime, 1 gm IV every 8 hr until 2–3 days or clinical improvement, *then* cefixime, 400 mg PO bid, or ciprofloxacin, 500 mg PO b.i.d. to complete 7–10 days of therapy

IV, Intravenously; PO, orally; b.i.d., twice a day.
From Medical Knowledge Self-Assessment Program (MKSAP). Rheumatology 1993, Table 40, p 154. Used by permission of S Karger AG, Basel.

TABLE 53–7. Recommendations for Lyme Disease Treatment by Disease Stage

STAGE	DRUG REGIMEN
I, Early infection	Doxycycline,* 100 mg b.i.d. × 10–30 days, *or*
	Amoxicillin, 500 mg q.i.d. × 10–30 days
II, Disseminated	Ceftriaxone, 2 gm IV daily × 14–30 days, *or*
	Aqueous penicillin G, 20 × 10⁶ U IV daily 14–30 days, *or*
	Chloramphenicol, 250 mg IV q.i.d. × 14–30 days
III, Persistent	Ceftriaxone, 2 gm IV daily × 14–30 days, *or*
	Aqueous penicilin G, 20 × 10⁶ U IV daily 14–30 days

*Doxycycline should not be given to children or pregnant women.
IV, Intravenously; b.i.d., twice a day; q.i.d., four times a day.
From Medical Knowledge Self-Assessment Program (MKSAP). Rheumatology 1993, Table 41, p 157. Used by permission of S Karger AG, Basel.

NONSTEROIDAL ANTI-INFLAMMATORY DRUGS

Nonsteroidal anti-inflammatory drugs or salicylates are the first line of therapy in patients with RA and osteoarthritis. These drugs are used almost uniformly during all stages of these disorders unless complications develop or the potential for adverse reactions precludes their use (discussed later). These drugs are also used for other painful conditions of the musculoskeletal system, such as regional pain syndromes (i.e., bursitis, tendinitis, and backache). Because of the prevalence of these disorders in general practice, it is no wonder that these drugs are frequently prescribed. Present estimates suggest that more than 100 million prescriptions for NSAIDs are written by physicians every year. At least 21 different preparations with different pharmacokinetic profiles from six chemical categories are approved by the Food and Drug Administration for clinical use (Table 53–8).

The gold standard against which all of the newer NSAIDs are compared is acetylsalicylic acid, or aspirin. This has been used extensively during the past century as an analgesic, antipyretic, and anti-inflammatory drug; however, the newer NSAIDs are easier to take and may have fewer side effects. On the other hand, NSAIDs are much more expensive than aspirin, with some preparations costing as much as $75 per month.

Mechanism of Action and Pharmacology

Nonsteroidal anti-inflammatory drugs inhibit inflammation by interfering with the metabolism of arachidonic acid to the terminal prostaglandins, a reaction that is mediated by cyclooxygenase. Cyclooxygenase is a very important enzyme complex that may exist in two forms: (1) constitutively expressed cyclooxygenase, which is present in many tissues including the gastric mucosa, and (2) inducible cyclooxygenase, which is present only at sites of active inflammation. Unfortunately, most available NSAIDs probably inhibit both forms of cyclooxygenase, thus producing a plethora of adverse reactions together with the desired reduction in prostaglandin-induced inflammation. Nonsteroidal anti-inflammatory drugs have been shown to have other biologic effects that may be equally as important. These include effects on neutrophil aggregation/activation, leukotriene synthesis, lysosomal enzyme release, lymphocyte function, and rheumatoid factor production. Most of these effects are biologic or in vitro observations, and thus they may have little clinical significance.

TABLE 53–8. Nonsteroidal Anti-inflammatory Drugs and Dose Ranges by Chemical Classification

CHEMICAL CATEGORY	DRUG (TRADE NAME)	DAILY INITIAL RECOMMENDED ADULT DOSE (mg)	PLASMA HALF-LIVES (hr)
Carboxylic acids	Acetylsalicylic acid (aspirin)	750 q.i.d.	4–15
	Choline magnesium salicylate (Trilisate)	750 b.i.d.	4–15
	Salsalate (Disalcid)	750 b.i.d.	4–15
	Diflunisal (Dolobid)	500 b.i.d.	7–15
Propionic acids	Ibuprofen (Motrin)	400 q.i.d.	2
	Naproxen (Naprosyn)	250 b.i.d.	13
	Fenoprofen (Nalfon)	300 q.i.d.	3
	Ketoprofen (Orudis)	50 t.i.d.	2
	Flurbiprofen (Ansaid)	100 b.i.d.	3–9
	Oxaprozin (Daypro)	1200 daily	40–50
Acetic acids	Indomethacin (Indocin)	25 t.i.d.	3–11
	Tolmetin (Tolectin)	200 q.i.d.	1
	Sulindac (Clinoril)	150 b.i.d.	16
	Diclofenac (Voltaren)	50 b.i.d.	1–2
	Etodolac (Lodine)	200 t.i.d.	2–4
	Ketorolac (Toradol)*	10 q.i.d.	2
Fenamic acids	Mefenamic acid (Ponstel)†	250 q.i.d.	2
	Meclofenamate sodium (Meclomen)	50 q.i.d.	2–3
Enolic acids	Piroxicam (Feldene)	20 daily	30–86
Naphthyalkanones	Nabumetone (Relafen)	1000 daily	19–30

*Used for management of acute pain (not recommmended for use for more than 21 days).
†Used for management of pain or dysmenorrhea (not recommended for more than 7 days).
b.i.d., Twice a day; t.i.d., 3 times a day; q.i.d., 4 times a day.
From Medical Knowledge Self-Assessment Program (MKSAP). Rheumatology 1993, Table 10, p 73. Used by permission of S Karger AG, Basel.

Pharmacologically, most NSAIDs are readily absorbed from the gastrointestinal tract and are almost completely bound by serum proteins, a factor that must be considered when prescribing other protein-bound drugs. The plasma half-lives are highly variable (see Table 53–8), perhaps because of individual patients' differences in hepatic metabolism and renal excretion. Plasma drug pharmacokinetics may have little relation to clinical effectiveness; however, NSAIDs with a longer plasma half-life may be more toxic for the elderly or infirm.

Clinical Uses

Well-controlled trials comparing specific NSAIDs with salicylates have not demonstrated a significant difference in efficacy for patients with RA. However, most rheumatologists agree that for an individual patient, major differences in the effectiveness of NSAIDs may be clinically apparent. The whole notion of the standard pyramid approach to antirheumatic therapy for patients with RA is now under scrutiny. Although NSAIDs and salicylates have traditionally been used as the first step in this pyramid, some authorities now suggest that disease-modifying antirheumatic drug therapy (i.e., gold, hydroxychloroquine, methotrexate, and others) be initiated earlier in the disease course.

Although NSAID use for patients with osteoarthritis accounts for 50% of prescriptions written by physicians, studies have shown that acetaminophen may be as effective as some NSAIDs in the management of osteoarthritis pain. Indeed, other investigators have suggested that NSAIDs may adversely affect the chondrocyte in biologic systems. Occasionally, however, osteoarthritis has an inflammatory component, which may respond better to NSAIDs than simple analgesics. The long-term efficacy of NSAIDs for patients with osteoarthritis has never been adequately studied. Nonsteroidal anti-inflammatory drugs have never been shown to be chondroprotective and thus should be prescribed with full knowledge of the potential for toxicity. Nonpharmacologic strategies such as weight control and exercise prescription should be considered despite the fact that in most cases patients expect a physician to provide a drug for relief. Finally, inhibition of the cardinal signs of inflammation (redness, swelling, effusion) in patients with either osteoarthritis or RA is frequently but not always accompanied by a reduction in pain. Pain amplification (because of sleep disturbance or depression) or pain due to mechanical factors may occasionally complicate the assessment of NSAID effectiveness.

TABLE 53–9. Effects of Nonsteroidal Anti-inflammatory Drugs on Gastrointestinal and Renal Physiology

Gastrointestinal
Decreases gastrointestinal blood flow
Increases gastric acid production
Decreases the production of gastric mucus
Decreases the rate of cellular proliferation of the gastric mucosa
Decreases gastroesophageal sphincter tone
Renal
Reduces medullary blood flow
Reduces glomerular filtration rate
Potentiates antidiuretic hormone effects
Reduces renin release
Increases osmotic force for water absorption
Increases tubular reabsorption of sodium chloride

From Medical Knowledge Self-Assessment Program (MKSAP). Rheumatology 1993, Tables 12 and 13, p 77. Used by permission of S Karger AG, Basel.

Toxicity

The major toxicities of NSAIDs involve the gastrointestinal tract and the kidneys. These toxicities presumably are due to prostaglandin inhibition and the resultant deleterious effects on gastrointestinal and renal physiology (Table 53–9). Nonsteroidal anti-inflammatory drugs are known to cause a peculiar gastropathy characterized by a diffuse gastritis or multiple shallow gastric erosions usually localized near the antrum of the stomach. They may also cause ulcers at any location in the gastrointestinal tract, including the small and large bowel. This syndrome frequently produces no symptoms, making estimation of its prevalence difficult. Many patients present silently with a significant anemia and occult gastrointestinal blood loss. However, patients with a perforated viscus have also been reported.

Treatment of endoscopically proven erosive gastritis is controversial; however, at the very least, most authorities suggest discontinuing the NSAID. The use of misoprostol (100–200 μg three to four times per day) may reduce the risk of developing gastric ulcers and gastritis in some patients. However, it may cause significant diarrhea, may precipitate spontaneous abortions, and probably should be coupled with effective contraception in women of childbearing age. Histamine$_2$ blockers may improve symptoms of dyspepsia and probably heal duodenal disease, but they have never been proved to improve NSAID-induced gastric lesions.

Nonsteroidal anti-inflammatory drugs also have profound effects on renal function. The most commonly encountered adverse reaction in the kidneys involves reversible reduction in renal blood flow and glomerular filtration rate, which is clinically manifested as renal failure of various degrees. This problem is most commonly noted in elderly patients with other significant comorbid diseases, such as diabetes, heart failure, or dehydration. Nonsteroidal anti-inflammatory drugs may also precipitate heart failure or may interfere with blood pressure management by virtue of their effects on sodium and water retention. Significant hyperkalemia has been observed, especially in patients taking potassium-sparing diuretics. Occasionally, NSAIDs may affect tubular function, thus producing interstitial nephritis and nephrotic range proteinuria.

Finally, NSAIDs have significant interactions with other drugs, and clinicians should familiarize themselves with these potential interactions. Nonsteroidal anti-inflammatory drugs should not be administered with warfarin, because coadministration of these two drugs can result in significant prolongation of the prothrombin time or gastrointestinal bleeding.

REFERENCES

Arnett FC. The seronegative spondyloarthropathies (editorial overview). Curr Opin Rheumatol 1991;3:559.

Arkfield DG, Leibling MR, Michelini GA, et al. Identification of *Neisseria gonorrhoeae* in synovial fluid using the polymerase chain reaction. Arthritis Rheum 1991;34:S33.

Berardi VE, Weeks KE, Steere AC. Serodiagnosis of early Lyme Disease: Analysis of IgM and IgG antibody responses by using an antibody-capture enzyme immunoassay. J Infect Dis 1988;158:754.

Benjamin R, Parham P. HLA-B27 and disease: A consequence of inadvertant antigen presentation? Rheum Dis Clin North Am 1992;18:11.

Brooks P, Day R. Nonsteriodal antiinflammatory drugs—differences and similarities. N Engl J Med 1991;324:1716.

Bradley J, Brandt K, Katz B, et al. Comparison of an antiinflammatory dose of ibuprofen, an analgesic dose of ibuprofen, and acetaminophen in the treatment of patients with osteoarthritis of the knee. N Engl J Med 1991;325:87.

Chiang T-Y, Hunder GG, Ilstrup DM, et al. Polymyalgia rheumatica: A 10 year epidemiologic and clinical study. Ann Intern Med 1982;97:672.

Chou CT, Schumacher HR. Clinical and pathologic studies of synovits in polymyalgia rheumatica. Arthritis Rheum 1984;13:322.

Clive D, Stoff J. Renal syndromes associated with nonsteroidal antiinflammatory drugs. N Engl J Med 1984;310:563.

Dattwyler RJ, Halperin JJ, Volkman DJ, Luft BJ. Treatment of late Lyme borreliosis—randomized comparison of cephtriaxone and penicillin. Lancet 1988;1:1191.

Espinoza LR, Aguilar JL, Berman A, et al. Rheumatic manifestations associated with human immunodeficiency versus infection. Arthritis Rheum 1989;32:1615.

Felson DT. Osteoarthritis. Rheum Dis Clin North Am 1990;16:499.

Fries J, Williams CA, Bloch DA. The relative toxicity of non-steroidal antiinflammatory drugs. Arthritis Rheum 1991;34(11):1353.

Goldenberg DL. Bacterial arthritis. In: Kelley WN, Harris ED Jr, Ruddy S, Sledge CB (eds). Textbook of Rheumatology. 3rd ed. Philadelphia: WB Saunders, 1989.

Harris ED. Rheumatoid arthritis (editorial overview). Curr Opin Rheumatol 1993;5:167.

Harris ED. Rheumatoid arthritis: Pathophysiology and implications for therapy. N Engl J Med 1990;322:1277.

Ho G. Bacterial arthritis. Curr Opin Rheumatol 1991;3(4):603.

Khan MA. An overview of clinical spectrum and heterogeneity of spondyloarthropathies. Rheum Dis Clin North Am 1992;8:1.

Koopman W. Host factors in the pathogenesis of arthritis triggered by infectious organisms: Overview. Rheum Dis Clin North Am 1993;19:279.

O'Brien JP, Goldenberg DL, Rice PA. Disseminated gonococcal infection: A prospective analysis of 49 patients and a review of the pathophysiology and immune mechanisms. Medicine 1983;62:395.

Panagi GS, Lauchburg JS, Kingsley GH. The importance of the T cell in initiating and maintaining the chronic synovitis of rheumatoid arthritis. Arthritis Rheum 1992;35:729.

Pritchard C, Berney SN. Septic arthritis caused by penicillinase producing *Neisseria gonorrhoeae*. J Rheumatol 1988;15:719.

Roth SH. Misoprostol in the prevention of NSAID-induced gastric ulcer: A multicenter, double-blind, placebo-controlled trial. J Rheumatol 1990;17(Suppl 20):20.

Sandler DP, Burn F, Weinberg CR. Nonsteroidal antiinflammatory drugs and the risk of chronic renal disease. Ann Intern Med 1991;115:165.

St. Clair EW, Haynes BF. The future of rheumatoid arthritis treatment. Bull Rheum Dis 1993;42:1.

Schmid FR. New developments in bacterial arthritis. Bull Rheum Dis 1992;41:1.

Scopelitis E, Matinez-Osuna P. Gonococcal arthritis in infectious arthritis. Rheum Dis Clin North Am 1993;19(2):363.

Steere AC. Lyme disease. N Engl J Med 1989;321:586.

Weyand CM, Xie C, Goronzy JJ. Homozygosity for the HLA-DRB1 allele selects for extra-articular manifestations in rheumatoid arthritis. J Clin Invest 1992;89:2033.

Wilske K, Healy L. Remodeling the pyramid—a concept whose time has come. J Rheumatol 1989;16:565.

54

Connective Tissue and Autoimmune Diseases

Margaret Seton and Richard Polisson

The autoimmune and connective tissue diseases represent a highly variable spectrum of illness in which clinical and pathogenetic features exhibit considerable overlap. The general pathogenetic concept is that the immune system, the human body's first defense against injury, infection, malignancy, and allografts, directly or indirectly attacks host tissues. The exact cause of these aberrations is unknown at present. However, the production of autoantibodies, immune complexes, and growth factors; the stimulation of fibroblasts; and the generation of immunocompetent cells with affinity for host antigens are examples of proposed pathogenetic mechanisms. These illnesses exhibit clinical and serologic features that wax and wane and as a result can challenge the diagnostic abilities of many practitioners. When to initiate evaluation for a potential connective tissue or autoimmune disease is always problematic and must be approached in a consistent and rational manner. Many results of serologic studies are difficult to interpret apart from the clinical setting and the context of other laboratory values. Rheumatology remains one field in which the insight, time, and expertise of the physician are quintessential. This is so because the evolution of these diseases varies tremendously in each patient, as does the degree of emotional and physical impairment. The complexity of the pathophysiology of these diseases, their immunogenetic basis, and their variable extra-articular manifestations underscore why this is true. The drama in rheumatology tends to be the impact of the disease on the self-esteem and independence of the woman.

SYSTEMIC LUPUS ERYTHEMATOSUS

Pathogenesis and Epidemiology

Systemic lupus erythematosus (SLE) is a systemic inflammatory disease of unknown cause, characterized by profuse autoantibody production and multisystem visceral involvement. Whether the pathophysiology results from a defect in suppressor cell function, autonomous B-cell autoantibody production, or virally induced autoantibody excess in the susceptible host is not understood. Systemic lupus erythematosus may represent a heterogeneous group of disorders with similar clinical manifestations, a theory supported by observations of murine lupus. Whatever the cause of SLE in any one individual, it is probable that disease expression is further modulated by hormonal, genetic, and environmental factors. Each woman presents with her own history and laboratory abnormalities, describes variable patterns of exacerbation and remission, and presents different psychological concomitants. Each woman, however, has recognizable SLE that will persist throughout her lifetime, leaving her vulnerable to infection, susceptible to complications during pregnancy, and at risk for significant morbidity and early mortality.

The incidence of SLE is estimated to be 5 per 100,000 per year, but epidemiologic studies are hampered by racial biases and inconsistent diagnostic criteria. Clearly, SLE is a disease of women, who represent almost 90% of documented cases. Most of these women are in their reproductive years. Although SLE may run a mild course characterized by fatigue, photosensitivity, and arthralgias, it may also present as a fulminant disease with life-threatening renal failure due to immune-complex glomerulonephritis or it may present with a devastating neurologic event such as stroke, organic brain syndrome, psychosis, or transverse myelitis. Epidemiologic studies today describe a tendency toward more severe disease in African Americans and Asians.

Clinical Features

The clinical manifestations of SLE are protean (Table 54–1). A history of a photosensitive rash,

TABLE 54–1. Frequency of Clinical Symptoms in Systemic Lupus Erythematosus

SYMPTOMS	PERCENTAGE
Fatigue	80–100
Fever	>80
Weight loss	>60
Arthritis, arthralgia	95
Skin	>80
Butterfly rash	>50
Photosensitivity	<58
Mucous membrane lesion	27–41
Alopecia	<71
Raynaud's phenomenon	17–30
Purpura	15
Urticaria	8
Renal	50
Nephrosis	18
Gastrointestinal	38
Pulmonary	0.9–98
Pleurisy	45
Effusion	24
Pneumonia	29
Cardiac	46
Pericarditis	8–48
Murmurs	23
Electrocardiographic changes	34–70
Lymphadenopathy	50
Splenomegaly	10–20
Hepatomegaly	25
Central nervous system	25–75
Functional	Most
Psychosis	5–52
Convulsions	15–20

From Kelley WN, Harris ED Jr, Ruddy S, Sledge CB (eds). Textbook of Rheumatology. 4th ed. Philadelphia: WB Saunders, 1993, Table 61–1, p 1018.

classically malar in location, should be sought, as should the presence of hair loss or alopecia, recurrent oral or nasal ulcers, serositis, Raynaud's phenomenon, arthralgias or arthritis, fever, weight loss, and systemic malaise. The possibility of a lupus anticoagulant or antiphospholipid antibody should prompt the physician to ask for a history of venous or arterial thromboses or difficulties in carrying a pregnancy to term. A family history of SLE or other autoimmune disease should be elicited. A history of recurrent abdominal surgery for an acute abdomen may signal episodes of abdominal serositis. No organ system is uniformly spared by SLE; it is essential that a thorough history taking and physical examination be performed, so that proper staging of the illness may be determined.

Evaluation of a patient suspected of having SLE is similar to that of a patient with rheumatoid arthritis (RA) (see Chapter 53). However, evaluation of vital signs and review of the urine sediment are mandatory in a patient suspected of having SLE.

Urgent consultation should be sought for any patient showing signs or symptoms of major organ involvement, including the central nervous system (transverse myelitis, seizures, stroke syndromes, psychosis/organic brain syndrome), kidneys (renal insufficiency, active urine sediment), or hematologic system (thrombocytopenia, leukopenia, hemolytic anemia). The differential diagnosis of SLE is extensive, and the laboratory tests show variable sensitivity and specificity. It is critical not to burden a patient with a diagnosis of SLE on the basis of a positive antinuclear antibody test result. The import of the laboratory findings may be ascertained only in the context of a thorough history, physical examination, and careful observation through time.

Antiphospholipid Antibody Syndromes

The antiphospholipid antibody syndrome describes a clinical pattern of recurrent arterial or venous thrombosis and measurable antiphospholipid antibodies in the context of recurrent fetal wastage or other autoimmune, hematologic, or neurologic phenomena. These autoantibodies are thought to be related to the thrombotic events, either by binding to activation complexes in the coagulation pathway or by a direct effect on endothelial cells or platelet membranes. However, the setting in which these antibodies promulgate a thrombotic vasculopathy is unclear.

It is estimated that 1 to 2% of the general population and more than 25% of patients with SLE have measurable antiphospholipid antibodies. In asymptomatic persons, the significance of these autoantibodies is unclear. In symptomatic persons, the significance of the antibody titer and antibody isotype in disease activity is likewise unclear. High titers of anticardiolipin antibodies are thought to imply a poor prognosis, but suppression of these titers (when and if possible) does not clearly alter this prognosis. There is no evidence that prophylactic therapy is indicated in the absence of a thrombotic event.

The hypercoagulable state clinically described by the antiphospholipid syndrome was first characterized in the laboratory as the lupus anticoagulant in two patients with SLE. It was defined by prolongation of the activated partial thromboplastin time. Although an anticoagulant in its ability to slow the clotting process in vitro and frequently associated with thrombocytopenia, the lupus anticoagulant soon proved a herald to thrombotic tendencies rather than bleeding diatheses. The effect on the clotting pathway was shown to be due to impaired formation of the prothrombin activator complex secondary to an antibody complexed with endogenous phospholipid in association with β-2 glycoprotein-1. Other assays used to identify this antiphospholipid antibody included Russell's viper venom test and kaolin clotting time, both of which may be more sensitive than the standard activated partial thromboplastin time in a given patient. False positive serologic tests for syphilis (Venereal Disease Research Laboratories or rapid plasma reagin) may also signal the presence of antiphospholipid antibodies. Enzyme-linked immunosorbent assays have been developed to measure immunoglobulin G and immunoglobulin M anticardiolipin titers. In an individual with recurrent thrombosis, none, one, or several of these assays may have positive results. It has been suggested that these immunoglobulins may be consumed during a thrombotic event, giving rise to false negative results.

Although initially described in patients with SLE, the antiphospholipid syndrome includes more than 50% of persons with no systemic rheumatic disease as documented by American College of Rheumatology criteria. These patients are diagnosed as having a primary antiphospholipid syndrome. The clinical spectrum of the antiphospholipid syndrome is broad, and many putative syndromes are ascribed to this noninflammatory vasculopathy. Certainly, recurrent venous and arterial thromboses are hallmarks of the disease, as well as placental insufficiency secondary to vascular disease. Thrombocytopenia, hemolytic anemia, livedo reticularis, digital gangrene, and leg ulcers are reported. Valvular heart disease and pulmonary hypertension are well-described manifestations of the antiphospholipid syndrome, and the association with myocardial infarction in young persons is being investigated. The central nervous system seems particularly vulnerable in this disease, with recurrent stroke and transverse myelopathy as recognized manifestations; migrainous states, seizures, movement disorders, and psychoses remain tentative associations.

A study of 70 patients with the antiphospholipid syndrome found that "the site of the first event (arterial or venous) tended to predict the site of subsequent events." Mitigating the risk of thrombosis by eliminating concurrent risk factors (such as estrogens or cigarette smoking) or treating with aspirin or low-dose warfarin was not protective in many cases. Rosove and Brewer conclude that only intermediate- to high-dose warfarin seems to offer protection against recurrent thromboses.

Antiphospholipids secondary to acquired immunodeficiency syndrome or chlorpromazine do not seem to impart risk for thrombosis, but this is not true of other drug-induced lupus syndromes.

In pregnant women, prospective studies reviewed by Love and Santoro suggest that "there is significantly higher incidence of fetal loss (60%) in patients with systemic lupus erythematosus who have lupus anticoagulant or anticardiolipin than in those without antiphospholipid antibodies." This association is noted particularly in women with prior spontaneous abortions(s) or thrombotic events. Identifying patients at risk and delineating the treatment for venous versus arterial lesions remain difficult, however.

Given the information available at this time, it is reasonable to anticoagulate fully all those patients with documented thrombosis and positive antiphospholipid antibodies. Therapy may need to be indefinite if the site of the initial thrombosis is either life threatening (as in pulmonary emboli) or catastrophic to the integrity of the individual (as in stroke). Any factors that contribute to the risk of thrombosis should be delineated and modified, if possible. Women who have a history of recurrent spontaneous abortion and who wish to conceive should be monitored in a high-risk obstetric practice, preferentially in an academic center where the risks and benefits of treatment can be analyzed. The use of glucocorticoids to treat antiphospholipid antibodies currently is not advised in pregnant women without SLE and is controversial in patients with the disease.

Treatment

The initial treatment of SLE usually involves nonsteroidal anti-inflammatory drugs (see Chapter 53) for treatment of arthritic complaints and serositis. It should be noted that some of these nonsteroidal anti-inflammatory drugs rarely may cause aseptic meningitis in certain patients and that they may be contraindicated in the presence of evolving renal insufficiency. Fatigue is an overwhelming complaint of most patients with SLE, but in the absence of renal failure or hemolytic anemia, treatment is problematic. The use of low doses of glucocorticoids should be reserved for patients with refractory arthritis or serositis. Patients must be taught to avoid the sun and to wear a broad-brimmed hat and sunscreen. Hydroxychloroquine is an antimalarial drug that has been shown to be an effective therapy for skin and joint manifestations of SLE but should be administered with the assistance of a rheumatologist or dermatologist. Although exceedingly rare, hydroxychloroquine has been associated with a maculopathy; therefore, periodic eye examinations should be performed by an ophthalmologist.

The optimal therapy for lupus nephritis and central nervous system lupus is still a matter of considerable debate but generally involves the use of high-dose glucocorticoids (1 mg/kg/day of prednisone or equivalent) in conjunction with immunosuppressive agents (i.e., cyclophosphamide). Because of the risk of hemorrhagic cystitis, malignancy, opportunistic infections, and early gonadal failure, the latter should be instituted only with assistance from a rheumatologist experienced in the use of this highly toxic medication.

IDIOPATHIC INFLAMMATORY MYOPATHIES

Pathogenesis and Epidemiology

Heterogeneous in both pathologic and clinical presentation, the inflammatory myopathies include polymyositis, dermatomyositis, and inclusion body myositis, as well as polymyositis associated with underlying malignancy and polymyositis associated with other connective tissue diseases. The pathogenesis of these disorders is unknown, but increasing evidence shows autoimmune mechanisms in the perpetuation of disease expression. Initially thought to reflect a spectrum of disease activity, dermatomyositis may now be characterized serologically and histopathologically as distinct from polymyositis. In dermatomyositis, the muscle is relatively acellular on histologic examination. A perivascular cellular infiltrate is noted, predominantly B cell in origin. The early lesion in this disease may be the complement C5b-9 attack complex, which localizes to capillary walls, causing a microangiopathy with subsequent loss of capillaries and ischemia of the surrounding muscle. By comparison, in polymyositis and inclusion body myositis, antigen-specific cytotoxicity may be the more predominant pathologic mechanism. Histologically, these are true inflammatory diseases of striated muscle, characterized by mononuclear cell infiltration of muscle fibers with attendant necrosis. The cellular infiltrates are characterized as CD8 + cytotoxic T cells and macrophages, which target the class I histocompatibility antigens. These are expressed on muscle fibers both within and distant from the inflammatory site and are not expressed on muscle fibers of normal persons. In addition to this evidence of up-regulated autoimmunity, various autoantibodies have been identified in the idiopathic inflammatory myopathies, some of which are myositis specific. Of these, the most clinically interesting is the Jo-1 antibody, which recognizes the histidyl transfer ribonucleic acid synthetase enzyme. This autoantibody is found in as many as 50% of patients with

polymyositis and dermatomyositis and is associated with an increasing frequency of intersitial lung disease, nonerosive arthritis, and Raynaud's phenomenon. The Jo-1 antigen has been reported to share homologies with picornavirus ribonucleic acid, prompting further studies to determine the role of viruses in triggering the idiopathic inflammatory myopathies.

The idiopathic inflammatory myopathies are rare diseases of muscle, with incidence estimates of 1 to 8 cases per million annually. Polymyositis and inclusion body myositis are predominantly diseases of adults, whereas dermatomyositis presents in children as well. Except for inclusion body myositis, which has a male preponderance, the inflammatory myopathies are more common in women. Evidence suggests that at least in cases of dermatomyositis, patients seem to have a heightened risk of concurrent malignancy and an increased risk of dying of that malignancy.

Clinical Features

Whatever the differences in pathophysiology, polymyositis and dermatomyositis share a distressing clinical picture of progressive, symmetric proximal muscle weakness with or without muscle tenderness or pain. More distal involvement or involvement of the fine motor function of the hands should suggest inclusion body myositis or perhaps a neuropathic disorder. Asymmetric presentations, ocular involvement, or a positive family history of myopathies all argue against the diagnosis of an idiopathic inflammatory myopathy.

The history of dermatomyositis or polymyositis tends to be subacute, measured in months rather than in the years that characterize the history of inclusion body myositis and the muscular dystrophies. Lifting her head from the pillow, combing her hair, and rising from a chair become increasingly difficult for a woman, reflecting the early involvement of the neck flexors, shoulder, and pelvic girdle. In severe cases, nasal regurgitation or difficulty swallowing and respiratory insufficiency may occur. Some patients with dermatomyositis complain of an erythematous facial and truncal rash and occasionally of swelling and purplish discoloration about the eyes. Other extra-articular manifestations of rheumatic disease should be sought by taking a history, such as photosensitivity, arthralgias, or Raynaud's phenomenon, which would suggest an overlap syndrome or the more accurately termed undifferentiated connective tissue disease with features of an inflammatory myopathy. Further, a careful review of systems and physical examination eliciting specific signs or

TABLE 54–2. Differential Diagnosis of Inflammatory Myopathies

Drug- and toxin-induced	Colchicine, D-penicillamine, cimetidine, antimalarials, zidovudine, lovastatin, clofibrate, ipecac, amphetamines, ethanol, corticosteroids, heroin, cocaine, pentazocine	
Endocrinopathies	Hypothyroidism, hyperthyroidism/thyroiditis, hypoparathyroidism, acromegaly, Cushing's syndrome, Addison's disease	
Electrolyte disorders	Hypokalemia, hypercalcemia, hypocalcemia, hypomagnesemia	
Infections	Viral:	Coxsackievirus B, adenovirus type 2, hepatitis B, influenza A and B, human immunodeficiency virus, echovirus, rubella
	Bacterial:	Legionnaires' disease, *Staphylococcus, Streptococcus,* clostridia
	Fungi/parasites:	*Borrelia,* trichinosis, *Mycobacterium, Toxoplasma gondii,* leprosy
Genetic	Metabolic:	Complete or partial deficiencies of phosphorylase (McArdle's disease), phosphofructokinase, acid maltase, carnitine and carnitine palmitoyl transferase, myoadenylate deaminase deficiency
	Mitochondrial:	Complete or partial deficiencies of cytochrome oxidase, cytochrome reductase, ubiquinone reductase
Neuromuscular disorders	Neuropathies (Guillain-Barré and other polyneuropathies, diabetes mellitus, porphyria), myasthenia gravis, Eaton-Lambert syndrome, amyotrophic lateral sclerosis, myotonic dystrophy, familial periodic paralysis, spinal muscular dystrophy	

From Medical Knowledge Self-Assessment Program (MKSAP). Rheumatology 1993, Table 28, p 125. Published by S Karger AG, Basel.

symptoms of malignancy are indicated because the idiopathic inflammatory myopathies have an association with malignancy.

Vital signs should be noted, with specific attention to respiratory rate and chest wall excursion. The skin should be inspected for the presence of a heliotrope rash on the eyelids and an erythematous rash over the neck and shoulders in a shawl-like distribution. Discoloration of the knuckles with raised violaceous papulosquamous lesions that spare the phalanges (Gottron's papules), cuticular overgrowth, and enlarged capillary loops in the nail beds may also be present. The head and neck are examined for signs of other connective tissue disease and endocrinopathy—specifically, dry eyes and mouth, palpable salivary glands, an enlarged thyroid, or the presence of adenopathy. Flexion of the neck against resistance, shoulder abduction, and thigh flexion should be tested, and muscle bulk and tone noted. The presence or absence of muscle tenderness and neurologic findings should be carefully noted. Pulmonary or cardiac involvement, subcutaneous calcifications, and joint contractures also may be present.

Evaluation of a patient with an idiopathic inflammatory myopathy includes laboratory studies, electrophysiologic studies, and a muscle biopsy. Aldolase and creatinine kinase determinations, complete blood count, sedimentation rate, liver function studies, electrolyte values, creatinine levels, blood urea nitrogen, and stool guaiac testing all should be included in the initial screening. A chest radiograph, electrocardiogram, blood gas determinations, thyroid function studies, mammogram, and specific autoantibody tests may be indicated as well. An electromyographic study is performed to document insertional irritability with fibrillation potentials at rest and short-wave, low amplitude, polyphasic potentials with contraction. Biopsy of a muscle not used in the electromyographic study is important. This should be performed by a surgeon competent in delivering the specimen in a nontraumatic way to the pathologist and should be reviewed by a pathologist anticipating the specimen so that the muscle may be properly prepared for special stains and electron microscopy. Inattention to any one of these details makes the diagnosis more difficult, given the spectrum of abnormalities in these diseases and the nonuniformity of the muscle involvement.

The differential diagnosis of the idiopathic inflammatory myopathies is extensive (Table 54–2), and the diseases are rare. A family history of myopathies should be sought, and medications such as the cholesterol-lowering drugs, hydroxychloroquine, penicillamine, and zidovudine should be excluded along with trauma, alcoholism, toxins, concurrent infections, and other connective tissue diseases. The concern about an underlying malignancy, particularly in an adult with dermatomyositis, is real. A detailed physical examination should suggest the appropriate workup, because little evidence supports an unfocused approach. Routine blood work, guaiac screening of the stool, a chest radiograph, and a mammogram should also be completed. Dalakas points out that in patients with dermatomyositis, cancers have been discovered by abnormal findings and not by randomly ordered radiographic studies.

Treatment

High-dose glucocorticoids (1 mg/kg/day of prednisone or equivalent) is the initial therapy of

TABLE 54–3. Clinical Findings in Scleroderma: Limited Cutaneous Disease Compared with Diffuse Cutaneous Disease

CLINICAL FINDINGS	LIMITED CUTANEOUS DISEASE	DIFFUSE CUTANEOUS DISEASE
Raynaud's phenomenon	May antedate other symptoms by years	Onset associated with other symptoms within 1 year
Skin changes	Distal to elbow/wrist	Spread proximal to elbow, involvement of trunk, tendons
Telangiectasias, digital ulcers, calcinosis	Frequent	Rare
Visceral symptoms	Pulmonary hypertension	Renal, myocardial, intestinal disease, pulmonary fibrosis
Nail fold capillaries	Dilated	Dilated with dropout
Autoantibodies	Anticentromere (44–98%)	Antitopoisomerase 1 (Scl$_{70}$) (25–75%) and others
10-year survival	>50%	<50%

From Medical Knowledge Self-Assessment Program (MKSAP). Rheumatology 1993, Table 26, p 118. Published by S. Karger AG, Basel.

choice for the idiopathic inflammatory myopathies and should be undertaken in consultation with a rheumatologist to determine the dose and duration. Treatment failures are common with too rapid a reduction in steroids and particularly in the setting of inclusion body myositis. Methotrexate has been shown to reduce the need for steroids in some individuals. The prognosis is probably worsened by delay in appropriate treatment; therefore, urgent consultation with a rheumatologist should be sought. Although the mortality from these diseases has diminished during recent years, the morbidity continues to be profound and the need for psychosocial support is essential.

SCLERODERMA AND FIBROSING DISORDERS

Pathogenesis and Epidemiology

Scleroderma, a rare systemic disorder of unknown cause, presents with progressive thickening of the skin and vascular hyperactivity manifested by cold-induced spasm of vessels. Interest in the role of tryptophan metabolism in the pathophysiology of this disease was raised during the toxic oil scandal in Spain and the worldwide eosinophilia-myalgia epidemic. Drugs, vinyl chloride, and other immunotoxins have been implicated as a cause of scleroderma. Studies on the incidence of scleroderma in patients with silicone breast implants have reopened the issue of causality in this disease. However, its rare occurrence makes epidemiologic studies difficult to perform and still harder to interpret when associations are being sought. In the case of silicone breast implants, silicone fragments have been found in the cells of the immune system distant from the breast im-

plant. There are reports that the progressive fibrosis of systemic sclerosis has regressed in some patients who have undergone removal of the silicone implants. The latter are anecdotal observations and are subject to bias and confounding. Epidemiologic studies of disease causation have not been completed. The decision to remove the implants surgically should be made only after education of and careful deliberation with a patient.

Clinical Features

Scleroderma exists in both limited and diffuse forms. The limited form, which generally has a more favorable prognosis, is characterized by calcinosis cutis, Raynaud's phenomenon, esophageal dysmotility, sclerodactyly, and telangiectasias and is often known by the eponym CREST or limited cutaneous disease (Table 54–3). Although Raynaud's phenomenon can be an isolated medical problem in many women without other sequelae, a careful history and physical examination searching for evidence of systemic disease should always be undertaken in these patients. Studies have suggested that the CREST syndrome may be characterized serologically by the anticentromere antibody and that this marker may identify a smaller group of patients at risk for early pulmonary hypertension. The diffuse form of progressive systemic sclerosis is characterized by many of the previously mentioned findings, but the dermal fibrosis is much more extensive and the vascular hyperreactivity with fibrosis seems to involve the internal organs of the body as well. Serologically, the marker for this disease when present is anti-Scl 70, an antibody to a topoisomerase. Irreversible impairment of respiratory exchange, dysrhythmias and myocardial dysfunction, and accelerated hypertension and renal failure all are manifestations of systemic disease.

Treatment

Treatment of limited scleroderma is symptomatic. Avoidance of cold is not enough. Active measures to remain warm are important, especially in northern climates or southern air-conditioned environments. Treatment of progressive systemic sclerosis has been discouraging to date. A few patients may respond to penicillamine, but it is a toxic and poorly tolerated drug, and no randomized controlled trials have proved its efficacy. The practical therapy is directed primarily at the complications of scleroderma, including gastrointestinal dysfunction, heart failure, renal crises, and Raynaud's phenomenon. Oral antibiotics may improve malabsorption states due to bacterial overgrowth. The newer prokinetic agents are being tried to improve gut dysmotility. Histamine$_2$ blockers and omeprazole may be effective at reducing symptomatic gastroesophageal reflux, which is common in patients who have scleroderma with esophageal fibrosis and a patulous gastroesophageal junction. Calcium channel blockers (particularly nifedipine) may reduce the frequency and severity of Raynaud's episodes. Most importantly, converting enzyme inhibitors are now the drugs of choice for potentially fatal scleroderma renal crises with malignant hypertension. Consultation with a rheumatologist is necessary for any of these therapeutic decisions.

POLYMYALGIA RHEUMATICA

Pathophysiology and Epidemiology

The pathophysiology of polymyalgia rheumatica is unknown. It may well be one manifestation of giant cell arteritis. This view is supported by the occasional finding of biopsy-proven granulomatous inflammation in the temporal artery of patients with polymyalgia rheumatica even in the absence of clinical signs or symptoms of arteritis. Against this concept, however, are the following observations: (1) negative biopsy findings in many patients with ''pure'' polymyalgia rheumatica; (2) the finding of synovitis in the girdle joints of patients with polymyalgia rheumatica, but with no histologic evidence of arteritis in these joints; and (3) in elderly men, a presentation of polymyalgia rheumatica more consistent with seronegative RA than with a systemic vasculitis. Some patients with polymyalgia rheumatica eventually suffer a peripheral synovitis, which has many of the characteristics of RA. This observation suggests that polymyalgia rheumatica may actually be a subset of RA and that the pathophysiologic mechanisms in both disorders may be similar (see Chapter 53).

When current and inactive cases are counted, prevalence estimates in the United States are 500 cases per 100,000 persons age 50 years or older. Initially described as a disease of white women, this observation has been brought into question by a chart review study of 27 patients with polymyalgia rheumatica or giant cell arteritis in which 13 were African American. Polymyalgia rheumatica is primarily a disease of women, affecting four women for every man.

Clinical Features and Differential Diagnosis

Polymyalgia rheumatica is characterized by profound axial stiffness, shoulder and hip girdle pain that increases with movement, systemic malaise, and a salient elevation in the erythrocyte sedimentation rate (ESR). The hallmark of the disease is the dramatic overnight response to low-dose glucocorticoids. The symptoms of shoulder and hip pain are usually symmetric and are occasionally sudden in onset. Patients may at times present with a bursitis syndrome that evolves to the typical polymyalgia rheumatica stigmata with time. Constitutional features, including malaise, weight loss and poor sleep, define this syndrome as a systemic inflammatory disease and not a local process. Because of the age group involved, the differential diagnosis is extensive and includes occult malignancy, other connective tissue disease (i.e., SLE or RA), thyroid disease, depression, or fibromyalgia.

A thorough history and physical examination should include palpation of the temporal arteries for evidence of tenderness or swelling. The patient should be queried about headache, sudden visual loss, and jaw claudication. The latter is sometimes difficult to differentiate from temporomandibular joint pain. Adenopathy and abdominal masses should be sought, and rectal examination with stool guaiac analysis should be performed. Laboratory testing should include a complete blood count, ESR, rheumatoid factor, antinuclear antibodies, chemistries, thyroid function tests, chest radiograph, and mammogram.

Whether polymyalgia rheumatica is one expression of giant cell arteritis or is merely associated with the latter disease remains speculative. Because of recognized concurrence of the two diseases and the potential consequence of giant cell arteritis (blindness), it is unclear whether a temporal artery biopsy specimen should be obtained in every case of polymyalgia rheumatica or whether all patients should be treated empirically with high-dose glucocorticoids. This question has been examined clinically and using formal methods of decision analysis. Blindness must be weighed against the morbidity of a benign surgical procedure and the toxicity of high-dose glucocorticoids. The current recommendations are to treat polymyalgia rheumatica with low-dose prednisone alone. The morbidity of high doses of glucocorticoids in these patients outweighs the possible benefits when a history of giant cell arteritis is missing. If localized scalp tenderness, headache, visual disturbances, or jaw claudication ensues, a temporal artery biopsy is indicated. The likelihood of positive temporal artery biopsy findings in this setting is high. Because giant cell arteritis may present at any point with polymyalgia rheumatica, physicians should educate patients about the symptoms of giant cell arteritis so that the emergence of this disease will be noted promptly and treated appropriately.

Treatment

Polymyalgia rheumatica by itself is a disabling disease but one that is very amenable to therapy. Prednisone, 10 to 15 mg daily, is the recommended starting dose, tapering to 7.5 mg daily and then to alternate-day therapy as tolerated. The symptoms of morning stiffness and shoulder and hip pain with movement, as well as the ESR, generally improve promptly and dramatically with low doses of glucocorticoids. A lack of response should prompt a physician to consider other diagnoses, such as giant cell arteritis or malignancy. Nonsteroidal anti-inflammatory drugs typically only partially alleviate symptoms. In the absence of giant cell arteritis, polymyalgia rheumatica tends to run a benign course lasting a variable period with a range from 2 to 8 years. Were it not for the association with giant cell arteritis and the attendant risk of blindness, the diagnosis of polymyalgia rheumatica would be a simpler task, as would be the choice of therapy. Because the presentation of giant cell arteritis may be subtle, all patients with suspected giant cell arteritis should be referred to a rheumatologist and monitored until in a sustained clinical remission on low doses of glucocorticoids. There is no justification for resuming higher doses of glucocorticoids on the basis of a rise in ESR alone. In the future, bone-sparing glucocorticoids or concurrent use of calcitonin or the bisphosphonates with prednisone therapy may provide some protection from accelerated

osteoporosis. For now, rapid reduction in the steroid dose and early use of a steroid-sparing agent may be tried.

TEMPORAL ARTERITIS AND THE VASCULITIDES

Pathophysiology and Epidemiology

Giant cell arteritis (or temporal arteritis) affects primarily large to medium-sized arteries that branch from the arch of the aorta. Although many of the great vessels may be involved, most of the clinically apparent vasculopathy involves the cranial arteries. Biopsy specimens of an involved temporal artery demonstrate destruction of the elastic lamina and infiltration of the media and intima with inflammatory cells and multinucleated giant cells. The walls of affected vessels become thickened with resultant occlusion, ischemia, and necrosis of tissue. Some studies have shown immunoglobulin deposits in the walls of affected vessels. Likewise, histologic analysis has revealed that the predominant inflammatory cell is the helper T cell, thus suggesting that immunologic mechanisms are somehow involved in the pathogenesis of this disease.

Because the inflammation may involve the vessel sporadically, the size of the biopsy sample taken and the number of cuts reviewed are important in securing a diagnosis of giant cell arteritis. These factors contribute to the difficulty in estimating the true frequency of giant cell arteritis. The Mayo Clinic has estimated a prevalence of approximately 130 cases per 100,000 in people 50 years of age and older. Although properly conducted epidemiologic studies are lacking in culturally diverse populations, present data suggest a higher frequency in whites.

Clinical Features

Initial manifestations of giant cell arteritis are listed in Table 54–4. Although the disease may present acutely, more often it is subtle and insidious. Patients should be questioned about weight loss, malaise, low-grade fever, and poor appetite. A more focused history directed at the vasculopathic features should aim to identify temporal or occipital headaches, scalp tenderness, and jaw claudication. Finally, involvement of the ophthalmic or ciliary arteries may produce transient visual loss, a decrease in acuity, diplopia, or at times sudden and irreversible blindness. The

TABLE 54–4. Initial Clinical Manifestations in Patients with Giant Cell Arteritis (%)

Headache	32
Polymyalgia rheumatica	25
Fever	15
Visual symptoms without loss	7
Weakness/malaise/fatigue	5
Tenderness over arteries	3
Myalgias	4
Weight loss/anorexia	2
Jaw claudication	2
Permanent loss of vision	1
Tongue claudication	1
Sore throat	1
Vasculitis on angiogram	1
Stiffness of hands and wrists	1

Adapted from Kelley WN, Harris ED Jr, Ruddy S, Sledge CB (eds). Textbook of Rheumatology. 4th ed. Philadelphia: WB Saunders, 1993, Table 65–1, p 1105.

polymyalgia rheumatica syndrome may be present in as many as 50% of patients with giant cell arteritis. The physical examination findings may be remarkably normal. However, clinicians should specifically palpate the temporal arteries and seek scalp tenderness. Because this is a systemic illness, laboratory workup is usually extensive but frequently reveals only an elevated ESR (commonly in the 60–100 mm/hour range) and a normochromic-normocytic anemia. If giant cell arteritis is suspected, prednisone (40–60 mg daily) should be initiated immediately and a biopsy of the temporal artery scheduled within the next 72 hours. For the most part, a temporal artery biopsy is an outpatient procedure that can be performed under local anesthesia with little attendant risk. It is imperative that an adequate sample be obtained, because the vessel inflammation is sporadic. In the ideal situation, a 4 to 6 cm length of artery should be obtained by an interested and experienced surgeon, and the pathologist should be encouraged to examine multiple sections along the entire length. If the initial biopsy findings are negative yet the index of suspicion for the disease is still high, the opposite artery should be sampled as well. After a week of glucocorticoid therapy, biopsy specimens are infrequently diagnostic.

Treatment

High-dose glucocorticoids (1 mg/kg/day prednisone or equivalent) are the mainstay of treatment, although studies are now under way to evaluate steroid-sparing regimens. Treatment of biopsy-proven giant cell arteritis should be carried out with the assistance of an experienced rheuma-

tologist. Mistakes are made during the taper of steroids. After 2 to 4 weeks of high-dose prednisone, the clinical features, laboratory abnormalities, and risk of catastrophic events are usually minimized sufficiently that the taper can begin. Eight to 12 weeks of high-dose prednisone therapy usually does not improve outcome and frequently increases the potential for adverse reactions in the typically older female patients. Finally, steroid dose should not be determined solely on the basis of the ESR. As with any laboratory test (especially with one so prone to nonspecific elevations in older patients), the ESR should be interpreted by virtue of the company that it keeps.

Other Systemic Necrotizing Vasculitides

The other vasculitides tend to be grouped according to clinical syndromes and the vessel size involved. A simple classification of these may be noted in Table 54–5. Some of these diseases, involving small to medium-sized arteries (i.e., polyarteritis nodosa, Wegener's granulomatosis), are life-threatening disorders. Appropriate therapeutic approaches are still unclear, as is an understanding of their pathophysiology. For this reason, all patients with systemic necrotizing vasculitis should be cared for in concert with a rheumatologist, immunologist, or nephrologist. All biopsy findings and pathology reports in these cases, including antineutrophil cytoplasmic antibody, should be reviewed by the attending physician with the pathologist to establish a coherent approach to therapy.

GLUCOCORTICOIDS

Glucocorticoids, initially introduced for therapeutic purposes in the late 1940s by Hench and colleagues, are powerful inhibitors of inflammation and the immune response. As a class of drug, they are the mainstay of immunosuppressive therapy for patients with connective tissue diseases. In high doses (i.e., 1 mg/kg/day of prednisone or equivalent), they are used alone and in concert with other immunosuppressive drugs (i.e., methotrexate, cyclophosphamide, azathioprine, and others) for life- or organ-threatening autoimmune disorders, such as lupus nephritis, cerebritis, or systemic necrotizing vasculitis. In lower doses (i.e., 5–10 mg/day of prednisone or equivalent), they are used in the management of the inflammatory arthropathies, such as RA or polymyalgia rheumatica. Although these drugs are very potent

TABLE 54–5. Partial Classification of Vasculitic Syndromes by Pattern of Common Features

DISEASE ENTITY	CLINICAL	PATHOLOGY
Polyarteritis	Multiple organs	Fibrinoid necrosis of the small and medium arteries
Kawasaki's disease	Infants, mucocutaneous involvement, coronary arteritis	Fibrinoid necrosis of the small and medium arteries
Mixed cryoglobulinemia	Purpura, cryoglobulins, hepatitis B antigen	Fibrinoid necrosis of the small and medium arteries
Churg-Strauss vasculitis	Asthma, eosinophilia	Granulomatous small vessel vasculitis
Wegener's granulomatosis	Upper and lower respiratory tract involvement	Granulomatous small vessel vasculitis
Granulomatous angiitis of the central nervous system	Central nervous system involvement	Granulomatous small and medium vessel vasculitis
Hypersensitivity vasculitis	Drug induced, purpura	Small vessel leukocytoclastic vasculitis
Henoch-Schönlein purpura	Children, purpura	Small vessel leukocytoclastic vasculitis (IgA)
Hypocomplementemic cutaneous vasculitis	Hypocomplementemia, urticaria	Small vessel leukocytoclastic vasculitis
Giant cell arteritis	Elderly, polymyalgia rheumatica, cranial artery involvement	Giant cell arteritis of the medium and large arteries
Takayasu's arteritis	Young person, ischemic symptoms from artery involvement	Giant cell arteritis of the medium and large arteries
Cogan's syndrome	Interstitial keratitis, audiovestibular dysfunction	Small, medium, and large artery involvement
Buerger's disease	Young, smokers, peripheral artery involvement	Occlusive inflammatory nonnecrotic involvement of the small and medium arteries
Goodpasture's syndrome	Pulmonary hemorrhage, glomerulonephritis	Glomerulonephritis

From Schumacher HR Jr. Primer on the Rheumatic Diseases. 9th ed. Atlanta: Arthritis Foundation, 1988, Table 22–1, p 124. Used by permission of the Arthritis Foundation.

anti-inflammatory agents, they also exhibit significant toxicity, especially at high doses, and should be carefully administered.

Mechanism of Action and Pharmacology

Glucocorticoids gain access to target cells through the cell membrane and then bind to cytosolic high-affinity glucocorticoid receptors, thus activating the receptor-ligand complex. This complex in turn enters the nucleus and, depending on the physiologic capability of the cell, interacts with deoxyribonucleic acid and modifies (either inhibits or stimulates) transcription of messenger ribonucleic acid. The eventual result is modification of translation and protein synthesis that ultimately is expressed by the biologic activity of glucocorticoids. This proposed molecular mechanism of action may explain the plethora of therapeutic and adverse effects induced by glucocorticoids. These drugs have dramatic effects on the immune and inflammatory response, including (1) redistribution of mononuclear cells (especially monocytes/macrophages and T lymphocytes); (2) accelerated release (from bone marrow) and demargination of neutrophils; (3) inhibition of neutrophil accumulation at sites of inflammation; (4) alteration in HLA-DR expression; (5) suppression of delayed-type hypersensitivity; (6) inhibition of cytokine (especially interleukin-1) secretion; and (7) inhibition of prostaglandin and leukotriene production.

The anti-inflammatory potency of glucocorticoids is dramatically affected by minor changes in chemical structure. For example, dexamethasone differs from hydrocortisone by virtue of a methyl and fluorine group at the 16 and 9 position, respectively, yet it is 30 times more potent and has an extended half-life. The bioavailability of glucocorticoids is somewhat variable, depending on the preparation used. They are 90% bound to cortisol-binding globulin and 10% bound (weakly) to albumin; thus, patients with hypoalbuminemic states may be subject to more drug effects at lower doses. They are metabolized in the liver and excreted in the urine.

Clinical Uses

For patients with severe autoimmune disease, including SLE (especially nephritis, cerebritis, or severe cytopenia), active dermatomyositis or poly-

TABLE 54–6. Glucocorticoid Side Effects

Very common and should be anticipated in all patients
  Osteoporosis
  Increased appetite
  Centripetal obesity
  Impaired wound healing
  Increased risk of infection
  Suppression of hypothalamic-pituitary axis
  Arrest of normal growth in children
Frequent
  Myopathy
  Osteonecrosis
  Hypertension
  Plethora
  Thin fragile skin, striae, purpura
  Edema
  Hyperlipidemia
  Psychiatric symptoms, particularly euphoria
  Diabetes mellitus
  Posterior subcapsular cataracts
Uncommon but important to recognize early
  Glaucoma
  Benign intracranial hypertension
  "Silent" intestinal perforation
  Peptic ulcer disease
  Gastric hemorrhage
  Hypokalemic alkalosis
  Hyperosmolar nonketotic coma
Rare
  Pancreatitis
  Hirsutism
  Panniculitis
  Secondary amenorrhea
  Impotence
  Epidural lipomatosis
  Allergy to synthetic corticosteroids

From Behrens TW, Goodwin JS. Glucocorticoids. In: McCarty D, Koopman W. Arthritis and Related Conditions. 11th ed. Philadelphia: Lea & Febiger, 1989.

myositis, active systemic necrotizing vasculitis (polyarteritis nodosa, Wegener's, giant cell arteritis), high doses are frequently required. However, the ultimate goal of therapy always should be reduction to the lowest dose necessary to maintain control of the disease. High steroid doses for long periods are associated with a high risk of infection, avascular necrosis, and other adverse reactions. A structured algorithm for steroid tapering does not exist, but general guidelines include (1) no abrupt discontinuation of glucocorticoids; (2) slow and methodic tapering, with the largest decrements occurring at the highest doses and the smaller decrements occurring at the lower doses; (3) slow change to alternate-day dosing; and (4) consideration of steroid-sparing drugs (i.e., methotrexate) if prolonged use becomes necessary. The lower doses (i.e., 5–15 mg/day prednisone equivalent) are advocated for polymyalgia rheumatica and RA. In the former case, the dose of glucocorticoids can gradually be reduced and eventually discontinued over the course of 12 to 24 months while monitoring clinical symptoms and ESR. For patients with RA, low doses of glucocorticoids are used frequently as bridge therapy while awaiting the effects of disease-modifying drugs, such as parenteral gold or methotrexate. Regardless of the dose, consultation with a rheumatologist is advised to implement and manage glucocorticoid dosing in patients with an inflammatory or autoimmune disease.

Toxicity

The adverse reactions of glucocorticoids are numerous (Table 54–6). Glucocorticoid use is associated with significant osteoporosis, especially in physically incapacitated or immobilized women with an inflammatory disease. The loss of bone mass occurs early in therapy and is likely due to a decrease in bone formation and an increase in bone resorption. No specific therapies for preventing glucocorticoid-induced bone loss have been devised, although current wisdom suggests that at the very least vitamin D (400 IU/day) and elemental calcium (1000–1500 mg/day) be administered orally and that parenteral calcitonin be considered.

REFERENCES

Alarcon-Segovia D, Deleze M, Oria CV, et al. Antiphospholipid antibodies and the antiphospholipid syndrome in systemic lupus erythematosus. Medicine 1989;68:353.

Bengtsson B, Malmvall B. The epidemiology of giant cell arteritis including temporal arteritis and polymyalgia rheumatica. Arthritis Rheum 1981;24(7):899.

Boumpas D, Chrousos GP, Wilder RL, et al. Glucocorticoid therapy for immune-mediated diseases: Basic and clinical correlates. Ann Intern Med 1993;119:1198.

Chang RW, Fineberg HV. Risk-benefit considerations in the management of polymyalgia rheumatica. Med Decis Making 1983;3(4):459.

Cronin ME, Plotz PH. Idiopathic inflammatory myopathies in epidemiology of rheumatic diseases. Rheum Dis Clin North Am 1990;16(3):655.

Dalakas M. Treatment of polymyositis and dermatomyositis. Curr Opin Rheumatol 1989;1:443.

Dalakas M. Inflammatory myopathies. Curr Opin Neurol Neurosurg 1990;3:689.

Dalakas M. Polymyositis, dermatomyositis and inclusion-body myositis. N Engl J Med 1991;325(21):1487.

Galve E, Ordi J, Barquinero J, et al. Valvular heart disease in the primary antiphospholipid syndrome. Ann Intern Med 1992;116:293.

Germaine BF. Silicone breast implants and rheumatic disease. Bull Rheum Dis 1991;41(6):1–5.

Gonzalez EB, Varner WT, Lisse JR, et al. Giant cell arteritis in the southern United States. Arch Intern Med 1989;149:1561.

Grob JJ, Bonerandi JJ. Thrombotic skin disease as a marker of the anticardiolipin syndrome. J Am Acad Dermatol 1989;20:1063.

Hart FD. Polymyalgia rheumatica. Its correct diagnosis and treatment. Drugs 1987;33:280.

Hughes, Graham RV. The antiphospholipid syndrome: Ten years on. Lancet 1993;342:341.

Jimenez SA, Sigal SH. A 15-year prospective study of treatment of rapidly progressive systemic sclerosis with D-penicillamine. J Rheumatol 1991;18(10):1496.

Lavalle C, Pizarro S, Drenkard C, et al. Transverse myelitis: A manifestation of systemic lupus erythematosus strongly associated with antiphospholipid antibodies. J Rheumatol 1990;17:34.

Love LA, Leff RL, Fraser DD, et al. A new approach to the classification of idiopathic inflammatory myopathy: Myositis-specific autoantibodies define useful homogeneous patient groups. Medicine 1991;70(6):360.

Love PE, Santoro SA. Antiphospholipid antibodies: Anticardiolipin and the lupus anticoagulant in systemic lupus erythematosus (SLE) and in non-SLE disorders. Ann Intern Med 1990;112:682.

Michet CJ. Polymyalgia rheumatica/giant cell arteritis and other vasculitides. Rheum Dis Clin North Am 1990;16(3):667.

Montanaro A. Rheumatic diseases from non-prescriptive biologic agents and silicone implants. Prim Care Rheumatol 1992;2(3):12.

Petri M, Rheinschmidt M, Whiting-O'Keefe Q, et al. The frequency of lupus anticoagulant in systemic lupus erythematosus. Ann Intern Med 1987;106:524.

Rosove MH, Brewer MC. Antiphospholipid thrombosis: Clinical course after the first thrombotic event in 70 patients. Ann Intern Med 1992;117:303.

Sigurgeirsson B, Lindelof B, Edhag O, et al. Risk of cancer in patients with dermatomyositis or polymyositis. N Engl J Med 1992;326(6):363.

Steinberg A (moderator). NIH Conference, Systemic Lupus Erythematosus. Ann Intern Med 1991;115(7):548.

Varga J, Schumacher R, Jimenez SA. Systemic sclerosis after augmentation mammoplasty with silicone implants. Ann Intern Med 1989;111(5):377.

Fibromyalgia and Regional Pain Syndromes

Margaret Seton and Richard Polisson

Fibromyalgia is a common chronic rheumatic disorder, characterized by generalized muscle tenderness, nonrestorative sleep, fatigue, and axial skeletal pain. True articular disease and inflammation are absent. The clinical picture of this disorder has only evolved in recent years. Many clinicians are skeptical about the existence of fibromyalgia because of the lack of a well-defined pathologic lesion or laboratory abnormality. However, fibromyalgia should be considered in any woman presenting with chronic pain that is diffuse and unexplained.

EPIDEMIOLOGY

It is estimated that 15 to 20% of patients referred to rheumatology clinics and 3 to 10% of patients seen in internal medicine clinics have fibromyalgia. In 1904, Gowers first called the clinical syndrome fibrositis, and noted it to be "aching, stiffness, a readiness to feel muscular fatigue, interference with free muscular movement and very often a want of energy and vigor." Terminology has varied since then, because the inflammatory condition implied by fibrositis has not been found. Fibromyalgia, tension myalgia, and generalized rheumatism are generally recognized epithets for this disorder.

Predominantly a disease of women, fibromyalgia usually presents in the fourth to fifth decades, although it has been reported in children and the elderly. Primary fibromyalgia is a diagnosis of exclusion—that is, other connective tissue diseases are not present. Secondary fibromyalgia suggests that the evolution of this chronic pain syndrome is a consequence of other illness (i.e., rheumatoid arthritis). Stress, trauma, surgery, and infectious diseases all have been implicated as causes of this syndrome, but these remain only associations at this time.

The argument has also been made that fibromyalgia is not a disease but an "unwellness" within the spectrum of normal aches and pains of everyday life. Certainly the subjective impairment far outweighs the clinical and laboratory evidence of rheumatic disease in these patients. But this concept of unwellness and the allegation that this represents psychogenic rheumatism fail to account for the consistency of presentation and the level of distress in many of these patients.

CLINICAL PRESENTATION

The history is characterized by the diffuse quality of the pain and the broad constellation of systems. Headaches, temporomandibular jaw dysfunction, nonrestorative sleep, generalized stiffness and muscle discomfort, dysesthesias or paresthesias, depression, inattention, irritable bowel syndrome, cold intolerance, dry eyes, and functional disability all are frequent concurrent symptoms that may be elicited. Routine activities of daily living become insurmountable because of muscle fatigue and pain; workplace modifications or job changes are not uncommon for these patients. The impact on the family remains largely unexplored, although this is also a significant health and economic issue.

The physical examination usually reveals a well but uncomfortable-appearing patient with normal vital signs. Patients do not have an antalgic gait and do not have muscle spasm or true loss of range of motion. Findings on the joint examination remain objectively normal, and the nail beds and skin are benign. Auscultation and percussion of heart, lungs, and abdomen reveals no abnormalities. Neurologic findings are normal in detail. It is only when pressure points are sought in a deliberate fashion that the history and physical examination develop cogency and a diagnosis of fibro-

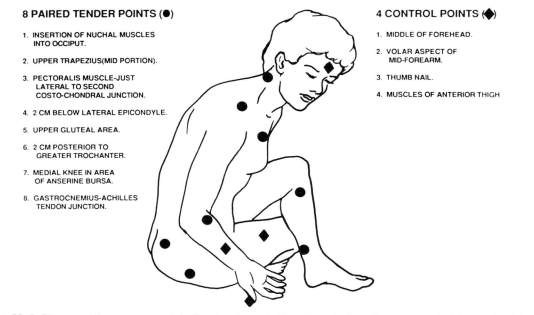

8 PAIRED TENDER POINTS (●)

1. INSERTION OF NUCHAL MUSCLES INTO OCCIPUT.

2. UPPER TRAPEZIUS(MID PORTION).

3. PECTORALIS MUSCLE-JUST LATERAL TO SECOND COSTO-CHONDRAL JUNCTION.

4. 2 CM BELOW LATERAL EPICONDYLE.

5. UPPER GLUTEAL AREA.

6. 2 CM POSTERIOR TO GREATER TROCHANTER.

7. MEDIAL KNEE IN AREA OF ANSERINE BURSA.

8. GASTROCNEMIUS-ACHILLES TENDON JUNCTION.

4 CONTROL POINTS (◆)

1. MIDDLE OF FOREHEAD.

2. VOLAR ASPECT OF MID-FOREARM.

3. THUMB NAIL.

4. MUSCLES OF ANTERIOR THIGH.

Figure 55–1. Fibromyolgia pressure points. The tender point locations in fibrositis are remarkably constant from patient to patient. Multiple locations have been described; the eight paired tender points shown represent frequently occurring points in a wide distribution. Most patients with fibrositis usually have seven or more tender points. Control points are not unduly tender; their examination should be interspersed with that of the tender points. (From Bennett RB. Fibrositis. In: Kelley WN, Harris ED Jr, Ruddy S, Sledge CB (eds). Textbook of Rheumatology. 3rd ed. Philadelphia: WB Saunders, 1989, p 543.)

myalgia becomes evident. The pressure points are illustrated in Figure 55–1, and current diagnostic criteria of the American College of Rheumatology are listed in Table 55–1. Pressure points should be sought by applying firm pressure with the thumb over the sites indicated. Control points, such as the tip of the thumb or the forehead, may also be tested.

No diagnostic laboratory abnormality exists. Results of blood studies tend to be unremarkable, and muscle enzymes and sedimentation rates are within the normal range. Tests of antinuclear antibody and rheumatoid factor are negative, and results of thyroid function tests are also unremarkable. No indication is found for more extensive laboratory evaluations in most of these individuals, nor do expensive radiographic studies or electromyography have a role. The salient clinical features of fibromyalgia are outlined in Table 55–2.

TABLE 55–1. American College of Rheumatology Classification Criteria: Fibromyalgia

1. Widespread pain for more than 3 months, on both sides of the body, above and below the waist, and axial skeleton (cervical spine, anterior chest, thoracic pain, or low back)
2. Tenderness to palpation in 11 of 18 bilateral sites

PATHOPHYSIOLOGY

The cause of fibromyalgia is undetermined. Yunus theorized that the primary defect in fibromyalgia is neurohormonal. Abnormal concentrations of neurotransmitters, in conjunction with hormonal disturbances, are believed to contribute to an aberrant central pain mechanism that becomes amplified by regional musculoskeletal dysfunction and central affective disturbances.

The initial dysregulation of painful stimuli may originate in the spinal cord, with aberrant recording of stimuli carried from involved dermatomes. Normally, delta and C fibers are nerve fibers that carry painful stimuli from peripheral nociceptors to the dorsal horn area of the spinal cord. The neurotransmitter substance P is thought to be important in this synapse, before the decussation of fibers to the contralateral spinothalamic tract. Modulation of the transmission of these afferent fibers may occur presynaptically via touch or pressure sensations carried by type A beta fibers. Alternatively, descending inhibitory pathways in the spinal cord itself may influence the gating of the dorsal horn impulses. Theoretically, either a deficiency of inhibitory neurotransmitters on the one hand, such as serotonin or somatostatin, or an excess of stimulatory neurotransmitters on the other,

TABLE 55–2. Salient Clinical Features of Fibromyalgia

History	Patient complains of chronic diffuse pain in articular and nonarticular areas. No history of joint swelling, redness
Constitutional symptoms	Fatigue, sleep disturbance, but no fever or major weight loss
Joint examination	Pain on full motion may be present, but no joint effusion or deformities
Muscle examination	Tenderness at certain muscle-tendon junctions and muscle bellies (see Fig. 55–1) but no muscle weakness or atrophy
Neurologic examination	No characteristic positive findings and no sensory or motor abnormalities
Laboratory studies	No characteristic positive findings; normal complete blood count, erythrocyte sedimentation rate, muscle enzymes, thyroid function, and serologic profile

From Goldenberg DL, Diagnostic and therapeutic challenges of fibromyalgia. Hosp Prac 1989; 9A:35.

such as cholecystokinin or substance P, may modulate the expression of pain.

In support of this theory of amplified pain is the finding in animal models that serotonin works to enhance sleep and inhibit the afferent signals of pain and that depressed levels of this neuroamine and its metabolites have been reported in some patients with fibromyalgia. It has been shown that serotonin enhances sleep in animal studies. Thus, a deficiency of serotonin could contribute to the sleep abnormalities described in these patients. Certainly, abnormalities of sleep have been described in fibromyalgia, classically as an abnormal alpha-wave intrusion into slow-wave, non–rapid-eye-movement sleep recorded by electroencephalography. These periods of slow-wave sleep correspond to times when growth hormone is secreted in normal individuals. Subnormal secretion of somatomedin C during non–rapid-eye-movement sleep, blunted diurnal fluctuations in plasma cortisol levels, and increased concentrations of substance P in the cerebrospinal fluid of patients with fibromyalgia have been noted. Subtle immune abnormalities, evidence of antecedent or concurrent infection, autonomic dysfunction, cumulative ischemic microtrauma to muscles, and associated metabolic imbalances all are described in the medical literature in association with fibromyalgia.

Whatever the biochemistry of aberrant pain in fibromyalgia, the clinical expression is one of an evolving state of depression, anxiety, physical deconditioning, and generalized pain. The significance of the cognitive response in the pathophysiology of fibromyalgia as expressed in affective mood and behavior is unclear. Antecedent or concurrent affective disorders are noted in many patients with fibromyalgia, as well as in relatives of these patients; however, not all patients may be characterized so succinctly by psychological testing. The emotional response to pain certainly has a role in the expression of fibromyalgia and contributes to amplification of the symptoms of chronic pain. Psychiatric illness, however, cannot at this time be identified as causative in this disorder. Nevertheless, Littlejohn believes that whatever triggers fibromyalgia or regional pain syndromes, the treatment must be aimed at the psychological issues in evidence.

What is attractive about the theory of a neurohormonal dysregulation underlying this chronic pain syndrome is that it allows for the plasticity observed in the expression of fibromyalgia. That is, it supports the observation that these patients do not have uniformity in the intensity of their pain, disability, or psychological status, although they all show some degree of consistency in meeting the diagnostic criteria for the fibromyalgia syndrome. This theory of neurohormonal dysfunction also accounts for the absence of inflammation and the absence of microscopic or macroscopic structural abnormalities noted in most tissue biopsy specimens. It accounts for the observation that musculotendinous junctions, which are rich in nociceptors, are the sites of tender pressure points in these patients. It suggests why anti-inflammatory drugs are often ineffective in easing symptoms of fibromyalgia. Finally, by implicating modulation of the disease by the endocrine system, this theory may account for the prevalence in women and the exacerbation of the disease in the premenstrual period.

DIFFERENTIAL DIAGNOSIS

The differential diagnosis of fibromyalgia is broad (Table 55–3), and the nonspecific nature of the complaints makes it difficult to distinguish fibromyalgia from other systemic diseases. The following observations are useful: (1) The muscle fatigue and weakness often suggest a myopathy, but muscle bulk, strength, and tone remain normal in these patients, as do results of laboratory tests of muscle enzymes. (2) Arthralgias, fatigue, and morning stiffness simulate an inflammatory connective tissue disease. What is important to differentiate here is the diffuse rather than discrete articular localization of the complaints, the prolonged

TABLE 55–3.   Differential Diagnosis of Fibromyalgia

Seronegative spondyloarthropathy
Rheumatoid arthritis
Systemic lupus erythematosus
Polymyositis or dermatomyositis
Polymyalgia rheumatica
Hyperthyroidism or hypothyroidism
Hyperparathyroidism
Affective disorder
Occult malignancy

morning stiffness without variation in quality, the frequently associated history of weight gain rather than weight loss, the absence of synovitis on physical examination, and the normal findings on complete blood count, Westergren sedimentation rate, and urinalysis. (3) Axial stiffness, low back pain, and loss of full range of motion in the lumbar spine often mimic neurologic disease or muscle strain, although patients with fibromyalgia lack an antalgic gait or list. Muscle findings are symmetric, and palpation elicits more tenderness than spinal motion. Neurologic abnormalities are absent, and radiographic findings are generally benign. (4) When patients present with listlessness, cold intolerance, and pronounced fatigue, hypothyroidism becomes an important diagnostic consideration. (5) Patients with primary fibromyalgia occasionally have a focus of their pain that suggests a regional pain disorder, such as costochondritis, epicondylitis, or anserine bursitis. However, a careful musculoskeletal examination may reveal widespread pressure points in the usual fibromyalgia areas. (6) Other confounding complaints may be dry eyes, urinary urgency or frequency, chest pain, or dry cough. These complaints, too, when pursued with a more detailed history taking and diagnostic studies and monitored over time, have no objective basis that can be defined by current practice.

THERAPY

The symptoms of fibromyalgia become amplified over time by the interplay of fatigue, diffuse pain, and physical deconditioning. Therapy for fibromyalgia is complex and needs to be directed at many fronts. Psychotherapy in conjunction with a cardiovascular reconditioning program and judicious pharmacologic intervention is currently the best approach. For women newly presenting with fibromyalgia, amitriptyline (or a similar mildly sedating tricyclic medication), 10 to 25 mg (occa-

sionally advancing to 50 or 75 mg) at bedtime, or diphenhydramine, 25 to 50 mg at bedtime, is a reasonable medication to attempt to improve the quality of sleep. Exercise programs such as stretch aerobics or aquatic programs are useful. A formal cardiovascular health program may be ideal for some, although few insurance companies cover this therapy under the diagnosis of fibromyalgia. Individualization of these recommendations and for psychiatric intervention is imperative. Some women fare well in self-help groups, in which their sense of isolation is relieved and they can gain validity and understanding of the disease. Others have the insight, time, and money to profit from more intensive private psychotherapy. Still others find biofeedback programs useful. Rather than obsess about the specific medication, activity, or therapy prescribed, attention needs to be focused on the aims of the therapy, which are improved sleep, improved physical conditioning, and an improved sense of well-being.

For those patients who fail to respond to initial drug therapies, studies have suggested that alprazolam with ibuprofen may be more useful than either agent alone and that cyclobenzaprine may help some patients. Nonsteroidal anti-inflammatory drugs may or may not be useful adjunctive therapy in other settings as well. Psychotherapists may recommend higher doses of antidepressants or other psychoactive medications, which may improve affect, outlook, and ultimate ability to function. There is no simple approach. Treatment of fibromyalgia requires time, determination, and education on the part of both the patient and the physician. No role has been found for glucocorticoids or other immunoregulatory drugs.

Measuring the clinical effectiveness of any single agent or therapeutic modality is a current area of study in fibromyalgia. Proposed criteria for treatment response are physician global assessment, patient sleep score, and tender point score as outlined by Simms and colleagues. The reliability of these preliminary criteria is important in weighing the relative importance of psychiatric, pharmacologic, physical, and homeopathic interventions in the treatment of this disease.

The combination of psychotherapy, physical reconditioning, improvement of sleep, and education enables patients to live with the disease. Many patients with fibromyalgia are concerned that a diagnosis is being missed or that their physician does not believe fibromyalgia is a real disease. The latter concern is often reiterated by family members or friends. The visual cues of illness are wanting in this disorder, and the malaise always seems disproportionate to the clinical findings. Validating the diagnosis through discourse and education, although time-consuming, is an important therapeutic modality. Patients must take an active role in mitigating the symptoms of their disease. Although workplace modifications may be useful, withdrawing a patient from the workplace is not usually indicated and sometimes fosters an illness behavior that prevents further clinical improvement.

Fibromyalgia newsletters or other sources of information that may be obtained through the Fibromyalgia Association of Texas (5650 Forest Lane, Dallas, TX 75230) should be made available during the first or second office visit. This early emphasis on diagnosis and its implications may spare a patient visits to neurologists, orthopedists, and other subspecialists in her effort to establish the cause of her distress. This approach may also spare her unneeded diagnostic studies or medications.

MEDICOLEGAL ISSUES

The theory of neurohormonal dysregulation attempts to address the pathophysiology of fibromyalgia but fails to address causality. It is important for physicians to take an active role in these medicolegal issues today because they affect the health of individuals in their offices. Thus, in an effort to do no harm, a physician must weigh the subjective distress of an individual against the consequences of disability and try to find an enabling pathway for the patient.

Because the cause of fibromyalgia is unknown, physicians must respect the limits of scientific knowledge and try to remain neutral on issues of causality. This attitude has ramifications for the individual as well as for society. An analysis of patients with fibromyalgia looked at the outcome of those with reactive fibromyalgia secondary to trauma, medical, or surgical stress versus those with primary fibromyalgia. In this limited study, 70% of patients with reactive fibromyalgia lost employment, as compared with 12% of those with primary fibromyalgia; and 34% of patients with reactive fibromyalgia received disability, compared with 1% of those with primary fibromyalgia. These numbers suggest that litigation and promise of compensation are poor prognostic factors in this disease state. Certainly, this pattern is seen in studies of low back pain, an axial musculoskeletal complaint that shares many patterns of chronic pain perception or disability with fibromyalgia. A physician who supports the notion of reactive fibromyalgia may actually be supporting a less healthy outcome for an individual.

The background for these concerns is a description in the medical literature by Littlejohn of an epidemic of arm and neck pain, attributed to repetitive motion strain in the workplace, that occurred in Australia in the 1980s. No proof that ergonomic factors were causal was uniformly found, but the linking of the workplace to the musculoskeletal discomfort led to an escalation of concern by unions, physicians, public health officials, and lawyers. Despite modifications in the workplace, many individuals did not improve or return to work. Littlejohn estimated in his report of the epidemic that in some workplaces, ''up to 30% of previously asymptomatic staff missed work with persisting pain and disability,'' despite the fact that no pathologic lesion was identified.

Discomfort in the arm, neck, shoulder, and lower back is common. The point at which these ailments become compensable diseases remains undefined. Although a few patients with fibromyalgia seem disabled by their disease and quite refractory to therapy, a disability status is difficult to obtain for them on the basis of their diagnosis. The most useful approach for most patients is to encourage them to see themselves not as disabled but as resourceful, enduring, and able.

When viewed from both socioeconomic and medical perspectives, fibromyalgia and other regional pain syndromes are not benign disorders. Despite the absence of crippling deformities and end-organ damage often noted in other rheumatic diseases, these chronic pain syndromes result in considerable functional disability, personal stress, and medicolegal costs.

CHRONIC FATIGUE SYNDROME

Many patients who present with chronic fatigue syndrome actually suffer from fibromyalgia. Goldenberg's studies have shown that 70% of patients with chronic fatigue syndrome meet criteria for fibromyalgia. Indeed, the revised Centers for Disease Control and Prevention criteria include fibromyalgia in the definition of chronic fatigue syndrome, raising the question of whether a true distinction between patients with fibromyalgia and chronic fatigue syndrome is possible. Two discriminating features of chronic fatigue syndrome may be the history of an antecedent viral illness and the presentation of disease in the third decade of life, somewhat younger than the mean age of onset of fibromyalgia. The problem remains that in the absence of diagnostic clinical or laboratory tests, both syndromes are descriptive in nature.

The Centers for Disease Control and Prevention has published criteria for the diagnosis of chronic fatigue syndrome in an attempt to identify distinct cases. The two major criteria of chronic fatigue syndrome that must be met are as follows:

1. New onset of persistent or relapsing, debilitating fatigue in a person without a previous history of such symptoms that does not resolve with bed rest and that is severe enough to reduce or impair average daily activity to less than 50% of the patient's premorbid activity level for at least 6 months

2. Fatigue that is not explained by the presence of other evident medical or psychiatric illness

These major criteria, along with six or more symptoms and two or more signs listed in Table 55–4, need to be present to diagnose this condition.

REGIONAL PAIN SYNDROMES

Myofascial pain syndromes continue to be included in the discussion of chronic pain syndromes, although their definition varies from one of localized fibromyalgia to tension myalgia to any regional soft tissue pain disorder. What commonly identifies these disorders is the regional clustering of tender musculotendinous sites, with characteristic referral of pain into the tender area on palpation of the trigger points. Treatment is dependent on many of the same principles used in the treatment of fibromyalgia. Physical therapy, reassurance, workplace modification, and education about repetitive motion injury may be useful. Chiropractic care and acupuncture may have a role as well. The prognosis is contingent on many of the same factors that influence the outcome of fibromyalgia.

TABLE 55–4.   Clinical Features of Chronic Fatigue Syndrome

PHYSICAL SIGNS	SYMPTOMS
Low-grade fever	Mild fever or chills
Nonexudative pharyngitis	Sore throat
Palpable or tender anterior or posterior, cervical or axillary lymph nodes	Painful adenopathy (posterior or anterior, cervical or axillary)
	General muscle weakness
	Myalgias
	Prolonged generalized fatigue after previously tolerated levels of physical activity
	Generalized headaches
	Migratory arthralgia without swelling or redness
	Neuropsychological complaints
	Sleep disturbance
	Main symptom complex developing over a few hours to a few days

---

A cursory look at other forms of regional pain concludes this chapter. This includes carpal tunnel syndrome (hand pain), impingement syndrome and rotator cuff syndromes (shoulder pain), patellofemoral pain syndromes (knee pain), trochanteric bursitis (hip pain), and low back pain.

Carpal Tunnel Syndrome

Carpal tunnel syndrome is a common disorder caused by compression, irritation, or infiltration of the median nerve at the wrist. The entity is more common in women and frequently occurs bilaterally, often with no predisposing cause. Carpal tunnel syndrome is considered epidemic in the workplace, where overuse activities involving repetitive flexion at the wrist or repetitive pincer motion may precipitate this syndrome (see Chapter 75). It is also encountered in systemic disorders, such as diabetes mellitus, myxedema, amyloidosis, acromegaly, systemic lupus erythematosus, or rheumatoid arthritis. In women, a self-limited form of this disease presents during pregnancy and subsides after delivery (see Chapter 43).

Whatever the insult to the nerve as it passes through the bony canal of the wrist, the symptoms are a predictable consequence of median nerve dysfunction distal to this site. Patients complain of numbness and tingling in the thumb, the index and middle fingers, and sometimes the lateral aspect of the fourth finger. Nocturnal pain, pain radiating up into the proximal forearm, and some associated swelling in the fingers or wrist may be concomitant findings. Patients frequently show little evidence of intercurrent disease at presentation. The physical examination may reveal Tinel's sign (percussion over the median nerve at the wrist reproducing symptoms), Phalen's sign (complete flexion at the wrists for 30–60 seconds reproducing symptoms), or demonstrable sensory loss in the distribution of the median nerve; or the findings on examination may be benign. Evidence of thenar atrophy should be sought and noted if present.

Screening blood studies might include a complete blood count, Westergren sedimentation rate, urinalysis, thyroid function studies, and rheumatoid factor test, depending on the clinical picture. Unless thenar wasting is evident, conservative measures of splinting the wrist in the neutral position and nonsteroidal anti-inflammatory drugs are indicated. Electrophysiologic studies should be deferred unless surgery is being considered or the site of entrapment seems unclear. Refractory cases or those associated with other rheumatic complaints should be referred to a rheumatologist or orthopedist. When treated nonoperatively, a patient must be monitored for thenar atrophy or muscle weakness in the opponens or abductor of the thumb. These findings do constitute indications for surgery.

Shoulder Pain

The shoulder is a complex joint that derives its extensive range of motion from the shallow articular surface formed by the glenoid and the head of the humerus (Fig. 55–2). The head of the humerus is stabilized within the joint by the short rotator cuff muscles, and further dynamic stability and strength are provided by the overlying strap muscles of the shoulder girdle. Additional degrees of motion are provided by the articulation of the acromioclavicular joint and the movement of the scapula. Each or several of these sites may give rise to shoulder pain or contribute to loss of range of motion of the shoulder.

Shoulder pain is common. The differential may be divided among those processes affecting periarticular structures, those due to true lesions of the glenohumeral joint, and those due to referred pain. Some knowledge of the anatomy of the shoulder joint, coupled with a detailed history, helps guide the clinician in his or her physical examination and diagnosis.

Examination of a patient should be carried out with the patient's upper torso bared. Careful inspection for incongruities in muscle bulk, tone, and carrying angle of the shoulder can then be noted. Palpation of the articular margins of the shoulder, as well as the long head of the biceps and the subacromial bursa, may reveal point tenderness in bursitis or tendinitis. A painful arc of abduction or an impingement sign may be elicited. Cervical range of motion testing and a detailed neurologic examination are important components of this examination. Pain within a few degrees of passive range of motion suggests an intrinsic lesion of the glenohumeral joint. Table 55–5 outlines some distinguishing features of common shoulder conditions.

Plain radiographs are useful in defining abnormalities of bone, degenerative changes of the acromioclavicular or glenohumeral joint, and the presence of calcific tendinitis. Ultrasonography, magnetic resonance imaging, and arthrograms all have a role in the diagnosis of lesions of the shoulder, but the indications for each vary, as does the expertise in interpretation. Articular lesions should be referred to a rheumatologist or orthopedist, as should refractory shoulder pain. Bursitis or tendinitis is generally responsive to glucocorticoid injections (20 mg depot methylprednisolone) or non-steroidal anti-inflammatory drugs coupled with a graded physical therapy program. A precise diagnosis, education about movements that exacerbate the condition, reassurance about the benign nature of the lesion, and a reasonable exercise program all are indicated. Modifications in the workplace or time off from work may be appropriate. In a shoulder with full range of motion, without evident musculoskeletal findings, referred causes of shoulder pain should be remembered.

Patellofemoral Pain Syndromes (Chondromalacia Patellae)

Patellofemoral pain syndrome, including chondromalacia patellae, is a distinctive problem affecting the anterior compartment of the knee. Classically found in women more often than in men, it is characterized by knee discomfort that is exacerbated by going up and down stairs and by prolonged sitting. The pathogenesis of this disorder likely is inappropriate tracking of the patella within the patellofemoral groove. This may be associated with a high-riding patella, lateral subluxation of the patella, or other incongruities of the patellofemoral joint. Physical examination is remarkable for pain localized to the anterior portion of the knee, worsened by compression of the patella against the femoral condyles. Crepitance may be present, although the joint margins are generally nontender and typically no joint effusion is present. Therapy is based on strengthening the supportive muscles of the knee (especially the quadriceps and vastus medialis) and avoiding positions that overload the knee in a flexed position. Nonsteroidal anti-inflammatory drugs may be useful. Intra-articular glucocorticoids have no proven value. Refractory cases may be referred for orthopedic consultation.

Trochanteric Bursitis

Trochanteric bursitis is another common ailment that seems to affect women slightly more often than men and often presents in midlife or later. The chief complaint is pain in the hip. This pain is localized to the lateral aspect of the hip (Fig. 55–3) and may be aggravated by the patient's lying in bed, thus causing her to sleep on the unaffected side. Walking, too, may provoke the discomfort, which may extend down into the lateral thigh, resembling a lumbar radiculopathy. Because concurrent musculoskeletal disease is the rule (e.g., osteoarthritis of the lumbosacral spine, sciatica, or

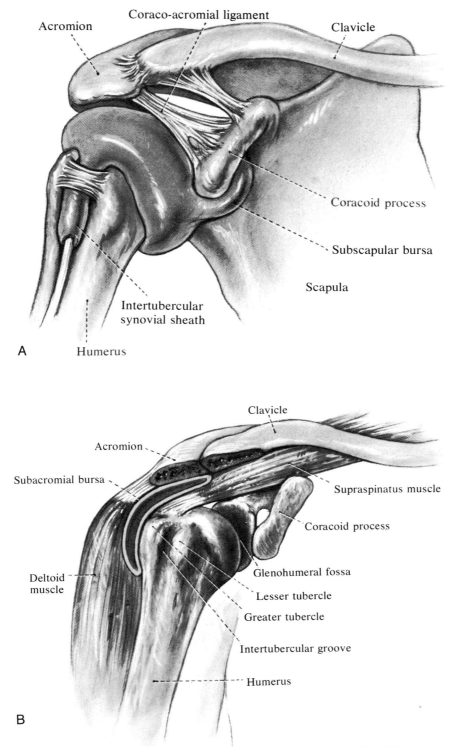

Figure 55–2. *A,* Anterior aspect of the shoulder joint showing the distribution of the distended synovial membrane of the glenohumeral joint and its relationship to adjacent bony structures. *B,* Anterior aspect of the shoulder joint showing palpable landmarks and their relationship to the subacromial bursa. (From Polley HF, Hunder GG. Rheumatologic Interviewing and Physical Examination of the Joints. 2nd ed. Philadelphia: WB Saunders, 1978, pp 62, 63.)

TABLE 55–5. Clinical Features of Common Painful Shoulder Conditions

CONDITION	CLINICAL FEATURES
Glenohumeral joint disorder	Generalized shoulder pain; crepitation or inflammatory signs; possible painful limitation in all planes including internal and external rotation.
Acromioclavicular and sternoclavicular joint disorders	Shoulder arc painful but limited only during mid to late range of abduction. Joint tender and prominent compared with contralateral side if separation, osteophytes, or effusion is present.
Referred shoulder pain from cervical area (e.g., C5 radicular pain from nerve root encroachment)	Shoulder motion shows painless complete arc: no specific periarticular shoulder tender point. Muscle spasm may be present. Neck rotation or neck compression testing may trigger radicular pain.
Subacromial bursitis and noncalcific supraspinatus tendinitis	Painful shoulder motion especially between 60 and 120 degrees of active abduction; tender subacromial region. Anesthetic subacromial infiltration can minimize pain during movement.
Bicipital tendinitis	Localized anterior shoulder pain over long head of biceps tendon with forearm supination. Tendon sheath is tender with thumb rolling. Shoulder motion normal.
Impingement syndrome	Impingement typically begins at 60 to 70 degrees and is maximum between 100 and 120 degrees of abduction. Recurrent pain from compression of subacromial tissue also occurs at 90 and 100 degrees of forward flexion.
Rotator cuff tear or rupture	After trauma in the young; abrupt pain and weak or absent active abduction. More gradual onset of pain and weakness with tears in older people. Anesthetic subacromial infiltration reduces pain, but absent or weak resisted abduction at 90 degrees persists. Small tears may mimic tendinitis symptoms.
Adhesive capsulitis (frozen shoulder)	Gradual onset of diffusely painful shoulder, markedly restricted passive *and* active motion in all planes.

From Medical Knowledge Self-Assessment Program (MKSAP). Rheumatology, 1993, p 192. Used by permission of S Karger AG, Basel.

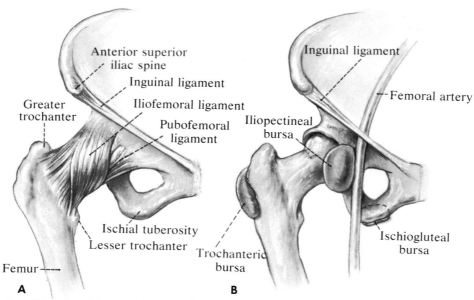

Figure 55–3. *A,* Diagram of the anterior aspect of the hip joint and adjacent bony structures. The fibers of the iliofemoral and pubofemoral ligaments fuse with those of the underlying articular capsule. The synovial membrane lines the inner surface of the articular capsule. *B,* Diagram of the relationship of distended iliopectineal, trochanteric, and ischiogluteal bursae to the hip joint and adjacent structures. (From Polley HF, Hunder GG. Rheumatologic Interviewing and Physical Examination of the Joints. 2nd ed. Philadelphia: WB Saunders, 1978, p 183.)

true arthritis of the hip joint), the history and clinical examination become important in identifying this bursal component of inflammation. Palpation of the trochanteric area discloses focal tenderness at rest, unrelated to movement of the lower extremity or lumbar spine. In severe cases, injection of glucocorticoids (40 mg depot methylprednisolone) locally, a walking and weight loss program, and reassurance are indicated.

Low Back Pain

It is estimated that 60 to 80% of adults suffer from low back pain at some time in their lives. Most of these cases improve in a week, 90% in a month. However, given the numbers of individuals involved, the loss of function and impaired mobility, and the individual distress, the socioeconomic consequences are staggering. Most of the cost of treating low back pain is incurred by the 7% of individuals who continue to suffer from chronic low back pain 6 months after the initial event. Nachemson reports in a review of the problem that ''psychosocial factors, including insurance benefits, have been demonstrated to be more important than biomechanical workload not only for acute but also for chronic low back pain patients who are unable to work.''

The etiology of much low back pain remains obscure. In the young, spondylolisthesis is implicated as a cause of low back pain, although the pathogenetic mechanisms by which this spinal instability causes pain is unclear. In the elderly, spinal stenosis often contributes to the syndrome of low back pain. More often than not, however, the objective findings are few or nonspecific. Serious lesions are precluded, and the diagnosis of muscle tenderness, facet arthritis, ligamentous instability, or strain is made. This diagnostic problem should besiege epidemiologists more than clinicians because the majority of low back pain conditions truly have benign outcomes.

Some women suffer from herniated intervertebral disks. These tend to be young people in their work years, ages 25 to 45 years. Many are involved in an occupation that requires lifting. In particular, nurses and nurses' aides who often lift while twisting (e.g., movements involved in repositioning a patient in bed) are at high risk for low back pain syndromes. Truck drivers and other laborers subject to constant vibration, perhaps exacerbated by the fixed position imposed by driving, are also subject to an increased frequency of low back pain and episodes of sciatica. The signs and symptoms of lumbar radiculopathy are noted in Table 55–6.

It is important in evaluating low back pain to observe the patient. The ease of moving from sitting to standing, the gait, and the unguarded face are useful diagnostic impressions. Listing, muscle spasm, and the use of alternate muscles to accomplish a simple movement about the shoulder all should be noted. Lumbar flexion, extension, and lateral flexion may be measured and the findings of the straight leg raising test documented. A detailed neurologic examination is required. As the physical examination dictates, special attention to the sacroiliac joints or hips may be useful.

Plain radiographs of the lumbosacral spine are reasonable in evaluating a person with low back pain, although in the absence of trauma they may be of low yield. This is particularly true in young women, who should be protected from unnecessary pelvic irradiation unless they have a history of trauma or some atypical presentation that suggests an abnormality diagnosable by radiographs. Computed tomographic scans or magnetic resonance imaging with or without myelography may be useful in those suspected of having bony lesions or disk herniations. Magnetic resonance imaging may offer more information if a soft tissue abnormality is suspected. Nerve conduction studies are useful in documenting a radiculopathy suspected on clinical grounds. All of these studies are expensive and time-consuming, however, and

---

TABLE 55–6.   Signs and Symptoms of Lumbar Radiculopathy

ROOT	PAIN NUMBNESS	SENSORY LOSS	MOTOR LOSS	REFLEX LOSS
L4	Anterior thigh and medial leg	Medial leg to medial malleolus	Anterior tibialis	Patellar
L5	Lateral leg and dorsum of the foot	Lateral leg and dorsum of the foot	Extensor hallucis longus	Posterior tibial
S1	Lateral foot	Lateral foot	Peroneus longus and brevis	Achilles reflex

From Medical Knowledge Self-Assessment Program (MKSAP). Rheumatology, 1993, p 190. Used by permission of S Karger AG, Basel.

some are invasive, and for the most part they should be ordered by a consulting orthopedist or neurosurgeon when surgery is being considered.

It needs to be stated again that the majority of low back pain syndromes resolve in 4 weeks no matter what therapy is prescribed. This should argue for prudence in diagnostic testing and the expectation of improvement. Six weeks of bed rest has not proved effective therapy for sciatica and tends to accentuate the physical deconditioning and depression often associated with loss of function. An aggressive, graded physical therapy program is indicated with consideration of a back-to-work rehabilitation program for manual laborers. Chiropractic therapy and acupuncture are alternative but unproven interventions. Nonsteroidal anti-inflammatory drugs, muscle relaxants, analgesics, ice or heat applied to the lumbar area, and low doses of benzodiazepines for severe cases of muscle spasm all are useful adjunctive therapies. Whatever is prescribed, some reassessment in 3 to 4 weeks in mandatory. Little evidence shows that protracted therapy offers any benefit to patients.

REFERENCES

Bennett RB. Fibrositis. In: Kelley WN, Harris ED Jr, Ruddy S, Sledge CB (eds). Textbook of Rheumatology. 3rd ed. Philadelphia: WB Saunders, 1989, pp 541–553.

Bennett RM. Fibromyalgia and the facts: Sense or nonsense. Rheum Dis Clin North Am 1993;19:45.

Block SR. Fibromyalgia and the rheumatisms: Common sense and sensibility. Rheum Dis Clin North Am 1993;19:61.

Goldenberg DL. A review of the role of tricyclic medications in the treatment of fibromyalgia syndrome. J Rheumatol 1989;16(Suppl A):137.

Goldenberg DL. Diagnostic and therapeutic challenges of fibromyalgia. Hosp Pract 1989;9A:39.

Goldenberg DL. Fibromyalgia and other chronic fatigue syndromes: Is there evidence for chronic viral disease. Semin Arthritis Rheum 1988;18:111.

Goldenberg DL. Fibromyalgia syndrome: An emerging but controversial condition. JAMA 1987;257:2782.

Goldenberg DL. Fibromyalgia, chronic fatigue and myofascial pain syndromes. Cur Opin Rheumatol 1992;4(2):247.

Greenfield S, Fitzcharles M, Esdaile JM. Reactive fibromyalgia syndrome. Arthritis Rheum 1992;35:678.

Hawley DJ, Wolfe F. Pain, disability, and pain/disability relationships in seven rheumatoid disorders: A study of 1522 patients. J Rheumatol 1991;18:1552.

Hudson JI, Goldenberg DL, Pope HG, et al. Comorbidity of fibromyalgia with medical and psychiatric disorders. Am J Med 1992;92:363.

Littlejohn CO. Fibrositis/fibromyalgia syndrome in the work place. Rheum Dis Clin North Am 1989;15(1):45.

McCain GA, Bell DA, Mai FM, Halliday PD. A controlled study of the effects of a supervised cardiovascular fitness training program on the manifestations of primary fibromyalgia. Arthritis Rheum 1988;31:1135.

Nachemson AL. Newest knowledge of low back pain: A critical look. Clin Orthop Rel Res 1992;279:8.

Polisson RP. Sports medicine for the internist. Med Clin North Am 1986;70:469.

Schluederberg A, Straus, SE, Peterson P, et al. Chronic fatigue syndrome research: Definition and medical outcome assessment. NIH Conference. Ann Intern Med 1992;117:325.

Simms RW, Felson DT, Goldenberg DL. Development of preliminary criteria for response to treatment in fibromylagia syndrome. J Rheumatol 1991;18:1558.

Smythe H. Fibrositis syndrome: A historical perspective. J Rheumatol 1989;16(Suppl 19):2.

Smythe HA. Nonarticular rheumatism and psychogenic musculoskeletal syndromes. In: McCarty DJ (ed). Arthritis and Allied Conditions. Philadelphia: Lea & Febiger, 1989, pp 1241–1254.

Wolfe F. Fibromyalgia in the elderly: Differential diagnosis and treatment. Geriatrics 1988;43:57.

Wolfe F. Fibromyalgia: The clinical syndrome. Rheum Dis Clin North Am 1989;15:1.

Wolfe F. Fibromyalgia. Rheum Dis Clin North Am 1990;16:681.

Yunus MB. Towards a model of pathophysiology of fibromyalgia: Aberrant central pain mechanisms with peripheral modulation. J Rheumatol 1992;19:846.

COMMON MEDICAL PROBLEMS IN WOMEN

56

Irritable Bowel Syndrome

Debra F. Weinstein

Irritable bowel syndrome (IBS) is a chronic or relapsing digestive disorder that affects approximately 15% of the population in developed countries.[1] It is manifested as disturbed bowel function, usually with associated abdominal pain and often with abdominal distention and a sense of incomplete evacuation. Extraintestinal manifestations may also be part of the symptom complex.

The cause of IBS is uncertain and is probably multifactorial. Abnormal gut motility and an increased perception of bowel distention are thought to be pathophysiologically important. Psychological factors have a role in symptom manifestation and health care seeking. In some patients, dietary and hormonal factors may be involved as well.

Although the disorder is usually chronic, it is generally not progressive and does not involve serious outcomes. The severity of symptoms is quite variable, however, and in a few patients may be disabling.

No reliable physiologic or structural testing has been devised for IBS, because no markers of the disorder have been identified. Attempts have been made to develop clinical criteria that would allow a positive diagnosis, but such efforts have had limited success. Evaluation of patients with suspected IBS is challenging: When the disorder is suggested by a characteristic constellation of symptoms, some testing for alternative diagnoses is often appropriate but must be applied judiciously.

Therapy is empirical and is developed on an individual basis, based on the predominant symptom. None of the many interventions studied has been convincingly demonstrated to confer benefit.

EPIDEMIOLOGY

Irritable bowel syndrome is frequently encountered in a primary care setting and accounts for between 2.4 and 3.5 million physician visits in the United States annually[2] and for nearly one half of patients referred to gastroenterologists.[3] Numerous epidemiologic studies have attempted to define the prevalence of IBS in the general population and in clinical populations (i.e., consumers of medical care). Results of these studies depend on the diagnostic criteria applied, which vary between investigations. Prevalence rates between 8 and 37% have been reported[4] and are highest in the 45- to 65-year-old age group.[2] One third[5] to one half[6] of those with symptoms of IBS present for medical care. Psychological factors play a part in determining which patients seek care,[7, 8] as does the presence of abdominal pain[6, 9]; data regarding whether age and the number of symptoms experienced are important determinants are conflicting.[5, 6]

Irritable bowel syndrome is generally thought to be more common in women, and most[2] but not all[10] epidemiologic studies have supported this observation. Heaton and colleagues found that IBS in a British community had a prevalence of 13% among women and 5% among men[6]; this correlates with Everhart and Renault's finding of a 2.4 to 1 female predominance in a survey of U.S. office practice.[4] The question of whether this represents an actual difference in disease prevalence or a higher rate of reporting among women has not been adequately studied. Women tend to be diagnosed at a younger age than men,[4] and female predominance is more marked before age 65 years.[2] A racial difference has also been noted: Pooled data from several large national health surveys show prevalence in whites to be fivefold higher than in blacks.[2]

CLINICAL PRESENTATION

Patients with IBS are heterogeneous with respect to their presenting complaints and the frequency and severity of symptoms. The syndrome is characterized by abdominal pain and disordered bowel function, involving diarrhea, constipation, or both. Any of these symptoms may be the dominant complaint. No universally accepted definition has been developed, but consensus panels have defined criteria for IBS[11, 12] that have greater utility in a research setting than in clinical practice.

The pain of IBS may be migratory or multicentric or may be fixed in any location within the abdomen. The left lower quadrant is most frequently involved.[13] The pain is usually intermittent and crampy in nature, although some patients describe continuous achy discomfort with periodic exacerbations. The abdominal pain of IBS is often relieved by defecation.

A history of alternating diarrhea and constipation is classic for IBS but is actually elicited in a minority of patients.[5] Often only diarrhea or constipation occurs, commonly associated with abdominal bloating or distention. Diarrhea may be described as loose or watery, and in some patients the complaint represents an increased frequency of apparently normal stools. Generally, the stool volume is not markedly increased. The complaint of constipation often reflects difficulty associated with bowel movements, including a sense of incomplete evacuation, with or without a significant decrease in the frequency of bowel movements. To a modest extent, the prevalence of specific symptoms may be age related: Urgency, incomplete evacuation, and straining to complete a bowel movement are reported more frequently in older than in younger women.[6]

The timing of symptoms in IBS is also variable. Symptoms may occur at night but generally do not awaken a patient from sleep. Patients often report that meals precipitate symptoms of pain or diarrhea, but in only a minority are specific offending foods identified. Emotional stress has a role in precipitating or exacerbating symptoms among a subset of patients.

Some studies have found that upper gastrointestinal symptoms such as dyspepsia, nausea, and vomiting are more common in patients with IBS than in healthy controls,[14, 15] although not all studies have upheld this association.[16] Extraintestinal symptoms including back pain, lethargy, headache, and urinary frequency are often associated with IBS.[17, 18] Sexual dysfunction and manifestations of autonomic dysfunction (e.g., diaphoresis, labile hypertension, syncope) have also been observed in patients with IBS.[5] The presence of these associated symptoms may help to distinguish IBS from other organic gastrointestinal disorders.[19]

The great variability in IBS has prompted investigators to examine whether or not a distinct syndrome as described does exist. Whitehead and colleagues found (in a study of women) that indeed bowel symptoms do cluster in a pattern consistent with this syndrome.[16]

ETIOLOGY

The etiology of IBS is not well understood and is probably multifactorial. There are several putative contributing factors.

Motor Abnormalities

Investigators have sought to determine whether patients with IBS have abnormalities in baseline intestinal motor or myoelectric function, abnormalities under certain circumstances (e.g., stress, hormonal stimulation, meal stimulation), or heightened visceral perception. Many abnormalities have been identified; some have been reproducible, but few have been shown to correlate with the symptoms of IBS.

Overall, no consistent basal motor abnormalities of the colon have been demonstrated.[20] Snape and co-workers reported a decreased frequency of slow wave contractions in diarrhea- and constipation-predominant patients with IBS versus normal controls,[21, 22] but subsequently this pattern was also observed in psychiatric patients without bowel symptoms.[23] Other investigators found a marked increase in high-amplitude pressure waves in patients with painful IBS and normal or decreased pressure waves in those with painless diarrhea.

Studies of small bowel motor function have demonstrated dysmotility in IBS under basal and stimulated conditions.[20, 24] Speed of small bowel transit seems to correlate with symptoms of diarrhea (faster than controls) or constipation-pain (slower than controls).[25] Some evidence also suggests that ileocecal transit and cecal distensibility may relate to symptoms in IBS.[20]

Patients with IBS have been found to have altered gut motility in response to stimulation with intravenous cholecystokinin,[26] colonic perfusion with deoxycholic acid,[27] and rectal or sigmoid distention.[28] The gastrocolonic response was also observed to be abnormal in IBS, in that patients may exhibit a delayed or blunted onset and prolonged occurrence of colonic motor activity.[22] Studies have yielded conflicting results in terms of whether stress induces abnormal motor responses in IBS, but most suggest that it does.[20] In some studies, stimulated abnormal motor responses have been accompanied by symptoms,[22, 29] and balloon distention at various sites including the colon, rectum, and small bowel has been shown to provoke typical symptoms in patients with IBS.[20]

Motor abnormalities noted in the waking state in patients with IBS disappear during sleep,[30] suggesting a pathophysiologic role for the central nervous system. A finding of increased proportion of rapid eye movement sleep in patients with IBS versus healthy controls is consistent with this hypothesis.[30a]

Abnormal visceral perception probably contributes to symptoms in IBS, along with altered motility. Several studies have noted a lower threshold for perception or discomfort relating to intestinal contraction or distention[31] in patients with IBS versus controls, but such findings have not always been reproducible.[32] This heightened visceral sensitivity does not seem to be part of a generalized decrease in pain threshold.[20]

In summary, it is likely that motor abnormalities of the small bowel or the colon combined with altered visceral perception contribute to symptoms in IBS.

Hormonal Factors

Progesterone appears to have several effects on gastrointestinal motility, including inhibition of colonic contractions. This may have a role in cyclic symptoms, as well as in the constipation apparent during pregnancy (especially in the second and third trimesters).[33]

It is not clear whether hormonally mediated changes in tone or motility account for the perception of increased bowel symptoms at the onset of menstruation, as reported in 34% of control women, 47% of patients with IBS, and 50% of nonpatients with symptoms of IBS.[34] Elevated levels of prostaglandin E_2 and $F_2\alpha$ in menstrual fluid present a potential but probably incomplete explanation.

An association between IBS and hysterectomy has been repeatedly observed. Women with IBS have a higher rate of hysterectomy than the national average (21% versus 5%).[34] This observation might suggest that surgery has been performed for undiagnosed pain or perhaps that surgery somehow induces or unmasks IBS. Because some patients attribute symptoms of IBS to a prior hysterectomy, a prospective study was performed to assess IBS symptoms preoperatively and postoperatively in a group of women undergoing hysterectomy.[35] Prior and colleagues found that preoperatively 22% of women had symptoms suggestive of IBS. After surgery, 33% of this group became symptom free, 27% improved, and 20% noted an increase in symptoms at 6 months. Ten percent of women who were asymptomatic preoperatively developed symptoms of IBS (at least once per week) after hysterectomy; most of these women had predominant constipation. Possible explanations include autonomic denervation of the distal colon during surgery, hormonal changes following oophorectomy, or decreased prostaglandins after hysterectomy.[35]

Luminal Factors

Luminal factors implicated in the pathophysiology of IBS include exogenous and endogenous components. Many patients and some physicians have suspected that symptoms of IBS may be precipitated by dietary factors, and numerous investigations have explored this possible relationship.

Adverse reactions to food can be categorized as food allergy (hypersensitivity) or food intolerance. Food allergy is probably a very infrequent cause of IBS-type symptoms in adults, more likely to occur in the diarrhea-predominant group and in atopic individuals, and the diagnosis may be difficult to pinpoint. Skin testing of food antigens can be used to assess for immediate hypersensitivity reactions, but a positive test result does not in itself confirm this diagnosis (a negative response, however, has a very high [approximately 99%] negative predictive value).[36, 37] A double-blind placebo-controlled food challenge (after a period of improvement on an elimination diet) remains the most convincing evidence.

Food intolerance, on the other hand, is quite common. Lactose intolerance (due to lactase deficiency and lactose malabsorption) is estimated to occur in 10 to 25% of whites and 45 to 80% of blacks in the United States; substantially higher rates are noted in Asians and African blacks.[38] The disorder can present with any combination of abdominal pain, diarrhea, flatulence, and distention. It can be symptomatically indistinguishable from IBS. Lactose intolerance can be easily distinguished from IBS, however, by history, an avoidance trial, and (if necessary) by performing a lactose hydrogen breath test or a lactose tolerance test. The extent to which lactose intolerance may cause or be mistaken for IBS is debated because of conflicting results in trials of exclusion diets.[39] Other food intolerances, although less prevalent, may be more likely to escape detection and be classified as IBS. Investigators have claimed that specific foods can reproduce symptoms in IBS patients and that a significant subset of patients with IBS achieve symptomatic benefit by food avoidance, but this claim is debated.[40]

A physiologic mechanism for the production of symptoms has been defined for some foods. Caffeine in doses of 75 to 300 mg per day causes net secretion in the jejunum and ileum in healthy subjects[3, 41]; in patients with IBS, 1000 mg or more of caffeine per day may cause diarrhea. Fructose and sorbitol have been studied for a potential etiologic role in IBS. As with lactose, malabsorption of these compounds can cause abdominal pain, bloating, and diarrhea.[42] These carbohydrates are found in fruits and other foods and are used in higher concentrations as artificial sweeteners in gum, soft drinks, and diabetic food substitutes. Malabsorption of the combination seems to occur with smaller amounts than with either component alone.[42] A controlled study[43] demonstrated that fructose-sorbitol malabsorption (as detected by a hydrogen breath test) is no more common in patients with IBS than in healthy controls; patients with IBS were, however, more likely to report symptoms during the test. It is important to note that a minority of patients in this study were of the diarrhea-predominant type.

Idiopathic bile acid malabsorption (i.e., occurring in the absence of ileal resection or disease) may be underdiagnosed as a cause of chronic diarrhea and may present with symptoms consistent with IBS.[44] Whether this is considered etiologic in a subset of diarrhea-predominant IBS patients or whether it is an independent (organic) diagnosis may be a matter of semantics.

An excess of short- or medium-chain fatty acids is less frequently sought or described as a cause of diarrhea but has been observed to cause colonic contraction. Further study is necessary to define a potential role in IBS.

Psychological Factors

Psychological factors may have a role at several levels in the expression and recognition of IBS, including the onset and exacerbation of symptoms, the perception of symptoms, and the reaction to symptoms, such as whether or not a patient seeks medical care.[7, 8] It has been postulated that the pathophysiologic connection between psychologi-

cal factors and the gut relates to the effect of acute psychological stress on gastrointestinal motility.[1]

Patients with IBS manifest certain psychological features more frequently than non-IBS controls, including hypochondriasis, depression, and hysteria.[7] Somatization, anxiety, hostility, phobia, and paranoia are also more common in patients with IBS. In fact, several studies have demonstrated that psychiatric diagnoses are made in a majority of patients with IBS.[8] Investigators have explored whether psychiatric diagnoses or anxiety-provoking situations preceded the onset of functional bowel disease and found that in a majority of patients they did.[45] Of note, a high prevalence of a history of sexual and physical abuse is found in women with functional gastrointestinal disorders, and this history is associated with increased symptom reporting.[46]

Drossman and associates[7] found that people who meet criteria for IBS but have not sought medical attention (i.e., nonpatients) are psychosocially closer to normals than to patients with IBS. They conclude that psychosocial factors previously associated with IBS are not part of the syndrome itself but rather characterize the subset of affected individuals who become patients. Thus, psychological factors are important in determining which patients will present for medical care.

DIAGNOSIS

Manning's Criteria

The goal of patient evaluation is to arrive at a diagnosis using the fewest diagnostic tests with the least risk and the lowest cost. Unfortunately, IBS has no pathognomonic clinical feature, and because no structural or biochemical defect has been identified, no specific diagnostic test is available. Thus, IBS has traditionally been considered a diagnosis of exclusion.

In a landmark study published in 1978, Manning and colleagues began to focus attention on a positive diagnosis of IBS, based on clinical (historic) features.[47] The investigators studied a group of 109 patients presenting with complaints of abdominal pain, constipation, or diarrhea. The patients were asked about the presence or absence of 15 other symptoms that might be helpful in diagnosing IBS. Among the 106 patients assessed 17 to 26 months later, 14 were excluded because of diverticular disease, 32 were diagnosed with IBS, and 33 had organic disease defined. Chi-squared analysis showed that patients with IBS were more likely to have (1) visible abdominal distention, (2) pain relief with bowel movements, (3) more frequent stools with the onset of pain, and (4) looser stools with the onset of pain, compared with patients with organic disease. Ninety-one percent of the patients with IBS (versus 30% of those with organic disease) had two or more of these symptoms. Two other symptoms, the passage of mucus and a sensation of incomplete evacuation, were more common in patients with IBS. Although the difference was not statistically significant, these additional symptoms are often considered part of Manning's criteria. The researchers acknowledged that these criteria are relevant only to the subset of patients with painful IBS, because three of four defining symptoms involve abdominal pain. Despite methodologic flaws, this study was helpful in beginning to define clinical criteria for the diagnosis.[47]

Other investigators have sought to validate and refine Manning's criteria. Thompson reported that Manning's criteria distinguished IBS from peptic ulcer disease but were less reliable in distinguishing IBS from inflammatory bowel disease.[48] Smith and colleagues[49] investigated whether six psychosocial factors (anxiety, depression, stress, lack of social support, somatization, and abnormal illness behavior) often noted in patients with IBS were helpful in distinguishing IBS from organic disease, and found that they were not.

Talley and associates[50] assessed the value of Manning's criteria in distinguishing IBS from health, from nonulcer dyspepsia, and from organic disease. They found that, as expected, the presence of at least three of six of Manning's criteria identified painful IBS more reliably than the painless subgroup (sensitivity of 61 versus 19%); no significant difference in sensitivity was noted between diarrhea and constipation-predominant subgroups. In this study, the symptom of loose or watery stools (at least 25% of the time) improved the discrimination when added to the other criteria. The researchers found that the more Manning's criteria that were present, the greater the likelihood of IBS. The predictive value was greatest in younger patients and in women. Overall, the sensitivity and specificity of Manning's criteria in discriminating IBS from organic gastrointestinal disease were 58% and 74% and were 65% and 86% in identifying IBS from among healthy controls.

Another study found that Manning's criteria correlated with the presence of IBS overall and in the subgroup of women. Notably, however, no correlation was found in men with IBS.[49]

Although Manning's criteria remain useful, at least in women, their sensitivity and specificity are not adequate to use these criteria as a sole diagnostic tool. Kruis and colleagues evaluated a scoring system incorporating selected symptoms assessed by patient questionnaire (e.g., bowel irregularity, flatulence, and abdominal pain), physical examination findings, and simple laboratory data (hemoglobin, white blood cell count, and erythrocyte sedimentation rate). The investigators reported a specificity of 99% using a cutoff of sensitivity at 64%.[51] Although this low sensitivity would lead to one third of patients with IBS having additional tests to preclude organic disease, the high specificity indicates that few patients would receive a false diagnosis of IBS using these criteria. This scoring system has not been widely accepted. Further prospective validation is necessary to help define its usefulness. At least one other tool, a 46-symptom bowel disease questionnaire, has been developed and is reported to distinguish between functional and organic gastrointestinal disease,[52, 53] but this too lacks extensive validation and is likely to prove more useful in research than in clinical settings.

Initial Evaluation of Suspected Irritable Bowel Syndrome

Manning's criteria and other features are helpful in suggesting IBS and in assessing the pretest probability of this diagnosis (Table 56–1), but almost all patients warrant some degree of testing. It is important, however, that a strategy of ruling out organic disorders with symptoms that may overlap those of IBS be undertaken judiciously. No single list of differential diagnoses applies to all patients. Specific diagnoses should be entertained as suggested by an individual's symptoms and the clinical setting.

In all patients, the primary evaluation of IBS consists of a careful history and physical examination, along with a few selected tests (phase I— Table 56–2). During the interview, it is important to ascertain the duration, frequency, and associations of symptoms, with careful questioning about

---

TABLE 56–1.   Features Suggestive of Irritable Bowel Syndrome

- Abdominal pain associated with defecation (relieved or exacerbated by bowel movements or relieved by flatus)
- Abdominal pain precipitated by meals
- Onset of pain correlated with a change in stools (usually looser and more frequent)
- Sense of incomplete evacuation
- Passage of mucus per rectum
- Sense of bloating with or without visible abdominal distention
- Long duration of symptoms with a fairly consistent pattern

TABLE 56–2. Evaluation of Irritable Bowel Syndrome: Phase I

History, with emphasis on:
  Specific symptom characterization
  ?Presence of symptoms incompatible with irritable bowel
    syndrome
  Diet (including lactose, fructose, sorbitol, caffeine, ethanol;
    ?specific symptom precipitants)
  Medications
  Prior abdominal surgery
  Family history

Physical examination, with special attention to:
  Abdominal examination
  Rectal examination
  Pelvic examination

Laboratory:
  Complete blood count
  Erythrocyte sedimentation rate
  Depending on symptoms: liver function tests, amylase
  Fecal occult blood testing

Other testing:
  Lactose avoidance trial for diarrhea or pain/bloating/
    flatulence
  Flexible sigmoidoscopy, with biopsy for diarrhea; may
    defer in young women without diarrhea
  Stool ova and parasites if diarrhea is present
  Consider barium enema or colonoscopy in older (>50 yr)
    patients with new onset of constipation
  Phenolphthalein test if suspicious of surreptitious laxative
    use in patient with diarrhea
  Metabolic evaluation (see text) if indicated based on history
    and physical examination
  Human immunodeficiency virus testing in patients who
    have diarrhea and are at risk

potential foods (especially artificial sweeteners, high-lactose foods, caffeine, and alcohol) or emotional precipitants. A careful medication history is important because IBS symptoms can occur as adverse effects of medication, and a history of abdominal surgery is certainly relevant. It is also important to have patients detail which, if any, therapies have been tried previously in response to the symptoms. Features incompatible with IBS should be specifically sought: Weight loss, fever, anorexia, occult or clinical gastrointestinal bleeding, and diarrhea or pain that awakens a patient from sleep are not explained by IBS. The onset of symptoms in later life is not incompatible with a diagnosis of IBS, but it is uncommon and should increase the index of suspicion for organic disorders. A family history of colorectal neoplasm, inflammatory bowel disease, or other gastrointestinal illness may be useful in assessing a patient's risk of organic disease. In addition, it is useful to gain perspective about a patient's concerns regarding the symptoms and her coping strategies. Recent emotional stress or evidence of an affective disorder may have relevance to the gastrointestinal complaints.

A thorough physical examination should be performed so that clues to possible alternative diagnoses (e.g., hypothyroidism causing constipation) are not overlooked. Particular attention should be paid to the abdominal examination; organomegaly, a mass, or shifting dullness suggesting ascites would suggest organic disease. Patients with constipation should have a careful assessment of sphincter tone and strength of voluntary contraction; rectal prolapse should be sought during a Valsalva maneuver. Perianal sensation can be checked and an "anal wink" reflex elicited. Stool guaiac tests are an important adjunct to the physical examination. Whether guaiac testing should be done at the office visit (risking dietary false positives) or through mail-in cards (risking noncompliance or delay-dependent false negatives) is controversial. Findings inconsistent with IBS (Table 56–3) should prompt investigation for an alternative unifying diagnosis or an additional (intermediate) diagnosis, such as hemorrhoids or fissures causing hematochezia in a patient with constipation, or depression leading to weight loss.

Simple laboratory tests, including a complete blood count, erythrocyte sedimentation rate, and (in some patients) liver function tests should be

TABLE 56–3. Elements Suggestive of Organic Disease

HISTORY	PHYSICAL EXAMINATION	LABORATORY
Bleeding	Fecal occult blood	Anemia
Weight loss	Cachexia	Leukocytosis
Fever	Fever	Elevated erythrocyte sedimentation
Nocturnal symptoms	Ascites	rate
Large-volume diarrhea	Abdominal mass	(Laboratory test results are normal in
Diarrhea persists with fast		patients with irritable bowel
Progressive course		syndrome)
Abrupt change in symptoms		

part of the initial evaluation. Almost all patients warrant flexible sigmoidoscopy (with biopsy if chronic diarrhea is prominent) to evaluate for possible inflammation or a structural abnormality. The occasional finding of melanosis coli may also be helpful as a reflection of significant cathartic use or abuse. In selected patients, additional tests may be indicated as part of the initial evaluation (see Table 56–2). Abnormal laboratory values or endoscopic-radiologic test results should be pursued appropriately. Further investigation is guided by the predominant symptom (Tables 56–4 to 56–6), the specific findings on presentation, and the clinical setting (i.e., age and family history), which help determine the risk of serious disease.

Differential Diagnosis and Further Diagnostic Evaluation

In pursuing this approach, no single list of differential diagnoses applies to all patients. Specific diagnoses should be entertained as suggested by an individual patient's symptoms and the clinical setting (see Tables 56–4 to 56–6). In many patients—especially young women, with a low suspicion of organic disease—a tentative diagnosis can be made without further testing, subject to the outcome of a therapeutic trial. In others, when the diagnosis remains uncertain at this stage or when a therapeutic trial is unsuccessful, more extensive evaluation may be necessary.

To a large extent, the differential diagnosis relates to the chief complaint, although there is certainly overlap (e.g., many disorders can cause both abdominal pain and diarrhea). In patients with predominant diarrhea, infectious causes (particularly parasites, likely to be chronic), lactose intolerance, inflammatory bowel disease, bile salt or other causes of malabsorption (such as sprue, bacterial overgrowth, etc.), collagenous or microscopic colitis and possible neoplasm should be considered. Endocrine causes of diarrhea are also possible. Thus, stool examination for ova and parasites (arguably stool culture and sensitivity tests) and *Clostridium difficile* toxin assay if a patient has a history of antibiotic therapy are indicated in most patients. Chronic nonbloody diarrhea has an extremely broad differential diagnosis that is not reviewed here; in a minority of patients, further testing is necessary (see Table 56–4), and in such cases a gastroenterology consultation may be helpful.

Patients with a complaint of constipation may fulfill several of Manning's criteria (such as abdominal pain, bloating, and a sense of incomplete evacuation) and appear to have IBS; however,

TABLE 56–4. Evaluation of Diarrhea-Predominant Irritable Bowel Syndrome (Initial History, Physical Findings, and Laboratory Results Unrevealing)

Evaluation: Phase II
(If not yet done)
- Inspection of stool for leukocytes
- Stool ova and parasites 3 times
- Stool culture and sensitivity tests and *Clostridium difficile* toxin assay, if applicable
- Flexible sigmoidoscopy with biopsy
- Lactose-avoidance trial
- Phenolphthalein test (if laxative abuse suspected)
In addition:
- Thyroid function tests (rule out hyperthyroidism)
- Stool collection to document high output; if positive, repeat with 24–48 hr fast

Evaluation: Phase III
(the sequence and tests selected relate to the individual presentation, likelihood of various diagnoses, and availability of testing)
- Further evaluation for malabsorption: albumin, iron/total iron-binding capacity, vitamin B_{12}, carotene, folate; Sudan stain of stool for fat
  Consider: d-xylose test and/or 72-hr fecal fat
- String test or duodenal aspirate for *Giardia* (vs. empirical trial of metronidazole if suspicion is high)
- Small bowel barium study (for ?short gut, blind loop, Crohn's, lymphoma, mucosal disease)
- Endoscopy with small bowel biopsy (for ?sprue, Whipple's disease, and so forth if suspected) and jejunal aspirate for ova and parasites
- Therapeutic trial of cholestyramine
- Further endocrinologic evaluation if indicated (e.g., urine 5-hydroxyindoleacetic acid for ?carcinoid, thyroid scan/calcitonin for ?medullary carcinoma of the thyroid, gastrin for ?Zollinger-Ellison syndrome, cortisol and electrolytes for ?Addison's, vasoactive intestinal polypeptide for VIP-oma)
- Consider barium enema or colonoscopy (? neoplasm, Crohn's, fistula, other)

these symptoms all may be attributable to constipation.[54] Such patients often have complete resolution of symptoms when the constipation is adequately treated. They probably do not have the same underlying pathophysiology as others with more diverse symptoms of IBS. Neoplasm, intestinal pseudo-obstruction, and pelvic floor dysfunction are differential diagnostic considerations in patients with severe or refractory constipation; metabolic causes such as hypothyroidism and hypercalcemia are other possibilities. Although a flexible sigmoidoscopy is usually indicated, it may be unnecessary in a young woman who responds promptly to a therapeutic trial. Older patients or those with refractory symptoms generally warrant a barium enema or colonoscopy to preclude neoplastic disease. Metabolic assays (thyroid-stimulating hormone, calcium) may be part of the initial evaluation if historic clues or physical findings

TABLE 56–5.   Evaluation of Constipation-Predominant Irritable Bowel Syndrome (Initial Evaluation Unrevealing, Including Flexible Sigmoidoscopy)

Evaluation: Phase II

Age >50* and/or
(1) significant family history of colorectal neoplasm
or (2) features suggestive of organic disease
Barium enema (or colonoscopy);
if negative—
Thyroid function; serum calcium;
lead level if at risk;
if negative—
Therapeutic trial;
if unsuccessful—
Radiopaque marker study†

Age <50*
Flexible sigmoidoscopy, if not yet done
Therapeutic trial;
if unsuccessful—
Thyroid function; serum calcium;
lead level if at risk;
if negative—
Barium enema;
if negative—
Radiopaque marker study†

*Some authorities recommend visualizing the colon in patients older than 40 years.
†If normal, no further evaluation; if abnormal, further study as noted in text.

suggest a particular disorder. An algorithm for the second phase of evaluation in constipation-predominant patients is proposed in Table 56–5.

Patients with severe refractory constipation and no structural abnormality on sigmoidoscopy and barium enema (or colonoscopy) require further evaluation. Metabolic causes of constipation should be sought if not investigated previously. Other testing can be pursued to assess intestinal transit and, if it is delayed, to determine whether the problem is one of colonic inertia or outlet obstruction. A colonic transit study using radiopaque markers is simple to accomplish. It may well demonstrate normal transit in a patient complaining of constipation. If results are abnormal, it can demonstrate segmental or diffuse delay or normal passage to the rectum with accumulation of markers there. Further evaluation with anorectal manometry, defacography, or electromyography can better define the abnormality and guide proper therapy. Again, a gastroenterologic consultation may be helpful in selected patients.

When pain is the prominent symptom, biliary disease, peptic ulcer disease, inflammatory bowel disease, diverticular disease, and neoplasm are important considerations. Chronic pancreatitis may rarely be mistaken for IBS; if it is not suggested by history, pancreatic enzyme abnormalities or pancreatic calcification on an abdominal radiograph can lead to the diagnosis. Liver disease is usually distinguished from IBS by history or physical examination and—if not—would be apparent on laboratory examination. In Manning and colleagues' original series,[47] the patients found to have an organic cause of abdominal pain (with or without disturbed bowel function) were found to have peptic ulcer (46%), inflammatory bowel disease (15%), gastroesophageal reflux (12%), gallstones (6%), colon carcinoma (6%), and miscellaneous gastrointestinal disorders (15%).

Some clinical examples may be helpful. A woman who has episodic diarrhea and abdominal bloating with symptoms related to food or meals should have a lactose avoidance trial (or lactose

TABLE 56–6.   Phase II Evaluation of Abdominal Pain: Selected Diagnostic Considerations

SYMPTOM	SUSPECTED DIAGNOSIS	TEST
Distinct episodes of RUQ or epigastric pain; may awaken from sleep	Gallstones/biliary pain	RUQ ultrasonography
Epigastric location; relieved by meals	Peptic disease	Upper endoscopy or upper gastrointestinal series
Protracted episodes of LLQ pain; fever or leukocytosis	Diverticulitis	Barium enema or colonoscopy (not during acute episode)
Nausea/vomiting; abdominal distention	Obstruction	Abdominal plain film and upright
Epigastric/LUQ pain	Chronic pancreatitis	Plain abdominal radiograph (?calcification); pancreatic enzymes; ?endoscopic retrograde cholangiopancreatography
Elderly; vascular disease; diarrhea and weight loss	Mesenteric ischemia	Angiography
Dark urine; personality change	Acute intermittent porphyria	Porphyria screen
With constipation; lead exposure	Lead poisoning	Serum lead level

RUQ, Right upper quadrant; LLQ, left lower quadrant; LUQ, left upper quadrant.

hydrogen breath test) to assess the possibility of lactose intolerance. She should also undergo stool examinations for ova and parasites to look, in particular, for *Giardia*—especially in cases of a known potential exposure (e.g., work in a daycare center). Laboratory findings suggesting malabsorption should prompt evaluation for specific causes, such as sprue.

A woman whose pain tends to occur in the right upper quadrant or epigastrium, possibly with radiation to the back, should be investigated for gallstones or peptic ulcer disease, depending on other features of the history and physical examination findings. If gallstones are present, given their high prevalence, it may still be difficult to determine whether symptoms are due to biliary colic or to IBS.

The importance of clinical setting is easily illustrated by the example of a 65-year-old woman who presents with abdominal pain and a change in bowel habits and whose family history is notable for a primary relative with colon cancer. The threshold to pursue a colonoscopy (or barium enema and flexible sigmoidoscopy) in this patient certainly would be much lower than in a 25 year old with no risk factors for neoplasm—despite identical symptoms and physical examination findings.

It should be emphasized that because IBS is common, it may certainly coexist with other disorders, or a second problem may be superimposed on a background of chronic IBS. For this reason, it is important to be alert to changes in symptoms that are sudden, unexplained, or inconsistent with the diagnosis. Although limiting the initial work-up is usually reasonable, it may be appropriate to undertake further testing at a later time. However, repeating the evaluation periodically without a change in clinical findings (which are by definition chronic or recurrent) is not indicated.

THERAPEUTIC INTERVENTIONS

A wide variety of therapeutic approaches have been claimed to benefit patients with IBS. Drug trials have included antispasmodic agents such as mebeverine and trimebutine, anticholinergic-barbiturate combinations, antidepressants, tranquilizers, dopamine antagonists, carminatives (peppermint oil), opioids, and bulking agents (psyllium, wheat bran, ispaghula).[55] Psychotherapy, biofeedback, and exclusion diets have also been studied as treatments for IBS. Unfortunately, despite the large number of published studies, effectiveness has not been convincingly demonstrated for any intervention.[55] Several problems plague the IBS

literature. First, no objective measurements of improvement have been devised. Various symptoms scales or subjective patient assessments are used. Second, given the variability of IBS manifestations and severity, nonrandomized controlled studies are suspect and randomized studies must be interpreted in light of the entry criteria, because they may be applicable to only certain subgroups of patients with IBS. Heterogeneity within IBS may also explain the lack of proven benefit of several therapies commonly used with a high degree of anecdotal success in individual patients. Studies failing to show a benefit in a broad spectrum of patients with IBS might have efficacy if studied in the symptom subset most likely to respond. Finally, studies that are not placebo controlled must be interpreted with care in light of the high rate of placebo response (up to 84% [56]) in IBS.

Therapy in IBS is directed at controlling symptoms. Because no single therapy has been proved to have overall efficacy in IBS and because the symptoms are quite variable, an individualized approach is appropriate. Therapeutic trials should be selected on the basis of the predominant complaint and modified according to the symptomatic response. In general, drug therapy should be held in reserve until other methods have failed, because the condition is chronic, cost and side effects are deterrents, and high placebo response rates may be misleading.

Predominant Constipation

Treatment is most straightforward in patients with constipation. Fiber supplementation is a mainstay of therapy. Dietary fiber can be classified as soluble (including psyllium) or insoluble (contained in many cereals and whole grains). Fiber can increase stool volume by (1) holding water on its hydrophilic sites (especially soluble), (2) increasing bacterial proliferation associated with fermentation of fibers, and (3) adding to the volume of indigestible material (especially insoluble); the increased distention from greater stool bulk stimulates peristalsis and decreases transit time. Through its gel-forming capacity, fiber also serves to lubricate the stool.[57]

Fiber supplementation with bran (e.g., unprocessed miller's bran beginning at a dose of 1 tablespoon one to three times per day) or a bulking agent such as psyllium (3–4 gm one to three times per day) with adequate fluid intake is often efficacious in mild constipation. Patients should be cautioned that bloating or distention may occur (or worsen) for the first 1 to 2 weeks after initiation of therapy and usually resolves thereafter. This effect may be mitigated by beginning with a modest dose and increasing gradually; 30 gm of fiber per day may be necessary to achieve benefit. If constipation is severe, fiber supplementation should follow an initial enema clean-out.

Nonresponders may benefit from the addition of stool softeners (such as docusate salts) or osmotic cathartics (e.g., magnesium citrate, mixed electrolyte solutions, lactulose). Stimulant laxitives should be avoided as a long-term approach. Cisapride, a prokinetic agent, has become widely available, and its role in treating constipation will be defined with further experience. Behavioral approaches including habit training and biofeedback may be appropriate in selected patients. Rare patients with colonic inertia require surgery.

Abdominal pain accompanying constipation frequently responds to the successful treatment of constipation and in most cases should not be specifically treated until the constipation is under control.

Predominant Diarrhea

As previously noted, patients with diarrhea warrant an early therapeutic trial of lactose avoidance; other exclusion diets may be indicated on the basis of a careful history and review of a symptom diary. In the setting of a negative diagnostic evaluation (and in part as further evaluation), other therapeutic trials can be pursued. These might include a course of metronidazole for the possibility of giardiasis (250 mg three times a day for 7 days), unless it has been ruled out by a string test or duodenal aspirate, and a trial of cholestyramine (4 gm two to four times a day) for possible idiopathic bile salt malabsorption.

Patients with diarrhea due to IBS often benefit from bulk-forming agents (see the previous section on therapy for constipation). If this is unsuccessful, then loperamide (2–4 mg as needed, not to exceed 8 mg per day) can be used to diminish symptoms of frequency, loose stools, and abdominal cramping[58] after organic disease has been satisfactorily precluded. Diphenoxylate is an alternative but is likely to have more frequent systemic side effects. Anticholinergics may occasionally be helpful in treating the diarrhea of IBS.

Predominant Pain

Nondrug therapy of abdominal pain in IBS is preferable and can be successful in a significant proportion of patients. Specific exclusion diets are helpful if offending foods can be identified. Patients who have pain associated with bloating or flatulence may respond to measures aimed at reducing intestinal gas. These include (1) avoidance of gas-producing foods, such as legumes and cabbage, and (2) minimizing air swallowing by avoiding carbonated beverages, smoking, and gum chewing and by eating slowly. In addition, simethicone, activated charcoal, or oral microbial α-galactosidase (Beano) can be tried, although they do not confer predictable benefit.

The use of psychological therapy is discussed next. When antidepressants are prescribed for IBS, low-dose therapy with gradual increase as needed is appropriate. It is important to note that tricyclics may cause or exacerbate constipation.

In patients with postprandial pain, when heightened visceral perception and an abnormal gastrocolic reflex may be playing a part, low doses of anticholinergics (e.g., begin at 7.5 mg of propantheline bromide or 10 mg of dicyclomine 30–60 minutes before meals and adjust to individual patient needs) may relieve symptoms.[59] Combined tranquilizer-anticholinergic agents have also had anecdotal success. When anxiolytics are necessary, they should be used only for brief periods.

As noted earlier, when pain and constipation coexist, constipation should be treated before approaching therapy directed at abdominal pain.

Psychological Treatments

Several psychological approaches have been studied in IBS, including pharmacotherapy (with antidepressants or anxiolytics), psychotherapy, hypnotherapy, and behavioral therapy. Antidepressant medications have been demonstrated to have some success in patients with pain and/or diarrhea, but whether they confer a statistically significant benefit is debated.[60] It is not clear whether improvement on antidepressants is attributable to a reduction in psychological symptoms (which was noted to occur) mediated by the antidepressant effects or through direct antimuscarinic effects on bowel motility.[60]

Trials of psychotherapy for IBS have produced some encouraging results,[61] although once again the mechanism of improvement is not entirely clear. A controlled trial demonstrated benefit in patients refractory to medical therapy; patients with overt psychiatric symptoms and those with stress-induced symptom episodes were most likely to benefit.[62] It is important to consider that a long duration of treatment may be necessary before improvement is noted and that this approach is costly. Psychotherapy is appropriate for patients in whom an independent psychiatric diagnosis is evident or in whom significant psychological issues accompany refractory IBS.[60]

Hypnotherapy is an interesting approach to IBS that has undergone limited study, showing some benefit in patients with refractory symptoms.[63] Behavioral therapy, including relaxation training, group therapy, and biofeedback, has been assessed in small, mostly uncontrolled trials, and further research is needed to define its role.

Overall, psychological approaches to the treatment of IBS are appropriate to pursue in patients who have not responded to other measures (especially in the setting of predominant pain) and those who manifest overt psychiatric symptoms. Antidepressant therapy probably has the largest role.

Finally, the importance of the therapeutic relationship must be emphasized. Patients with IBS are facing a chronic, possibly lifelong disorder whose etiology is poorly understood and whose therapy may be a series of best guesses, all without any guarantee of success. Intensive efforts at patient education are an important component of therapy for every patient with IBS. Patients may draw comfort from understanding that IBS is a recognized disorder, that it is common, and that a number of nonsurgical therapeutic alternatives may be used in order to arrive at a program that maximally controls symptoms. Drawing out, acknowledging, and addressing patients' fears about underlying organic disease, progression to malignancy, and so forth are a key part of the interaction. In fact, it has been suggested that the high placebo response rate in IBS is attributable to the doctor-patient relationship.[60]

It is also important to help patients achieve realistic expectations and understand that IBS is a chronic or relapsing condition. Failure to respond to an initial treatment plan (or failure to respond completely to any treatment plan) does not negate the diagnosis. Reassurance is an important component of therapy in this disorder.

PROGNOSIS

Few investigators have systematically assessed the long-term prognosis in patients diagnosed with IBS.[13, 64, 65] Harvey and colleagues obtained follow-up after a mean of 5.6 years on 97 of 104 sequential patients treated at a gastroenterology clinic. Patients in this group had been initially treated with a bulking agent, a high-fiber diet, and a brief course of an antispasmodic. The results demonstrate that at first follow-up (5–9 weeks after the initial visit), 31% were symptom free and 27% were considerably improved. Six months after the initial visit, 83% were asymptomatic or had minor

symptoms. At 5 to 7 years of follow-up, 68% were asymptomatic or had only occasional minor symptoms. Factors predicting a better response to therapy included (1) male sex, (2) a short duration of symptoms, (3) predominant constipation, (4) bowel disturbance beginning in the setting of an acute illness, and (5) a good initial response to therapy. It is interesting to note that in no patient was the diagnosis of IBS revised.[13]

An earlier study found that only 12% of IBS sufferers had improved at 12-month follow-up.[64] Differences between these findings may in part relate to the populations under study and the methods used. It is likely, however, that we have become better at correctly identifying patients with IBS and are now able to achieve durable symptomatic improvement in most patients with flexible application of various interventions.

When patients do respond to therapy, a question arises about the optimal duration of treatment. This has not been well studied, but at least one small, nonblinded controlled trial has assessed the role of maintenance therapy in IBS.[66] Misra and co-workers randomized IBS sufferers who had become asymptomatic on an anticholinergic drug plus a bulking agent to continued therapy versus placebo, and they assessed symptoms at monthly intervals. After 4 months, a significantly greater proportion of patients taking a placebo had become symptomatic, and the majority of these had resolution when therapy was reinstituted. These results suggest that maintenance therapy reduces the likelihood of symptom recurrence, and therefore it seems reasonable to continue therapies that are well tolerated and inexpensive (such as dietary modification and bulking agents). Because most recurrences can be effectively treated, however, one should consider discontinuing (or using only as needed) most drug treatments after achieving a prolonged symptom-free period.

SUMMARY

Irritable bowel syndrome remains a challenging disorder to recognize, identify, and treat. In women, who are affected more frequently than men, the diagnosis is more likely to be made earlier in life and the symptoms may be more difficult to control. A combination of abnormal gut motility, abnormal visceral perception, hormonal factors, luminal factors, and psychological profile may be etiologically important.

An algorithm for patient evaluation has been proposed here as a general guide, but the approach to each patient clearly must be individualized in light of the great heterogeneity of this disorder. Likewise, therapy is tailored to the individual, based on the specific symptoms, and often involves a series of therapeutic trials. Detailed reviews of the evaluation of diarrhea, constipation, or abdominal pain may be helpful and are available elsewhere. Consultation with a gastroenterologist may be of benefit for patients in whom the diagnosis is unclear or response to therapy is unsatisfactory.

Although IBS presents challenges and frustrations for both physicians and patients, its successful management can be rewarding and in fact can be achieved in the great majority of patients.

REFERENCES

1. Almy T, Rothstein R. Irritable bowel syndrome: Classification and pathogenesis. Annu Rev Med 1987;38:257.
2. Sandler R. Epidemiology of irritable bowel syndrome in the United States. Gastroenterology 1990;99:409.
3. Bayless TM, Harris ML. Inflammatory bowel disease and irritable bowel syndrome. Med Clin North Am 1990;74(1):21.
4. Everhart J, Renault P. Irritable bowel syndrome in office-based practice in the United States. Gastroenterology 1991;100(4):998.
5. Jones R, Lydeard S. Irritable bowel syndrome in the general population. Br Med J 1992;304:87.
6. Heaton KW, O'Donnell LJ, Braddon FE, et al. Symptoms of irritable bowel syndrome in a British urban community: Consulters and nonconsulters. Gastroenterology 1992;102:1962.
7. Drossman D, McKee DC, Sandler RS, et al. Psychosocial factors in the irritable bowel syndrome. A multivariate study of patients and nonpatients with irritable bowel syndrome. Gastroenterology 1988;95(3):701.
8. Smith RC, Greenbaum DS, Vancouver JB, et al. Psychosocial factors are associated with health care seeking rather than diagnosis in irritable bowel syndrome. Gastroenterology 1990;98:293.
9. Sandler RS, Drossman DA, Nathan HP, McKee DC. Symptom complaints and health care seeking behavior in subjects with bowel dysfunction. Gastroenterology 1984;87:314.
10. Talley NJ, Zinsmeister AR, VanDyke C, Melton LJ. Epidemiology of colonic symptoms and the irritable bowel syndrome. Gastroenterology 1991;101:927.
11. Thompson W, Dotevall G, Drossman DA, Heaton KW. Irritable bowel syndrome: Guidelines for diagnosis. Gastrointest Int 1989;2:92.
12. Drossman D, Funck-Jensen P, Janssens J. Identification of subgroups of functional gastrointestinal disorders. Gastroenterol Int 1990;3:159.
13. Harvey RF, Mauad EC, Brown AM. Prognosis in the irritable bowel syndrome: A 5-year prospective study. Lancet 1987;1:963.
14. Whorwell PJ, McCallum M, Creed FH, Roberts CT. Non-colonic features of irritable bowel syndrome. Gut 1986;27:37.
15. Svedlund J, Sjodin I, Dotevall G, Gillberg R. Upper gastrointestinal and mental symptoms in the irritable bowel syndrome. Scand J Gastroenterol 1985;20:595.
16. Whitehead WE, Crowell MD, Bosmajian L, et al. Existence of irritable bowel syndrome supported by factor analysis of symptoms in two community samples. Gastroenterology 1990;98:336.
17. Whorwell PJ, Lupton E, Erduran D, Wilson K. Depression and functional bowel disorders in gastrointestinal outpatients. Gut 1986;27(9):1025.
18. Maxton DG, Morris JA, Whorwell PJ. Irritable bowel syndrome in the gynecological clinic. Survey of 798 new referrals. Dig Dis Sci 1989;34(12):1820.
19. Maxton D, Morris J, Whorwell P. More accurate diagnosis of irritable bowel syndrome by the use of 'non-colonic' symptomatology. Gut 1991;32:784.
20. Lind C. Motility disorders in the irritable bowel syndrome. Gastroenterol Clin North Am 1991;20:279.
21. Snape W, Matarazzo S, Cohen S. Effect of eating and gastrointestinal hormones on human colonic myoelectrical and motor activity. Gastroenterology 1978;75:373.
22. Sullivan M, Cohen S, Snape W. Colonic myoelectrical activity in irritable bowel syndrome: Effect of eating and anticholinergics. N Engl J Med 1978;298:878.
23. Latimer P, Sarna S, Campbell D. Colonic motor and myoelectrical activity: A comparative study of normal subjects, psychoneurotic patients, and patients with irritable bowel syndrome. Gastroenterology 1981;80:893.
24. Kellow JE, Phillips SF, Miller LJ, Zinsmeister AR. Dysmotility of the small intestine in irritable bowel syndrome. Gut 1988;28:1236.
25. Cann P, Read N, Brown C, et al. Irritable bowel syndrome: Relationship of disorders in the transit of a single solid meal to symptom patterns. Gut 1983;24:405.
26. Harvey R, Read A. Effect of cholecystokinin on colon motility and symptoms in patients with the irritable bowel syndrome. Lancet 1973;1:1.
27. Taylor I, Basu P, Hammond P, et al. Effect of bile acid perfusion on colonic motor function in patients with the irritable colon syndrome. Gut 1980;21:843.
28. Whitehead WE, Holtkotter B, Enck P, et al. Tolerance for rectosigmoid distention in irritable bowel syndrome. Gastroenterology 1990;98:1187.
29. Snape W, Carlson G, Matarazzo S. Evidence that abnormal myoelectrical activity produces colonic motor dysfunction in the irritable bowel syndrome. Gastroenterology 1977;72:383.
30. Kellow J, Gill R, Wingate D. Prolonged ambulant recordings of small bowel motility demonstrate abnormalities in the irritable bowel syndrome. Gastroenterology 1990;98:1208.
30a. Kumar D, Thompson PD, Wingate DL, et al. Abnormal REM sleep in the irritable bowel syndrome. Gastroenterology 1992;103(1):12–17.
31. Prior A, Maxton D, Whorwell P. Anorectal manometry in irritable bowel syndrome: Differences between diarrhea and constipation predominant subjects. Gut 1990;31:458.
32. Kendall GPN, Thompson DG, Day SJ, Lennard-Jones JE. Inter- and intraindividual variation in pressure-volume relations of the rectum in normal subjects and patients with the irritable bowel syndrome. Gut 1990;31:1062.
33. Baron T, Ramirex B, Richter J. Gastrointestinal motility disorders during pregnancy. Ann Intern Med 1993;118(5):366.
34. Whitehead WE, Cheskin LJ, Heller BR, et al. Evidence for exacerbation of irritable bowel syndrome during menses. Gastroenterology 1990;98:1485.
35. Prior A, Stanley KM, Smith ARB, Read NW. Relation between hysterectomy and the irritable bowel syndrome. Gut 1992;33:814.
36. Schmidt M, Floch M. Food hypersensitivity and the irritable bowel syndrome (editorial). Am J Gastroenterol 1992;87(1):18.
37. Mullin GE. Food allergy and irritable bowel syndrome. JAMA 1991;265(13):1736.

38. Simoons F. The geographic hypothesis and lactose malabsorption. Am J Dig Dis 1978;23:963.
39. Lisker R, Solomons MW, Briceno RP, Mata MR. Lactase and placebo in the management of the irritable bowel syndrome: A double-blind, cross-over study. Am J Gastroenterol 1989;84(7):756.
40. Nanda R, James R, Smith H, et al. Food intolerance and the irritable bowel syndrome. Gut 1989;30:1099.
41. Wald A, Back C, Bayless TM. Effect of caffeine on the human small intestine. Gastroenterology 1976;71:738.
42. Rumessen JJ, Gudmand-Hoyer E. Functional bowel disease: Malabsorption and abdominal distress after ingestion of fructose, sorbitol, and fructose-sorbitol mixtures. Gastroenterology 1988;95:694.
43. Nelis G, Vermeeren M, Jansen W. Role of fructose-sorbitol malabsorption in the irritable bowel syndrome. Gastroenterology 1990;99:1016.
44. Merrick M, Eastwood M, Ford M. Is bile acid malabsorption underdiagnosed? An evaluation of accuracy of diagnosis by measurement of SeHCAT retention. Br Med J 1985;290:665.
45. Ford MJ, Miller PMcC, Eastwood J, Eastwood MA. Life events, psychiatric illness and the irritable bowel syndrome. Gut 1987;28:160.
46. Drossman DA, Leserman J, Nadiman G, et al. Sexual and physical abuse in women with functional or organic gastrointestinal disorders. 1990;113(11):828.
47. Manning A, Thompson WG, Heaton KW, Morris AF. Towards a positive diagnosis of the irritable bowel. Br Med J 1978;2:653.
48. Thompson W. Gastrointestinal symptoms in the irritable bowel compared with peptic ulcer and inflammatory bowel disease. Gut 1984;25:1089.
49. Smith RC, Greenbaum DS, Vancouver JB, et al. Gender differences in Manning criteria in the irritable bowel syndrome. Gastroenterology 1991;100:591.
50. Talley NJ, Phillips SF, Melton LJ, Mulvihill C, Wiltgen CM, Zinsmeister AR. Diagnostic value of the Manning criteria in irritable bowel syndrome. Gut 1990;31:77.
51. Kruis W, Thieme C, Weinzierl M, et al. A diagnostic score for the irritable bowel syndrome. Gastroenterology 1984;87:1.
52. Talley NJ, Phillips SF, Melton J, et al. A patient questionnaire to identify bowel disease. Ann Intern Med 1989;111:671.
53. Talley N, Phillips SF, Wiltgen CM, et al. Assessment of functional gastrointestinal disease: The bowel disease questionnaire. Mayo Clin Proc 1990;65:1456.
54. Marcus S, Heaton K. Irritable bowel-type symptoms in spontaneous and induced constipation. Gut 1987;28:156.
55. Klein K. Controlled treatment trials in the irritable bowel syndrome: A critique. Gastroenterology 1988;95:232.
56. Milo R. Use of the peripheral dopamine antagonist, domperidone, in the management of gastro-intestinal symptoms in patients with irritable bowel syndrome. Curr Med Res Opin 1980;6:577.
57. Friedman G. Nutritional therapy of irritable bowel syndrome. Gastroenterol Clin North Am 1989;18(3):513.
58. Conn P, Read NW, Holdsworth CD, Barends D. Role of loperamide and placebo in the management of irritable bowel syndrome. Dig Dis Sci 1984;29:239.
59. Friedman G. Treatment of the irritable bowel syndrome. Gastroenterol Clin North Am 1991;20(2):325.
60. Creed F, Guthrie, E. Psychological treatments of the irritable bowel syndrome: A review. Gut 1989;30:1601.
61. Svedlund J, Ottosson JO, Sjodin I, Dotevall G. Controlled study of psychotherapy in irritable bowel syndrome. Lancet 1983;2:589.
62. Guthrie E, Creed F, Dawson D, Tomenson B. A controlled trial of psychological treatment for the irritable bowel syndrome. Gastroenterology 1991;100:450.
63. Whorwell P, Prior A, Faragher EB. Controlled trial of hypnotherapy in the treatment of severe refractory irritable bowel syndrome. Lancet 1984;2:1232.
64. Waller SL, Misiewicz JJ. Prognosis in the irritable bowel syndrome: A prospective study. Lancet 1969;2:753.
65. Chaudhary N, Truelove S. The irritable colon syndrome. Q J Med 1962;31:307.
66. Misra S, Thorat VK, Sachdev GK, Anand BS. Long-term treatment of irritable bowel syndrome: Results of a randomized controlled trial. Q J Med 1989;73(270):931.

Bibliography

Camilleri M, Prather CM. The irritable bowel syndrome: Mechanisms and a practical approach to management. Ann Intern Med 1992;116:1001.

Drossman DA, Richter JE, Talley NJ, et al (eds). The Functional Gastrointestinal Disorders: Diagnosis, Pathophysiology and Treatment—A Multinational Consensus. Little, Brown & Co., 1994.

Drossman DA, Thompson WG. The irritable bowel syndrome: Review and a graduated multicomponent treatment approach. Ann Intern Med 1992;116:1009.

Lynn RB, Friedman LS. Irritable bowel syndrome. N Engl J Med 1993;329:1940.

Gallbladder Disease

James M. Richter

In the United States, approximately 1 million people, most of whom are women, are annually diagnosed with cholelithiasis. About half of these are symptomatic, and in 1991, 600,000 patients underwent cholecystectomy. In addition to the morbidity of cholelithiasis, the disease results in an estimated cost of more than $5 billion per year for hospitalization for biliary tract disease plus lost productivity at work and home.

GALLSTONE FORMATION

In North America and Europe, most gallstones are composed principally of cholesterol. The factors contributing to the formation of cholesterol gallstones can be divided into three phases: first, cholesterol supersaturation in bile; second, nucleation of cholesterol crystals; and third, alteration in gallbladder motility and contractility.

Cholesterol is highly insoluble in aqueous solution and is solubilized in bile by a combination of bile salts and lecithin. Several factors may conspire to raise biliary cholesterol concentrations beyond those that can be effectively solubilized, including obesity, age, drugs, and hormones such as estrogen. Estrogens are thought to increase lipoprotein receptors B and E, leading to increased hepatic cholesterol uptake.[1, 2] Progesterone is thought to inhibit hepatic acyl coenzyme A and choline cholesterol acyltransferase, leading to decreased conversion of cholesterol to cholesterol esters. Disease entities that decrease bile salt availability also predispose to cholesterol stone formation. These may include ileal disease or resection, congenital bile acid synthesis deficiency, cirrhosis, or chronic cholestasis.

Supersaturated bile, however, is quite common and is not sufficient for the formation of stones. Nucleating factors, which are believed to be biliary proteins, facilitate vesicle aggregation and fusion and crystal growth in supersaturated, metastable bile. Other factors such as calcium bilirubinate, carbonate, or phosphate complexes are often found in cholesterol gallstones. Exactly how these interact to form cholesterol gallstones is unknown.

Decreased gallbladder contractility predisposes to cholesterol gallstone formation by allowing supersaturated metastable bile or crystals to stay in the gallbladder long enough to form macroscopic stones. Perhaps weak gallbladder motility may fail to pass tiny nascent stones that would otherwise be passed before becoming clinically significant. Pregnancy and the use of oral contraceptives seem to predispose women to cholelithiasis, a phenomenon that may be explained by progesterone's inhibition of gallbladder motility.

Approximately 20% of gallstones in North America are primarily composed of biliary pigment. Black pigment stones occur in the setting of chronic hemolysis such as sickle cell disease, hereditary spherocytosis, thalassemia, or cardiac valvular devices. They also occur with chronic liver disease, such as cirrhosis, and long-term total parenteral nutrition. With increased excretion or hydrolysis of conjugated bilirubin, an insoluble pigment polymer with calcium phosphate and calcium carbonate is formed. Brown pigment gallstones are composed of calcium bilirubinate and calcium soaps formed by bacterial hydrolysis of conjugated bilirubin.

EPIDEMIOLOGY

More than 20 million people in the United States have gallstones. The prevalence of cholesterol stones varies in different racial groups. Native Americans, particularly the Pima Indians, have the highest prevalence of gallstones. European Americans have a lower prevalence; African Americans and Asians have an even lower prevalence.[3] Mexican Americans, a racially mixed group, have a prevalence intermediate to that of American Indians and whites. These racial differences are partially dietary. When African American or Asian people eat a Western diet, the prevalence of cholesterol gallstones increases. The prevalence of gallstones increases with age, and in a study from Malmo, Sweden, gallstones were found in 55% of all adult women. Although the prevalence of pigment stone disease is the same in males and females, cholesterol stones are two to three times more common in women than in men.[4] This gender difference in cholesterol gallstone disease prevalence begins at puberty, increases until menopause, and then subsequently declines.

Obesity increases the risk of gallstone disease, at least in part, by increased gallbladder bile cholesterol saturation.[5-7] Bernstein assessed the risk of more than 6000 American women and found a strong correlation between the risk of gallstone disease and the degree of obesity. Overweight women between the ages of 20 and 29 years had a 6.75-fold increased risk of gallstones compared with women of normal weight and of the same age.[8] Dietary factors such as fat intake and total caloric intake have not been demonstrated to correlate with the incidence of gallstones. Historically, a correlation has been noted between parity and gallstones in women, although this has not been uniformly observed and appears to be less important than obesity. Oral contraceptives do not appear to increase the incidence of gallstones but may facilitate their development at a younger age.

Significant rapid weight loss, however, does substantially increase the risk of developing gallstone disease. This has been observed both in patients who have undergone surgical therapy for morbid obesity and in those who comply with rigorous hypocaloric diets. It may be that patients effectively mobilizing calories from adipose tissue present the liver with a very highly saturated fat energy source, resulting in supersaturated bile. Furthermore, the decrease of oral caloric intake results in relative gallbladder stasis.

NATURAL HISTORY

Most stones in the gallbladder are asymptomatic and remain so.[9, 10] Gallstones discovered incidentally on abdominal ultrasonography are associated with symptomatic cholelithiasis in 1 to 4% of patients per year. Some evidence suggests that the risk of becoming symptomatic is greater immediately after the development of gallstones. No concomitant medical conditions seem to either increase or decrease the rate at which cholelithiasis becomes symptomatic. The vast majority of patients developing symptoms develop abdominal pain, sometimes called biliary colic. Most patients with biliary colic continue to have intermittent abdominal pain. Complications such as acute cholecystitis and choledocholithiasis occur much less

frequently. Rarely, acute cholecystitis develops without antecedent transient abdominal pain.

BILIARY PAIN

Gallstones most often become apparent clinically as abdominal pain, which is often called biliary colic or a gallstone attack.[11] Traditionally, this occurs when a gallstone obstructs the cystic duct. Most patients experience a severe aching or gripping pain in the epigastrium or right upper quadrant of the abdomen. Pain may radiate to the back, the left upper quadrant, or the precordium and may be associated with diaphoresis or vomiting. Although referred to as colicky, the pain usually increases in intensity for 15 minutes to an hour, then remains steady in intensity for 1 to 8 hours, and then slowly improves and resolves in its entirety. Pain that does not resolve or is associated with fever suggests acute cholecystitis or pancreatitis. Some patients find that attacks occur after large or fatty meals, often in the evening or shortly after retiring to bed. More often, however, no clear precipitant is identified, and the pain may recur at uncertain and unpredictable intervals. Physical examination findings of patients with biliary colic are normal except when examination is performed during an attack, at which time tenderness is often noted in the region of the gallbladder.

Dyspepsia, which includes flatulence, fatty food intolerance, bloating, pyrosis, and nausea, is often observed in patients with cholelithiasis but has not been shown to be more frequent or severe in patients with cholelithiasis than in similar, unaffected persons. Because cholelithiasis does not cause these dyspeptic symptoms, it is not surprising that they do not improve with removal of the gallbladder.

ACUTE CHOLECYSTITIS

Acute cholecystitis is the second most common manifestation and complication of cholelithiasis. Unremitting obstruction of the cystic duct results in inflammation of the gallbladder. The inflammation appears to be due to mechanical pressure and chemical damage to the compromised gallbladder wall by bile components. Bacterial infection of the gallbladder is a late and secondary event. Acute cholecystitis occasionally develops in the absence of gallstones, principally in the setting of recent major surgery, extensive trauma, or critical illness.

Most patients with acute calculous cholecystitis have had a previous attack of biliary pain. Acute cholecystitis often begins with pain similar to that

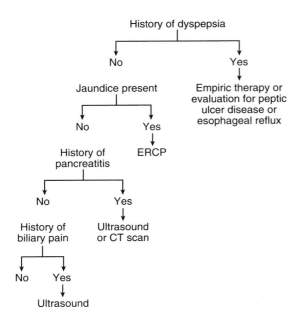

Figure 57–1. Algorithm for evaluation of suspected cholelithiasis. ERCP, Endoscopic retrograde cholangiopancreatography; CT, computed tomography.

of biliary colic, but the pain increases in intensity and is unremitting. Fever, vomiting, and local tenderness are usual. Murphy's sign, an abrupt, involuntary arrest of inspiration due to pain from direct palpation of the right upper quadrant, may be present. In some elderly, chronically ill, or immunocompromised patients, fever, pain, and tenderness may be less marked or absent.

Obstructive jaundice occurs when a gallstone passes through the cystic duct into the common bile duct and becomes impacted at the papilla, obstructing the flow of bile into the duodenum. Patients with choledocholithiasis often have a history of biliary colic but may be pain free. Patients often observe jaundice, pruritus, dark urine, or clay-colored stools. Physical examination is usually significant for jaundice but no stigmata of chronic liver disease. The gallbladder is usually not distended or palpable. When bile flow is obstructed by common duct stones and contaminated with bacteria derived from normal intestinal flora, ascending cholangitis may follow. In ascending cholangitis, signs of obstructive jaundice are accompanied by sepsis and even shock. Treatment is circulatory support, re-establishment of the normal flow of bile, and broad-spectrum, enteric coverage antibiotics.

Choledocholithiasis is also a common cause of acute pancreatitis and the most common cause of acute pancreatitis in women. It is postulated that as gallstones pass through the papilla, the pancreatic duct is transiently occluded, producing chemical or mechanical injury to the pancreatic duct and acute pancreatitis. This may or may not occur with other evidence of acute common bile duct obstruction or jaundice.

LABORATORY EVALUATION

Patients suspected of having symptoms due to gallstones undergo radiologic or ultrasonographic studies to confirm their presence (Fig. 57–1). Although virtually all outpatients and most inpatients with symptomatic gallbladder disease have ultrasonographic or radiographic evidence of stones, not all patients with stones have symptomatic gallbladder disease. Hence, careful clinical assessment and judgment are required to ascertain which patients have symptoms caused by stones. This is made more difficult by the fact that most patients with biliary pain or colic have normal levels of bilirubin and hepatic enzymes and normal responses on other serologic studies of liver function.

Ultrasonography

Ultrasonography has emerged as the principal diagnostic test to be used in cases of suspected cholelithiasis.[12, 13] The procedure requires no preparation, although it is best performed in a fasting state to ensure distention of the gallbladder. The presence of liver disease or jaundice does not affect the performance of the examination, and concomitant disease, such as dilation of the common bile duct, pancreatic disease, and urinary tract abnormalities, can be detected. The presence of echogenic material and shadowing in the dependent part of the gallbladder is the most reliable criterion for the diagnosis of gallstones. Echogenic material that does not move or shadow is less reliable and may represent an incidental gallbladder polyp. Sludge in the gallbladder is not an abnormal finding but must be interpreted with caution because it may decrease the echogenic contrast around the gallstone and diminish detection.

Oral Cholecystography

Oral cholecystography was developed in 1924. Although it remains a valuable test, because of the need for patient preparation with iodinated materials and ionizing radiation, it has largely been supplanted by ultrasonography. Oral cholecystography cannot be used in jaundiced patients because of impaired bile excretion. In approximately 20% of patients who are properly prepared for oral cholecystography and who have gallstones, the gallbladder does not concentrate sufficient contrast to opacify. This is generally interpreted as an abnormal study result but is not as reliable as an oral cholecystogram showing opacification and filling defects or dependent echogenic material with shadowing on ultrasonography. Oral cholecystography is most commonly used now to assess the patency of the cystic duct and function of the gallbladder for the selection of patients for nonsurgical treatment of gallstones.

Other Studies

Plain radiography of the abdomen may provide valuable information by demonstrating the presence of radiopaque stones in the right upper quadrant. This study has the greatest value when used for the evaluation of a patient with acute abdominal pain to investigate the possibility of air in the peritoneum, distention of the large and small bowels, and calcification of the pancreas, as well as calcified renal stones and gallstones. It is of little value in evaluating patients with suspected, currently asymptomatic biliary colic. Computed tomography is a reliable technique for demonstrating the presence of gallstones. When compared with ultrasonography, however, it is an inefficient use of an expensive technology unless one is equally interested in investigating the health of adjacent solid organs such as the liver, pancreas, and kidneys.

Radionuclide materials that are concentrated in the bile, such as derivatives of iminodiacetic acid (e.g., HIDA, DESIDA), have been developed for imaging of the biliary tree. Their images are generally not sufficiently discriminating to visualize or to rule out a filling defect, but they can clearly demonstrate normal gallbladder filling. Because acute cholecystitis is often associated with occlusion of the cystic duct by a stone, failure of the gallbladder to opacify in an acutely ill patient suggests the presence of acute cholecystitis. Knowledge of the presence of stones in a patient with historical and clinical findings of acute cholecystitis is, however, often sufficient for diagnosis and therapy.

Ultrasonography, cholecystography, and computed tomography are much less useful in evaluating patients with suspected obstructive jaundice. The stones themselves are rarely detected in the extrahepatic bile ducts. The suspicion of obstruction is supported by the observation of proximal dilation of the ductal system. Dilation itself is dependent on the degree and duration of the obstruction, and patients with low-grade or partial obstruction may have normal-caliber ducts. In addition, the observation of dilation does not distinguish between stones, stricture, or tumor. Consequently, direct radiographic visualization of the bile duct with either endoscopic retrograde cholangiography or percutaneous transhepatic cholangiography is usually necessary. Currently, the expertise to perform these tests is widely available and the success rates for ductal opacification are greater than 90%. Endoscopic retrograde cholangiopancreatography also permits opacification of the pancreatic duct and removal of the common bile duct stones after papillotomy.

GALLBLADDER CANCER

Gallbladder cancer develops in a small number of patients with long-standing cholelithiasis. It consequently occurs most frequently in older patients who developed stones at a young age, such as Native Americans or Hispanic Americans. Patients with calcified or porcelain gallbladders or large calcified stones seem to be at higher risk, but not sufficiently to recommend prophylactic surgery for most patients. Patients with gallbladder cancer present with right upper quadrant abdominal pain, jaundice, weight loss, or a mass. Gallbladder cancer may be cured when cholecystectomy is performed for symptomatic gallstones and incidental small tumors are discovered. Virtually no other patients with this cancer are cured.

THERAPY AND EXPECTANT MANAGEMENT

Patients with symptoms clearly referable to cholelithiasis should be treated. Infrequent exceptions may be pregnant women or patients with serious comorbid diseases whose aggregate risk of complications might be reduced by delayed therapy (Table 57–1). Patients without symptoms clearly referable to the biliary tree should not be treated.[10, 14] Possible exceptions are young diabetic patients who may be at risk for serious morbidity from the complications of biliary tract disease or otherwise well people with calcified stones or porcelain gallbladder who are at an increased risk for developing carcinoma of the gallbladder.

Oral Bile Acids

Since the early 1970s, chenodeoxycholic acid and ursodeoxycholic acid have been available. When taken orally, they increase the concentration of bile acids and thus the solubility of cholesterol in gallbladder bile. In patients with cholesterol stones and functioning gallbladders in which bile acids may enter and concentrate, cholesterol stones may be solubilized or dissolved. Patients are good candidates for oral bile acid therapy when they have stones that are less than 5 mm in diameter, that float, that have small surface-to-volume ratios, and that are rich in cholesterol.[15]

Six to 24 months of therapy is required for most patients. The use of chenodeoxycholic acid has been limited by significant diarrhea and concerns about liver damage. Only 5 to 15% of patients with symptomatic gallstones are good candidates for oral dissolution therapy, and the efficacy in these patients may be only 70%. Recurrence rates are high, with up to one half of patients having recurrent gallstones within 5 years. The proportion of these recurrent stones that will give rise to symptoms is unknown. Whether hydroxymethylglutaryl coenzyme A reductase inhibitors or nonsteroidal anti-inflammatory drugs will facilitate dissolution therapy or whether bile acids should be used to prevent recurrence is unknown.[16] Currently, oral dissolution therapy with bile acids is limited to patients who are poor surgical risks and those who strongly desire to avoid surgery.

Contact Dissolution Therapy

Oral bile acids are weak cholesterol solvents. Agents such as methylterbutyl ether are much more potent but must be instilled directly into the gallbladder, usually by a percutaneous transhepatic catheter. The solvent may be delivered by hand with a syringe, or an automatic peristaltic pump. Cholesterol stones may be fully dissolved in hours to days. Stones that contain a substantial amount of noncholesterol elements or those that are calcium bilirubinate stones cannot be dissolved. This technique remains available only on an experimental basis and seems to be applicable only to patients who are at very high risk for surgery. Little information about recurrence rates is available. Monooctanoin is a less potent contact solvent that is approved by the Food and Drug Administration and may be infused directly into the common bile duct over a period of days via endoscopic or transhepatic catheter to dissolve retained common bile duct stones.

Extracorporeal Shock Wave Lithotripsy

Extracorporeal shock wave lithotripsy was developed and widely popularized for the fragmen-

---

TABLE 57–1. Comparison of Treatment Modalities for Cholelithiasis

THERAPY	ADVANTAGES	DISADVANTAGES
Oral bile acids	Safe Painless	Slow Ineffective
Contact dissolution (methylterbutyl ether)	Quick Nonsurgical	Uncertain toxicity Moderately high recurrence rate
Extracorporeal shock wave lithotripsy	Effective Quick	Expensive High recurrence rate
Open cholecystectomy	Effective No recurrence Low complication rates	Painful Slower recuperation
Laparoscopic cholecystectomy	Less painful Inexpensive Rapid recuperation	Uncertain complication rates

tation of renal calculi. It was then applied to gallbladder stones with variable effectiveness depending on the amount of energy delivered to the stone and the concomitant use of oral bile acid therapy. The originators of the technique in Munich have demonstrated stone clearance by ultrasound in more than 90% of symptomatic patients who have solitary noncalcified stones less than 20 mm in diameter and who have functioning gallbladders as defined by oral cholecystogram.[17] By including patients with stones up to 3 cm in diameter or with three stones, total stone clearance rates fall to about 60%. Only 16% of all patients with symptomatic gallstone disease have a functioning gallbladder and noncalcified stones of appropriate size and number necessary to be lithotripsy candidates. Significant numbers of patients undergoing lithotripsy experience increased biliary colic after therapy. The frequency of recurrence after lithotripsy has not been determined exactly but is significant. Whether the stones can be prevented by further use of oral bile acids and whether these stones may cause significant symptoms are uncertain.

Open Cholecystectomy

Conventional open, operative cholecystectomy has been used by surgeons for more than 100 years and is successful for treating symptomatic gallstones.[18, 19] At surgery, an incision is created sufficient to allow clear visualization of the gallbladder, bile ducts, and blood vessels, as well as safe dissection, ligation of vessels and ducts, and removal of the gallbladder. The procedure may be extended to include common bile duct exploration and removal of bile duct stones. The rate of common bile duct exploration varies from 3 to 20%, depending on the surgeon's judgment of the likelihood of common duct stones. This evaluation is based on a history of jaundice or pancreatitis, elevated alkaline phosphatase levels, or a dilated common bile duct on ultrasonography. Major complications are infrequent but include bile duct injury, bleeding, bile leak, and local infections. Pneumonia and pulmonary embolism are more significant sequelae. This procedure has been performed by a large number of surgeons and for a long period, and it must be considered the standard with which other treatments are compared. Currently, most patients are hospitalized for 3 to 5 days and have their activities restricted for at least 1 month afterward.

Laparoscopic Cholecystectomy

During the past 5 years, the technology permitting removal of the gallbladder through a laparo-scope has been developed.[20, 21] The peritoneal cavity is distended with an infusion of carbon dioxide gas. Laparoscopic imaging and surgical instruments are advanced, usually through 1-cm incisions in the abdominal wall, for visualization of the gallbladder and surrounding structures. The operation proceeds similarly to open cholecystectomy, using the laparoscope for visualization. The instruments used for dissection, isolation, and division of the cystic duct and artery, as well as for removal of the gallbladder, are controlled percutaneously through the small incisions. The gallbladder is removed through one of the incisions, and the incisions are then closed with sutures and covered. General anesthesia is usually used and entails the same risk as with conventional open cholecystectomy; however, patients undergoing laparoscopic cholecystectomy report much less pain after the operation and experience shorter hospital stays and convalescence. Approximately 5% of the procedures must be converted to conventional open cholecystectomy because of intraoperative difficulties. Common bile duct injuries after laparoscopic cholecystectomy occur more often than after open cholecystectomy, but the frequency of these injuries and their importance have not yet been determined. This technique has assumed a rapid and astounding popularity, and more than half of cholecystectomies are now performed laparoscopically. To be proficient with laparoscopic cholecystectomy, most surgeons should perform 20 procedures with supervision and continue to perform at least one monthly. Although clinicians would find the data quite valuable, no randomized trials comparing laparoscopic with open cholecystectomy have been performed, and it appears unlikely that such a study will be undertaken in the United States.

Almost all patients who are candidates for cholecystectomy because of biliary colic are potential candidates for laparoscopic cholecystectomy unless they have significant local pathology such as portal hypertension, adhesions, or coagulopathy. Patients with complications of acute cholecystitis, such as peritonitis, septic shock due to ascending cholangitis, or pancreatitis, may not be good candidates for laparoscopic cholecystectomy. Many patients with resolving acute cholecystitis or pancreatitis may undergo laparoscopic cholecystectomy. Most patients with cardiopulmonary disease may successfully undergo laparoscopic cholecystectomy rather than open cholecystectomy, recognizing that the infusion of carbon dioxide intraperitoneally may result in hypercarbia and acidosis. Laparoscopic cholecystectomy may be the preferred technique for operating on very obese patients if the instruments can reach the area of dissection and can be adequately controlled.

Treatment of Cholelithiasis During Pregnancy

Although pregnancy is a significant risk factor for the development of cholelithiasis, biliary pain and acute cholecystitis are relatively unusual, perhaps because of hormonal suppression of biliary contractility. When symptomatic cholelithiasis is suspected, the clinician should be particularly careful about firmly establishing the diagnosis with ultrasonography. Pharmacologic agents for the treatment of cholelithiasis, such as bile acids and methylterbutyl ether, have not been studied for fetal safety and should not be used. Most patients with biliary pain and some patients with milder forms of acute cholecystitis can be treated supportively. With technical advances in surgery, anesthesia, and obstetrics, cholecystectomy appears to be safe, but the optimal threshold for intervention is uncertain.[22, 23] If treatment is necessary, operative cholecystectomy remains the preferred technique. Laparoscopic cholecystectomy has potential advantages but should be avoided during the third trimester because of the potential for injuring the uterus with the laparoscopic instruments.

PREVENTION OF CHOLELITHIASIS

Clinically significant obesity occurs in approximately 20% of women in the United States. Obesity is associated with high cholesterol saturation in bile and a two- to four-fold increased risk of cholelithiasis. To diminish this risk, as well as other serious health problems, weight control is strongly recommended.[24] However, it has been documented that cholesterol saturation may increase and gallbladder motility may decrease during caloric restriction, further predisposing to gallstone formation during weight reduction and dieting. To determine whether this risk could be mitigated, patients beginning a 500 kcal per day weight loss diet were randomized to receive ursodiol, aspirin, or placebo for 16 weeks. They were monitored by ultrasonography and duodenal drainage for cholesterol crystals, and it was demonstrated that ursodiol diminishes the lithogenic changes in formation of gallstones in obese patients on weight loss diets. This unique finding is perhaps the best indication for the current clinical use of oral bile acids in the treatment of cholelithiasis. Low-fat, higher-fiber diets and aspirin may

help prevent cholelithiasis but are unproven. They can, however, be recommended for other, better established health goals.

REFERENCES

1. Scragg RKR, McMichael AJ, Seamark RF. Oral contraceptives, pregnancy, and endogenous oestrogen in gall stone disease—a case control study. Br Med J 1984;288:1795.
2. Lynn J, Williams L, O'Brien J, et al. Effects of estrogen upon bile; implications with respect to gallstone formation. Ann Surg 1973;178:514.
3. Williams CN, Johnston JL. Prevalence of gallstones and risk factors in Caucasian women in a rural Canadian community. Can Med Assoc J 1980;120:664.
4. Barbara L, Sama C, Labate AMM, et al. A population study of the prevalence of gallstone disease: The Sirmione study. Hepatology 1987;7:913.
5. Stampfer MJ, Maclure KM, Colditz GA, et al. Risk of symptomatic gallstones in women with severe obesity. Am J Clin Nutr 1992;55:652.
6. Maclure KM, Hayes KC, Colditz GA, et al. Weight, diet, and the risk of symptomatic gallstones in middle-aged women. N Engl J Med 1989;321:563.
7. Liddle FA, Goldstein RB, Saxton J. Gallstone formation during weight reduction dieting. Arch Intern Med 1989;149:1750.
8. Sichieri R, Everhart JE, Roth H. A prospective study of hospitalization with gallstone disease among women: Role of dietary factors, fasting period, and dieting. Am J Public Health 1991;81:880.
9. Gracie WA, Ransohoff DF. The natural history of silent gallstones: The innocent gallstone is not a myth. N Engl J Med 1982;307:798.
10. Friedman GD, Raviola CA, Fireman B. Prognosis of gallstones with mild or no symptoms: 25 years of follow-up in a health maintenance organization. J Clin Epidemiol 1989;42:127.
11. Jorgensen T. Abdominal symptoms and gallstone disease: An epidemiological investigation. Hepatology 1989;9:856.
12. Burrell MI, Zeman RK, Simeone JF, et al. The biliary tract: Imaging for the 1990's. AJR 1991;157:223.
13. Carroll BA. Preferred imaging techniques for the diagnosis of cholecystitis and cholelithiasis. Ann Surg 1989;210:1.
14. Ransohoff DF, Gracie WA, Wolfenson LB, Neuhauser D. Prophylactic cholecystectomy or expectant management for silent gallstones: A decision analysis to assess survival. Ann Intern Med 1983;99:199.
15. Weinstein WC, Coley CM, Richter JM. Medical management of gallstones: A cost effectiveness analysis. J Gen Intern Med 1990;5:277.
16. Broomfield PH, Chopra F, Sheinbaum RC, et al. Effects of ursodeoxycholic acid and aspirin on the formation of lithogenic bile and gallstones during loss of weight. N Engl J Med 1988;319:1567.
17. Sackman M, Delius M, Sauerbruch T, et al. Shock-wave lithotripsy of gallbladder stones: The first 175 patients. N Engl J Med 1988;318:393.
18. Glenn F, McSherry CK, Dineen P. Morbidity of surgical treatment for non-malignant biliary tract diseases. Surg Gynecol Obstet 1968;126:15.
19. McSherry CK. Cholecystectomy: The gold standard. Am J Surg 1989;158:174.
20. Cheslyn-Curtis S, Russell RCG. New trends in gallstone management. Br J Surg 1991;78:143.

21. The Southern Surgeons Club. A prospective analysis of 1518 laparoscopic cholecystectomies. N Engl J Med 1991;324:1073.
22. Landers D, Carmona R, Crombleholme W, Lim R. Acute cholecystitis in pregnancy. Obstet Gynecol 1987;69:131.
23. McKellar DP, Anderson CT, Boynton CJ. Cholecystec-

tomy during pregnancy without fetal loss. Surg Gynecol Obstet 1992;174:465.
24. Diehl AK, Haffner SM, Hazuda HP, Stern MP. Coronary risk factors and clinical gallbladder disease: An approach to the prevention of gall stones? Am J Public Health 1987;77:841.

Headache

Nagagopal Venna

MIGRAINE

Migraine is the most common type of recurring headache and is especially prevalent in women. The American Migraine Study[1] found that 18% of women suffer from migraine compared with 6% of men. It is estimated that about 18 million females older than 12 years have migraine, half of them experiencing moderate to severe disability from the headaches. The female preponderance appears at puberty, peaking in the early forties to 3.3 times the prevalence in men but persisting at a ratio of 2.5 to 1 up to the age of 70 years.

Definite but complex relationships exist between migraine onset, remissions, relapses, and reproductive phases. The onset is most often in adolescence and young adulthood, gradually fading at or after menopause. There is, however, no sound evidence that oophorectomy or hysterectomy decreases migraine. Rarely, menopause may be associated with exacerbations or activation of long-dormant migraine. Estrogen therapy at the time of menopause has been reported to worsen migraine. Interaction of menstruation and migraine has long been recognized: About 60% of patients experience worsening of headaches in the premenstrual period. Rarely, some women experience migraine exclusively during menstruation or in the immediate perimenstrual period. This form appears to be linked to a decline in the blood levels of estradiol. Menstrual migraine is usually of the common variety, although classic or complicated syndromes of migraine may also occur. Pregnancy, as a rule, ameliorates migraine, especially beyond the first trimester, but in about a third it may precipitate or aggravate migraine. Common migraine may evolve to complicated migraine with visual or other neurologic aura for the first time during pregnancy. Oral contraceptive drugs have definite but unpredictable and variable effects on migraine: Migraine may appear for the first time when a woman takes the pill, especially in persons with a family history of migraine, and tends to occur in the early cycles of pill use. Preexisting migraine is frequently exacerbated by oral contraceptive use; moreover, the pattern of migraine may change. For instance, visual aura or other neurologic accompaniments may occur with the headache for the first time after beginning oral contraceptives. New onset of migraine, however, may occur after prolonged use of the pill. Similarly, discontinuation of the drug may not lead to rapid disappearance of migraine. On the other hand, in some, the contraceptive pill may lead to clear improvement of migraine, underscoring the marked variability of migraine response to different hormonal perturbations. Among patients receiving estrogens for gynecologic indications, nearly half experienced more frequent migraine headaches, the frequency decreasing with lower doses of estrogen.

Pathophysiology of Migraine

Despite extensive investigation, a cogent theory of the pathogenesis of migraine has not yet been developed.[2] However, it is clear that migraine diathesis is inherent in some people and is periodically provoked by various external and internal psychological, chemical, physical, and biologic triggers. The neurologic substrate of migraine is increasingly being understood. The trigeminal nervous system, through its connections to the extensive vascular bed of the head and face, is involved in mediating vascular headaches as well as neurogenic vascular inflammation. Strong evidence also demonstrates that the brain stem serotonin neural system and its extensive cerebral and descending networks have a central role in the production of pain and other manifestations of migraine. It is interesting that most antimigraine drugs have serotonin agonist activity. The neurologic accompaniments of migraine are likely to be mediated by the brain stem norepinephrine-producing locus caeruleus system, with its extensive network to the entire brain and its microvasculature.

Clinical Picture

Various phenomena occur in migraine sufferers as a group (Table 58–1). Family history of migraine is present in about 60% of cases, often in the mother. Childhood antecedents such as cyclic vomiting, recurrent benign abdominal pain, motion sickness, and recurrent benign vertigo are common in the histories of patients with migraine and are considered migraine equivalents. An association is noted between migraine and mitral valve prolapse, Prinzmetal's angina, Raynaud's phenomenon (syndromes with autonomic instability), left-handedness, and polycystic ovarian disease. Various vasoactive drugs may precipitate or exacerbate migraine. Reserpine does so predictably, as do nitroglycerin and less commonly hydralazine, prazosin, nifedipine, captopril, and atenolol. Antipeptic ulcer drugs such as cimetidine and ranitidine and the anti-inflammatory drug indomethacin are other notable examples that induce migraine. The influence of oral contraceptives and estrogens has already been mentioned. The onset of essential hypertension may trigger migraine in certain patients, as may head trauma and certain foods.

Characteristics of Episodes of Migraine

Headache is the dominant part of migraine and evolves over many minutes to an hour but rarely is explosive (thunderbolt headache). It does not awaken a patient from sleep but may occur on awakening. It is predominantly hemicranial, not only left- or right-sided but at times in the anterior or posterior half of the head, and it may switch sides in different attacks. The pain is typically pounding but is frequently steady and lasts from a few hours to a day or two. In some patients, discrete startling jabs of pain (icepick headaches) over the orbits and scalp occur during or, more often, between the migraine attacks. Tenderness over the scalp of the temple and rarely subcutaneous swelling from serious effusion in the temple secondary to sterile vascular inflammation may accompany severe attacks.

Headache Accompaniments

Although headache is the most distressing part of migraine, various regional, systemic, and neurologic disturbances frequently accompany the episodes and are diagnostically more useful than the headache itself. Nausea, anorexia, and vomiting are the rule. Patients may occasionally experience abdominal discomfort and diarrhea. Skin pallor and cold and clammy extremities are common. Fluid retention followed by brisk diuresis at the end of attacks is frequent. Various neurologic and behavioral alterations are common attendants, but patients often do not report them unless specifically questioned. Patients describe a general heightening of all perceptions: Photophobia and sonophobia are routine; others describe odorophobia as well as intolerance to touch. Patients typically lie down in a quiet, dark room and try to fall asleep. For some patients, sleep regularly terminates the headache. A prodrome of fatigue, depression, lethargy, euphoria, or craving for candy frequently precedes the headache. Older patients may develop periorbital ecchymoses in severe attacks.

Neurologic Accompaniments

About 90% of patients suffer no elementary neurologic accompaniments and are said to have common migraine. About 10% of patients experience a characteristic aura, usually a visual disturbance, preceding the onset of headache. The episodes of this classic type of migraine begin with a visual hallucination in the form of flashing lights, zigzag lines (fortification spectra), circles, stars, or scintillating scotomata. A pathognomonic but not invariable feature is buildup of these hallucinations from the center of vision to the periphery, rarely in the reverse, at a deliberate pace for 20 to 30 minutes. As the scintillations regress, hemianopia or total blindness may follow in their wake, along with a throbbing headache. Less common accompaniments are hemiplegia, aphasia, complex symptoms of brain stem dysfunction, ophthalmoplegias and amaurosis due to retinal ischemia, and paresthesia of the hand, face, and mouth. In these cases, the neurologic symptoms resolve over a few min-

---

TABLE 58–1.   Migraine Diathesis

Family history of migraine
Childhood motion sickness
Cyclic vomiting of childhood
Cyclic abdominal pain of childhood
Benign recurrent vertigo of youth
Onset at puberty
Accentuation by menstrual periods
Modulation by pregnancy and oral contraceptive pills
Amelioration after menopause
Aggravation by vasoactive drugs such as nitroglycerin, reserpine, and prazosin
Association with vasospastic conditions: Raynaud's phenomenon, Prinzmetal's angina

utes to hours, followed by abatement of the headache.

Diagnosis

A detailed and focused history is the cornerstone of diagnosis, because laboratory test results and clinical findings are typically normal. A useful way of eliciting the details of the episodes is to ask a patient to describe the most recent headache from the onset. Helpful direction can be given by asking for a description of the pain, as well as regional (head, neck, or face), neurologic, mental, behavioral, and systemic accompaniments around the headache to determine whether the episodes are consistent with migraine. Hemicranial headaches that alternate sides in different episodes, typical behavior of lying down in a quiet place, termination of the headache by sleep, and normal health between episodes are particularly suggestive.

The next step is to support this diagnosis by documenting the longitudinal course of the syndrome over the life of the patient. A single headache with visual disturbances and nausea is not necessarily migraine. The episodic symptom complex should be supported by a history of headaches in the family, the influence of puberty, oral contraceptive use, pregnancy, menstruation, vasoactive drugs, and childhood migraine equivalents. The interval neurologic examination should yield normal findings, with particular attention given to visual fields, gait, optic fundi, and behavior.

Brain imaging by magnetic resonance imaging or computed tomography (CT) scan with contrast is not routinely necessary but is appropriate in the first episodes of migraine with visual, hemiplegic, ophthalmoplegic, or brain stem accompaniments, especially in the absence of the pathognomonic crescendo development and regression of symptoms and when the headaches and neurologic abnormalies have not resolved and when the neurologic symptoms are always on the same side of the body. Persistent neurologic abnormalities and change in the character of the usual migraine also merit such imaging: Patients with migraine are not immune to other intracranial causes of headache, including arteriovenous malformation, aneurysm, and tumors. Electroencephalography is helpful in patients who experience headache and visual symptoms resembling migraine and in whom confusion, automatisms, or alteration of consciousness also occurs and are key to identifying occipital lobe epilepsy.

In the occasional instance when migraine has an explosive thunderbolt-like onset, a lumbar puncture is needed to rule out subarachnoid hemorrhage if a brain CT scan yields normal results. The general medical evaluation may occasionally make it appropriate to determine the erythrocyte sedimentation rate and the serum antinuclear antigen because migraine-like syndrome has been described in systemic lupus erythematosus.

Consultation with a neurologist is appropriate if the diagnosis is uncertain and in cases of unusual variants of migraine (such as basilar artery or ophthalmoplegic migraine) and in patients with headaches intractable to therapy.

Treatment

Pharmacotherapy

ACUTE ATTACKS. Treatment of acute episodes of migraine is readily available to suit the wide range of severity of headaches commonly encountered (Table 58–2). Mild attacks of migraine respond to standard doses of aspirin, acetaminophen, or nonsteroidal anti-inflammatory drugs such as ibuprofen or naproxen. Moderately severe episodes may need more potent medications such as ketorolac. Ergotamine, often combined with caffeine (e.g., Cafergot), has a time-honored role in aborting migraine and is especially useful in infrequent cases. Most patients tolerate oral medication, but others may require suppositories or sublingual preparations if they are subject to vomiting. Patients with intense, prolonged episodes of migraine often require urgent therapy: Parenteral administration of dihydroergotamine combined with metoclopramide and prochlorperazine is often effective.[3] The serotonin agonist sumatriptan has been approved by the Food and Drug Administration for the treatment of migraine. It appears to be an effective and easily administered treatment for infrequent severe migraine, although clinical experience is not extensive.[4] It can be administered by either a physician or the patient at the onset of the headache at a dose of 6 mg subcutaneously using the preset autoinjector. About 70% of patients experience relief or a marked decrease in pain within 1 hour. Nausea and photophobia are also relieved. Side effects are mild and consist of a sense of heaviness in various parts of the body and flushing. Sumatriptan appears to be a highly effective abortive treatment that can be administered by a patient at home after initial dosing under medical supervision. It is best avoided in migraine associated with visual or other neurologic symptoms. Recurrence of headache within 24 hours after one or two injections is reported by one third of patients. If the headache recurs, it should be

TABLE 58–2. Treatment of Acute Attacks of Migraine

ORAL MEDICATIONS
Analgesics

Aspirin	325-mg tablets: 2 tablets at onset. Repeat every 6 hr as needed.
Acetaminophen	500-mg tablets: 2 tablets at onset. Repeat every 6 hr as needed.

Nonsteroidal anti-inflammatory drugs

Ibuprofen	800-mg tablets: 1 tablet at onset. Repeat every 6 hr as needed.
Naproxen sodium	275-mg tablets: 3 tablets at onset. Repeat 2 tablets every 8 hr as needed.
Ketorolac	10-mg tablets: 2 tablets at onset. Repeat 1 tablet every 12-hr as needed.

Ergot Compounds

Ergotamine, 1 mg, with caffeine	2 tablets at onset. Repeat 1 tablet every 30 min as needed; maximum of 6 tablets/day and 10 tablets/week.
Ergotamine suppositories, 1 mg with caffeine	1 suppository at onset. Repeat 1 suppository at 1 hr; maximum 6/day and 10/week.
Corticosteroids	Useful for occasional intractable migraine. Prednisone, 60 mg/day for 4–7 days. Dexamethasone, 4–8 mg/day for 4–7 days.

PARENTERAL THERAPY

Dihydroergotamine (DHE-45)	
Intramuscular(ly) (IM)	1 mg (1 ml) IM at onset. Repeat 1 ml at 1 hr as needed. Maximum 3 ml.
Intravenous(ly) (IV)	1 ml (1 mg) of DHE-45 and 2 ml (10 mg) of prochlorperazine. Slow IV push over 2 min.

Phenothiazines

Prochlorperazine	10 mg by slow IV injection over 2 min.

Serotonin Receptor Agonists

Sumatriptan, 6 mg dose in autoinjection device	6 mg, subcutaneously at onset. Repeat once at 1 hr if needed. Can be self-administered by patient.

treated by the alternatives listed in Table 58–2. Intravenous chlorpromazine or prochlorperazine is also effective.[5]

PREVENTIVE THERAPY. In many patients, episodic occasional migraine may become more frequent, from fewer than two attacks a month to nearly daily episodes. In these circumstances, prophylactic therapy is indicated. Various drugs have proved to be helpful (Table 58–3). The β-blocker propranolol has an established role as a generally well-tolerated and effective drug. Its usual dose is 20 to 40 mg four times a day. After achieving an initial response, it can be administered in the long-acting form in a once-daily dose.

Some patients cannot tolerate propranolol because of side effects, ineffectiveness, or pulmonary or cardiac contraindications. Calcium channel blockers can also alleviate frequent migraine. The most widely used is verapamil in doses of up to 360 mg per day. A long-acting form is also available. Extensive experience has proved the powerful beneficial effects of tricyclic antidepressant drugs in the prophylaxis of migraine. These drugs have been effective and devoid of serious side effects in patients with migraine and its frequent combination with muscle contraction headache and depression. The drug most widely used is amitriptyline, which is especially useful in patients with coincident insomnia or signs of an agitated depression. Desipramine, nortriptyline, doxepin, and nontricyclic antidepressants such as trazodone and fluoxetine have also been useful in this context. An addition to the armamentarium is the antiepileptic drug valproate, in a dose of up to 1200 mg per day.[6]

Nonpharmacologic Treatments of Migraine

Migraine is intimately woven into the life of patients and is often brought to the surface by predictable triggers. These include sleep deprivation, hunger, emotional stress, and certain foods. Identification of these factors by a carefully taken history and their avoidance are a mainstay of therapy. Because emotional stress is an all-too-common exacerbating factor that often transforms occasional headaches into nearly daily episodes, methods of relaxation have long been tried and in some patients are clearly beneficial. Biofeedback has been used and studied most extensively in this context. Relaxation training, focusing on relaxa-

TABLE 58–3. **Prophylaxis of Migraine**

PHARMACOLOGIC TREATMENT
Tricyclic Antidepressants

Amitriptyline	Start with 10 mg at bedtime. May need incremental increases up to 100 mg/day
Nortryptyline	Start with 10 mg; incremental increases up to 100 mg/day
Doxepin	Start with 10 mg at night. Increase as needed up to 100 mg/day
Fluoxetine	20 mg/day

β-Blockers

Propranolol	Start with 40 mg t.i.d. Increase up to 320 mg/day. If successful, can be conveniently given in single daily dose in the long-activating form
Atenolol	50–100 mg/day
Nadolol	40–240 mg/day
Timolol	10–30 mg/day

Calcium Channel Blockers

Verapamil	240–720 mg/day
Nifedipine	30–180 mg/day
Diltiazem	120–360 mg/day

Serotonin Modulators

Methysergide	2–8 mg/day, in divided doses up to 14 mg/day

Antihistamines

Cyprohepatadine	2–4 mg q.i.d.

Anticonvulsants

Valproic acid	250 mg t.i.d.

Antiprostaglandins

Aspirin	325 mg/day
Naproxen sodium	550 mg/day

NONPHARMACOLOGIC MEASURES
Biofeedback
Relaxation techniques
Ergonomic correction at work
Aerobic exercises

t.i.d., 3 times a day; q.i.d., 4 times a day.

tion of the entire body, has been helpful. Extensive literature indicates that biofeedback and relaxation techniques are best used in combination. They are clearly helpful as adjuncts to medical treatment, giving patients better control of the pain and decreasing the need for drugs. They are best suited for younger patients who have frequent attacks and who are well motivated.[7]

Menstrual Migraine

Menstrual migraine is an uncommon variety of migraine in which the headache syndrome occurs exclusively or predominantly in the perimenstrual phase, usually beginning a few days before the onset of menses, persisting through the menstruation, and remitting between the periods. The headache syndrome usually has the characteristics of common migraine, but classic migraine with visual aura may occasionally occur. The headaches tend to be severe and add to the distress of the premenstrual syndrome, and treatment is often difficult. Many drugs conventionally used for acute treatment of migraine can also be effective in this context and are started a few days before the expected onset of menses and continued through the period of menstruation (Table 58–4). Nonsteroidal anti-inflammatory drugs are often effective. Menstrual migraine is associated with an increase in prostaglandin synthesis, and the effectiveness of the nonsteroidal anti-inflammatory drugs may be related to their powerful inhibition of prostaglandin synthesis. Ergotamine at a dose of 1 mg once at bedtime or 1 mg twice a day for the duration of the menstrual period can also be markedly effective. Short perimenstrual courses of prednisone at a dose of 60 mg a day may be helpful.

Not infrequently, menstrual migraine may be resistant to conventional treatments. In selected patients, hormonal therapy may be indicated and is best given in consultation with a patient's gynecologist. Most of these treatments are based on the clinical experience of physicians specializing

TABLE 58–4.   **Treatment of Menstrual Migraine**

Perimenstrual Period Medication	
Ergotamine with caffeine	1 tablet at bedtime or 1 tablet b.i.d.
Propranolol	40 mg t.i.d.
Nonsteroidal anti-inflammatory drugs	As in Table 58–2
Hormonal Drugs	
Estradiol gel	
Estradiol implants	
Estradiol cutaneous patch	
Ethinyl estradiol with methyltestosterone	
Danazol	200–600 mg/day
Tamoxifen	5–15 mg/day
Prednisone	60 mg/day
Bromocriptine	2.5–5 mg/day

b.i.d., 2 times a day; t.i.d., 3 times a day.

in headache treatment, anecdotal accounts, and open label trials in small numbers of patients, rather than on large systematic controlled trials. Because evidence shows that a decrease in estrogen levels occurs during the late luteal phase of the menstrual cycle and that this decrease is a likely trigger of menstrual migraine, various short courses of estrogen treatment before the onset of menstruation have been tried and have generally been helpful. Various combinations and routes of administration have been used, and there is no standard method. Oral estrogen in the form of ethinyl estradiol at a dose of 0.05 mg combined with methyltestosterone 2 mg a day was anecdotally reported to be effective.[8] Percutaneous estradiol gel perimenstrually has been shown to be beneficial in two double-blind studies.[9, 10] Danazol, a synthetic androgen, has been reported to alleviate menstrual migraine.[11] This drug inhibits ovarian steroid production and suppresses the pituitary-ovarian axis by binding to androgen and progestin receptors. It is given in a dose of 200 to 600 mg a day in the perimenstrual period. Tamoxifen has been used successfully in resistant cases of menstrual migraine without adverse side effects.[12] It is given in a dose of 5 to 15 mg a day for days 7 to 14 during the luteal phase of the menstrual cycle. Tamoxifen is an antiestrogen drug that acts by binding to cellular estrogen receptors. It has other complex effects on ovarian function and decreases prostaglandin synthesis. Bromocriptine is an agonist of brain D2 dopamine receptors and is a potent inhibitor of prolactin secretion. It is used regularly in the treatment of prolactinomas and Parkinson's disease and has occasionally been used in the treatment of menstrual migraine. It is given in a dose of 2.5 to 5 mg a day during the luteal phase as an adjunctive, and it is also known to alleviate other symptoms of premenstrual syndrome.[13] After the

first dose, a patient should be checked for postural hypotension, which can occasionally occur.

Migraine Associated with Menopause

Estrogens are currently being increasingly prescribed for menopausal and postmenopausal women. In some patients, this treatment may aggravate migraine headaches significantly. The headaches can be improved by empirical fine-tuning of estrogen therapy.[13] The suggested manipulations are decreasing the dose of estrogen or switching from conjugated estrogens to pure estradiol, ethinyl estradiol, or pure estrone. In one study, oral estropipate decreased the headaches whereas ethinyl estradiol worsened them.[14] Another modification of estrogen therapy that reduces headaches is the change from intermittent to continuous lower-dose estrogen therapy.[15] Finally, amelioration of estrogen-induced headache was also found when oral estrogen was replaced by parenteral estradiol and the addition of testosterone.[16] A modality of treatment more readily acceptable to patients is the estradiol patch, which was anecdotally reported to be associated with fewer headaches. The patch does provide steady levels of estrogen and a more physiologic ratio of estradiol to estrone.[17]

In contrast to the estrogen-aggravated or estrogen-provoked migraine, some women experience worsening of migraine in the menopause that improves with estrogen therapy alone or in combination with testosterone.[16] A double-blind study confirmed this effect, but another published in the same monograph did not find a similar benefit.[18]

Oral Contraceptives in Migraine

In patients with common migraine or migraine with visual aura, oral contraceptives are permissible. However, it is prudent to avoid them if the pill triggers migraines accompanied by other neurologic symptoms such as aphasia or hemiparesis, although no studies have been performed to establish an increased risk of permanent neurologic sequelae in these circumstances.[19]

Stroke in Migraine

Stroke with permanent neurologic sequelae due to brain infarction is a rare but documented complication of migraine.[20] As expected, most patients are women and most have had classic or complicated chronic migraines with episodic visual and neurologic symptoms. Many experience prodromes of increasing frequency and severity of the migraine before the stroke. However, stroke without other known cause has occurred in common migraine as well as recent-onset migraine. As can be expected, most strokes are in the posterior cerebral artery distribution in the occipital-medial temporal lobes, with hemianopia. The question whether oral contraceptive drugs enhance the risk of stroke when used in patients with migraine is not clearly answered, although the Colloborative Group for the Study of Stroke in Young Women found no evidence that migraine increases the risk of stroke in women using oral contraceptives.[21]

TENSION HEADACHE

The epidemiology of tension headache has not been systematically studied, although clinical experience shows that tension headache is nearly universal. The pathophysiology of the syndrome is not well understood, but sustained excessive contraction of scalp and cervical muscles appears to be the final common pathway. Acute and chronic psychological stresses, anxiety states, and especially depression often express themselves in this manner, presumably through the limbic inputs into the craniocervical muscular tone maintenance mechanisms. Tension headache does, however, appear as an idiopathic syndrome without any apparent physical or psychiatric disorder in some persons. Tension headaches not infrequently merge into migraine or vise versa, and current thinking favors the view that they are a part of the spectrum of migraine.[22]

Clinical Picture

Acute Tension Headache

Most of these headaches do not reach a physician's attention because of their self-limited course and the moderate intensity of pain. However, they can be of disabling severity. The pain is generalized, with a predilection for bilateral frontotemporal and occipital regions. It develops over hours and may last hours to days. It is described as an ache, pressure, tightness, or heavy weight sensation. Some patients describe it as a feeling of the head being pressed in a vise, a tight skull cap, or crawling sensations. Excessive sensitivity to touch on combing the scalp and touching the temples is often mentioned. Nausea, vomiting, photophobia, sonophobia, visual scintillations, and other neurologic symptoms do not occur. A sense of fatigue is a common accompaniment. Pain may spread to the shoulders and upper back. Results of physical examination including neurologic examination are normal except for generalized tenderness over the temples or neck. An acute life stress situation can usually be identified by a carefully taken history.

Chronic Tension Headache

Chronic tension headache is one of the most common and difficult to treat headache syndromes. Pain characteristics are the same as in the acute type described earlier, but the pain is present continuously for days, weeks, or even months at a time, patients being unaware of the headaches only in sleep, although intensity may fluctuate. The physical examination findings are again normal, including the results of neurologic and craniocervical and facial regional examinations.

Diagnosis is chiefly based on a carefully taken and detailed history. A comprehensive history of life stress, job stress, anxiety, and especially depression should be diligently sought. This often requires several visits and the establishment of an empathic relationship with the patient. A work history with particular regard to prolonged uncomfortable positions at video terminals and computers should be obtained. A thorough general physical and neurologic clinical examination is needed, with careful evaluation of the optic fundi and visual fields. One should look for evidence of temporal giant cell arteritis in older women. A brain CT scan may be a reasonable test to add further support to the clinical diagnosis by ruling out structural lesions and providing a measure of reassurance to both the provider and the patient. Particular attention should be paid to the pituitary fossa, perisellar regions, sphenoid sinuses, and ventricular pathways, looking for obstructive lesions such as colloid cysts of the third ventricle, all of which can produce nondescript headaches without other clinical signs. A careful follow-up clinical examination is essential to evaluate psychosocial and physical abnormalities. A history of excessive use of caffeine, analgesic drugs with or without caffeine, and ergotamine should be sought, because such use may have the paradoxical effect of worsening the headache.

Treatment

Acute tension headaches are self-limited and respond to analgesic drugs and resolution of acute stresses. Chronic tension headaches are a challenging problem and constitute at least 50% of referrals to specialized headache clinics. Underlying psychological problems should be identified, the most common being depression. Anxiety and occupational and marital stresses are frequent. Psychiatric evaluation and psychological counseling are needed in some cases. Behavioral modification using relaxation techniques and biofeedback is often of major long-term benefit in well-motivated patients. Withdrawal of excessively used analgesics, ergotamine, and caffeine can be of substantial benefit. The most consistently effective pharmacologic treatment of chronic tension headache is tricyclic antidepressant therapy with amitriptyline, desipramine, or nortriptyline in doses of 10 to 100 mg a day. These drugs are effective at doses much smaller than those needed for major depression. In most instances, treatment using these drugs in conjunction with biofeedback, relaxation techniques, and appropriate counseling is adequately and indeed optimally carried out in a primary care setting. For intractable cases, referral to a neurologist with particular expertise in headaches or to regional headache clinics with multidisciplinary units is advisable.

MIXED HEADACHE SYNDROMES

Another common cause of chronic daily headaches usually affecting 30- to 50-year-old women is the mixed headache syndrome.[22] Most patients have had several years of episodic migraine that then becomes continuously painful for weeks or months. A background generalized pressure-like tension headache merges with superimposed throbbing headaches of the migraine type. Patients typically are taking multiple analgesics, tranquilizers, and migraine medications. General physical and neurologic examinations and brain imaging by CT or magnetic resonance imaging yield normal results. Psychological evaluation often reveals depression. Evaluation should also focus on the triggers and contributing factors that transform episodic migraine into the continuous daily headaches with the addition of a tension headache com-

ponent. Psychological stresses on the job or at home, anxiety, and depression in various combinations are often the undercurrents, although patients may be unaware of these or may not realize their relationship to the ongoing head pain. The headache syndrome may be worsened or perpetuated by new-onset hypertension, introduction of the oral contraceptive pill, and use of excessive amounts of analgesic drugs (e.g., >30 tablets a month) or ergotamine and caffeine-containing preparations, including over-the-counter drugs as well as drugs introduced for intercurrent illness, such as nitroglycerin, nifedipine, reserpine, cimetidine, and ranitidine.

Treatment is challenging and involves many modalities (Table 58–5). It is critically important to reassure patients that the pain syndrome is a combination of migraine and tension headaches, has a benign nature, and can be alleviated. Tricyclic antidepressant drugs such as amitriptyline are important, combined with behavioral modification techniques in the form of biofeedback and relaxation techniques, especially in motivated persons. Excessively used analgesics and chronically used ergotamine should be withdrawn because both can cause rebound headaches.[23] Addition of β-blocker drugs such as propranolol may act synergistically with amitriptyline. Referral to headache clinics is sometimes helpful for comprehensive advice that can be implemented over the long term by the primary physician.

HEADACHES RELATED TO SEXUAL ACTIVITY

A benign recurrent headache syndrome related to sexual activity has become increasingly recognized.[24] The headache is believed to be mediated by transient systemic hypertension and excessive craniocervical muscle contraction associated with

---

TABLE 58–5.   Treatment Modalities in Chronic Tension and Mixed Headaches

---

Pharmacologic
  Prophylaxis with amitriptyline as for migraine
  Propranolol as for migraine
  Withdrawal of analgesics, caffeine, and ergotamine

Behavior Therapies
  Psychological counseling
  Psychiatric consultation in selected cases
  Biofeedback
  Relaxation techniques
  Physical exercise program
  Optimization of physical work environment (ergonomics)

---

sexual intercourse and masturbation. Although more common in men, the syndrome is also documented in women. A prior history of episodic migraine or tension headache is present only in some patients. Headache of moderate to explosive intensity begins during sexual activity and is usually located over the occipital area but can be generalized and fades gradually after a few hours. The first attacks simulate spontaneous subarachnoid hemorrhage. Findings of interval neurologic and systemic examinations are normal, as are results of a brain CT scan. Headaches tend to recur for several months to a few years but gradually remit spontaneously. Reassuring patients about the benign nature of the headaches after conducting a neurologic examination and brain imaging considerably allays the understandable anxiety engendered by this disturbing phenomenon. Prophylaxis with β-blocker drugs such as propranolol is generally effective. Patients may also prevent the headaches by using nonsteroidal anti-inflammatory medications or propranolol about an hour before sexual activity.

PSEUDOTUMOR CEREBRI

Pseudotumor cerebri, also called benign intracranial hypertension, is an important cause of recurrent headaches.[25] More than 80% of affected patients are women, usually between the ages of 16 and 45 years. However, this sex predilection is not noted in children. In rare cases, a self-limited form of the syndrome develops in girls at menarche and resolves spontaneously within a few weeks.[26] Pseudotumor cerebri has also been described in association with pregnancy.[27] It appears in the first half of pregnancy, remits spontaneously after delivery, and may occasionally recur with subsequent pregnancies. In young women with this condition, obesity and menstrual irregularities are the rule, but no other etiologic factor can be discerned in 90% of patients. Rare cases have been associated with hypervitaminosis A, tetracycline use, steroid use or withdrawal, thyroid replacement, and nalidixic acid therapy.

The pathogenesis of the intracranial hypertension remains elusive. It is currently believed that the mechanisms for the absorption of the cerebrospinal fluid (CSF) by the arachnoid granulation tissues in the region of the superior sagittal sinus are impaired, leading to excessive resistance to the flow of CSF and consequent elevation of the intracranial pressure. Estrone, whose secretion by adipocytes is increased in obese persons, stimulates CSF production and may contribute to the elevation of intracranial pressure. In rare instances, this condition is familial. By definition, patients have no intracranial mass lesions, hydrocephalus, or other mechanisms for their intracranial hypertension. An extraordinary feature of this syndrome is that despite the chronic, moderately severe elevations of CSF pressure to greater than 400 mm of water, the functions of the brain are not affected, the only neurologic consequences being papilledema and sixth nerve palsies.

Clinical Picture

This syndrome is typically encountered in obese young women seeking advice for recurrent headaches. The headaches are nondescript and have features overlapping episodic tension and migraine headaches. They are generalized, throbbing, and can be severe, and they sometimes are associated with nausea. Worsening of the headaches by Valsalva maneuver, as in coughing or straining, as well as by sudden changes in body position is the only other suggestive feature. Patients may experience such a recurring headache for weeks to months or years. Transient bilateral visual obscurations occur in about 70% of patients and are a manifestation of the high intracranial pressure and disk edema. Characteristic is a brief, sudden loss of vision for a few seconds in one or both eyes. Sparkles or flashes of light seen in front of both eyes may suggest a migraine type of headache. Some patients complain of double vision along with headaches due to sixth nerve palsies. About 10% of patients may present with progressive unilateral or bilateral diminution of vision. Findings on neurologic examination are normal except for papilledema and occasionally sixth nerve palsies. Optic nerve disk edema may be subtle or florid. Visual acuity is preserved in most cases, but examination of the visual fields shows enlargement of the blind spot, and in some instances, perimetric examination reveals various field defects. The earliest and most characteristic abnormality is a defect in the inferior nasal quadrant of the visual field. However, later in the course, this can extend to produce concentric constriction of the visual fields and eventually blindness. Brain imaging by CT or magnetic resonance imaging scans shows a normal appearance except for an occasional patient with slit-like ventricles. Some patients also show an enlarged sella that is filled with CSF, known as the empty-sella syndrome. This is not associated with pituitary endocrine dysfunction. Diagnosis requires a lumbar puncture that reveals high CSF pressure, often to greater than 400 mm of water. The protein may be low, but otherwise, results of CSF analysis by definition are normal. Extensive endocrinologic evaluations in these patients have been nondiagnostic.

In more than 90% of patients, the course is benign, with spontaneous remission and rarely relapses without permanent visual sequelae, even in patients with visual obscurations. In about 10% of patients, however, progressive visual failure ensues. Chronic systemic arterial hypertension is the single most important risk factor identified for visual impairment.

Treatment

Treatment is tempered by the knowledge of the benign natural history of the condition in most patients with or without specific therapy. It is best coordinated by a neurologist and ophthalmologist. Long-term control of systemic arterial hypertension is important in preventing blindness. Careful monitoring of visual symptoms and perimetric examination of the visual fields are important, not relying on visual central acuity or tangent screen examinations, which tend to be unaffected until late in the course of the disease. Any defect in the inferior nasal field and any progressive worsening of vision, the principal serious complications of this condition, demand aggressive treatment. At present, the best therapy is surgical optic nerve sheath fenestration, which helps relieve the headaches and preserve optic nerve integrity and vision.[28] A less effective, alternative approach is placement of a lumbar peritoneal CSF shunt.

In the usual situation of recurrent headaches and papilledema without visual impairment, various treatments have been advocated and tried. No controlled studies have been conducted, however, and no reliable ways have been found to predict which treatment is best suited for an individual patient. Thus, a trial-and-error approach is required. Some patients experience permanent or long-lasting remissions with a 2- to 4-week course of prednisone or dexamethasone. Others seem to respond to the carbonic anhydrase inhibitor Diamox, presumably because of its effects in reducing the production of CSF. Some patients experience a lasting remission with one or two lumbar punctures. Others may need repeated lumbar punctures based on recurrence of the headaches and visual changes.

REFERENCES

1. Stewart WF, Lipton RB, Colentano DD, et al. Prevalence of migraine headache in the United States: Relation to age, income, race and other sociodemographic factors. JAMA 1992;267:64.
2. Lance JW. Current concepts of migraine pathogenesis. Neurology 1993;43(suppl 3):511.
3. Callaham M, Raskin NH. A controlled study of dihydro-ergotamine in the treatment of acute migraine headache. Headache 1986;26:168.
4. Ferrari MD, Melamed E, Garvell MJ, et al. Treatment of migraine attacks with sumatriptan. N Engl J Med 1991;325:316.
5. Jones J, Sklar D, Dougherty J, et al. Randomized double-blind trial of intravenous prochlorperazine for the treatment of acute headache. JAMA 1989;261:1174.
6. Sorensen KU. Valproate: A new drug in migraine prophylaxis. Acta Neurol Scand 1988;78:346.
7. Diamond S. Biofeedback and headache. Neurol Clin 1983;1:479.
8. Silberstein SD. The role of sex hormones in headache. Neurology 1992;42(suppl 2):37.
9. DeLegineres B, Vincens M, Mauvais-Jarvis P, et al. Prevention of menstrual migraine by percutaneous estradiol. Br Med J 1986;293:1540.
10. Dennersten L, Morse C, Burrows G, et al. Menstrual migraine: A double-blind trial of percutaneous estradiol. Gynecol Endocrinol 1988;2:113.
11. Calton GJ, Burnett JW. Danazol and migraine. N Engl J Med 1984;310:721.
12. O'Dea JPK, Davis EH. Tamoxifen in the treatment of menstrual migraine. Neurology 1990;40:1470.
13. Silberstein SD, Merriam GR. Estrogen, progestins, and headache. Neurology 1991;41:786.
14. Aylward M, Holly F, Parker KJ. An evaluation of clinical response to piperazine estrogen sulphate (Harmogen) in menopausal patients. Curr Med Res Opin 1974;2:417.
15. Kudrow L. The relationship of headache frequency to hormone use in migraine. Headache 1975;15:36.
16. Greenblatt RB, Bruneteau DW. Menopausal headache—psychogenic or metabolic? J Am Geriatr Soc 1974;283:186.
17. Judd H. Efficacy of transdermal estradiol. Obstet Gynecol 1987;156:1326.
18. Campbell S. Double-blind psychometric studies of the effects of natural estrogens in post-menopausal women. In: Campbell S (ed). The Management of the Menopause and Postmenopausal Years. Baltimore: University Park Press, 1975, pp 149–158.
19. Ryan RE. A controlled study of the effect of oral contraceptives in migraine. Headache 1978;17:250.
20. Featherstone HJ. Clinical features of stroke in migraine: A review. Headache 1986;26:128.
21. Collaborative Group for the Study of Stroke in Young Women. Oral contraceptives and stroke in young women. JAMA 1975;231:718.
22. Featherstone HJ. Migraine and muscle contraction headaches: A continuum. Headache 1985;25:194.
23. Matthew NT, Kurman R, Perez F. Drug-induced refractory headache: Clinical features and management. Headache 1990;30:634.
24. Porter M, Jankovic J. Benign coital cephalgia. Differential diagnosis and treatment. Arch Neurol 1981;38:710.
25. Ahlskog EJ, O'Neill BP. Pseudotumor cerebri. Ann Intern Med 1982;97:259.
26. Greer M. Benign intracranial hypertension. IV. Menarche. Neurology 1964;14:569.
27. Powell JL. Pseudotumor cerebri and pregnancy. Obstet Gynecol 1972;40:713.
28. Kelman SE. Optic nerve decompression surgery improves visual function in patients with pseudotumor cerebri. Neurosurgery 1992;30:391.

Anemia

Ina Ratner

Anemia is a common problem encountered in primary care practice. Because it is a sign of disease and not a final diagnosis, an underlying cause must be determined. Anemia is defined as a reduction in either the red blood cell (RBC) volume (hematocrit) or the concentration of hemoglobin in the blood. The normal ranges for hematocrit and hemoglobin vary with age,[1] sex, race,[2, 3] and stage of pregnancy. The most current representative sample of hematologic reference data for the United States is available from the Second National Health and Nutritional Examination Survey, 1976–1980.[4] The cutoffs for hematocrit and hemoglobin recommended in Table 59–1 represent the age-specific fifth percentile values for healthy people from this sample. Tobacco use and residing at high altitudes affect hematocrit levels.

Residing at high altitudes increases the hematocrit and hemoglobin values.[5, 6] People living at altitudes above 3300 feet tend to have higher hematocrit levels than those living at sea level.[6] The body compensates for a decrease in the partial pressure of oxygen saturation in the blood at high altitudes by increasing the production of RBCs to provide adequate oxygen delivery at the tissue level. Cigarette smoking also increases the hematocrit.[5, 6] Inhalation of carbon monoxide increases carboxyhemoglobin, a form of hemoglobin that has no oxygen-carrying capacity. This, in turn, causes an upward shift of the hematocrit and hemoglobin distribution curves. The proper diagnosis of anemia for smokers or for those living at higher altitudes requires an upward adjustment of the hematocrit and hemoglobin cutoffs (Tables 59–2 and 59–3).[6] The effects of smoking cigarettes and living at high altitude are additive.[6]

SCREENING FOR ANEMIA

The three potential reasons to screen in an outpatient setting are (1) to identify specific treatable causes of mild, asymptomatic anemias, (2) to prevent adverse outcomes for asymptomatic individuals with anemia, and (3) to enable early detection and treatment of an underlying disease (e.g., malignancy).[7] Although it is often routine to obtain a complete blood count on patients, such screening is of value only in specific situations. Available data suggest that screening for anemia is not an efficient way to detect a serious underlying disorder. Nor has it been found to be important to treat mild asymptomatic anemias. No difference in mortality or morbidity has been found between women with and without mild anemia.[7] Treating specific, mild anemia may not improve a patient's well-being, especially if the patient is asymptomatic.

No evidence suggests that the complete blood count should be used to screen for anemia in the general population. It may be beneficial to screen specific subgroups in which the prevalence of anemia is high (e.g., pregnant women), but this has yet to be established.

Once anemia has been detected, clinicians tend to evaluate women if the hematocrit is less than 34.[8] Most people with anemia deserve some degree of evaluation. Anemia results from a decreased production of RBCs, an increased destruction or loss of RBCs, or a combination of both. A complete blood count with RBC indices, a peripheral smear, and reticulocyte count are quite effective at directing the initial anemia evaluation. If the white blood cell and platelet counts are abnormal in addition to the hematocrit, ineffective hematopoiesis affecting all blood lines is implicated and a bone marrow evaluation is mandated.[8, 9]

Anemia can be classified as microcytic (mean corpuscular volume [MCV] <80), macrocytic (MCV >100), or normocytic based on the RBC indices[9, 10] (Table 59–4). Red blood cell indices are calculated values reflecting the average characteristics of a certain RBC population. They are reliable indicators when the RBC population is homogeneous.[11] Homogeneity of RBC populations is reflected on RBC volume distribution width (RDW), which measures the variability of RBC size (anisocytosis).[12–14] The RDW appears to

TABLE 59–1. General Hemoglobin and Hematocrit Cutoffs*

SEX	AGE (years)	HEMOGLOBIN (gm/dl)	HEMATOCRIT (%)
Both sexes	1–1.9	11.0	33.0
	2–4.9	11.2	34.0
	5–7.9	11.4	34.5
	8–11.9	11.6	35.0
Female	12–14.9	11.8	35.5
	≥15.0	12.0	36.0
Male	12–14.9	12.3	37.0
	15–17.9	12.6	38.0
	≥18.0	13.6	41.0

*For children, men, and nonpregnant women.
From Centers for Disease Control and Prevention criteria for anemia in children and childbearing-aged women. MMWR 1989;38:400.

TABLE 59–2. Altitude Adjustments for Hemoglobin and Hematocrit Cutoffs

ALTITUDE (ft)	HEMOGLOBIN (gm/dl)	HEMATOCRIT (%)
<3,000	0.0	0.0
3000–3999	+0.2	+0.5
4000–4999	+0.3	+1.0
5000–5999	+0.5	+1.5
6000–6999	+0.7	+2.0
7000–7999	+1.0	+3.0
8000–8999	+1.3	+4.0
9000–9999	+1.6	+5.0
>10,000	+2.0	+6.0

From Centers for Disease Control and Prevention criteria for anemia in children and childbearing-aged women. MMWR 1989;38:400.

change early in anemias, even before the MCV, probably in part because of small RBCs entering the periphery as an anemia develops.

It is useful when possible to check a peripheral smear. Certain anemias can be characterized and identified by specific aberrations in RBC structure.[10] Sickled cells, for example, are diagnostic of sickle cell disease. Spherocytes suggest hereditary spherocytosis or hemolysis, and elliptocytes represent hereditary elliptocytosis. Schistocytes (RBC fragments) can help make the diagnosis of hemolysis from a mechanical valve. Burr cells characteristically are found in uremic patients. Bite cells are suggestive of glucose-6-phosphate dehydrogenase deficiency.[8, 10]

The corrected reticulocyte count is useful to assess bone marrow response to the anemia. Reticulocytes are immature RBCs that circulate for approximately 24 hours before maturing. The normal reticulocyte count is about 1% of the total RBC population. To obtain a more accurate measure of reticulocyte production, one has to correct the count for the degree of anemia compared with a normal hematocrit (e.g., 45%), as follows[7, 9]:

$$\text{Corrected reticulocyte count} = \text{measured reticulocyte count} \times \text{hematocrit}/45$$

Increased RBC loss or destruction causes the reticulocyte count to become elevated. A decrease in RBC production leads to a lower than expected reticulocyte count.

MICROCYTIC ANEMIA

The differential diagnosis of microcytic anemias includes iron deficiency, thalassemia, anemia of chronic disease, sideroblastic anemia, lead poisoning, and hemoglobin E disorders.[9–11] Iron deficiency and thalassemia are the anemias most commonly encountered in a primary care practice. The algorithm in Figure 59–1 can help direct the workup of a microcytic anemia.

The initial step is to check the corrected reticulocyte count. If elevated, it suggests a hemoglobinopathy with shortened RBC survival. This subsequently may be diagnosed with a hemoglobin electrophoresis.[10, 16] For example, increased amounts of fetal hemoglobin and hemoglobin A_2 imply β-thalassemia. α-Thalassemia is more difficult to diagnose and is often a diagnosis of exclusion.[8, 10, 16] It was thought that the RDW would be a useful index to differentiate iron deficiency from other microcytic anemias, but this has not been the case. The RDW does increase early in iron deficiency, but not exclusively.[17] It may be elevated in thalassemia, hemolytic anemia, and other hemoglobinopathies.

If the reticulocyte count is normal or low, serum ferritin determination can be quite helpful. A low ferritin level (<20 μg/dl) is quite specific for identifying iron deficiency.[17–19] However, the useful-

TABLE 59–3. Smoking Adjustments for Hemoglobin and Hematocrit Cutoffs

CHARACTERISTIC	HEMOGLOBIN (gm/dl)	HEMATOCRIT (%)
Nonsmoker	0.0	0.0
Smoker (all)	+0.3	+1.0
½–1 pack/day	+0.3	+1.0
1–2 packs/day	+0.5	+1.5
>2 packs/day	+0.7	+2.0

From Centers for Disease Control and Prevention criteria for anemia in children and childbearing-aged women. MMWR 1989;38:400.

TABLE 59–4.   Common Causes of Anemia

MICROCYTIC	NORMOCYTIC	MACROCYTIC
Iron deficiency	Anemia of chronic disease	Vitamin B_{12} deficiency
Hemoglobinopathy	Endocrinopathy	Folate deficiency
Anemia of chronic disease	Renal failure	Liver disease
Sideroblastic anemia	Hemolysis	Alcohol use
Lead poisoning	Hemorrhage	Reticulocytosis
	Hypersplenism	Myelodysplasia
		Antimetabolite drugs
		Antifolate drugs

ness of ferritin determination can be limited because ferritin can be an acute-phase reactant,[19] and ferritin level can be elevated with liver disease, chronic infection, inflammation, or malignancy. Ferritin levels can rise rapidly during iron replace- ment therapy; thus, iron treatment should be stopped for at least 1 week before measuring fer- ritin.[18]

If the ferritin value is normal or high, checking serum iron level, total iron-binding capacity

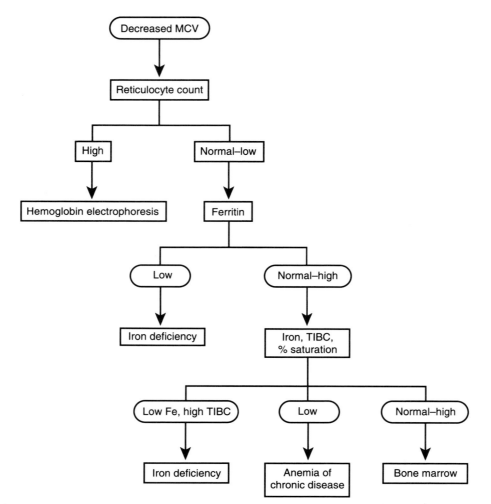

Figure 59–1. Evaluation of microcytic anemia. MCV, Mean corpuscular volume; TIBC, transferrin binding capacity; % saturation, saturation of transferrin sites; Fe, serum iron.

([TIBC] i.e., transferrin level), and transferrin saturation may be useful. If all these values are low, an anemia of chronic disease is suggested. If the TIBC is elevated and the transferrin saturation is low (<15%), iron deficiency is suggested (Table 59–5).[17, 20]

It may be difficult to distinguish iron deficiency from anemia of chronic disease, and an empirical course of iron therapy may be warranted. Documenting a rise in the reticulocyte count and hematocrit is diagnostic of an iron-deficient state. If the diagnosis remains unclear, a bone marrow evaluation can assess iron stores as well as look for ringed sideroblasts.[17]

Often it is not possible to check laboratory data in a stepwise fashion, because it is time-consuming and impractical for patients. After discovering a microcytic anemia, a reticulocyte count, ferritin value, serum iron level, TIBC, and transferrin saturation can be measured simultaneously, eliminating repeated blood drawing. With those data, one should be able to diagnose most microcytic anemias while reserving the most expensive and possibly invasive tests for cases in which they are indicated.

The most common cause of microcytic anemia in young women is iron deficiency secondary to blood loss from menses or pregnancy. In such women, any evaluation can be deferred pending the response to empirical therapy.

Healthy women of childbearing age with mild anemias (hematocrit >30), low MCVs, elevated RDWs, normal white blood cell counts, and normal platelets can be treated empirically with iron replacement. This assumes the anemia is due to iron deficiency resulting from menses or pregnancies. If no improvement is noted after a few months, further search for the cause of the anemia must be initiated.

IRON DEFICIENCY ANEMIA

Like anemia, iron deficiency is a sign of disease, not a complete diagnosis. The cause of the iron deficiency should be considered. Iron is a nutrient that is primarily absorbed in the duodenum.[17, 21]

The stomach's acidity promotes the reduction of iron from its ferric (Fe^{3+}) to ferrous (Fe^{2+}) state, which is better absorbed.[22] The daily dietary intake of iron in the United States typically is about 10 to 20 mg, of which only 10% is absorbed.[23] Within the circulation, iron is bound entirely to transferrin, a transport protein of which one third is saturated with iron. Iron is stored in the bone marrow as ferritin or hemosiderin.[18] The serum ferritin level is often used as an accurate measure of total body iron stores.

Ideally, in healthy adults, the amount of iron absorbed equals the amount lost physiologically through the shedding of cells (approximately 1 mg/day).[21] Pregnancy and menstruation increase daily intake needs and can create diminished iron stores. Typically women lose 10 to 20 mg of iron with each menstrual period. Iron loss per pregnancy ranges from 500 to 1000 mg.[17] In premenopausal women, it is reasonable to conclude that iron deficiency is due to menstruation or pregnancy. In postmenopausal women, gastrointestinal pathology is the most common cause of iron deficiency. Dietary iron deficiency can cause an anemia in infants but rarely in adults,[17, 21] because foods are often fortified.[22] Malabsorption of iron can occur in people with partial gastrectomies, celiac sprue, or Crohn's disease.[17] Most often, chronic gastrointestinal blood loss is the cause of an iron deficiency state.[10] Gastritis due to chronic nonsteroidal anti-inflammatory drug use, peptic ulcer disease, angiodysplasia, and colon cancer all can underlie an iron deficiency.

Once the diagnosis of iron deficiency is made, treatment should be initiated, even while searching for an underlying disorder. Oral iron therapy with ferrous salts is preferred, because it is the best absorbed, safest, and least expensive treatment.[16, 22] Enteric coated and sustained-release preparations are better tolerated but release iron too distal in the gastrointestinal tract for maximal absorption.[16, 23] The standard therapeutic dose is 60 mg of elemental iron three times a day. Ferrous sulfate, for example, contains 60 mg of elemental iron in its usual 325-mg dose.[17] Approximately 15 to 20% of patients experience gastrointestinal side effects.

TABLE 59–5. Comparison of Microcytic Anemias

	SERUM IRON	TOTAL IRON-BINDING CAPACITY	SATURATION (%)	FERRITIN
Iron deficiency	Low	High	Low	Low
Thalassemia	Normal–high	Normal	Normal	Normal
Anemia of chronic disease	Normal–low	Normal–low	Normal–low	Normal–high

Gastric irritation can be decreased by slowly increasing the dose and ingesting it with meals. Large amounts of ascorbic acid (>200 mg) may help to increase the absorption of iron,[22] whereas antacids may interfere by increasing gastric pH.[17] If a patient is unable to tolerate or absorb any oral iron preparations, parenteral iron dextran may be given intravenously. This treatment should be reserved for clear indications because of the small but significant incidence of anaphylaxis.[17, 22]

Once treatment is initiated, a response occurs quickly. The reticulocyte count rises in 4 to 7 days, and the anemia should be corrected in 4 to 8 weeks.[22] It is important to treat for at least 6 months, the time required to replete iron stores.[17]

THE THALASSEMIAS

Another major type of anemia is the hereditary microcytic anemias. Fortunately, the severe form, thalassemia major, is rare. More often, thalassemia minor (the carrier state) is encountered.[16] The thalassemias are hereditary anemias caused by defects in the production of the alpha or beta globin chains. The resultant RBCs have a normal life span, but the concentration of hemoglobin is diminished.

Human hemoglobin typically consists of two alpha and two beta chains.[9, 13] Individuals typically inherit two alpha chain genes and one beta chain gene from each parent. β-Thalassemia is caused by a defect in the expression of one of the two beta globin genes.[11] A failure to produce normal amounts of beta globin chain results in an excess of alpha chains. These alpha chains combine with either delta chains to form an increased amount of hemoglobin A_2 or with gamma chains to form fetal hemoglobin.[16] Most often, β-thalassemia is diagnosed by demonstrating increased amounts of hemoglobin A_2 on hemoglobin electrophoresis (Table 59–6).[8, 9, 16]

β-Thalassemia occurs mainly in people of Mediterranean decent (Italian and Greek),[11] in whom the gene frequency approaches 10%.[16] The heterozygote state, or β-thalassemia trait, is a benign, asymptomatic disease characterized by a mild microcytic anemia. Homozygous disease, or β-thalassemia major, is a severe childhood anemia characterized by hemolysis, severe hepatomegaly, and secondary hemosiderosis resulting from multiple blood transfusions.[16] It is rare for affected individuals to survive into adulthood.

α-Thalassemia is caused by a defect, usually a deletion, in two of four alpha globin genes.[11] Unlike β-thalassemia, no alpha-like chains can combine with the surplus beta chains. Deletion of all four alpha genes results in only gamma chains, which form tetramers (Bart's hemoglobin). These cannot support life and cause hydrops fetalis.[16] This condition afflicts Southeast Asians and causes a brisk hemolytic anemia and hypersplenism. If only one alpha gene is available and three are deleted, excess beta chains abound and form tetramers, creating hemoglobin H.[16] This is also most often encountered in Southeast Asians.

More commonly, only one or two alpha genes are missing and little (if any) hemoglobin H is made. This form of α-thalassemia occurs in approximately 3% of the American black population because many have only one alpha locus instead of two.[10] In these more common forms of α-thalassemia trait, little to no hemoglobin H is made, and the diagnosis of α-thalassemia becomes difficult to make except with sophisticated biomedical tests such as globin chain analysis.

Patients with thalassemia minor are usually asymptomatic and do not require treatment. It is reasonable to make the diagnosis to avoid further work-up and inappropriate treatments, as well as for genetic counseling implications.[9, 16]

MACROCYTIC ANEMIA

Macrocytosis is defined as an elevated RBC MCV (MCV >100). The incidence of macrocytosis in the adult population noted on an automated cell blood count varies from 1.7 to 3.6% as reported in several series.[24] Approximately 60% of patients with macrocytosis do not have an associated anemia. However, because an elevated MCV often precedes the development of anemia, the isolated elevated MCV should be evaluated.[24]

Probably the most common cause of an isolated macrocytosis is alcohol use, followed by vitamin B_{12} (cobalamin) and folate deficiencies.[9, 15] Other causes include chemotherapy, other drug effects, hemolysis or bleeding, liver dysfunction, myelodysplasia, and hypothyroidism. Approximately 10% of patients have unexplained macrocytosis after the laboratory evaluation.[24]

In evaluating macrocytosis, it is useful to obtain an accurate history to help determine its cause. Specific questions about diet, alcohol intake, medications, and past operations can direct the work-up and often suggest the diagnosis.[15] For example, strict vegetarians who do not eat any animal protein including dairy products and eggs are at risk for vitamin B_{12} deficiency.[9, 24] Although folate is widely distributed in nature, especially in green leafy vegetables, it is heat labile and can be destroyed by excessive cooking.[21] People with marginal diets who subsist mainly on carbohydrates

TABLE 59–6. **Comparison of Thalassemias**

	HEMOGLOBIN ELECTROPHORESIS	ETHNIC GROUP
β-Thalassemia		
Heterozygote β°/β	↑ Hemoglobin A_2 ($\alpha_2 \delta_2$)	Mediterranean (Italian, Greek)
Homozygote β°/β°	↑ Hemoglobin F ($\alpha_2 \gamma_2$)	
α-Thalassemia		
Silent carrier α°α/αα	Normal	
α Trait α°α/α°α or α°α/αα	Normal (↓ hemoglobin A_2)	African Americans
Hemoglobin H disease α°α°/α°α	↑ Hemoglobin H (beta chain tetramers)	Southeast Asians
Hydrops fetalis α°α°/α°α°	↑ Bart's hemoglobin (gamma tetramers)	Southeast Asians

°, Deletion.

are at risk for folate deficiency.[25] Antineoplastic agents such as methotrexate, hydroxyurea, and cyclophosphamide can cause macrocytosis. Azidothymidine causes a macrocytosis in the majority of patients taking it.[24] Anticonvulsants (phenytoin, primidone, phenobarbital) as well as oral contraceptive pills and sulfamethoxazole-trimethoprim can cause an elevated MCV by altering folate metabolism.[24, 25] Alcohol causes direct marrow toxicity and interferes with folate metabolism.[21] Partial or total gastrectomies can decrease intrinsic factor synthesis and thereby cause a vitamin B_{12} deficiency.

A physical examination is often not revealing or helpful in determining the cause of an elevated MCV.[15, 26] Neurologic findings of lower extremity weakness, diminished vibratory and proprioceptive sensation, and ataxic gait, which are classically associated with vitamin B_{12} deficiency, are rare. Folate deficiency is not associated with any particular neurologic findings.[7, 24]

The initial step in evaluating macrocytosis is to determine if it is megaloblastic (i.e., impaired deoxyribonucleic acid synthesis) or nonmegaloblastic (Fig. 59–2).[9–11] A megaloblastic peripheral smear has oval macrocytes, hypersegmented neutrophils (any with six or more nuclear segments or greater than 5% of neutrophils with five segments), and possibly giant platelets and leukopenia.[25] Megaloblastic changes are mainly encountered with vitamin B_{12} and folate deficiencies, although they can be caused by antifolate or antimetabolite drugs. Once the anemia is determined to be megaloblastic, serum vitamin B_{12} and folate levels should be checked. Both are sensitive tests, and levels are frequently decreased before the development of macrocytosis.[24, 25] The serum folate level is relatively labile and quite sensitive to short-term changes in folate balance. An erythrocyte folate level can often be useful because it reflects the average blood folate levels during the previous weeks.[8] In patients with an oval macrocytic anemia, normal serum levels of vitamin B_{12} and folate, and no history of chemotherapy, a bone marrow aspiration and biopsy are indicated. This may reveal myelodysplasia.[15]

If no megaloblastic changes are observed on the peripheral smear, the next step is to proceed with a corrected reticulocyte count. An elevated reticulocyte count can elevate the MCV and suggests hemolysis or acute blood loss as the cause of anemia. If the reticulocyte count is low or normal, thyroid and liver function tests should be performed. If these tests still do not reveal an answer, a bone marrow evaluation is indicated.

VITAMIN B_{12} AND FOLATE DEFICIENCIES

Both vitamin B_{12} and folic acid are essential cofactors for the synthesis of deoxyribonucleic acid.[21] Vitamin B_{12} is ubiquitous in the diet. After vitamin B_{12} enters the stomach, it is bound to intrinsic factor, and the complex is absorbed in the terminal ileum.[24, 25] Vitamin B_{12} has large total body stores, which exceed daily use by more than a thousandfold. Years must pass before a deficiency state develops after ceasing vitamin B_{12} intake. Pernicious anemia, a gastric mucosal defect that impairs the synthesis of intrinsic factor, is the most common cause of vitamin B_{12} deficiency. Other causes include gastrectomy, ileitis, and fish tapeworm infestation.[8, 12, 24]

Unlike vitamin B_{12} deficiency, folate deficiency is often nutritional, mainly because the amount of dietary folate does not greatly exceed nutritional requirements and total body folate stores are relatively small.[24] Folate deficiency can develop within months after folate intake is ceased. Folate

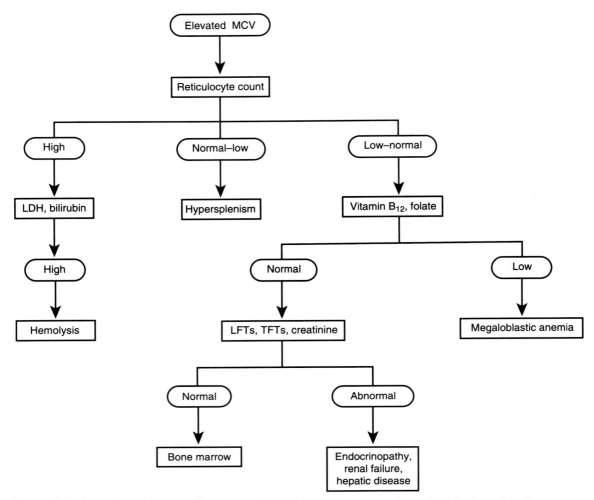

Figure 59–2. Evaluation of macrocytic anemia. MCV, Mean corpuscular volume; LDH, lactose dehydrogenase; LFTs, liver function tests; TFTs, thyroid function tests.

is also absorbed in the small intestine, and diseases that affect the jejunum can interfere with its absorption.[21] Other major causes of folate deficiency include pregnancy, which causes increased folate requirements, and drugs, including anticonvulsants, oral contraceptives, and methotrexate.[24, 25]

If the underlying disorder cannot be determined by history alone, other tests can be useful. Schilling's test is recognized as the standard test for evaluating vitamin B_{12} deficiency. It differentiates pernicious anemia from a malabsorptive disorder. Schilling's test is typically performed in two stages. In stage 1, radioactive B_{12} is given orally at the same time a dose of unlabeled B_{12} is administered intramuscularly to correct any underlying deficiency. A 24-hour urine sample is then collected to measure B_{12} excretion. Values less than 7% are suggestive of pernicious anemia.[24]

In the second stage, radioactive B_{12} and intrinsic factor are administered simultaneously. The remainder of the test is the same. Pernicious anemia is diagnosed if the urinary excretion is normal in stage 2 but low in stage 1. If both stages are low, malabsorption is suggested.[24]

An updated version of Schilling's test consists of administering B_{12} and a B_{12}–intrinsic factor complex simultaneously but labeled with different isotopes.[21] Patients with pernicious anemia excrete only the B_{12}–intrinsic factor complex. Patients with malabsorption do not excrete either, and those with dietary deficiency of B_{12} excrete both.[21] As with the older version, the underlying B_{12} deficiency must be corrected before performing the test.

If results of the Schilling's test are equivocal, anti–intrinsic factor antibodies may be checked.

These antibodies are specific for pernicious anemia but are present in only 60% of cases.[24]

A D-xylose test to identify proximal small bowel malabsorption may also be useful. A 25-gm oral dose of labeled xylose is administered. A 5-hour urinary excretion is measured, as well as peak blood levels at 1 and 2 hours. Low urinary excretion and low blood levels signify malabsorption. A small bowel biopsy is also occasionally needed to diagnose malabsorption. It is worthwhile to pursue the underlying disorder, because it can often be treated.

NORMOCYTIC ANEMIA

Normocytic anemia (normal MCV) is the other major category of anemia. The reticulocyte count is helpful in differentiating the underlying causes (Fig. 59–3). An elevated reticulocyte count represents acute blood loss or peripheral destruction of RBCs. A normal or lower than anticipated reticulocyte count is inappropriate in the anemic state and implies either bone marrow dysfunction or inhibition of the normal marrow hematopoiesis.[15]

An elevated reticulocyte count points to one of three causes: acute blood loss, hypersplenism, or hemolysis. Acute blood loss is usually apparent with menorrhagia or gastrointestinal bleeding, but sometimes it is more subtle, as in a retroperitoneal bleed. Hypersplenism causes premature destruction of RBCs and splenic pooling.[9] To cause a noticeable decrease in blood volume, the spleen must be three to four times its normal size and can be detected on physical examination.[15]

Hemolysis is evident when lactate dehydrogenase and indirect bilirubin levels are elevated and serum haptoglobin (a free hemoglobin-binding protein) level is decreased. Hemolytic anemias are classified as either congenital or acquired.[15] Congenital hemolytic anemias include disorders of RBC membranes, such as hereditary spherocytosis, hemoglobinopathies, and RBC enzyme deficiencies such as pyruvate kinase and glucose-6-phosphate dehydrogenase deficiencies.[15] The peripheral blood smear can often aid in this differentiation by identifying characteristic cells such as spherocytes and elliptocytes.[11] Hemoglobin electrophoresis can identify hemoglobinopathies. Specific enzyme activity assays diagnose glucose-6-phosphate dehydrogenase and pyruvate kinase deficiencies.

Acquired hemolytic anemias include mechanical hemolysis (from a prosthetic heart valve or disseminated intravascular coagulation), immune-mediated hemolysis, or paroxysmal nocturnal hemoglobinuria.[8, 15] The peripheral smear can often

reveal schistocytes, RBC fragments. Immune-mediated hemolysis due to warm-reactive immunoglobulin G antibodies or cold-reactive immunoglobulin M antibodies[15] is caused by collagen vascular diseases, infections, or neoplasms, or it can be idiopathic. Results of a direct Coombs' test are often positive, helping to identify immune-mediated hemolysis. Paroxysmal nocturnal hemoglobinuria is rare and can be precluded if no hemosiderin is found in the urine. The diagnosis can be confirmed with the acid hemolysis test.[11, 15]

When the corrected reticulocyte count is normal or low in the setting of normocytic anemia, bone marrow dysfunction or inhibition of marrow hematopoiesis needs to be considered. With concomitant leukopenia and thrombocytopenia, a bone marrow aspiration and biopsy are indicated to rule out aplastic anemia. If the other cell lines are normal, systemic diseases causing anemia should be considered. Renal insufficiency as well as endocrinopathies (thyroid, adrenal, and pituitary hypofunction) can cause an anemia.[9, 11, 15] The anemia of renal failure is due to decreased erythropoietin production and shortened RBC survival. The degree of the anemia is directly proportional to the degree of renal failure. It can often be alleviated by treatment with recombinant erythropoietin.[9]

Erythropoietin, a hematopoietic growth factor that stimulates the growth of erythroid precursor cells, is produced in the interstitial cells of the renal cortex.[27] Recombinant erythropoietin is primarily used to treat the anemia of renal disease. It has been shown to be of some benefit in the treatment of anemias due to inflammatory processes such as rheumatoid arthritis and malignancy. It remains difficult to predict which patients will respond to this therapy.[9] The benefits of parenteral recombinant erythropoietin therapy are sustained elevations in the hemoglobin and hematocrit levels, reducing transfusion requirements. Patients also report an improved sense of well-being. This therapy has few side effects except in renal patients, whose hypertension may be exacerbated.[27]

ANEMIA OF CHRONIC DISEASE

If no systemic disorder is identified, the anemia of chronic disease should be considered. This is a broad category of anemia with several characteristic features. The degree of the anemia is usually mild (hematocrit between 30 and 40), and patients are not symptomatic.[21, 28] It typically is normocytic but can become microcytic. The main three underlying disorders are chronic infections such as endocarditis, chronic inflammatory conditions such as rheumatoid arthritis, and neoplasms. However,

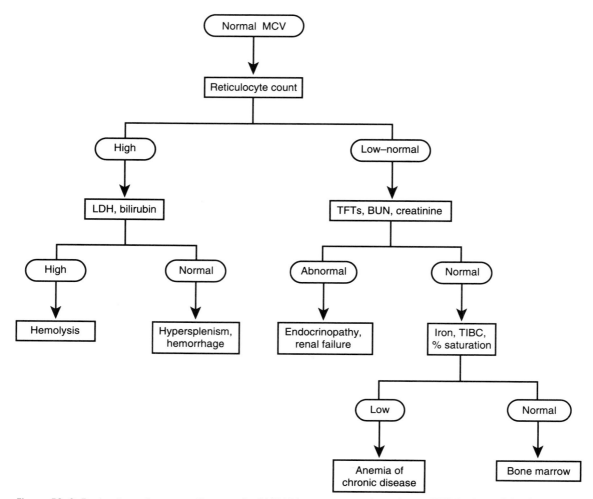

Figure 59–3. Evaluation of normocytic anemia. MCV, Mean corpuscular volume; LDH, lactose dehydrogenase; TFTs, thyroid function tests; BUN, blood urea nitrogen; TIBC, transferrin binding capacity; % saturation, saturation of transferrin sites.

25% of patients with anemia of chronic disease have no known systemic diseases.[28]

Abnormalities of iron distribution are the most consistent and concrete characteristics of the anemia of chronic disease.[27, 28] The serum iron level, the transferrin level (TIBC), and the percent saturation of transferrin typically are decreased, and the ferritin level is normal or elevated.[27–29] The ferritin level is often used to distinguish iron deficiency anemia from the anemia of chronic disease.[17, 19] In uncomplicated iron deficiency, the ferritin level is less than 20 μg per ml, whereas in anemia of chronic disease the ferritin level is usually elevated (>100 μg/ml).[20] The bone marrow has an increased amount of storage iron in the reticuloendothelial system but a diminished amount of iron-containing erythroblasts (RBC precursors).[20, 28] The reticuloendothelial cells have an impaired ability to release iron from previously phagocytosed RBCs for heme synthesis. The exact mechanism of this impairment is not known.[28] The end result is decreased production of RBCs. Because anemia of chronic disease usually does not cause symptoms, there is no specific therapy beyond treatment of the underlying disease.

It is important to remember that multifactorial anemias can arise, especially in sick or hospitalized patients. Determining the cause of the anemia is not as straightforward as presented in the foregoing algorithms. For example, a patient with celiac sprue may be deficient in iron as well as folate, potentially creating a normocytic picture on the peripheral smear. If the work-up is nondiagnostic, bone marrow evaluation is indicated and can be especially helpful in distinguishing iron deficiency, anemia of chronic disease, and marrow suppression as the reason for the anemia.

REFERENCES

1. Yip R, Johnson C, Dallman P. Age-related changes in laboratory values used in the diagnosis of anemia and iron deficiency. Am J Clin Nutr 1984;39:427.
2. Dallman P, Barr G, Allen C, Shinefield H. Hemoglobin concentration in white, black, and Oriental children: Is there a need for separate criteria in screening for anemia? Am J Clin Nutr 1978;31:377.
3. Cresanta J, Hyg MS, Croft J, et al. Racial difference in hemoglobin concentration of young adults. Prev Med 1987;16:659.
4. Dallman P, Yip R, Johnson C. Prevalence and causes of anemia in the United States, 1976 to 1980. Am J Clin Nutr 1984;39:437.
5. Nordenberg D, Yip R, Binkin N. The effect of cigarette smoking on hemoglobin levels and anemia screening. JAMA 1990;264(12):1556.
6. Centers for Disease Control and Prevention. CDC criteria for anemia in children and childbearing-aged women. MMWR 1989;38:400.
7. Shapiro M, Greenfield S. The complete blood count and leukocyte differential count. Ann Intern Med 1987;106:65.
8. Means R Jr. Anemia: When—and how aggressively—to work it up. Hosp Med 1992;10:84.
9. Welborn J, Meyers F. A three-point approach to anemia. Postgrad Med 1991;89(2):179.
10. Brown R. Determining the cause of anemia. Postgrad Med 1991;89(6):161.
11. Djulbegovic B, Hadley T, Pasic R. A new algorithm for diagnosis of anemia. Postgrad Med 1989;85(5):119.
12. Thompson W, Meola T, Lipkin M Jr, Freedman M. Red cell distribution width, mean corpuscular volume, and transferrin saturation in the diagnosis of iron deficiency. Arch Intern Med 1988;148:2128.
13. Guyatt G, Patterson C, Ali M, et al. Diagnosis of iron-deficiency anemia in the elderly. Am J Med 1990;88:205.
14. Stander P. Anemia in the elderly. Postgrad Med 1989;85:85.
15. Brown R. Normocytic and macrocytic anemias. Postgrad Med 1991;89(8):125.
16. Beutler E. The common anemias. JAMA 1988;259(16):2433.
17. Massey A. Microcytic anemia. Med Clinics North Am 1992;76(3):549.
18. Yip R, Dalman P. The roles of inflammation and iron deficiency as causes of anemia. Am J Clin Nutr 1988;48:1295.
19. Lipschitz D, Cook J, Finch C. A clinical evaluation of serum ferritin as an index of iron stores. N Engl J Med 1974;290(22):1213.
20. Lipschitz D. The anemia of chronic disease. J Am Geriatr Soc 1990;38:1258.
21. Krause J. The bone marrow in nutritional deficiencies. Hematol Oncol Clin North Am 1988;2(4):557.
22. Farley P, Foland J. Iron deficiency anemia. Postgrad Med 1990;87(2):89.
23. Mohler E Jr. Iron deficiency and anemia of chronic disease. Postgrad Med 1992;92(4):123.
24. Colon-Otero G, Menke D, Hook C. A practical approach to the diagnosis and evaluation of the adult patient with macrocytic anemia. Med Clin North Am 1992;76(3):581.
25. Beck W. Diagnosis of megaloblastic anemia. Annu Rev Med 1991;42:311.
26. Nardone D, Roth K, Mazur D, McAfee J. Usefulness of physical examination in detecting the presence or absence of anemia. Arch Intern Med 1990;150:201.
27. Damon L. Anemias of chronic disease in the aged: Diagnosis and treatment. Geriatrics 1992;47(4):47.
28. Sears D. Anemia of chronic disease. Med Clin North Am 1992;76(3):567.
29. Henry D. Changing patterns of care in the management of anemia. Semin Oncol 1992;19(3) (Suppl 8):3.

MENOPAUSE

Menopause

Gail A. Greendale and Howard L. Judd

Menopause is defined as the cessation of ovarian function resulting in permanent amenorrhea. A period of 12 months of amenorrhea usually signifies cessation of ovarian function; identification of menopause is therefore necessarily retrospective. The climacteric is the term used to describe the clinical symptoms and the physiologic changes that are associated with the change from reproductive to nonreproductive status. The symptoms and syndromes associated with menopause and the climacteric are summarized in Table 60–1. These are divided into symptoms with an onset in the perimenopausal and early postmenopausal period (− 5 to 5 + years around menopause), those that occur somewhat later after the menopause (5 + to 10 + years), and those that become apparent many years postmenopausally.

Climacteric symptoms include hot flushes, genitourinary atrophy, and possibly alterations in mood. In addition, asymptomatic physiologic changes related to the hypoestrogenemic postreproductive state are associated with the development of cardiovascular disease and osteoporosis. Although clinically apparent heart disease or fractures do not increase in frequency until 10 to 15 years after menopause, their prevention should be considered as a part of perimenopausal and early postmenopausal health maintenance.

This chapter discusses the etiology and treatment of the clinical climacteric symptoms. Because the effectiveness of hormonal and nonhormonal interventions varies by indication, the approach to each of the climacteric symptoms is discussed separately. Chapter 61 discusses hormone dosage, schedules, and safety monitoring. Osteoporosis is discussed in Chapter 62. Cardiovascular diseases are discussed in Chapters 50 to 52.

PHYSIOLOGY OF THE MENOPAUSE TRANSITION

The beginning of the menopausal transition is signaled by changes in the menstrual pattern and the trophic hormones that regulate it. In the earliest phase of the transition, which occurs about 10 years before menopause, menstrual cycle length shortens, the length of the follicular phase decreases, and follicle-stimulating hormone levels become relatively higher than those of younger women. The overtly perimenopausal menstrual pattern consists of varying short cycles and long intermenstrual intervals. Perimenopausal menstrual cycles can be either ovulatory (accompanied by luteal phase progesterone secretion) or anovulatory. Estradiol and progesterone levels of transitional cycles are lower than those of younger women, and levels of follicle-stimulating hormone are relatively higher (>25 mIU/ml).

The average age at which menopause occurs is 50 years. When menses cease, the secretion of steroid hormones and gonadotropins changes. The level of estradiol is substantially lower than during the premenopausal period. Estradiol levels are higher than estrone levels in premenopausal women, and this ratio reverses postmenopausally. After menopause, estradiol and estrone are no longer principally derived from the ovaries; they arise from the peripheral conversion of other steroid hormones. The sources of estrone are androstenedione and testosterone. The adrenal glands supply about 80% and the ovaries about 20% of the postmenopausal androstenedione. Overall, androstenedione levels are roughly half those of premenopausal women. The ovaries continue to make the same amount of testosterone as they did during the premenopause. Dehydroepiandrosterone and

TABLE 60–1. Symptoms and Syndromes That May Be Associated with Menopause and the Postreproductive State

PERI- AND EARLY POSTMENOPAUSE (−5 to 5+ YR)	MID POSTMENOPAUSE (5+ to 10+ YR)	LATER POSTMENOPAUSE (10+ YR)
Irregular menses	Stress incontinence	Cardiovascular disease
Hot flushes	Sensory-urge incontinence	Osteoporosis
Dysphoric mood	Urinary urgency	
Mild memory impairment	Dysuria	
Interrupted sleep	Dyspareunia	
	Atrophic vaginitis	
	Increased susceptibility to bacterial vaginitis	
	Epidermal thinning	

dehydroepiandrosterone sulfate continue to be made by the adrenal glands. The levels of these hormones decrease after the age of 30 years, unrelated to changes in ovarian function.

CLIMACTERIC SYNDROMES AND THEIR TREATMENT

Hot Flushes

Hot flushes are experienced as an initial sensation of pressure in the head, followed by a feeling of warmth in the head and upper trunk, that may then spread over the rest of the body. Perspiration occurs in the affected regions, and a chill often follows. Hot flushes can be objectively documented by measuring elevated skin temperature, diminished skin resistance (due to perspiration), and decreased core temperature (due to peripheral vasodilation and subsequent cooling).

Hot flushes are common and may not be unique to the perimenopause and postmenopause. In longitudinal population-based studies, 10 to 20% of women report hot flushes in their 40s, during which time their menstrual cycles are still regular. The incidence of flushes clearly increases at the menopausal transition, with 40 to 58% of women noting flushes within the 2-year period around their final menses. Flushes decrease as time from menopause increases. Most women experience them for a few years, but 29 to 50% of women in clinical samples report hot flushes for longer than 5 years.

TREATMENT OF HOT FLUSHES. Randomized placebo-controlled trials have demonstrated the effectiveness of both hormonal and nonhormonal therapies for hot flushes. Estrogens reduce both perceived and objectively measured hot flushes. Higher doses of estrogen are associated with increasing degrees of hot flush suppression. For example, hot flushes are decreased by about 50% when 50 μg of estradiol-17β is used, and 100 μg reduces their frequency by about 70%. Therefore, the dose of estrogen for hot flushes should be adjusted to control symptoms. Although the time required to achieve the maximum hot flush suppression by a given estrogen dose has not been formally studied, at least 4 weeks' elapse between dose adjustments seems reasonable. Women who require high doses of estrogen early in menopause usually tolerate later dose reduction, because hot flushes decrease with time from menopause.

Alternatives to estrogen are available for the treatment of hot flushes. Progestins, such as 20 mg of medroxyprogesterone acetate or 20 to 40 mg of megestrol acetate, diminish hot flushes by approximately 25 to 75%. Methyldopa, 250 mg orally three times a day, reduces hot flushes by about 30%; side effects can be troublesome, however, with 60% of subjects noting dizziness, nausea, and fatigue. Clonidine also achieves a dose-related decrease in hot flushes, ranging from a 20 to 45% reduction when doses of 100 to 400 μg per day are used. At the higher end of the dose range, the side effects of dry mouth, insomnia, and syncope are frequent.

Lower Urinary Tract

The female lower urinary tract and genital tract derive from a common precursor, the urogenital sinus. Atrophic changes occur in the urethra and periurethral tissue in association with the menopause, similar to those that occur in the genital tract. The urethral epithelial layer regresses, and the urethra becomes thinner. Atrophy of the periurethral tissues and blood vessels also occurs. These atrophic changes lead to a decrease in the normal upward pressure generated by the urethra and surrounding tissues, termed the urethral factor. Decreased urethral factor can contribute to stress incontinence, or the involuntary loss of small amounts of urine with maneuvers that increase abdominal pressure, such as coughing or stepping down off a curb.

Estrogen receptors have been isolated from the trigone and bladder; thus, postmenopausal hypoestrogenemia may have a role in the pathobiology of lowered sensory threshold to void. The consequence of lowering the sensory voiding threshold is sensory-urge incontinence, a particular form of urge continence. Urge incontinence is the loss of urine because of inability to delay voiding once bladder fullness is sensed. Urge incontinence can be caused by detrusor hyperrelexia (a hyperreactive bladder) or the sensory-urge mechanism, which is urge incontinence without detrusor overactivity.

In some women, loss of pelvic tone and decreased pelvic support (pelvic descent) lead to prolapse of the urethrovesicular junction. This can contribute to incontinence, because the intra-abdominal location of the urethrovesicular junction is another important aspect of bladder control. However, the relative contributions of aging, hypoestrogenemia, and obstetric stress to pelvic descent remain uncertain.

Dysuria, urgency, and frequency, without overt incontinence, may also occur in relation to atrophic postmenopausal changes in the lower urinary tract. These three symptoms have been called the senile urethral syndrome. Dysuria is attributed to urine coming in close contact with exposed urethral sensory nerves, causing noninfectious pain on urination. Frequency is ascribed to atrophic trigonitis, and urgency to an aberrant sensory feedback loop with abnormal urethral relaxation.

LOWER URINARY TRACT TREATMENT. Postmenopausal stress incontinence has been treated with estrogens to improve urethral anatomy and tone, with α-agonists to increase urethral sphincter pressure, and with combination therapy. In uncontrolled studies, oral conjugated equine estrogens have improved urethral pressure profiles and decreased the occurrence of stress incontinence. Similar improvements in pressure profiles and symptoms have been reported with the use of intravaginal estrogen cream. The combination of phenylpropanolamine and oral or vaginal estriol has produced a 40% cure rate of stress incontinence in uncontrolled trials.

Similar encouraging preliminary results have been observed with the use of estrogen for urge incontinence in postmenopausal women. One small clinical trial of estradiol and estriol found a 40% cure rate of urge-incontinent symptoms. A second study, which compared oral and vaginal estrogen alone or in combination with phenylpropanolamine, reported the greatest benefit, a 50% decrease in the number of urge-incontinent episodes, in women treated with combination therapy.

Therapeutic interventions for the senile urethral syndrome have not been formally studied. Estrogen is often used in clinical practice, and noninfectious dysuria and urgency often appear to respond to estrogen therapy. However, systematic study of this problem is needed.

Postmenopausal Genital Atrophy

The postmenopausal decrease in estrogen levels is associated with atrophy of the lower genital tract. Subepithelial vaginal changes produce a loss of vaginal elasticity, shortening of the vaginal canal, and loss of rugae. The vaginal epithelium also regresses, leading to a pale-appearing vaginal surface. With increasing degrees of vaginal atrophy, the epithelial surface can become easily friable and may ultimately ulcerate. Glycogen content of vaginal epithelial cells also decreases in association with vaginal atrophy. The resultant increase in pH of the vagina may decrease host resistance to bacterial vaginitis. In contrast to the natural history of hot flushes, genital atrophic changes of the menopause tend to increase in frequency and severity with time from menopause. Some postmenopausal women develop atrophic vaginitis, clinical symptoms that occur in association with the physical findings of an atrophic vagina. The symptoms of atrophic vaginitis include vaginal dryness, pruritus, and dyspareunia.

The cervix also atrophies; ultimately, it becomes flush with the vaginal wall. The squamocolumnar junction migrates upward into the cervical canal, and stenosis of the external and internal ora may occur. These anatomic cervical alterations often impede the performance of Papanicolaou smears in older women.

TREATMENT OF GENITAL ATROPHY. Vaginal atrophy is generally responsive to systemic estrogen administration. However, genital symptoms are sometimes incompletely resolved when usual systemic estrogen doses are used. Rather than increasing the systemic dose, a small amount (1 gm of conjugated equine estrogen every third day) of vaginal estrogen cream may be added. Daily use of very low-dose topical therapy (vaginal conjugated equine estrogen, 0.5 gm, for 1 month) also restores vaginal cytology and is not associated with increased systemic levels of estradiol or estrone. This form of therapy is regarded by many experts as local treatment and thus is considered safe for use by women in whom systemic estrogens are contraindicated. Because the commercially available vaginal applicator is graded in 1-gm (rather than 0.5 gm) markings, daily low-dose therapy is more conveniently prescribed as 1 gm every second or third day. It is important to note that there are no data on this regimen of low-dose vaginal estrogen use for longer than a month. Whether systemic absorption would increase or decrease over time remains unknown.

Psychological Changes

The existence of a possible association between psychological symptoms and menopause has been controversial. In part, the difficulty in studying this question has been methodologic. Older studies used unstandardized and unvalidated scales of menopausal complaints. Also, most information was derived from cross-sectional surveys of community-based or large general medical practice–based populations. This type of survey is subject to the problem of responder bias from more symptomatic women. Nonetheless, an increased prevalence of symptoms such as irritability, dysphoria, and nervousness early in the menopausal transition was suggested.

Results from new community-based longitudinal studies of midlife women are refining knowledge in the area of mood, mentation, and menopause. These studies use standardized scales, collect extensive psychosocial data in addition to menstrual status, and use sophisticated analyses. The initial longitudinal results of a United States–based cohort find increased nonspecific symptom reporting at the menopause. In a Canadian cohort, depressive symptoms were common during the menopausal transition. Half of the subjects screened positive for depression at least once during a 3-year follow-up period. Depression on more than two serial interviews was noted in 26% perimenopausal women. Perceived health was most strongly related to depression. These findings are consistent with the concept of variability in response to the menopause; individual characteristics and self-perceptions appear to be important determinants of each woman's experience of the climacteric. The relationship between each woman and her reaction to menopause has been termed the vulnerability model. The vulnerability model holds that the presence of adverse sociodemographic or psychosocial factors makes some women vulnerable to the development of physical and psychological symptoms. The onset of affec-

tive or cognitive symptoms may not be simultaneous with the cessation of menses; some women may find the perimenopause more distressing than the menopause itself.

Several mechanisms of menopause-associated affective or cognitive complaints have been proposed, including a primary central nervous system cause (i.e., an alteration in brain amines). Opioid antagonist studies have demonstrated that estrogen deficiency is associated with low levels of endogenous opioid activity and that estrogen supplementation increases opioid activity. These findings support the hypothesis that estrogen-related alterations in neurotransmitters may contribute affective/cognitive complaints. A second mechanistic hypothesis postulates that hot flushes and nighttime awakenings cause loss of sleep and that irritability, fatigue, and cognitive impairment are secondary events.

PSYCHOLOGICAL EFFECTS OF HORMONE THERAPY. Available evidence does not support a relationship between clinical depression or anxiety disorders and the menopause. These conditions should not be primarily treated with estrogens. However, improvements in self-reported irritability, mild anxiety, and dysphoria have been found in double-masked studies of estrogen alone or combined with progestin. Beneficial effects of estrogen on self-reported memory and anxiety have been specifically noted in women without hot flushes or sleep disturbance, suggesting an effect independent of improved sleep and decreased discomfort from hot flushes. Estrogen has also been found to improve mood in surgically menopausal women who were neither depressed nor having hot flushes at baseline. Knowledge of estrogen's affective and cognitive effects is based on small numbers of women; additional research is needed before conclusions can be drawn. At present, a trial of estrogen is reasonable for the complaints of irritability, anxiety, diminished concentration, or dysphoria associated with the perimenopause or postmenopause. Other medical and psychosocial causes of these symptoms should also be considered, evaluated, and specifically treated as appropriate.

REFERENCES

Bergman A, Brenner PF. Alterations in the urogenital system. In: Mishell DR (ed). Menopause Physiology and Pharmacology. Chicago: Year Book Medical Publishers, 1987, pp 67–76.

Bolli P, Simpson FO. Clonidine and menopausal flushing: A double blind trial. N Z Med J 1975;82:196.

Cardozo L. Role of estrogens in the treatment of female urinary incontinence. J Am Geriatr Soc 1990;38:326.

Chang RJ, Judd HL. The ovary after menopause. Clin Obstet Gynecol 1981;24:181.

D'Amico JF, Greendale GA, Lu JKH, et al. Induction of hypothalamic opioid activity with transdermal estradiol administration in postmenopausal women. Fertil Steril 1991; 55:754.

Dennerstein L, Burrows GD. A review of the studies of the psychologic symptoms found at the menopause. Maturitas 1978;1:55.

Ditkoff EC, Crary WG, Cristo M, et al. Estrogen improves psychological function in asymptomatic postmenopausal women. Obstet Gynecol 1991;78:991.

Erlik Y, Meldrum DR, Lagasse LD, et al. Effect of megestrol acetate on flushing and bone metabolism in postmenopausal women. Maturitas 1981;3:167.

Hinton P, Tweddell AL, Mayne C. Oral and intravaginal estrogens alone and in combination with alpha adrenergic stimulation in genuine stress incontinence. Int Urogynecol J 1990;1:80.

Holte A. Influences of natural menopause in health complaints: A prospective study of healthy Norwegian women. Maturitus 1992;14:127.

Hunter MS. Psychological and somatic experience of the menopause: A prospective study. Psychosom Med 1990;52:357.

Hunter MS. Emotional well-being, sexual behavior, and hormone replacement therapy. Maturitus 1990;12:299.

Ingelman-Sundberg A, Rosen J, Gustafsson SA, et al. Cytosol estrogen receptors in the urogenital tissues in stress-incontinent women. Acta Obstet Gynecol Scand 1981;60:585.

Iosif CS, Batra S, Sek A, et al. Estrogen receptors in the human female lower urinary tract. Am J Obstet Gynecol 1981;141:817.

Judd HL. Menopause. In: Hacker NF, Moore JG (eds). Essentials of Obstetrics and Gynecology. Philadelphia: WB Saunders, 1986, pp 436–443.

Judd HL, Judd GE, Lucas WE, et al. Endocrine function of the postmenopausal ovary: Concentration of androgens and estrogens in ovarian and peripheral vein blood. J Clin Endocrinol Metab 1974;39:1020.

Kaufert PA, Gilbert P, Tate R. The Manitoba Project: A re-examination of the link between menopause and depression. Maturitus 1992;14:143.

Kinn A-C, Lindskog M. Estrogens and phenylpropanolamine for stress urinary incontinence in postmenopausal women. Urology 1988;32:273.

Loprinzi CL, Michalak JC, Auella SK, et al. Megestrol acetate for the prevention of hot flashes. N Engl J Med 1994;331:347.

Lu JKH, Judd HL. The neuroendocrine aspects of menopausal hot flushes. Prog Basic Clin Pharmacol 1991;6:83.

Marslaw U, Christiansen C. Desogestral in hormone replacement therapy: Long-term effects on bone, calcium, and lipid metabolism, climacteric symptoms, and bleeding. Eur J Clin Invest 1991;21:601.

Matthews KA, Wend PR, Kuller LH, et al. Influences of natural menopause on psychological characteristics and symptoms of middle-aged healthy women. J Consult Clin Psychol 1990;58:345.

McKinlay SM, Brambilla PJ, Posner JG. The normal menopause transition. Maturitus 1992;14:103.

McKinley S, Jeffreys M. The menopausal syndrome. Br J Prev Soc Med 1974;28:108.

Metcalf MG, Livesey JG. Gonadotrophin excretion in fertile women: Effect of age and the onset of the menopausal transition. J Endocrinol 1985;104:357.

Notelovitz M. Gynecologic problems of menopausal women. Changes in genital tissues. Geriatrics 1978;33:24.

Ouslander JG, Bruskewitz R. Disorders of micturition in the aging patient. Adv Intern Med 1989;34:165.

Schiff I, Tulchinsky D, Cramer D. Oral medroxyprogesterone in the treatment of postmenopausal symptoms. JAMA 1980;244:1443.

Scotti RJ, Ostergard DR. The urethral syndrome. Clin Obstet Gynecol 1984;27:515.

Sherman BM, Korenman SG. Hormonal characteristics of the human menstrual cycle throughout reproductive life. J Clin Invest 1975;55:699.

Sherman BM, West JH, Korenman SG. The menopausal transition: Analysis of LH, FSH, estradiol and progesterone concentrations during menstrual cycles of older women. J Clin Endocrinol Metab 1976;42:629.

Sonnedecker EUW, Polakow ES. Effects of conjugated equine estrogens with and without the addition of cyclical medrogestone on hot flushes, liver function, blood pressure, and endocrinological indices. S Afr Med 1990;77:281.

Steingold KA, Laufer L, Chetkowski RJ, et al. Treatment of hot flashes with transdermal estradiol administration. J Clin Endocrinol Metab 1985;61:627.

Tulandi T, Samarthji L. Menopausal hot flush. Obstet Gynecol Surv 1985;40:553.

Voda AM. Climacteric hot flush. Maturitus 1981;3:73.

61

Hormone Therapy in the Menopause

Gail A. Greendale and Howard L. Judd

OVERVIEW OF NONCONTRACEPTIVE ESTROGEN PRESCRIBING PATTERNS

Postmenopausal estrogen use has vacillated in popularity among both professionals and lay people in the United States during the past 30 years. Initial enthusiasm during the 1960s stemmed from uncontrolled studies of estrogen's apparent benefit in preventing epidermal, vaginal, and breast atrophy, as well as dowager's hump, hypertension, and atherosclerosis. During the next decade, scientific reports of the adverse consequences of unopposed estrogen use, specifically an increased risk of endometrial cancer, caused millions of physicians to stop prescribing postmenopausal estrogens and women to discontinue using them. In the 1980s, reports of the benefits of postmenopausal estrogen again began to proliferate. Prevention of bone loss and osteoporotic fractures and prevention of cardiovascular disease were described in several large cohort studies. These positive findings, in conjunction with the development of combined estrogen and progestin regimens to protect the endometrium, led to a resurgence of interest in postmenopausal hormones.

The current decade brings with it a burgeoning interest in women's health. Careful investigation of the benefits and risks of hormone therapy has increased, yet much remains to be learned. However, decisions about hormone therapy are based on evidence currently available; refinements and revisions of these recommendations will inevitably occur as knowledge increases.

INTRODUCTION TO MENOPAUSE TREATMENT

Hormone use in the menopause can be directed at symptom relief, such as the treatment of urogenital atrophy, or at prophylaxis, such as prevention of osteoporosis. The Food and Drug Administration has given formal approval for the use of estrogens to treat hot flushes and urogenital atrophy and for specific estrogen preparations to prevent osteoporosis. These and other clinical conditions for which estrogen therapy is in common clinical use are summarized in Table 61–1.

A medical history, with attention to specific contraindications and precautions related to hormone therapy, should be completed before initiating therapy. A general physical examination, gynecologic examination, Papanicolaou smear, and mammogram should also be performed. The choice of a particular hormone regimen or a nonhormonal therapy must then be based on each woman's treatment goals, benefit-risk analysis, and medical history. Re-evaluation in 3 months to assess therapeutic effectiveness and the occurrence of any side effects is recommended. Annual follow-up is sufficient thereafter, if no problem arises. Patients who decide to take hormone therapy should be counseled about what type of bleeding pattern to expect and advised to report any deviation from the expected pattern.

ESTROGEN

Estrogen can be administered daily or with a 1-week interruption of therapy at the end of each

TABLE 61–1. Clinical Conditions Commonly Treated with Noncontraceptive Estrogens

Hot flushes	Dysphoric mood
Atrophic urethritis	Dyspareunia
Stress incontinence	Decreased sexual motivation
Sensory-urge incontinence	Osteoporosis (prevention)
Atrophic vaginitis	Cardiovascular disease (prevention)

From Greendale GA, Judd HL. The menopause: Health implications and clinical management. J Am Geriatr Soc 1993; 41:426.

635

TABLE 61–2. Serum Estrone and Estradiol Levels by Doses and Types of Oral* and Nonoral† Estrogen

ESTROGEN TYPE AND DOSE	SERUM ESTRONE (PG/ML)	SERUM ESTRADIOL (PG/ML)
Conjugated equine estrogen		
0.3 mg	76	19
0.625 mg	153	40
1.25 mg	200	60
Piperazine estrone sulfate		
0.6 mg	125	34
1.2 mg	200	42
Micronized estradiol		
1 mg	150	40
2 mg	250	60
Estradiol valerate		
1 mg	160	50
2 mg	300	60
Estradiol, 17β, by transdermal system		
50 μg	51	72
100 μg	57	120

*Adapted from Lobo A. Clin Obstet Gynecol 1987.
†Adapted from D'Amico JF, et al. Fertil Steril 1991.
From Greendale GA Judd HL. The menopause: Health implications and clinical management. J Am Geriatr Soc 1993;41:426.

month. Uninterrupted or continuous administration of estrogen is preferable because no benefit is conferred by the interrupted or cyclic regimen. In addition, cyclic estrogen therapy may cause decreased compliance because of symptom recurrence during medication interruption. The cyclic estrogen regimen is also more complex, and therefore, it may be more difficult to remember.

The lowest estrogen dose that affords relief of symptoms or achieves disease prevention should be administered. Using the minimum effective dose minimizes estrogen-related side effects, such as breast tenderness, and may also diminish potential toxicities. For example, the possible increased risk of breast cancer with estrogen, if real, appears to be related to the dose and duration of estrogen use. Therefore, while awaiting further data on this question, it is advisable to minimize risk by using the lowest effective estrogen dose. The incidence of endometrial hyperplasia also increases with higher doses of estrogen. Conversely, caution directed at minimizing toxicity should not prompt the use of ineffective preventive regimens. Effective doses of estrogens for osteoporosis prevention can be estimated from randomized trials. Of the estrogens available in the United States, conjugated equine estrogens (0.625 mg), 50 μg of transdermal estradiol-17β, 0.1 mg of oral estradiol-17β, and 1.2 mg piperazine estrone sulfate have been approved by the Food and Drug Administration for osteoporosis prevention. In cohort studies of osteoporotic fracture prevention in the United States, most women were using conjugated equine estrogens in doses of at least 0.625 mg daily. Car-

diovascular risk reduction in association with non-contraceptive estrogen use has been demonstrated in cohort studies in which women reported using similar amounts of oral estrogens.

Table 61–2 lists the estrogen preparations in common use, along with the usual dose range for each. The average serum levels of estrone and estradiol achieved with each dose and formulation are also summarized.

PROGESTIN REGIMENS

In clinical practice, progestins are added to estrogen regimens to prevent endometrial hyperplasia and, probably, endometrial cancer. Progestins are associated with the unpleasant side effects of headache, fatigue, bloating, and menstrual cramps, but the exact incidence of these side effects has not been well studied. Progestins also induce vaginal bleeding, another action that is usually unwelcome. Continuous low-dose progestin regimens have been developed in an attempt to minimize the uncomfortable side effects and vaginal bleeding associated with standard cyclic therapies.

Progestins can be broadly classified into the 19-nortestosterone compounds and the 17α-hydroxyprogesterones. The 19-nortestosterone family includes first-, second-, and third-generation compounds. First-generation compounds (estranes) are related to norethindrone and its derivatives. Norgestrel and its derivatives compose the second-generation compounds, or gonanes. Estranes and gonanes are relatively androgenic. These compounds are infrequently used in the United States for postmenopausal therapy. Newer, third-generation 19-nortestosterones, such as desogestrel, are less androgenic than the earlier derivatives. Little research has been directed at third-generation 19-nortestosterones in postmenopausal women, and these have only recently been approved for use in the United States as oral contraceptives. The most common 17α-hydroxyprogesterone compound used for noncontraceptive hormone therapy is medroxyprogesterone acetate. This progestin is less androgenic and therefore affects lipids less than the 19-nortestosterone compounds. It is commonly used for postmenopausal hormone therapy in the United States, although not approved for that specific purpose.

Progesterone, in a micronized formulation, is active when given orally. Early reports suggest that micronized progesterone may have no adverse lipid effect. It is not approved for any use in the United States at this time.

Progestins may be administered cyclically (for part of each month) or continuously. Progestins, given cyclically, have been used for several years; thus, experience with this regimen is extensive. The occurrence of endometrial hyperplasia is extremely rare when 10 mg of medroxyprogesterone is prescribed for at least 12 days of each month, along with estrogen. Lower doses and durations of progestins used cyclically (e.g., 2.5–5.0 mg of medroxyprogesterone for 7–11 days) decrease the rate of hyperplasia compared with unopposed estrogen use but do not eliminate it completely. Because the higher dose given for 12 days is associated with a very low risk of hyperplasia, it is the cyclic regimen most commonly recommended. Most researchers believe that it is not necessary to perform routine baseline or surveillance endometrial biopsies when the 12-day cyclic progestin regimen is used, unless problematic vaginal bleeding develops. Approximately 80% of women experience vaginal bleeding with cyclic progestin, and bleeding should commence after day 9 of the progestin cycle.

Progestin regimens that use daily 2.5 or 5.0 mg of medroxyprogesterone acetate provide a new approach that is intended to decrease uncomfortable side effects and to diminish bleeding. Continuous use of both estrogens and progestins also makes regimens simpler to explain and remember, perhaps enhancing compliance. In many small studies that have used various estrogen preparations and different low-dose continuous progestins, amenorrhea has been accomplished in 70 to 90% of women who remained on therapy at 1 year. However, almost all women experience light bleeding

for the first 6 months of low-dose combination therapy. Although bleeding is lighter, consisting of 1 to 3 days of spotting to light flow, it is also unpredictable. Daily conjugated estrogens, 0.625 mg, in conjunction with either 2.5 or 5.0 mg of medroxyprogesterone daily, have been tested in two large multicenter studies. Reports from these studies suggest no endometrial hyperplasia at 1 year with the 5.0-mg continuous progestin dose. Hyperplasia rates of approximately 1% have been reported with use of continuous combined therapy at the 2.5-mg dose of medroxyprogesterone acetate. When 5.0 mg of medroxyprogesterone acetate was given continuously, no hyperplasia was seen. Although the incidence of hyperplasia did not differ statistically between the 2.5 mg and the 5.0 mg progestin groups, more conservative practice would be to use 5.0 mg of medroxyprogesterone acetate. In one study 84% of women taking 2.5 mg and 89% using 5.0 mg of medroxyprogesterone daily were amenorrheic at 1 year. In the other large trial, 40% of the women using 2.5 mg medroxyprogesterone acetate were amenorrheic for the last 6 months of the study. Continuous use of 2.5 or 5.0 mg of medroxyprogesterone is therefore considered safe, and routine baseline and surveillance biopsies are not recommended with this regimen.

The use of oral micronized progesterone is promising because it appears to produce fewer side effects and may be preferable from a cardiovascular standpoint. The endometrial safety of this formulation has not been extensively evaluated, however. Until the dose and schedule of micronized progesterone that demonstrate endometrial protection have been established, its use does not eliminate the need for endometrial surveillance.

Progestin use by women without a uterus is not recommended because a nonandrogenic progestin offers no specific benefit except endometrial protection. Progestins may mitigate, at least in part, estrogen's cardioprotective effects. In addition, the uncomfortable side effects of progestins make regimens that include them less desirable for many women.

A schematic summary of our recommendations for hormone therapy is shown in Figure 61–1. The cyclic schedule of estrogen for 25 days and progestin for days 12 to 25 is not recommended because it is more cumbersome and results in more breakthrough symptoms.

MONITORING THE ENDOMETRIUM

The requirement for performing an endometrial biopsy depends on the hormone regimen used and

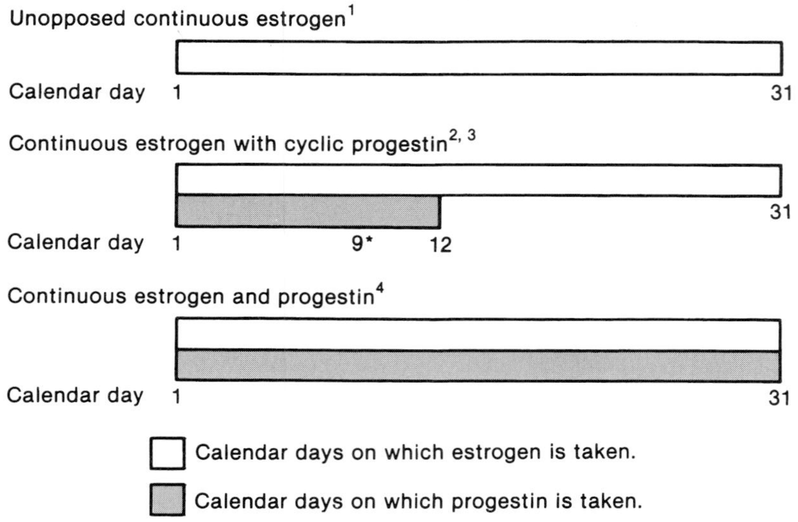

Unopposed continuous estrogen[1]

Calendar day 1   31

Continuous estrogen with cyclic progestin[2, 3]

Calendar day 1   9*   12   31

Continuous estrogen and progestin[4]

Calendar day 1   31

☐ Calendar days on which estrogen is taken.

▨ Calendar days on which progestin is taken.

Figure 61–1. Recommended hormone therapy schedules.

[1]For use in women without a uterus. If uterus is present, biopsy surveillance must be performed.

[2]There is no specific benefit from interrupted estrogen therapy. In women with a uterus, cyclic estrogen does not prevent endometrial cancer.

[3]Ten mg of medroxyprogesterone acetate (MPA) for 12 calendar days at the beginning of each month. Older combination regimens used estrogen for days 1–25 and progestin for days 15–25 each month. This was more complex and cumbersome.

[4]MPA, 2.5 or 5.0 mg, is given daily along with estrogen.

*Vaginal bleeding should commence after day 9 of cyclic progestin.

the bleeding pattern observed. In women who have a uterus and who wish to take unopposed estrogen (without a progestin), biopsies should be performed before treatment and annually thereafter. An additional endometrial sampling is recommended if vaginal bleeding or uterine growth occurs on the unopposed estrogen regimen. If endometrial hyperplasia is observed on biopsy, estrogen-only therapy should be discontinued.

When combination estrogen and progestin therapy is used, the expected bleeding pattern depends on the progestin dose and regimen. If 12 days of cyclic progestin is prescribed, bleeding is expected to start after day 9 of progestin use. Earlier bleeding onset may indicate hyperplasia and warrants evaluation. With continuous (daily) use of 2.5 or 5.0 mg of medroxyprogesterone acetate, the expected bleeding pattern is erratic spotting and light bleeding of between 1 and 5 days' duration for the first year of therapy. The necessity of a surveillance biopsy can, therefore, be difficult to determine. A biopsy is recommended if the bleeding is heavier or more prolonged than the usual pattern established by each individual. There are no data available to guide the need for biopsy after 1 year of therapy; the Postmenopausal Estrogen Progestins Intervention (PEPI) Trial is expected to provide this information in the near future.

The development of flexible cannulas to obtain endometrial biopsies has facilitated the performance of office-based endometrial sampling. Advances in vaginal ultrasonography may ultimately make it possible to perform endometrial surveillance noninvasively. In women not taking estrogen, an endometrial thickness of less than 4 mm has been associated with the absence of hyperplasia or carcinoma. Further studies of this test are necessary, particularly in the setting of hormone intervention, before it can be accepted as a substitute for endometrial sampling.

CONTRAINDICATIONS AND PRECAUTIONS

The absolute contraindications to estrogen use are undiagnosed vaginal bleeding, suspected breast or endometrial carcinoma, and active thrombotic disease. In general, women with a history of breast or endometrial cancer are not advised to use estrogen, but this view is under debate and re-evaluation. Few data define the safety of noncontraceptive estrogen use in those populations. Because women with successfully treated early breast and endometrial tumors often enjoy a long survival, the consequences of hypoestrogenemia can substantially affect their health and quality of life. Similarly, the effect of estrogen on malignant melanoma is uncertain. Estrogen receptors have been isolated from this tumor, and concern about stimulation of melanoma growth by noncontraceptive estrogens is warranted.

The low doses of estrogens used in noncontraceptive regimens generally do not stimulate growth of uterine leiomyomas or endometriosis, although patients with a history of these disorders should be specifically counseled about this unlikely event. The size of leiomyoma can be monitored by clinical examination, but there is no easy way to monitor for regrowth of endometriosis or to monitor endometrial implants for the development of hyperplasia. Therefore, some experts recommend prescribing progestins for women who do not have a uterus but who have a history of endometriosis; however, no consensus has been reached on this point. Prior gallbladder disease is also a relative concern, because oral estrogen causes increased bile saturation of cholesterol. Studies to evaluate the role of nonoral estrogens in women with gallbladder disease are under way; the use of nonoral estrogen may avoid increase in cholesterol saturation.

Estrogen may be a hypotensive agent in women who are both normotensive and mildly hypertensive before therapy. Several small trials have found reductions in systolic and diastolic blood pressure of between 5 and 10 mm Hg with use of oral and transdermal noncontraceptive estrogen doses. There is limited and opposing evidence of estrogen's effect on migraine. Patients should therefore be advised to report worsening of symptoms should they occur. The standard National Cholesterol Education Program guidelines should be followed with respect to cholesterol screening in postmenopausal women. Women with significant baseline elevations of triglycerides should be monitored for a further increase when oral estrogen is prescribed. Elevations in triglycerides do not result from the use of nonoral estrogen. Thrombosis has not been shown to be associated with noncontraceptive estrogen use. However, a dose-related increase in some procoagulants and anticoagulants is noted with use of oral conjugated equine estrogens. Transdermal estrogen elicits no change in the levels of clotting and anticlotting factors known to change with oral contraceptives. Women with a history of oral contraceptive or pregnancy-related thrombosis should be counseled about these findings. Caution should also be expressed in women with a recent history of thromboembolic disease. In general, nonoral therapy should be used in women with a higher risk of thrombosis.

TABLE 61–3. Absolute and Relative Contraindications to the Use of Noncontraceptive Estrogens

Absolute Contraindications
Undiagnosed vaginal bleeding
Suspected breast cancer
Suspected endometrial cancer
Active venous thrombosis
History of breast cancer*
History of endometrial cancer*
Malignant melanoma*
Relative Contraindications†
Uterine leiomyoma
Endometriosis
History of cholelithiasis
History of migraine
Hypertriglyceridemia
History of pregnancy-related thrombosis
History of oral contraceptive–related thrombosis
Liver disease

*Under debate at present. Some women who have these conditions and who strongly wish to take estrogen are being treated.
†Patients should be counseled about the specific consequences of taking estrogen if they have any of these conditions.
From Greendale GA, Judd HL. The menopause: Health implications and clinical management. J Am Geriatr Soc 1993; 41:426.

Table 61–3 summarizes the absolute and relative contraindications to the use of postmenopausal estrogens. Based largely on incorrect extrapolation from the oral contraceptive literature, some misconceptions remain about estrogen being contraindicated in women who smoke, are hypertensive, or have coronary artery disease. In fact, estrogen's cardiac benefit extends to smokers, and no apparent increase in toxicity has been found. Estrogen does not elevate blood pressure in normotensive and hypertensive women. Finally, the misplaced concern about using estrogen in women with coronary artery disease may arise from some unsuccessful results at secondary prevention in men. Coronary artery disease is not a contraindication to estrogen use in women.

COMPLICATIONS OF HORMONE THERAPY

Unopposed stimulation of the endometrium by estrogen is associated with the development of endometrial hyperplasia. Hyperplasia ranges in grade, in increasing degree of severity, from simple, to complex, to atypical simple, and to atypical complex. Atypical complex hyperplasia is associated with a significant (23–57%) risk of developing endometrial adenocarcinoma. Several large observational studies have also reported an increased risk of endometrial cancer in women who were taking unopposed estrogen. The complication of hyperplasia can be prevented by using appropriate doses and durations of progestin. Advanced hyperplasia can also be avoided by performing regular endometrial biopsies on women who wish to use estrogen only.

Postmenopausally, breast tissue regresses and women who have had benign breast cysts and cyclic breast swelling and tenderness tend to be relieved of these symptoms. The use of noncontraceptive estrogens sometimes causes resurgence of breast swelling, breast nodularity, and a sense of breast fullness or pain. Although these findings are not medically dangerous, patients sometimes choose to cease therapy to relieve severe breast fullness or pain. Annual mammographic surveillance is mandatory for all estrogen-treated women, and dominant masses should be evaluated in the same manner as in untreated women (see Chapter 17).

Whether the use of current doses of noncontraceptive estrogens increases the risk of breast cancer is an unresolved question. The overall risk of breast cancer with ever-use of estrogen does not appear to be increased. However, high doses, specific formulations, and long durations of use may be important variables that increase risk. For example, one meta-analysis found that breast cancer risk was not increased when doses of 0.625 mg or less of conjugated equine estrogens were used. The increased risk evidenced in European studies may be related to the use of estrogen preparations not used in the United States. In some long-term observational studies as well as in some data summaries, a modest (20–30%) but not always statistically significant increase in breast cancer risk is noted with greater than 10 to 15 years of estrogen use. Very few long-term follow-up studies have been conducted; as follow-up accrues in enrolled cohorts, enough data may accumulate to confirm or refute this suggested duration effect. At present, there is insufficient evidence on which to base an opinion about the effects of noncontraceptive progestin therapy on breast tissue.

APPROACH TO THE HORMONE THERAPY DECISION PROCESS

A postmenopausal woman must address several questions in the hormone therapy decision process. The major ones are whether or not to use hormones, which hormones to use, and how long to use hormones. The approach presented here builds on the information presented in Chapters 52, 60, and 62. This strategy represents one method of assisting women with the decision process.

SHOULD I USE HORMONES? It is helpful to elicit a patient's short- and long-term treatment goals. Relatively short-term goals can include the relief of hot flushes, therapy of genital atrophic conditions, and possibly treatment of mood and memory disorders associated with the perimenopause and early postmenopause. *Because many women are concerned about the potential long-term toxicities of estrogens and progestins, clarifying the short-term nature of the planned therapy may relieve these concerns.*

Although other therapies are available for hot flushes, estrogen is generally the most effective and the best tolerated. For the majority of women, flushes abate in 1 to 2 years; therefore, if used solely for this purpose, hormone therapy can be discontinued in a relatively short time.

In contrast to hot flushes, genital atrophy progresses rather than resolves with time. However, if longer-term therapy is not desired, treatment of genital atrophy and related conditions can be approached in a short-term fashion. Short courses (1–2 months) of oral hormone therapy can be used to relieve symptoms and then can be repeated when symptoms recur. (It should not be assumed that intermittent unopposed systemic estrogen is safe in women who have an intact uterus; the same approach as outlined later under ''Which hormones should I use?'' should be applied.) Very low dose vaginal estrogen used for 1 month also restores vaginal cytology without measurable systemic estrogen absorption. (The main shortcoming in our knowledge is whether longer-term use of mini-dose therapy produces higher systemic levels.) One approach is to prescribe 1 month of low-dose vaginal therapy to alleviate symptoms and then to periodically prescribe another month when symptoms recur.

The mood disruption that may be associated with the menopause appears to be a transitional phenomenon; again, a 1- to 2-year course may be adequate to address this problem.

Long-term goals include prevention of cardiovascular disease and osteoporosis. Whether women who are at higher risk for cardiovascular disease benefit to a greater extent from hormone therapy is unknown. Available information suggests that cardiovascular protection is greater for current than for former users of estrogen; in this case, a short-term approach would not apply.

Some data are available to help a woman understand her risk of osteoporosis. All research has been conducted entirely in Caucasian populations. Models have been formulated to extrapolate the risk of hip fracture in the seventh and eighth decades of life to the bone density in the fifth decade of life. If these models are accurate, a single perimenopausal bone density measurement should stratify a woman into high, average, or low risk (see Chapter 62). In a woman whose decision hinges entirely on her osteoporosis risk, bone density measurement may clarify her decision.

WHAT HORMONES SHOULD I USE? Unopposed estrogen, estrogen plus progestin, and oral versus nonoral therapy are the major choices women must consider. Unopposed estrogen may be a better choice if (1) a woman has had intolerable side effects from progestins; (2) a woman wishes to *possibly* maximize her cardiovascular benefit, noting that the lipid effect is far from the complete mechanism underlying cardiac protection (see Chapter 60); or (3) a woman wishes to avoid vaginal bleeding (although if she develops hyperplasia and is treated with progestins, she will likely have heavy bleeding at that time).

Combined therapy is preferred if a woman does not wish to undergo surveillance biopsies. Cyclic progestins induce predictable bleeding, an advantage to some. Continuous progestins provoke 6 to 12 months of erratic spotting and bleeding in most users, but amenorrhea eventually occurs. For some, the initial unpredictable and fairly constant bleeding is intolerable; others are comfortable with the initial bleeding for ultimate freedom from it.

Transdermal estrogen has the potential advantage of requiring only twice-weekly application. In a woman without a uterus, this mode of administration can obviate the need for pill taking. The relative effectiveness of transdermal estrogen for osteoporosis prevention appears to be equal to oral estrogen. Whether the cardiovascular benefit is equivalent to the oral route is more difficult to determine. Total cholesterol and low-density lipoprotein cholesterol are reduced by the patch; high-density lipoprotein is unchanged. Again, the currently postulated mechanisms of estrogen's vascular effect are much broader than for lipids; caution is advised in inferring too generally from lipid comparisons.

HOW LONG SHOULD I USE HORMONES? In women who are apprehensive about long-term use, the duration of use should be guided by the reason for treatment as discussed earlier. For long-term prevention of osteoporosis and cardiovascular disease, there is now no rationale for discontinuation.

THE BENEFIT-RISK EQUATION: THEORY AND PRACTICE. Formal decision analyses have concluded that the benefit of hormone use (in this case unopposed estrogen, *even in women who have a uterus*) outweighs the risk. This equation is driven by the substantial reduction of mortality from cardiovascular disease, even if some cases of endometrial cancer and breast cancer result. However, in clinical practice, the valence, or relative importance that each woman attaches to the potential benefits and risks of hormones, varies enormously. For example, some women with a personal grave concern about breast cancer cannot tolerate the absence of a randomized controlled trial with breast cancer outcomes; until the data are known, hormones are not for them. Other women opt for combined hormone therapy, including the bleeding that accompanies it, because the risk of endometrial hyperplasia, although relatively less important with respect to mortality than the prevention of heart disease, has a high negative valence for them. Health care providers must assist each woman by providing her with accurate information, including what is unknown as well as what is known about benefits and risks. It is important to respect the variations in priorities that individual patients place on various aspects of the decision process.

REFERENCES

ACOG Technical Bulletin. April 1992;166.

American College of Physicians. Guidelines for counseling postmenopausal women about preventive hormone therapy. Ann Intern Med 1992;117:1038.

Archer DF, Pickar JH, Bottiglioni F, et al. Bleeding patterns in postmenopausal women taking continuous combined or sequential regimens of conjugated estrogens with medroxyprogesterone acetate. Obstet Gynecol 1994;83:686.

Barrett-Connor E. Postmenopausal estrogen replacement and breast cancer. N Engl J Med 1989;321:319.

Barrett-Connor E, Bush TL. Estrogen and coronary heart disease in women. JAMA 1991;265:1861.

Bush TL, Miller VT. Effect of pharmacologic agents used during the menopause: Impact on lipids and lipoproteins. In: Mishell DR (ed). Menopause Physiology and Pharmacology. Chicago: Year Book Medical Publishers, 1987, pp 187–208.

Chetkowski RJ, Meldrum DR, Steingold KA, et al. Biologic effects of transdermal estradiol. N Engl J Med 1986;314:1615.

Clisham PR, Cedars MI, Greendale GA, et al. Long term estradiol therapy: Effects in endometrial histology and bleeding patterns. Ostet Gynecol 1992;79:200.

Creasman WT. Estrogen replacement therapy: Is previously treated cancer a contraindication? Obstet Gynecol 1991;77:308.

Dupont WD, Page DL. Menopausal estrogen replacement and breast cancer. Arch Intern Med 1991;151:67.

Gelfand MM, Ferenczy A. A prospective one-year study of estrogen and progestin in post-menopausal women: Effects in the endometrium. Obstet Gynecol 1989;74:398.

Genant HK, Baylinh DJ, Gallagher JC, et al. Effect of estrone sulfate on postmenopausal bone loss. Obstet Gynecol 1990;76:579.

Gibbons WF, Judd HL, Moyer D, et al. Evaluation of sequential versus continuous estrogen/progestin replacement therapy on uterine bleeding patterns and endometrial histology (abstract 490). Annual Meeting of the Society for Gynecologic Investigation, San Antonio, Texas, March 20–23, 1991.

Grady D, Rubin S, Petitti DB, et al. Hormone therapy to prevent disease and prolong life in postmenopausal women. Ann Intern Med 1992;117:1016.

Granberg S, Wikland M, Karlson B, et al. Endometrial thickness as measured by endovaginal ultrasonography for identifying endometrial abnormality. Am J Obstet Gynecol 1991;164:47.

Gusberg SB. The individual at high risk for endometrial carcinoma. Am J Obstet Gynecol 1976;126:535.

Hasager C, Riis BJ, Guyene TT, et al. The long-term effect of oral and percutaneous estradiol on plasma renin substrate and blood pressure. Circulation 1987;76:753.

Kiel DP, Felson DT, Anderson JJ, et al. Hip fracture and the use of estrogens in postmenopausal women: The Framingham Study. N Engl J Med 1987;317:1169.

Kurman RJ, Kaminski PE, Norris HE. The behavior of endometrial hyperplasia. Cancer 1985;56:403.

Lindsay R. Estrogen therapy in the prevention and management of osteoporosis. Am J Obstet Gynecol 1987;156:1347.

Lobo RA. Absorption and metabolic effects of different types of estrogens and progestins. Clin Obstet Gynecol 1987;14:143.

Meade TW, Dyer SA, Howarth DJ, et al. Antithrombin III and procoagulant activity: Sex differences and effects of the menopause. J Hematol 1990;74:77.

Padwick ML, Pryse-Davies J, Whitehead MI. A simple method for determining the optimal dosage of progestin in postmenopausal women receiving estrogens. N Engl J Med 1986;315:930.

Pang SCE, Lozano K, Cedars MI, et al. Two-year prospective randomized study of transdermal estradiol use with and without cyclic progestin in postmenopausal women. 37th Annual Meeting of the Society for Gynecological Investigation, St Louis, Missouri, March 21–24, 1990.

Shoupe D, Mishell DR. Therapeutic regimens. In: Mishell DR (ed). Menopause Physiology and Pharmacology. Chicago: Year Book Medical Publishers, 1987, pp 335–351.

Steinberg KK, Thacker SB, Smith SJ, et al. A meta-analysis of the effect of estrogen replacement therapy on the risk of breast cancer. JAMA 1991;265:1985.

Stevenson JC, Cust MP, Gangar KF, et al. Effects of transdermal oral hormone replacement therapy on bone density in spine and proximal femur in postmenopausal women. Lancet 1990;336:265.

Walsh BW, Sacks FM, Caine Y, et al. Conjugated equine estrogens induce a dose-dependent activation of the coagulation system in postmenopausal women. 39th Annual Meeting of the Society for Gynecologic Investigation, San Antonio, Texas, March 18–21, 1992.

Walsh BW, Schiff I, Rosner B, et al. Effects of postmenopausal estrogen replacement on the concentrations and metabolism of plasma lipoproteins. N Engl J Med 1991;325:1196.

Welch KMA, Darnley D, Simkins RT. The role of estrogen in migraine: A review and hypothesis. Cephalalgia 1984;4:227.

Whitehead MI, Fraser D. Controversies concerning the safety of estrogen replacement therapy. Am J Obstet Gynecol 1987;156:1313.

Whitehead MI, Hillard TC, Crook D. The role and use of progestogens. Obstet Gynecol 1990;75(Suppl):59S.

Whitehead MI, Siddle L, Lane G, et al. The pharmacology of progestogens. In: Mishell DR (ed). Menopause Physiology and Pharmacology. Chicago: Year Book Medical Publishers, 1987, pp 335–351.

Wingo P, Layde PM, Lee NC, et al. The risk of breast cancer in postmenopausal women who have used estrogen replacement therapy. JAMA 1987;257:209.

Woodruff JD, Pickar JH, et al. Incidence of endometrial hyperplasia in postmenopausal women taking conjugated estrogens (Premarin) with medroxyprogesterone acetate or conjugated estrogens alone. Am J Obstet Gynecol 1994;170:1213.

Wren BG, Roultedge AD. The effect of type and dose of estrogen on the blood pressure of postmenopausal women. Maturitus 1983;5:135.

Osteoporosis

Karen M. Freund

SCOPE OF THE PROBLEM

Osteoporosis is a major medical and public health issue for women in the United States. Osteoporosis not only is a major cause of mortality in elderly women but is associated with significant morbidity from chronic pain and decreased functional ability in previously active women. In the United States, 1.3 million fractures yearly are attributable to osteoporosis, including 500,000 vertebral fractures and 250,000 hip fractures in women. The lifetime risk of a vertebral fracture is 40% for women who live to be 80 years of age. Fifteen percent of women who reach age 80 years will suffer a hip fracture. The 1-year mortality from a hip fracture is 12 to 20%, and 15 to 25% of survivors previously living independently require institutional care as a result of their fracture. Annual health care expenditures for osteoporosis-related conditions exceed $7 billion.

PATHOPHYSIOLOGY

Osteoporosis is defined pathologically as bone of normal architecture but with an absolute decrease in the amount of bone. Bone strength develops rapidly at adolescence after bone growth is complete. Most data show that bone density can increase until the third decade and is responsive to environmental factors including activity and diet. Bone density then begins to decrease after the fourth decade, in two patterns described as type I and type II osteoporosis.[1] Type I osteoporosis occurs after menopause, is characterized by rapid resorption of bone (2–4% bone loss per year for 5–8 years after menopause), and involves mainly trabecular bone. Type II osteoporosis includes both trabecular and cortical bone and generally begins in the fourth decade. It is characterized by slow bone resorption and bone loss. In both types of osteoporosis, increased osteoclast activity or bone resorption and decreased osteoblast activity

of bone formation at the sites of resorption occur. Over time, this leads to not only thinning of existing trabeculae but also loss of entire trabeculae (Fig. 62–1). When trabeculae are only thinned but still present, therapeutic intervention can theoretically reverse the resorption-formation imbalance and normal bone density can be restored. However, once trabeculae are lost, no template on which to rebuild this bone remains, so that even with effective therapy to alter the balance of formation to resorption, this bone cannot be restored. This observation underscores the increased effectiveness of early prevention.

CLINICAL RELEVANCE OF RISK FACTORS

Well-defined risk factors, medications, and chronic conditions predispose to osteoporosis (Table 62–1). Patients with renal disease and inflammatory bowel disease should always be considered at increased risk owing to abnormalities in calcium and vitamin D metabolism. Those who have been taking chronic corticosteroids, thyroxine, anticon-

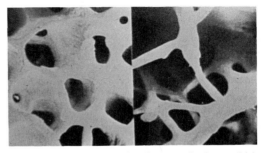

Figure 62–1. Normal and osteoporotic bone histology. (From Dempster DW, Shane E, Horbert W, Lindsay R. A simple method for correlative tight and scanning electron microscopy of human iliac crest bone biopsies: Qualitative observations in normal and osteoporotic subjects. J Bone Miner Res 1986;1:15.)

TABLE 62–1.   Risk Factors for Osteoporosis

Diseases	Thin body habitus
	Asian, Caucasian race
	Family history
	Menopause before age 45 years
	Smoking
	Alcohol use
	Low dietary calcium
	Sedentary lifestyle
	Hyperthyroidism
	Hyperparathyroidism
	Cushing's disease
	Chronic obstructive lung disease
	Intestinal malabsorption
	Renal dysfunction
	Rheumatoid arthritis
	Disability resulting in immobility
	Diabetes mellitus
Drugs	Corticosteroids
	Thyroid hormone
	Anticonvulsants
	Heparin
	Aluminum-containing antacids
	Loop diuretics
	Tetracycline
	Isoniazid

vulsants, or loop diuretics are also at increased risk.

The other known risk factors for osteoporosis explain only 25% of the variance seen in bone density. Thus, they are limited in their clinical utility to assess which patients are at greatest risk for fracture and would most benefit from empirical therapy.[2] The peak bone mass attained during the premenopausal years is an important determinant of subsequent bone mass, and the menstrual history is a prime determinant of this peak bone mass. It is well established that amenorrhea due to either weight loss such as in anorexia nervosa[3] or athletic amenorrhea[4] has a negative effect on bone density. This effect is believed to be related to low estrogen levels and possibly low progesterone levels in these women. Drinkwater and colleagues[5] found that low body weight was a stronger predictor of low bone density than menstrual oligomenorrhea or amenorrhea in young athletes and that the two factors together accounted for 43% of the variation in bone density in this group. Nonovulatory cycles with either anovulation or a short luteal phase have at least a short-term adverse effect on bone density.[6] The use of combination oral contraceptives increases bone mass.[7] Bone density drops transiently during lactation but returns to previous levels within 12 months.[8] Menopause before age 45, due to either natural or surgical means, is also a risk factor for osteoporosis. Increased body mass appears to be protective against osteoporosis sec-

ondary to production of estrogen in peripheral fat tissue. Body mass may also have an independent protective effect against hip fractures, serving to cushion falls and distribute the energy of the fall into the soft tissue.

A family history of osteoporosis is a known risk factor for osteoporosis. Reduced bone mass has been noted in daughters and other first-degree relatives of women with osteoporosis.[9, 10] Twin studies found a higher correlation of bone mass in monozygotic than in dizygotic twin pairs and a higher correlation of bone density at the spine than at the proximal femur, suggesting a greater environmental component of hip strength and fracture risk.[11] It can be difficult to assess the family history of osteoporosis, because vertebral fractures often remain unrecognized, and the kyphosis due to compression fractures in elderly women is often considered to be normal.

Obtaining an accurate history of lifetime alcohol consumption, smoking, calcium intake, and weight-bearing exercise can also be difficult. High alcohol consumption has been noted to increase bone loss, and one study found that even one drink daily increased the risk of hip and forearm fractures in thin women.[12] Smoking has been found to be a risk factor in most studies, with one study of monozygotic female twin pairs estimating a 5 to 10% bone density loss with smoking one pack daily through adulthood.[13] Data from the Framingham study showed that in postmenopausal women, smoking eliminates the protective effect of estrogens on the risk for hip fracture.[14] Evaluation of the benefits of lifelong exercise are confounded by low weight and menstrual disorders in young women. However, a number of studies have been able to demonstrate a 5 to 12% increased bone density in physically active premenopausal women compared with sedentary controls.[15]

Lifetime calcium intake may be of prime importance in attainment of peak bone mass, an area for primary prevention given that less than half of American women consume the recommended daily allowance for calcium. One study of two regions in Croatia with high- and low-calcium diets found that a lifetime high-calcium diet was associated with higher bone density as well as lower hip fracture rates at age 55 years and thereafter, most notably in women.[16] Retrospective assessment of calcium intake can be difficult. A history of lactose intolerance or low dairy intake (less than two servings per day) may signal low calcium intake.

Race has been shown to be a strong predictor of bone density and fracture risk. Black women in the United States have half the rate of hip fractures of white women.[17] Although part of this difference

TABLE 62–2. **Methods of Bone Density Assessment**

TYPE	SITE	ACCURACY	PRECISION
Single-photon absorptiometry	Radius	4–5%	1–2%
Dual-photon absorptiometry	Spine	3–6%	2–4%
	Hip	3–4%	4%
Quantitative computed tomography	Spine	5–10%	4%
Dual x-ray absorptiometry	Spine and hip	3–4%	1–2%

is due to the higher average body weight of black women, studies controlling for body weight continue to find that black women have greater bone density.[18, 19] In multivariate analysis, body mass was a stronger predictor of bone density than was race.[19] The mechanism of these differences in bone density is unclear. Bone density before puberty is the same in black and white girls, and differences become apparent in later stages of adolescence.[20] Studies of premenopausal women suggest that black women both achieve a higher peak bone mass and have a delayed onset of bone loss.[18] Possible differences in vitamin D metabolism remain to be elucidated. One study has shown lower bone turnover in blacks and postulates that lower rates of resorption and formation may result in less bone loss.[21] The usefulness of race alone, however, as a determinant of risk of osteoporosis is limited. The heterogeneity of both the African American and white populations in this country results in significant overlap in bone density measurements between the two groups, and other factors including body mass appear to be stronger predictors. One study found similar risk factors for black women as in previous studies on white women.[22] Race alone cannot be used to predict who is at risk for osteoporosis.

Given the limitations of traditional risk factor assessment in defining a subgroup for whom the risk of hip fracture is the greatest, biologic or gene markers would be extremely helpful. It is hoped that in the future such gene markers can more accurately stratify by risk.

CURRENT TECHNOLOGIES FOR SCREENING

Given the limitations of risk factors in identifying women at risk for fractures, the silent nature of osteoporosis until fractures occur, the substantial morbidity and mortality associated with fractures, and the relative merit of early intervention, osteoporosis is a disorder ideally suited to screening for asymptomatic disease. Screening has the ability of more precisely defining high- and low-

risk groups of women based on their actual physiology rather than their risk profile.

Screening tests studied to date have included both assessment of current bone density and measures of rate of bone turnover. Measures of bone density have received the most attention. Four methods are currently available to assess bone density. Table 62–2 summarizes the differences between the methods. The ability to assess bone mineral content accurately compared with a known standard (accuracy) and the reproducibility of the result on repeat measure (precision) are compared. Single-photon absorptiometry uses a single-photon beam with differential photon absorption between bone and soft tissue, allowing for determination of bone density in grams per centimeter. It can only be used at peripheral sites. Dual-photon absorptiometry uses two different energies that allow direct assessment of the hip and spine. However, it is limited by a lack of precision and accuracy. Quantitative computed tomography (CT) has been used principally to assess the lumbar spine and can distinguish between trabecular and cortical bone, although accuracy is a problem. Dual-energy x-ray absorptiometry currently has the highest precision and is able to study both femur and lumbar spine sites.

Those methods using direct measurement of the spine and femur have a greater correlation with risk of site-specific fractures, although measures from single-photon absorptiometry of peripheral sites are also predictive of fractures in other locations. The ability to separately assess cortical versus trabecular bone may be of some benefit but requires further study. The usefulness of any technique for follow-up is limited by its precision. To assess changes of 1 to 2% between readings, a precision greater than 99% is required. Dual-energy x-ray absorptiometry is the only modality capable of this precision for repeat measures.

No single fracture threshold or bone density value at which point risk of fracture sharply increases has been identified; instead, what is noted is a continuous curve of increasing risk with decreasing bone strength (Fig. 62–2). Therefore, deciding what is high versus normal risk is by defi-

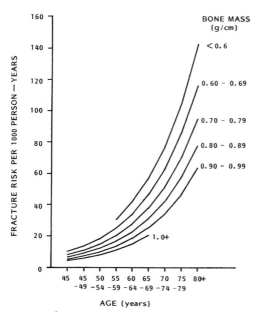

Figure 62-2. Estimated incidence of fracture as a function of bone mass. (Reproduced from Hui SL, Slemenda CW, Johnston CC Jr. Age and bone mass as predictors of fracture in a prospective study. J Clin Invest 1988;81:1804–1809, by copyright permission of The Society for Clinical Investigation.)

nition arbitrary. Some use sixty-fifth or ninetieth percentile for one's age group. Others have considered absolute bone density values to assess risk. One study gave normal risk being greater than 1.0 gm per cm, 0.8 to 1.0 gm per cm as moderate risk, and less than 0.8 gm per cm as high risk, whereas another study considered measures greater than 0.8 gm per cm to be normal risk, 0.6 to 0.8 gm per cm to be moderate risk, and less than 0.6 gm per cm to be high risk.

The appropriate frequency of screening and the site to screen are other areas without a consensus. Evaluation at one point in time does not demonstrate rapid bone loss. For patients currently normal or at moderate risk, bone loss could be rapid, and this increased risk could be missed with one observation. This observation suggests that repeat measures would be of value. However, only dual-energy x-ray absorptiometry can measure the magnitude of changes expected over a 1- to 2-year period. Biochemical markers of bone turnover may in the future provide an adjunct to screening. Rather than obtaining two bone density readings over time to demonstrate the rate of bone loss, future screening with bone density plus a measure of bone turnover may allow prediction of the future rate of bone loss at a single point in time. The site or sites to be screened are also undetermined. All bone density measures provide some estimate

of fracture risk at other sites, although the strongest associations are site specific. Therefore, hip and spine measures appear preferable to peripheral sites. Whether one needs to assess both sites is not determined. Because vertebral bone loss represents the first manifestation of osteoporosis, spinal measurements may be more sensitive. If the main outcome of importance is hip fracture, screening at this site will be more specific.

Cost-effectiveness analyses before introduction of dual-energy x-ray absorptiometry argued against the value of screening, in part based on poor precision.[23] Subsequent reports found that across a wide range of assumptions, bone density screening was cost-effective when compared with other preventive strategies used for other diseases.[24] It is reasonable to consider screening when these results are likely to affect treatment recommendations or a patient's acceptance or rejection of these recommendations. One study has shown both adverse and positive effects of bone density screening. Of women surveyed after screening, more than half reported taking some preventive steps to avoid bone loss or falls, and 95% of women labeled as having below normal bone density reported such changes. Although most of these interventions were positive, including increased use of calcium, vitamin D, or estrogen, other interventions were less positive. One quarter of women with below normal density reported decreasing their activity as a means of preventing falls.[25] Thus, although positive effects of screening were noted, appropriate education and follow-up are necessary.

Specific algorithms for screening depend on the type of screening services available to patients. For patients with known risk factors such as chronic corticosteroid use, thyroxine therapy, or parathyroid disease, bone density assessment is clearly important. The decision to screen menopausal women should be based on the likelihood that the results of screening will change pharmacologic management. For example, in a woman who has already decided whether or not to use estrogen therapy after menopause, screening will not alter this management and may therefore be of less value. However, for those women whose individual risk is unclear or when a provider's estimate of risk is substantial but a patient is reluctant to consider therapy, a single bone density study at menopause may help determine the course of treatment. In women who have normal bone density and who choose not to take estrogen, repeat of this measure in 1 to 2 years is dependent on availability of technology that can detect 1 to 4% changes in density.

TABLE 62–3. Calcium Content of Certain Foods

FOOD	SERVING SIZE	CALCIUM CONTENT (mg)
Parmesan cheese, grated	1 ounce	390
Collards, cooked from frozen, chopped	1 cup	357
Sardines, canned in oil	8 medium	354
Rhubarb, cooked, added sugar	1 cup	348
Yogurt (lowfat, fruit-flavored)	8 ounces	345
Gruyere cheese	1 ounce	308
Milk, skim	1 cup	303
Blackstrap molasses	2 tablespoons	274
Figs, dried	10 figs	269
Spinach, cooked from raw	1 cup	245
Cheddar cheese (American)	1 ounce	211
Creamed cottage cheese	1 cup	211
Broccoli, cooked, drained	1 spear, medium	205
American cheese, processed	1 ounce	195
Salmon, canned (pink)	3 ounces	167
Tofu	1 piece (1″ × 2½″ × 2¾″)	108

From The Medical Letter on Drugs and Therapeutics, November 17, 1989, vol. 31 (issue 805), p 102, adapted from Pennington JAT, Church HN. Bowes and Church's Food Values of Portions Commonly Used. 13th ed. New York: Harper & Row, 1980; and Gebhardt SE, Matthews RH. Nutritive Value of Foods. Washington DC: Government Printing Office, US Dept of Agriculture, 1981.

PREVENTIVE MEASURES

Lifestyle modification should be reviewed as an aspect of osteoporosis prevention for women of all age groups, including exercise, calcium intake, and habit modification. Weight-bearing exercise has been shown to be of benefit in increasing and maintaining bone strength and preventing fractures in both pre- and postmenopausal women with and without existing osteoporosis. Regular weight-bearing exercise, such as walking, cycling, or aerobics for 20 minutes three times weekly should be recommended to women of all ages.

Adequate intakes of calcium and vitamin D are a prerequisite to bone development. Cross-sectional data comparing fracture rates in two communities, one with a diet low in calcium and the other with high dietary calcium, suggest that much osteoporosis could be prevented with adequate diet early in life. Estimates from the National Health and Nutrition Examination Surveys demonstrate that 56% of American girls and women do not take in sufficient calcium to meet their recommended daily allowance.[26] The current recommendations for calcium are 1500 mg daily for adolescents, 1000 mg daily for premenopausal women, and 1500 mg for postmenopausal women, with a 50% increase recommended for pregnant and lactating women. The increased requirement for adolescents relates to bone growth during that time. The increase for menopausal women is necessary because of decreased absorption of calcium in this group. Evidence suggests that increasing dietary calcium can increase bone strength in women until at least age 30 years; therefore, this preventive suggestion should be part of routine counseling.

Because dairy products make up the major source of calcium in Western diets, assessment of dairy intake is the easiest way to estimate a woman's calcium intake. One can multiply the average daily number of dairy servings by 300 mg to estimate usual calcium intake, with a serving being 1 cup of milk, yogurt, ice cream, or cottage cheese or 2 to 4 ounces of cheese (Table 62–3). Because so many adults have difficulty increasing their dairy consumption owing to the extra calories or cholesterol contained in them or because of lactose intolerance, the use of supplements is recommended, especially when the calcium deficit is 300 mg or more daily. Although calcium citrate may be better absorbed, calcium carbonate is readily available and inexpensive. Sudden supplementation with 1000 mg or more may lead to constipation; therefore, one should advise patients to increase the dose gradually or use stool softeners.

In addition to calcium supplementation, the need for vitamin D to prevent osteomalacia should be addressed. For active women, skin production is sufficient during the warmer months, but with less production in colder climates due to the low angle of sunlight and filtering of ultraviolet radiation,[27] this is often not adequate in winter months. Although milk is fortified with vitamin D, the amounts often vary widely from what is reported.[28] Therefore, supplementation with vitamin D, especially in older women and women with little exposure to direct sunlight, is important.

Cigarette smoking and excessive alcohol intake promote bone loss, and counseling directed at eliminating these additional risk factors should be instituted for all women. Low weight should be addressed with young women as a risk for inadequate bone development. Women with oligomenorrhea or amenorrhea related to low weight and strenuous exercise should be counseled on the detrimental effects this may have on their bone health. In this group, in whom changes in either weight or exercise pattern are difficult to achieve, consideration of the use of oral contraceptives to provide the necessary hormonal stimulation will be of benefit.

PHARMACOLOGIC APPROACHES FOR PREVENTION AND TREATMENT

Because osteoporosis consists of defects in both increased resorption and decreased formation of bone, therapy would ideally be aimed at both defects. To date, all therapeutic modalities decrease bone resorption but none increases bone formation. They all maintain bone at its current density or increase the density by a few percent. Pharmacologic therapy is most effective before trabeculae are lost. Treatment of late osteoporosis, once fractures are manifested, can at best maintain bone at that suboptimal level.

The goal of any pharmacologic therapy is prevention of fractures. Although many studies of therapies look at intermediate outcomes of bone density, these measures do not always correlate with the fracture rate. Currently, only estrogen is approved for the prevention of osteoporosis, but both estrogen and calcitonin are approved for treatment. Calcitonin, bisphosphonates, fluoride, and calcitriol are under investigation as preventive and therapeutic modalities.

Estrogen therapy after menopause has been shown not only to stabilize and slightly increase bone density but also to reduce the rate of vertebral and hip fractures in women. A dose of 0.625 mg daily has been shown to be effective for most women.[29] (Details on prescribing estrogens, the other health benefits and risks, and monitoring while on estrogens are found in Chapter 61.) Most authorities recommend beginning treatment within the first year of cessation of menses. Some data suggest that in the years before total cessation of menopause, when menses are irregular, accelerated bone loss has already occurred. However, given the difficulties in monitoring abnormal uterine bleeding, unless a patient is known to be at very high risk or has established osteoporosis, most recommend waiting until menses have ceased to begin preventive therapy.

The usefulness of initiating therapy in older women is not yet well established. On the one hand, a rapid rate of bone loss has already occurred by the seventh decade. As women age, however, the risk increases. Thus, prevention and treatment at this point may be of particular use. Lindsay and colleagues have shown that bone density can be benefited by starting estrogen therapy at any time before age 70 years.[30] Others have also shown that estrogen therapy begun later in life can benefit bone density and fracture rate.

For therapy to be of benefit when begun in early menopause, it must be continued for at least 5 to 8 years. Felson and associates[31] examined longitudinal estrogen use and bone fracture. Long-term use of estrogen has its greatest effect in spine fracture prevention, with a lesser effect on hip fracture rate. The use of less than 7 years of therapy provided no benefit in later life.

Calcitonin is approved for the treatment of existing osteoporosis. Its mechanism of action is to reduce the rate of bone turnover, and it results in a 2 to 5% increase in bone density. Studies to demonstrate a fracture reduction from its use are yet in progress. The drug is currently available only in a parenteral formulation (50 U subcutaneously three times weekly), although an intranasal formulation is currently under investigation. Side effects of the medication include gastrointestinal pain in 8 to 10%, which can be ameliorated by giving the dose 4 to 5 hours after the last meal of the day. Flushing occurs in 2 to 5% and local pruritic reactions in 10% of patients; these symptoms tend to wane with continued administration and respond to prophylactic antihistamine use 30 minutes before administration. There appears to be an escape phenomenon after roughly 2 years of therapy, limiting the duration of use. The combination of parenteral administration, side effects, expense, and limited period of use, plus the lack of data about fracture rate reduction, have resulted in limited use of this medication. Calcitonin has an additional benefit in the treatment of acute pain due to osteoporotic fractures.[32] Typical dosages for the treatment of skeletal pain are 100 U subcutaneously daily 5 days per week.

Bisphosphonates are one of the new classes of drugs under investigation for the treatment of osteoporosis. They also reduce bone resorption by inhibiting osteoclastic activity. Etidronate is the only drug currently available; however, it has been approved by the Food and Drug Administration only for the treatment of Paget's disease. Continuous use of etidronate as used to control Paget's disease exacerbates bone loss in osteoporosis. Clinical trials of intermittent cyclic therapy are under way, using 5 mg per kg or 400 mg daily for 2 weeks, followed by a 13-week hiatus before the next cycle is administered. Preliminary data have shown that this therapy does increase bone mass.[33] However, data are too premature to show a decrease in fracture rate.

Initial studies of the use of fluoride to increase bone strength appeared promising, with as much as twofold increases in bone mass noted. However, randomized controlled trials of daily sodium fluoride use did not show decreased vertebral fracture rates, and an increase in hip fracture rate actually resulted.[34] It appears that although the bone is denser, it is structurally less sound. In the absence of adequate calcium intake, impairment of mineralization can also occur. Therefore, fluoride is not currently recommended for the treatment of osteoporosis. Preliminary studies suggest that a slow-release fluoride formulation may be useful for fracture reduction.[35]

Thiazide diuretics lower the urinary excretion of calcium, improve calcium balance, and are associated with increased bone density. However, diuretics may also lead to hypotension, syncope, and falls, potentially increasing the risk of fractures. Case-control studies conflict in their results, with one showing a one third decrease in hip fracture rate[36] and another showing a 60% increase in hip fracture risk.[37] A randomized trial of diuretic use is needed to address this issue. In the interim, the use of thiazide diuretics should be based on considerations other than bone density.

EVALUATION OF OSTEOPENIA OR BONE FRACTURE IN ELDERLY WOMEN

Osteopenia is identified either directly through bone density measurements, incidentally on plain radiographs obtained for other reasons, clinically by episodes of vertebral or hip fracture, or radiologically by evidence of prior vertebral fracture. Once osteopenia is identified, secondary causes should be ruled out before assuming the cause is primary osteoporosis. Medical and medication risk factors should be reviewed. Osteomalacia should be identified with a 25(OH)D level in all elderly women, especially those with limited mobility and those unlikely to see much sunlight. An alkaline phosphatase level should be obtained to evaluate for other metabolic bone disorders. A normal alkaline phosphatase level precludes other bone abnormalities including hyperparathyroidism, and further evaluation is not indicated. A baseline assessment of renal function to identify renal causes of bone disease and thyroid-stimulating hormone for hyperthyroidism should also be obtained.

PREVENTION OF FALLS IN THE ELDERLY

Hip fractures are the greatest source of morbidity and mortality resulting from osteoporosis. An assessment of risk for hip fracture should address not only bone density but also the risk of falling. One study evaluating the risk of hip fracture identified characteristics of the falls associated with fractures, including falls to the side, the energy of the fall, and a low body mass index. These factors were as important in predicting hip fracture as femoral neck bone density.[38] Interventions targeted at such factors may do as much to reduce morbidity as efforts aimed at strengthening bone.

Tinetti and colleagues have identified risk factors for falling.[39] Thirty percent of ambulatory persons older than 65 years fall each year, and nearly

---

TABLE 62–4. Risk Factor Reduction for Falls

Postural hypotension	Behavioral measures—arising slowly especially in morning and after meals, avoiding hot baths or showers, adequate hydration
	Medication review—diuretics, antihypertensives, nitrates, antidepressants
Sedatives	Medication review—benzodiazepines, alcohol, sleep medications
	Nonpharmacologic management of sleep
Other medications	Centrally acting antihypertensives, nitrates, diuretics, H_2-blockers, nonsteroidal anti-inflammatory drugs
Environmental safety	Trip hazards, lighting, structural additions such as grab bars
	Evaluation of transfers to tub and toilet
Foot problems	Antalgic gait due to toenail pain, calluses, bunions, and toe deformities
Strength and balance	Evaluation of transfers, balance, strength. Range of motion, strengthening exercise

Adapted from Tinetti ME, Baker DI, Garrett PA, et al. Yale Ficsit: Risk factor abatement strategy for fall prevention. J Am Geriatr Soc 1993;41:315.

one quarter of those who fall suffer serious injuries, including 6% who are afflicted with fractures. The highest risk of falls was associated with the use of sedatives, cognitive impairment, the presence of a palmomental reflex, foot problems including bunions, toe deformities, ulcerations or nail deformities, lower extremity disability, and balance and gait disorders. Randomized trials to assess the usefulness of interventions aimed at reducing those risk factors that are modifiable are in progress, including exercise, balance and resistance training, nutritional supplementation, and protective garments worn on the hip joint area.[40] One trial found that efforts to reduce those factors that can easily be modified through an office visit assessment or a physical and occupational therapy home consultation resulted in a 25% decrease in falls[41] (Table 62–4).

REFERENCES

1. Riggs BL, Melton LJ III: Heterogeneity of involutional osteoporosis: Evidence for two osteoporosis syndromes. Am J Med 1983;75:899.
2. Melton LJ, Wahner HW, Richelson LS, et al. Osteoporosis and the risk of hip fracture. Am J Epidemiol 1986;124:254.
3. Rigotti NA, Nussbaum SR, Herzog DB, Neer RM. Osteoporosis in women with anorexia nervosa. N Engl J Med 1984;311:1601.
4. Drinkwater BL, Bruemner B, Chesnut CH. Menstrual history as a determinant of current bone density in young athletes. JAMA 1990;263:545.
5. Drinkwater BL, Nilson K, Chesnut CH, et al. Bone mineral content of amenorrheic and eumenorrheic athletes. N Engl J Med 1984;311:277.
6. Prior JC, Vigna YM, Schechter MT, Burgess AE. Spinal bone loss and ovulatory distrubances. N Engl J Med 1990;323:1221.
7. Kleerekoper M, Brienza RS, Schultz LR, et al. Oral contraceptive use may protect against low bone mass. Arch Intern Med 1991;151:1971.
8. Sowers M, Corton G, Shapiro B, et al. Changes in bone density with lactation. JAMA 1993;269:3130.
9. Seeman E, Hopper JL, Bach LA, et al. Reduced bone mass in daughters of women with osteoporosis. N Engl J Med 1989;320:554.
10. Evans RA, Marel GM, Lancaster EK. Bone mass is low in relatives of osteoporotic patients. Ann Intern Med 1988;109:870.
11. Popcock NA, Eisman JA, Hopper JL, et al. Genetic determinants of bone mass in adults. J Clin Invest 1987;80:706.
12. Hemenway D, Colditz GA, Willett WC, et al. Fractures and lifestyle: Effect of cigarette smoking, alcohol intake, and relative weight on the risk of hip and forearm fractures in middle-aged women. Am J Public Health 1988; 78:1554.
13. Hopper JL, Seeman E. The bone density of female twins discordant for tobacco use. N Engl J Med 1994;330:387.
14. Kiel DP, Baron JA, Anderson JJ, et al. Smoking eliminates the protective effect of oral estrogens on the risk for hip fracture among women. Ann Intern Med 1992;116:716.
15. Drinkwater BL. Physical exercise and bone health. In Swartz DP (ed). Hormone Replacement Therapy in the Ovarian Deficient Woman. Baltimore, MD: Urban and Schwarzenberg Medical Publishers, 1991.
16. Matkovic V, Kostial K, Simonovic I, et al. Bone status and fracture rates in two regions of Yugoslavia. Am J Clin Nutr 1979;32:540.
17. Farmer ME, White LR, Brody JA, Bailey KR. Race and sex differences in hip fracture incidence. Am J Public Health 1984;74:1374.
18. Liel U, Edwards J, Shary J, et al. The effects of race and body habitus on bone mineral density of the radius, hip, and spine in premenopausal women. J Clin Endocrinol Metab 1988;66:1247.
19. Luckey MM, Meier DE, Mandeli JP, et al. Radial and vertebral bone density in white and black women: Evidence for racial differences in premenopausal bone homeostasis. J Clin Endocrinol Metab 1989;69:762.
20. Gilsanz V, Roe TF, Mora S, et al. Changes in vertebral bone density in black girls and white girls during childhood and puberty. N Engl J Med 1991;325:1597.
21. Weinstein RS, Bell NH. Diminished rates of bone formation in normal black adults. N Engl J Med 1988;319:1698.
22. Grisso JA, Kelsey JL, Strom BL, et al. Risk factors for hip fracture in black women. N Engl J Med 1994;330:1555.
23. Cummings SR, Black D. Should perimenopausal women be screening for osteoporosis? Ann Intern Med 1986;104:817.
24. Tosteson ANA, Rosenthal DI, Melton J, Weinstein MC. Cost effectiveness of screening perimenopausal white women for osteoporosis: Bone densitometry and hormone replacement therapy. Ann Intern Med 1990;113:594.
25. Rubin SM, Cummings SR. Results of bone densitometry affect women's decisions about taking measures to prevent fractures. Ann Intern Med 1992;116:990.
26. Preliminary Finding of the First Health and Nutrition Examination Survey, United States, 1971–1972, Anthropometric and Clinical Findings. DHEW Publication No. (HRA) 75–1229. Rockville, MD: US Department of Health, Education, and Welfare Public Health Service, 1975.
27. Holick MF. Photosynthesis of vitamin D in the skin: Effect of environmental and lifestyle variables. Fed Proc 1987;46(5):1876.
28. Holick MF, Shao Q, Liu WW, Chen TC. The vitamin D content of fortified milk and infant formula. Bone Research Laboratory, Boston University School of Medicine. N Engl J Med 1992;326(18):1178.
29. Lindsay R, Hart DM, Clarke DM. The minimum effective dose of estrogen for prevention of postmenopausal bone loss. Obstet Gynecol 1984;63:759.
30. Lindsay R, Hart DM, Forrest C, Baird C. Prevention of spinal osteoporosis in oophorectomised women. Lancet 1980;2:1151.
31. Felson DT, Zhang Y, Hannan MT, et al. The effect of postmenopausal estrogen therapy on bone density in elderly women. N Engl J Med 1993;329:1141.
32. Avioli LV. Calcitonin therapy in osteoporotic syndromes. JAMWA 1990;45:103.
33. Storm T, Thamsborg F, Steniche T, et al. Effect of intermittent cyclical etidronate therapy on bone mass and fracture rate in women with postmenopausal osteoporosis. N Engl J Med 1990;322:1265.
34. Riggs BL, Hodgson SF, O'Fallon WM, et al. Effect of fluoride treatment on the fracture rate in postmenopausal women with osteoporosis. N Engl J Med 1990;323:416.
35. Pak CY, Sakhaee K, Piziak V, et al. Slow-release sodium fluoride in the management of postmenopausal osteoporosis. Ann Intern Med 1994;120:625.
36. LaCroix AZ, Wienpahl J, White LR, et al. Thiazide diuretic agents and the incidence of hip fracture. N Engl J Med 1990;322:286.

37. Heidrich FE, Stergachis A, Gross KM. Diuretic drug use and the risk for hip fracture. Ann Intern Med 1991;115:1.
38. Greenspan SL, Myers ER, Maitland LA, et al. Fall severity and bone mineral density as risk factors for hip fracture in ambulatory elderly. JAMA 1994;271:128.
39. Tinetti ME, Baker DI, Garrett PA, et al. Yale Ficsit: Risk factor abatement strategy for fall prevention. J Am Geriatr Soc 1993;41:315.
40. Ory MG, Schechtman KB, Miller JP, et al. Frailty and injuries in later life: The FICSIT trials. J Am Geriatr Soc 1993;41:283.
41. Tinetti ME, Baker DI, McAvay G, et al. A multifactorial intervention to reduce the risk of falling among elderly people living in the community. N Engl J Med 1994;331:821.

Urinary Incontinence

Joan Bengtson

Urinary incontinence affects approximately 10 million adults in the United States at a cost conservatively estimated at $10 billion annually.[1] The U.S. Department of Health and Human Services published a Clinical Practice Guideline on urinary incontinence in adults.[2] This effort acknowledges the importance of the condition and the need to educate both the public and the health care profession about it. Despite recent attention, urinary incontinence remains too frequently underreported by patients and underdiagnosed by physicians.

The reported prevalence of incontinence varies from 8 to 50%, depending on the gender composition and age of the population studied.[1] Women are affected twice as frequently as men.[3] Among older community-dwelling women, it is estimated that 15 to 30% have significant symptoms. Incontinence will be increasingly important as the proportion of older individuals in society grows. It is not an inevitable consequence of aging, however, and all reasonable efforts should be made to diagnose and treat the condition in older patients.

Parity is another established risk factor, but women having had only one delivery are as likely to be incontinent as those having had two or three deliveries.[4] It had been hoped that the declining parity of this generation might result in lower rates of incontinence in the future, but the data argue against such a trend.

It is estimated that only about half of affected individuals consult a physician. Reasons cited by women after prolonged delay in seeking help include embarrassment, acceptance of the condition as normal for aging, and belief that prognosis for treatment is poor.[5] Many patients live in social isolation, suffering a sense of stigmatization as a result of incontinence. Physicians, especially those in primary care, must be cognizant of incontinence and the options for treatment if they are to help reduce its enormous costs.

ANATOMY AND PHYSIOLOGY

The lower urinary tract functions to store urine until a socially acceptable opportunity occurs for efficient and complete excretion. The two phases of function, storage and emptying, require reciprocal activity of two structural components, the bladder and the urethra.

The bladder is a highly distensible muscular-walled viscus. It changes shape and its superior relations in the pelvis as it fills with urine. The smooth muscle fibers composing the wall form a syncytium, called the detrusor muscle, designed to effect coordinated contractions. The bladder dome is covered with a loose adventitia and the visceral peritoneum, which accommodate bladder distention and contraction.

The urethra in an adult woman is approximately 4 cm in length. It is positioned between the pubic symphysis and the anterior vaginal wall. It is relatively fixed in this position and intimately attached to the vagina, a position maintained by the investing layers of connective tissue called the endopelvic fascia and by the medial portions of the levator ani muscle.[6] This relationship is important in the continence mechanism.

During the storage phase, continence is maintained because at all times the pressure in the urethra exceeds the pressure in the bladder. The detrusor muscle is relaxed, allowing the bladder to accommodate a wide range of volume under low pressure. Concurrently, the urethra is contracted. During the emptying phase, these relationships must be simultaneously and completely reversed. The detrusor contracts while the urethra relaxes so that urine passes through a low-pressure conduit out of the body.

The mechanism of continence has been difficult to discern because the urethra lacks an anatomically discrete, circumferential sphincter. Instead, several components contribute to continence (Table 63–1). Smooth muscle tissue in the proximal urethral wall contiguous with fibers from the bladder form an involuntary sphincter that maintains resting tone during filling. Skeletal muscle fibers of the sphincter urethrae muscles add an element of voluntary control to urethral closure. The ure-

TABLE 63–1. Components of the Urethral Sphincter Mechanism

> Smooth muscle
> Skeletal muscle
> Urethral mucosa
> Ligaments and fascia

thral mucosa also contributes to continence by forming a watertight seal when the walls coapt. The walls must be soft and pliable to allow closure. However, the most important elements of the sphincter mechanism, especially during stress, are the ligamentous and fascial supports. They allow the urethra to be fixed against the upper vagina and compressed by the pressure forces.

Bladder and urethral function are mediated by both the autonomic and central nervous systems. During infancy, the bladder functions primarily as a reflex organ. As it fills, stretch receptors in the wall are stimulated, and these in turn stimulate afferent nerves traveling to the sacral spinal cord segments S2 to S4. Efferent nerves return to the bladder and cause detrusor contraction and urethral relaxation. Toilet training brings this reflex under voluntary control. Inhibitory signals arising in the cerebral cortex stifle the sacral micturition reflex until a socially acceptable time and place for emptying are available. Proper function depends on intact sensory nerves that allow one to perceive bladder fullness.

The bladder contracts with parasympathetic stimulation through release of acetylcholine. The urethra contracts with sympathetic stimulation of α-adrenergic receptors in the smooth muscle of the bladder neck. Thus, the parasympathetic system stimulates the emptying phase of bladder function and the sympathetic system contributes to the storage phase.

PATHOPHYSIOLOGY

Incontinence is defined as involuntary loss of urine of sufficient magnitude to create a social or hygienic problem.[1] It is a failure of the storage phase of bladder function. Recalling the two components of the lower urinary tract, it can result from defects in bladder function, urethral function, or both. A useful differential diagnosis based on the etiology of urine loss follows:

1. Incompetence of the urethral sphincter mechanism
   a. Urethral hypermobility
   b. Intrinsic sphincteric deficiency
2. Detrusor instability
   a. Idiopathic
   b. Secondary
3. Overflow incontinence
   a. Obstructive
   b. Neurogenic
4. Extraurethral incontinence
   a. Congenital
   b. Acquired
5. Other

Urethral Sphincter Incompetence

Continence is maintained during normal storage because urethral pressure exceeds bladder pressure even during episodes of marked elevation in intra-abdominal pressure such as with the Valsalva maneuver, sneezing, coughing, and laughing. Elevations in intra-abdominal pressure during these periods of stress are passively transmitted across the bladder wall, causing bladder pressure to rise. However, if the urethra maintains its normal anatomic relations, the pressure rise is simultaneously transmitted across its wall and its lumen is pressed closed. Bladder pressure rises, urethral pressure rises concomitantly, urethral pressure remains higher than bladder pressure, and the individual remains dry.

Urethral hypermobility can interfere with this mechanism (Fig. 63–1). Pressure transmission to the urethral lumen does not occur if the ligaments that fix it snugly between the anterior vaginal wall and the posterior surface of the pubic bone are weakened or ruptured. This is the major cause of stress incontinence. Conditions contributing to poor ligamentous support include connective tis-

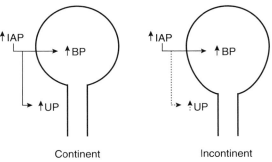

Figure 63–1. An increase in intra-abdominal pressure (IAP) is transmitted equally across the walls of both the bladder and the urethra in the continent state so the relationship UP>BP is maintained. If the urethral supports are inadequate, pressure transmission to the urethra is poor. During an increase in intra-abdominal pressure, BP rises in excess of UP and incontinence occurs. UP, Urethral pressure; BP, bladder pressure.

sue disease, obstetric trauma, and aging. As expected, stress incontinence often occurs in conjunction with other manifestations of poor pelvic support such as cystocele, rectocele, and uterine prolapse.

However, normal anatomic alignment alone does not ensure continence. If the intrinsic components of the sphincter mechanism malfunction, urethral incompetence may also occur. For example, it was previously mentioned that the mucosal layer of the urethra contributes to continence by forming a watertight seal. If the pliability and turgor of the urethral tube are lost through atrophic changes associated with estrogen deprivation or scarring from prior surgery, incontinence may result. Similarly, if the strength of the sphincter urethrae muscles or the resting tone of the smooth muscle component is lost, a person is prone to leakage.

Detrusor Instability

Detrusor instability is a mechanism of incontinence involving bladder dysfunction rather than urethral dysfunction. It occurs when the detrusor muscle inappropriately contracts during the storage phase. The pressure rises in the bladder, and a patient often perceives a subjective sense of urgency. If the pressure rises sufficiently to exceed urethral pressure, leakage results.

Most cases of detrusor instability occur without apparent cause.[7] Idiopathic detrusor instability is likely a functional disorder and may be thought of as a partial or incomplete loss of the toilet training skills achieved in childhood. Other cases of detrusor instability result from an underlying disease. Two categories to consider are local processes and neurologic diseases. Among the local diseases, urinary tract infection is most common. Bacterial cystitis can cause detrusor instability by inciting local irritation. Other local conditions to consider are bladder stones, dysplastic mucosal lesions, and polyps. When detrusor instability results from a discernible neurologic lesion, the term bladder hyperreflexia is applied. The lesion is located in the upper motor neurons, above the sacral micturition center. Dysfunction of the inhibitory neurons in the cortex or cord releases the bladder from normal suppression, and hyperreflexia results. Examples of diagnoses leading to bladder hyperreflexia include cerebrovascular accidents, multiple sclerosis, and trauma.

Overflow Incontinence

Overflow incontinence is leakage from an over-distended bladder. The bladder does not empty at normal volumes, and intravesical pressure rises as filling exceeds physiologic limits. When bladder pressures rise above urethral pressure, incontinence results. Urine retention may result from either outlet obstruction or bladder atony. Women (unlike older men with prostatism) rarely suffer from outlet obstruction. However, this mechanism should be remembered in the setting of trauma, recent vaginal delivery, and pelvic surgery.

Bladder atony results from neurologic dysfunction of lower motor neurons. The sacral spinal cord roots S2 to S4 and the peripheral pelvic nerves innervating the detrusor stimulate contraction. Damage to these nerves from cauda equina lesions, diabetic neuropathy, and pelvic surgery, for example, can result in atony. Atony is often accompanied by deficits in the ability to perceive bladder filling.

Extraurethral Incontinence

Extraurethral incontinence results from a conduit that bypasses the normal sphincter mechanism. The conduit may be a congenital anomaly such as an ectopic ureter, or it may result from an acquired defect such as a fistula. Fistulas should be considered in the setting of prior pelvic surgery or irradiation.

Other

Incontinence may occur in patients with an intrinsically intact urinary tract if an additional impairment keeps them from exercising their normal continence mechanisms. For example, elderly patients with limited mobility may not be able to get to a bathroom or commode in time to stay dry if assistance is not readily available. Many medications impair urinary tract function and result in incontinence in patients who were previously dry. Patients with psychiatric disorders may lack normal social awareness necessary to maintain continence. The differential diagnosis should not fail to include consideration of factors such as these.

The relative frequency of these disorders has been estimated in a typical gynecologic practice.[8] Fifty to 75% of patients have sphincter incompetence leading to stress incontinence, 10 to 30% have isolated detrusor instability, and 5 to 15% have mixed stress incontinence and detrusor instability. Bladder hyperreflexia, overflow, and fistulas account for the remaining 5 to 10% of cases. Mixed incontinence is important to emphasize, because patients may have more than one pathophysiologic mechanism.

CLINICAL EVALUATION OF PATIENTS WITH INCONTINENCE

The initial evaluation of a patient with incontinence attempts to assess her general health, the severity of the symptom, and associated pathology. Efforts should be made to confirm incontinence objectively. The mechanism cannot be determined without observing a patient's complaint. The basic evaluation includes history, physical examination, urinalysis and culture, and simple urodynamic tests.

The history is a crucial component of the evaluation. Complaints related to the symptom of incontinence can be extensive. Prepared questionnaires such as the one developed by Hodgkinson may be used (Fig. 63–2).[9] Affirmative answers to questions in group 1 suggest intrinsic urinary tract disease such as cystitis or a fistula. Group 2 ques-

tions elicit symptoms associated with neurologic disorders and detrusor instability. Positive responses to group 3 questions suggest stress incontinence. However, questionnaires should never preclude direct discussion between a patient and her physician. One must confirm that questions and answers are properly interpreted and that a patient has the opportunity to explain the significance of her symptoms.

Although a thorough history is important, symptoms alone are poor predictors of the mechanism of incontinence. Most patients with genuine stress incontinence state that they leak with stressful stimuli (95% sensitivity). However, this symptom is only 50 to 70% specific and cannot be relied on to establish the diagnosis or to direct therapy.[10] In addition, one would expect that patients with detrusor instability would complain of urgency, but as many as 40 to 60% of women with urodynami-

Group 1

1. Have you had treatment for urinary tract disease, such as stones, kidney disease, infections, tumors, or injuries?	Yes	No
2. Have you had repeated bouts of pyelitis?	Yes	No
3. Is your urine ever bloody?	Yes	No
4. Is the volume of urine you usually pass large, average, small, or very small? (Please check one.)		
5. When you lose your urine accidentally, are you ever not aware that it is passing?	Yes	No
6. Do you always have a severe sense of urgency before you lose your urine?	Yes	No
7. Do you lose urine as a constant drip from your vagina?	Yes	No
8. Is it usually painful to pass your urine?	Yes	No

Group 2

1. As a child, did you wet the bed?	Yes	No
2. Do you wet the bed now?	Yes	No
3. Have you ever had paralysis, polio, multiple sclerosis, a serious injury to your back, a cyst or tumor on your spine, tuberculosis, a stroke, syphilis, diabetes, or pernicious anemia?	Yes	No
4. Does the sound, the sight, or the feel of running water cause you to lose urine?	Yes	No
5. Is your loss of urine a continuous drip so that you are constantly wet?	Yes	No
6. Are you ever not aware that you are losing urine or are about to lose urine?	Yes	No
7. Is your clothing slightly damp, wet, or soaking wet, or do you leave puddles on the floor? (If yes, check the proper one.)	Yes	No
8. Have you had an operation on your spine, brain, or bladder?	Yes	No
9. Do you find it necessary to have your urine removed by means of a catheter because you are unable to pass it?	Yes	No

Group 3

1. Do you lose urine by spurts during coughing, sneezing, laughing, or lifting?	Yes	No
2. Do you lose urine when you are lying down?	Yes	No
3. Do you lose urine when you are sitting or standing erect?	Yes	No
4. When you are urinating, can you stop the flow?	Yes	No
5. Did your urine difficulty start after delivery of an infant?	Yes	No
6. Did it follow an operation? What type of operation? _____		
7. If your menstrual periods have stopped, did the menopause make your condition more severe?	Yes	No
8. Is your control of urine good unless you cough, sneeze, laugh, or strain?	Yes	No
9. Do you have difficulty holding urine if you suddenly stand erect from a sitting or lying-down position?	Yes	No
10. Do you find it necessary to wear protection because you get wet?	Yes	No

Figure 63–2. Urologic questionnaire. (Modified from Hodgkinson CP. Stress urinary incontinence—1970. Am J Obstet Gynecol 1970;108:1141–1168.)

cally proven unstable bladders do not. Therefore, the history should be regarded as a screening tool, and its utility is in directing further evaluation.

The physical examination of incontinent women includes careful abdominal and pelvic examinations with special emphasis on neurologic assessment of the sacral nerve roots. First, the mucosal surfaces of the lower genital tract are inspected for integrity and evidence of estrogen deprivation. A bimanual examination after a patient voids is necessary to preclude pelvic masses that might exert extrinsic compression on the bladder. It may also demonstrate bladder distention, suggesting overflow incontinence.

Sphincter incompetence due to loss of ligamentous support is one manifestation of the more generalized process of pelvic relaxation. Patients with incontinence often suffer from uterine prolapse, cystocele, rectocele, and enterocele. These conditions should be specifically and systematically sought. Pelvic relaxation is evaluated by using a Sims's speculum or by disarticulating a bivalve speculum and inserting only the posterior blade into the vagina. While depressing the posterior vaginal wall, the physician asks the patient to strain and assesses the anterior wall supports. The speculum is then repositioned to retract the anterior vaginal wall while the rectovaginal septum is evaluated for evidence of rectocele and enterocele. If the patient complains of a sensation of pelvic pressure but no prolapse is demonstrated in the lithotomy position, she should be reassessed while standing.

The proximal urethral supports are further assessed by the Q-Tip test. In a woman at rest in the lithotomy position, the urethra normally courses beneath the pubic bone parallel to the horizontal plane. Its position is marked by placing a sterile, lubricated cotton swab in the urethra. The patient is asked to strain and then to cough several times. If the proximal urethra is well supported, there is little mobility downward away from the pubis. Therefore, the distal end of the Q-Tip is only minimally displaced upward. However, with loss of support, straining causes hypermobility of the proximal urethra downward, resulting in significant upward displacement of the distal urethra and Q-Tip. A positive test is defined as an upward deflection of the distal Q-Tip of 30 degrees or more.

The Q-Tip test provides an objective measure of urethral mobility. It is not diagnostic of incontinence, which is a functional not an anatomic diagnosis.[11] It is relevant, however, especially in patients who are considering surgical treatment. The standard surgical procedures used to treat incontinence are urethropexies. They are designed to ele-

vate and fix the proximal urethra to various pelvic supports. In the absence of demonstrable urethral hypermobility, the likelihood of improving a patient's symptoms by this surgical maneuver is low. Bergman and colleagues[12] reported a fivefold increase in failure rates (from 10–50%) for urethropexies in patients with a negative Q-Tip test result compared with those with a positive result.

The neurologic examination tests spinal segments S2 to S4. The bulbocavernosus and anal sphincter reflexes depend on intact afferent and efferent limbs. They are occasionally difficult to elicit in neurologically intact individuals because patients quickly accommodate to touch. It is best to test them at the very beginning of the physical examination. To elicit the bulbocavernosus reflex, the area of the clitoral hood is stroked and a contraction of the vaginal constrictor muscles should occur. Similarly, a contraction of the anal sphincter should follow lightly stroking the skin near the anus.

Sensory function of the sacral roots is judged by testing for responses to touch and pinprick in the sacral dermatomes (perineum, posterior thigh, and lateral foot). Motor function is tested by asking the patient to resist the maneuvers of plantar flexion of the foot and eversion and inversion of the ankle. Ankle reflexes, plantar reflexes, and anal sphincter tone are checked. Any significant deficit in sensory or motor function should prompt a more thorough neurologic evaluation.

All patients with urinary tract symptoms should have a screening urinalysis. The presence of bacteria or leukocytes on microscopy indicates the need for a clean voided specimen for culture. It has been suggested that even asymptomatic bacteriuria can affect bladder function.[13] Hematuria is associated with urinary tract cancer, calculi, and infection. Urine cytologic study, cystoscopy, and radiologic evaluation of the upper urinary tract by intravenous pyelogram may be indicated.[14]

The mechanism of incontinence cannot be determined by history and physical examination alone. Although function often follows form, a one-to-one correlation is not always noted between anatomy and pathophysiology. A patient with significant urethral hypermobility may be incontinent as a result of detrusor instability and may not leak because of sphincter incompetence as one might first suspect. Urodynamic tests are required to establish the pathophysiology by allowing a clinician to reproduce a patient's symptoms under observation. Simple urodynamic tests can be performed in the office without special equipment.

The simplest yet most important urodynamic test is the stress test.[15] A patient is examined with a full bladder in the lithotomy and standing positions. She is asked to increase intra-abdominal pressure first by Valsalva maneuver, then by rapid, forceful coughing. A spurt of urine lost simultaneously with stress defines a positive response and confirms urethral sphincter incompetence. If leakage is delayed or persists after the time of increased intra-abdominal pressure, detrusor instability is suggested.

Another simple but important test is measurement of postvoid residual volume. The most accurate technique is catheterization after the patient spontaneously voids. An alternative is ultrasonographic assessment of residual volume,[16] which normally does not exceed 50 ml. Overflow incontinence is suspected in the presence of excessive postvoid residual volumes.

At this point in the evaluation, a patient may need to be referred, because additional urodynamic testing requires special equipment. Cystometry assesses detrusor function by simulating the storage phase of bladder function. A pressure transducer placed in the bladder records while the bladder is filled with warm, sterile water via a urethral catheter. The bladder is filled at a rate of 50 ml per minute, and the patient is questioned about symptoms. If only a single intravesical pressure transducer is placed (single-channel cystometry), caution must be used in interpreting the results because the pressure measured in the bladder represents the sum of pressure generated by detrusor activity plus intra-abdominal pressure passively transmitted across the bladder wall. To overcome this difficulty, multichannel systems are used to measure intravesical pressure and intra-abdominal pressure simultaneously via a rectal or vaginal transducer. Changes in ambient intra-abdominal pressure as measured by the second transducer are electronically subtracted from intravesical pressure, yielding true detrusor pressure.

Four parameters of bladder function are determined by cystometry: bladder compliance ($\Delta V/\Delta P$), bladder capacity, bladder sensations, and detrusor stability. The bladder normally functions as a low-pressure reservoir with good compliance. Baseline pressures remain at about 10 to 15 cm H_2O over the normal range of volume. Maximum bladder capacity ranges from 300 to 600 ml. Patients usually report a first sensation of filling between 100 and 200 ml. Sensation is then suppressed until fullness is reported at capacity. During normal filling, the detrusor muscle should be stable. Detrusor instability is defined as involuntary detrusor contractions that occur during filling and that the patient cannot completely suppress.[17]

Urethral pressure profilometry measures urethral pressure both at rest and with exertion. The resting urethral pressure profile curve (Fig. 63–3) is a plot of pressure measured along the length of the urethra. It is determined by inserting a specialized catheter equipped with two pressure transducers into the bladder. One transducer is at the tip of the catheter and remains within the bladder throughout the test. The second transducer is located about 6 cm from the tip. The proximal transducer is pulled through the urethra at a constant rate by a motorized mechanism while pressures are recorded. The dynamic urethral pressure profile is obtained by asking the patient to cough or strain while the transducers monitor bladder and urethral pressures simultaneously. The urethral pressure is monitored at the location of maximum pressure. If the bladder and maximum urethral pressures equalize during stress, sphincter incompetence is suggested.

Urethral pressure profilometry is useful in research, but clinically it fails to discriminate the mechanism of incontinence. Values overlap among stress-incontinent and non–stress-incontinent women.[18] In one study, however, the value for maximum urethral closure pressure was correlated with surgical outcome.[19] Women with a low-pressure urethra, defined as a maximum urethral closure pressure of less than 20 cm H_2O, were less likely to be helped by a retropubic urethropexy procedure.

Uroflowmetry assesses the emptying phase of bladder function by generating a curve of urine flow rate versus voiding time. It is not diagnostic of incontinence that is a defect in the storage phase. It can, however, identify patients with abnormal voiding patterns that might be associated with overflow incontinence, but it cannot distinguish detrusor atony from outflow obstruction.

Videourodynamics combines pressure measurements with simultaneous visualization of bladder function by fluoroscopy. It requires sophisticated

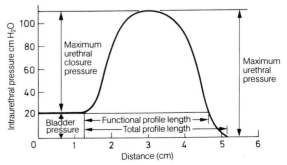

Figure 63–3. Schematic representation of urethral pressure profile. (From Stanton SL. Investigation of incontinence. In: Stanton SL, Tanagho EA [eds]. Surgery of Female Incontinence. 2nd ed. New York: Springer-Verlag; 1986; p 36.)

equipment and specially trained personnel, and thus its use is limited to patients with complex problems.

Cystoscopy allows visualization of the bladder and urethral mucosa. Its role in evaluating incontinence is limited. However, it is used to diagnose mucosal lesions, foreign bodies, and diverticuli. Cystoscopy is indicated in patients with hematuria and abnormal urine cytologic findings. It should be considered in patients with new or acute onset of urgency, especially elderly patients who are at increased risk of bladder neoplasia.

Electromyography of the pelvic floor muscles using either surface electrodes or needle electrodes has been described for evaluating voiding disorders. It is indicated to diagnose detrusor-sphincter dyssynergia, in which the normal reciprocal function of the bladder and sphincter is lost. Muscle activity is usually measured in conjunction with a cystometrogram.

TREATMENT

Treatment is prescribed only when the pathophysiology is well understood, because it depends on the mechanism of incontinence. An improperly applied therapy may not only be ineffective but could worsen a patient's symptoms. Several options for treatment are available for each type of incontinence. The appropriate approach is to reserve invasive treatments for patients who fail to be helped by conservative therapy. In all cases, a patient participates in the choice of treatment through a process of informed consent.

Although the goal is to achieve complete continence in all patients, this sometimes is not possible. Incontinence appliances should be provided for patients who decline treatment, who are not candidates for it, or who fail to respond. Absorbent pads and garments are available. In addition, external collecting devices for women are being developed but have not been perfected. Indwelling catheters should be avoided because of the risk of infection.[20]

Urethral Sphincter Incompetence

The nonsurgical options for the treatment of urethral sphincter incompetence exploit the multifaceted nature of the sphincter complex. In general, they attempt to improve the intrinsic strength of the sphincter, not hypermobility.

The urethral mucosa is an estrogen-dependent tissue. Improved bladder control has been reported with estrogen therapy in postmenopausal women.[21]

The mechanisms proposed for this effect include an increase in the suppleness of the urethral tube, allowing better hermetic closure; increased periurethral blood flow, which increases resistance along the tube; and improved sphincter muscle responsiveness.[22] However, the lack of objective changes in urethral parameters suggests that the primary benefit may derive from an effect on the sensory threshold of the lower urinary tract tissues.[23] Use of estrogens requires consideration of the usual contraindications.

α-Adrenergic agonists have been used to improve the resting tone of the smooth muscle component of the sphincter mechanism. Phenylpropanolamine has been the most extensively studied. In placebo-controlled trials using a dosage of 50 mg twice a day, cure rates were only 0 to 14%. However, rates of subjective improvement in symptoms ranged from 30 to 60%.[24] Side effects include anxiety, insomnia, and headaches. Phenylpropanolamine has a potential for causing or aggravating hypertension and cardiac arrhythmia and should be used with caution, especially in older patients.

The combination of α-agonists and estrogens has also undergone limited evaluation. Estrogens may enhance the number or reactivity of the α-receptors so that the drugs may act synergistically. In four studies reviewed for the Department of Health and Human Services Clinical Practice Guideline, the results with this combination were improved compared with either drug used alone.[25]

Physiotherapy by pelvic floor exercises can improve the continence mechanism by strengthening the striated muscle component of the sphincter. Resting tone is improved, and reflex contraction in response to stress is also enhanced. Kegel is credited with initially describing the technique.[26] Modifications that have been recommended combine the basic exercises with biofeedback techniques and with electric stimulation.

The success of pelvic floor exercises depends on proper performance. A clinician must instruct a patient to identify and contract the correct muscles by performing a digital vaginal examination.[27] Once a patient knows which muscles to exercise, she is asked to contract them vigorously for 5 to 10 seconds. Between contractions, she rests for 10 seconds. Sets of 10 contractions are performed three times a day and increased to five times incrementally. It may be best to perform the exercises every other day rather than daily. Improvement may take 2 months or more, and the exercises may need to be continued indefinitely. Efficacy has been demonstrated, however, with improvement in as many as 67% of patients.[28] Many patients have been instructed to perform pelvic floor exercises while voiding by interrupting the stream of urine. This is an inappropriate way to perform the exercises and should be discouraged.

When conservative measures fail in the treatment of urethral sphincter incompetence, surgical intervention is indicated. The choice of procedure depends on the anatomic findings, the presence of associated pathology, the morbidity of the procedure, and the general health of a patient.

Many operations have been described as correcting urethral hypermobility. All are urethropexies—that is, they are procedures designed to elevate and fix a pathologically hypermobile and descended proximal urethra. The operations vary by the surgical approach to the periurethral tissues and by the structure used in the fixation. Retropubic urethropexies approach the periurethral tissues through an incision in the anterior abdominal wall. The retropubic space of Retzius is developed, and the urethrovesical junction is identified. In the Marshall-Marchetti-Krantz procedure, the periurethral tissues are sutured to the posterior surface of the pubic bone.[29] In Burch's procedure, the urethra is elevated on a sling created by suturing the paravaginal tissues to the Cooper ligament.[30] Cure rates averaged 78% when results from 31 studies were reviewed.[31] Advantages of this approach are the excellent results and the ability to combine the procedure with other operations requiring laparotomy (e.g., large uterine fibroids). Complications include osteitis pubis and occasionally troublesome retropubic bleeding.

Needle urethropexies (e.g., Stamey's, Raz-Pereyra, and Gittes's procedures) avoid the need for a large abdominal incision. Special long needles are used to pass sutures from the periurethral tissues through the retropubic space using a vaginal approach.[32] The sutures elevate the periurethral tissues by securing the knot above the rectus abdominus fascia on the abdominal side. Because the sutures are not placed under direct visualization, cystoscopy is performed to ensure that the bladder and urethral lumina are not violated. Needle suspensions are readily combined with vaginal hysterectomy if indicated. Some studies have suggested that the cure rate for needle procedures is somewhat less than for the abdominal retropubic procedures.[33] When outcomes from more than 1300 patients were reviewed, however, cure rates were 84%.[34]

Patients with urethral incompetence but no urethral hypermobility have an intrinsically deficient sphincter. Surgical options for treatment include sling procedures, artificial sphincters, and periurethral bulking injections. Several different sling procedures have been described.[35] Some use autologous material for the sling such as fascia, and others use synthetic materials. A tunnel is created under the urethra, and the sling is passed through it and attached above the pubis. The sling is intended to compress the urethra closed against the pubic bone. The resulting obstruction sometimes precludes normal voiding, and patients require chronic intermittent self-catheterization. Patients must be carefully counseled about this possibility preoperatively.

Artificial sphincters consist of an inflatable cuff that is implanted around the urethra.[36] A pump is used to fill the cuff during urine storage to compress the urethra extrinsically. A valve allows the cuff to be deflated for voiding. Although successful at controlling incontinence, the complication rate is high. Complications include serious sequelae such as infection and cuff erosion.

Attempts have been made to provide extrinsic urethral compression using injections of Teflon or collagen into the periurethral tissues.[37, 38] The obvious advantage is the ability to treat in the office under local anesthesia. Success rates are lower, however, and Food and Drug Administration approval has not yet been granted. One concern is the possibility of migration of foreign material from the site of injection.

Detrusor Instability

The treatment modalities for detrusor instability include behavior therapy, drugs, electric stimulation, and surgery. Local processes should be treated or precluded before initiating therapy for idiopathic detrusor instability. In addition, treatment should proceed in consultation with a neurologist if bladder hyperreflexia is suspected.

Behavior therapy attempts to re-establish inhibitory control of the cerebral cortex over the sacral micturition reflex. Bladder retraining by scheduled voiding is the basis of most programs. Intense patient education and support are important components. Patients are asked to suppress any urge to void until a prescribed time interval has passed. The interval is initially set low, with the intention that it is increased gradually as a patient is successful at controlling symptoms. She then voids on schedule regardless of urge to reinforce her control. Bladder training can achieve cure rates of up to 90%.[39]

Several classes of drugs have been used to treat detrusor instability. Anticholinergics block the action of acetylcholine on the detrusor muscle, helping to suppress uninhibited contractions. Propantheline is efficacious, but its use is limited by often intolerable anticholinergic side effects including xerostomia, dry eyes, and blurred vision.

It is contraindicated in patients with narrow-angle glaucoma. Oxybutynin is a smooth muscle relaxant that also has anticholinergic action. Subjective improvement compared with placebo has been demonstrated,[40] but anticholinergic side effects are common. They may be controlled by starting patients on low doses and gradually increasing as tolerated. Tricyclic antidepressants have been used with success to treat detrusor instability. The mechanism of action may again depend on anticholinergic properties, although direct smooth muscle effects and central nervous system effects may also contribute to efficacy.[41] Calcium channel blockers, local anesthetics, nonsteroidal anti-inflammatory agents, and β-agonists all have been used for the treatment of detrusor instability. However, data from clinical trials are inadequate to fully evaluate efficacy and safety at this time.[42]

Electric stimulation to control detrusor instability has been studied, but extensive clinical experience is lacking. It is based on the theory that stimulation of the pelvic floor muscles will induce reflex relaxation of the detrusor muscle.[43]

Two types of surgical procedures have been recommended for detrusor instability.[41] They are reserved for the most severe, intractable cases after nonsurgical approaches have failed and thus are only rarely indicated. Augmentation cystoplasty attempts to improve symptoms by increasing bladder capacity. Bladder denervation procedures attempt to control symptoms by interrupting motor and sensory fibers to the detrusor.

Overflow Incontinence

The treatment of overflow incontinence depends on whether it is due to detrusor atony or outflow obstruction. Transient detrusor atony due to acute overdistention or anesthesia is managed by catheter drainage for 24 to 48 hours. Drugs with cholinergic activity are sometimes used to assist in restoration of bladder tone. Chronic atony usually requires intermittent catheterization for management.

Outflow obstruction in women may occur either as a postoperative complication or secondary to severe pelvic prolapse. Acute obstruction due to soft tissue edema usually resolves with temporary catheter drainage. Nontransient causes usually require surgical relief of obstruction.

Extraurethral Incontinence

Surgical correction is indicated for fistulas and congenital defects. In severe cases, urinary diversion may be required.

REFERENCES

1. National Institutes of Health. Consensus development conference statement: Urinary incontinence in adults. Bethesda, Md, October 3–5, 1988.
2. Urinary Incontinence Guideline Panel. Urinary Incontinence in Adults: Clinical Practice Guideline. AHCPR Publication 92-0038. Rockville, MD: Agency for Health Care Policy and Research, Public Health Service, US Department of Health and Human Services, 1992.
3. Consensus Conference. Urinary Incontinence in Adults. JAMA 1989;261:2685.
4. Thomas TM, Plymat KR, Blannin J, Meade TW. Prevalence of urinary incontinence. Br Med J 1980;281:1243.
5. Norton PA. Prevalence and social impact of urinary incontinence in women. Clin Obstet Gynecol 1990;33:295.
6. Delancy JOL. Anatomy and physiology of urinary incontinence. Clin Obstet Gynecol 1990;33:298.
7. Wise BG, Cardozo LD. The treatment of detrusor instability. Int Urogynecol J 1992;3:229.
8. Walters MD. The history and physical examination in women with urinary incontinence. American Uro-Gynecology Society Quarterly Report, January, 1989;7:1.
9. Hodgkinson CP. Stress urinary incontinence. Am J Obstet Gynecol 1970;108:1149.
10. Summitt RL, Stovall TG, Bent AE, Ostergard DR. Urinary incontinence: Correlation of history and brief office evaluation with multichannel urodynamic testing. Am J Obstet Gynecol 1992;166:1835.
11. Karram MM, Bhatia NN. The Q-tip test: Standardization of the technique and its interpretation in women with urinary incontinence. Obstet Gynecol 1988;71:807.
12. Bergman A, Koonings PP, Ballard CA. Negative Q-tip test as a risk factor for failed incontinence surgery in women. J Reprod Med 1989;34:193.
13. Bergman A, Bhatia NN. Urodynamics: Effect of urinary tract infection on urethral and bladder function. Obstet Gynecol 1985;66:366.
14. Sutton JM. Evaluation of hematuria in adults. JAMA 1990;263:2475.
15. Kadar N. The value of bladder filling in the clinical detection of urine loss and selection of patients for urodynamic testing. Br J Obstet Gynaecol 1988;95:698.
16. Ireton RC, Krieger JN, Cardenas DD, et al. Bladder volume determination using a dedicated portable ultrasound scanner. J Urol 1990;143:909.
17. Abrams P, Blaivas JG, Stanton SL, Andersen JT. Standardization of terminology of lower urinary tract function. Neurourol Urodyn 1988;7:403.
18. Summitt RL. Investigative techniques, assessment of incontinence, and urodynamics. Curr Opin Obstet Gynecol 1992;4:548.
19. Sand PK, Bowen LW, Panganiban R, Ostergard DR. The low pressure urethra as a factor in failed retropubic urethropexy. Obstet Gynecol 1987;69:399.
20. Warren JW, Damron D, Tenney JH, et al. Fever, bacteremia, and death as complications of bacteriuria in women with long term urethral catheters. J Infect Dis 1987;155:1151.
21. Walter S, Kjaergaard B, Lose G, et al. Stress urinary incontinence in postmenopausal women treated with oral estrogen (estriol) and an alpha-adrenoceptor stimulating agent (phenylpropanolamine): A randomized double-blind placebo-controlled study. Int Urogynecol J 1990;1:74.
22. Hilton P, Stanton SL. The use of intravaginal oestrogen cream in genuine stress incontinence. Br J Obstet Gynecol 1983;90:940.
23. Fantl JA, Wyman JF, Anderson RL, et al. Postmenopausal urinary incontinence: Comparison between non-estrogen

supplemented and estrogen-supplemented women. Obstet Gynecol 1988;71:823.

24. Urinary Incontinence Guideline Panel. Urinary Incontinence in Adults: Clinical Practice Guideline. AHCPR Publication 92-0038. Rockville, MD: Agency for Health Care Policy and Research, Public Health Service, US Department of Health and Human Services, 1992, p 44.

25. Urinary Incontinence Guideline Panel. Urinary Incontinence in Adults: Clinical Practice Guideline. AHCPR Publication 92-0038. Rockville, MD: Agency for Health Care Policy and Research, Public Health Service, US Department of Health and Human Services, 1992, p 47.

26. Kegel AH. Progressive resistance exercise in the functional restoration of the perineal muscles. Am J Obstet Gynecol 1948;56:238.

27. Bo K, Larsen S, Oseid S, et al. Knowledge about and ability to correct pelvic floor muscle exercises in women with urinary stress incontinence. Neurourol Urodyn 1988;7:261.

28. Henalla SM, Kirwin P, Castleden CM, et al. The effect of pelvic floor exercises in the treatment of genuine urinary stress incontinence in women at two hospitals. Br J Obstet Gynaecol 1988;95:602.

29. Marshall VF, Marchetti AA, Krantz KE. The correction of stress incontinence by simple vesicourethral suspension. Surg Obstet Gynecol 1949;88:509.

30. Burch J. Urethrovaginal fixation to Cooper's ligament for correction of stress incontinence, cystocele and prolapse. Am J Obstet Gynecol 1961;81:281.

31. Urinary Incontinence Guideline Panel. Urinary Incontinence in Adults: Clinical Practice Guideline. AHCPR Publication 92-0038. Rockville, MD: Agency for Health Care Policy and Research, Public Health Service, US Department of Health and Human Services, 1992, p 55.

32. Cornella JL, Ostergard DR. Needle suspension procedures for urinary stress incontinence. A review and historical perspective. Obstet Gynecol Surv 1990;45:805.

33. Bergman A, Ballard CA, Koonings PP. Comparison of three different surgical procedures for genuine stress incontinence: Prospective randomized study. Am J Obstet Gynecol 1989;160:1102.

34. Urinary Incontinence Guideline Panel. Urinary Incontinence in Adults: Clinical Practice Guideline. AHCPR Publication 92-0038. Rockville, MD: Agency for Health Care Policy and Research, Public Health Service, US Department of Health and Human Services, 1992, p 55.

35. Hohenfellner R, Petri E. Sling Procedures. In: Stanton SL, Tanagho EA (eds). Surgery of Female Incontinence, 2nd ed. New York: Springer-Verlag, 1986, pp 105–113.

36. Diokno AC, Hollander JB, Alderson TP. Artificial urinary sphincter for recurrent female urinary incontinence: Indications and results. J Urol 1987;138:778.

37. Beckingham IJ, Wemyss-Holden G, Lawrence WT. Long-term follow up of women treated with periurethral Teflon injections for stress incontinence. Br J Urol 1992;69:580.

38. Appell R, McGuire E, DeRidder P, et al. Updated multicenter study on the use of Gax-collagen for female type III stress urinary incontinence (abstract). Int Urogynecol J 1992;3:268.

39. Fantl JA, Wyman JF, Harkins SW, Hadley EC. Bladder training in the management of lower urinary tract dysfunction in women. J Am Geriatr Soc 1990;38:329.

40. Tapp AJS, Cardozo LD, Versi E, Cooper D. The treatment of detrusor instability in post-menopausal women with oxybutynin chloride: A double-blind placebo controlled study. Br J Obstet Gynecol 1990;97:521.

41. Wall LL. Diagnosis and management of urinary incontinence due to detrusor instability. Obstet Gynecol Surv 1990;45:1S.

42. Urinary Incontinence Guideline Panel. Urinary Incontinence in Adults: Clinical Practice Guideline. AHCPR Publication 92-0038. Rockville, MD: Agency for Health Care Policy and Research, Public Health Service, US Department of Health and Human Services, 1992, pp 40–43.

43. Tanahgo EA. Electrical stimulation. J Am Geriatr Soc 1990;38:352.

Health Care of the Elderly Woman

Patricia P. Barry

In the United States, the population older than 65 years has been projected to double in the next 50 years; those older than 85 years are increasing in number most rapidly. In particular, health concerns of older women are a significant component of medical practice in most of the countries of Western Europe and North America, where the elderly population is predominantly female owing to a preponderance of surviving women, especially older than 75 years. Higher male mortality begins at birth and continues throughout the life span, with much of the early difference due to infection and accidents. Coronary heart disease is the leading cause of death among older persons of both sexes, but deaths in men occur about 10 years earlier than in women. Although this sex differential in coronary disease is a major cause of higher mortality in older men, male mortality rates are also higher for many other diseases as well. As a result, by the age of 85 years, there are 225 women for every 100 men in the United States, and female life expectancy at birth is 7 years longer than for males. Seventy percent of women older than 75 are widows; the same percentage of men are married. About 85% of those in U.S. nursing homes are women, and 25% of women older than 85 years reside in nursing homes. Fifty percent of women older than 75 live alone, although a majority live close to families. The typical older American woman outlives her husband, maintains an independent residence, remains in contact with her family, and survives through her 70s. Older women also frequently serve as caregivers for their husbands or other family members.

Although at a lower rate, older women die of the same diseases as older men—heart disease, cancer, and cerebrovascular disease. Older women, however, are more likely to suffer from chronic diseases such as arthritis, diabetes, osteoporosis, urinary incontinence, and hypertension, which may affect their functional status and their ability

to live independently. Thus, despite their lower mortality rates, older women as a group have greater morbidity, including more limitations in self-care.

ASSESSMENT

Although the majority of elderly women are in good health, a significant number suffer from multiple illnesses and disabilities. Because physical, mental, and social aspects of illness are closely interrelated, the diagnosis-oriented approach has significant limitations and may not correlate well with overall health and functional status. In order to evaluate and plan appropriately for the long-term health care of frail elderly patients, information must be obtained and organized regarding five basic domains: performance of activities of daily living, physical health, mental health, socioeconomic resources, and the environment. Because the interrelationship among these factors is especially important, a coordinated multidimensional multidisciplinary approach, referred to as geriatric assessment, has evolved.

The Consensus Development Conference on Geriatric Assessment Methods for Clinical Decision-Making, sponsored by the National Institutes of Health, noted that the goals of assessment are to improve diagnostic accuracy, guide selection of interventions to restore or preserve health, recommend an optimal environment, predict outcomes, and monitor clinical change. These goals are often interdependent. Thus, diagnostic accuracy leads to more appropriate interventions and better use of available services, resulting in improved level of function and optimal placement. Geriatric assessment can be performed in many different clinical settings, both institutional and community, and is especially useful at the time of initial evaluation; with any change of location, such as institutionalization or hospital discharge; when planning for service provision in the home; and to assist in monitoring treatments and effects of medication, therapy, or assistive devices.

The Consensus Statement points out that two aspects of geriatric assessment are particularly important. First is the need to target assessment to those persons most likely to benefit, especially those who are frail but not terminally ill, those at critical transition points such as when nursing home placement is being considered, and those at times of decline in both health and function. Second is the need to link assessment with care management and follow-up services, in order to implement the recommendations resulting from assessment. Geriatric assessment is thus a process involving referral, collection of information, assessment, and development and implementation of a care plan, with periodic reassessment and modification of that plan.

Geriatric assessment often involves several health care professionals, including a physician, nurse, and social worker. Well-designed studies have demonstrated the value of assessment in improving diagnostic and therapeutic outcomes in settings such as geriatric inpatient and outpatient units. Multidisciplinary teams carry out such assessment, usually with follow-up case management. Although several studies have demonstrated that geriatric assessment in the office and hospital practice of an individual physician can identify previously unsuspected problems, the impact on outcome depends on the ability to target appropriate patients for assessment and to identify resources and services necessary for follow-up care.

Physical Health

A standard medical history and physical examination probably provide the most useful clinical evaluation of physical health, although they do not allow for overall measures of health status, indicators of severity, or an older woman's perceptions of illness. Extra time may be required, and the information may need to be collected during several visits. The examiner needs to speak clearly and distinctly and to allow a patient time for a complete response. The chief complaint may not be a classic symptom of a specific disease but rather a vague or nonspecific problem such as fatigue or confusion; the past medical history may be complex and detailed. Specific questions about nutrition, exercise, vision and hearing, ambulation, sexual function, sleep pattern, falls, incontinence, and immunizations are especially important in evaluating older women. All medications (pre-

scription and over-the-counter) should be brought to the appointment, including any medication that was prescribed for someone else and that the patient may be taking.

Common physical manifestations of aging include gray hair, thinning hair, wrinkles, shortening of stature, thinning of skin, mild kyphosis, and redistribution of fat to the abdomen and hips. Presbycusis (high-frequency hearing loss) and presbyopia (farsightedness) are common aging changes, as are loss of vibratory sensation in the lower extremities and diminished ankle jerks. Normal values for laboratory studies are essentially unchanged with age, except for nonspecific elevations of the sedimentation rate and slight elevations in serum glucose levels.

In general, a focus on recent changes and identification of any illness that is treatable and affects function is especially useful in evaluating elderly women. In addition, a woman's values and advance directives regarding end-of-life decisions should be elicited and documented in the medical record.

Functional Competence

Good medical care is an essential component of geriatric management. However, diagnosis and treatment of diseases is only the first step in helping an elderly woman to achieve maximum independence and quality of life. Attention to her functional status and ability to provide self-care is essential. In order to evaluate function, measurements of activities of daily living are necessary, including critical items of self-care: bathing, toileting, feeding, dressing, and ambulating.

In community-residing elderly women, assessment of instrumental activities of daily living, which require a higher level of function, may identify impairment at an earlier stage. Instrumental activities of daily living usually include the following: managing finances, managing medication, preparing meals, housekeeping, shopping, using a telephone, and arranging transportation. Of interest is that these are activities customarily performed by women.

To determine which services are needed for assistance, it is useful to categorize performance of activities of daily living and instrumental activities of daily living into three levels: (1) independent, (2) need for some assistance, and (3) unable to perform (even with assistance). Women who need mechanical aids but do not require caregiver assistance may be considered independent.

Mental Status

Both cognition and affect should be assessed; some elderly women may require further psychiatric, neurologic, or neuropsychological evaluation. Cognition includes orientation, memory, perception, judgment, and intelligence, as well as psychomotor skills; measures of cognition are used to identify impairment such as that caused by delirium or dementia. Brief tests, such as Folstein's mini-mental state (Table 64–1), have been widely used and validated in the clinical setting.

Affective measures usually attempt to identify depression, which is common, treatable, and an important cause of dysfunction in elderly women. Although evaluation by a skilled psychiatrist remains the gold standard for this diagnosis, routine use of one of several instruments is justified in patients at risk of this disorder; the Geriatric Depression Scale (Table 64–2), developed by Yesavage and colleagues, has been shown to be useful in a clinical setting.

Socioeconomic Status

Identification of social resources is particularly important for appropriate clinical care, especially noting those caregivers available to provide help and their willingness and ability to do so, the strength of interpersonal relationships, and the sources of stress and support for the caregiver. Community resources available may include services such as daycare, respite care, home health care, and homemakers. Information about financial resources is necessary to determine eligibility for programs such as Medicaid and to assess the ability to pay for needed services not otherwise able to be provided.

Environment

Descriptions of the living environment are an important part of an elderly woman's assessment and include such factors as convenience, safety, and availability of services and social supports. A home visit by a physician or other health care professional may provide essential information to determine the need for specific interventions, which may include physical equipment (ramps, grab bars), special services (homemakers, meals), and increased social activity (visitors, daycare).

PHYSICAL HEALTH

Older women have several major health problems that either do not affect older men or are much more prevalent and serious in older women: breast cancer, osteoporosis and associated fractures, urinary incontinence, and gynecologic malignancies such as endometrial, ovarian, and vulvar cancers (see Chapters 9, 14, 15, 17, 18, 62, and 63). As noted, older women also have many of the same health problems as older men and die of many of the same causes. Heart disease (see Chapter 52) is by far the leading cause of death in women older than 75 years (270,000 in 1988), cancer is the second most common cause (85,000), and cerebrovascular disease the third (68,000). The common cancers in elderly women are breast cancer, lung cancer, colon cancer, and gynecologic cancers.

Lung Cancer

The leading cause of cancer death in women of all ages combined and in women of ages 55 to 74 years is now lung cancer, which has a 5-year survival rate of less than 20%. Because of the dramatic increase since 1960 in this cause of cancer death in women, half of their survival advantage may be lost by the end of this century. Ferguson and colleagues found differences between men and women with this disease: Women had a greater proportion of adenocarcinomas than men; men were more likely to be cigarette smokers and to have a higher consumption of cigarettes. Women also appeared to have a slight survival benefit, controlling for age, cell type, and stage of disease. Older patients in general may have more localized disease and earlier detection, owing to case finding from routine chest radiographs taken for other purposes. Whether the result is actual survival benefit, as opposed to simply an earlier diagnosis of this fatal disease, is not clear.

Lung cancer is usually divided histologically into the two major groups of non–small cell and small cell. Non–small cell includes squamous cell, adenocarcinoma, and large cell carcinoma and constitutes about 75% of all lung cancers. Staging is aimed at establishing resectability, because surgery is the only potentially curative treatment. Surgical therapy may be limited, however, by cardiac or pulmonary comorbidity or age bias in older women. Small cell cancers are treatable by chemotherapy, with or without radiation therapy, and treatment should be considered for elderly women, regardless of age, based on presumed ability to benefit.

Cerebrovascular Disease

As noted, earlier, cerebrovascular disease is the third leading cause of death in women older than

TABLE 64–1. **"Mini-Mental" State**

I. Orientation (Maximum Score 10)		
"What is the _____ ?"	Date	(1)
	Month	(1)
	Day	(1)
	Season	(1)
	Year	(1)
"What is the name of this hospital?"	Hospital	(1)
"What floor are we on?"	Floor	(1)
"What town (or city) are we in?"	Town/city	(1)
"What county are we in?"	County	(1)
"What state are we in?"	State	(1)

II. Registration (Maximum Score 3)

Say "ball," "flag," "tree" clearly and slowly, about one second for each. After you have said all three words, ask the patient to repeat them. This determines the score (1–3). Keep repeating them (up to six trials) until the patient can repeat all three words. If all three are not learned, recall cannot be meaningfully tested.	Ball	(1)
	Flag	(1)
	Tree	(1)

III. Attention and Calculation (Maximum Score 5)

Ask the patient to begin at 100 and count backward by 7, stopping after five subtractions. Score one point for each. *Or*, if the patient cannot or will not perform this task, ask her to spell the word "world" backward (D,L,R,O,W).	"93" or "D"	(1)
	"86" or "L"	(1)
	"79" or "R"	(1)
The score is one point for each correctly placed letter.	"72" or "O"	(1)
	"65" or "W"	(1)

_____ (5)

    D   L   R   O   W

IV. Recall (Maximum Score 3)

Ask the patient to recall the three words you previously asked her to remember:	"ball"	(1)
	"flag"	(1)
	"tree"	(1)

V. Language (Maximum Score 9)

Naming: Show the subject a wristwatch and a pencil and ask "What is this?" Score one point for each item.	"watch"	(1)
	"pencil"	(1)
Repetition: Ask the patient to repeat, "No if's, and's, or but's."		
Score one point if correct.	Repetition	(1)
Three-stage Command: Give the subject a piece of blank paper and say, "Take the paper in your right hand, fold it in half, and put it on the floor." Score one point for each action performed correctly.	Takes in rt hand	(1)
	Folds in half	(1)
	Puts on floor	(1)
Reading: On a blank piece of paper, print the sentence "Close your eyes" in large letters. Ask the patient to read it and do what it says. Score if she actually closes her eyes.	Closes eyes	(1)
Writing: Give the patient a blank piece of paper and ask her to write a sentence. It must contain a subject and verb and make sense. Ignore grammar, spelling, and punctuation.	Writes sentence	(1)
Copying: On a clean piece of paper, draw intersecting pentagons, each side about 1 inch, and ask the patient to copy it exactly as it is. All 10 angles must be present, and 2 must intersect to score 1 point.	Draws pentagons	(1)
	Total score	(30)

Adapted with permission from Folstein MF, Folstein ME, McHugh PR. "Mini-mental state": A practical method for grading the cognitive state of patients for the clinician. J Psychiatr Res 1975;12:189, Elsevier Science Ltd., Pergamon Imprint, Oxford, England.

75 years and the proportion of strokes as a cause of death in women rises with advancing age, although men are at higher risk of stroke at virtually all ages. Use of aspirin for the prevention of stroke in women does not appear to have the same benefit demonstrated in men; other risk factors do not appear to differ between the sexes. Atrial fibrillation is a major risk factor in both sexes, conferring a highly significant risk of stroke that increases with age, according to the Framingham Study. Anticoagulation appears to be effective in reducing stroke risk in elderly men and women with atrial fibrillation.

Arthritis

Musculoskeletal diseases are the leading cause of functional disability in the elderly and affect more women than men. The most common form of arthritis in the elderly is osteoarthritis, which in women causes more symptoms but less disability than in men. Women have a higher prevalence of osteoarthritis of the extremities (hands, knees, ankles, and feet), compared with more common truncal (spine and hip) disease in men. The strongest risk factor for osteoarthritis is age; wear and tear appears to be the most important additional risk

---

TABLE 64–2. Geriatric Depression Scale: Forced

Yes/No Choice
1. Are you basically satisfied with your life?
2. Have you dropped any of your activities or interests?
3. Do you feel that your life is empty?
4. Do you often get bored?
5. Are you hopeful about the future?
6. Are you bothered by thoughts you can't get out of your head?
7. Are you in good spirits most of the time?
8. Are you afraid that something bad is going to happen to you?
9. Do you feel happy most of the time?
10. Do you often feel helpless?
11. Do you often get restless and fidgety?
12. Do you prefer to stay at home rather than go out and do new things?
13. Do you frequently worry about the future?
14. Do you feel you have more problems with memory than most?
15. Do you think it is wonderful to be alive now?
16. Do you often feel downhearted and blue?
17. Do you feel pretty worthless the way you are now?
18. Do you worry a lot about the past?
19. Do you find life very exciting?
20. Is it hard for you to get started on new projects?
21. Do you feel full of energy?
22. Do you feel that your situation is hopeless?
23. Do you think that most people are better off than you are?
24. Do you frequently get upset over little things?
25. Do you frequently feel like crying?
26. Do you have trouble concentrating?
27. Do you enjoy getting up in the morning?
28. Do you prefer to avoid social gatherings?
29. Is it easy for you to make decisions?
30. Is your mind as clear as it used to be?
A score of 11 has been shown to be useful in the diagnosis of depression.

Adapted with permission from Yesavage JA, Brink TL, Rose TL, et al. Development and validation of a geriatric depression scale: A preliminary report. J Psychiatr Res 1982;17:37–49, Elsevier Science Ltd., Pergamon Imprint, Oxford, England.

---

factor. In addition, obesity is an important risk factor for knee arthritis, and an inverse relationship between osteoarthritis and osteoporosis has been found in some studies. Many elderly persons have radiographic changes of osteoarthritis but remain asymptomatic. At present, treatment of such silent disease does not appear to be beneficial.

Falls

A fall is an unintentional change in position, occurring in circumstances in which normal homeostatic mechanisms should preserve stability; it represents an interaction between the individual and her environment. Approximately 35 to 50% of persons older than 65 years fall each year, usually without suffering injury. However, 5% of falls re-

sult in fractures, and 1 to 2% in hip fractures, especially in women older than 80 years, in whom the risk of this serious complication is significantly increased.

Intrinsic factors that contribute to the risk of falls include age-related physiologic changes such as decreased overall postural stability, cervical articular mechanoreceptor degeneration, basal ganglion atrophy and loss of dopaminergic neurons, and sensory changes in proprioception and vision. Disease-related risk factors include perceptual deficits, arthritis and other musculoskeletal conditions, neuromuscular diseases, and side effects of medications. Falls have multiple pathologic and etiologic factors and frequently represent an atypical presentation of an underlying disease. The risk of falls increases with increased disability.

Prevention of falls and injury includes identification of those at risk, especially those having suffered a previous fall. Identified predisposing factors include use of sedative-hypnotic medications, cognitive impairment, lower extremity disability, balance and gait abnormalities, and foot problems. Interventions include treatment of diseases that increase risk and referral to physical therapy for rehabilitation, gait training, muscle-strengthening exercises, and possible use of assistive devices. Identification of extrinsic or environmental risk factors may be facilitated by a home visit. The overall goal is to minimize risk while preserving activity and improving function. In general, use of restraints has not been shown to decrease the risk of falls.

Dementia

In the past 10 to 15 years, physicians have learned that senility (loss of cognitive function) is not a component of normal aging but is in fact a symptom of an underlying disease. Loss of intellectual capacity severe enough to interfere with social or occupational functioning in a mature adult constitutes a dementia, which usually develops gradually, is progressive, and occurs in persons with appropriate social skills. The most common form is senile dementia of the Alzheimer type, which appears to have a prevalence of 10% in persons older than 65 and nearly 50% in those older than 85 years, according to one study. This dementia has a major impact on elderly women, who constitute nearly two thirds of the population older than 85 years; in addition, some studies demonstrate a higher age-adjusted prevalence in women. Data from the Framingham Heart Study found a prevalence of moderate to severe dementia of 48.2 per 1000 for women and 30.5 per 1000 for men; prevalence of Alzheimer-type dementia was

30.1 per 1000 for women and 11.7 per 1000 for men and increased significantly with advancing age. The female to male ratio for the cohort older than 75 years was 1.8 for all causes of dementia and 2.8 for probable Alzheimer-type dementia.

The *Diagnostic and Statistical Manual of Mental Disorders*, fourth edition, has revised the criteria for the diagnosis of dementia from a single category to three major categories: dementia of the Alzheimer's type, vascular dementia, and dementia due to other general medical conditions. These categories share the following criteria:

A. Memory impairment
B. Impairment of at least one of the following:
   1. Aphasia
   2. Apraxia
   3. Agnosia
   4. Executive functioning (organizing, abstracting)
C. Significant interference with work or social activities and significant decline from previous level of functioning
D. Not occurring only in the course of delirium

A number of conditions can cause reversible or potentially reversible cognitive decline or chronic confusion, including myxedema, normal-pressure hydrocephalus, Korsakoff's psychosis, vitamin B_{12} deficiency, intracranial masses, and central nervous system syphilis. The so-called pseudodementia of severe depression is a common, treatable cause of cognitive impairment; however, persons with dementia can also be depressed, especially if they have insight into their condition. Chronic alcoholism has also been associated with the development of a dementing illness.

The most common irreversible primary brain disease is Alzheimer's disease, which constitutes 60 to 70% of all cases of dementia and is a leading cause of death among elderly persons in the United States. This dementia often occurs in people who are otherwise initially normal and progresses relentlessly, with deterioration of intellect, speech, memory, and judgment. Death usually occurs within 5 to 10 years, although some studies have documented survival of as long as 15 years. The second most common cause of dementia is multi-infarct dementia, due to multiple occlusions of small cerebral arteries over a wide area, usually related to hypertension, arteriosclerotic cardiovascular disease, or diabetes and generally accompanied by other evidence of arterial disease such as small strokes. This dementia, which is more common in men than women, progresses slowly in a sporadic stepwise fashion and often causes dysarthria, an abnormal gait, and other focal neurologic abnormalities. Unusual causes of irreversible dementia include Pick's disease, Huntington's chorea, and Creutzfeldt-Jakob syndrome.

Systematic multidisciplinary evaluation of 300 elderly persons presenting with cognitive impairment was conducted by Larson's group at the University of Washington. Most treatable diagnoses were at least suspected on the basis of the history and physical examination. Persons with treatable disorders were younger, had significantly shorter duration of symptoms and less severe mental status deficits, and were receiving more drug therapy. The investigators concluded that few dementias were completely reversible; the most common treatable conditions were drug toxicity, depression, and metabolic disturbances; and important medical or psychiatric comorbidity was frequently identified. Improvement (but not total reversal) of symptoms was noted after treating coexisting medical, psychiatric, or pharmacologic disorders. Analysis of the components of the diagnostic evaluation resulted in suggestions for a limited number of diagnostic tests (complete blood count and determinations of glucose, electrolytes, calcium, creatinine, and thyroid-stimulating hormone), and the recommendation that other tests, including brain imaging with computed tomography or magnetic resonance imaging, should be ordered selectively based on the results of history and physical examination.

Larson has pointed out the need to identify treatable conditions causing or aggravating dementia rather than to continue the overemphasis on potentially curable dementia. The risk of other undetected, treatable diseases (comorbidity) in demented elderly individuals is high because of the inability to provide an accurate history of symptoms, social isolation, atypical presentations, and multiple illnesses associated with increased age. Undiagnosed chronic and acute medical illness is present in as many as two thirds of demented patients and in at least one half contributes to cognitive dysfunction. Expectation of cure or total reversibility is probably unrealistic. Useful diagnostic strategies include an open-minded, carefully conducted history and physical and neuropsychiatric evaluation, a nondrug trial, and selective tests based on clinical judgment, because multiple diagnostic tests may lead to incidental and false positive results.

Goals of treatment by the physician and other care providers include maintenance of a patient's social and functional skills and provision of effective support and care for the caregiver. It may be helpful to meet with the caregiver separately and acknowledge her burden. Medical problems (comorbidity) can affect cognition and function and may also be a source of anxiety and stress for the caregiver. The physician's important role in health maintenance consists of frequent observation and an organized medical evaluation during regularly scheduled office visits, which also provide opportunities to monitor the status of the caregiver's support. In addition to a physical examination, special attention is needed to assess a patient's functional status, mental status, vision, and hearing. Immunization against pneumonia, influenza, and tetanus should be current, and a baseline tuberculin skin test should be performed. Selected laboratory studies should be based on clinical indications, and use of screening tests should be selected on the basis of likelihood of benefit (Table 64–3).

Primary care of older women with dementia also includes appropriate referrals to community services, including the Alzheimer's Association and its support groups, an excellent source of information and help for families. Special daycare programs provide caregiver respite as well as appropriate social and cognitive activity for patients. Many communities have institutional respite programs available for short-term care, to allow for family vacations and other needs. Local agencies on aging, councils on aging, and Alzheimer's association groups may be contacted for information about other services available in the community.

The 1987 National Institutes of Health Consensus Conference on the Differential Diagnosis of Dementing Disease recommended that medical emphasis should be on

1. Diagnosis and treatment of coexisting medical and psychiatric conditions
2. Special concern for medications and toxicity
3. Preservation of function
4. Good preventive care—immunizations, nutrition
5. Attention to the support system—especially caregiver needs and stress
6. Attention to advance directives for medical treatment

These simple principles provide excellent guidance for the care of older women afflicted with dementia, as well as for many others with chronic disabling diseases.

Adverse Drug Reactions and Iatrogenesis

Although the elderly constitute only 12% of the U.S. population, they consume more than 25% of prescription medications. Some studies show that adverse drug reactions are not only more common in older persons but may also differ according to gender. Exclusion of women and elderly subjects from most drug trials has seriously limited the data available for consideration when prescribing medications for older women. The risk of adverse drug reactions appears to be dependent on the number of medications taken rather than on age alone. Other risk factors include the number and severity

---

TABLE 64–3 Diagnostic Evaluation of Suspected Dementia

Evaluation for All Patients:

History	Medications
	Alcohol use
	Functional status
	Onset and progression of illness
Physical examination	Active medical problems
	Neurologic examination
	Mental status
	Affect
Laboratory studies	Complete blood count
	Electrolytes
	Renal function
	Calcium, phosphorus
	Thyroid-stimulating hormone
	Vitamin B_{12}, folate
	Venereal Disease Research Laboratories (VDRL) or rapid plasma reagin (RPR)

Evaluation for Specific Condition:

Human immunodeficiency virus	Risk based on history
Cerebrospinal fluid analysis	If focal findings
Erythrocyte sedimentation rate	Based on physical findings
Electroencephalogram	If focal findings or history of seizures
Computed tomography/magnetic resonance imaging	If focal findings
Neuropsychological testing	Uncertain diagnosis

of illnesses, which increase the use of medications and may cause altered responses to drug therapy. Most studies have surveyed hospital admissions or inpatient populations, and few data are available on adverse drug reactions in outpatients.

Important physiologic changes occur with increasing age, resulting in alterations in pharmacokinetics and pharmacodynamics. Diminished reserves, secondary to disease or physiologic decline, result in a decreased ability to tolerate stress and to respond to medications appropriately. Deficits in memory, sensation, and function may impair the ability to comply with complex schedules. Increased prevalence of disease results in the need for more diagnostic and therapeutic interventions. Atypical or unusual presentations of many diseases may result in more extensive evaluations to obtain a diagnosis. Finally, physicians (and other health care providers) are often unaware of the foregoing factors and thus prescribe and treat elderly women in an inappropriate manner.

Elderly women absorb orally administered drugs appropriately but may have altered distribution and clearance of medications due to physiologic changes that occur as a result of aging. Body composition may be altered, resulting in decreased body water, decreased muscle mass, and increased body fat. In addition, elderly women have a larger proportion of body fat than elderly men, potentially resulting in an increased half-life of lipid-soluble drugs. For example, some benzodiazepines appear to have an increased half-life, and thus prolonged activity, in elderly women. Other studies have also suggested that women may have decreased protein binding and increased effects of certain drugs. In elderly persons of both sexes, hepatic blood flow may be reduced, and hepatic enzyme activity involved in phase I metabolism (oxidation or reduction by the cytochrome P-450 system) may be diminished. Renal blood flow and glomerular filtration frequently decline, and creatinine clearance is decreased, but this may not be reflected by the serum creatinine level because creatinine production is also decreased with age.

Pharmacodynamics, which depend on drug action at the receptor site, may also be altered in the elderly, although this effect has not generally been well studied. β-Receptors have been shown to be less responsive in the elderly, and it is possible that central nervous system receptors may be more sensitive, especially in patients with dementia.

Adverse drug reactions include idiosyncratic and allergic reactions (which do not appear to be more frequent in the elderly), toxicity, and side effects. Polypharmacy increases the risk of individual adverse reactions and the likelihood of drug-drug interactions. Prescribing errors, such as

incorrect dosages, are more likely to occur, and patients themselves have more difficulty with compliance if multiple drugs are prescribed and regimens are complex. Illnesses that appear to increase the risk of adverse drug reactions include sensory loss, cognitive dysfunction, and diseases of the kidneys, liver, and heart. Risk also depends on the specific medication being used; within certain classes of drugs, some medications have been found to be more appropriate for use in the elderly. Physicians need to be aware of those drugs likely to cause problems in elderly women. General guidelines for use of medications include the following:

1. Obtain a thorough medication history—have the patient bring all medications to the appointment.
2. Prescribe only when necessary—consider alternatives to medications whenever possible.
3. Choose carefully, considering toxicity, drug and disease interactions, compliance, and cost.
4. Give careful instructions—verbal and written.
5. Initiate therapy one drug at a time.
6. Titrate dosage carefully.
7. Monitor effects and toxicity closely—measure levels when appropriate.
8. Stop nonessential medications.
9. Review indications for all drugs.
10. Review evidence of efficacy of all drugs.
11. Always consider drugs as a cause of morbidity and toxicity.

Sexual Dysfunction

Sexual problems are more common among elderly women than among men or younger women and primarily involve the lack of a partner. The remarriage rate for women older than 65 years is only one sixth that of men, and older men usually marry younger women. Societal stereotypes of older women as sexless have resulted in little concern for older women's sexuality, although studies show that many older women, especially those who have partners, maintain strong interest in sexual activity. The physiologic effects of menopause, including changes in the levels of sex steroids and their decreased effects on genital tissues, apparently result in slowed and diminished (but not absent) sexual response. However, the effects of chronic diseases, side effects of medications, and results of operative procedures may be even more important. Physicians may be unaware of the importance of such factors and often do not inquire about or encourage discussion of sexual activity in women with chronic disabling conditions. For example, women with cardiovascular disease appear to be counseled less frequently about sexual activity than men. Chronic obstructive pulmonary disease, with symptomatic dyspnea and use of corticosteroids, may affect the feasibility of intercourse. Diabetic women may suffer from vaginal and urinary tract infections, and symptomatic arthritis, especially of the hips, may interfere with coitus. Cancer surgery, especially mastectomy, hysterectomy, and ostomy, may lead to poor self-image and subsequent sexual dysfunction.

Physicians should encourage their older women patients to discuss their concerns about sexual activity. Treatment of atrophic vaginitis with estrogen, aggressive management of the symptoms of chronic conditions, attention to psychosocial factors, and appropriate referral for counseling all may be beneficial to older women with sexual difficulties.

MENTAL HEALTH

Alcoholism

Substance abuse in older women is underdiagnosed owing to denial by patients and families, lack of awareness by health care providers, and attribution of symptoms to advancing age. Although alcohol abuse is less common in elderly women than in elderly men, older women seem to be more susceptible to the toxic effects of alcohol at the same consumption level and thus may be at higher risk of complications. Women are less likely to be identified as abusers than men and in some studies have been shown to be more likely to abuse prescription drugs (benzodiazepines) than alcohol. As cohorts of women with higher alcohol consumption grow older, the prevalence of alcoholism in elderly women is likely to increase.

Elderly alcoholic patients are more likely to be found among those presenting for medical and psychiatric care, and efforts at case finding will be more productive among those populations. Clinicians who combine a reasonable index of suspicion, use of psychosocial screening instruments, careful examination for symptoms and signs of chemical dependence, and evaluation of biochemical markers may be better able to diagnose substance abuse and refer their patients to appropriate treatment.

Treatment of chronic alcoholism can result in long-term improvement (abstinence for more than 1 year) in approximately 25% of all alcoholic persons. The recommended approach includes nonjudgmental confrontation and detoxification, fol-

lowed by intense inpatient or outpatient educational and therapeutic experiences, including introduction into Alcoholics Anonymous. Elderly women should have recovery rates at least equal to those of the general population, once they are brought into treatment.

Depression

The most common mental disorder in older women, depression may be difficult to diagnose and may also result in greater alcohol consumption. Depression may be mistaken for dementia and may be exacerbated by medications such as central nervous system depressants and medical illness such as hypothyroidism, malignancy, stroke, and other diseases of the central nervous system. Depression may present with physical complaints, and its symptoms may be accepted by elderly women as a normal manifestation of aging. Older women generally respond to treatment, but administration of antidepressant medications may cause side effects, especially if drugs with significant anticholinergic properties are used. Careful prescribing of the least toxic medications, in low doses, with careful follow-up, is necessary.

SUMMARY

Appropriate care of elderly women requires attention to many aspects of health, including some not traditionally considered in the patient-physician encounter. The distinction between physical, mental, and social aspects of health becomes less clear, requiring an open-minded approach to assessment and consideration of any intervention that will improve an elderly woman's well-being and quality of life.

REFERENCES

Applegate WB. Use of assessment instruments in clinical settings. J Am Geriatr Soc 1987;35:45.

Bachman DL, Wolf PA, Linn R, et al. Prevalence of dementia and probable senile dementia of the Alzheimer type in the Framingham Study. Neurology 1992;42:115.

Barnett HJ. Stroke in women. Can J Cardiol 1990;6:11B.

Barry PP. The demented elderly patient: Evaluation and management. J Fla Med Assoc 1991;78:767.

Barry PP. Chemical dependency in the elderly. In: Hazzard WR, Andres R, Bierman EL, Blass JP (eds). Principles of Geriatrics and Gerontology. 3rd ed. New York: McGraw-Hill, 1993.

Barry PP, Ibarra M. Multidimensional assessment of the elderly. Hosp Pract 1990;15:117.

Boring CC, Squires TS, Tong T. Cancer statistics, 1992. CA Cancer J Clin 1992;42:19.

Clarfield AR. The reversible dementias: Do they reverse? Ann Intern Med 1988;109:476.

Consensus Conference: Differential diagnosis of dementing diseases. JAMA 1987;258:3411.

Consensus Development Panel—Solomon D (Chairman). National Institutes of Health Consensus Development Conference Statement: Geriatric assessment methods for clinical decision-making. J Am Geriatr Soc 1988;36:3422.

Council on Scientific Affairs (AMA). Elder abuse and neglect. JAMA 1987;257:966.

Davis MA. Epidemiology of osteoarthritis. Clin Geriatr Med 1988;4:241.

Ferguson MK, Skoskey C, Hoffman PC, Golomb HM. Sex-associated differences in presentation and survival in patients with lung cancer. J Clin Oncol 1990;8:1402.

Folstein MF, Folstein ME, McHugh PR. "Mini-mental state": A practical method for grading the cognitive state of patients for the clinician. J Psychiatr Res 1975;12:189.

Ganz PA. Age and gender as factors in cancer therapy. Clin Geriatr Med 1993;9:145.

Greenblatt DJ, Sellers EM, Shader RI. Drug disposition in old age. N Engl J Med 1982;306:1081.

Gurwitz JH, Avorn J. The ambiguous relation between aging and adverse drug reactions. Ann Intern Med 1991;114:956.

Health and Public Policy Committee, American College of Physicians. Comprehensive functional assessment for elderly persons. Ann Intern Med 1988;109:70.

Itri L. Women and lung cancer. Women's Health. Public Health Rep 1987;(Suppl):92.

Jarvik L, Winograd C (eds). Treatments for the Alzheimer Patient. New York: Springer, 1988.

Kase CS. Epidemiology of multi-infarct dementia. Alzheimer Dis Assoc Disord 1991;5(2):71.

Larson EB, Lo B, Williams ME. Evaluation and care of patients with dementia. J Gen Intern Med 1986;1:116.

Lew EA, Garfinkel L. Mortality at ages 75 and older in the Cancer Prevention Study (CPS I). CA Cancer J Clin 1990;40:210.

Maletta G. Management of behavior problems in elderly patients with Alzheimer's disease and other dementias. Clin Geriatr Med 1988;4:719.

Mooradian AD, Grieff V. Sexuality in older women. Arch Intern Med 1990;150:1033.

O'Malley TA, Everitt DE, O'Malley HC, Campion EW. Identifying and preventing family-mediated abuse and neglect of elderly persons. Ann Intern Med 1983;98:998.

Rubenstein LZ, Robbins AS, Schulman BL, et al. Falls and instability in the elderly. J Am Geriatr Soc 1988;36:266.

Tinetti ME, Speechley M. Prevention of falls among the elderly. N Engl J Med 1989;320:1055.

Wolf PA, Abbott RD, Kannel WB. Atrial fibrillation: A major contributor to stroke in the elderly. Arch Intern Med 1987;147:1561.

Yesavage JA, Brink TL, Rose TL, et al. Development and validation of a geriatric depression scale: A preliminary report. J Psychiatr Res 1982;17:37.

PSYCHOSOCIAL ISSUES
Addiction

65

Smoking Cessation

Karen M. Freund

Women have taken up smoking in large numbers since the 1940s, and the effects of this habit on the health of women are now evident. Coronary artery disease is the number one cause of death in women, and one half of all coronary events are attributable to cigarette smoking.[1] Lung cancer is the most common cause of cancer death in women, and 80% of cases are attributable to smoking.[2] A number of other important common problems in women, including obstructive pulmonary disease; cancers of the cervix, lung, and oropharynx; peptic ulcer disease; osteoporosis; premature menopause; and wrinkling of the skin, are also increased in women who smoke.[2–6]

The delay in the prevalence of cigarette smoking among American women compared with that among men reflected the social taboos of smoking in public for women. At the turn of the century, only educated women and women who were social leaders commonly smoked. There are few reliable estimates of the prevalence of smoking in women before 1934.[7] With the onset of World War II and a generation of younger, primarily urban women entering the work force, the smoking rate increased to 18.1% of women in 1935, 24.5% of women in 1955, and it peaked at 33.3% in 1965. The concerns about health and smoking resulted in fewer women taking up the habit after that time. Currently, about one in four adult women smoke, or about 21.6 million women.[8]

Although men have always outnumbered women smokers, it is a disturbing fact that adolescent girls now make up the largest group of new smokers, with 27% of all female high school students reporting current cigarette use.[9] Cigarette ad-

vertising has been effective in specifically targeting minors and especially minor girls, portraying smoking peers as happy, slim, physically active, and attractive to their male peers. The specific targeting of female minors by the tobacco industry has been criticized by the U.S. Surgeon General and other public health advocates.[10]

This chapter outlines current knowledge of the pharamacology of smoking addiction and withdrawal and of smoking cessation patterns in women. Based on the knowledge of how women succeed in quitting, the chapter focuses on the physician's role in counseling on smoking cessation. It also reviews pharamacologic aids used in smoking cessaton as well as nonpharmacologic approaches to stopping smoking.

DO WOMEN HAVE A HARDER TIME QUITTING?

The general perception prevails that women have a more difficult time quitting smoking than men. This perception is in large part based on the conclusion of the 1980 surgeon general's report on smoking in women.[7] The report's conclusion that women have lower quit rates than men was drawn from clinical trial data and some population-based data, both of which have been criticized by some investigators.[11, 12] The clinical trial data have been criticized for their limited generalizability to the overall population. As most smokers quit on their own, participants in clinical trials often represent the most recalcitrant smokers and select groups of mainly women smokers. The population studies that concluded that women quit at lower rates than men have been criticized for their analyses, which considered pipe smokers as nonsmokers rather than as continued smokers who only switched their delivery system for nicotine. Because pipe and cigar smoking remained socially acceptable alternatives for men only, these data suggested more men had quit smoking than in fact had. Reanalysis of these population data,[12] as well as analysis of other cohort studies,[11] suggests that women and men have equal success at quitting.

THE STAGE MODEL OF SMOKING CESSATION

The stage model of smoking cessation, initially proposed by Prochaska and DiClemente,[13] is useful for providers to consider when counseling smokers to quit (Table 65–1). This model suggests that smokers go through a number of stages before they try to quit, and movement from one stage to the next indicates progress even before the patient first tries to quit on her own. The model also has stages following the actual quit date, with clinical implications on how to assist smokers beyond this point. The model begins with the precontemplator, the smoker who is not considering quitting. Before attempting to quit, this smoker goes through a phase of contemplating cessation, in which she begins to consider how she would cope with quitting and when she might try to quit. Action is the next phase, usually defined as the first 3 months after quitting, when the physical and psychological withdrawal symptoms are the most severe and the chances for relapse the greatest. Following this

acute action period comes a period of maintenance, during which time relapse is less common but continues to occur. When a smoker relapses back to regular cigarette use, she begins again at the contemplator phase before her next quit attempt.

PREDICTORS OF SMOKING CESSATION IN WOMEN

Once a woman becomes a regular smoker, a number of factors have been shown to influence the likelihood of success at a given quit attempt. Increasing age and level of education are predictors of successful quitting.[11] The most powerful predictor of quitting smoking in women is the number of cigarettes smoked, with heavy smokers of two or more packs daily having the most difficult time quitting.[11] The presence of social support is one of the most important predictors of successful quitting. Women who live with nonsmokers have an easier time quitting than those with smokers in the house.[14] Also the presence of support in terms of nonsmoking colleagues and nonsmoking areas in the workplace can be crucial in supporting a smoker trying to quit.[15] Women seem to report less concern about developing smoking-related illnesses than men; the possibility of developing such illnesses appears to be less of a motivator to quitting in women than in men.[16] This observation may be related to the fact that much of the data on detrimental health effects of smoking have been targeted toward men and diseases perceived to be diseases of men, such as lung cancer and coronary heart disease. However, several studies have shown that once a woman develops a smoking-related condition, she is more likely to try to quit smoking.[11, 17]

Weight and weight gain are cited as one of a woman's major concerns when considering quitting smoking.[18] Even as early as 1928, advertising targeted at women encouraged women to "reach for a Lucky instead of a sweet,"[7] linking cigarette smoking to slimness. Nicotine is known to increase the metabolic rate, and a physiologic effect of smoking results in a decrease in weight that is reversed when the smoker quits.[19] However, the magnitude of the effect is small, usually between 3 to 5 pounds. Other factors have been hypothesized to account for the larger gain in weight noted by a minority of quitters. These include an increase in smell and resulting increase in appetite for food and the use of food as a substitute for cigarettes when cravings occur. For all women, the health benefits of quitting smoking far outweigh

---

TABLE 65–1. Physician's Role in Counseling by Stage of Smoking

STAGE OF SMOKING*	PHYSICIAN'S ROLE AT STAGE
Precontemplation	Encourage to consider quitting
	Discuss personal health effects of smoking
Contemplation	Anticipate quit attempt problems
	Set quit date
Action	Pharmacologic aids
	Specific follow-up to discuss problems in quitting
Maintenance	Continue to address cessation for 1–2 years after quitting
Relapse	Discuss reasons for relapse
	Anticipate next quit attempt
	Set next quit date

*Data from Prochaska JO, Norcross J, DiClemente CC. Changing for Good. New York: William Morrow & Co; 1994.

the risks of weight gain. However, given the social pressure on women to be slim in our society, this issue must be addressed directly with women who are contemplating quitting smoking.

Some data suggest that women may make more attempts at quitting cigarettes and have more relapses before they successfully quit than men.[11] Most data show that the majority of smokers do not quit on their first attempt and the ultimate success at long-term cessation improves with each new quit attempt. Useful information appears to be gained about how to quit smoking, even during attempts in which relapse to smoking occurs. This fact can be of use in counseling women who are discouraged by their inability to quit after one or more attempts.

The one factor known to specifically influence minors against smoking, and to a lesser degree committed smokers, is the cost of cigarettes.[20] The recent move by several states to sharply raise the sales tax on cigarettes should provide the greatest public health benefit in the number of minors who do not start smoking as a result.

THE PHARMACOLOGY OF NICOTINE

It is useful to consider the pharmacology of nicotine, the main addictive substance in cigarette smoke. The psychoactive properties of nicotine are complex. It can act both as a stimulant, increasing one's sense of concentration, and as a relaxant during stressful times. Both these effects are described anecdotally by smokers who find that smoking helps them concentrate while working and helps them relax at other times.

The smoker with a physical addiction to nicotine is usually smoking at least 20 cigarettes, or one pack, daily. She will most often smoke within 30 minutes of awakening and will continue to smoke except during more serious illnesses. Distinguishing the addicted from the nonaddicted smoker is useful in preparing her for what to anticipate when she quits smoking and in providing suggestions for managing the anticipated withdrawal from nicotine.

The withdrawal syndrome from smoking usually begins within 3 to 4 hours after abstinence from smoking. Symptoms include cravings for cigarettes, difficulty concentrating, anxiety, irritability, increased appetite, dizziness, tightness in the chest, constipation, and sleep disturbance.[21] The syndrome usually diminishes after 2 weeks of cessation, although some researchers argue that withdrawal can extend for up to 6 weeks.[22] The psychological withdrawal and craving extend beyond

this point and are the main reasons for relapse beyond the first month.

THE PHYSICIAN'S ROLE IN SMOKING CESSATION

There are two compelling reasons for physicians to play an active role in helping women to quit. Data indicate that more than 75% of all smokers see a physician at least yearly.[23] Therefore, physicians have access to the majority of smokers. Second, there is evidence now from 40 controlled trials to indicate that brief counseling by physicians on smoking cessation is effective in helping smokers to quit.[24] This chapter describes what aspects of brief counseling have been found to be effective.

Of the current smokers, more than 80% state that they would like to quit smoking, and two thirds have tried to quit at least once.[25] It is clear, then, that the role of the provider need not be to convince the smoker of the importance of quitting but rather to become a partner in her efforts to quit.

It has been documented that efforts in counseling need not be lengthy and that even the briefest of discussions is beneficial. One controlled study showed that physicians who only advised smokers to quit at each visit led to a 1% quit rate.[26] Other studies have found that 2 to 5 minutes of counseling can result in up to 5% of smokers quitting yearly.[24] Although increasing quit rates of 1 to 5% per year seem like a modest result, the impact of this short intervention on the 21.6 million women who smoke can result in 1 million women quitting smoking over a 5-year period.

The protocol of counseling on smoking cessation can be considered in the following five steps:

1. Discuss smoking at every visit.
2. Personalize the health message to the patient.
3. Anticipate a quit attempt.
4. Ask the patient to set a quit date.
5. Provide follow-up.

DISCUSSION OF SMOKING. Part of the initial evaluation of all patients should be questioning on current smoking status. For the patient who smokes, this should be noted as a problem in her medical record and referred to at all visits. Some researchers advocate reminder systems, such as separate stickers on the front of charts of all smoking patients, to cue the physician to discuss smoking at each visit.

PERSONALIZE THE HEALTH MESSAGE. Most patients are concerned about the health effects of smoking, have heard about the detrimental effects, and want to quit. Therefore, a detailed lecture about the ill effects of smoking is not necessary and may be detrimental to the physician-patient relationship. As smoking becomes more socially unacceptable, smokers may experience shame and blame when confronted with their smoking habit. Assuming that all smokers have some interest in quitting and providing encouragement around their previous plans and efforts may be the most effective strategies in reassuring the patient that she has an ally in this process.

Despite the global knowledge of the harmful effects of smoking, many women in particular feel less personally susceptible to the hazards of cigarettes. Pointing out those aspects of the patient's examination in which the effects of smoking may be noted or areas in which the patient may be at higher risk for illness is effective. For younger women, this may include discussing decreased exercise tolerance, an episode of bronchitis, or the increased risk of early aging and wrinkling of the skin. For the woman presenting with concerns about chest pain, discussion of the immediate cardiac benefits of quitting smoking may be useful.

A special comment should be made about counseling pregnant women on quitting smoking. Educating pregnant women regarding the harmful effects on the fetus is effective, with 21% of pregnant smokers quitting during the pregnancy and another 36% cutting back on their smoking while pregnant.[27] However, the relapse rate among mothers following delivery is as high as 82%.[28] Discussion that includes the personal health benefits of quitting to the mother and the ongoing risks of parental smoking to young children in the development of bronchitis and other upper respiratory infections should be provided.

ANTICIPATE A QUIT ATTEMPT. For most smokers, anticipating quitting begins with a discussion of their previous quit attempts, because two thirds of smokers have tried quitting at least once. Opening a dialogue on what made the last attempt difficult and how the next attempt could be better supported is important. Asking the woman who has never tried to quit to anticipate her difficulties will begin the process of contemplation before quitting.

It is useful to ask patients who have tried to quit how long they were successful and what circumstances led to the relapse. The circumstances around relapse usually fall into two broad categories. The first is stressful situations, in which the calming effect of nicotine has been helpful to the person in the past. The second is an environment in which one previously smoked, such as meeting a group of friends for a drink where others are smoking. After identifying an area of difficulty with a past quit attempt, ask the patient to consider what alternatives might have been useful to avoid this situation. Women usually have ideas of what would personally help them, from finding other resources for stress reduction to avoiding social situations in which smoking is occurring in the early days and weeks of quitting.

Weight concerns with quitting should be discussed. On average, women smokers gain between 3 and 5 pounds when they quit, mainly because of changes in basal metabolic rate with the elimination of nicotine. However, given the weight consciousness of women in the United States, many find even this small gain objectionable, and this concern is best dealt with directly. For those who have used smoking as an appetite suppressant to cope with eating difficulties, greater weight gain can be anticipated, and dealing with the weight issues simultaneously may be crucial if long-term cessation is to be achieved. Having low-calorie snacks on hand during cravings and using exercise to reduce both food and nicotine cravings can be suggested. Patients who have experienced serious weight gain during past attempts to stop smoking may benefit from nutritional counseling before their quit date.

SETTING A QUIT DATE. Ask each patient who expresses interest in quitting if she wishes to set a quit date. Requesting a specific date reinforces the provider's concern about smoking and encourages the patient to begin to think concretely about her plans even if she is not yet ready to quit. Some researchers advocate writing out the anticipated quit date as a prescription or a written agreement between the patient and the physician to further reinforce the patient's commitment to quitting.[29]

A smoker should be encouraged to set a specific date to quit smoking all forms of tobacco products. The method of tapering to fewer and fewer cigarettes to quit is less effective. Most smokers absorb less than 10% of the nicotine in a cigarette. By decreasing to lower nicotine brands or fewer cigarettes, smokers often compensate by smoking cigarettes more thoroughly to maintain their nicotine level.

FOLLOW-UP. Each smoker who does choose a quit date optimally requires follow-up shortly after that time. This allows the provider to become aware of any problems she is experiencing and any slips to further cigarette use and to provide further help that may be needed. This follow-up can be a phone call or an office visit and can be handled by support staff in the office.

AIDS TO SMOKING CESSATION

Most smokers, including most women smokers, wish to and are successful at quitting on their own without the help of groups or prescription aids. However, a minority of quitters, especially those with a number of unsuccessful quit attempts, become discouraged about their ability to quit and can benefit from assistance.

The only medication approved for prescription use for smoking cessation is nicotine in alternative delivery systems. Currently nicotine is available in a polacrilex gum, or as a transdermal patch, with a nasal spray form of delivery currently under study. Because nicotine is not absorbed through the gastric mucosa, alternative delivery systems require absorption through skin or buccal or nasal mucosa. The theory behind the use of these nicotine replacement systems is to separate the habit of smoking from the withdrawal symptoms; thus, the smoker stops the habit immediately, and the nicotine is tapered through another system to minimize or eliminate the withdrawal symptoms.

The nicotine gum, which contains 2 mg of nicotine per piece, has been available for several years. Its effectiveness is dependent on the provider giving proper instructions for its use. Because the nicotine is absorbed from the buccal mucosa, the patient should be advised to "chew and park," allowing the gum to stay in contact with the side of the gums. Chewing vigorously and swallowing may lead to stomach upset from the nicotine. The patient should be advised to use the gum on a regular basis for the first week; this usually consists of 9 to 15 pieces daily for addicted smokers, with a maximum recommended 30 pieces daily. Because the gum takes 10 to 20 minutes to reach peak serum nicotine concentrations, compared with 3 to 5 minutes for a cigarette, smokers may find that the gum does not stop the urge to smoke if used on an "as needed" basis. Some studies have found that for heavy smokers 2-mg gum does not provide nicotine doses similar to that of smoking and that 4-mg gum, available in other countries and expected to be approved soon in the United States, provides better nicotine levels for heavy smokers. It is strongly recommended that patients stop cigarette smoking altogether before starting the gum; tapering the number of cigarettes smoked using the gum is an ineffective method of cessation. However, studies of individuals who both use the gum and smoke cigarettes find that nicotine levels rarely exceed baseline levels when smoking only, implying that smokers adjust both the gum and smoking to maintain steady nicotine levels.

Disadvantages of the nicotine gum are the diffi-culty in teaching and learning proper use. Many object to the taste. Also, because the gum is hard, it can cause problems with teeth or dental fillings. In addition, absorption of nicotine requires a basic medium, and because salivary pH falls after drinking coffee or carbonated beverages, the gum is ineffective for about 20 minutes after oral intake. Other side effects include hiccups, oral discomfort, heartburn, nausea, and upset stomach. There is no evidence that use of the gum exacerbates preexisting cardiac disease. One major advantage of the gum is the ability of the quitter to titrate the dose of nicotine during the day, using increased amounts at times when withdrawal symptoms are more severe. The gum is approved for use for up to 3 months. Many investigators argue for tapering use of the gum for as long as 6 months in an attempt to prevent early relapses.

Studies comparing the effectiveness of nicotine gum with that of placebo gum found fewer withdrawal symptoms and short-term improvement in cessation rates for up to 6 months with use of the nicotine gum. Data on use of gum in smoking cessation clinics have shown that the gum has a greater effect than when it is prescribed in an internist's office, with the difference being ascribed to the importance of proper counseling on the gum's use.[30] Data comparing gum use with other methods after 1 year show that the gum has little long-term benefit. This is as expected, because the goal of the gum is to assist women over the immediate withdrawal symptoms from nicotine, not to address the problem of relapse months after physical withdrawal symptoms are eliminated.

The introduction of the nicotine transdermal patch in 1992 was accompanied by an unprecedented direct marketing campaign to consumers. Its advantage over nicotine gum is ease of use. The patch is replaced on a daily basis. Produced by four different pharmaceutic firms, the patches come in two or three different strengths, with the highest dose providing serum nicotine levels similar to those from smoking two packs daily. The patch should be used in the context of overall smoking cessation counseling, in which the patient picks a quit date, stops smoking cigarettes altogether, and begins to use the patch daily. Current data suggest that the recommended time for use is 6 to 8 weeks, tapering from the highest dose patch in 2 to 5 weeks and tapering every 2 weeks thereafter. The main advantages of use are the convenience to the patient and the decreased instruction on use compared with that required with the gum. The patch also maintains a more constant serum nicotine level, which theoretically can prevent withdrawal symptoms. Another potential advantage is that levels of nicotine are maintained overnight, providing early morning protection when withdrawal symptoms are often most severe. Disadvantages of the patch include insomnia and abnormal dreams in 3 to 5%, presumably due to the overnight level of nicotine. One manufacturer has produced a 15-hour patch to be removed at bedtime to eliminate this problem, but any of the patches can be removed overnight by the minority of patients who experience sleep disturbance. The most common side effect is skin irritation from the nicotine in the patch itself, occurring in about one third of users. Rotating the patch to different sites, avoiding sun exposure at patch sites, and applying topical steroids can usually prevent the need to discontinue use for this reason.

Preliminary evidence exists on the usefulness of the patch. A number of trials have shown benefits of the patch over placebo patches for 3 to 6 months of cessation.[31] Again, the benefits over placebo are diminished at 1 year, when relapse of all successful quitters is based less on physical withdrawal symptoms than on psychological factors.

Concurrent use of the patch and gum has not been studied, but anecdotal descriptions of patients who benefitted from use of the gum above the patch have been documented. It may be advantageous for certain patients to use the patch and to chew the gum in certain stressful situations.

Neither the nicotine patch nor the nicotine gum has been approved for use in pregnancy, and both have been classified by the Food and Drug Administration as Category D (positive evidence of human fetal risk). It has been argued that one must weigh the relative hazards of smoking, with nicotine, carcinogens, and carbon monoxide, against the hazards of nicotine alone in pregnant women who smoke.[32] Nicotine itself has been implicated in birth defects, and there are no data on whether continuous low doses from the patch may be more or less harmful to the fetus than the intermittent peaks of nicotine that occur with smoking. All pregnant women who smoke should be encouraged to quit without the assistance of nicotine replacement. However, for those who smoke heavily or for those who have tried unsuccessfully to quit, nicotine replacement at the lowest dose for a brief period might be considered the lesser of two hazards.

Media reports of a cluster of myocardial infarctions in patch users have prompted a study of this issue. A review of these cases found no increased risk of myocardial infarction in patch users.[31] Studies of individuals with stable coronary artery disease have not shown an increased risk of problems. Given that smoking is a major risk factor for developing coronary artery disease, cessation using all methods available should be strongly urged for all women.

Clonidine has been studied for its potential benefit in smoking cessation. As it has been shown to

---

TABLE 65–2.   Fagerstrom's Tolerance to Nicotine Questionnaire

QUESTION	RANGE	SCORE
1. How soon after you wake up do you smoke your first cigarette?	<30 min	1
	>30 min	0
2. Do you find it difficult to refrain from smoking in places where it is forbidden (e.g., office, church, cinema)?	Yes	1
	No	0
3. Which cigarette would you hate most to give up?	First in the morning	1
	Any other	0
3. How many ciagrettes per day do you smoke?	15 or less	0
	16–25	1
	26 or more	2
5. Do you smoke more frequently during the first hours after awakening than during the rest of the day?	Yes	1
	No	0
6. Do you smoke if you are so ill that you are in bed most of the day?	Yes	1
	No	0
7. What is the nicotine level of your usual brand of cigarette?	<1.0 mg	0
	1.0–1.2 mg	1
	>1.3 mg	2
8. Do you inhale?	Never	0
	Sometimes	1
	Always	2

A score of 6 or more indicates a smoker who is strongly addicted to nicotine and likely to experience withdrawal symptoms on quitting.

Reprinted from Fagerstrom KO. Measuring degree of physical dependence to tobacco smoking with reference to individualization of treatment. Addict Behav 1978;3:235–241, copyright 1978, with kind permission from Elsevier Science Ltd, The Boulevard, Langford Lane, Kidlington 0X5 1GB, UK.

decrease withdrawal symptoms caused by other drugs, the theory is that it would eliminate nicotine withdrawal symptoms and promote cessation of smoking. Several controlled trials have not found any benefit from clonidine in quit rates, although it does appear to decrease withdrawal symptoms.[33] One study found a benefit in quit rates in women only, especially those with depressive symptoms.[34] The value of antidepressants or benzodiazepines in smoking cessation is unproven, and they should not be used.

Nicotine replacement is of greatest value among smokers most likely to have nicotine withdrawal symptoms and those unsuccessful at quitting in the past. The Fagerstrom index of addiction provides an easy means of assessing addiction (Table 65–2).[35] In general, those who smoke at least one pack daily or require a cigarette within 30 minutes of awakening are addicted smokers. Women who smoke less than this are unlikely to benefit from nicotine replacement. Most experts do not recommend pharmacologic aids for the first quit attempt, as many women making such an attempt will quit on their own.

Patients may also request advice and referral for nonpharmacologic interventions for cessation. These include support groups, behavioral therapy, and hypnosis. Controlled trials have shown that all these methods are of some benefit.[36] These adjuncts may be of greatest value to the smoker who has failed several attempts at quitting and lacks a supportive network to assist her in efforts to quit. The expense (none of these methods is covered by third-party payers) and time commitment limit the usefulness of these groups to a small number of smokers.

PROMOTING NONSMOKING IN THE OFFICE

In addition to the specific advice given to smoking patients, the physician can also promote nonsmoking in the office. Brochures with information and practical suggestions are available from many organizations (Table 65–3) and provide useful information to reinforce the message of the office visit. Physician's offices can also provide an example by becoming smoke free, not only for patients but also for all physicians and support staff. Lists of periodicals without cigarette advertising are published, and this choice of publication can be stated to patients to demonstrate support for all efforts against smoking.[37] Unfortunately, many ''women's'' magazines rely on cigarette advertising for revenue and therefore rarely have published articles discussing the health effects of

TABLE 65–3. Sources of Adjuvant Materials to Help Smokers Quit

National Cancer Institute	(800) 4CANCER
American Academy of Family Physicians	(800) 274–2237
American Cancer Society	(212) 315–8700
National Heart, Lung and Blood	(301) 951–3260
Minnesota Heart Health Program	(612) 887–9603

smoking on women.[38] Finding women's magazines that are able to forego cigarette advertising and therefore publish articles on smoking and women is beneficial.

Of all the preventive measures undertaken in office practice, none has as much potential benefit as smoking cessation counseling. All providers who care for women should determine the smoking status of their patients, advise smokers to quit, and be able to provide brief counseling on techniques of cessation.

REFERENCES

1. Willet WC, Green A, Stampfer MJ, et al. Relative and absolute excess risks of coronary heart disease among women who smoke cigarettes. N Engl J Med 1987;317:1303.
2. Report of the Surgeon General. Reducing the Health Consequences of Smoking: 25 Years of Progress. Publication CDC 90–8416. Washington, DC: US Department of Health and Human Services, 1989.
3. Freund KM, Belanger AJ, D'Agostino RB, Kannel WB. The health risks of smoking: The Framingham study. Ann Epidemiol 1993;3:417.
4. Jick H, Porter J, Morrison AS. Relation between smoking and age of natural menopause. Lancet 1977;1:1354.
5. Allen HB, Johnson BL, Diamond SM. Smokers' wrinkles. JAMA 1973;225:1067.
6. Daniell HW. Smoker's wrinkles. A study in the epidemiology of ''crow's feet.'' Ann Intern Med 1971;75:873.
7. Report of the Surgeon General. The Health Consequences of Smoking for Women. Washington, DC: US Department of Health and Human Services, 1980.
8. Centers for Disease Control. Cigarette smoking among adults—United States, 1990. MMWR 1992;41:354.
9. Centers for Disease Control. Tobacco, alcohol and other drug use among high school students—United States, 1991. MMWR 1992;41:698.
10. Broder S. Cigarette advertising and corporate responsibility. JAMA 1992;268:782.
11. Freund KM, Belanger AJ, D'Agostino RB, et al. Predictors of smoking cessation: The Framingham study. Am J Epidemiol 1992;135:957.
12. Jarvis M. Gender and smoking: Do women really find it harder to give up? Br J Addict 1984;79:383.
13. Prochaska JO, DiClemente CC. Stages and processes of self-change of smoking: Toward an integrative model of change. J Consult Clin Psychol 1983;51:390.
14. Cohen S, Lichtenstein E, Mermelstein R, et al. Social support interventions for smoking cessation. In: Gottlieb BH (ed). Marshalling Social Support: Formats, Processes and Effects. New York: Sage, 1988.
15. Sorensen G. Occupational and worksite norms and attitudes about smoking cessation. Am J Public Health 1986;76:544.

16. Sorensen G, Pechacek TF. Attitudes toward smoking cessation among men and women. J Behav Med 1987;10:129.

17. Ockene JK, Hosmer DW, Williams JW, et al. Factors related to patient smoking status. Am J Public Health 1987;77:356.

18. Piric PL, McBride CM, Hellerstedt W, et al. Smoking cessation in women concerned about weight. Am J Public Health 1992;82:1238.

19. Perkins KA, Epstein LH, Marks BL, et al. The effect of nicotine on energy expenditure during light physical activity. N Engl J Med 1989;320:898.

20. Warner KE. Smoking and health implications of a change in the federal cigarette excise tax. JAMA 1986;255:1028.

21. Cummings KM, Giovino G, Jaen CR, Emrich LJ. Reports of smoking withdrawal symptoms over a 21 day period of abstinence. Addict Behav 1985;10:373.

22. Cummings KM, Jaen CR, Giovino G. Circumstances surrounding relapse in a group of recent exsmokers. Prev Med 1985:14:195.

23. Report of the Surgeon General. Nicotine Addiction. Publication No. CDC 88–8406. Washington, DC: US Department of Health and Human Services, 1988.

24. Kottle TE, Battista, RN, DeFriese GH, Brekke ML. Attributes of successful smoking cessation interventions in medical practice. JAMA 1988;259:2882.

25. US Department of Health and Human Services. Tobacco Use in 1986. Methods and Basic Tabulations from Adult Use of Tobacco Survey. Publication No. 90–2004. Washington, DC: US Department of Health and Human Services, Public Health Service, CDC, 1990.

26. Russell MA, Wilson C, Taylor C, Baker CD. Effect of general practitioners' advice against smoking. BMJ 1979;2:231.

27. National Center for Health Statistics, Schoenborn CA. Health promotion and disease prevention: United States, 1985. In: Vital and Health Statistics, 1988, Series 10, no. 163. DHHS Publication No. (PHS) 88–1591. Rockville, Md.

28. Harris JE. Smoking during pregnancy: Preliminary results from the National Clearinghouse on Smoking and Health, 1975 prevalence data. September 1979.

29. Cummings SR, Coates TJ, Richard RJ, et al. Training physicians in counseling about smoking cessation. Ann Intern Med 1989;110:640.

30. Lam W, Sze PC, Sacks HS, Chalmers TC. Meta-analysis of randomized controlled trials of nicotine chewing gum. Lancet 1987;2:27.

31. Fiore MC, Jorenby DR, Baker TB, Kenford SL. Tobacco dependence and the nicotine patch. Clinical guidelines for effective use. JAMA 1992;268:2687.

32. Benowitz NL. Nicotine replacement therapy during pregnancy. JAMA 1991;266:3174.

33. Prochazka AV, Petty TL, Nett L, et al. Transdermal clonidine reduced some withdrawal symptoms but did not increase smoking cessation. Arch Intern Med 1992; 152:2065.

34. Glassman AH, Stetner F, Walsh BT, et al. Heavy smokers, smoking cessation, and clonidine: Results of a double-blind, randomized trial. JAMA 1988;259:2863.

35. Fagerstrom KO. Measuring degree of physical dependence to tobacco smoking with reference to individualization of treatment. Addict Behav 1978;3:235.

36. Fiore MC, Novotny TE, Pierce JP, et al. Methods used to quit smoking in the United States: Do cessation programs help? JAMA 1990;263:2760.

37. Magazines without tobacco advertising (news). JAMA 1991;266:3099.

38. Warner KE, Goldenhar LM, McLaughlin CG. Cigarette advertising and magazine coverage of the hazards of smoking. A statistical analysis. N Engl J Med 1992;326:305.

Alcohol and Substance Abuse

Booker Bush

The abuse of alcohol, cocaine, sedatives, and heroin has been increasing among women over the past 2 decades. Women now experience problems with all of these substances both as bystanders and as addicts themselves. Although the physical effects produced by the use of these substances are similar in both men and women, the symptoms, signs, and treatment can differ in a number of ways.

Although cocaine, sedative, and narcotic abuse are major problems for women, alcohol still remains the major addiction. The amount of information concerning alcohol and women is large and still growing. Much of the literature on cocaine and sedative abuse in women is descriptive. Specific studies are hindered by the fact that many women are polysubstance abusers: Cocaine is used in combination with sedatives (alternating the stimulatory mood swing with a depressant mood swing), and alcohol may be combined with benzodiazepines.

Medical providers frequently need to help their patients determine whether use of alcohol or other substances represents merely "social" use or has become abuse. Medical texts and training reveal the medical and social consequences of alcohol ingestion; recent literature has assessed possible "healthy" aspects of moderate alcohol use, such as a reduction in cardiovascular risk. All providers should be able to help their patients determine when alcohol use is safe, the dangers of cocaine and benzodiazepine abuse, what constitutes abuse of alcohol or another substance, and the physiologic changes that alcohol may cause in women. Strategies for further evaluation and treatment recommendations for women who abuse or are dependent on alcohol and other substances are other considerations.

ALCOHOL ABUSE

It is estimated that 6 million American women have an alcohol disorder.[1, 2] Younger women are more likely to drink and to be heavy drinkers than older women. Trends in the data suggest that the differences between men and women in terms of alcohol and drug abuse behaviors are shrinking. Although drinking patterns in the general population have not changed from 1965 through 1990, the number of younger women who are heavy drinkers (defined as more than five drinks per day) has increased. Earlier studies suggested large differences in alcohol use in women from different cultural and ethnic groups. More recent research has suggested that Hispanic women entering new social and work arenas are displaying drinking patterns similar to those of white women. African American women drink in equal proportion to white women but report fewer alcohol-related personal and social problems than white women. A greater proportion of African American women, however, experience alcohol-related health problems.

ALCOHOL-RELATED MORBIDITY

Women are subject to all the illnesses from alcohol that affect men. Cirrhosis, pancreatitis, gastritis, cardiomyopathy, and neurologic diseases, both central and peripheral, can occur. One major difference in women is that these physiologic disorders may occur at a much younger age and after a briefer drinking history than those seen with men. This brief or "telescopic"[1] history of alcohol-related problems may be due to higher blood alcohol levels in women than in men who have ingested similar amounts of alcohol or a reduced threshold for the development of alcohol-induced injury. Women have lower levels of alcohol dehydrogenase in their gastric mucosa than men, which allows more alcohol to pass unmetabolized into the circulation.[3] Also, because the volume of distribution of alcohol is in water, and because women have a higher ratio of fat to water, they develop higher serum alcohol levels than men.

ALCOHOL AND HORMONAL CHANGES

Although it is well understood that alcohol is a direct gonadal toxin in men, there has been little research until recently on the effects of alcohol on female gonadal function. Because alcohol inhibits testosterone biosynthesis by a direct toxic effect on the testes, testicular atrophy, low testosterone levels, gynecomastia, impotence, and diminished sexual interest occurs in some alcoholic men. The effect of alcohol on hypothalamic and pituitary function in men is controversial and is only beginning to be studied in women.[4]

In women studied on a metabolic ward, 60% of heavy drinkers (seven to eight drinks per day on average in this study) and 50% of "social" drinkers who consumed more than three drinks per day had significant derangements of the menstrual cycle. A few of these women developed hyperprolactinemia, and others had delayed ovulation and anovulatory cycles. These menstrual cycle disorders appear to be dependent on alcohol dose. There was no evidence of menstrual cycle dysfunction or abnormal hormone levels in occasional drinkers or in women who consumed less than an average of three drinks per day.

Alcohol may have either stimulatory or suppressive effects on pituitary and gonadal hormones, depending on the duration of alcohol administration (acute vs. chronic) and the status of gonadotropin stimulation. This is a complex problem, and it is difficult at present to describe a clear mechanism to explain why alcohol intoxication or intake induces derangements of the menstrual cycle.

ALCOHOL AND PREGNANCY

Although there are adverse effects of alcohol on menstrual cycle function, chronically alcoholic women do become pregnant and their children may be afflicted with physical abnormalities, abnormal brain function, and pre-and postnatal retardation of growth and development.[5]

Because alcohol freely diffuses across the placental barrier, the fetus is exposed to the same dose of alcohol as the mother. It remains unclear what the range of doses of alcohol are that cause the fetal alcohol syndrome. It is also unclear whether the fetal abnormalities in the syndrome are due to the direct toxic effect of alcohol on the developing fetus or are secondary to hormonal, vascular, or structural changes that occur to the mother from alcohol (or other substances such as marijuana or cocaine) ingested during the pregnancy.

ALCOHOL AND THE MENOPAUSE

In postmenopausal women, alcohol appears to cause a mild increase in serum estradiol concentrations.[6] This may be secondary to alcohol's stimulatory effect on the adrenal gland to produce both estrone and estradiol along with an increase in the conversion of androgens to estrogens. Alcohol, when it causes liver disease, also may cause an elevation in the level of serum estrogens because of a decrease in hepatic metabolism. It is unclear whether this mild increase in estrogen levels is of any biologic or psychological value to normal postmenopausal women. Although the benefit from alcohol on cardiovascular disease in women may be secondary to an increase in estrogen as well as beneficial effects on high-density lipoprotein cholesterol, it is unclear whether moderate alcohol consumption is associated with positive changes in bone density or with reducing the risk of breast or endometrial cancer. Indeed, there are case-control studies to suggest that alcohol increases the risk of breast cancer and osteoporosis in women.

DIAGNOSIS

Addiction is a special case of dependence. It is a compulsive use of a substance and an inability to control intake despite negative consequences. The life of the addicted person revolves around obtaining, using, and recovering from the effects of the substance despite medical complications, failure in life roles, or interpersonal difficulties. Drugs produce addiction in the setting of individual vulnerability (genetics, development, preexisting psychiatric disorders, and stress) and sociocultural factors (drug availability, peer and family pressure).

The *Diagnostic Manual of Statistical and Psychiatric Disorders* (3rd ed.), or DSM-III, offers the gold standard criteria for the diagnosis of alcohol abuse or dependence. Many treatment specialists find it useful to consider four parameters when considering the diagnosis of alcoholism.[7] It is also important to diagnose problem drinking as well as alcohol dependence because problem drinking may respond better to simple interventions.

Chronic Use of Large Quantities of Alcohol

Although the National Council on Alcoholism and the DSM-III both agree that alcoholism exists when a 70-kg person drinks more than a *fifth of hard liquor (approximately 17–20 drinks) per day* for a prolonged period of time, this definition is not helpful in assessing alcohol use in women. A similar dose of alcohol in women will lead to higher blood alcohol levels than in a similar-sized man. Levels of intake considered safe for men can be unsafe for women. (There is less agreement about what level of alcohol intake suggests abuse.) Most would consider a patient's report of drinking "a pint or more" when drinking (roughly equivalent to nine drinks) a problem even in the absence of other symptoms. Consumption of more than *four drinks per day* is cause for concern.

Physiologic Changes Related to Alcohol Use

Tolerance is an early sign of alcohol abuse. Tolerance means that the patient appears to be sober even though she may have an intoxicating level of alcohol in her blood stream. Tolerance is not an improved ability to metabolize alcohol, only an adaptation of the neurologic system to appear to function normally despite intoxicating levels of alcohol.

Blackouts are short-term memory deficits that occur while drinking. Women who cannot remember how they got home after drinking or incidents that occurred while drinking are suffering blackouts. There is no actual loss of consciousness or effect on long-term memory; indeed, the patient might function quite normally during a blackout.

Sleep disturbance occurs after heavy drinking because alcohol, like other sedative drugs, can disrupt rapid eye movement (REM) sleep. People report falling asleep easily but awakening at 2:00 or 3:00 A.M., tossing and turning, and then usually falling asleep. Needless to say, taking another drink at the time of the arousal also induces sleep. This sleep disturbance does not represent alcohol withdrawal; however, that syndrome also prompts arousal due to an increase in autonomic discharge.

Peptic symptoms occur that are due to gastric acid secretion stimulated by alcohol, along with dissolution of the gastric mucosal barrier, which is also prompted by alcohol.

High blood pressure and hypertension are direct results of alcohol use. There is a direct correlation between alcohol intake and elevation in blood pressure. Six to 8 weeks after cessation of alcohol use, blood pressure will fall.

Tremor and delirium tremens occur, and the latter is diagnostic of alcohol dependence. Tremor is also evidence of alcohol withdrawal and can be reversed with alcohol or benzodiazepines.

Chronic Loss of Control of Alcohol

The essence of an addiction or a problem with drinking is loss of control. Women may report a number of episodes of quitting drinking or multiple attempts to "cut down" on their alcohol use. It is never part of social drinking to use alcohol before going to a party or to "get in the mood." Drinking quickly to get an alcohol effect would also be evidence of trouble. Craving is a classic symptom of addiction; however, it is rare for a person to report this symptom until they are in recovery. In the same sense, drinking alone is a well-known attribute of alcohol abuse in women, and many women are unlikely to report it.

Social or Physical Damage Resulting from Alcohol Abuse

The clinician should try to make a diagnosis of alcohol abuse before damage occurs. Unfortunately, the majority of problems come to attention late in the course of the problem.

Family losses occur early with alcohol use. Separation, divorce, loss of children, or estrangement from parents can all be the result of an addiction.

Job loss may also occur because of alcohol. Asking about performance at work and relationships with peers, supervisors, and others can be helpful in making a diagnosis.

The rate of success of an intervention for alcohol abuse is dependent on the existence of a family and a job. Patients without work or family have a much lower rate of response to treatment, which indicates that early intervention is important.

Trauma formerly referred to falls, automobile accidents, and other physical incidents that occur because of alcohol abuse. However, for women, trauma can also mean physical abuse from companions or family, and the association with alcohol is high. Evaluation of a woman who has been physically or sexually abused should always include a history of alcohol and substance abuse.

Psychiatric disorders such as depression, bipolar disorder, panic disorder, and other character disorders can be mimicked and "treated" with alcohol and other drugs of abuse. *Dual diagnosis,* or the coexistence of an addictive disorder along with a primary psychiatric disorder is more frequent in women. A primary psychiatric disorder can be diagnosed only after a patient has been evaluated after being free of alcohol for at least 3 months. The clinician should be careful about making a primary psychiatric or dual diagnosis early in a patient's evaluation.

Cirrhosis, pancreatitis, cardiomyopathy, and *organic dementias* are well-known consequences of alcohol abuse, and their existence requires the diagnosis of alcohol dependence. These topics are better covered elsewhere, but it is important to recognize that these complications can occur much earlier in the patient's drinking history in women than in men. However, the relatively poor prognosis for treatment when these complications occur is similar in both men and women.

DRUG ABUSE

More than 5 million Americans have used heroin at least once.[8] Opiate use has increased at a greater rate among women than men, and a greater proportion of women abuse barbiturates, sedatives, and amphetamines.[9] Before the 1970s, drug abuse among women was relatively infrequent, with women accounting for less than 20% of addicts. Currently 25 to 30% of addicts are women.[9] Among adolescents, there are fewer gender-related differences in illicit drug use. Younger addicts are more likely to experiment with a wider range of drugs before heroin use and are more often multiple concurrent drug abusers. Women are more frequently initiated into drug use by a male companion, often in the context of an intimate relationship. In addition, women's spouses or common-law partners are more likely to have been daily narcotic users. This pattern is uncommon in men.

Women initiate drug use for more diverse reasons than men, including curiosity, relief for a crisis situation, relief of physical pain (generally for older women), and pleasure. The mean age of first narcotic use for women averages 19 to 20. Women are more frequently on welfare or disability and are less likely to be employed than men. Women use more nonnarcotic drugs than men but less marijuana and alcohol. Other patterns around drug use also differ by gender. Women tend to be less involved in criminal activity, are less likely to be incarcerated, and are less frequently involved in dealing drugs.[9] Women who become addicted do so in a shorter time interval (the time from initiation to narcotic use to addiction) and have a larger habit than men who have been addicted for

a similar period of time. Heavier use for women is often brought on by a personal problem.[8]

These patterns of initiation and use have implications for intervention for women. Drug prevention efforts for women should focus on interpersonal relationships, including the avoidance of involvement with an addicted man and the severance of relationships that promote drug use. Economic deficiencies, including lack of job training and employment experience, may encourage the dependence of women on male partners. Social support for stressful life events is also clearly important for women.[8]

DRUG-RELATED MORBIDITY

Ten percent of all inner-city hospital admissions are addiction related.[10] The use of diluents results in variable concentrations of drug and the risk of overdose. It is estimated that 1% of addicts die each year from drug overdose. Men appear to have a threefold higher risk of death from overdose than women.[11] Seizures, generally grand mal, result from respiratory depression and hypoxia. The diluents themselves are also sources of morbidity. Quinine is associated with chemical abscesses at injection sites, cardiac arrhythmias, and the growth of anaerobic organisms such as *Clostridium tetani.*[10]

Myriad infections are seen among drug addicts, including soft tissue infections, mycotic aneurysms, thrombophlebitis, septic arthritis, lower respiratory tract infections, osteomyelitis, and endocarditis. The skin flora of the drug addict is generally felt to be the source of most common bacterial infections.[10] The rapid transmission of the human immunodeficiency virus (HIV) among intravenous drug users has alarmed health officials and placed addicts at risk for all of the infectious complications of acquired immunodeficiency syndrome (AIDS).

The sequelae of intravenous drug use include thrombus, particulate embolization, vascular insufficiency, pneumothorax or hemothorax, pseudoaneurysm, deep venous thrombosis, endarteritis, and arteriovenous fistulas. Skin popping results in lymphatic obstruction and lymphedema. Pulmonary complications include acute noncardiac pulmonary edema, bronchospasm, septic emboli, and community-acquired pneumonia. Chronic sequelae such as talc granulomatosis, interstitial fibrosis, and bullous disease are also described. Renal abnormalities such as myoglobinuria, glomerulonephritis with endocarditis or hepatitis, hypertension, diabetes insipidus, and end-stage renal failure can also occur. Hepatitis generally occurs in the first year of use, with 1 to 10% of drug users becoming chronic carriers of hepatitis B surface antigen.[10] There is no evidence to suggest that the morbidity of drug abuse is different for women than for men.

DRUG USE AND PREGNANCY

The frequency of drug abuse during pregnancy has paralleled the rise in society throughout the 1980s. It is estimated that the overall rate of substance abuse among pregnant women is approximately 11%.[12] This figure is higher for women who have not sought prenatal care. More detail regarding the specific effects of narcotics, cocaine, marijuana, and benzodiazepines during pregnancy is found in Chapter 34.

OFFICE MANAGEMENT: IDENTIFICATION AND TREATMENT

Screening tests to identify problem drinking or drug abuse in the office include standard laboratory studies and verbal or written questionnaires. The Michigan Alcoholism Screening Test, or MAST questionnaire, is a good diagnostic tool. However, it was defined using a cohort of men entering an alcoholism treatment facility.[13, 14] Many of the questions lack sensitivity and specificity when used with women: a past history of physical fights while using alcohol or arrests for driving under the influence of alcohol. Because women seen in primary care settings are less likely to have experienced the social and legal consequences of alcohol or drug use, the traditional screening questionnaires such as the MAST may be less useful. The CAGE questionnaire (Table 66–1) is an excellent and fast questionnaire for screening, although it can be problematic because many women experience guilt about alcohol or drug use whether they have alcohol- or drug-related problems or not.[15–17] A more general approach is provided by the questions in Table 66–2. A nonthreatening and supportive approach is critical in whatever technique the clinician uses for screening. It is often difficult to screen every pa-

TABLE 66–1. CAGE Questionnaire

Have you ever CUT down on alcohol?
Does anyone ANNOY you about your drinking?
Do you feel GUILTY about your drinking?
Do you use alcohol as an EYE-OPENER?

From Ewing FA. Diagnosis and treatment of alcoholism: The CAGE questionnaire. JAMA 1984;252:1905–1907. Copyright 1984, American Medical Association.

TABLE 66–2. Screening for Potential Drug and Alcohol Problems

1. How many drinks does it take for you to feel high (>3 = tolerance)?
2. Have you felt you should cut down on your use of alcohol, medications, or drugs?
3. Has anyone close to you been affected by your use of alcohol, medications, or drugs?
4. Do you ever use more alcohol, medications, or drugs than you intended?
5. Do you ever use alcohol, medications, or drugs to relieve problems?
6. Do you think you have had a past problem with alcohol, medications, or drugs (patients with a current problem are often willing to admit to a past problem)?

tient for alcohol- and drug-related problems, but women with the signs or symptoms listed in Table 66–3 are at particular risk and should receive specific questions about alcohol and drug use.

The laboratory evaluation for a patient suspected of an addiction should include a complete blood cell count because alcohol can cause myelosuppression, thrombocytopenia, and macrocytosis. So-called liver function tests, which measure aspartate transaminase (serum glutamic-oxaloacetic transaminase [SGOT]), alanine transaminase (serum glutamic pyruvate transaminase [SGPT]), alkaline phosphatase, bilirubin, protein, and albumin, give evidence of alcoholic hepatitis or cirrhosis. A very low blood urea nitrogen can suggest alcohol-related malnutrition (or an eating disorder). A serum magnesium and calcium should also be obtained because alcohol can prompt a magnesium diuresis; without magnesium, parathyroid hormone is suppressed, causing hypocalcemia. Perhaps the most useful blood test is the gamma-glutamyl transpeptidase (GGTP). The GGTP is a part of the P-450 microsomal oxidase system of the liver and is induced by alcohol. However, this test may offer poor specificity because it is also

TABLE 66–3. Potential Warning Signals of Substance Abuse

1. Stressful events such as divorce, financial problems, employment issues
2. Depression, insomnia, suicidal ideation, self-mutilation
3. Anxiety, panic disorders, hyperventilation
4. Menstrual cycle dysfunction
5. Requests for tranquilizers, narcotics, or sedatives
6. Chronic pain

induced by many drugs metabolized by the liver. High-density lipoprotein cholesterol can also be raised with alcohol.

These laboratory tests may have a low sensitivity for alcoholism. As many as 40% of patients whose MAST test results were positive for alcoholism had normal results on laboratory tests.

Initiating Treatment

It is important first to define the role of the physician in the treatment of alcoholism and other addictive disorders. All physicians and health care providers should know how to screen, recognize, diagnose, and refer to treatment individuals with addictive disorders.[14] Many clinicians, however, should not plan to do the actual treatment of the addiction. Referral to Alcoholics Anonymous (AA) and other 12-step programs or addiction-related counseling is appropriate along with arranging to continue to monitor the patient's treatment. The provider should make clear to the patient that he or she will remain involved, but treatment of the addiction requires time and expertise not available to most clinicians. It is not unlike referral to a mental health specialist, surgeon, or a medical subspecialist. Simply taking a careful, nonjudgmental history from a patient begins the treatment process. Motivating the patient to accept the diagnosis and to begin active treatment is the next step.

Treatment professionals describe two kinds of denial from the addicted patient. The first type of denial is that a problem exists: "I can't be an alcoholic; I still have a job," "I don't get drunk," and similar statements. When the provider discusses the problem with the patient, the data obtained during the patient's assessment must be offered in a straightforward fashion along with concern for the patient. Although the data to be transmitted contradict the patient's self-image, the manner in which they are offered need not be confrontational. The physician should be clear in stating the findings: "Everything you have told me and that I find on my examination shows that alcohol is a problem." When the clinician takes a complete history and offers the patient's words back to the patient along with the clinician's observations, most patients can see that there is a problem.

When the patient chooses not to accept the diagnosis, a plan should be offered to help both the provider and the patient work to an agreement. The provider may suggest a trial of "controlled drinking" or a period of abstinence to let both the patient and provider see if symptoms or signs change over time. Sometimes a referral to a specialist or an invitation to members of the family to come in for a visit helps the patient see how alcohol affects her life.

The second type of denial is when the patient accepts the diagnosis but she feels that she can treat the addiction on her own and does not need assistance in regaining control of her life. This is frequently a more difficult problem for the provider. In a sense, it is no different from treating the obese diabetic or the tobacco-addicted asthmatic. Both the doctor and the patient agree that there is a problem, but the behavioral changes necessary usually require active treatment—treatment the patient may choose to avoid. Patients sometimes must learn for themselves that help is necessary; arguments should be avoided. If a patient agrees to a trial of abstinence, a contract can be made that the patient will pursue treatment if unable to abstain.

In some cases, intervention is necessary. This is a technique in which a number of family members, friends, individuals from the workplace, and health care providers under the guidance of a facilitator or treatment specialist meet together with the patient to describe the impact of the addiction on all of their lives. The meeting usually ends with a plan or contract for the patient to enter treatment as part of the intervention.

Treatment Options

12-Step Programs

Alcoholics Anonymous, Al-Anon, Narcotics Anonymous (NA), and Alateen are all community-based support programs for people with addictions and family members and friends affected by addicted people.[18] All of these organizations serve to break feelings of isolation that many addicted women experience. They also educate people about the diseases of alcohol and drug addiction. Because much of the treatment of addiction is behavioral, these organizations provide vital information about new socialization skills, assistance with relapses, and filling the time that was formerly spent dedicated to a drug or alcohol. In many communities there are "women only" meetings of AA and other 12-step groups to help prospective patients find a group that speaks to their concerns.

Perhaps most important, these groups offer significant hope for recovery. By hearing and meeting other people who share their experiences with addiction and recovery, the addict can see that recovery is possible for herself. A practitioner must be familiar with these groups and with what they provide to prescribe them for appropriate patients.

The best way for a health care provider to learn about 12-step groups is to visit an AA or Al-Anon meeting.

Whereas AA is for people who are in trouble with alcohol, Al-Anon and Alateen are for family members or friends affected by alcoholism.

Counseling

Many patients require individual counseling in addition to group and 12-step work. Intensive psychoanalysis is usually not helpful in early recovery. However, supportive psychotherapy can be quite useful. One-on-one counseling is critical in patients with defined or suspected dual diagnosis.

Inpatient Treatment

Inpatient treatment of an addictive disorder is indicated in cases of life-threatening health problems, major psychiatric illness (including suicidal ideation), failure to maintain sobriety despite appropriate outpatient treatment, or no stable social supports at home. The most common indication for hospitalization is alcohol withdrawal that is resistant to outpatient treatment with benzodiazepines. An inpatient treatment program is sometimes essential to coordinate treatment modalities and to involve the patient's family with treatment.

Specific Treatment Issues For Women

Clinicians who care for women with addictions find it necessary to develop referral networks for additional problems that are special to women.[1, 19]

Child Care Services

A major difficulty in caring for addicted women is arranging for adequate support for the family while the woman receives treatment. Child care and financial issues frequently complicate treatment; very few treatment programs offer onsite child care. Women may also be concerned about the loss of child custody if they publicly acknowledge their alcohol or drug disorder. Knowledge of both the patient's family supports and the community's child care agencies is important to keep the patient in treatment.

Violence Counseling

Because abuse is more common in women with alcohol and drug problems, counseling for such women is essential. The clinician should have such resources available for patients. Referrals for women who have been raped, survivors of incest, and women who have been battered should be provided.

Legal and Vocational Assistance

Both civil and criminal issues may need resolution during the course of the addict's treatment (e.g., child custody, divorce). Job training and job-seeking support are helpful for women in recovery because financial stability is part of rebuilding self-esteem and independence.

Social Supports

Social supports for addicted women may be nearly absent when they enter treatment. It may be important to offer programs to bolster supports, especially programs that encourage healthy relationships with other women, avoid overdependency on partners who may also be substance dependent, and offer training in financial management.

Services for Women Infected with the Human Immunodeficiency Virus

Many HIV-infected women will have issues with addictions. Coordination between providers for persons infected with HIV and providers for treatment of addiction is important for keeping the patient in treatment for both issues.

Many women have problems related to alcohol and other substances. There are a number of medical, social, and psychiatric problems that may occur due to addictions; all of them are more responsive to treatment early in the disease. A concerned, nonjudgmental approach to data gathering and negotiation for treatment is important in motivating the patient to accept the diagnosis of an addictive disorder and to enter treatment. A number of specific barriers to treatment may impair a woman's ability to remain in treatment that can be managed effectively by appropriate planning and referrals.

REFERENCES

1. Lane PA, Burge S, Graham A. Management of addictive disorders in women. In: Fleming MF, Barry KL: Addictive Disorders. St. Louis: Mosby Year Book, 1992.
2. Epidemiology; Population subgroups. In: Secretary of Health and Human Services: Alcohol and Health. Washington, D.C.: US Department of Health and Human Services, 1990, p 24.
3. Frezza M, DiPadova C, Pozzato G, et al. High blood alcohol levels in women: The role of decreased gastric alcohol dehydrogenase and first pass metabolism. N Engl J Med 1990;322:95.

4. Mello NK, Mendelson JH. Alcohol and neuroendocrine function in women of reproductive age. In: Mendelson JH, Mello NK (eds). Medical Diagnosis and Treatment of Alcoholism. New York: McGraw-Hill, 1992, p 575.

5. Fetal alcohol syndrome and other effects of alcohol on pregnancy outcome. In: Alcohol and Health. Washington, DC: US Department of Health and Human Services, 1990, p 154.

6. Gavaler JS. Alcohol effects in postmenopausal women: Alcohol and estrogens. In: Mendelson JH, Mello NK (eds). Medical Diagnosis and Treatment of Alcoholism. New York: McGraw-Hill, 1992, p 623.

7. Armor DJ, Polich JM, Stambul HB. Perspectives on alcoholism and treatment. In: Alcoholism and Treatment. New York: Wiley Interscience, 1978, p 11.

8. Anglin DA, Hser YI, McGlothlin WH. Sex differences in addict careers. 2. Becoming addicted. Am J Drug Alcohol Abuse 1987;13:59.

9. Hser YI, Anglin MD, McGlothlin WH. Sex differences in addict careers. 1. Initiation of use. Am J Drug Alcohol Abuse 1987;13:33.

10. Stein MD. Medical complications of intravenous drug use. J Gen Med 1990;5:249.

11. Harlow KC. Patterns of rates of mortality from narcotics and cocaine overdose in Texas, 1978–87. Public Health Rep 1990;105:455.

12. Cartwright PS, Schorge JO, McLaughlin FJ. Epidemiologic characteristics of drug use during pregnancy: Experience in a Nashville hospital. South Med J 1991;84:867.

13. Selzer ML. The Michigan alcoholism screening test: The quest for a new diagnostic instrument. Am J Psychiatry 1971;127:1653.

14. Brown RL. Identification and office management of alcohol and drug disorders. In: Fleming MF, Barry KL. Addictive Disorders. St. Louis: Mosby Year Book, 1992, p 29.

15. Ewing JA. Detecting alcoholism: The CAGE questionnaire. JAMA 1984;252:1905.

16. Bush B, Shaw S, Cleary P, et al. Screening for alcohol abuse using the CAGE questionnaire. Am J Med 1987;82:231.

17. Halliday A, Bush B, Cleary P, et al. Alcohol abuse in women seeking gynecologic care. Am J Obstet Gynecol 1986;68:322.

18. Schulz J, Barry KL. Alcohol and drug treatment and role of 12-step programs. In: Fleming MF, Barry KL. Addictive Disorders. St. Louis: Mosby Year Book, 1992, p 77.

19. Haliday A, Bush B. Women and alcohol abuse. In: Barnes HN, Aronson MD, Delbanco TL. Alcoholism: A Guide for the Primary Care Physician. New York: Springer-Verlag, 1987, p 176.

Obesity

George Blackburn and Zoe Miner

Obesity is one of the most common diet-related problems in the United States, affecting 34 million people aged 20 to 74.[1] This population, which represents one in five Americans, is 20% or more above ideal body weight; it also includes 12 million individuals who are 40% or more above ideal body weight.[2, 3] Trends toward obesity also appear among children and adolescents in the United States. In addition, the incidence and prevalence of obesity may be underestimated, as sustained use of hypocaloric diets in the healthy overweight population may mask obesity.[4]

The purpose of this chapter is to clarify the disease of obesity, to review its associated health risks, to examine public and health professional perceptions of body weight, and to consider intervention strategies for this illness.

Although the increased incidence of obesity is seen in both males and females, it is an especially distressing trend for women not only because more women (19 million) than men (15 million) are obese,[5] but also because the social stigma associated with obesity has a larger effect on women. The highest rates of obesity are seen in poor and minority women; 24.6% of white women, 45.1% of African American women, and 39.0% of Mexican American and Puerto Rican American women are obese.[5] The greatest weight increase in women occurs between the early twenties and early thirties, but weight continues to rise throughout all ages, reaching a peak in 65 to 74 year olds. Indeed, the alarming increase in the incidence of obesity, the poor treatment success rates, and the significant comorbidity (including hypertension, diabetes, and cardiovascular disease) associated with obesity prompted the National Institutes of Health to sponsor a Technology Assessment Conference to review the American perspective on weight loss.[4]

Obesity is a chronic disease that results from multiple and complex causes. The definition of obesity is imprecise but is usually stated as a 20% excess over desirable weight or a body mass index above the eighty-fifth percentile. Desirable weight is based on height and body build; body mass index is defined as body weight in kilograms divided by height in meters squared and can be obtained from the nomogram in Figure 67–1. More precisely defined medical classifications of obesity in women are shown in Table 67–1.

ADIPOSE TISSUE DISTRIBUTION

In the 1950s, a French investigator reported a distinction in male and female body fat distribution.[6] The sex-specific characteristics of adipose tissue lead to its subcutaneous (peripheral) deposition in women and its intra-abdominal (central or android) deposition in men (Fig. 67–2). In addition, women exhibit specific enlargement of gluteofemoral adipocytes for fat storage, giving rise to the gynoid fat distribution pattern. Obese women usually continue to deposit excess fat into the peripheral and gluteofemoral depots. Most women do not deposit fat into intra-abdominal stores until a severe degree of obesity is reached, although a small percentage of obese women do exhibit a central localization of fat tissue.[7–11]

Regional adipose tissue depots demonstrate differences in metabolic activity. Tissue isolated from the gluteofemoral region of premenopausal women exhibited greater activity from lipoprotein lipase, an enzyme necessary for triglyceride deposition into adipocytes, than tissue isolated from subcutaneous abdominal depots. Lipoprotein lipase activity in the femoral fat depot increases during pregnancy but decreases during lactation. The latter observation suggests that triglycerides are rerouted to other tissues, possibly the mammary gland for milk production. These regional variations in lipoprotein lipase activity appear to be regulated by reproductive hormones, glucocorticoids, and possibly other factors. In fact, women with Cushing's syndrome show increased abdominal fat deposition, implying corticosteroids can increase lipoprotein lipase activity in adipocytes in this region.[10]

NOMOGRAM FOR BODY MASS INDEX

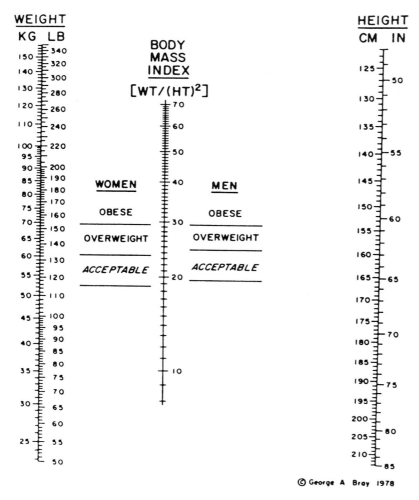

Figure 67–1. Relationship of height and weight to body mass index (BMI). The BMI may be determined by the BMI line intersect of a line drawn connecting weight and height of an individual. (From Bray GA. Obesity in America. NIH publication No. 79–359. Washington, DC: US Government Printing Office, 1979. George A. Bray, M.D., copyright 1978).

© George A. Bray 1978

TABLE 67–1. **Medical Classification of Obesity Using Body Mass Index**

DESIRABLE WEIGHT (%)	DEFINITION	GRADE OF OBESITY	EXCESS FAT (LB/KG)	BMI (KG/M²)
Women				
245	Super morbid obesity	6	158/72	≥50
220	Morbid obesity	5	131/59	45
195	Super obesity	4	103/47	40
170	Medically significant obesity	3	76/34	35
145	Obesity	2	49/22	30
120	Overweight	1	22/10	25
100	Desirable weight	0	0	21
75	Medically significant starvation	−3	−20/−9*	15

The relationship of percentage of desirable body weight, definition of obesity, grade of obesity, and excess body fat to BMI. Morbidity and mortality increase sharply when BMI is >35. Excess fat (lb) assumes 90% of excess body weight is fat.

*Assuming 75% of weight loss in simple semi-starvation is body fat.

% Desirable weight, % desirable body weight ÷ 120 lb for (64 in) Reference Woman (1980 Recommended Dietary Allowance Table). BMI, body mass index (weight/height²).

From Kanders BS, Forse RA, Blackburn GL. Obesity. In: Rakel RE (ed). Conn's Current Therapy. Philadelphia: WB Saunders, 1991. Developed by the Nutrition/Metabolism Laboratory, Cancer Research Institute, Boston, Mass.

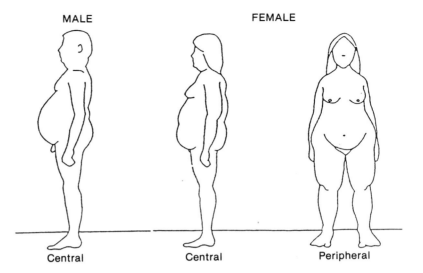

Figure 67–2. The male and female central (android or intra-abdominal) fat distribution pattern and the peripheral (gynoid) pattern most often seen in women. Health risks appear to be associated with the android distribution pattern. (From Greenwood MRC, Pittman-Waller V. Weight control: A complex, various and controversial problem. In: Frankle RT, Yang M (eds). Obesity and Weight Control: The Health Professional's Guide to Understanding and Treatment. Rockville, Md: Aspen Publications, 1988, p 9. Reprinted with permission of Aspen Publications, Inc., © 1988.)

MALE   FEMALE

Central   Central   Peripheral

Evidence for gender-specific determinants of adipose tissue distribution in women (and men) is inconclusive owing to the multifactorial aspect of this phenomenon. The role of reproductive hormones is suggested by the appearance of centrally located adipose tissue in boys coincident with androgen production, and the gluteofemoral profile appears in girls at the time of enhancement of estrogen production.[10] However, a cause-effect relationship has not been established.

Recent findings have shown that the health hazards of obesity are often associated with the android (central) body fat distribution pattern. Correlations between android obesity and non–insulin-dependent diabetes mellitus (NIDDM) as well as android obesity and coronary heart disease are well documented,[10–18] although a mechanism to explain these correlations remains unknown.

Thus, for the primary care physician, it becomes important to identify not only the degree of obesity but also the fat distribution pattern of the obese patient. Although women typically demonstrate a gynoid (peripheral) pattern of fat distribution, which appears not to have a strong association with the comorbidity of obesity,[19] an absence of health risks with this type of fat distribution has not been confirmed. The ratio of waist circumference (measured at the umbilicus) to hip circumference (measured at the widest point of the buttocks), known as waist to hip ratio, can be used to assess risk; in women, a ratio greater than 0.8 generally indicates increased risk for comorbidity.

GENETICS AND HUMAN OBESITY

Knowledge of the genetic aspects of obesity has increased substantially in the past decade. Al-though obesity is a multifaceted disease with hereditary and environmental aspects, researchers are becoming increasingly convinced of the strong role of genetics. Determining the individual genetic components that control the amount and distribution of body fat, adipose tissue metabolism, thermoregulation, and appetite satiety are exciting areas of research in this field. Familial obesity has been demonstrated by several studies that correlated body mass index within family members. These studies indicate that heritability estimates of obesity among family members range from approximately 0.40 to 0.60. This suggests that genes are responsible for approximately half of the phenotypic variations of obesity that are observed. Twin studies have confirmed the findings of the family studies.[20] The genetic aspects of changes in adipose tissue metabolism associated with obesity have also been studied. Results in both family and twin studies indicate a strong genetic effect for the examined parameters.[21]

Genetically altered obese rodents have been engineered whose offspring are also obese. Although the genes responsible for the obese phenotype in rodents remain elusive, researchers are actively pursuing their discovery. Identification of these genes will begin to elucidate the genetic pathway or pathways to obesity.

Although diet and exercise undoubtedly play a role in obesity, they do so within the confines set by genetic constraints. The body usually maintains its weight within a narrow range, resisting major weight changes of both increasing and decreasing amounts. Even obese people have a stable weight, although at a higher set-point than the nonobese. Knowledge of the genes responsible for maintenance of this weight set-point in the context of nutrition and exercise will greatly improve the treatment of obesity.

OBESITY-RELATED HEALTH RISKS

Obesity is associated with five of the ten leading causes of death (heart disease, some types of cancer, stroke, diabetes, and atherosclerosis) and with many other diseases (gallstones, sleep apnea, gout, and degenerative joint disease of the hips and knees).[17, 22] Symptoms of these diseases can appear in even mildly overweight individuals[23] and have been shown to disappear with weight loss.

Non–Insulin-Dependent Diabetes Mellitus

Eighty to 90% of patients with NIDDM are obese.[24, 25] Obesity is a contributing factor, increasing the risk for developing NIDDM 2.3- to 3.0-fold.[24, 26] Data from the Nurses Cohort Study indicate that the risk for developing NIDDM increased with weight gain after the age of 18. This study also showed that the relationship between the development of NIDDM and body mass index was continuous in women and that the risk increased to 17.3 for a weight gain of 35 kg.[27] Weight loss in the obese diabetic patient can sometimes ameliorate the condition.[28] In one small short-term study, a 6% weight loss in obese subjects with newly diagnosed NIDDM increased insulin sensitivity and reduced fasting plasma glucose levels.[29] Another larger long-term study found that a 20% weight loss resolved diabetes in 34% of patients.[14]

Hypertension

A strong correlation exists between obesity and hypertension.[30] Obesity increases the risk of hypertension threefold, with the risk in persons 20 to 44 years of age reaching almost sixfold.[26] As with NIDDM, insulin resistance is thought to play a causal role in increasing blood pressure, although further evidence to support this theory must be obtained.[31] In addition, increased blood volume found in the obese patient may also be a determinant in hypertension. In any event, even modest weight loss can lower blood pressure. In one study, 58% of the obese men and women participants who had maintained a 20% weight loss at 18 months experienced a resolution or improvement of their hypertension.[14]

Coronary Artery Disease

Although convincing evidence has been shown to correlate obesity with hypertension and hyperlipidemia, evidence implicating obesity as an independent risk factor in coronary artery disease (CAD) has been conflicting.[32] Most data, however, suggest that obesity is linked to increased mortality and morbidity from CAD.[23, 33–35] When the presence of abdominal obesity is used in correlation studies, a strong relationship to CAD has been shown in several studies.[23, 32, 33, 36, 37] In one Swedish study of 1462 women, the risk ratio between the highest and the lowest waist to hip ratio quintiles was 8.2 for myocardial infarction, 3.8 for stroke, and 2.0 for death of any cause.[36]

One study of 101 women showed a decrease in cardiovascular risk factors (blood pressure, cholesterol, triglycerides) following reductions in weight and waist to hip ratio.[38] Other studies have confirmed this observation.[39]

Cardiac structure and function are altered considerably in morbidly obese patients, resulting in cardiomegaly with both preload and afterload elevations, increased cardiac output, and increased risk of congestive heart failure.[40] Changes in cardiac electrophysiology are known to occur with obesity, and evidence has shown a specific electrocardiographic change with increasing abdominal obesity in premenopausal obese women. In one study of 27 women, elongation of the Q–Tc interval was associated with abdominal obesity independently of general obesity and other cardiovascular risks.[41] Such an electrocardiographic change may increase the risk of cardiac arrhythmias and sudden death.

Changes in cardiac structure and function in the morbidly obese are the reason why very low calorie treatment programs for weight loss in these patients should be undertaken in conjunction with medical monitoring. The clinician should be aware of the effects of electrolyte and micronutrient imbalances, rapid weight and fluid loss, continued use of antihypertensive medications, and other factors that may affect the cardiac-compromised obese patient during weight loss.

Cancer

An association between obesity and cancer was observed at the beginning of this century.[42] For obese women, this association has been shown to be especially strong for cancer of the breast[32, 43–48] and endometrium[45, 49–52] in addition to cancer of the uterus, cervix, and ovary.[44]

Obesity increases the risk of developing breast

cancer 1.25- to 1.5-fold in postmenopausal women. Studies examining the role of obesity in breast cancer prognosis, morbidity, and mortality indicate that in postmenopausal obese women, obesity increases the recurrence and mortality of breast cancer.[53, 54] In one large study by the American Cancer Society, breast cancer mortality was 50% higher in the most obese postmenopausal women.[55]

In one study, the relative risk of developing endometrial cancer was 17.7 in women weighing 190 or more pounds compared with women weighing less than 130 pounds.[51] Although the association between endometrial cancer and obesity has been noted by several investigators,[32, 49, 50, 52] one epidemiologic study examined data from 56,111 women and determined that only women who were greatly obese as teenagers had a higher risk (1.62) of developing endometrial cancer.[49] However, mortality ratios for cancer of the endometrium calculated by another investigator indicate increasing mortality with increasing weight; women who were 140% or more over the ideal body weight showed a 5.42 mortality ratio for this cancer site,[45] with similar increases in uterine (4.65), cervical (2.39), and ovarian (1.63) cancer.

Gallbladder Disease

In the obese patient, cholesterol turnover may be increased, which can lead to an increase in biliary excretion of cholesterol. Gallstone formation may result from these events and give rise to the increase in gallbladder disease. In an epidemiologic study, the age-adjusted risk for symptomatic gallstone formation in women was 7.0 with a body mass index greater than 45 kg/m^2, 6.0 with a body mass index greater than 32 kg/m^2, 1.7 with a body mass index of 24.0 to 24.9 kg/m^2, and 1.0 with a body mass index less than 20 kg/m^2.[56–58]

PREGNANCY AND THE OBESE WOMAN

Pregnancy can be a diabetogenic state for all women and definitely more so for obese women who may already be compromised in their glucose metabolism.[59] It has been suggested that hormones produced during pregnancy (placental lactogen, estrogen, progesterone, and cortisol) have anti-insulin effects that exacerbate the insulin resistance found in many obese women. As a consequence, increased maternal serum glucose, free fatty acids, triglycerides, and other substrates result in fetal hyperinsulinemia and organomegaly.[60, 61] Obese

women also give birth to heavier babies than do normal-weight women and have increased neonatal macrosomia independent of excessive weight gain during pregnancy. Because increasing body weight results in elevated estrogen production and subsequently multiple ovulation, obese women also bear more dizygotic twins, with the associated risk of preterm birth.[62, 63]

Because prevention of obesity is of concern to the medical community, identification of situations resulting in large weight gain is important. Pregnancy is a time of high risk for development of obesity in many women. One Swedish study determined that 1 year after delivery the average weight increase was 1.1 ± 7.9 pounds in 1423 women.[64] In a retrospective study by the same investigator, weight retention exceeded 22 pounds 1 year after delivery in 128 severely obese women.[65] Another investigator reported that pregnancy-associated weight gain contributed significantly to later development of obesity in 50% of the women examined.[66] Thus, women at risk for obesity (genetic factors, previously overweight, or at-risk nutrition patterns or lifestyle) should be carefully monitored before and after delivery. Appropriate weight gain during pregnancy to ensure maternal and fetal well-being in the obese patient is lower than in the nonobese woman, usually 15 to 20 pounds.[67]

SOCIAL PRESSURES

The obese woman not only suffers from poor self-image but also experiences discrimination in employment, education, and marriage.[68] Most people view obesity in a negative way as indicating a lack of willpower. Many assume that people are overweight because they overeat; however, little evidence supports this assumption.[69]

Obese women bear the additional burden of not conforming to the accepted American standard of female beauty. Even the nonobese woman has difficulty attaining the ideal body shape as it becomes more and more thin. By comparison with 1990s standards, the ''beautiful women'' of the 1950s would be considered overweight. Explanations of this trend toward extreme thinness abound in the popular literature, as do diet and exercise plans to achieve ideal weight. The seriousness of this trend is reflected in the preoccupation of women with weight and dieting and in the associated increase in eating disorders. A survey published in a popular magazine showed that 25% of the persons striving to lose weight through self-help, over-the-counter liquid diet food, or commercial weight loss centers were of normal weight.[70]

The weight-loss industry is a multibillion dollar

business that promotes books about dieting, over-the-counter medications for dieters, weight-loss clinics, and diet foods. Women tend to use the products and services of the weight-loss industry to a greater extent than do men, not only because more women than men are overweight, but also because the social pressure to be thin is greater for women than for men. Although more men than women (44% versus 35%) exercise to lose weight, more women attend organized diet programs such as Weight Watchers (46% of women versus 10% of men),[71] attempt fad diets, and consume diet pills as a means to weight loss.

The obese woman is in a situation that encourages two patterns present in eating disorders that are used to achieve and to sustain weight loss: an unhealthy reduction in food intake and the adoption of compensatory mechanisms to offset the effects of eating. It has been observed that after a large weight loss, obese individuals often display high rates of binge eating; have lower caloric maintenance requirements; and suffer from depression, impaired concentration, and preoccupation with weight and food.[72]

INTERVENTION OPTIONS

Overview

Views on successful weight loss treatments vary, and, in fact, the issue of whether to treat obesity is debated today. The debate arises from the challenges encountered in providing treatment. The obese patient may not remain in treatment for a sufficient length of time and may be discouraged by the amount and rate of weight loss. If the patient loses weight, maintaining the weight loss is even more difficult. Regaining lost weight can initiate weight cycling, which is a repeated pattern of weight loss followed by a gain greater than the initial loss. Severe weight cycling (>20 lb) is associated with adverse health, metabolic, and psychological consequences.[73–77] Health professionals who oppose the treatment of obesity believe the health risks of weight cycling outweigh the health benefits of weight loss.

Health professionals who do feel that the treatment of obesity is a necessity usually use current intervention methods. They believe that success depends on determining the correct treatment for each individual and suggest slight alterations in our perceptions of effective treatment. Weight loss intervention should incorporate the concept that prevention of obesity must be undertaken by every individual, lean or obese, and that prevention of weight gain may be viewed as the initial, and

minimum, treatment for all stages of obesity. In addition, improved health status may be achieved with a weight loss of 10%. For the obese, a 10% weight loss is attainable, whereas losing enough weight to be considered lean might not be. Success can be achieved if treatment focuses on reducing the health risks associated with obesity. Continued weight loss must be achieved gradually through serial weight loss interventions. Due to the difficulty of losing large amounts of weight and the risk of subsequent weight cycling, the obese patient should not lose more weight than she is able to keep off. This loss rarely exceeds 10% per year. Treatment must continue indefinitely until a cure for obesity is identified. Obese patients and those at risk for becoming obese must make a lifetime commitment to good nutrition, exercise, and modified behaviors.

Overweight and obesity classifications (see Table 67–1) are best treated by using conservative therapy that produces a 1% weight loss per week through dietary change, nutrition education, behavior modification, and exercise. Treatment choices for medically significant and super obesity are less clear. Very low calorie diets in conjunction with behavior therapy have been used successfully in some cases, but more research is needed to determine optimal treatment.[78] Morbid and super morbid obesity places patients at high risk for many weight-related disorders; bariatric surgery is recommended for treatment of this group.[78]

Assessment and Treatment Planning

Physician monitoring is central to the treatment of medically significant obesity.[79] Although comprehensive treatment of obesity may require a team approach that includes a physician, nurse, dietitian, and psychologist specializing in weight control, the best initiation of therapy takes place in the primary care physician's office in collaboration with a consulting clinical dietitian. Also, when necessary, an exercise physiologist, psychiatrist, or social worker can be consulted.

At the first appointment, the physician (or dietitian or nurse) interviews the patient to document her medical and nutritional history with particular emphasis on family history of obesity, eating habits, environmental influences, symptoms of eating disorders, attitudes toward weight loss, and prior weight cycling patterns and dieting attempts.[80] The initial evaluation also includes a comprehensive physical examination and laboratory tests to determine the presence of health risks or contraindications to a specific weight loss intervention. Body composition and fat distribution should also be assessed at this time. Goals are discussed with the patient to discourage unrealistic expectations and to focus on an achievable target weight that reduces health risks (usually 10–20% of body weight). The patient is also made aware at this time of the chronic and complex nature of obesity, the treatment of which requires a lifelong plan of weight maintenance and lifestyle change.

The dietitian also meets with the patient to obtain information on nutrient intake and dietary patterns and to discuss lifestyle changes that are required: lower calorie and fat consumption, increased activity, and modification of eating habits. The nutritionist teaches the patient how to keep 3-day food diaries, in which the type, amount, and time of consumption of all foods eaten during the scheduled period (including 1 weekend day) are recorded. The dietitian provides the patient with nutrition information, sample menus, and low-fat recipes and should instruct the patient to begin a walking program, beginning with a minimum of three to five 15-minute sessions per week.

The psychologist is not always an active member of the initial screening team unless the patient is experiencing significant stress or depression. The team psychologist may administer psychological tests to assess possible eating disorders, teach coping mechanisms and stress management, and become a member of the patient's support network.

The patient is instructed to begin a nutrient-balanced deficit diet. The low-fat diet provides approximately 1200 calories for women plus 2 liters of water or caffeine-free low-calorie beverages per day. The patient's motivation and commitment to weight loss can be evaluated the following week by her efforts to keep detailed food and activity records. If the patient cannot comply with these recommendations, she will probably be best served by waiting to undergo a weight-loss regimen until diet readiness is achieved.

If the multidisciplinary team and she determine that she is ready and motivated to lose weight, a 4- to 6-week program is designed that may include diet, exercise, behavior modification, and adjunctive pharmacotherapy or surgery. The selection of adjunctive therapy is based on the patient's excess body weight, her diet and weight cycling history, her physical and mental health status, and her preferred lifestyle. Team members monitor for any associated health risks during weight loss and record changes in weight, body composition, fat distribution, vital signs, biochemical tests, and metabolic tests. It is important that the patient establish a good working relationship with the intervention team so that future problems in motivation, compliance, or health can be easily discussed and the team can become a part of the patient's support network.

Dietary Intervention

LOW-CALORIE DIET. Low-calorie diets are based on food exchanges and provide 1000 or more calories per day. Daily caloric intake is based on the patient's initial weight. Low-calorie diets are safe and are best suited for overweight and mildly obese patients (body mass index of 25–30). Dietary intervention succeeds in reducing weight most often when weekly or monthly monitoring and support are provided. The primary care physician may assume this responsibility or may recommend weight loss support groups in the community.

As part of a low-calorie diet, patients may be encouraged to engage in fat-gram counting to monitor fat intake.[81] With fat-gram counting, patients restrict their fat intake (approximately 55 gm fat/day or <25% kcal) by using lists of low- and high-fat foods in each food category (found in commercially available books) and by learning how to modify food preparation, food selection, and recipes to reduce fat intake. Patients learn quickly which foods are low or high in fat and become quite adept at counting their daily fat-gram intake, which in turn reduces calorie levels without the need for formal calorie counting. The use of fat-gram counting techniques has been shown to be successful in producing weight loss in both mildly and morbidly obese patients.

VERY LOW CALORIE DIET. Very low calorie diets provide 800 or fewer calories per day and are sometimes referred to as semistarvation diets or supplemented fasts. Because some risk is associated with the use of these extremely low calorie diets (cardiac arrhythmias, excessive loss of lean body mass), they should be limited to women who are minimally 30% or 50 pounds overweight and should be undertaken only with physician supervision; use of a very low calorie diet outside a medical setting can result in injury and possibly death and may initiate weight cycling. Very low calorie diets are useful in certain situations, such as when weight must be lost quickly to reduce urgent health problems and when patients are very obese (body mass index >32).

The initial screening physical examination should be much more rigorous for patients considering a very low calorie diet and should include an electrocardiogram and blood tests to monitor electrolytes, liver function, urea nitrogen, creatinine, and other metabolic parameters. To limit cardiac problems that may result from the loss of lean body mass, a very low calorie diet should last no longer than 12 to 16 weeks.[72] Exclusion criteria are listed in Table 67–2.

The very low calorie diet provides 1.2 to 1.5 gm of protein per kg of ideal body weight and is adjusted to restrict the loss of lean body mass to less than 15% of weight loss. Commercial liquid diets include Optifast, HMR, and Medifast. Morbidly obese patients should supplement these diets with 3 to 4 ounces of lean meat, fish, or fowl daily. These diets are relatively expensive, with weekly costs ranging from $75 to $100.[82] Patients enrolling in these diets must be willing to attend weekly meetings on lifestyle change for 3 to 4 months and then monthly meetings on weight maintenance for an additional 6 to 12 months.[83]

The protein-sparing modified fast offers an alternative form of very low calorie diet that provides 1.5 gm of protein per kg of ideal body weight per day in the form of lean meat, fish, or fowl. No other food is allowed, so vitamin and mineral supplements are essential, and the consumption of 2 to 3 liters of fluid per day is recommended. Supplementation of folic acid, potassium, calcium, sodium chloride, and magnesium may be needed. As with a liquid very low calorie diet, physician supervision is mandatory for patients using a protein-sparing modified fast, which is suitable for persons weighing at least 50 pounds more than their ideal weight.[84]

Clinical research has shown that patients who use very low calorie diets without behavior modification instruction regain 55 to 67% of their lost weight in the year following therapy.[85] Even with behavior modification, patients regain weight, although a lesser amount (≤33%).[85] Because most of the research on weight relapse has used a very low calorie diet as the dietary intervention, outcome data for other diets are unavailable for comparison.

TABLE 67–2. Exclusion Criteria for a Very Low Calorie Diet

Advanced age
Cerebrovascular disease
Recent myocardial infarction (within 3 mo)
Insulin-dependent diabetes mellitus
Young age
Malignancy
Hepatic disease
Renal disease
<30% above desirable weight

The physician may also want to include a history of weight cycling in a patient as an exclusion criterion.

Additional Treatment Components

PHYSICAL ACTIVITY. Although a necessary component of a weight loss regimen, the exercise component need not and should not entail an extreme, rapid increase in physical activity. Exercise must be emphasized, however, not only because it has been shown to produce weight loss in the absence of caloric restriction but also because studies have shown that patients who exercise and diet are better able to maintain their weight loss than those who do not exercise.[86, 87] Walking briskly for 30 to 60 minutes a day improves both weight loss efforts and overall health. Patients can begin with 10 minutes a day and increase their time until they achieve at least 30 minutes. Increasing routine physical activity, such as taking the stairs instead of an elevator or parking farther away from a destination than usual, also helps in weight control efforts.

BEHAVIOR MODIFICATION. Although a complete discussion of the field of behavior modification is beyond the limits of this chapter, problem behaviors are identified, and efforts to modify them or to find alternative behaviors are undertaken. A goal-oriented approach is used that clearly defines measurable objectives, such as eating 1200 calories per day, eating 20% of calories from fat, or walking 20 minutes per day. Observing and recording behaviors are the primary components of behavior modification, and group support is often used.[80]

Pharmacologic Intervention

Appetite suppressants are the primary type of pharmacologic agents used to treat obesity. Amphetamine, an adrenergic agonist, is probably the best known but least used of these. Because of substantial abuse potential, emphasis has been placed on finding a replacement for this drug that is as effective in suppressing appetite but that has no potential for abuse. Several drugs have since been synthesized that also mimic norepinephrine, including mild sympathomimetic drugs such as phenylpropanolamine hydrochloride (Dexatrim) and phentermine hydrochloride (Ionamin), which reduce appetite and lower food intake but also have stimulant properties.

A second type of appetite suppressant acts via the serotonin pathway without producing stimulant side effects. Serotoninergic agents include fenfluramine (Pondimin), which acts by inhibiting serotonin uptake and by stimulating the release of serotonin from nerve endings, and fluoxetine hydrochloride (Prozac, Lovan), which acts by inhibiting serotonin uptake. Clinical trials have demonstrated the efficacy of these drugs as well as other potential benefits, such as improved glucose tolerance.

New pharmacologic agents for obesity treatment are also under investigation. The manipulation of body fat can be undertaken by several different mechanisms: inhibition of gastric emptying, blockage of carbohydrate digestion, blockage of lipid digestion, stimulation of lipid oxidation, and increase in thermogenesis. Drugs that incorporate these mechanisms are currently being studied in clinical trials. In addition, new approaches to drug therapy include the use of combined low-dose therapy of both a noradrenergic agent, such as phentermine, and a serotoninergic agent, such as fenfluramine.[88]

Obstacles to the pharmacologic treatment of obesity still exist, many of them due to misperceptions of drug therapy by both the patient and the physician. The first obstacle is related to the public perception of obesity as an indication of lack of willpower. In this case, resorting to drug therapy is seen as additional evidence of the inability of the patient to lose weight by willpower alone. The second obstacle is failure to realize that drug therapy is an adjunctive treatment of obesity. Patients are predisposed to gain weight when the drug is removed if other dietary and behavior modification are not used in combination with the drug. The result is that physician and patient both report that the drug is not useful in obesity treatment. The third obstacle is the limitation of pharmacologic treatment time. Due to the chronic nature of obesity, a lengthy or possibly even a lifetime of drug intervention may be required as with other chronic diseases, such as hypertension.[89] No prescription should be given without a physical examination, without indication of prior compliance to diet and exercise regimens, or without prior involvement in behavior modification and group support.

Surgical Intervention

The morbidly obese patient (body mass index of 45) who has failed to respond to medically supervised obesity treatment may become a candidate for surgical intervention.[90, 91] Treatment begins approximately 6 to 8 weeks before surgery and comprises major lifestyle changes in preparation for the surgery, including smoking cessation as well as all interventions discussed previously. This preoperative weight loss should decrease total body water, decrease stroke work in the right side of the heart, ease breathing, and decrease hepatic glycogen and thus improve surgery outcome and reduce morbidity and length of hospital stay. Following surgery, treatment continues with behavior modification, nutrition education, moderate exercise, patient support, and weight loss monitoring with an emphasis on preserving lean body mass and preventing vitamin and mineral deficiencies.

Vertical banded gastroplasty is the simplest and most often performed surgical intervention. In this procedure, the receptive ability of the stomach is reduced to a small (15 ml) pouch with a 10-mm diameter opening. The rationale is that prolonged emptying time of the pouch after eating leads to overdistention and causes "satiety," nausea, discomfort, or pain. The procedure also limits the amount of food that can be ingested at any one time; a few months following surgery, 1 cup of food can be ingested in 20 minutes with small bites and maximal chewing, and liquids can be ingested in larger amounts.[92] The patient may experience vomiting if she does not chew extremely carefully or if she consumes liquids with meals or soon thereafter (<2–3 hr).[92]

The immediate postoperative course of recovery is usually uneventful. The most serious complication is perforation of the digestive tract, which occurs in 0.6% of patients. Early detection of perforation with subsequent emergency operation and closure (or drainage) results in a rapid recovery with a median postoperative stay of 12 days. Delayed detection of perforation with resulting peritonitis has a more complicated and lethal course. The mortality rate after vertical banded gastroplasty is less than 0.3%.[92]

Two flaws are associated with this surgical procedure that can affect weight loss. Soft calorie syndrome refers to the excessive consumption of easily dissolved high-calorie foods (cake, cookies, ice cream), which can pass unimpeded through the pouch. In addition, repeated overdistention expands pouch capacity and thus permits increased dietary intake.[93] Long-term metabolic complications have not been found with use of vertical banded gastroplasty.[94]

Gastrointestinal bypass, the Roux-en-Y gastric bypass, is the second most frequently used surgical intervention for obesity. In this operation, one limb of the Y-shaped reconstructed jejunum is used to drain a small (15–30 ml) stomach pouch, and the other limb is used to drain bile and pancreatic juice. The remaining stomach and duodenum are bypassed.[95]

Gastric bypass has a slightly higher operative risk and increased long-term complications, mostly from bowel obstruction and acid peptic ulceration. Gastric leaking with peritonitis is the most common postoperative complication, occurring in 0.6 to 1.2% of patients.[95] A "dumping syndrome" can occur after high-carbohydrate intake due to the loss of osmoreceptors in the duodenum that allow hypertonic fluids to enter the small bowel. The patient may complain of weakness, sweating, and palpitations with excess consumption of carbohydrates. Diarrhea is also common and is easily remedied with antidiarrheal medication or dietary counseling. Malabsorption of iron, calcium, and other vitamins and minerals (particularly vitamin B_{12} and folate) occurs in 15 to 30% of bypass patients; in women, the loss of calcium increases the risk of osteoporosis at an earlier age.[94] Micro- and macronutrient malabsorption should be monitored, especially in women who have undergone bariatric surgery and subsequently become pregnant.[4] With time, the pouch, stoma, and adjacent jejunum may expand, causing the patient to eat more, gain weight, and need another operation[92,93]; this expansion occurs in 1 to 6% of patients.[92,96]

Weight loss results are better with gastric bypass than with gastroplasty procedures. With gastroplasty, patients lost 40% of excess weight 3 years after surgery, whereas bypass patients lost 66%.[94] Another report showed that 5 years after surgery, patients undergoing gastroplasty maintained a loss of 50 to 60% of excess weight, and patients undergoing bypass maintained a loss of 48 to 74% of excess weight.[97] Substantial weight loss continues for 18 to 24 months following surgery, with some weight regain appearing at 2 to 5 years.[92,96,98-100] Improvement or resolution of obesity-related health risks is seen in a significant percentage of surgical patients.[97-103]

Commercial Products and Services

DIET PILLS. Both Acutrim and Dexatrim contain phenylpropanolamine hydrochloride, which is similar to amphetamine, an appetite suppressant. One survey determined that less than 5% of the people who tried these over-the-counter drugs were successful in weight loss and maintenance.[70]

MEAL REPLACEMENTS. Meal replacements include shakes (diet, instant breakfast), bars, snacks, and frozen and shelf-stable entrees designed to replace whole-food meals.[82] Meal replacements promote portion control and provide balanced nutrition. Meal-replacement shake labels recommend obtaining physician approval for use by pregnant and lactating women, by consumers younger than 18 years old, by consumers with existing health problems, and by consumers who want to lose more than 30 pounds or 15% of their weight. Meal replacements can be incorporated into a balanced low-calorie diet designed to produce gradual, moderate weight loss.

DIET CENTER. This commercial weight-loss clinic requires physician approval for enrollment of clients more than 40% or 50 pounds overweight or for those with existing health problems. The cost is approximately $50 per week during the reducing phase. A minimum of 1000 kcal per day is provided during the reducing phase, and vitamin-mineral supplements are taken daily. Nutrition education, behavior modification, and exercise are minimally addressed, usually not by health professionals.[82]

DIET WORKSHOP. This commercial weight-loss clinic requires physician approval for clients with existing health problems. The cost includes a $14 registration fee and a $9 weekly fee. The reducing phase provides 900 to 1000 kcal per day that are based on food units; use of vitamin-mineral supplements is recommended. Counselors are not health professionals.[82]

JENNY CRAIG WEIGHT LOSS CENTER. This commercial weight-loss clinic requires physician approval for clients with existing health problems. The cost is $185 for membership and approximately $65 per week for food purchased from the center. Initially, clients rely completely on prepackaged foods. The reducing phase provides 1000 kcal per day, and the use of vitamin-mineral supplements is not addressed. Counselors are not health professionals.[82]

WEIGHT WATCHERS. This commercial weight-loss clinic requires a client to be more than 10 pounds overweight. The cost is approximately $20 for the registration fee and $10 per week. The reducing phase allows 1000 to 1400 kcal per day based on a system of food exchanges, and weight loss is not allowed to exceed 1% of body weight per week. Counseling is done by formerly overweight clients, not by health professionals. Group counseling is used exclusively.[82]

OVEREATERS ANONYMOUS. This self-supporting, volunteer organization requires only that participants "desire to stop eating compulsively." This 12-step program is patterned after Alcoholics Anonymous and is not staffed by health professionals. Members include those who are obese or who have eating disorders or both. There are no food plans, and obese members are encouraged to seek outside medical assistance for help with weight loss. Members pay no fees (funded through donations). Members attend meetings as often as desired and are assigned a mentor who can act as support.

TAKE OFF POUNDS SENSIBLY (TOPS). This motivational and support program encourages members to attend weekly meetings. Nutritional and dietary issues are not addressed at these meetings. The cost of this program is minimal, less than $5 a week.

SUMMARY

Obesity is a chronic and complex disease that affects millions of American women. Obesity-related health risks include hypertension, diabetes, cardiovascular disease, gallbladder disease, cancer, and pregnancy complications. Negative public perception of the obese woman adds an additional burden, as does treatment for cosmetic reasons and failure to diagnose eating disorders. Treatment must focus on medically significant obesity by use of special diets or pharmacologic or surgical adjunct interventions. Treatment must also recognize the chronic nature of obesity and emphasize the health benefits of moderate weight loss.

REFERENCES

1. US Department of Health and Human Services. Public Health Service. Surgeon General's Report on Nutrition and Health. DHHS (PHS) Publication No. 88–50210. Washington, DC: US Government Printing Office, 1988.
2. Najjar MF, Rowland M. Anthropometric Reference Data and Prevalence of Overweight, United States, 1976–1980. Vital and Health Statistics, Series 11, No. 238. DHHS Pub. No. (PHS) 87–1688. Washington, DC: US Government Printing Office, October 1987.
3. Van Itallie TB. Health implications of overweight and obesity in the United States. Ann Intern Med 1985;103:983.
4. Methods for Voluntary Weight Loss and Control. NIH Technology Assessment Conference. Ann Intern Med 1992;116:942.
5. Kucsmarski RJ. Prevalence of overweight and weight gain in the United States. Am J Clin Nutr 1992;55:495S.
6. Vague J. The degree of masculine differentiation of obesitites: A factor determining predisposition to diabetes, atherosclerosis, gout and uric calculous disease. Am J Clin Nutr 1956;4:20.
7. Ailhaud G, Amri E, Bardon S, et al. Growth and differentiation of regional adipose tissue: Molecular and hormonal mechanisms. Int J Obes 1991;15:87.
8. Björntorp P. Adipose tissue distribution and function. Int J Obes 1991;16:67.
9. Björntorp P. Classification of obese patients and complications related to the distribution of surplus fat. Nutrition 1990;6:131.
10. Bouchard C, Deprés J-P, Mauriège P. Genetic and non-genetic determinants of regional fat distribution. Endocr Rev 1993;14:72.
11. Bouchard C, Déprés J-P, Mauriège P, et al. The genes in the constellation of determinants of regional fat distribution. Int J Obes 1991;15:9.
12. Déprés J-P. Lipoprotein metabolism in visceral obesity. Int J Obes 1991;15:45.
13. Hartz AJ, Rupley DC, Kalkhoff RD, et al. Relationship of obesity to diabetes: Influence of obesity level and body fat distribution. Prev Med 1983;12:351.
14. Kanders BS, Peterson FJ, Lavin PT, et al. Long term effects associated with significant weight loss: A study of the dose-response effect. In: Blackburn GL, Kanders BS (eds). Obesity: Pathophysiology, Psychology and Treatment. New York: Chapman & Hall, 1994, p 167.
15. Kaplan N. The deadly quartet: Upper body obesity, glucose intolerance, hypertriglyceridemia, and hypertension. Arch Intern Med 1989;149:1514.
16. Kissebah AH. Insulin resistance in visceral obesity. Int J Obes 1991;15:109.
17. Sjöstrom LV. Mortality of severely obese subjects. Am J Clin Nutr 1992;55:516S.
18. Weinsier RL, Norris DJ, Birch R, et al. The relative contribution of body fat and fat pattern to blood pressure level. Hypertension 1985;7:578.
19. Rössner S. Towards a new policy for obesity treatment. In: Björntorp P, Rössner S (eds). Obesity in Europe 88. London: John Libbey & Company Ltd, 1989, pp 29–34.
20. Meyer JM, Stunkard AJ. Genetics and human obesity. In: Stunkard AJ, Wadden TA (eds). Obesity Theory and Therapy. New York: Raven Press Ltd, 1993, pp 137–149.
21. Bouchard C. Inheritance of fat distribution and adipose tissue metabolism. In: Vague J, Björntorp P, Guy-Grand B, et al. (eds). Metabolic Complication of Human Obesities. New York: Elsevier Science Publishing Company, 1985, pp 87–96.
22. Berg F. Part I: Risks of obesity. In: Health Risks of Obesity. 2nd ed. Hettinger, ND: Obesity and Health, 1993, pp 9–33.
23. Kannel WB, Cupples LA, Ramaswami R, et al. Regional obesity and risk of cardiovascular disease: The Framingham study. J Clin Epidemiol 1991;44:183.
24. Felber J-P, Acheson KJ, Tappy L. From Obesity to Diabetes. New York: John Wiley & Sons, 1993, pp 213–231.
25. Olefsky JM. Obesity. In: Wilson JD, Braunwald E, Isselbacher KJ, et al. (eds). Principles of Internal Medicine. New York: McGraw-Hill, 1991, p 411.
26. Robbins SL, Kumar V. In: Basic Pathology. 4th ed. Philadelphia: WB Saunders, 1987, p 250.
27. Colditz GA, Willett WC, Stampfer MJ, et al. Weight as a risk factor for clinical diabetes in women. Am J Epidemiol 1990;132:501.
28. Kanders BS, Blackburn GL. Reducing primary risk factors by therapeutic weight loss. In: Wadden TA, Vanltallie TB (eds). Treatment of the Seriously Obese Patient. New York: The Guilford Press, 1992, pp 213–230.
29. Bak JF, Møller N, Schmitz O, et al. In vivo insulin action and muscle glycogen synthase activity in Type 2 (non–insulin-dependent) diabetes mellitus: Effects of diet treatment. Diabetologia 1992;35:777.
30. Sims EAH, Berchtold P. Obesity and hypertension: Mechanisms and implications for management. JAMA 1982;247:49.
31. Istfan NW, Plaisted CS, Bistrian BR, et al. Insulin resistance versus insulin secretion in the hypertension of obesity. Hypertension 1992;19:385.
32. Pi-Sunyer FX. Health implications of obesity. Am J Clin Nutr 1991;53:1595S.
33. Kannel WB, Zhang T, Garrison RJ. Is obesity-related hypertension less of a cardiovascular risk? The Framingham Study. Am Heart J 1990;120:1195.
34. Manson JE, Colditz GA, Stampfer MJ, et al. A prospective study of obesity and risk of coronary heart disease in women. N Engl J Med 1990;322:882.
35. Rissanen A, Knekt P, Heliövaara M, et al. Weight and mortality in Finnish women. J Clin Epidemiol 1991;44:787.

36. Lapidus L, Bengtsson C, Larsson B, et al. Distribution of adipose tissue and risk of cardiovascular disease and death: A 12-year follow-up of participants in the population study of women in Gothenburg, Sweden. BMJ 1984;289:1257.

37. Peiris AN, Sothmann MS, Hoffmann RG, et al. Adiposity, fat distribution, and cardiovascular risk. Ann Intern Med 1989;110:867.

38. Wing RR, Jeffery RW, Burton LR, et al. Change in waist-hip ratio with weight loss and its association with change in cardiovascular risk factors. Am J Clin Nutr 1992;55:1086.

39. Raison J, Bonithon-Kopp C, Guy-Grand B, et al. Body fat distribution and metabolic parameters in a healthy French female population in comparison with obese women. In: Björntorp P, Rössner S (eds). Obesity in Europe 88. London: John Libbey & Company Ltd, 1989, pp 43–48.

40. Heymfield SB, Jain P, Ortiz O, et al. Cardiac structure and function in markedly obese patients before and after weight loss. In: Wadden TA, Vanltallie TB (eds). Treatment of the Seriously Obese Patient. New York: The Guilford Press, 1992, pp 136–162.

41. Peiris AN, Thankur RK, Sothmann MS, et al. Relationship of regional fat distribution and obesity to electrocardiographic parameters in healthy premenopausal women. South Med J 1991;84:961.

42. Simopoulos AP. Obesity and carcinogenesis: Historical perspective. Am J Clin Nutr 1987;45:271.

43. Brinton LA, Williams RR, Hoover RN, et al. Breast cancer risk factors among screening program participants. J Natl Cancer Inst 1979;62:37.

44. de Waard F, Cornelis JP, Aoki K, et al. Breast cancer incidence according to weight and height in two cities of the Netherlands and Aichi Prefecture, Japan. Cancer 1977;40:1269.

45. Garfinkel L. Overweight and cancer. Ann Intern Med 1985;103:1034.

46. Helmrich SP, Shapiro S, Rosenberg L, et al. Risk factors for breast cancer. Am J Epidemiol 1983;117:35.

47. Hershcopf RJ, Bradlow HL. Obesity, diet, endogenous estrogens, and the risk of hormone-sensitive cancer. Am J Clin Nutr 1987;45:283.

48. Paffenbarger RS, Kampert JB, Chang H-G. Characteristics that predict risk of breast cancer before and after menopause. Am J Epidemiol 1980;102:258.

49. Blitzer PH, Blitzer EC, Rimm AA. Association between teen-age obesity and cancer in 56,111 women: All cancers and endometrial carcinoma. Prev Med 1976;5:20.

50. Dunn LJ, Bradbury JT. Endocrine factors in endometrial carcinoma. Am J Obstet Gynecol 1967;97:465.

51. Henderson BE, Casagrande JT, Pike MC, et al. The epidemiology of endometrial cancer in young women. Br J Cancer 1983;47:749.

52. MacMahon B. Risk factors for endometrial cancer. Gynecol Oncol 1974;2:122.

53. Herbert JR, Augustine A, Barone J, et al. Weight, height, and body mass index in the prognosis of breast cancer: Early results of a prospective study. Int J Cancer 1988;42:315.

54. Tretli S. Height and weight in relation to breast cancer morbidity and mortality. A prospective study of 570,000 women in Norway. Int J Cancer 1980;44:23.

55. Lew EA, Garfinkel L. Variations in mortality by weight among 750,000 men and women. J Chronic Dis 1979;32:563.

56. Maclure KM, Hayes KC, Colditz GA, et al. Weight, diet, and the risk of symptomatic gallstones in middle-aged women. N Engl J Med 1989;321:563.

57. Stampfer MJ, Maclure KM, Colditz GA, et al. Risk of symptomatic gallstones in women with severe obesity. Am J Clin Nutr 1992;55:652.

58. Weinsier RL, Ullmann DO. Gallstone formation and weight loss. Obesity Res 1993;1:51.

59. Cousins L. Insulin sensitivity in pregnancy. Diabetes 1991;40(supp 2):39.

60. Kalkhoff RK. Impact of maternal fuels and nutritional state on fetal growth. Diabetes 1991;40(suppl 2):61.

61. Naeye RL. Maternal body weight and pregnancy outcome. Am J Clin Nutr 1990;52:2724.

62. Naeye RL. Maternal body weight and pregnancy outcome. Am J Clin Nutr 1990;52:273.

63. Siiteri P. Adipose tissue as a source of hormones. Am J Clin Nutr 1987;45:277.

64. Öhlin A, Rössner S. Maternal body weight development after pregnancy. Int J Obes 1990;14:159.

65. Rössner S. Pregnancy, weight cycling and weight gain in obesity. Int J Obes 1992;16:145.

66. Bradley PJ. Pregnancy as a cause of obesity and its treatment. Int J Obes 1992;16:935.

67. Steinfeld JD, Cohen AW. Obstetrical problems in the obese patient. In: Stunkard AJ, Wadden TA (eds). Obesity Theory and Therapy. New York: Raven Press, 1993, pp 327–334.

68. Gortmaker SL, Must A, Perrin JM, et al. Social and economic consequences of overweight on adolescence and young adulthood. N Engl J Med 1993;329:1008.

69. Frank A. Futility and avoidance—Medical professionals in the treatment of obesity. JAMA 1993;269:2131.

70. Losing weight—What works. What doesn't. Consumer Rep June 1993, p 347.

71. Jeffry RW, Adlis SA, Forster JL. Prevalence of dieting among working men and women: The healthy worker project. Health Psychol 1991;10:274.

72. Goodrick GK, Foreyt JP. Why treatments for obesity don't last. J Am Dietetic Assoc 1991;91:1243.

73. Blackburn GL, Wilson GT, Kanders BS, et al. Weight cycling: The experience of human dieters. Am J Clin Nutr 1989;49:1105.

74. Froidevaux F, Schutz Y, Christin L, et al. Energy expenditure in obese women before and during weight loss, after refeeding, and in the weight-relapse period. Am J Clin Nutr 1993;57:35.

75. Jeffery RW, Wing RR, French SA. Weight cycling and cardiovascular risk factors in obese men and women. Am J Clin Nutr 1992;55:641.

76. Kayman S, Bruvold W, Stern JS. Maintenance and relapse after weight loss in women: Behavioral aspects. Am J Clin Nutr 1990;52:800.

77. Wooley SC, Garner DM. Obesity treatment: The high cost of false hope. J Am Dietetic Assoc 1991;91:1248.

78. Stunkard AJ. An overview of current treatments for obesity. In: Wadden TA, Vanltallie TB (eds). Treatment of the Seriously Obese Patient. New York: The Guilford Press, 1992, pp 33–43.

79. Blackburn GL. Comparison of medically supervised and unsupervised approaches to weight loss and control. Ann Int Med 1993;119:714.

80. Wadden TA. The treatment of obesity. In: Stunkard AJ, Wadden TA (eds). Obesity Theory and Therapy. New York: Raven Press, 1993, pp 197–217.

81. Buzzard IM, Asp EH, Chlebowski RT, et al. Diet intervention methods to reduce fat intake: Nutrient and food group composition of self-selected low-fat diets. J Am Diet Assoc 1990;90:42.

82. Dwyer JT, Lu D. Popular diets for weight loss: From nutritionally hazardous to healthful. In: Stunkard AJ, Wadden TA (eds). Obesity Theory and Therapy. New York: Raven Press, 1993, pp 231–252.

83. Atkinson RL. Medical evaluation and monitoring of patients treated by severe caloric restriction. In: Wadden TA, VanItallie TB (eds). Treatment of the Seriously Obese Patient. New York: The Guilford Press, 1992, pp 273–289.

84. Pagli A, Read JL, Greenberg I, et al. Multidisciplinary treatment of obesity with a protein-sparing modified fast: Results in 668 outpatients. Am J Public Health 1985;75:1190.

85. Wadden TA, Van Itallie TB, Blackburn GL. Responsible and irresponsible use of very-low-calorie diets in the treatment of obesity. JAMA 1990;263:83.

86. O'Neil PM, Jarrell MP. Psychological aspects of obesity and dieting. In: Wadden TA, VanItallie TB (eds). Treatment of the Seriously Obese Patient. New York: The Guilford Press, 1992, pp 252–270.

87. Wadden TA, Letizia KA. Predictors of attrition and weight loss in patients treated by moderate and severe caloric restriction. In: Wadden TA, VanItallie TB (eds). Treatment of the Seriously Obese Patient. New York: The Guilford Press, 1992, p 399.

88. Weintraub M, Sundaresan PR, Madan M, et al. Long-term weight control studies I–III. Clin Pharmacol Ther 1992;51:586.

89. Bray GA. Drug treatment of obesity. Am J Clin Nutr 1992;55:538S.

90. Forse A, Benotti PN, Blackburn GL. Morbid obesity: Weighing the treatment options—Surgical intervention. Nutr Today 1989;Sept/Oct:10.

91. Kral JG. Overview of surgical techniques for treating obesity. Am J Clin Nutr 1992;55:552S.

92. Mason EE, Doherty C. Surgery. In: Stunkard AJ, Wadden TA (eds). Obesity Theory and Therapy. New York: Raven Press, 1993, pp 313–325.

93. Kral JG. Surgical treatment of obesity. In: Wadden TA, VanItallie TB (eds). Treatment of the Seriously Obese Patient. New York: The Guilford Press, 1992, pp 496–506.

94. Halverson JD. Metabolic risk of obesity surgery and long-term follow-up. Am J Clin Nutr 1992;55:602S.

95. Sugerman JH, Kellum JM, Engle KM, et al. Gastric bypass for treating severe obesity. Am J Clin Nutr 1992;55:560S.

96. Linner JH, Drew RL. Reoperative surgery—Indication, efficacy, and long-term follow-up. Am J Clin Nutr 1992;55:606S.

97. Brolin RE. Critical analysis of results: Weight loss and quality of data. Am J Clin Nutr 1992;55:577S.

98. Gleysteen JJ. Results of surgery: Long-term effects on hyperlipidemia. Am J Clin Nutr 1992;55:591S.

99. Pories WJ, MacDonald KG, Morgan EJ, et al. Surgical treatment of obesity and its effect on diabetes: 10-y follow-up. Am J Clin Nutr 1992;55:582S.

100. Sugerman JH, Fairman RP, Sood RK, et al. Long-term effects of gastric surgery for treating respiratory insufficiency of obesity. Am J Clin Nutr 1992;55:597S.

101. Benotti PN, Bistrian B, Benotti JR, et al. Heart disease and hypertension in severe obesity: The benefits of weight reduction. Am J Clin Nutr 1992;55:586S.

102. Charuzi I, Lavie P, Peiser J, et al. Bariatric surgery in morbidly obese sleep-apnea patients: Short- and long-term follow-up. Am J Clin Nutr 1992;55:594S.

103. Gastrointestinal surgery for severe obesity: National Institutes of Health Consensus Development Conference Statement. Am J Clin Nutr 1992;55:615S.

Eating Disorders

Elizabeth R. Woods

Case reports of patients who voluntarily starve themselves have been noted in medical literature for centuries.[1, 2] However, the striking increase in the prevalence of anorexia nervosa to 0.5 to 1.0% of the adolescent population in affluent societies is a phenomenon of the second half of the twentieth century.[3–6] Anorexia nervosa, the "relentless pursuit of thinness,"[7] is primarily a disorder of modern-day adolescents and young adult women. Although patients may state that they feel well or even euphoric, significant morbidity and mortality are associated with eating disorders.

The most common eating disorder of modern society is obesity, which is discussed in Chapter 67. In addition, 20 to 40% of obese patients may have significant problems with compulsive overeating or binge eating.[8] A surprisingly large percentage (3–19%) of young women who are of normal weight or are overweight binge and purge.[3–6, 9–11] The prevalence of bulimia nervosa is 1 to 4%, using the stricter criteria given in the fourth edition of the *Diagnostic and Statistical Manual of Mental Disorders* (DSM-IV).[3–6, 11] Patients' feelings of guilt and the secretiveness associated with bulimia often lead to a delay in diagnosis and treatment.

EPIDEMIOLOGY

The DSM-IV criteria for anorexia nervosa (Table 68–1) include a weight of 15% below that expected for height, an intense fear of gaining weight, a distorted body image, and amenorrhea for three or more cycles. Ninety-five percent of anorexia nervosa patients are female, with 85% presenting between the ages of 13 and 20 years of age. A small subgroup (22%) are premenarcheal, and they have a worse prognosis. Most patients (50–75%) with anorexia nervosa are depressed, and 10 to 15% have obsessive-compulsive disorder at presentation.[5]

The DSM-IV criteria for bulimia nervosa include persistent overconcern with body shape and weight and recurrent episodes of binging or eating of large amounts of food in a discrete period of time, followed by activities to prevent weight gain, such as fasting, self-induced vomiting, diuretic or laxative abuse, or exercise. Binging must be present twice weekly for 3 months, and feelings of loss of control are accompanied by the binges.

Symptoms of bulimia nervosa are even more common (1–19% for high school and college students) than those of restrictive anorexia nervosa.[3–6, 9–11] Bulimia patients are frequently older than those with anorexia and have normal or high weights. Using stricter DSM-IV criteria, the prevalence of bulimia nervosa is 1 to 4%.[3–6, 11] Other impulsive behaviors such as substance abuse, stealing, overspending, promiscuity, and self-mutilation are associated with bulimia.[5] Many investigators have noted a high rate of sexual abuse (20–50%); however, this rate may not be different from that of other psychiatric populations,[5] and many studies have not selected appropriate control groups.[12]

There is a fine line between the symptoms of an eating disorder and the behavior of some athletes and some patients who adhere to fad diets.[13, 14] Some marathon runners and vegetarians may meet the criteria for eating disorders but are overlooked because of their professed devotion to these activities.

The DSM-IV criteria for anorexia and bulimia nervosa are more similar and overlap more than their previous versions because hyperexercising and fasting are now listed as purging responses to binge eating (see Table 68–1). Frequently patients oscillate between the two diagnoses over time. The new DSM-IV criteria for these disorders differentiate between the restricting type and the binge eating and purging type of anorexia nervosa and the purging type and nonpurging type of bulimia nervosa. There is an additional diagnostic category entitled "eating disorders not otherwise specified" for patients who do not fit into either of the anorexia or bulimia categories.

TABLE 68–1.   DSM-IV Criteria for Anorexia Nervosa and Bulimia

ANOREXIA NERVOSA

A. Refusal to maintain body weight over a minimal normal weight for age and height, e.g., weight loss leading to maintenance of body weight 15% below that expected; or failure to make expected weight gain during period of growth, leading to body weight 15% below that expected.

B. Intense fear of gaining weight or becoming fat, even though underweight.

C. Disturbance in the way in which one's body weight, size, or shape is experienced, e.g., the person claims to "feel fat" even when emaciated, believes that one area of the body is "too fat" even when obviously underweight.

D. In females, absence of at least three consecutive menstrual cycles when otherwise expected to occur (primary or secondary amenorrhea). (A woman is considered to have amenorrhea if her periods occur only following hormone, e.g., estrogen, administration.)

Specify type:

Restricting Type: during the current episode of Anorexia Nervosa, the person has not regularly engaged in binge-eating or purging behavior (i.e., self-induced vomiting or the misuse of laxatives, diuretics, or enemas)

Binge-Eating/Purging Type: during the current episode of Anorexia Nervosa, the person has regularly engaged in binge-eating or purging behavior (i.e., self-induced vomiting or the misuse of laxatives, diuretics, or enemas)

BULIMIA NERVOSA

A. Recurrent episodes of binge eating (rapid consumption of a large amount of food in a discrete period of time).

B. A feeling of lack of control over eating behavior during the eating binges.

C. The person regularly engages in either self-induced vomiting, use of laxatives or diuretics, strict dieting or fasting, or vigorous exercise in order to prevent weight gain.

D. A minimum average of two binge eating episodes a week for at least three months.

E. Persistent overconcern with body shape and weight.

Specify type:

Purging Type: during the current episode of Bulimia Nervosa, the person has regularly engaged in self-induced vomiting or the misuse of laxatives, diuretics, or enemas.

Nonpurging Type: during the current episode of Bulimia Nervosa, the person has used other inappropriate compensatory behaviors, such as fasting or excessive exercise, but has not regularly engaged in self-induced vomiting or the misuse of laxatives, diuretics, or enemas

From American Psychiatric Association. Diagnostic and Statistical Manual of Mental Disorders. 4th ed. Washington DC: American Psychiatric Association, 1994.

RISK FACTORS

The original description of eating disorders was derived from patients in upper-class families, which may have reflected the population that presented initially for medical care—one of academically driven adolescents with successful parents. As time passed, however, patients of all ages from a broad socioeconomic background and educational level have presented with eating disorders.[4, 5, 15, 16] Nonetheless, for food to become the focus of struggle within the family, sufficient resources must be available to afford an adequate food supply. With the present social pressures to be thin, the prevalence of eating disorders in the general population has reached epidemic proportions.[10] Halmi and colleagues showed in a survey of U.S. college women that the self-reported prevalence of bulimia was 13%, subclinical anorexia nervosa 5%, and anorexia nervosa 1%.[9] The magnitude of these numbers represents the impact of the present social climate on women's view of the ideal female figure.

Previous obesity and peer teasing about weight are important triggers for an adolescent in the development of an eating disorder. A family history of obesity, eating disorders, depression, or substance or alcohol abuse is also frequently present.[5] In an adolescent population, a history of laxative abuse or parental alcohol abuse was associated with poorer general functioning and depression at presentation.[16] The start of the eating disorder often followed a mild illness with weight loss, the death or illness of a close relative, or a recent change in family constellation. The loss of a parent to cancer or a wasting illness appears to be a particularly potent trigger for eating problems. The young adolescent normally struggles with body image issues, and this easily becomes an extreme obsession within the context of a stressful family situation.

The interaction of depression and stress with the noradrenergic, serotonergic, and dopaminergic systems has an important relationship with the development of an eating disorder.[3, 4] The fact that some patients develop secondary amenorrhea before they lose weight suggests a close connection among depression, the neuroendocrine system, and the hypothalamic appetite center.[13, 17, 18] Patients with bulimia are particularly sensitive to increased stress and treatment with antidepressants, which are serotonergic agonists.[5] The euphoric and addictive quality of anorexia nervosa related to self-starvation and hyperexercising may increase central nervous system endorphins (opiates) and counterbalance the patient's intrinsic depression.

CLINICAL FEATURES

Many patients with anorexia nervosa are high achievers and are engaged in strenuous physical activity. Weight loss is the result of self-imposed dietary restriction in the range of 500 to 800 calories per day. Patients do not complain of weight loss and deny that they are ill. Other common features include a high rate of depression (50–75%),[5] obsessive-compulsive behaviors (25% lifetime risk),[5] an interest in preparation of food for others, and a pervasive sense of inadequacy. Some have been abused sexually. There is often a history of digestive disorders, food struggles, and "picky eating" as a child, but this may be due to recall bias of a patient presenting with eating problems.

Patients with bulimia have a poor sense of self-esteem and are excessively concerned about weight and food intake. Binge eating is the primary feature of the disorder. The food binging may be followed by purging via self-induced vomiting or laxative or diuretic abuse. In contrast to the anorectic patients, who take pride in their rigid control of food intake, bulimic patients are distressed that their eating is out of control. The binging and purging are usually done secretly, and those who live with the patient may be unaware of the severity of the symptoms. The patients feel guilty and unhappy with their binging and may seek medical help themselves. Patients who present for treatment have a high rate of comorbid disorders including chemical dependency (49%), alcoholism (25%), anxiety (43%), bipolar disorders (12%), personality disorders (50–75%), and borderline personality (2–60%).[5, 11]

SYMPTOMS

Patients with anorexia nervosa and bulimia can present with a variety of symptoms (Table 68–2).[4, 11, 19–22] Many of the complaints are nonspecific, so the diagnosis of eating problems can be difficult, with the exception of the anorexia nervosa patient who has very low weight. In light of the high prevalence of these illnesses, providers should have a high index of suspicion and might consider using screening questions and tools for eating disorders in their practices.[11]

Delayed and impaired growth, amenorrhea, and interruption of puberty are secondary to hypogonadotropic hypogonadism due to self-starvation. Patients are often not concerned about amenorrhea and poor growth because of their ambivalence about becoming or being an adult and having these obvious signs of maturity. However, prolonged amenorrhea often is associated with irreversible reduction of bone density and increased risk of fractures.[23, 24]

A wide variety of gastrointestinal complaints are secondary to self-starvation, vomiting, laxative abuse, and the patient's distorted body image. Patients often offer complex explanations for these complaints, which can delay the recognition of the true cause of these symptoms. A surprising number of patients present with the chief complaint of fainting at school. Patients with very little oral intake can be extremely constipated and can develop lactose intolerance, which can cause increased symptoms with refeeding. Hypervomiting can cause severe esophagitis and even esophageal rupture on occasion. Laxative abuse can enhance the patient's constipation, which may alternate with diarrhea secondary to laxative intake. Prolonged laxative abuse can make reestablishment of a normal bowel regimen difficult even with the assistance of stool softeners, fiber supplements, and mild bowel stimulants.

The most common metabolic findings in bulimia nervosa are hypokalemic, hypochloremic, and metabolic alkaloses due to poor intake, vomiting, laxative abuse, or a combination of these, which can cause muscle weakness and cramps. These findings are detected in the most extreme cases; however, because of the life-threatening nature of these findings, patients with eating problems should be screened and followed for these changes on a regular basis. Often the provider first detects a high serum total CO_2, a low chloride, or both; these findings should be recognized as a serious warning for further electrolyte changes. Low potassium levels also cause decreased platelet function, leading to easy bleeding and bruising. Bruising can also be caused by vitamin K deficiency due to poor intake. Patients who water load can develop marked hyponatremia. Many patients are also deficient in calcium, phosphorus, magnesium, zinc, and vitamins.[4, 14] Starvation and electrolyte abnormalities can contribute to the cardiac symptoms of irregular heartbeat and, rarely, sudden death.[25, 26]

TABLE 68–2. Symptoms of Anorexia Nervosa and Bulimia Nervosa

ANOREXIA NERVOSA	BULIMIA NERVOSA
Endocrine Complaints	
Amenorrhea (primary or secondary)	Menstrual irregularities
Short stature	
Delayed puberty	
Osteoporosis	
Euthyroid sick syndrome	
Gastrointestinal Complaints	
Cramping, abdominal pain	Mouth sores
Lactose intolerance	Salivary gland enlargement
Constipation, diarrhea	Dry mouth
Vomiting	Pharyngeal irritation or trauma
Decreased gastric emptying	Dental caries and enamel erosion
Bloating	Heartburn
Early satiety	Esophagitis
	Chest pains
	Acute gastric dilation
	Mallory-Weiss tears
	Esophageal or gastric rupture
	Dissection of the mediastinum
	Diarrhea, bloody diarrhea (in laxative abusers)
Systemic Complaints	
Fainting	Fainting
Cold intolerance	Weakness
Weakness	Muscle weakness or cramps
Muscle weakness or cramps	
Cardiovascular Complaints	
Bradycardia	Symptoms of ipecac poisoning
Hypotension	Congestive heart failure
Orthostatic hypotension	Orthostatic hypotension
Arrhythmias	Arrhythmias
Cardiac arrest or sudden death	Cardiac arrest or sudden death
Hematologic Complaints	
Bruising	Bruising, bleeding
Petechiae, purpura	Petechiae, purpura
Anemia	
?Increased infections	
Hair and Skin Changes	
Cold, dry, scaly skin	Calluses on knuckles
Scalp hair loss	Mouth sores or calluses
Lack of shine	Facial petechiae from vomiting
Thin and brittle hair or nails	Cheilosis (sores at mouth corners)
Lanugo hair	
Loss of subcutaneous fat	
Hypercarotemia	
Pulmonary	
	Aspiration pneumonia

PHYSICAL EXAMINATION

In addition to supportive findings associated with the previously listed complaints, there are many possible physical findings, although patients are unaware of them. However, with the exception of low weight in the anorectic patient, the physical examination is often of limited usefulness in detecting bulimia.

Patients with anorexia nervosa may present with dry, coarse, yellowed skin (carotenemia) and hypertrichosis (lanugo hair). Their extremities may be cold and cyanotic. Their vital signs are frequently depressed (bradycardia, hypotension, and orthostatic hypotension). These symptoms may be due to a functional hypothyroidism, which is a physiologic adaptation that promotes conservation of energy in the starvation state. Patients may also have atrophic vaginitis and breasts secondary to low estrogen levels. Rarely, a patient may present with pitting edema, particularly on refeeding.

One third of patients have new cardiac murmurs that are often related to mitral valve prolapse. Arrhythmias and prolonged Q–Tc intervals secondary to the effects of hypokalemia, starvation, or both can be of particular concern and can contribute to the risk of sudden death.[25, 26] Most deaths of patients with eating disorders are due to cardiac arrest or suicide.[4, 5] Bulimic patients can also have severe morbidity and mortality from rupture of the esophagus with possible dissection into the mediastinum.[19]

DIFFERENTIAL DIAGNOSIS

Many female patients present with signs and symptoms of eating problems, including a distorted body image and a reluctance to gain weight so that the diagnosis does not present much of a dilemma. However, other less common diagnoses can be extremely subtle and can masquerade as an eating disorder. An occasional patient presents with an eating problem who in fact has a pituitary tumor or an inflammatory bowel disease. Patients with severe persistent headaches even after eating more regularly, neurologic signs or symptoms, prepubertal presentation, or severely delayed development may warrant a cranial magnetic resonance imaging scan. Patients with persistent amenorrhea may be followed regularly with bone density measurements and should be considered for calcium supplementation and estrogen replacement if there is no indication of an early remission of their symptoms.[5, 13, 23, 24]

BASIC EVALUATION

A careful history and physical examination, including a 24-hour dietary history, height, weight, growth chart, and vital signs including temperature and orthostatic changes are essential at presentation. The initial laboratory evaluation is described in Table 68–3, and results are frequently unremarkable. Many abnormal results on laboratory tests may be found in patients with anorexia nervosa, including electrocardiographic abnormalities, hypovitaminosis A, hypercarotenemia, low levels of luteinizing and follicle-stimulating hormones, glucose intolerance, hypoglycemia, elevated cortisol levels, abnormal xylose excretion, blood urea nitrogen elevation (dehydration) or decrease (poor intake of protein), leukopenia, bone marrow hypoplasia, and thyroxine and triiodothyronine decrease, plus myriad rarer abnormalities.[4, 19–21] A detailed description of the range of medical complications of eating disorders can be found elsewhere.[4, 19–21]

Although only 50% of patients with inflammatory bowel disease have an elevated erythrocyte

TABLE 68–3. Basic Laboratory Evaluation

Complete blood count, differential, erythrocyte sedimentation rate (if elevated consider evaluation for inflammatory bowel disease), platelet count
Urinalysis with specific gravity
Blood chemistries including blood urea nitrogen, electrolytes, creatinine, glucose, calcium, magnesium, phosphorus (with refeeding may go into cells and further decrease to critical levels [<2 mg/dl])
Thyroid function tests, prothrombin time and partial thromboplastin time (for bruising), stool for occult blood (if indicated)
Electrocardiogram if bradycardia, arrhythmia, or antidepressant therapy to be prescribed
Consider densitometry of the spine (dual energy x-ray absorptiometry, dual photon) if prolonged amenorrhea
Consider cranial magnetic resonance imaging scan for possible hypothalamic tumor if neurologic symptoms present
Evaluate amenorrhea if atypical or not responding to improved weight and sense of well-being after 6–12 mo
Blood sugar if symptoms of hypoglycemia present

sedimentation rate, an elevated rate in a patient with an eating disorder warrants further evaluation because most patients with anorexia nervosa have an extremely low erythrocyte sedimentation rate. In response to starvation, patients can have remarkable bone marrow suppression of any or all of the cellular lines but most commonly leukopenia.

Amenorrhea often persists for 6 to 12 months after stabilization of the patient's weight and improvement in the sense of well-being. The provider should check a urine pregnancy test to be sure that the patient is not also pregnant. However, if the amenorrhea is atypical or is associated with increasing headaches, the provider should consider further evaluation, which includes a cranial magnetic resonance imaging scan and prolactin, luteinizing hormone, follicle-stimulating hormone, and thyroid function tests to evaluate for hypothalamic-pituitary tumors and other endocrine diseases. If the patient shows signs of androgen excess, such as hirsutism, severe acne, or clitoromegaly, or has a high luteinizing hormone to follicle-stimulating hormone ratio, then tests of dehydroepiandrosterone sulfate, testosterone, and free testosterone levels may be helpful. A measure of blood glucose and electrolyte levels can also assist in the diagnose of diabetes, diabetes insipidus, and Addison's disease. If the patient has significant short stature compared with those in her family, the provider should consider chromosomal evaluation for Turner's syndrome even if the patient does not have the expected elevation of luteinizing hormone and follicle-stimulating hormone, because these can be suppressed during the starvation phase. Bulimia and anorexia nervosa may complicate the management of endocrine disorders such as diabetes mellitus, hyperthyroidism, Turner's syndrome and any illness requiring oral medication.

Prolonged amenorrhea in athletes and patients with eating disorders has been shown to contribute to decreased bone density and increased fractures due to the hypoestrogen state and poor calcium intake.[5, 6, 13, 23, 24] Because of the potential negative impact on bone density in later life, concern is increasing about patients who have hypoestrogenic amenorrhea of longer than 1 year and no immediate hope for remission.[5, 6, 13, 23, 24] If the patient has prolonged amenorrhea, the provider may consider estrogen replacement with cyclic conjugated estrogen and medroxyprogesterone acetate or a combined hormone (oral contraceptive) pill. Estrogen replacement plus increasing calcium dietary intake or supplementation may reduce the long-term deleterious effects of eating disorders on bone density.[13, 23]

Other psychiatric disorders including affective, obsessive-compulsive, and thought disorders can manifest with a component of eating problems. Treating the premorbid and comorbid disorder can greatly improve the degree of nutritional insufficiency and purging activities.

OUTPATIENT TREATMENT

Optimal management of a patient with an eating disorder requires a multidisciplinary team consisting of a medical provider, individual therapist, family therapist for patients in the adolescent age group, and nutritionist. In addition, many patients improve with medication for symptoms of associated depressive, obsessive-compulsive, or anxiety disorders.

Role of the Medical Provider

Long-term follow-up by a medical provider is essential to monitor the patient's stability and to reduce the morbidity and mortality associated with eating disorders. Patients who are not monitored medically are at increased risk for developing sudden death and arrhythmias. The medical provider is essential for evaluating the validity of the diagnosis and for screening for alternative diagnoses and complications. This person should follow the patient regularly to ensure adequate nutrition and medical safety.

Frequently, the medical provider coordinates the multidisciplinary care and sets clear limits for admission (Table 68–4). Providers must be consistent in following any guidelines that have been set. Often one is wiser to avoid giving an exact weight that requires admission because patients can look more medically stable than expected when they reach the designated weight. Vital signs and electrolyte guidelines can be firm, and the provider can maintain some latitude to evaluate the weight trend at the time of considering admission or readmission.

The outpatient plan should be clear, with gradual changes expected to give the patient an increasing sense of control over her eating and weight. The provider should express concern about the severity and life-threatening nature of the illness at the first visit. Patients with low weight should be expected to gain a minimum of 1 pound per week if possible. Weight gain should be gradual so that the patient develops a sense of control over her eating and weight.[5] Bulimic patients should be encouraged to stabilize their weight and control purging. Once this is accomplished, overweight patients can consider losing a maximum of 1 to 2 pounds per week. A target weight range is desirable so that the patient does not rigidly cling to one weight. If a patient gains weight too quickly, she may panic and return to a severely restricted diet or resort to purging.

Frisch and colleagues showed that women must obtain a minimum weight for height to achieve menarche (Table 68–5).[27] Patients with low weight should be given a minimum weight range associated with maintenance or regaining of menses from the Frisch tables (see Table 68–5) of the tenth percentile plus 10 pounds (approximately the tenth to the twenty-fifth percentile for age and height).[27] If a patient attains this weight range and

---

TABLE 68–4.   Admission Guidelines

Physiologic instability:
  Hypotension or orthostatic hypotension
  Bradycardia
  Hypothermia
  Syncope or arrhythmia
Severe electrolyte abnormality:
  Potassium <3.0 mEq/L
  Phosphorus <2.0 mg/dl
Critically low weight:
  Weight loss of 40% of body weight
  Weight loss of 25–30% in less than 3 months
Failure to make progress as an outpatient:
  Unable to eat, uncontrollable binging/purging
  Unable to cooperate with the outpatient program
  Extremely depressed or suicidal
  Requiring intensive family intervention

TABLE 68–5.   Approximate Minimum Weight Associated with Menarche in a 13-Year-Old Girl and the Reestablishment of Menses in an 18-Year-Old Woman (10th Percentile for Height) in Patients with Average Build (Interpreted from Frisch Growth Curves[27])

	MENARCHE	REESTABLISHMENT OF MENSES
Inches	Pounds	Pounds
4'11"	82	91
5'1"	86	97
5'3"	91	102
5'5"	97	108
5'7"	102	114
5'9"	106	119
5'11"	111	125

improves psychologically, then she is likely to regain her menses. The optimal range for a patient may need to be adjusted depending on the individual's bone structure, activity level, and muscle mass. This low range is less threatening to the patient than the fiftieth percentile and usually results in medical stability with the eventual return of menses.

If a patient has just presented with severe eating problems or she is doing poorly, the medical provider may want to see the patient weekly until she is stabilized. Orthostatic vital signs, weight in a gown after voiding, and urine specific gravity should be performed at each visit. The provider should check the urine specific gravity for water loading. Electrolytes should be checked every one to two visits and as indicated. Nutritional supplements can be added to the diet gradually if the patient is unable to eat the required amount of food. The outpatient program should be intensified in all aspects to avoid admission, but the provider should be consistent about the need for admission. If the patient improves, the interval for appointments and blood tests can be slowly increased as the patient maintains a stable weight. The patient and family should understand from the beginning the need for long-term medical monitoring at regular intervals.

Role of the Nutritionist

The nutritionist is a key member of the team. The adolescent frequently overestimates the number of calories she is eating and underestimates the nutritional requirements needed for exercise. The nutritionist should perform an initial diet evalua-

tion including the intake of vitamins and minerals. The nutritionist should work with the medical provider to develop a diet plan for slow weight gain for the anorectic patient or a loss or maintenance program for the bulimic patient. This may include supplementation with balanced calorie drinks, multivitamins, iron, and calcium. The nutritionist plays a key role in education and in monitoring the progress of patients with eating disorders.

Individual Psychotherapy

Although medical follow-up is essential for the safety of the patient, the real progress is made through individual and supportive family therapy. Patients younger than 18 years can experience greater improvement with family therapy than with individual therapy, whereas older anorexia nervosa patients improve more with individual therapy.[5] An initial psychosocial evaluation is essential for diagnosis and planning the individualized treatment program.[8] Frequently, the family dynamics of eating disorder patients are dysfunctional, and the patient's presenting symptoms may be an outlet for the family's stresses. The initial evaluation includes an assessment of the family constellation and a history of psychiatric disorders, depression, and substance use. Initially the psychosocial evaluation should include an assessment of the role that the eating disorder plays in the family dynamics.[15]

Most patients require individual therapy. As the patient's medical status is stabilized, more progress occurs during therapy. Initially, therapy should focus on the patient as an individual and enhancement of her sense of self. Later issues for therapy include the patient's ability to express anger, need for control, awareness of body signals, ambivalence toward parents and independence, and relationships.[15]

Family Support

Many families require family therapy, support, individual therapy, or a combination of these for other members of the family. The patient's therapist should usually be someone other than the family's therapist to enhance the patient's trust. Often the family needs supportive counseling as well as assistance in setting consistent limits. Parents and family groups can be very helpful to families of patients of all ages who frequently feel isolated and overwhelmed by the illness.[5, 15]

Medications

A psychopharmacology consultation can be extremely helpful in patients with more severe illness. Many medications have been used successfully. Tricyclic antidepressants (desipramine, imipramine, or amitriptyline) or monoamine oxidase inhibitors (phenelzine or isocarboxazid) have been studied in double-blind studies and are particularly effective in bulimia patients.[5, 28, 29] Maintaining a tyramine-free diet can be very difficult for adolescents. Medications to treat obsessive-compulsive disorder such as fluoxetine (20–80 mg/day) and sertraline (50–200 mg/day) can be extremely helpful for some patients with anorexia nervosa.[5] Antianxiety medications can be useful before meals or previously identified stressful times.[5] Other medications for treating associated bipolar and thought disorders can be effective for a subgroup of severe patients.[5] Frequently, medications early in the treatment program or during a recurrence can relieve the symptoms sufficiently to allow continued progress in psychotherapy.

INPATIENT CARE

A patient may require admission on diagnosis or when her outpatient program is insufficient to stabilize her course. There is a limited role for a medical admission to stabilize fluids, electrolytes, and nutritional condition and to evaluate the severity of the illness. Behavioral modification at the start of refeeding is also important.[30] Initially, the patient should stay at bed rest until vital signs have been stabilized. Increasing activity can be used as a reward for weight gain. A reasonable inpatient goal is 0.2 kg per day with increasing caloric intake (starting at 1250 kcal/day and increasing 250 calories every 1–2 days), plus supplements and no advance in activity unless sufficient weight gain is accomplished. If supplements are refused after 15 minutes with a nasogastric tube in front of the patient, a nasogastric tube must be placed for nutritional support.[30] Many patients need intravenous fluids for rehydration or electrolyte imbalance. Intravenous fluids should be given slowly because edema is inevitable and patients can even develop congestive heart failure.[26] Arrhythmias can be precipitated by large shifts in potassium and phosphorus. The maximum tolerated in a peripheral intravenous infusion is 20 mEq of potassium chloride and 20 mEq of K-Phos per liter, with a three fourths maintenance fluid rate of one fourth to one half normal saline. Potassium should be added only if the patient is voiding. The electrolytes and phosphorus levels should be monitored daily. Intracellular potassium replenishment lags behind the serum levels and should be continued 1 to 2 days past the day the serum levels become normal. Abuse of oral potassium can be life threatening and should be avoided in the adolescent age group.[30] Neutra-Phos, 250 mg to 2 gm per day, divided in four doses, in capsules or packets can be used for oral phosphorus replenishment. Phosphorus can drop extremely low with refeeding. Patients are at the greatest risk of myocardial decompensation during the refeeding and rehydration phases.[26]

Patients should be encouraged to join peer group activities when possible. Individual and family therapy should be initiated or continued while in the hospital. If the patient continues to have a difficult time eating and vital signs and electrolytes have been stabilized, then a combined psychiatric, medical, psychopharmacologic, and nutritional admission is optimal.[30] Programs that have other eating-disordered patients of a similar age range are preferable. This admission allows for more intensive psychotherapy plus time to stabilize the family situation and allow for home visits with close monitoring.[31] Admission to a combined psychiatric-medical program can be extremely helpful in changing the patient's and family's understanding and approach to the eating disorder in an efficient manner.

After such an admission, most patients can return home directly. A voluntary change in residence, placement in a residential school for adolescents, group independent living for adults, or a long-term treatment program may be necessary for some patients.[31] Many day programs are developing and offer long-term treatment while the patient is still living at home.[32] Ultimate prognosis is better if the eating disorder is of short duration and the circumstances leading to the eating problems can be ameliorated quickly.

PROGNOSIS

A significant mortality rate estimated between 0 and 22% is associated with eating disorders.[4, 5, 30] The mortality rate is higher for patients who fail to comply with medical follow-up and treatment programs. The mortality rate is primarily due to cardiorespiratory arrest and suicide. Patients who are thin and purge by vomiting or using diuretics or laxatives are at greatest risk for sudden death or arrhythmias.

Long-term follow-up (5 years) of hospitalized patients reveals that one third are symptom free, one third have some symptoms but are functioning well, and one third have poor outcomes with incapacitating chronic symptoms.[33, 34] Other studies show that 71 to 86% of patients treated on a general adolescent medical service have a satisfactory outcome at short-term follow-up (2 years).[5, 16, 33, 35] Poor outcome is more likely if the illness has lasted for more than 1 year, if multiple hospitalizations have been necessary, if onset is at an older age or before menarche, if symptoms include vomiting or laxative abuse or both, if weight at presentation is extremely low, if patient overestimates her own body size or if patient has premorbid psychological problems.[33–35] Young postmenarcheal adolescents who are ill for less than 1 year and who have no bulimia or premorbid symptoms have the best prognosis. Older patients with a chronic course including multiple admissions, severe symptoms, accompanying psychiatric diagnoses, and purging have the worst prognosis.[5]

SUMMARY

Anorexia and bulimia nervosa can be life-threatening diseases with significant morbidity. Early diagnosis and intervention are essential for optimal outcome. Patients and family members should understand the seriousness of these illnesses in spite of the patient's professed feelings of well-being. Frequently the struggles over food have evolved from a stressed or dysfunctional family environment. Individual therapy for all patients and family involvement for adolescent patients are essential to interrupt the symptoms of starvation or binging and purging. Medical and nutritional evaluation are necessary to limit the morbidity and mortality of these diseases. Modern society should develop more realistic and healthy images of successful women to reduce the prevalence of eating disorders.

REFERENCES

1. Gull W. Anorexia nervosa. Lancet 1888;1:516.
2. Silverman JA. Richard Morton, 1637–1698, limner of anorexia nervosa: His life and times. JAMA 1983;250:2830.
3. Chaum E, Herzog DB. New directions in anorexia nervosa and bulimia nervosa. Curr Opin Pediatr 1990;2:641.
4. Fisher M. Medical complications of anorexia and bulimia nervosa. Adolescent Medicine: State of the Art Reviews, 1992;3(3):487.
5. American Psychiatric Association. Practice guideline for eating disorders. Am J Psychiatry 1993;150:212.
6. Lucas AR. The eating disorder ''epidemic'': More apparent than real? Pediatr Ann 1992;21:752.
7. Bruch H. Eating Disorders: Obesity, Anorexia Nervosa and the Person Within. New York: Basic Books, 1973.
8. Williamson DA. Assessment of eating disorders. In: Williamson DA (ed). Obesity, Anorexia and Bulimia Nervosa. New York: Pergamon Press, 1990.
9. Halmi HA, Falk FR, Schwartz E. Binge-eating and vomiting: A survey of a college population. Psych Med 1981;11:697.
10. Casper RC, Offer D. Weight and dieting concerns in adolescents: Fashion or symptom. Pediatrics 1990;86:384.
11. Freund KM, Graham SM, Lesky LG, Moskowitz MA. Detection of bulimia in a primary care setting. J Gen Intern Med 1993;8:236.
12. Pope HG, Hudson JI. Is childhood sexual abuse a risk factor for bulimia nervosa? Am J Psychiatry 1992;149:455.
13. Mansfield MJ, Emans SJ. Anorexia nervosa, athletics and amenorrhea. Pediatr Clin North Am 1989;36:533.
14. Schebendach J, Nussbaum MP. Nutrition management in adolescents with eating disorders. Adolescent Medicine: State of the Art Reviews 1992;3(3):541.
15. Eliot AO. More than anorexia: An example of an integrated treatment approach for adolescents. In: Lemberg R (ed). Controlling Eating Disorders with Facts, Advice and Resources. Phoenix: Oryx Press, 1992, pp 134–137.
16. Eliot AO. Disorders of consumption: A follow-up study of the anorexia nervosa and associated disorders clinic. Ph.D. dissertation, Simmons College School of Social Work, 1988.
17. Golden NH, Shenker IR. Amenorrhea in anorexia nervosa: Etiology and implications. State of the art reviews. Adolesc Nutr Eating Disorders 1992;3(3):503.
18. Litt IF, Glader L. Anorexia nervosa: Athletes and amenorrhea. J Pediatr 1986;109:150.
19. Mitchell JE, Harold SC, Colon E, et al. Medical complications and medical management of bulimia. Ann Intern Med 1987;107:71.
20. Palla B, Litt IF. Medical complications of eating disorders in adolescents. Pediatrics 1988;81:613.
21. Spack NP. Medical complications of anorexia nervosa and Bulimia. In: Emmett SW (ed). Theory and Treatment of Anorexia Nervosa and Bulimia: Biomedical, Sociocultural and Psychological Perspectives. New York: Brunner/Mazel, 1985.
22. Herzog DB, Copeland PM. Eating disorders. N Engl J Med 1985;313:295.
23. Rigotti NA, Nussbaum SR, Herzog DB, et al. Osteoporosis in women with anorexia nervosa. N Engl J Med 1984;311:1601.
24. Emans SJ, Grace E, Hoffer FA, et al. Estrogen deficiency in adolescents and young adults: Impact of estrogen replacement therapy. Obstet Gynecol 1990;76:585.
25. Isner JM, Roberts WC, Heymsfield SB, et al. Anorexia nervosa and sudden death. Ann Intern Med 1985;102:49.
26. Kreipe RE, Harris JP. Myocardial impairment resulting from eating disorders. Pediatr Ann 1992;21:760.
27. Frisch RE, McArthur JW. Menstrual cycles: Fitness as a determinant of minimum weight for height necessary for their maintenance or onset. Science 1974;185:949.
28. Pope, MG, Hudson JI, Jonas JH, et al. Bulimia treated with imipramine: A placebo controlled double-blind study. Am J Psychiatry 1983;140(5):554.
29. Kaye, WH, Ebert MH, Raleigh M, et al. Abnormalities in CNS monoamine metabolism in anorexia nervosa. Arch Gen Psychiatry 1984;41:350.
30. Harper G. Eating disorders in adolescents. Pediatr Rev 1994;15(2):72.
31. Harper G. Varieties of parenting failure in anorexia ner-

vosa: Protection and parentectomy, revisited. J Am Acad Child Psychiatry 1983;22:134.

32. Danziger Y, Carcl CA, Varsano I, et al. Parental involvement in treatment of patients with anorexia nervosa in a pediatric day-care unit. Pediatrics 1988;81:159.

33. Kreipe RE, Uphoff M. Treatment and outcome of adolescents with anorexia nervosa. Adolescent Medicine: State of the Art Reviews 1992;3(3):519.

34. Thompson MG, Gans MT. Do anorexics and bulimics get well? In: Emmett SW (ed). Theory and Treatment of Anorexia Nervosa and Bulimia: Biomedical, Sociocultural and Psychological Perspectives. New York: Brunner/Mazel, 1985.

35. Nussbaum M, Shenker R, Baird D, Saravay S. Follow-up investigation in patients with anorexia nervosa. J Pediatr 1985;106:835.

Physical Abuse

69

Sexual Assault

Elizabeth Kling Handleman

Every medical practitioner working with women deals with patients who have been sexually assaulted, whether or not the clinician is aware of it. For this reason, it is important to understand the aftermath of sexual assault. Rape victims' utilization of health care increases after the assault and is higher than that of women who have not been criminally victimized.[1] Vital areas for every provider to understand include the assessment and acute management of sexual assault, the aftermath of sexual trauma and the ways it may affect a woman's behavior in the physician's office, the doctor-patient relationship, and methods to determine a history of sexual assault.

Sexual assault is a problem of great magnitude. A report based on a national telephone survey of 4008 randomly sampled adult women and 370 rape crisis centers indicates that 683,000 women were raped in 1990. This incidence of rape is more than five times higher than government estimates; the 1990 Federal Bureau of Investigation's Uniform Crime Report (based on police reports) estimated only 102,560 rapes, and the 1990 Justice Department's National Crime Survey estimated 130,000 women were raped. Respondents in the telephone survey described reluctance to report rape because of fears of (1) their families finding out, (2) people blaming them, (3) other people finding out, and (4) their names being reported in the media. These responses indicate that it is likely that the telephone survey provides a more accurate report.[2] In fact, a 1987 survey of 6159 college students corroborates the finding by indicating that 15% of respondents reported having been raped.[3] The telephone survey found that approximately 13% of women, or one in eight, are raped in their lifetimes. Twenty-nine per cent of these rapes happen to girls younger than 11 years, 32% to girls aged 11 to 17, and 22% to women aged 18 to 24. At that point the rates drop dramatically, with 7% of rapes occurring to women aged 25 to 29 and 6% to women 30 and older.[2]

There are two reasons why these numbers may seem high. One is the secrecy that tends to surround sexual victimization. The second reason is the limited understanding of rape. "Sexual assault" connotes to many the idea of victimization by a stranger. In fact, only 22% of rapes are perpetrated by strangers. Ten per cent of rapes are committed at the hands of boyfriends or former boyfriends, 29% are committed by other nonrelative friends or acquaintances, 9% by husbands or former husbands, 11% by fathers or stepfathers, and 16% by other relatives. Three per cent of rapists were not identified by category.[2] A broader definition of sexual assault includes any unwanted sexual contact in which an unwilling participant is coerced by physical force, violence, threats of violence, or threats (whether explicit or implicit) of abandonment or financial or emotional punishment. Harmful and often traumatic sexual experiences include sexual contact, even if it is "consensual," between people in a relationship in which a power differential exists in their roles, that is, between a caregiver and a child or teenager or between two adults when one is in a position of power and authority. Consent cannot be considered freely given, even from an adult, when it occurs in relation to an authority figure, such as a clergy member, psychotherapist, or physician. All of these types of assault are painful and can be traumatic. Patients may be suffering from the damage caused by sexual assaults that they do not define for themselves as rape because they do not fit the stereotype: there was no stranger, no dark alley, no weapon, not even a fight. The absence of those factors does not diminish the intensity of the impact or the pain, although the victim's awareness of the damage may be limited.

ACUTE MANAGEMENT OF SEXUAL ASSAULT

The sexual assault victim presents with parallel medical and psychological trauma. The physician

713

is also placed in the position of collecting legal evidence because the patient is the victim of a crime, and evidence may be found on her person. Attending to the patient's medical condition, to her emotional and psychological state, and to legal issues is a complex and challenging task.[4]

Helplessness, terror, and isolation are core aspects of the traumatic experience, resulting in feelings of loss of control, connection, and meaning.[5] When the patient arrives for care she is likely to be overwhelmed. Although at one level she may recognize that she has reached a safe place, in other ways she may still be feeling helpless and in danger. It is crucial in working with the traumatized patient to provide her with both information and choices to offset her sense of powerlessness. The patient may be so distraught that she is unable to process the information she receives. Furthermore, she may be feeling more overwhelmed than she appears. Care should be taken to present information as clearly and as simply as possible. In addition, instructions and information should be provided in written as well as oral form.

The sense of degradation by unwanted intrusion is profound for victims of sexual assault; it contributes to feelings of helplessness and creates shame. Some of the medical and legal procedures are also intrusive; they would be unpleasant under the best of circumstances but are potentially traumatic in the wake of sexual assault. It is important that the procedures not be experienced as beyond the victim's control. Even history taking may seem intrusive and perhaps blaming. This can be addressed by explaining to the patient the medical reasons for asking about her menstrual history, contraceptive use, and recent intercourse. It is important to provide her with privacy to avoid prolonging the sense of exposure and its concomitant humiliation.

Profound feelings of helplessness on the part of the patient may contribute to an inability to make decisions. The caregiver should present choices as simply as possible, explaining the risks and benefits of each option. The patient may make choices that she thinks will please her care providers or, alternatively, make another choice in an attempt to regain her independence. She may also feel so terrorized that she is unable to challenge the physician by refusing procedures. Although the physician may be understandably invested in gaining the patient's consent for medically beneficial procedures, this should not be achieved at the cost of the patient's sense of control over her life. Thus, the physician may want to give the patient an opportunity to consent as each step of a procedure is initiated.

Supplying social support is another critical aspect of care. Trauma leads to the disruption of the basic sense of trust in others.[5] To avoid feelings of abandonment, the patient should be asked whether there are friends or family members who could be called for support and asked to bring a change of clothing.[6] If this is not possible, a staff member should remain with the patient at all times, especially during physical examination, to both provide support and serve as a witness. Delays in attending to the patient should be avoided.[4, 6]

The medical history should include a menstrual and contraceptive history, including the first day of the last period and information about contraceptive use to determine the likelihood of pregnancy resulting from the assault. The date of most recent intercourse must also be established to evaluate postcoital contraceptive options. The physician has four major tasks to accomplish: collection of evidence, if consent is granted; treatment of the patient's injuries; assessment of the possibility of pregancy; and assessment of the potential for sexually transmitted diseases.[4, 6]

Documentation

The medical record may be used as a legal document. Therefore, it must be a detailed, complete, and legible record of the patient's report as well as observable facts. The record may be read in court and is likely to be more influential than the patient's verbal testimony. It should include a detailed report of the attack using the patient's own words, including a description of threats made, weapons or restraints used, and all physical contact, violence, and resistance. A detailed description of all sexual acts attempted or completed is necessary, including oral, rectal, and vaginal penetration. The patient should be asked whether the assailant ejaculated, used a condom, penetrated her with foreign objects or performed other degrading acts.[4]

The physician should record in detail physical signs that corroborate the patient's account of the assult. These include observable signs of penetration or force such as the condition of the patient's clothing (rips, blood or semen stains, mud, soil, leaves, carpet fibers, or other foreign matter), contusions or red marks around the wrists or neck, or scratches or bruises on the patient. In addition, the physician must inquire regarding any activity of the patient since the assault that would alter the physical evidence, such as washing herself or wiping herself off, douching, bathing, showering, inserting a tampon or contraceptive jelly, urinating, defecating, vomiting, brushing her teeth, or changing her clothes.[4] All of these must be documented carefully. In addition, the patient's emotional condition should be noted, including both the subjective report and objective observation. That is, the patient's description of her emotions should be recorded in her words, and objective signs of emotion, such as crying or trembling, should be noted. Information placed in the medical record regarding details of treatment should be recorded with the knowledge that the record can be subpoenaed by legal authorities.[4]

Collection of Samples

If the patient consents, the physician should collect the necessary physical evidence. The patient may be uncertain whether to press charges or may change her mind later; if evidence is collected, it does not have to be turned over immediately, and charges do not have to be pressed. However, if not collected, physical evidence is irretrievably lost. Nevertheless, it is up to the patient to decide whether to allow the collection of evidence as well as whether to report the incident to the police. Medical personnel must have the patient's written permission to release physical evidence to the police. It should be explained to the patient (and police officer) that written permission is required as a means of protecting the patient's right to confidentiality. It is very important that medical personnel not engage in verbal exchanges of information with persons not directly involved in the patient's immediate health care needs.[4]

Physical Examination

The physical examination is guided by the description of the attack. Signs of trauma such as bruises, lacerations, and fractures should be noted. The physician must carefully record the location, appearance, and size of all injuries in addition to treating them. The mouth, throat, wrists, arms, breasts, and thighs should be examined carefully, as they are the most common sites of extragenital trauma.[6] Bimanual examination, urethral, rectal, and oral cavity examinations should be conducted as necessary. Pelvic examination should be performed with a nonlubricated, water-moistened speculum. Vaginal secretions should be collected on swabs or aspirated, or saline should be instilled into the vagina and aspirated. A wet-mount sperm examination should be conducted, and if sperm are detected, their motility and number per field should be documented.[6] Absence of sperm does not exclude the possibility of assault, but vaginal aspirate should be sent to a forensic laboratory to

test for acid phosphatase or p30. The results of these tests can be particularly important if semen is not detected.[6] When appropriate, the mouth and rectum should be swabbed for semen and acid phosphatase as well.

It is crucial that the patient's clothing, if it is that worn at the time of the assault, not be altered. Existing holes, rips, or stains should not be cut through. Clothing must be collected carefully and not shaken out to avoid the loss of microscopic evidence.[4] The patient should stand on examination table paper as she undresses to collect falling debris, hair, or fibers. When feasible, she should be the only one to handle her clothing to reduce the possibility of contamination.[6] Foreign materials such as leaves, fibers, or hairs found on the patient's body or clothes should be collected, and samples should be taken of any dry or damp blood, semen, or saliva stains.[4] The perianal area and inner thighs should be examined with a Wood's lamp to detect semen stains.[6] Legal protocol for the collection of evidence varies according to state guidelines. Likely to be included are oral swabs and smears, a saliva sample to determine secretor status, fingernail scrapings, head hair combing and collection of samples, pubic hair combing and collection of samples, external genital swabbings, vaginal swabs and smears, perianal swabbings, anorectal swabs and smears, blood sample, and collection of clothing worn at the time of the assault.[7] Rape kits can be obtained from forensic crime laboratories, and each step of evidence collection should be documented to ensure a chain of evidence that will be admissable in a court of law.[6]

Laboratory specimens must be collected to test for sexually transmitted diseases. Cultures should be taken from the cervix, rectum, pharynx, and vagina, as appropriate, to test for *Neisseria gonorrhoeae* and *Chlamydia*. A rapid plasma reagin test should be drawn as a baseline for syphilis; patients with active syphilis require further treatment. If there is a possibility of early pregnancy previous to the assault, blood may be drawn for a serum human chorionic gonadotropic β-subunit assay. Prophylactic treatment for gonorrhea and chlamydial infection should be initiated (Table 69–1).[4]

Patients may be concerned about the possibility of infection with the human immunodeficiency virus. Currently the risk of human immunodeficiency virus infection due to sexual assault is unknown. In other circumstances, the risk of transmission from a single sexual encounter with an infected partner is very low; bleeding in the genital area may increase the likelihood of transmission, but there are no data at this time to assess the risk. Patients should be given information

TABLE 69–1. Options for Prophylactic Treatment of Sexually Transmitted Diseases

FOR GONORRHEA AND INCUBATING SYPHILIS		FOR CHLAMYDIAL INFECTION		FOR *TRICHOMONAS* AND BACTERIAL VAGINOSIS		FOR HEPATITIS B
125 mg IM ceftriaxone *or* 2 gm IM spectinomycin	*plus*	100 mg p.o. doxycycline b.i.d. for 7 days *or* 1 gm p.o. azithromycin,* single dose	*plus*	2 gm p.o. metronidazole, single dose	*plus*	Initiate hepatitis B vaccine†

*Not yet recommended by the Centers for Disease Control and Prevention. Ineffective for syphilis; advantage of short course of therapy.
†This is given for an exposed person who has not been vaccinated and whose source of potential infection has not been tested or is unknown.
IM, Intramuscularly; p.o., orally; q.i.d., four times a day; b.i.d., twice a day.
From Ryback VR, Lichter E, Diamond A. Guidelines for the care of female-male rape patients. Unpublished manuscript, Rape Crisis Intervention Program, Beth Israel Hospital, Boston, Mass.

about acquired immunodeficiency syndrome and other sexually transmitted diseases, and any questions should be answered and concerns addressed. The patient should be advised to seek counseling regarding acquired immunodeficiency syndrome and encouraged to consider human immunodeficiency virus testing 3 months, 6 months, and 1 year after the assault. She must receive this information both orally and in written form.[4]

Acute management also includes assessing the risk of pregnancy as a result of the rape and reviewing options for postcoital contraception with the patient. If the patient is midcycle at the time of the rape and is neither taking oral contraceptives nor using an intrauterine device, she should be considered unprotected. The incidence of pregnancy after one unprotected intercourse is 1 to 5%; nevertheless, alternatives must be reviewed, including postcoital hormonal contraception. Side effects of such contraception include nausea, vomiting, breast tenderness, delayed menses, and higher ectopic pregnancy rate should the treatment fail. There is a 0.03 to 0.30% risk that postcoital estrogen treatment will fail to prevent pregnancy. If such failure occurs, therapeutic abortion is recommended because treatment poses a risk to the fetus. A β subunit of human chorionic gonadotropin can rule out an existing pregnancy of more than 7 days after fertilization. If the decision to use hormone treatment is made, 2 pills of Ovral should be administered, followed by 2 pills in 12 hours. Prochlorperazine maleate (Compazine), 10 mg twice a day or 25 mg rectally, should be given with the hormone treatment to reduce discomfort from nausea and vomiting. The patient is told to

notify her health care provider if she vomits after taking the pills, as this may interfere with the action of the medication.[4]

If the patient is unprotected against pregnancy but does not want hormone treatment, she can return for a standard pregnancy test if she misses a period. Or, if she is quite distressed about the possibility of pregnancy, a β subunit of human chorionic gonadotropin can be drawn as soon as 3 days after the rape, but a span of 9 days after the rape is preferable to ensure maximum accuracy.[4] If the pregnancy test results are positive, the patient should receive counseling, including options for termination or continuation of pregnancy (see Chapter 26).

When the examination is completed, the patient should be allowed to ask any questions she may have and to voice any concerns. She should also be provided with the names and telephone numbers of her care providers so that she can contact them with questions or concerns which may arise after she has left. All instructions and information regarding treatment plans, medications, and side effects should be given to her in written form. Instructions should include a suggestion for gynecologic follow-up in 2 to 4 weeks and referral names and telephone numbers for follow-up psychological counseling, as well as telephone numbers for any rape crisis centers where she may receive further support and information. Care providers should ascertain that she has adequate transportation home and a safe place to stay. If not, they should help her to make such arrangements. If police have been notified, they may be willing to provide transportation.[4]

THE AFTERMATH OF SEXUAL ASSAULT

Sexual assault has both immediate and long-term consequences.[8] Overall, individual characteristics of the victim and of the attack tend to be poor predictors of how women will respond.[9] Nevertheless, there is some indication that younger victims[10] and married victims[11] may be more traumatized. Victims found to be the least distressed 3 months after the rape were less likely to have lost a close family member in the previous year and more likely to have had intimate, loving relationships with men before the rape.[9] In general, victims are extremely distressed for several weeks, but their distress begins to abate after a month and tends to show improvement 2 to 3 months after the assault.[8] Fear and anxiety can persist at that level for 3 years and longer, however.[12] In another study a significant minority (17–25%) described themselves as relatively symptom-free 1 year later.[13] Thus, a wide range of response does exist. When assault occurs in childhood, the victim has fewer internal resources for coping with the trauma, particularly if the perpetrator was a trusted adult. In that case, another factor is the response of other adults in the child's world, if indeed there is anyone in whom she feels she can confide. Retrospective studies suggest that those assaulted as children are more likely than those assaulted for the first time in adulthood to report major depression, drug or alcohol abuse or dependence, and phobias at some point after the assault.[10] Some long-term effects of childhood rape may develop over time as outgrowths of the untreated primary effects.

Posttraumatic stress disorder (PTSD) is a common consequence of sexual assault. This cluster of responses is more correctly understood as a syndrome, or a normal reaction to an extreme situation, than a disorder. The first diagnostic criterion for PTSD is the occurrence of an experience that would be markedly distressing to almost anyone and is outside the range of usual human experience.[14] Other criteria include reexperiencing the trauma through mechanisms such as intrusive recollections, nightmares, or flashbacks and avoiding reminders of the trauma or experiencing a generalized numbing. This may manifest itself through loss of interest in important activities, feelings of detachment or estrangement from others, and using dissociation as a coping response.[14] "Spacing out" into a neutral state, experiencing the circumstances or environment as unreal (derealization), experiencing oneself as different from one's "normal" or "usual" self (depersonalization), and experiencing oneself as observing one's body and behavior from the outside are forms of disso-

ciation that may be used to tolerate abuse or modulate affect.[15] Amnesia regarding the event and multiple personality disorder are more extreme forms of dissociation. The final major symptom of PTSD is a prolonged hyperarousal, which may be evident in sleep disturbances, irritability, poor concentration, hypervigilance, or an exaggerated startle response. The symptoms must endure for at least 1 month for a diagnosis of PTSD to be made.

The hallmark of PTSD is vacillation between the extremes of reexperiencing the trauma and avoidance or numbing; likewise, symptoms of trauma tend to be exhibited at either of those extremes. It may be useful to think in terms of areas of functioning that tend to be affected, remembering that dysfunction may occur in a variety of ways. One individual's behavior may vacillate between two extremes, whereas another's may tend toward one extreme or the other. For example, one victim's sexual behavior may fluctuate from phobic avoidance to promiscuity at different times in her life; others consistently avoid sex, and still others are uniformly promiscuous.

Sexual assault has physical, cognitive, emotional, behavioral, and interpersonal effects. Rape often profoundly influences a woman's relationship with her body. Particularly in response to ongoing sexual trauma such as incest, a victim may become alienated from her body, having reduced awareness of sensations such as hunger, cold, or pain. This alienation may lead to poor self-care and cause her to ignore or minimize symptoms of illness.[16] She may have trauma-specific physical symptoms. Unexplained nausea, gagging, or choking may occur in women who have been forced to perform oral sex or swallow semen.[16] Women who have been raped see themselves as less healthy, report more physical complaints, and engage in more injurious behaviors, such as smoking, drinking alcohol, and failing to wear safety belts, than women who have not been criminally victimized.[1] Sexual effects include decreased sexual activity, abstinence for months or years, lack of sexual feeling, inorgasmia, and distress in response to particular sexual acts or circumstances.[17] In one study, about 37% of rape victims described themselves as sexually recovered within months, another 37% within years, and 26% did not feel recovered 4 to 6 years after the rape.[17] Finally, long-term neurologic changes have been posited to explain the hyperarousal seen in PTSD and may be relevant for some rape victims.[18]

Perhaps the most dramatic cognitive effect that is a potential result of trauma is amnesia regarding the event. This can be total or partial, and when abuse is ongoing, especially during childhood, a woman may report large blanks in her memories of her past. Some women recover memories during therapeutic work, others at developmental milestones, such as a daughter's reaching the age of the patient when the assault occurred. Another major cognitive effect of trauma is to revise some or all of a woman's basic assumptions and expectations about herself and the world.[19] Events seem to be most traumatic to an individual when they contradict beliefs that are most central to her world view and when they are perceived as threatening. Ideas about the world as meaningful (just, predictable, and controllable) and about hope for the future are often destroyed and must be reshaped. A woman may no longer perceive herself as able to avoid harm, and she may develop difficulty taking essential risks or facing the world's inherent dangers. Trust in others and in herself, including her ability to assess others' characters, is often damaged. Trauma can affect the sense of control of oneself and one's environment as well as the sense of others and the self as basically good. These changes can lead to withdrawal from connection with others. The experience of sexual assault may dash many of a woman's beliefs and leave her searching for a new way to order her world. This internal work may preoccupy her mind, making it difficult to concentrate. If she is unable to establish new organizing beliefs, she may see herself as helpless and the future as hopeless, which can contribute to depression.[19]

Emotionally, a woman who has been sexually assaulted may experience a generalized numbing. This can include a constriction of emotions (such as inability to have loving feelings) and a feeling of detachment or estrangement from other people. Within the first month after rape, victims describe generalized distress and disrupted behavior. Three months later, they differ from nonvictims principally on reports of fear and anxiety; these differences remain for at least a year,[13] and some studies suggest that the fear and anxiety persist for as long as 3 years.[12] She might have panic attacks, characterized by intense physical symptoms and fear of dying, going crazy, or losing control (see Chapter 72). A victim may develop phobias or become dysthymic or depressed, including thinking about or attempting suicide.[12, 20] In addition, she is likely to derive less satisfaction from life and less enjoyment from activities for a year or more.[21] Finally, she could have a tendency to dissociate as a coping mechanism, particularly if she lived in a situation in which the trauma recurred over a period of time.

A variety of behavioral problems may result from the trauma of sexual assault. Most women report nightmares and sleeplessness.[21] Victims may develop compulsive disorders, such as substance abuse, compulsive spending, compulsive sexual acting out, or eating disorders. If victimization occurred in the home during childhood, she may have a history of running away or delinquent behavior. In adulthood she may tend to flee from relationships or have a pattern of abusive or destructive relationships. Women who have been violently victimized, sexually or not, are more likely than others to direct aggression against themselves. This occurs in many ways, from behaviors as simple as quiet resignation to repeated self-mutilation or suicide attempts.[22] Many women lose jobs in the year after they are raped due to severe dysfunction.[21] Finally, victims are likely to engage in some sorts of avoidance behavior, shunning situations that consciously or unconsciously remind them of the assault. Medical examinations can serve as such a reminder; some women report flashbacks when having pelvic examinations.[17]

The effects on interpersonal relationships are apt to be quite varied depending on the developmental phase when the assault took place and the relationship to the assailant. A woman may have profound distrust of and anger toward people in general, particularly if the perpetrator was someone she had trusted. Her fear and anger may be especially directed toward those she sees as similar to her attacker. A woman who was abused by trusted adults in childhood is apt to have great difficulty relating to authority figures as an adult. Any woman who has been sexually victimized is likely to carry a great deal of shame that may be triggered easily in difficult interpersonal interactions. Shame can be understood as the painful feeling caused by a loss of pride, self-respect, or self-image.[23] It seems to concern the state of the whole self as defective or deficient.

IDENTIFYING WOMEN WITH A HISTORY OF SEXUAL ASSAULT

A trauma history could come to the clinician's attention in a variety of ways. Reexperiencing the trauma could occur in the form of a flashback in the physician's office. A more avoidant victim may shun visiting the doctor's office completely. Hyperarousal may come to the physician's attention in the form of an exaggerated startle response, hypervigilance, or complaints of difficulties with sleep or concentration. Other effects of assault that may come to the health care provider's attention are stress-related disorders such as headaches, muscle tension, asthma, temporomandibular joint dysfunction, or functional gastrointestinal disorders. Sexual dysfunction or a history of early or repeated pregnancy is another possible indicator.

A patient with a sexually transmitted disease, particularly if her history is inconsistent with its acquisition, may have been infected during rape. In addition, the physician might notice a negative reaction to touch or see scars or injuries that reveal self-mutilation. Research indicates that there is a greater reporting of symptoms and use of health care among women with histories of physical or sexual abuse, or both, and that referred patients with chronic pain and functional gastrointestinal disorders frequently have abuse histories.[24, 25] Therefore, when patients manifest or present with vague symptoms that defy diagnosis, a history of sexual assault or other trauma should be explored.

Behavioral and emotional signs may also be present to alert the physician to prior sexual assault. These would include substance abuse, suicide attempts, and eating disorders. The latter can include bulimia, anorexia, or compulsive overeating. Emotional signs that may become evident to the physician are hypervigilance about physical symptoms, emotional numbing (obvious through a significant lack of affect), or dissociation. This can be subtle but is sometimes discerned by a patient's glazed eyes and limited responsiveness to the current situation. Other emotional complaints may be depression, phobias, or panic disorder.

Because sexual assault affects a woman's health significantly, it is important for the physician to have information about her history. Most women do not volunteer such information for a variety of reasons. They may not be aware that it is useful information for their health care providers. They may fear retribution from their assailants or be otherwise influenced, even years later, by the manner in which they were silenced when assaulted. They might fear being stigmatized or blamed and may well have had painful experiences with previous disclosures. Therefore, if the physician suspects a trauma history, direct, broadly phrased questions about such experiences should be asked.

A useful routine question is, ''Do you have any particular concerns about safety, modesty, or pain?'' The question elicits important information, whatever the source of the concerns. If there are past traumas, the patient need not mention them to make her physician aware of her concern. If the woman does indicate concerns and the physician wants further information and has time for discussion, other questions could be asked. ''Have you ever been raped?'' may elicit negative answers from women who do not define their experience as such, even for themselves. Instead, ''Have you had any sexual encounters when you didn't want to or because you were forced, threatened with force, or felt you had to?'' opens a wide range of experiences for discussion.

A woman may be suffering from the effects of a sexual relationship to which she consented but from which she should have been protected by professional boundaries. Physicians, psychotherapists, clergy, and others in the helping professions have a responsibility to (1) recognize that the patient role, heavy with transference, need, and relative lack of power, does not allow for free consent to a romatic or sexual relationship with the caregiver and (2) maintain their ability to make professional judgments in the patient's best interest by keeping the relationship on a strictly professional level. Asking about these cases is sensitive because, similar to cases involving incest, the woman might feel very special for having received such attention, may have received sexual pleasure, may have a strong desire to protect the perpetrator, and could be unaware that what occurred was the cause of the symptoms that followed. ''Has a caregiver with whom you had a professional relationship ever had a sexual relationship with you?'' may need to be asked quite directly. The physician has to determine when to elicit such information. It is important to understand the potential severity and consequences that can result from such abuse. The patient may need someone who can identify this problem for her.

Despite carefully worded inquiries, a woman may be unable to say ''yes'' the first time she is asked any of these questions. It is entirely appropriate to ask again at a later time, when the patient may be more prepared to respond. Whatever question is used, it is vital to listen to the answers that follow and to continue to offer respect, belief, and acceptance.

MANAGEMENT ISSUES

Several things should be borne in mind when interacting with a woman who has been sexually assaulted. It is important to approach her with a willingness to believe what she says, to accept her story as the truth about what happened to her and its effects on her. Until very recently, most disclosures of incest were met with disbelief, and most adult victims were blamed for the attack. It is painful to be aware of the prevalence of sexual assault and the scope of the devastation it causes and to be reminded of one's own vulnerability in the world. But to provide adequate care for patients, caregivers must be willing to confront these realities. Extra effort to create an alliance may be especially important with such a patient because her sense of the basic goodness of other people has been severely damaged.

The patient may engage in behaviors that make

it difficult for her doctor to establish a professional relationship. The degree of difficulty the patient creates in establishing the doctor-patient relationship is often directly proportional to the trauma she has experienced. Although her behaviors may not be reasonable in the current context, at an earlier time in her life these behaviors were sensible and useful for her well-being.

It is best to refrain from making assumptions about how the trauma has affected the patient. There is quite a wide range of reactions to assault, and each patient must be regarded as the expert on her own. Each woman experienced a particular trauma in the context of her unique life history and personality and will experience a singular response and recovery, despite commonalities shared with others who have been abused. However, the woman may not recognize the connection between her assault and some or all of her symptoms. Furthermore, although the patient must be allowed to make her own assessment of the damage that has been done to her, the doctor should remember that a victim often minimizes. Finally, victims of sexual assault have a tendency to blame themselves. It is vital for health care providers to keep firmly in mind that no behavior on the part of the victim justifies rape. If a woman places herself in dangerous circumstances or dresses or behaves provocatively, she may need to examine and change those behaviors. However, these behaviors in no way remove responsibility for the crime from the perpetrator.

Physical examination of patients with sexual assault histories must be handled sensitively. Considerations like those described earlier for an examination immediately after rape should be kept in mind. Especially during gynecologic examination the physician should explain each step of the examination and receive permission before doing it. The patient may prefer to forgo the use of a drape and to have her head and torso inclined so that she can see what the physician is doing. She should be offered the opportunity to be accompanied by a support person if she wishes. The physician must offer the patient the possibility of stopping the examination at any point and must comply immediately with that request if it is made.

There are times when the physician should make a referral for psychological services, and there are several elements to making such a referral. The physician should recognize when it is appropriate, suggest it to the patient, and explain why the referral is being made and what the patient might gain from it. Referral for psychological treatment is in order when a history of assault is acknowledged and the patient is distraught when discussing it or if the patient describes somatic symptoms characteristic of stress (e.g., temporomandibular joint dysfunction, irritable bowel) or psychiatric symptoms (e.g., disrupted sleep, difficulty concentrating).

When a patient refuses a mental health referral, the physician should respect her autonomy but not be reluctant to attempt to make the referral again in the future. Reading can be very beneficial for many people and may be attractive because it is private, inexpensive, and accessible. A popular book on the topic is *The Courage to Heal: A Guide for Women Survivors of Child Sexual Abuse*, by Ellen Bass and Laura Davis, published by Harper & Row in 1988. The book is written for those assaulted in childhood, but some of the recommendations apply equally to adult victims. Although it has received deserved criticism for its position on identifying women as incest survivors based on rather generic symptoms, it can nevertheless serve as a useful tool for women who have been assaulted and are not yet ready to talk about it. Bibliotherapy can provide support for the internal preparation to proceed with other types of treatment. Another way for a woman to get information while maintaining her sense of privacy is to write to or call any of the following organizations:

Incest Survivor Information Exchange (ISIE)
P.O. Box 3399
New Haven CT 06515

VOICES in Action, Inc.
P.O. Box 148309
Chicago IL 60614

Incest Resources
46 Pleasant Street
Cambridge MA 02139

Bay Area Women Against Rape
(510) 465-3890

REFERENCES

1. Koss MP, Koss PG, Woodruff WJ. Deleterious effects of criminal victimization of women's health and medical utilization. Arch Intern Med 1991;151:342.
2. Youngstrom N. Grim news from national study of rape. Am Psychol Assoc Monitor 1992;23(7):38.
3. Koss MP, Gidycz CA, Wisniewski N. The scope of rape: Incidence and prevalence of sexual aggression and victimization in a national sample of higher education students. J Consult Clin Psychol 1987;55(2):162.
4. Ryback VR, Lichter E, Diamond A. Guidelines for the care of female-male rape patients. Unpublished manuscript, Rape Crisis Intervention Program, Beth Israel Hospital, Boston, Mass.
5. Herman JL. Trauma and Recovery. New York: Basic Books, 1992.
6. Beebe DK. Emergency management of the adult female rape victim. Am Fam Physician 1991;43:2041.

7. Commonwealth of Massachusetts Sexual Assault Evidence Collection Kit Instructions.

8. Koss MP. Rape: Scope, impact, interventions, and public policy responses. Am Psychol 1993;48(10):1062.

9. Kilpatrick DG, Veronen LJ, Best CL. Factors predicting psychological distress among rape victims. In: Figley CR (ed). Trauma and Its Wake. New York: Brunner/Mazel, 1985, pp 113–141.

10. Burnam MA, Stein JA, Golding JM, et al. Sexual assault and mental disorders in a community population. J Consult Clin Psychol 1988;56(6):843.

11. Ruch LO, Chandler SM. Sexual assault trauma during the acute phase: An exploratory model and multivariate analysis. J Health Soc Behav 1983;24:174.

12. Kilpatrick DG. The sexual assault research project: Assessing the aftermath of rape. Response. J Center Women Policy Studies 1985;8:20.

13. Veronen LJ, Kilpatrick DG. Stress management for rape victims. In: Meichenbaum D, Jaremko ME (eds). Stress Reduction and Prevention. New York: Plenum, 1983, pp 341–374.

14. American Psychiatric Association. Diagnostic and Statistic Manual of Mental Disorders. 3rd ed., rev. Washington, DC: American Psychiatric Association, 1987.

15. Briere J. Therapy for Adults Molested as Children: Beyond Survival. New York: Springer, 1989.

16. Courtois CA. Healing the Incest Wound: Adult Survivors in Therapy. New York: WW Norton & Co, 1988.

17. Burgess AW, Holmstrom LL. Rape: Sexual disruption and recovery. Am J Orthopsychiatry 1979:49(4):648.

18. Van der Kolk BA, Greenberg MS. The psychobiology of trauma response: Hyperarousal, constriction, and addiction to traumatic reexposure. In: van der Kolk BA (ed). Psychological Trauma. Washington, DC: American Psychiatric Press, 1987, pp 63–87.

19. McCann IL, Pearlman LA. Psychological Trauma and the Adult Survivor: Theory, Therapy, and Transformation. New York: Brunner/Mazel, 1990.

20. Kilpatrick DG, Best CL, Veronen LJ, et al. Mental health correlates of criminal victimization: A random community survey. J Consult Clin Psychol 1985;53:866.

21. Ellis EM, Atkeson BM, Calhoun KS. An assessment of long-term reactions to rape. J Abnorm Psychol 1981;90(3):263.

22. Carmen E, Rieker PP, Mills T. Victims of violence and psychiatric illness. Am J Psychiatry 1984:141(3):378.

23. Lazare A. Shame and humiliation in the medical encounter. Arch Intern Med 1987;147:1653.

24. Grossman DA, Leserman J, Nachman G, et al. Sexual and physical abuse in women with functional or organic gastrointestinal disorders. Ann Intern Med 1990;113:828.

25. Koss MP, Woodruff WJ, Koss PG. Relation of criminal victimization to health perceptions among women medical patients. J Consult Clin Psychol 1990;58(2):147.

Domestic Violence

Karen M. Freund

Violence within the context of an intimate relationship has long been denied and ignored by society. Through the work of the women's movement and women in allied health and law-related fields, the problems of coercion, physical assault, and threats have become well known to the public. In many areas of the United States, homicides and assaults previously labeled as isolated problems, mutual arguments, or problems of a jealous partner are now acknowledged as part of a continuum of violence within the relationship.

Until recently, little was written in the medical literature on domestic violence. The field was one of family psychologists, social workers, and nonmedical health advocates. Now members of the medical profession have begun to see the needs of women who are threatened and assaulted by intimate partners to be a problem within the realm of medical care.

SCOPE OF THE PROBLEM

Domestic violence can be defined as intentional violent behavior by a person who is currently or has previously been in an intimate relationship with the victim. Spouse abuse, partner violence, battering, and wife beating are some other terms that have been used to describe this syndrome, each acknowledging the breadth of intimate relationships that may be involved, from dating relationships, in which the partners live separately, to married couples, who live at the same residence.

For this discussion, domestic violence encompasses actual physical assault by an intimate partner. These assaults are rarely isolated and are usually part of a constellation. This may include threats of death or physical injury to the woman or other family members, sexual assault or coerced sexual activity, economic control, verbal abuse, and progressive social isolation.

Data on the extent of domestic assault in our society are staggering. Data from anonymous telephone surveys indicate that 20 to 25% of all women have at one time been physically assaulted by an intimate partner.[1-3] By these estimates, between 2 and 4 million women are assaulted by intimate partners each year in the United States. The data on the prevalence of domestic violence among women seen in the clinical setting suggest that these women are more likely to seek out medical care than other women.[4] Several surveys within emergency department settings suggest that one in three women who present for care, including women presenting with medical complaints as opposed to those presenting for care of acute injuries, are victims of violence.[5-7] Those seeking emergency psychiatric care are overrepresented by violence victims, with as many as one in four women who attempt suicide reporting past intimate violence.[8] Among women seeking routine primary care, it is estimated that 10 to 15% report a history of domestic violence, with one third of these women having ongoing issues involving their safety.[9] Pregnant women also report high rates of violence, with as many as 4 to 24% of women presenting for prenatal care acknowledging violence if asked.[10-12] The mothers of abused children also constitute a high-risk group, with half of these mothers themselves in violent relationships.[13]

Women who appear to be at the greatest risk of violence within a relationship are younger women and women with mental or physical disabilities. Of note, violence against women is not more common among the racial minorities and the economically disadvantaged, although the perception that domestic violence predominates in these groups often results in selective inquiry by providers to their patients and thereby reinforces this stereotype. One practice with patients who were primarily upper middle class, educated, employed women found no differences in violence rates by race or education of the victim.[9]

DYNAMICS OF INTERPERSONAL VIOLENCE

Attempts to understand domestic violence by the study of its victims has been limited, as it tells little about the perpetrator of these violent acts.

Men who assault their partners often appear to be normal, without difficulty with violence or impulse control in other realms of their lives. This apparent normality of the perpetrator leads to much of the disbelief of the existence or the seriousness of the problem in our society. The majority of perpetrators are not mentally ill and do not exhibit the lack of impulse control and general violent behavior in other settings, as would be seen with most sociopathic personalities.

The dynamic issues for the perpetrator are not impulsiveness, loss of control, or a generalized tendency toward violence. The aim of the violent behavior is to assert and maintain power and control over one's partner. This may begin insidiously at the beginning of the relationship as jealousy of other relationships and pressure to limit other social contacts. Often young women have been taught to interpret such excess jealousy as affection rather than as a control issue. This is accompanied by economic control that prevents a woman from working outside the home or retaining any personal financial assets and continual scrutiny of her actions while at work or outside the home. Interactions with friends and family may become so uncomfortable that these potentially supportive persons in time lose touch with the victim and interpret her partner's behavior as her desire to sever relationships. Assaults and threats of assaults are then part of the coercion and control within the relationship. In at least half of all cases, threats or attempts to kill his partner are part of the control.[9] Threats of harm to prized possessions such as photographs or pets or threats against children or other family members are common. Sexual assault is also common. The pattern of violence is usually not relentless but may be cyclic, followed by behavior that appears to be apologetic and conciliatory in nature. However, even this conciliatory behavior is often coercive, including coerced intercourse in order to "make up." Violence tends to escalate over time, increasing in severity.

Drugs and alcohol may be a part of the general pattern of violence in as many as half of all cases; however, the relation to the assaults may be complex. In only a minority of cases is the violence a direct result of intoxication, and removing the alcohol or drug problem generally does not resolve the violence. More often, women report that partners would either drink at times when they planned on assaulting them or, in spite of an alcohol problem, only batter them when sober. Treatment of the alcohol problem in most cases does not address the violence and will not lead to its decrease, as the same control issues are still present for the perpetrator.[14] Although some data indicate that substance and alcohol abuse problems are more prevalent among victims of domestic violence,[15] at least one longitudinal review of emergency department records suggests that when alcoholism is a problem for the woman, it is preceded by violence rather than being a cause of the violence.[7]

OBSTACLES TO LEAVING

When the dynamics of domestic violence are viewed within the context of progressive exertion of power and control, with loss of autonomy and social isolation on the part of the victim, the obstacles that make it difficult for women to leave become comprehensible.

FEAR. Women are at the greatest risk of assault and homicide when they try to leave a violent relationship. Often women are threatened with the loss of their lives or the lives of their children and family if they attempt to flee. Homicide data indicate that most completed homicides are in the context of the woman trying to leave the relationship. The safety of the woman and her dependents is foremost among the reasons women often continue to tolerate intolerable abuse.

ECONOMIC CONSTRAINTS. To the extent that the perpetrator is successful in controlling the financial resources of the family, the woman has difficulty finding the necessary cash, credit cards, and other resources necessary to escape. For some women, even making plans to escape, such as telephone calls to arrange for shelter or for a cab, are difficult. This problem becomes much more acute for the woman with dependent children. To gather the resources to sustain a number of people can be difficult. Case examples testify to the problem, including a woman who chose to remain in a relationship for several years until she could save first month's rent and a security deposit before she moved her children out of their home. Without sufficient financial resources, many women fear that the dangers of homeless shelters or living on the street or at the mercy of charity may be more dangerous than the known and more predictable dangers at home.

SOCIAL ISOLATION. To the extent that the woman has become isolated from friends and family members, support for the practical necessities of leaving may be lacking. The availability of a friend or family member who will provide housing decreases not only with the potential threats against those providing such help but also with the reality that this entails housing and safekeeping for children.

ATTACHMENT TO THE PERPETRATOR. Herman describes the similarities of chronically abused women and hostages or prisoners of war.[16] Both are left socially isolated and often rely on their abuser as the sole source of their own emotional support. This problem is compounded for the battered woman as she chose the support within the relationship. This reliance on support and connection with the abuser can lead the woman to listen to her partner's admonitions about her behavior and question her own self-worth, ultimately making the self-reliance to leave difficult. The success of peer support groups is in part attributed to the improvement in self-esteem and development of outside supports.

PRESENTATION OF DOMESTIC VIOLENCE VICTIMS IN PRIMARY CARE

Unlike in the emergency setting, where many women present with acute injuries, women presenting to their primary care provider rarely have stigmata to identify them as abuse victims. However, many women present with a medical concern that has some relation to the abuse or previous assaults.

Evidence of an injury in which care was delayed or complications of an unattended injury should raise concern about abuse, including old fractures, infected burns, or unattended lacerations. The perpetrator may initially deny the seriousness of the injuries or fear that the cause of the injury will be discovered if she seeks help.

Women presenting with chronic pain syndromes and chronic somatic complaints are more likely to be victims of domestic violence. Evidence from a number of clinical studies in various populations has documented that domestic violence victims are more likely to present to chronic pain clinics with chronic pelvic pain, irritable or nonorganic bowel disease, headaches, hearing loss, and other neurologic concerns.[17–22] These complaints may represent somatic manifestations of depression and anxiety disorders or may reflect sequelae of previous trauma, including pelvic pain from sexual assault and neurologic complaints related to repeated head trauma. Such women may present with concerns that previous trauma has caused permanent damage, and, although not volunteering the full nature of the problem, may be looking for such information.

Patients may also present with symptoms of psychological illness. Most common among these are posttraumatic stress disorder, with hyperarousability, sleep disorder, palpitations, hyperventilation, and generalized anxiety.[23] This syndrome, first described in war veterans who faced the stress of battle combat, can affect anyone experiencing a life-threatening trauma, particularly a repeated one. These patients may present predominantly with their somatic concerns to a physician, with or without an understanding of the potential relation of their complaint to the abuse they have suffered. Women may also present with other psychiatric disorders, including depression, anxiety disorders, and previous suicide attempts.[24–26]

Alcohol and substance abuse deserve special mention. Alcohol abuse by the perpetrator is related to the violence in a complex fashion; however, alcohol abuse by the victim usually follows the onset of violence.[7] Therefore, rather than alcoholism in the victim being related to the dynamic of the abuse, it appears to be a maladaptive coping mechanism in severely abused women.

Pregnancy may be a condition when violence is more prevalent. Whether this reflects the fact that younger women are at greater risk or that issues of control become more acute in the setting of pregnancy is under debate. Women who present for prenatal care late in pregnancy should be questioned carefully about violence.

INTERVIEWING WOMEN ABOUT DOMESTIC VIOLENCE

Given the high prevalence of violence in our society across all social and economic groups and the lack of specific indicators of abuse based on history and physical examination, asking all patients as part of a routine periodic review of systems about violence is the only effective means of adequately detecting this problem. Women acknowledge that it is difficult to initiate discussion about partner violence, even with a trusted provider, but most are willing to discuss violence if asked by a physician.[27] In one study, 97% of women patients new to a practice were willing to respond to a question about domestic violence when asked as part of a history questionnaire.[9]

Interviews about violence and safety issues should always occur in private, away from any family members, including children and partners, no matter how caring the relationship appears. A single question can significantly improve detection of domestic violence as a problem. One should ask directly about violent behaviors. Asking general questions such as, "How are things at home?" may be useful to introduce the topic but are not sufficient to elicit a story of violence from most women. Because most women who have been assaulted by their partners do not define themselves as battered or abused, avoid using such personal descriptions. In one study, the addition of the single question "At any time, has a partner ever hit you, kicked you, or otherwise hurt you?'' improved identification from 0 to 12% of all new patients presenting to the practice.[9] Additional or repeated questioning at follow-up examinations may be useful for some patients when clinical suspicion is high, as some patients may be better able to disclose such information once further trust in their provider is established.

Once a woman acknowledges violence as a problem, specific information should be asked to assess the nature, scope, timing and duration, and severity of past threats and assaults (Table 70–1). Determining who is the perpetrator, their relationship, and their living arrangements is essential. Asking a woman to describe the first, the most recent, and the most serious episodes of violence allows one to gather data on how long the violence has been occurring, whether it is an ongoing problem, and whether threats or assaults are escalating in intensity. This inquiry allows the woman to piece together her story, especially women who are discussing the problem for the first time. Asking about medical care after assaults and about threats and attempts on the patient's life or on the lives of others in the family, particularly children, is difficult but provides crucial information.

In addition to a description of the violence, inquiry about steps taken to try to deal with the problem can help in terms of later safety plans.

TABLE 70–1. History Protocol for Domestic Violence

Screening questions of all patients
When you have arguments at home, what happens?
Has a partner every hit you, kicked you, or otherwise physically hurt or frightened you?
If response to these questions indicates violence in the relationship:
Who is hurting you?
Where does he live? With you?
How long has this been going on?
Describe the first, most recent, and worst time he hurt you.
What types of injuries have you had? Did you get medical help for them?
Has anyone else in the family been hurt?
Risk assessment
Has he tried to kill you?
Has he threatened to kill you?
Does he own a gun? have a criminal record?
Do you feel it's safe to go home now?
Safety planning
Who knows about this?
What steps have you taken to keep yourself safe?
　　Called police
　　Obtained restraining order
　　Called battered women's shelter
Do you know where to get legal advice and help?
If you needed to flee suddenly, where could you go?

Asking about use of protection or restraining orders, calls to police, or use of hotlines informs the physician of her knowledge of potential resources available in the community and her potential personal resources in terms of friends and family.

PHYSICAL EXAMINATION

Within most ambulatory settings, women do not present with acute injuries. However, women may present evidence of injury that did not require or receive acute medical care. Documentation of location of contusions or other evidence of trauma can be crucial in the future if the woman decides to prosecute. When injuries are not consistent with the patient's explanation or when there are multiple or bilateral injuries or delay in seeking care for the injury, these findings should be documented in the medical record and discussed in private with the patient. For the woman who seems reluctant to reveal the nature of the injury, acknowledgment by the provider that the history is inconsistent and that abused women may be afraid to discuss the problem may lead her to disclose the information at a later time.

RISK ASSESSMENT

Just as suicidal patients may be at risk of death from their own hands, the patient who is the victim of abuse from her partner may be at risk of homicide, and this risk requires assessment. In the case of the suicidal patient, details of specific plans as well as the patient's ability to agree not to carry them out are obtained. When the patient is a victim, one can discuss specific plans and threats by her partner to establish her potential risk. Women may minimize or deny the danger and benefit from the reflection and concern of an outside party. Women at increased risk of further serious injury or homicide are those who report an increase in the frequency or severity of assaults, an increase or new threats of homicide or suicide by their partner, and the availability of a firearm. The woman's own level of fear, even in the absence of these other factors, should also lead to concern regarding her increased risk.

INTERVENTION

Although the ultimate goal of intervention in domestic violence is to ensure the safety of the patient, this is not a task that can be undertaken unilaterally by the physician. Recognition of this fact is crucial to prevent physicians from becoming discouraged and disillusioned when the patient does not immediately leave her abusive partner or returns to him after a time. Domestic violence is a social problem that requires choices on the part of the victim and resources from multiple systems in the community and from the criminal justice system. However, physicians can play a critical role in identifying battered women who come to their offices and in providing support and access to the available community resources.

The goal of intervention by the physician is to communicate concern about the victim's welfare and provide for her a framework to seek out the resources she requires. It is her decision on how and when to make changes in her life that may ensure her safety. Although the impulse is often to do everything possible to prevent any risk of injury, such efforts can often in themselves be coercive to the patient and not provide her with a model of independent decision-making that she needs to escape the abusive relationship.

Informing a patient directly about your concerns for her safety can do much in a trusting patient-physician relationship to provide an alternative understanding of her situation. It is important to reinforce that domestic violence is a common problem, that she holds no responsibility for another person's violence, and that intentional assault, even by a partner, is unacceptable and criminal behavior.

Referral for counseling can be important but requires knowledge of resources in the community. Legal assistance and support within self-help groups or from battered women's advocates are avenues most likely to directly address the necessary issues of safety. For many victims of long-standing abuse, symptoms of depression, anxiety, and posttraumatic stress disorder may warrant referral for psychiatric assessment. However, to make such a referral the prime focus of intervention may have the unintended effect of reinforcing the false notion that the problem lies in the patient's psyche and not in the perpetrator's behavior.

Discussion of safer sex practices to prevent sexually transmitted diseases and unintended pregnancy is critical and requires that the provider explore whether sexual contact is coerced or forced. Screening and treatment for sexually transmitted diseases and counseling about contraceptive methods that do not require the partner's consent, including oral contraceptives, long-acting progesterone agents, female condoms, and postcoital contraception, may be useful.

SAFETY PLAN

Discussing a safety plan reinforces to the patient the provider's concern and sense of urgency and allows the patient to contemplate and plan for future action that she might take. Such initial planning might include referral to agencies that can more thoroughly advise her of her legal rights and the procedures necessary to obtain protective orders or to obtain an arrest. This should include phone numbers for battered women's shelters. Planning needs to be directed at practical issues: where she might go (family, friends, shelter), what resources she has for leaving (extra car keys, money for cab), and her access to resources required to live (own finances, clothing, medications, and important documents). This planning does not commit her to any specific course of action but provides her with information to make choices.

BARRIERS TO CARE

There are many barriers to the care of victims of domestic violence. A series of ethnographic interviews with primary care providers described a number of these barriers.[28] Physicians described inquiry about violence as "opening Pandora's box," unearthing a number of evils that they are uncomfortable with and ill-equipped to handle. Physicians reported feeling powerless and inadequate and without the resources to assist victims. Often these feelings are accompanied by a sense that the tools of medical care cannot stop violent behavior directly, and consequently their involvement in the situation is useless. Physicians cited frustration at their lack of control over the situation, and they viewed their patients as uncooperative when they did not leave a violent situation. Physicians cited fear of offending both patients and their partners in inquiring about domestic violence. Physicians have voiced concern that this is not a legitimate area of concern for physicians to probe and may be offensive to patients, with some physicians even suggesting that broaching the subject would damage the patient's trust in her physician.

Identification with one's patient or the lack thereof can have profound effects on one's willingness to accept violence as a possible problem. A patient of their own socioeconomic status may cause physicians to be reluctant to acknowledge domestic violence. As a result, women of higher socioeconomic status are often ignored and disbelieved by health care providers. Alternatively, women of color or women of lower economic means may be asked about domestic violence more readily. Although this may result in higher detection rates in some groups, viewing the problem as one of race and class may narrow the provider's view of interventions.

The last barrier often cited by providers is the lack of time and compensation to the primary provider who deals with this and other psychosocial issues. However, an alternative argument can be made that ignorance of these issues in the long run may delay and increase the cost of diagnosing complaints. Difficult cases may be less time consuming to the provider if the problems are dealt with in a direct manner.

DEFINING LOCAL RESOURCES

Legal and support services are locally based and require that providers seek out listings of these resources for their patients. A previously available national hotline number has been discontinued owing to lack of federal funding, although federal funding to reinstitute it has since been appropriated. Table 70–2 provides current contact numbers for each state.

Laws against violence within relationships vary from state to state. Domestic violence is a criminal offense in all states. The civil remedies of protection or restraining orders to prevent contact vary from state to state regarding availability, how they are obtained in emergency situations, and who may use them. Restraining orders have no standing outside the state in which they are issued, although a recently introduced bill is trying to establish a nationwide enforcement system. Battered women's shelters exist in nearly all locales within the United States. The network of shelters established by lay persons during the 1960s was one of the first services available to women. The locations of shelters remain confidential. Sufficient availability of beds, especially for women with dependent children, has been a problem with the loss of federal funding over the past decade.

The shelter system also provides support groups to women. These allow women to develop a network of relationships outside the abusive home, to

---

TABLE 70–2. Reference Phone Numbers by State for Domestic Violence Coalitions or Shelters

STATE	COALITION	24-HR SHELTER OR HOTLINE	STATE	COALITION	24-HR SHELTER OR HOTLINE
Alabama		(205) 793-5214*	Montana		(800) 834-8296
Alaska	(907) 586-3650		Nebraska	(402) 476-6256	(402) 475-7273*
Arizona	(602) 836-1239	(800) 352-3792	Nevada	(702) 358-1171	
Arkansas	(501) 663-4668	(800) 332-4443	New Hampshire	(603) 224-8893	(800) 852-3388
California		(415) 924-6616	New Jersey	(609) 584-8107	(800) 572-7233
Spanish (not 24 hr)		(415) 924-3456	New Mexico	(505) 247-4219	(800) 773-3645
Colorado	(303) 322-1831		New York		
Connecticut	(203) 524-5890		English		(800) 942-6906
Delaware		(302) 762-6110	Spanish		(800) 942-6908
District of Columbia		(202) 529-5991	New York City		(212) 274-3209
Florida		(305) 547-3170*	North Carolina		(919) 828-7740*
Georgia	(404) 524-3847	(404) 688-9436*	North Dakota	(701) 255-6240	(800) 472-2911
		(912) 234-9999*	Ohio	(614) 221-1255	(800) 934-9840
Hawaii	(808) 595-6370		Oklahoma		(800) 522-7233
Idaho		(208) 263-1241	Oregon	(503) 239-4486	(503) 235-5333*
Illinois	(217) 789-2830		Pennsylvania	(717) 545-6400	
Indiana	(317) 643-0200	(800) 332-7385	Rhode Island	(401) 723-3051	(401) 861-2760*
Iowa	(515) 281-7284	(800) 942-0333	South Carolina		(803) 531-6211*
Kansas	(316) 232-2757	(913) 841-6887*	South Dakota		(605) 224-7187*
Kentucky	(502) 875-4132		Tennessee	(615) 327-0805	(615) 297-8833*
Louisiana	(504) 389-3001	(800) 541-9706	Texas		(214) 941-1991*
Maine		(800) 537-6066*	Utah		(800) 893-LINK
Maryland		(410) 889-RUTH*	Vermont	(802) 223-1302	
Massachusetts	(617) 426-8492	(800) 992-2600	Virginia	(802) 221-0990	(800) 838-8238
Michigan		(800) JANE-DOE	Washington	(206) 352-4029	(800) 562-6025
Minnesota	(612) 646-6177	(612) 646-0994	West Virginia	(304) 765-2250	(800) 352-6513
Mississippi		(601) 435-1968	Wisconsin	(608) 255-0539	
Missouri	(314) 634-4161	(800) 548-2480*	Wyoming		(307) 235-2814*

Note: There is currently no national hotline number, but legislation and funding efforts to reinstate one are under way. Many states have one single crisis number; however, most are a coalition of shelters, each with its own 24-hr crisis line.

*One of a number of shelters in the state that provide 24-hr service; no statewide number.

reestablish self-esteem, and to benefit from the experience of others who have left similarly dangerous relationships. They can often be of great help to women in defining the problem and should be offered to all women in violent relationships, whether or not they feel ready to make changes in their lives.

REPORTING

Reporting laws on violent acts vary from state to state. In general, no state has mandatory reporting requirements when the victim is a competent adult, although some states require reporting of all firearm or stabbing injuries. Most states have reporting requirements when victims are minors, and many have reporting requirements when the victims are elderly or disabled.

Ultimately, domestic violence is a community problem, and the extent to which our society tolerates or condones such violence plays a large role in its occurrence. As respected professionals, physicians can play a role in advocating for their patients and supporting legislation to provide services and resources for victims and appropriate remedies within the judicial system.

REFERENCES

1. Straus M, Gelles R, Steinmetz SK. Behind Closed Doors: A Survey of Family Violence in America. New York: Doubleday, 1980.
2. Schulman MA. Survey of spousal violence against women in Kentucky. Harris Study #792801, 1979.
3. Szinovacz ME. Using couple data as a methodological tool: The case of marital violence. J Marriage Fam 1983;45:63.
4. Koss MP, Koss PG, Woodruff WJ. Deleterious effects of criminal victimization on women's health and medical utilization. Arch Intern Med 1991;151:342.
5. Goldberg WG, Tomlanovich MC. Domestic violence victims in the emergency department. JAMA 1984;251:3259.
6. McLeer SV, Anwar R. A study of battered women presenting in an emergency department. Am J Public Health 1989;79:65.
7. Stark E, Flitcraft A, Frazier W. Medicine and patriarchal violence: The social construction of a ''private'' event. Int J Health Serv 1979;9:461.
8. Carlile JB. Spouse assault on mentally disordered wives. Can J Psychiatry 1991;36:265.
9. Freund KM, Blackhall LS. Detection of domestic violence in a primary care setting. Clin Res 1990;38:738A.
10. McFarlane J. Battering during pregnancy: Tip of an iceberg revealed. Women Health 1989;15:69.
11. Helton AS, McFarlane J, Anderson ET. Battered and pregnant: A prevalence study. Am J Public Health 1987; 77:1337.
12. Hillard PJA. Physical abuse in pregnancy. Obstet Gynecol 1985;66:185.
13. McKibben L, DeVos E, Newberger EH. Victimization of mothers of abused children: A controlled study. Pediatrics 1989;84:531.
14. Gorney B. Domestic violence and chemical dependency: Dual problems, dual interventions. J Psychoactive Drugs 1989;21:229.
15. Kantor GK, Straus MA. Substance abuse as a precipitant of wife abuse victimizations. Am J Drug Alcohol Abuse 1989;15:173.
16. Herman JL. Trauma and Recovery. New York: Basic Books, 1992.
17. Schei B. Physically abusive spouse—A risk factor of pelvic inflammatory disease? Scand J Prim Health Care 1991;9:41.
18. Rapkin AJ, Kames LD, Darke LL, et al. History of physical and sexual abuse in women with chronic pelvic pain. Obstet Gynecol 1990;76:92.
19. Drossman DA, Leserman J, Nachman G, et al. Sexual and physical abuse in women with functional or organic gastrointestinal disorders. Ann Intern Med 1990;113:828.
20. Schei B. Psycho-social factor in pelvic pain:. A controlled study of women living in physically abusive relationships. Acta Obstet Gynecol Scand 1990;69:67.
21. Haber JD, Roos C. Effects of spouse abuse and/or sexual abuse in the development and maintenance of chronic pain in women Pain 1984;2:5187.
22. Schei B, Bakketeig LS. Gynaecological impact of sexual and physical abuse by spouse. A study of a random sample of Norwegian women. Brit J Obstet Gynecol 1989; 96:1379.
23. West CG, Fernandez A, Hillare JR, et al. Psychiatric disorders of abused women in a shelter. Psychiatr Q 1990;61:295.
24. Jaffe P, Wolfe DA, Wilson S, Zak L. Emotional and physical health problems of battered women. Can J Psychiatr 1986;31:625.
25. Kilpratick DG, Best CL, Veronene LJ, et al. Mental health correlates of criminal victimization: A random community survey. J Consult Clin Psychol 1985;53:886.
26. Bergman B, Brismar B. Suicide attempts by battered wives. Acta Psychiatr Scand 1991;83:380.
27. Friedman LS, Samet JH, Roberts MS, et al. Inquiry about victimization experiences: A survey of patient preferences and physician practices. Arch Intern Med 1992;152:1186.
28. Sugg NK, Inui R. Primary care physicians' response to domestic violence: Opening Pandora's box. JAMA 1992;267:3157.

PSYCHOLOGICAL ISSUES

71

Depression in the Primary Care Setting

B. Jeanne Horner

There is a significantly higher rate of depressive disorders in women. In a 1988 study by Barrett and colleagues, it was found that women were 10 times as likely to have symptoms suggestive of depression.[1] Likewise, women outnumbered men 2:1 with diagnosable depressive disorders. Although many epidemiologic studies suggest that women are twice as likely to develop major depression, a more recent study found that men and women had equal prevalence rates for major depression using criteria listed in the fourth edition of the *Diagnostic and Statistical Manual of Mental Disorders* (DSM-IV), but that women outnumbered men by 11.2:1.0 in all other categories of clinically significant depressive disorders.[2] More important, one in 10 women is at risk for developing a depressive disorder at some point in her lifetime. Numerous theories have attempted to account for this, and it is likely that the reasons are multifactorial.

Research into women's psychological development reports significant differences from traditional psychoanalytic theories of development. Current theories suggest that women develop their sense of self through their relationships and connections with others.[3, 4] Women and girls tend to focus much of their energy on the maintenance of relationships. They have a drive to nurture others and attempt to relate on a more affectual level. Because these traits are not highly valued within traditional society, women and girls may be at risk for valuing themselves less highly as well. Psychodynamically, depression is most often associated with the experience of loss, inhibition of anger and aggression, inhibition of action or assertiveness, and low self-esteem.[5]

Examination of the effects of marital status on rates of major depression have shown that marriage has a protective effect on men. However, rates of mental illness are higher in married women and lower in single, divorced, and widowed women. Further exploration revealed that this effect was decreased when women worked outside the home and when they reported having a confiding relationship with their husband.[6] These findings suggest that women experience the inability to maintain an empathic relationship with their spouse as a loss. This is especially significant if a woman is also feeling socially isolated because she must remain at home to provide child care or because she is involuntarily unemployed.

Despite the strides that the women's movement has made in providing more opportunities for women, real economic and social inequalities continue to exist.[6] Anger is a frequent result of the sense of powerlessness that women may experience within their social or occupational roles. Yet the expression of anger is frequently inhibited socially as well as interpersonally by the fear of disrupting important relationships.[5] This tendency to hold back the expression of anger may also lead to feeling disempowered and helpless, which can further erode one's self-esteem. As social change has occurred, women's expectations for themselves have increased, and this may lead to further intrapsychic conflict or frustration when the likelihood of making their aspirations real is inhibited.[6] Thus, in addition to any potential biologic predisposition to experience affective symptoms, women also seem to be at risk because of conflicting social, cultural, and intrapersonal values.

IMPORTANCE OF IDENTIFYING DEPRESSION

In the community, depressive symptoms reported via self-rating scales are estimated to have a prevalence of 13 to 20%.[7] In more structured studies, the prevalence of a depressive disorder classified according to the DSM-III-R is estimated to be from 3 to 9%.[2, 7, 8] Studies of medical inpatients and outpatients show that 22 to 32% have some form of depressive symptoms.[9–11] A more recent study of primary care practice populations found 10% of patients met research diagnostic criteria for depression and an additional 11.2% were felt to have significant depressive symptomatology but could not be classified with a specific disorder.[1] Despite the fact it is the most common reason for psychiatric hospitalization, up to 80% of all those with major depression are treated by nonpsychiatric caregivers or not at all.[12] These figures highlight the role of the primary care physician in being the first to recognize and begin treatment of patients with affective disorders. However, studies of primary care practice reveal that psychiatric disorders appear to be unreported even when medication for these disorders has been provided.[12] Perhaps of more concern has been the observation that primary care physicians consistently underdiagnose depressive disorders.[13–15] Schulberg and coworkers found only 44.4% of patients with depressive disorders (as defined by a structured interview) were diagnosed by primary care physicians.[16] It is clear that the reasons for this failure to diagnose are multifactorial and depend both on the patient's presentation as well as the physician's ability to recognize the symptoms of affective disease.[14]

There is a need to rectify this situation, as patients with untreated depression increase the rate of utilization of medical care with more outpatient visits and tests for somatic complaints, nonadherence, and increased lengths of stay when hospitalized.[17–20] Studies have shown increased mortality secondary to cardiovascular disease in depressed outpatients as well as an increase in adverse outcomes in patients undergoing cardiac surgery when patients were clinically depressed before surgery.[21, 22] The rate of suicide continues to rise, and is a major cause of mortality in affective disorders.[23] Affective disorders are also associated with increased rates of drug and alcohol abuse and

eating disorders, all of which have their own associated medical complications.[24–27] Studies of victims of both sexual assault or childhood sexual abuse also show an increase in risk for developing an affective disorder.[28, 29]

In women, untreated major depression may have effects on subsequent generations. Women are still the primary caretakers of children. In severe depression, there may be decreased ability to respond to a child's emotional or physical needs, which may lead to neglect or physical abuse.[30–32] A history of neglect or abuse in childhood contributes to the risk of affective disorder later in life, thereby perpetuating an intergenerational pattern of affective disorder.[33]

DIAGNOSIS OF AFFECTIVE DISORDERS

The diagnosis of affective disorders is based upon fulfillment of criteria from the DSM-IV. In this nosology, patients are classified as having either a major depressive episode, dysthymia, adjustment disorder with depressed mood, or mood disorder due to a general medical condition.[34] These criteria are presented in Table 71–1. The criteria for major depression include both neurovegetative symptoms of change in appetite and sleep patterns, loss of energy, psychomotor changes, as well as more cognitive-affective symptoms of loss of pleasure or interest, feelings of guilt or worthlessness, suicidal ideation, and decreased concentration.

Dysthymia differs from major depression by the decrease in severity of symptoms and the longer duration of symptoms. It is important to recognize that patients with dysthymia are at risk of developing major depression with any loss or increase in stress. A third major category in the spectrum of affective disorders is adjustment disorder with depressed mood. These patients present with an identifiable stressor in the prior 3 months and in general, symptoms are not as severe as in major depression. Physical illness or hospitalization is a common precipitant.[35]

The DSM-IV criteria appear to provide a useful model for evaluating depression in medical patients.[36] The presence of neurovegetative signs such as sleep disorders, anorexia, and fatigue may be confusing, as between 50 to 80% of medical inpatients may complain of these symptoms.[10, 35] In 1983, Cavanaugh and associates reported that affective and cognitive symptoms were better predictors of the severity of depression. These include (1) feeling like a failure, (2) loss of interest in others, (3) the sense of being punished, (4) indecision, and (5) suicidal ideation. In this study, somatic symptoms were not a good indicator, al-

TABLE 71–1. Diagnostic Criteria for Major Depressive Episode

A. Five (or more) of the following symptoms have been present during the same 2-week period and represent a change from previous functioning; at least one of the symptoms is either (1) depressed mood or (2) loss of interest or pleasure.

   Note: Do not include symptoms that are clearly due to a general medical condition, or mood-incongruent delusions or hallucinations.

   1. Depressed mood most of the day, nearly every day, as indicated by either subjective report (e.g., feels sad or empty) or observation made by others (e.g., appears tearful). **Note:** In children and adolescents, can be irritable mood.
   2. Markedly diminished interest or pleasure in all, or almost all, activities most of the day, nearly every day (as indicated by either subjective account or observation by others).
   3. Significant weight loss when not dieting or weight gain (e.g., a change of more than 5% of body weight in a month), or decrease or increase in appetite nearly every day. **Note:** In children, consider failure to make expected weight gains.
   4. Insomnia or hypersomnia nearly every day.
   5. Psychomotor agitation or retardation nearly every day (observable by others, not merely subjective feelings of restlessness or being slowed down).
   6. Fatigue or loss of energy nearly every day.
   7. Feelings of worthlessness or excessive or inappropriate guilt (which may be delusional) nearly every day (not merely self-reproach or guilt about being sick).
   8. Diminished ability to think or concentrate, or indecisiveness, nearly every day (either by subjective account or as observed by others).
   9. Recurrent thoughts of death (not just fear of dying), recurrent suicidal ideation without a specific plan, or a suicide attempt or a specific plan for committing suicide.

B. The symptoms do not meet criteria for a Mixed Episode.
C. The symptoms cause clinically significant distress or impairment in social, occupational, or other important areas of functioning.
D. The symptoms are not due to the direct physiologic effects of a substance (e.g., a drug of abuse, a medication) or a general medical condition (e.g., hypothyroidism).
E. The symptoms are not better accounted for by Bereavement, i.e., after the loss of a loved one, the symptoms persist for longer than 2 months or are characterized by marked functional impairment, morbid preoccupation with worthlessness, suicidal ideation, psychotic symptoms, or psychomotor retardation.

From American Psychiatric Association. Diagnostic and Statistical Manual of Mental Disorders. 4th ed. Washington, DC: American Psychiatric Association, 1994, p 327.

though the intensity of somatic complaints increased with the severity of depression.[37]

Patients with depressive disorders may also present with somatic complaints or with a mixture of anxious and depressive features. In a study of primary care patients, approximately 10% had a mixed depression-anxiety syndrome that did not meet any diagnostic criteria, but were frequently felt to be "depressed" by primary care providers.[1] It is this large group of patients who do not fit neatly into any diagnostic category that are most frequently seen by primary care physicians. There is speculation that these patients may represent a form of masked depression or may even be a separate diagnostic entity.[1] Although this group of patients is now recognized by researchers, there are still no data on the natural history of this condition nor controlled trials on the efficacy of antianxiety versus antidepressant medication.

Other patients present primarily with somatic complaints that may represent covert symptoms of depression.[33] Lesse noted that "masked depression" may also appear as a form of acting out such as drug or alcohol addiction, pain, and hypochondriasis. Common to many of these patients was the finding of covert anger and rage, often arising as a result of severe childhood trauma such as physical or sexual abuse, neglect, or abandonment.[33] As a result of being unable to express their anger adequately as a child, these adults frequently develop somatic complaints rather than finding more adaptive ways to express their anger (even if the anger is appropriate). Women with this background are more likely to experience abusive relationships, and a history of domestic violence should be sought, in addition to the investigation of depressive symptoms, in women with multiple or unexplained somatic complaints.

Likewise, somatic complaints may represent an unconscious continuation of the abuse or punishment they have experienced in the past. Those in whom pain and hypochondriasis exist often deny or minimize affective complaints while selectively focusing on their somatic complaints. Depressed patients who present primarily with somatic symptoms are likely to be overlooked initially because of the tendency of physicians to focus on physical illness as well as the patient's insistence on having a physical diagnosis. It is usually only after repeated unsuccessful attempts at treating the somatic complaint or after numerous diagnostic tests that the psychological aspect is ascertained. Because of their use of somatization, these patients are particularly hard to treat with traditional psychiatric techniques.

It appears that the relationship with the primary care physician is the key to management. Frequently these patients have a need to develop dependent relationships, and when these relational needs are met through frequent, regular office visits, the severity and frequency of somatic complaints is reduced. Selected use of antidepressants or anxiolytics may be helpful in the management of patients who have complaints of anxiety, sleep disorders, or chronic pain. For patients who agree to psychiatric treatment, it is of the utmost importance to continue to maintain close ties with their primary care provider.

Complaints of pain have long been associated with depression, though the reason for the association is far from clear. Whereas some researchers see pain as a symptom of masked depression, others suggest that depression may be secondary to experiencing chronic pain and that the two may have a common neurophysiologic basis.[38, 39] Recent studies show that the number of simultaneous pain complaints was positively correlated with the diagnosis of major depression.[40] A single complaint of pain, no matter how severe or persistent, did not show this correlation. There was an association with depression found in patients who had more than 7 pain-related disability days in 6 months.[40] Still other patients may present with behavioral changes such as medical noncompliance or refusal of medical treatment.[19]

Women also experience mood disorders related to the reproductive cycle. Attempts at definition of premenstrual mood changes under the proposed category of late luteal phase dysphoric disorder are controversial, as up to 40% of women may experience some premenstrual symptoms and this "diagnosis" may simply be a description of normal biologic phenomena.[41] In addition, many reports of mood changes are retrospective and may be superimposed on an underlying psychiatric disorder, as women who experience moderate to severe premenstrual symptoms also have higher rates of other affective disorders as well.[41] Pregnancy is associated with several psychiatric syndromes, notably postpartum blues, postpartum depression, and postpartum psychosis. Like premenstrual syndrome, the subject of menopausal mood disorders has been debated for years. However, most studies have shown no increase in the prevalence of depression during menopause.[42] Many of the mood changes appear to respond to hormonal replacement.[42] More severe symptoms need the same evaluation and treatment as those of any other affective disorder and may reflect a familial or personal predisposition rather than a direct relation to menopause.

When depression is suspected, it is important for the physician to take a careful history, noting any risk factors or precipitating events. If not volunteered, it may be necessary to ask direct questions to elucidate the presence or absence of symptoms that fulfill the DSM-IV criteria. Risk factors for major depression include a family history of major depression or bipolar disorder; a past psychiatric history, including a past history of major depressive episodes; a past history of abuse; and concurrent medical illness or chronic pain.[43] There appears to be a familial pattern of affective disorder in women with a history of alcohol abuse in first-degree relatives.[44] Although not included in the diagnostic criteria, the presence of a precipitating event, often a loss, also appears to increase the risk of developing an affective disorder.[2, 43] Other symptoms that may be associated with affective illness include a decrease in libido or sexual functioning, anxiety symptoms, somatic preoccupation, indecisiveness, chronic pain, lack of self-care, and social withdrawal.[43]

As with most psychiatric disorders, it is necessary to rule out any organic or medical causes of depressive symptoms (classified as mood disorder due to a general medical condition). This has been extensively reviewed by others, and most precipitants of delirium have also been associated with depression.[45–47] A list of potentially useful screening tests is included in Table 71–2. Deciding which tests to order depends largely on pertinent points of history such as age, concurrent medical problems, drug and alcohol use, and other somatic complaints. Unexplained weight loss or anorexia in addition to depressive symptoms such as fatigue may signal the presence of an occult malignancy or metastatic disease. Persons with pancreatic cancer commonly present with major depression before discovery of the tumor. The elderly are particularly susceptible to mental status changes as a result of infection, electrolyte disturbances, vitamin deficiency, and hypoxia. In addition, many patients with early dementias may present first with mood or behavior changes that may appear to be simply major depression secondary to other changes in their lives such as the loss of a spouse or friends, or retirement. Neuropsychiatric testing may be quite helpful in screening for both.

Women who present with a first episode of affective disorder at any age should be screened for endocrine disturbances, blood dyscrasias, electrolyte abnormalities, vitamin deficiencies and use of illicit drugs and alcohol. In younger women with primary complaints of fatigue and sleep disturbance, one may need to rule out sleep disorders,

TABLE 71–2.   Screening Tests Useful in Evaluating Organic Affective Disorder

SCREENING TESTS IN ANY PATIENT	ADDITIONAL TESTS (DEPENDENT ON HISTORY)
Complete blood count	NH_3
Electrolytes: include Ca^{2+}, Mg^{2+}	Human immunodeficiency virus
Blood urea nitrogen/ creatinine	Erythrocyte sedimentation rate
Glucose (fasting)	Urine: urinalysis, porphyrins
Liver function tests	Arterial blood gases
Thyroid function tests	CT or MRI scan
Serum cortisol	Lumbar puncture—cell counts, culture, cerebrospinal fluid protein
B_{12}	
Folate	Sleep study
Serology (RPR, VDRL)	Neuropsychologic testing
Electrocardiogram (if prescribing tricyclic antidepressants)	Toxic screen
Chest radiograph	Mono spot test for mononucleosis

RPR, Rapid plasma reagin; VDRL, Venereal Disease Research Laboratory; CT, computed tomography; MRI, magnetic resonance imaging.

TABLE 71–3.   Medications Associated with Mood or Energy Changes

Amphetamines
Antihypertensives: reserpine, methyldopa, thiazide, clonidine, quanethidine, hydralazine, procainamide
Oral contraceptives
Steroids or adrenocorticotropic hormone
Cimetidine
Cocaine
Barbiturates
β-blockers
Benzodiazepines
Antineoplastics
Opiates
Anti-inflammatory agents: ibuprofen, indomethacin
Neurologic: baclofen, carbamazepine, phenytoin

autoimmune disorders, infectious mononucleosis, or indolent infection such as chronic fatigue syndrome or hepatitis. Women who present with a history of changing symptoms or waxing and waning of pain or neurologic complaints should be evaluated for porphyria or multiple sclerosis. The presence of a drug use history or multiple sexual partners warrants investigation of a patient's human immunodeficiency virus status.

It is especially important to review all medications and drugs that a patient may be using, as many can cause changes in mood or energy (Table 71–3). Of special importance to clinicians are a number of neuropsychiatric disorders that may manifest with depressive symptoms. These include cerebrovascular accidents, Parkinson's disease, Huntington's disease, multiple sclerosis, and human immunodeficiency virus encephalopathy.[35, 48] Studies by Robinson and colleagues have shown that up to 60% of patients with right hemispheric strokes and 15% of patients with left hemispheric strokes develop a clinically significant depression that responds to appropriate antidepressant therapy.[49, 50] As with poststroke depression, the depression of the previously mentioned illnesses also responds to antidepressant treatment. For most other organic affective disorders the treatment largely depends on treating the underlying cause of the mental status changes.

MANAGEMENT

Once the diagnosis of an affective disorder is made, the next decision facing the primary care physician is if and when the patient should be referred to a psychiatrist or other mental health provider. Factors that influence this decision include the availability of psychiatric services, the nature and severity of the mood disorder, the willingness of the patient to accept referral, and the comfort of the treating physician in managing psychiatric illnesses. Emergency psychiatric evaluation and possible hospitalization should be sought for persons who present with suicidal ideation or in whom the affective disorder impairs their ability to function at home or work. For patients who are experiencing an adjustment disorder because of an acute stress or loss, a supportive, caring, and consistent relationship with their physician may be most useful in alleviating their symptoms. During this time it may be beneficial for the physician to schedule more frequent appointments with the express purpose of allowing the patient to discuss concerns and feelings as well as to monitor closely for signs of the development of a major depression. The evaluation of an affective disorder may uncover an eating disorder, alcohol abuse, drug abuse, or the presence of an abusive relationship. When these complications are found, they should be addressed directly with the patient and referrals for specific treatment made. It is mandatory that cases of suspected child neglect or abuse be reported to the proper state or local agencies.

In addition to those with a need for acute psychiatric services, those with major depression or dysthymia can benefit from insight-oriented psychotherapy. Addressing issues of low self-esteem, previous unresolved losses, or unexpressed anger can be of benefit to many with depression, whether or not pharmacotherapy is used. The decision to refer to a therapist often revolves around patient interest and motivation to discuss personal issues. A personal recommendation to a therapist by the primary care provider can often assist those initially reluctant to seek therapy and help to provide confidence in the treatment plan. The patient's financial resources often play a large role in the decision to refer, as insurance coverage for psychotherapy becomes more restrictive. The availability of a therapist in the community also affects the decision to seek therapy. Despite these realities, education and income level in themselves do not predict the usefulness of psychotherapy, and options should be explored with all patients who may potentially benefit. Many medical clinics may also have psychologists, psychiatric social workers, or nurses who are available to provide additional counseling or psychotherapy to patients with affective disorders. The decision on psychotherapy also depends on the patient's views and interest or aversion or contraindications to use of medications.

Many patients with major depression and dysthymia as well as organic affective disorders with neuropsychiatric etiologies respond to antidepressant medication. It is important for the primary care physician to begin treatment for their patients when the diagnosis is made. The neurovegetative symptoms of major depression may respond within 1 or 2 weeks to medication. This in turn may allow patients to return to a functioning level in their occupational or social roles, prevent a worsening of the depression, and decrease the rate of complications in their medical illness from appetite disturbances, nonadherence, or decrease in physical activity.

The list of medications used for the treatment of depression continues to grow as the neurobiologic mechanisms of mood disorders are better understood. This may pose a dilemma to the clinician who attempts pharmacologic treatment. The choice of a specific antidepressant is largely based on the patient's presenting complaints as well as the side effects to be avoided. It is helpful to have a history of previous treatment to determine which medications a patient may have taken in the past and their effectiveness. The drugs used for their antidepressant effect may be divided into tricyclic and heterocyclic compounds, monoamine oxidase inhibitors, and serotonergic agents.[51] Their effect is largely due to their ability to block the presynaptic reuptake of either norepinephrine or serotonin or the inhibition of monoamine oxidase. This results in a functional increase of these neurotransmitters and over time causes down-regulation at the postsynaptic receptor sites. It is for this reason that the antidepressant effect may not be appreciated until after several weeks of treatment.

Tricyclic and heterocyclic compounds (trazodone) and selective serotonergic reuptake inhibitors are now considered effective first-line agents. Because insomnia may be the most troubling presenting complaint for patients with major depression and because many of the tricyclics and trazodone are sedating, they may be a logical first choice. The sedative side effect is largely based on their antihistaminic property (affinity for the H_1 receptor). This property varies between tricyclics, with doxepin and amitriptyline being the most sedating and desipramine and protriptyline being the least sedating. An exception is trazodone, which is very sedating but has few antihistaminic effects. These compounds are generally most effective if given in a single dose at bedtime when their sedative properties are appreciated. The starting dose of most tricyclic compounds is 25 to 50 mg per day and can be increased gradually up to 150 mg. With outpatients, it is easiest and safest to increase the dose weekly to biweekly until the patient shows signs of a response or develops intolerable side effects. Initial prescriptions should provide only sufficient medication until the next scheduled visit, especially in those reporting suicidal ideation, given the seriousness of tricyclic overdoses. Factors that may limit their use are the emergence of side effects and concern about cardiovascular toxicity. The most bothersome side effects include orthostatic hypotension, anticholinergic side effects, and weight gain. It is important to review the patient's other medications before starting a tricyclic antidepressant to avoid use of multiple anticholinergic agents. Amitriptyline is one of the most anticholinergic, and patients have a hard time tolerating its side effects. The tertiary amines (amitriptyline, imipramine, doxepin) and trazodone cause more hypotension than the secondary amines (nortriptyline, desipramine, protriptyline). Elderly patients are particularly at risk for falls secondary to orthostatic hypotension, and tricyclic antidepressants should be used at low starting doses (10 mg) in this population. Dividing the dose throughout the day may also help to avoid this complication. Nortriptyline appears to cause less postural hypotension than other agents and is felt by some to be safer for use in the elderly.[52]

Much of the concern about cardiovascular toxicity comes from studies of tricyclic overdose.[53] More recent studies show them to be relatively safe medications as long as their cardiac effects are taken into account.[54, 55] Several studies have shown no adverse effects of tricyclic medications on left ventricular function, even in patients with existing congestive heart failure.[56, 57] Tricyclic antidepressants appear to resemble antiarrhythmic agents such as quinidine and to slow conduction through the atrioventricular node. Patients may show a lengthening of the P–R, QRS, and Q–T intervals.[56] This is generally not a problem for patients unless there is preexisting disease in the cardiac conduction system. For this reason, it is important to have a baseline electrocardiogram in patients older than 40 before starting either tricyclics or heterocyclic compounds such as trazodone. Trazodone is not felt to have the same effects on conduction, but there have been reports that suggest that it may increase ventricular ectopy in patients with underlying ventricular irritability.[56]

The class of selective serotonergic reuptake inhibitors (fluoxetine, paroxetine, sertraline) enhances serotonin transmission and produces downregulation of postsynaptic serotonergic receptors.[58] Studies show them to be as efficacious as tricyclic medications, and they are now considered to be first-line agents, especially in patients with concurrent medical problems. Their onset of action is similar to that of tricyclic antidepressants, and several weeks may be needed to produce an antidepressant effect. They have no sedative, orthostatic, or anticholinergic side effects.[58] Many patients find them energizing, which makes them a good choice in patients with fatigue and loss of energy. They are felt to be safe in patients with cardiac disease, and they produce little weight gain. Side effects that may limit their use include headache, nausea, vomiting, insomnia, anxiety, restlessness, and akathisia.[58] Most side effects appear to be dose related. Starting doses are 10 to 20 mg for fluoxetine and 20 mg for paroxetine, taken once a day. Because of their energizing effects, they should be taken in the morning to decrease the risk of sleep disruption. Even so, some patients continue to complain of insomnia, and the addition of a low-dose benzodiazepine may help with sleep. This effect on sleep frequently disappears within several weeks. Many patients respond at this starting dose, although the dose can be increased to 40 mg a day if needed. It is rarely necessary to go beyond this dose, as higher doses of fluoxetine have been associated with severe akathisia and anxiety. As with many medications, it is wise to start elderly patients on a low dose, such as 5 to 10 mg a day, and gradually increase the dose weekly as necessary. Sertraline, another serotonergic agent, is usually started at doses of 25 to 50 mg a day in the morning and can be increased to doses of 150 to 200 mg a day if needed to obtain a therapeutic effect.

Of particular note are the recent reports linking fluoxetine to suicide attempts.[59] Systematic study of these reports reveals that the emergence or worsening of suicidal or aggressive behavior has been reported with a variety of antidepressants and that this complication is relatively uncommon, affecting fewer than 5% of patients who are treated.[60] It has been hypothesized that this phenomenon may be a response to the side effect of akathisia that may develop with fluoxetine treatment, especially with higher or rapidly increasing doses.[61, 62] Patients should be informed of this side effect and instructed to stop the medication and notify their physician if it occurs.

Other medications useful in the treatment of affective disorders include monoamine oxidase inhibitors, clomipramine, and bupropion. Although these agents are not always thought of as first-line agents, primary care physicians should be familiar with them, as they may care for patients who are using them. Monoamine oxidase inhibitors are now considered safe and effective medications if their interactions with foods and other medications are taken into account to avoid a hypertensive crisis caused by eating tyramine-containing foods. Patients on these medications should be instructed carefully about dietary restrictions and avoidance of over-the-counter cold medications that may contain sympathomimetics. Monoamine oxidase inhibitors generally have no anticholinergic side effects and little effect on cardiac conduction but frequently produce orthostatic hypotension, which limits their use in the elderly. The orthostatic effect can be lessened by giving it in divided doses. The list of potential drug interactions is lengthy and should be reviewed for the patient taking these medications. Especially significant are the interactions with meperidine hydrochloride, anesthetic agents, short-acting muscle relaxants, levodopa, and many centrally acting antihypertensives.[63]

Clomipramine is chemically related to the tricyclic compounds, and its dosing and side effect profile is similar. However, many of its therapeutic effects appear to be related to its action as a nonspecific serotonergic reuptake inhibitor. It has been quite effective in treating obsessive-compulsive disorder.[64, 65] Bupropion's antidepressant effects appear to be related to effects on both the noradrenergic and dopaminergic system.[66] Like the selective serotonergic reuptake inhibitors, it has few anticholinergic, histaminic, or cardiovascular side effects, which make it a potentially useful medication for those who have medical problems.[67] Typical side effects include agitation, insomnia, headache, tremor, dry mouth, and constipation.

Antidepressant use has been associated with an increased risk of seizure activity. Reports vary from 0.1% in patients with no predisposition to 1% in all treated patients.[68, 69] This does not imply that antidepressants should not be used in patients with seizure disorders or head trauma if it is clinically warranted. However, it does affect the choice of medication and requires that it be used in the lowest effective dose. Monoamine oxidase inhibitors and trazadone appear to be least epileptogenic. Maprotiline, clomipramine, and bupropion show the highest potential for inducing seizures and should be used with caution or not at all in those patients with known seizures.[70]

Women of childbearing age should be cautioned about becoming pregnant while taking an antidepressant. It is prudent to avoid the use of antidepressants during pregnancy, especially during the first trimester. If pregnancy is suspected, it may be wise to discontinue the medication but continue close monitoring for the appearance of worsening symptoms that may require the patient to be psychiatrically hospitalized and reevaluated for medication use. Women who decide to breast-feed should be informed that antidepressants are excreted in milk, and breast-fed infants may have demonstrable blood levels as well as display side effects from these medications.[71,72] If psychotropic use is needed, it may be safer to refrain from breast-feeding.

In general, a therapeutic trial of medication requires that it be given at an effective dose and over an adequate length of time. The most common reason for nonresponse is often the lack of an adequate dose of medication. Further guidelines for effective doses of medication can be found in most psychopharmacology texts.[51] It is important to keep in mind that elderly patients may respond at much lower doses and are more sensitive to side effects. In patients who have been on higher doses of antidepressants without developing side effects or a response, it may be helpful to check blood levels of the medication for an indication of adequate absorption. However, drug levels of most antidepressants do not correlate with therapeutic response. The only medication with a proven therapeutic window is nortriptyline. If a patient has been on an appropriate dose of antidepressant medication for 4 to 6 weeks without a significant response, it is likely that little benefit will result from continuing the medication. Referral to a psychiatrist is appropriate at this time to reevaluate the diagnosis and to make more specific recommendations for treatment. Likewise, should any patient show an increase in the severity of the depressive symptoms, psychiatric evaluation is indicated. Referral for psychiatric evaluation and treatment is always appropriate if the primary care physician has a question about diagnosis or treatment. Although clinicians often worry that patients may resist referral, patients may be more amenable to the idea if the physician discusses the reasons for the referral, emphasizes the need for and the effectiveness of treatment, and makes it clear that the relationship with the primary care physician will continue. Referral to a specific psychiatrist rather than to a clinic may indicate that the physician has an ongoing relationship with and confidence in the psychiatric provider and may increase the chance that the patient will accept the referral and follow recommendations.

In patients with severe, life-threatening depression, often with delusions, who are refractory to other treatments, and who have concomitant medical problems, the psychiatrist may recommend electroconvulsive therapy (ECT). The primary care physician should be familiar with ECT to advise and support patients for whom this is recommended. Electroconvulsive therapy remains the most efficacious treatment for major depression. There are few contraindications, which makes it useful in patients with multiple medical problems. It is relatively free of side effects when performed in a monitored setting. Patients may experience some anterograde memory impairment, which usually improves in a few weeks.[73] Patients who respond to ECT are often successfully maintained on antidepressant medication or on short repeated courses of ECT.

REFERENCES

1. Barrett JE, Barrett JA, Oxman T, et al. The prevalence of psychiatric disorders in a primary care practice. Arch Gen Psychiatry 1988;45(12):1100.
2. Romanoski AJ, Folstein MF, Nestadt G, et al. The epidemiology of psychiatrist ascertained depression and DSM III depressive disorders. Psychol Med 1992;22:629.
3. Miller JB. Toward a New Psychology of Women. Boston: Beacon Press, 1976.
4. Kaplan AG. The self-in-relation theory: Implications for depression in women. Work in Progress 84:14. Wellesley, Mass: Stone Center Working Papers Series, 1983.
5. Miller JB. The construction of anger in women and men. Work in Progress 83:01, Wellesley, Mass: Stone Center Working Papers Series, 1983.
6. Weissman MM, Klerman GL. Sex differences and the epidemiology of depression. Arch Gen Psychiatry 1977;34(1):98.
7. Blazer D, Swartz M, Woodbury M, et al. Depressive symptoms and depressive diagnoses in a community population. Arch Gen Psychiatry 1988;45(12):1078.
8. Myers JK, Weissman MM, Tischler GL, et al. Six-month prevalence of psychiatric disorders in three communities. Arch Gen Psychiatry 1984;41(10):959.
9. Moffic HS, Paykel ES. Depression in medical in-patients. Br J Psychiatry 1975;126:346.
10. Schwabb JJ, Bialow M, Brown JM, et al. Diagnosing depression in medical in-patients. Ann Intern Med 1967;67:695.
11. Kathol RG, Petty F. Relationship of depression to medical illness. J Affect Disord 1981;3:111.
12. Regier DA, Goldberg ID, Taube CA. The de facto US mental health services system. Arch Gen Psychiatry 1978;35(6):685.

13. Schulberg HC, Burns BJ. Mental disorders in primary care: Epidemiologic, diagnostic and treatment research directions. Gen Hosp Psychiatry 1988;10:79.

14. Kirmayer LJ, Robbins JM, Dworkind M, et al. Somatization and the recognition of depression and anxiety in primary care. Am J Psychiatry 1993;150(5):734.

15. Nielson AC, Williams TA. Depression in ambulatory medical patients: Prevalence by self report questionnaire and recognition by non-psychiatric physicians. Arch Gen Psychiatry 1980;37:999.

16. Schulberg HC, Saul M, McClelland M, et al. Assessing depression in primary medical and psychiatric practices. Arch Gen Psychiatry 1985;42:1164.

17. Stoudemire A, Thompson TL. Medication noncompliance: Systematic approaches to evaluation and treatment. Gen Hosp Psychiatry 1983;5:233.

18. Katon W. Depression: Relationship to somatization and chronic medical illness. J Clin Psychiatry 1984;45:4.

19. Hankin JR, Steinwachs DM, Regier DA, et al. Use of general medical care services by persons with mental disorders. Arch Gen Psychiatry 1982;39:225.

20. Levenson JL, Hamer RM, Rossiter LF. Relation of psychopathology in general medical inpatients to use and cost of services. Am J Psychiatry 147(11):1498.

21. Rabins PV, Harris K, Koven S. High fatality rates of late-life depression associated with cardiovascular disease. J Affect Disord 1985;9:165.

22. Kimball CP. Psychological responses to the experience of open heart surgery, I. Am J Psychiatry 1969;126:248.

23. Hacket TP, Stern TA. Suicide and other disruptive states. In: Hacket TP, Cassem NH (eds). Massachusetts General Hospital Handbook of General Hospital Psychiatry. 2nd ed. Littleton, Mass: PSG Publishing Company, 1987, p 268.

24. Hudson JL, Pope HG, Yurgelun-Todd D, et al. A controlled study of lifetime prevalence of affective and other psychiatric disorders in bulimic outpatients. Am J Psychiatry 1987;144(10):1283.

25. Weissman MM, Myers JK. Clinical depression in alcoholism. Am J Psychiatry 1980;137(3):372.

26. Schuckit MA. Genetic and clinical implications of alcoholism and affective disorder. Am J Psychiatry 1986;143(2):140.

27. Rounsaville BJ, Anton SF, Carroll K, et al. Psychiatric diagnoses of treatment seeking cocaine abusers. Arch Gen Psychiatry 1991;48:43.

28. Winfield I, George LX, Swartz M, et al. Sexual assault and psychiatric disorders among a community sample of women. Am J Psychiatry 1990;147:335.

29. Browne A, Finklhor D. Impact of childhood sexual abuse: A review of the research. Psychol Bull 1986;99:66.

30. Anthony EJ. An overview of the effects of maternal depression on the infant and child. In: Morrison HL (ed). Children of Depressed Parents: Risk Identifications and Intervention. New York: Grune & Stratton, 1982.

31. Downey G, Coyne JC. Children of depressed parents: An integrative review. Psychol Bull 1990;108:50.

32. Zuckerman BS, Beardslee WR. Maternal depression: A concern for the pediatrician. Pediatrics 1987;79:110.

33. Lesse S. The masked depression syndrome—Results of a seventeen year clinical study. Am J Psychother 1983;37:456.

34. American Psychiatric Association. Diagnostic and Statistical Manual of Mental Disorders. 4th ed. Washington, DC: American Psychiatric Association, 1994.

35. Rodin GM, Voshart K. Depression in the medically ill: An overview. Am J Psychiatry 1986;143(6):696.

36. Cavanaugh SVA. Diagnosing depression in the hospitalized patient with chronic medical illness. J Clin Psychiatry 1984;45(3):13.

37. Cavanaugh SVA, Clark DC, Gibbons RD. Diagnosing depression in the hospitalized medically ill. Psychosomatics 1983;24(9):809.

38. Hendler N. Depression caused by chronic pain. J Clin Psychiatry 1984;45:30.

39. Swanson DW. Chronic pain as a third pathologic emotion. Am J Psychiatry 1984;141:210.

40. Dworking SF, Vonkorff M, LeResche L. Multiple pains and psychiatric disturbance. Arch Gen Psychiatry 1990;47:239.

41. Gitlin MJ, Pasnau RO. Psychiatric syndromes linked to reproductive function in women: A review of current knowledge. Am J Psychiatry 1989;146(11):1413.

42. Schmidt PJ, Rubinow DR. Menopause-related affective disorders: A justification for further study. Am J Psychiatry 1991;148(7):844.

43. Cameron OG. Guidelines for diagnosis and treatment of depression in patients with medical illness. J Clin Psychiatry 1990;51(7,suppl):49.

44. Winokur G, Coryell E. Familial alcoholism in primary unipolar major depressive disorder. Am J Psychiatry 1991;148:184.

45. Hall RCW (ed). Psychiatric Presentations of Medical Illness: Somatopsychic Disorders. New York: SP Medical and Scientific Books, 1980.

46. Cameron OG (ed). Presentations of Depression: Depressive Symptoms in Medical and Other Psychiatric Disorders. New York: John Wiley & Sons, 1987.

47. Derogatis LR, Wise TN. Anxiety and Depressive Disorders in the Medical Patient. Washington, DC: American Psychiatry Press, 1989.

48. Hintz S, Kuck J, Peterkin JJ, et al. Depression in the context of human immunodeficiency virus infection: Implications for treatment. J Clin Psychiatry 1990;51(12):497.

49. Robinson RG, Lipsey JR, Price TR. Diagnosis and clinical management of post-stroke depression. Psychosomatics 1985;26:769.

50. Robinson RG, Morris PLP, Federoff JP. Depression and cerebrovascular disease. J Clin Psychiatry 1990;51(7, suppl):26.

51. Karasu TB (ed). Treatments of Psychiatric Disorders. Washington, DC: American Psychiatric Association, 1989.

52. Thayssen P, Bjerre M, Kragh-Sorenson P, et al. Cardiovascular effects of imipramine and nortriptyline in elderly patients. Psychopharmacology 1981;74:360.

53. Williams RB Jr, Sherter C. Cardiac complications of tricyclic antidepressant therapy. Ann Intern Med 1971;74:395.

54. Glassman AH, Bigger JT. Cardiovascular effects of therapeutic doses of tricyclic antidepressants. Arch Gen Psychiatry 1981;38:815.

55. Roose SP, Glassman AH. Cardiovascular effects of tricyclic antidepressants in depressed patients. J Clin Psychiatry Monograph 1989;7(2):1.

56. Veith RC, Raskind MA, Caldwell JH, et al. Cardiovascular effects of tricyclic antidepressant in depressed patients with chronic heart disease. N Engl J Med 1982;306:954.

57. Roose SP, Glassman AH, Giardina ECV, et al. Cardiovascular effects of imipramine and bupropion in depressed patients with congestive heart failure. J Clin Psychopharmacol 1987;7:247.

58. Rickels K, Schweizer E. Clinical overview of serotonin reuptake inhibitors. J Clin Psychiatry 1990;51(suppl):9.

59. Teicher MH, Glad C, Cole JO. Emergence of intense suicidal preoccupation during fluoxetine treatment. Am J Psychiatry 1990;147(2):207.

60. Mann JJ, Kapur S. The emergence of suicidal ideation and behavior during antidepressant therapy. Arch Gen Psychiatry 1991;48:1027.

61. Rothschild AJ, Locke CA. Re-exposure to fluoxetine after serious suicide attempts by three patients: The role of akathisia. J Clin Psychiatry 1991;52:491.

62. Lipinski JF, Mallya G, Zimmerman P, et al. Fluoxetine induced akathisia: Clinical and theoretical implications. J Clin Psychiatry 1989;50:339.

63. Bernstein JG. Drug interactions. In: Hacket TP, Cassem NH (eds). Massachusetts General Hospital Handbook of General Hospital Psychiatry. 2nd ed. Littleton, Mass: PSG Publishing Company, 1987, pp 548–559.

64. Insel TR, Murphy DL, Cohen RM, et al. Obsessive-compulsive disorder. Arch Gen Psychiatry 1983;40:605.

65. Benkelfat C, Murphy DL, Zohar J, et al. Clomipramine in obsessive-compulsive disorder: Further evidence for a serotonergic mechanism of action. Arch Gen Psychiatry 1989;46:23.

66. Ferris RM, Cooper BR. Mechanism of antidepressant activity of bupropion. J Clin Psychiatry Monograph 1993; 11(1):2.

67. Settle E. Bupropion: General side effects. J Clin Psychiatry Monograph 1993;11(1):33.

68. Jick H, Binan B, Hunter JR, et al. Tricyclic antidepressants and convulsions. J Clin Psychopharmacol 1983;3:182.

69. Lowry MR, Dunner FJ. Seizures during tricyclic therapy. Am J Psychiatry 1980;137:1461.

70. Davidison J. Seizures and bupropion: A review. J Clin Psychiatry 189;50:256.

71. Matheson I, Pande H, Alertson AR. Respiratory depression caused by N-desmethyldoxepin in breast milk (letter). Lancet 1985;2:1124.

72. Stancer HC, Reed KL. Desipramine and 2-hydroxydesipramine in human breast milk and the nursing infant's serum. Am J Psychiatry 1986;143:1597.

73. Welch C. Electroconvulsive therapy in the general hospital. In: Hackett TP, Cassen NC (eds). Massachusetts General Hospital Handbook of General Hospital Psychiatry. 2nd ed. Littleton, Mass: PSG Publishing Company, 1987, pp 261–267.

Management of Anxiety

Alma Dell Smith

Anxiety ranks as the fifth most common reason for a visit to a primary care physician, outnumbered only by preventative examinations, hypertension, trauma, and sore throats.[1] Anxiety is the most frequently reported complaint among the general population, affecting approximately 10% of the population,[2, 3] and occurs even more frequently in women. The incidence of general anxiety disorders is twice as high in women as in men, and women constitute approximately 75% of agoraphobics with panic disorder.[4] Among agoraphobics who develop severe avoidance behavior, almost 90% are women.[5]

Anxiety is one of the emotional signs of stress and is often accompanied by other stress symptoms such as insomnia, gastrointestinal distress, palpitations, atypical chest pain, headaches and other muscle tension complaints, dizziness, shortness of breath, and excessive sweating, flushing, or chills. Chronic conditions such as hypertension or diabetes can be exacerbated by stress due to changes in metabolic activity or neglect of self-care during stressful times. When these conditions are included, anxiety-related complaints may reach as high as 75% of visits to a primary care practice.[1]

Treatment of the anxious patient can be time consuming. Frequent emergency telephone calls and urgent visits and vague, often shifting, complaints, coupled with the patient's need to talk at length about things other than health, can become irritating for the busy physician. Because many organic disorders have similar presenting symptoms, the physician must rule out health-threatening disease, without pursuing excessively expensive diagnostic tests when initial evaluations prove negative.

When no organic disorder is found, the physician's explanations for symptoms are sometimes as vague as the patient's complaint: "It's your nerves," or "It's stress." Although many patients will acknowledge that their symptoms are stress related, they are confused about how to feel better. If the physician attempts to minimize the seriousness of patients' complaints, they may only escalate descriptions of aches and pains. The visit often ends with the writing of a prescription. However, the prescription need not be for anxiolytic medication.

This chapter presents a biobehavioral model of care that focuses on specific techniques for symptom reduction and instructions for self-management of anxious feelings. This approach follows a model of women's health care that addresses psychosocial issues and treats the woman as an active, educated, and participating member of the health care team. Although this approach may be more time consuming initially, it provides genuine benefit to the patient and helps contain the overutilization of health care in the longer term.

WOMEN'S INCREASED VULNERABILITY TO ANXIETY DISORDERS

Several hypotheses have been generated from clinical experience and preliminary studies to account for the higher incidence of anxiety in women. First, women and young girls are more often targets of physical and sexual assault, domestic violence, and abuse than males. Jaffe and co-workers[6] found that battered women reported significantly more somatic complaints than women from nonviolent homes. Because women are smaller in build, they are more easily overwhelmed in physical confrontations with males. They are also less likely to learn self-defense skills such as assertiveness and personal protection. Childhood or adult experiences with fear as well as cultural role expectations shape the individual's beliefs and expectations about herself and the world. As a result, women and girls are also more likely to believe they are relatively helpless and to experience chronic apprehension over future events.

Other threats may be more economic or social in nature. Owing to income differences, women tend to have fewer economic resources to use to escape abusive situations. Goldstein and Chambless have found that agoraphobia almost always develops in a climate of marked interpersonal conflict.[7] Women with low levels of self-sufficiency or confidence are torn between a desire to escape an unsatisfactory dependent relationship on the one hand and fears of independence on the other. Several multiple case studies have noted that improvement in women treated for panic disorder has been marked by increased jealousy, pressure to return to the dependent role, and even suicide attempts by the husband.[8, 9]

Another hypothesis for the higher incidence of anxiety in women is that it is more culturally acceptable for women to express fear and to avoid going out in public. If a woman does not work outside the home, for example, she is not forced to face her travel fears by employment demands. In contrast, it has been suggested that males are more likely to inhibit admissions of fear and abuse alcohol and drugs at a higher rate than females as a form of self-medication for anxiety. Males may also be more likely to express anger, not fear, in the face of threat. It has been less acceptable for women to respond with anger when her well-being is threatened.

Fluctuations in endocrine or hormonal states due to either normal or abnormal processes may make some women more physiologically reactive to anxiety during these special times. Anecdotally, some women report that their first major anxiety episode occurred after delivery, in association with infertility treatments, or after gynecologic surgery. It is also commonly reported that anxiety episodes are worse during the premenstrual period. However, there are no controlled studies clearly confirming the hypothesis that endocrine imbalances contribute to anxiety disorders.

Finally, the morphology of the body may also contribute to the higher incidence of anxiety symptoms among women. Hyperventilation, which tends to escalate an anxiety episode into a panic attack, is more likely to occur in persons with a small chest cavity or in persons who wear binding clothing such as tight belts or brassieres, which hamper diaphragmatic breathing. Being short-waisted, having a narrow or shallow rib cage, or having postural habits that compress the chest cavity all tend to increase the possibility of hyperventilation.

THE NATURE OF ANXIETY

Anxiety is not a disease but part of a normal survival response to danger. Anticipation of danger and scanning the environment for signs of threat are normal and important survival responses. Normally, once danger passes, the individual returns to a sense of safety, relaxation, and homeostasis. Anxiety is classified as a disorder when the anxiety is seen by others and even the patient as extreme, irrational, or unwarranted.

The threat causing the anxiety may be physical or social, real or imagined. Internal sensations such as pain, racing heartbeat, or images of jumping off a bridge can be as frightening to the patient as any external threat. Unfortunately, some individuals have greater than normal experiences with danger, have learned to expect social or physical threat, have lives that are not secure, or have an augmented physiologic response to threat. Such individuals have difficulty returning to the sense of safety. A general anxiety pervades their lives, which is characterized by heightened muscle tension, autonomic hyperactivity, vigilant scanning of the environment for danger, and apprehensive expectation. Such chronic apprehension is uncomfortable and tiring. At its worst, it interferes with the course of daily life, affecting sleep and eating patterns and disturbing work or social relationships, and may eventually result in stress-related physical disorders.

All moods, including anxiety, have three manifestations: cognitive, physiologic, and behavioral. Cognitive style refers to beliefs, thoughts, or visual images about the world and oneself. Anxiety begins with a belief that a situation is threatening and that one does not have the skills to cope safely. The predominant cognitive style is one of hypervigilance. This results in frequent frightening thoughts, distractibility, difficulty concentrating, insomnia, irritability, or racing thoughts. Upsetting thoughts include worry, ''what if'' thinking, catastrophizing, or ''thinking the worst.'' These thoughts can be accompanied by powerful visual images of danger, abandonment, embarrassment, or even death. The thoughts may or may not be expressed verbally to others.

The threatening cognitions start and then maintain the cycle of physiologic arousal. Signs of chronic muscle tension are muscle aches, tension headaches, upper or lower back pain, teeth grinding, and fatigue. Shakiness, trembling, restlessness, inability to relax, and easy startle are also signs of muscular reactivity to stress. Autonomic hyperactivity is manifested as tachycardia, peripheral vasoconstriction, cold clammy hands, dry mouth, gastrointestinal upset, frequent urination, lump in the throat, flushing, or pallor. Chronic autonomic hyperactivity in combination with other factors may result in migraines, ulcers, irritable bowel, hypertension, or exacerbation of other illnesses.

Behavioral manifestations of anxiety are primarily attempts to relieve the unpleasant experiences of dread and hyperarousal and to restore a sense of control over oneself and the environment. These behaviors include avoidance of certain situations, seeking help, asking for reassurance, and deliberate calming of the body. Less adaptive behaviors may include phobic avoidance, drug or alcohol use, or manipulative attempts to control others.

DIAGNOSIS AND CLASSIFICATION OF ANXIETY DISORDERS

The classification of anxiety disorders continues to undergo revision as new research emerges. To date, the *Diagnostic and Statistical Manual of Mental Disorders* (DSM-IV)[10] has classified anxiety disorders into the following categories: simple phobias, social phobias, obsessive-compulsive disorder, posttraumatic stress disorder, panic disorder with or without agoraphobia, anxiety disorder due to medical condition, substance-induced anxiety disorder, and generalized anxiety disorder. All anxiety disorders share the characteristics of apprehensive expectation, heightened autonomic reactivity, and some degree of avoidance behavior. The particular focus of apprehensive expectation is what differentiates one anxiety disorder from another. In simple phobia, the patient is worried about encountering the feared object or situation. A person with social phobia worries about encountering embarrassment or social rejection. In obsessive-compulsive disorder, certain dangerous or unwanted thoughts or impulses are feared. The individual suffering from posttraumatic stress disorder fears a recurrence of the trauma. In panic disorder, the person fears a loss of control and the discomfort of internal sensations. Those with generalized anxiety disorder worry over multiple life circumstances, both major and minor. This chapter will focus on two common types of anxiety: general anxiety disorder and panic disorder.

Generalized Anxiety Disorder

Patients with generalized anxiety disorder usually report experiencing anxiety over a period of years, whereas patients report with panic disorder symptoms that may have lasted a few weeks or months. They see themselves as chronic worriers and may seek treatment only when their somatic symptoms become severe enough to interfere with functioning. There are usually several areas of worry, most commonly family, work, money, and

health. The question ''Do you worry about minor things?'' is more frequently answered yes by patients with general anxiety disorder than by patients with other anxiety disorders.[11] Patients with generalized anxiety disorder also report feeling anxious or worried more than half of an average day in contrast to those with panic disorder, for whom the feelings are quite intense but may last only a few minutes at a time.

Barlow found that 73% of anxiety patients also reported occasional panic attacks.[11] Unlike those with a primary diagnosis of panic disorder, they are not particularly worried about the panic attack itself but focus more on their life circumstances. For these individuals, stress triggers a feeling that life is getting out of control. Chronic worry maintains a chronic physiologic arousal. Rather than being mobilized to cope with the tasks at hand in an adaptive way, the anxious individual becomes preoccupied with the sense of being out of control and the potential negative outcomes (catastrophizing) and fails to act adaptively. For patients with multiple life stressors, the pressures may seem overwhelming and paralyzing, and energy is spent in worry, escape or rescue fantasies, or avoidance of the problem. These behaviors do little to solve problems.

Panic Disorder

Persons presenting with panic disorder offer a more dramatic picture than those with general anxiety. They typically present to the emergency department or physician's office reporting sudden onset of distressing physical symptoms. Symptoms can range from tachycardia, atypical chest pain, dizziness, and dyspnea to nausea, diarrhea, urinary urgency, sweating, and flushing. Other symptoms may be visual disturbances in spatial perception, tremulousness, a sense of weakness, or feeling faint. Particularly disturbing to some individuals is a sense of doom or impending death. Derealization (the feeling that things are not real) or depersonalization (a feeling of not being fully in the body) are frequently experienced but not reported, as they are often interpreted by the individual as signs that they may be going crazy. Cardiovascular symptoms are often interpreted as heart attacks, and dizziness may be thought to be a signal of impending fainting or a brain tumor. These worst-case thoughts serve to further escalate hyperarousal.

An automatic behavior at this point is for the individual to seek assistance and to escape the situation that seemed associated with the onset of panic, such as a stuffy room or potentially embarrassing social or public situation. Relief of symptoms often comes on reaching the emergency department or the safety of home or even at the moment that a decision is reached to retreat from the situation. This relief reinforces escape behaviors and sets the stage for avoidance of possible panic-producing situations. Avoidance behaviors may be mild, such as avoidance of airplanes or specific places, or may generalize to avoidance of all public places and, in extreme cases, retreat to a single room in the house.

Because her fears are not of an external event or object, the patient may deny a specific stressor. It often seems that the "attack" or episode came "out of the blue" while driving, at a social event, or on public transport. However, closer questioning usually reveals ongoing stress of a subacute nature, such as separation from a family member, marital conflict, or the need to make an important decision.

Panic episodes often occur because of a inner conflict or a sense of becoming trapped or potentially out of control. These are what may be called the primary anxiety situations. Once the panic and physical sensations begin to occur, the patient enters a far more upsetting "secondary anxiety" phase, that is, the "fear of fear." It is this fear of death or of impending loss of control that brings them to the health care system.

Predisposing Factors for Panic Disorder

Research studies and anecdotal clinical reports seem to point to several factors that contribute to the development of panic disorder. These include biologic factors, personality factors, and life events.

There is some evidence of a genetic predisposition to have an overly responsive autonomic nervous system among people who develop anxiety and panic disorders, although more of the variance can be accounted for by environmental factors.[12, 13] It has been shown that first-degree relatives of phobic patients have a far greater risk for the presence of an anxiety disorder than those of controls.[13] Among patients with panic plus agoraphobia (compared with those with panic disorder alone), a seven times higher incidence of avoidance behavior sufficient for a diagnosis of agoraphobia was found in first-degree relatives.[14] This partially confirms the hypothesis that cultural factors influence the development of avoidance behaviors but not necessarily the experience of panic.

Personality factors that may contribute to the development of panic include nonassertiveness and dependence, which contribute to feeling stuck or out of control in interpersonal relationships. Individuals with panic disorder may also have a tendency toward a vivid imagination, coupled with negative expectations of catastrophe. The vividness of negative thoughts creates a physical reaction as if the worst-case scenes were actually occurring, creating just the sensations that are so frightening.

Physiologic events have also been linked with onset of an initial panic attack. These have included the use of marijuana, LSD, cocaine, or anesthesia; an anaphylactic reaction; hormonal disruption; or even a severe viral infection. These have in common the experience of unusual bodily sensations that the individual cannot alter and that the individual fears may be threatening to life or sanity. Excessive caffeine use has also been associated with panic.

Evaluation and Treatment

A biobehavioral evaluation assesses all three aspects of anxiety: the cognitive, the physiologic, and the behavioral. An assessment includes questions about physiologic symptoms, possible stress situations, how the patient thinks about her situation and her symptoms, and what action (or nonaction) she is pursuing. Establishing the links among situations, thoughts, sensations, and actions early in treatment lays the groundwork for future interventions. The focus for treatment of anxiety is also threefold: challenging irrational beliefs and thoughts and substituting more realistic or accurate thinking, reduction of autonomic arousal, and directing action toward constructive solutions.

As in the treatment of other illnesses, the primary care physician is in a position for early intervention in the treatment of anxiety. In ideal circumstances, a behavioral therapist can be responsible for training patients in the self-regulation techniques. However, if referral sources are limited or if the patient is not amenable to a psychological referral, there are interventions that a physician or nurse practitioner can offer in a primary care setting that rely on a combination of medical expertise and self-regulating potential in individuals.

This model of treatment is based on stepwise interventions, which begin with fairly simple interventions and progress toward intensive therapy as needed. The mnemonic R-I-SS-T summarizes the steps of *R*eassurance, *I*nformation, *S*pecific *S*uggestions, and *T*herapy.

REASSURANCE THROUGH INFORMATION. The management of the individual with anxiety begins with the initial physical examination. Before the visit, she may have imagined all kinds of dread reasons for her symptoms. Having these explained begins to provide a sense of control and to counteract feelings of helplessness that contribute to the overall anxiety.

In patients with panic disorder, episodes of panic are escalated by catastrophic thoughts about the meaning of physical symptoms. Again, the physician can help the patient identify what her frightening thoughts are and begin to counteract them as soon as possible. Concrete information about the patient's body, how it functions, and how to interpret the sensations are of primary importance. For example, a racing pulse, skipped beats, or chest tightness is often interpreted by the patient as evidence of heart disease. Once a cardiac disorder is ruled out, a detailed explanation of the relationships among stress, adrenaline responses, and the increased heart rate that comes with physiologic hyperarousal should be given. It can be pointed out that the heart rate during a panic episode is no greater than it might be while climbing a flight of stairs or doing aerobics. It is often helpful to explain the differences between symptoms that suggest medical disease and those that indicate a stress response.

If she reports derealization or depersonalization, she should be reassured that these feelings are signs of severe anxiety, not signs that she is going to lose her sanity. Again, an explanation of the difference between schizophrenia and anxiety may be helpful.

If her symptoms are those associated with hyperventilation, such as feeling she is unable to take a breath, smothering sensations, dizziness, tingling in the hands or around the mouth, she may experience a great sense of dread, again thinking that she might pass out, die from lack of oxygen, or have a serious illness. Such thoughts further escalate her fears, increasing shallow breathing and maintaining the state of hyperventilation. A full explanation of the phenomenon of hyperventilation should be given, using ordinary terms. In particular, explain that the sensation of lack of air is actually a result of overbreathing and that the body will readjust itself if her breathing slows down. If necessary, the symptoms of hyperventilation can be created in the office by having her breathe as quickly as she can until she begins to feel dizzy. At this time she can also practice any of several methods to limit hyperventilation: holding her breath, cupping her hands over nose and mouth and rebreathing carbon dioxide–laden air, or slow breathing through the nose.

Finally, information should be offered about the role of caffeine in potentiating the effects of adrenaline. Caffeine has a half-life of 4 to 6 hours and has been demonstrated to escalate the physical symptoms of anxiety.

SPECIFIC SUGGESTIONS FOR TALKING BACK TO IRRATIONAL THOUGHTS. In patients with generalized anxiety, the primary goal of a cognitive-behavioral intervention is to redirect the focus of attention away from negative possibilities, or "what if" thoughts, and toward possible actions that might solve the worrisome problem. Patients are encouraged to notice their frightening thoughts and to "talk back" to their fears. For example, if the patient has financial concerns, they may have thoughts such as "What if I get further behind? What if I lose my income? I might end up homeless." These thoughts are followed by images of being on the street, frightened, and without hope. Talking back to these thoughts entails asking such questions as, "What is the likelihood you will lose your income? What other resources do you have? What are the actual steps you need to take to address your financial concerns?" These are commonsense approaches to someone who is not paralyzed with anxiety, yet quite helpful to someone who is. For many, the process of voicing their worst fears allows them to gain some distance and see how they might counteract them.

Beck recommends using a two-column written format in which the fearful thoughts are listed on the left side of the page and the positive or contradictory thoughts are listed on the right.[15] This technique has been shown to reduce both anxious and depressed feelings. Another strategy is called self-instruction. With this technique, patients remind themselves to slow down and take one step at a time, asking themselves, "What do I have to do next?" Thought stopping is another technique for interrupting worrisome thoughts. Whenever the patient realizes she is engaging in negative thinking, she is instructed to say "STOP!" and shift her thinking to a more productive channel, just as one changes channels on the television. Panic-producing thoughts can be stopped by focusing on the present, letting time pass, and facing the fear.

For those who can sit still for 20 minutes and for whom it holds appeal, meditation is another method of noticing thoughts without reacting to them. For individuals with a strong faith, prayer may serve a similar purpose. The primary care provider may not be the one to teach such methods but can serve as an encouraging educator about the links between peace of mind and physical health.

SPECIFIC SUGGESTIONS FOR REVERSING AUTONOMIC HYPERACTIVITY. The second goal of intervention is to teach the individual to reverse the body's autonomic hyperactivity and heightened muscle tension. The most powerful strategy for managing anxiety that we have to offer patients is a combination of progressive muscle relaxation, diaphragmatic breathing, and auto-suggestion.

Muscle Relaxation Techniques. With muscle relaxation, the patient is asked to sit back in a chair or other comfortable place, close her eyes if that feels comfortable, and begin to let herself relax. The instructor then asks her to alternately tense and relax different muscle groups throughout the body, beginning with the hands and arms and moving through the shoulders, neck, face, abdomen, and legs. The patient is instructed particularly to notice the differences between tense and relaxed muscles and how it feels to let go of muscle tension. As part of the relaxation exercise, she is also instructed to notice the rhythm of her breathing and to take several deep breaths, relaxing as she exhales. Finally, she is instructed to notice her thoughts, to let troublesome thoughts leave the mind, and to focus her attention on visualizing a beautiful and relaxing place such as a beach.

This exercise takes about 15 to 20 minutes to complete. It is usually tape recorded so that the patient can practice several times daily at home. Commercial tapes are available at bookstores or by mail order.

After mastering the longer technique of muscular tensing and relaxing, patients can be taught a short form of autosuggestion for relaxation. They are instructed to say short suggestive sentences to themselves such as, "Let my arms feel heavy and relaxed. Let my legs feel heavy and relaxed. Let my breathing be gentle and even. Let my mind be calm and quiet." They are to repeat these phrases slowly two to three times until they are calm. Another short relaxation technique is the "slump," or "rag doll," which involves letting go of tension throughout the body all at once.

As muscles relax, the rest of the body tends to slow down as well. It is easier to begin with muscle relaxation because it is under more voluntary control. Control of other systems are an indirect function of muscle relaxation and respiration.

As needed, a referral to a behavioral medicine specialist for specific interventions may be required. Individuals with more severe symptoms may require referral for specific biofeedback to the system at risk. The effectiveness of progressive muscle relaxation training in reversing autonomic hyperactivity has been well documented in the extensive biofeedback literature.[16] For example, those with muscle tension pain benefit from electromyograph biofeedback. Those with cardiovascular symptoms such as migraines, Raynaud's syndrome, or hypertension benefit more from a combination of electromyograph biofeedback and peripheral vasodilation or hand temperature biofeedback in conjunction with training in deep muscle relaxation.

Restoring Normal Breathing Patterns. One aspect of the general arousal syndrome is a quickening of the breath as part of the body's readiness to fight or flee. This increase in respiration is often achieved by an increase in upper chest breathing. When slower abdominal breathing is restricted, overbreathing may occur, leading to an increase in levels of oxygen in the blood and decreasing levels of carbon dioxide. If this occurs during strenuous exercise (such as actual flight), carbon dioxide levels return to normal. If not, respiratory alkalosis ensues as percent of carbon dioxide decreases. These effects are responsible for most of the physical changes that occur with hyperventilation: constriction of peripheral blood vessels (including to the brain) and slower release of oxygen to the tissue due to the increase in blood alkalinity. There is an increase in heart rate to pump more blood through the system. The transient reduction in oxygen release to the brain may produce dizziness, lightheadedness, confusion, visual distortions, and a sense of unreality. Peripherally, patients may experience cold hands and numbness and tingling in the extremities. The individual feels as if she is not getting enough air. Yet, because of hypocapnia, respiratory drive is decreased, providing a sensation of difficulty breathing. Most frightening for many patients is the feeling of being unable to breathe. Another frightening feeling is chest pressure or tightness, as if there is a tight band around the chest, which may be interpreted as heart failure.

Many patients deny overbreathing, and indeed, their pattern of breathing may be both habitual and difficult to detect, yet it maintains chronically low levels of carbon dioxide and higher blood alkalinity, making them more susceptible to the onset of symptoms during acute anxiety. The patient's understanding of the role of mild hyperventilation in the development of anxiety symptoms is an initial step toward reversing this process.

Primary care providers should note the breathing patterns among their anxious patients: failure to breathe while talking, occasional sighing or yawning as they begin to relax, and differential movements between upper chest and abdominal muscles. Postures that might restrict breathing may include hunched shoulders, folded arms, or sitting with legs crossed and turned in the chair.

A quick behavioral assessment of breath pattern can be done as follows: "On the count of three, I want you to take a quick, deep breath and hold it. Ready? One, two, three!" Note the relative movements of shoulders and upper chest to abdomen.

Some movement in the upper body is normal, but the greater motion should occur in the area of the diaphragm and stomach. Exaggerated shoulder, neck, and chest movements indicate automatic and habitual chest breathing. A distention of the abdomen indicates diaphragmatic breathing.

Training a habitual chest breather to engage in slow, deep breathing takes a few minutes in session and several weeks of home practice. The training serves two goals: an appropriate rate of breathing and mental concentration. A central aspect of most meditative disciplines is breathing awareness. Observing respiration is the simplest of meditations and disciplines the mind not to engage in worrisome thoughts.

To begin, have the patient stand leaning against a wall, sitting back in a chair, or lying on a table in a position so that she can see her hands laced across the abdomen. Instruct her to breathe slowly and deeply through her nose, pulling air in with the diaphragm and pushing out the abdomen. Have her observe the rise and fall of her hands. This is a type of visual feedback that helps her learn the internal sensations of correct breathing. It may be difficult at first and may seem unnatural. An alternate hand position is one hand on the chest and one on the abdomen, noting differential movements and noticing the internal sensations of pressure as well. If the patient cannot alter her breathing pattern, have her sit in a chair, both feet on the floor, elbows on her knees, and chin cupped in her hands. This position immobilizes the scalene muscles and shoulders. The only way to breathe in this position is with the diaphragm.

If the patient notices that her mind is wandering or she is having worrisome thoughts, she is instructed to let the thoughts drift away and return her attention to the slow and gentle sensations of her breath.

Diaphragmatic or deep breathing should be practiced twice daily for at least 10 minutes for several weeks. Initially, it should be practiced in a quiet comfortable spot. Later, practice should occur under many different conditions and eventually should be used during times of stress to slow both the body and the mind.

Autosuggestion. Simple forms of autosuggestion have been developed from the field of hypnotic suggestion, in which patients practice self-reassurance phrases. An image of a quiet place such as the beach or listening to music is paired with physical relaxation and can evoke the relaxation response under times of stress. These images are seen as ''brakes'' to counteract the ''accelerator'' effect of adrenaline.

Taking Action. Once patients have mastered these techniques, they should be encouraged to take small steps toward regaining control of their lives (Table 72–1). Any efforts should be encouraged. In solving problems, persistence pays off. Chronic worriers need to learn to focus on the problem, not possible catastrophic outcomes. Agoraphobics should begin traveling to previously avoided places on a gradual basis. They should be encouraged not to leave the situation until symptoms subside through time or self-regulation.

This combination of cognitive and behavioral interventions has shown promise for the long-term treatment of general anxiety. Butler and colleagues evaluated a program of tape-recorded relaxation instructions, control of upsetting thoughts through distraction and thought stopping, and encouragement of patients to actively take control of their lives.[17] Patients were also asked to note areas of their lives in which they were functioning well. The treatment group improved compared with the controls on all measures at 3-month and 6-month follow-up. At 1 year, two thirds of patients in the treatment group had had no further contact with their primary care physician.

BEHAVIORAL TREATMENT OF PANIC AND AGORAPHOBIA. Behavioral treatments that encourage self-paced, gradual entering of feared situations have repeatedly been demonstrated to be effective in reducing panic.[18, 19] These treatments can take anywhere from 8 weeks to 1 year, depending on the severity of the disorder. The controlled studies that have follow-up data have shown long-lasting effects, with improvement maintained for up to 2 years after cessation of treatment.[20, 21]

There are several key elements in a behavioral program. Patients learn to recognize the cycle of panic and to understand the body's emergency re-

---

TABLE 72–1. A Behavioral Prescription for Self-Management of Physical Symptoms

---

1. Record symptoms daily and any activity or situation that makes the symptom better or worse.
2. Rate anxiety on a scale of 1 to 10, with 1 being calm and 10 feeling panicky and out of control. This rating exercise will help you to become more aware of tension before you develop actual symptoms. Notice those activities that make you less anxious.
3. Record worried thoughts you are having. This will increase your awareness of the relationships among situations, thoughts, and symptoms. Find a positive thought or action that would counteract your worries.
4. Take a daily rest period for 15 to 20 min. Practice relaxing both the body and the mind. During this time practice slow, deep breathing and a positive frame of mind. The rest period may include listening to music or other relaxing activities that feel natural to you.

action to real and imagined threat. They learn and practice the skills that physically calm the body, such as diaphragmatic breathing, muscle relaxation, and cognitive control of catastrophic thoughts. Feared activities or situations are listed in order of difficulty, and patients learn to approach their goals in small yet persistent steps. This exposure to the feared stimulus gradually reduces learned or conditioned fear. Setbacks are used to further analyze their particular areas of difficulty and to identify needed situations for practice. Confidence is developed through a combination of minor successes and positive imagery of successful coping. A behavioral program may also include marital or relationship counseling, group therapy, cognitive restructuring, assertiveness training, and development of life skills to increase independence.

THERAPY: COGNITIVE BEHAVIORAL INTERVENTIONS WITH OR WITHOUT MEDICATION. If initial interventions do not result in a reduction of anxiety symptoms, more intensive therapy may be necessary. More in-depth cognitive-behavioral therapy may be needed to address long-standing personality or situational issues. Medication may also be an adjunct to such treatment.

A primary question in the treatment of anxiety disorders is the relative merits of behavioral versus medication therapy. Proponents of behavioral therapy cite the longer-lasting effects of behavioral treatments and a preference for drug-free treatments, which avoid the risks of side effects and possible drug dependency. With such treatments the client develops a sense of self-regulation, mastery, and self-efficacy, which in itself helps reduce anxiety. A comprehensive behavioral treatment also addresses any underlying situations that may have given rise to the development of anxiety episodes.

Evidence of rebound anxiety on discontinuance of medication has been documented. A strong placebo effect has been noted in many studies of drug effects on anxiety, illustrating the powers of suggestion. This effect can be seen clinically in patients who carry a few pills with them for months after treatment termination "just in case" they have a panic attack. Leaving the bottle behind can itself bring on a panic episode.

Feminist analysts have also pointed out the excessive use of tranquilizers in women compared with that in men. Because of the high prevalence of anxiety disorders among women, women have been the recipients of millions of prescriptions for mood-altering medication. Holding diagnosis constant, women receive more mood-modifying drugs than men and account for almost 70% of such

prescriptions written.[22] The risks to women have included physical addiction with rebound anxiety on abrupt withdrawal, psychological dependence, sedation, cognitive impairments of memory and attention, and impairments in driving.

The use of medication as the treatment of choice for anxious feelings may encourage women to continue in a dependent role, relying on external authority for solutions, with little directed change in their life circumstances. Medication may also cover a woman's concerns rather than address the underlying causes in her social and economic condition.

Advocates of medication therapy cite the genetic predisposition of persons with anxiety disorders, arguing for a "chemical imbalance" that must be adjusted through drug therapy, using epilepsy or hypertension as an analogy. Long-term maintenance on the medication is seen as acceptable should symptoms return when medication is discontinued.[23] Anxiolytics such as alprazolam are also seen as quick acting, inexpensive compared with psychotherapy, and easy for the physician to prescribe. Referral to a behavioral therapist may be seen as stigmatizing, time consuming, or impractical. For individuals who accept medication, it is seen as a ready solution.

Several studies have attempted to clarify these issues, not only comparing drug treatment with placebo and behavioral instruction, but also investigating the merits of combined treatments. The medications investigated have been primarily anxiolytics such as alprazolam and the tricyclic antidepressants such as imipramine.

Benzodiazepines. There have been many well-designed, double-blind, placebo-controlled studies of the effects of benzodiazepines on generalized anxiety disorder. A review of 78 double-blind studies concluded that in spite of occasional small effects in some studies, benzodiazepines had not been demonstrated to be more effective than placebo in any clinically meaningful way.[24] Another review of an additional nine studies totaling 1200 subjects concluded that there was a marked overlap between the medication groups and the placebo groups on scores of anxiety.[25] This overlap suggests that although there may be a statistically significant difference, these drugs offer little clinical benefit over placebo. Fifty percent of the studies reviewed found no significant differences on self-reported measures. Any therapeutic effects were also found to be short lived, disappearing within 1 to 6 weeks.

Measuring the effects of treatments for a subjective symptom such as anxiety is a complex process, and the same data can lead different investigators to contrasting conclusions. This has been particularly true in the evaluation studies of the effectiveness of alprazolam. One report on a multiple site panic study concluded that "alprazolam is effective in the short-term treatment of panic disorder and agoraphobia."[26, 27] However, others noted many limitations in methodology and outcome results that have led them to emphasize different conclusions.[28] These included a high dropout rate among those receiving placebo and an inability of raters to remain blind as to control group assignment. They agreed that alprazolam was more effective than placebo in the first 4 weeks but emphasized that by week 8 there were no significant differences. Moreover, at week 14, after a 4-week taper, patients receiving alprazolam were worse off than those receiving placebo in terms of panic, avoidance, and anxiety, reflecting severe discontinuation problems. Equally striking yet minimally noted in the original articles was the marked parallel improvement by week 8 in those subjects receiving placebo. Although the longest follow-up study on the effects of benzodiazepines[29] was 6 weeks, 48% of psychotropic drugs prescribed in general practice had been used for more than 2 years.[30] Benzodiazepines may be useful as a temporary tool to reduce some of the physiologic manifestations of anxiety during a stressful period. However, without cognitive and behavioral treatments, no long-term benefit can be expected.

Tricyclic Antidepressants. Similar limitations have marred studies of other medications, but the tricyclic antidepressants imipramine and clomipramine have shown the most promise. Although antidepressants do not prevent panic itself, they may reduce the overall levels of anxiety and depression that contribute to the development of panic and avoidance behaviors.

Telch and colleagues examined the effects of imipramine alone without exposure instructions to enter feared situations.[31] They found little or no improvement in panic attacks, phobic avoidance, or anxiety. However, some reduction in depressed mood was observed. Comparison groups who received exposure instructions or imipramine plus exposure instructions displayed marked improvement on the same measures. In this study, imipramine did seem to enhance the effects of in vivo exposure treatment. In another study, imipramine had superior anxiolytic effects compared to benzodiazepines for patients with general anxiety.[32]

Other studies have investigated the additive or interactive effects of behavioral instructions plus imipramine in the treatment of agoraphobia. Marks and co-workers found no advantage in adding imipramine to exposure instructions compared with placebo.[18] Mavissakalian and Michelson reported

statistically significant differences in favor of a combined behavior therapy and imipramine treatment.[19] They found that imipramine plus exposure-based treatment added some advantage at post-treatment measures, but this difference disappeared within 1 month of treatment termination. Drug relationships were found only for global measures, not for panic itself, and only at post-treatment. The additive effects of imipramine were not evident at 6-month follow-up.

Other tricyclics have fewer studies supporting their effectiveness. Desipramine in higher doses (200 mg per day) may be more likely to yield a positive response than it does in lower doses. Fluvoxamine, zimeldine hydrochloride, nortriptyline, amitriptyline, and doxepin have received preliminary study but have not demonstrated conclusively that they are more effective than placebo or behavioral self-regulation techniques.[27]

Certain other antidepressant drugs have been tested in clinical trials with panic disorder and agoraphobia. Phenelzine (a monoamine oxidase inhibitor) has been shown to have little additive effect to behavioral treatments. Trazodone, however, may be somewhat effective in the treatment of panic disorder.[33]

Other medications have also been evaluated for the treatment of general anxiety. β-blockers may be effective for individual patients, but have not been demonstrated to be more effective than placebo in controlled studies.[34] Buspirone has shown promise as a treatment for both cognitive and somatic symptoms of general anxiety but has not been shown to be effective with panic disorder.[35] Imipramine has not been as well studied as a treatment for general anxiety as it has for panic disorder. However, Kahn and associates noted significant antianxiety effects after 8 weeks.[32]

In summary, cognitive-behavioral treatments alone have been shown to be effective in the treatment of subjective anxiety, number and severity of panic attacks, and avoidance behaviors. Medication alone is marginally useful, particularly in long-term symptom reduction. Although imipramine may not have a direct effect on panic, the effect on mood elevation may increase the likelihood that patients will practice homework instructions more readily and evaluate their successes more positively. Imipramine may also decrease overall anxious apprehension and the somatic sensations that tend to cause panic. Combined behavior therapy and medication appear to be useful for certain individuals in the beginning stages of treatment if they are otherwise unable to benefit from behavioral practice owing to severe physiologic symptoms. In actual practice, the selection of medication often depends on the broad range of indi-

TABLE 72–2. Books and Self-Help Resources for Patients with Stress, Anxiety, and Panic Disorder

1. Pamphlets on panic disorder. National Institute for Mental Health Panic Campaign, Room 15C-05, 5600 Fisher Lane, Rockville MD 20857.
2. Weekes C. Peace from Nervous Suffering. New York: New American Library, 1990.
3. Jeffers S. Feel the Fear and Do It Anyway. New York: Ballantine, 1988.
4. Miller LH, Smith AD. The Stress Solution. New York: Pocket Books, 1993.
5. ADDA Reporter, a bimonthly newsletter. Anxiety Disorder Association of America, 6000 Executive Boulevard, Suite 200, Rockville MD 20852–3801.
6. National Panic/Anxiety Disorder Newsletter. 1718 Burgundy Pl, Suite B-2, Santa Rosa CA 95403.
7. Relaxation and stress management tapes. Thought Technology, 2180 Belgrave Ave, Montreal, Quebec H4A 2L8, Canada
8. Relaxation and stress management tapes. Biobehavioral Institute, 1415 Beacon Street, Brookline MA 02146.

vidual differences in the tolerance of side effects and patients' preferences for drug or nondrug treatments. In addition, many patients can benefit from reading about the causes and treatments of stress, anxiety, and panic disorder (Table 72–2).

REFERENCES

1. Marsland DW, Wood M, Mayo F. Content of family practice: A data bank for patient care, curriculum, and research in family practice—526,196 patient problems. J Fam Prac 1976;3:25.
2. Shepherd M, Cooper B, Brown AC, Kalton GW. Psychiatric Illness in General Practice. London: Oxford University Press, 1966.
3. Uhlenhuth EH, Baltzer MB, Mellinger GE, et al. Symptom checklist syndromes in the general population. Arch Gen Psychiatry 1983;40:1167.
4. Agras WS, Chapin HN, Oliveau DC. The natural history of phobia. Arch Gen Psychiatry 1972;26:315.
5. Sanderson WC, Rapee RM, Barlow DH. The DSM-III-Revised Anxiety Disorder Categories: Description and Patterns of Comorbidity. Paper presented at the annual meeting of the Association of Advancement of Behavior Therapy, Boston, 1987.
6. Jaffe P, Wolfe DA, Wilson S, Zak L. Emotional and physical health problems of battered women. Can J Psychiatry 1986;31:625.
7. Goldstein AJ, Chambless DL. A reanalysis of agoraphobia. Behav Ther 1978;9:47.
8. Hafner RJ. Agoraphobic women married to abnormally jealous men. Br J Med Psychol 1979;52:99.
9. Hudson B. The families of agoraphobics treated by behaviour therapy. Br J Soc Work 1974;4:51.
10. American Psychiatric Association. Diagnostic and Statistical Manual of Mental Disorders. 4th ed. Washington, DC: American Psychiatric Association, 1994.
11. Barlow DH. Anxiety and Its Disorders. New York: The Guilford Press, 1988, pp 576–577.
12. Eysenck HJ (ed). The Biological Basis of Personality. Springfield, Ill: Charles C Thomas, 1967.
13. Crowe RR, Noyes R, Pauls DL, Slymen DJ. A family study of panic disorder. Arch Gen Psychiatry 1983;40:1065.
14. Harris EL, Noyes R, Crowe RR, Chaudhry DR. Family study of agoraphobia. Arch Gen Psychiatry 1983;40:1061.
15. Beck AT. Cognitive Therapy and the Emotional Disorders. New York: International Universities Press, 1976.
16. Basmajian JV (ed). Biofeedback: Principles and Practice for Clinicians. 3rd ed. Baltimore: Williams & Wilkins, 1989.
17. Butler G, Cullington A, Munby M, et al. Exposure and anxiety management in the treatment of social phobia. J. Consult Clin Psychol 1984;52:642.
18. Marks IM, Grey S, Cohen SD, et al. Imipramine and brief therapist-sided exposure in agoraphobics having self exposure homework: A controlled trial. Arch Gen Psychiatry 1983;40:1153.
19. Mavissakalian M, Michelson L. Agoraphobia: Relative and combined effectiveness of therapist-assisted in vivo exposure and imipramine. J Clin Psychiatry 1986;47:117.
20. Clark DM, Salkovskis PM, Chalkley AJ. Respiratory control as a treatment for panic attacks. J Behav Ther Exp Psychiatry 1985;16:23.
21. Salkovskis PM, Jones DR, Clark DM. Respiratory control in the treatment of panic attacks: Replication and extension with concurrent measurement of behaviour and pCO_2. Br J Psychiatry 1986;148:526.
22. Cooperstock R. Sex differences in the use of mood-modifying drugs: An explanatory model. J Health Soc Behav 1971;12:238.
23. Ballenger JC. Toward an integrated model of panic disorder. Am J Orthopsychiatry 1989;59:284.
24. Solomon K, Hart R. Pitfalls and prospects in clinical research on antianxiety drugs: Benzodiazepines and placebos. J Clin Psychiatry 1978;39:823.
25. Barlow DH. Anxiety and Its Disorders. New York: The Guilford Press, 1988, p 585.
26. Klerman GL. Overview of the cross-national collaborative panic study. Arch Gen Psychiatry 1988;45:407.
27. Ballenger JC, Burrows GD, Dupont RL, et al. Alprazolam in panic disorder and agoraphobia: Efficacy in short-term treatment. Arch Gen Psychiatry 1988;45:423.
28. Marks IM. The ''efficacy'' of alprazolam in panic disorder and agoraphobia: A critique of recent reports. Arch Gen Psychiatry 1989;46:668.
29. Herman JL, Perry JC, Van der Kolk B. Childhood trauma in borderline personality disorder. Am J Psychiatry 1989;146:490.
30. Anderson RM. The use of repeatedly prescribed medicines. J R Coll Gen Pract 1980;30:609.
31. Telch MJ, Agras WS, Taylor CB, et al. Combined pharmacological and behavioral treatment for agoraphobia. Behav Res Ther 1985;23:325.
32. Kahn RJ, McNair DM, Lipman RS, et al. Imipramine and chlordiazepoxide in depressive and anxiety disorders. Arch Gen Psychiatry 1986;43:79.
33. Mavissakalian M, Perel JM, Bowler K, Dealy R. Trazodone in the treatment of panic/agoraphobia. Am J Psychiatry 1987;144:785.
34. Noyes R. Beta-adrenergic blocking drugs in anxiety and stress. Psychiatr Clin North Am 1985;8:119.
35. Rickels K, Wiseman K, Norstad N, et al. Buspirone and diazepam in anxiety: A controlled study. J Clin Psychiatry 1982;43:81.

SPECIAL ISSUES

The Disabled Patient

Susan Biener Bergman and Sandra Lee Welner

As medical care improves, more individuals are surviving catastrophic injuries and illnesses. Many are left with serious disabilities. There are currently approximately 18 million disabled women in the United States.[1] Only recently have women who are challenged with physical disabilities emerged as a separate group distinct from their male counterparts and able-bodied women. The disabled woman confronts discrimination as a result of both her gender and her disability, that is, she may be seen as "less than whole" by able-bodied men and women and viewed in sexist terms by disabled men.[1]

Primary care providers need to familiarize themselves with the medical issues and the physical and emotional challenges of disabled women. There is a need for specific research on the care of disabled women. Much of the available literature focuses on disabled men, primarily because men are more often victims of traumatic injury. Because more males populate rehabilitation units, research studies as well as rehabilitation programs are often oriented to their needs.

THE MEDICAL HISTORY

Caring for the disabled woman begins with history taking. The physician should create an appropriate environment to ensure the patient's comfort by obtaining permission to discuss personal areas.[2] The examiner will need more time for the examination and the postexamination care, and scheduling should be done accordingly. Specific attention should be paid to a careful functional assessment, social history, and sexual history.

THE FUNCTIONAL HISTORY

When caring for a disabled woman, it is vital to know how she goes about her activities of daily living (ADLs), the equipment she uses, and any areas with which she is having difficulty. Within each activity are several recognizable levels of function:

1. *Independent*—The patient is able to accomplish a task without equipment or assistance from another person.
2. *Independent with aids*—The patient is able to complete the task with a piece of equipment but does not need the assistance of another person.
3. *Requires assistance*—The patient needs another person's help to complete the task.
4. *Dependent*—The patient is unable to provide any useful physical effort to complete the task.[3]

Daily tasks to ask about can be divided as follows:

1. Mobility
   a. *Transfers*—Assessment includes how the patient gets out of bed, on and off the toilet, in and out of a wheelchair, and whether she uses adaptive equipment such as a sliding board (a polished wood or plastic board over which one can slide from one surface to another) or a pneumatic lift.
   b. *Wheelchair mobility*—Assessment includes whether the patient uses a wheelchair, and if so, whether it is manual or power driven. Physicians should ask whether she can propel a manual chair independently and for what length of time. Users of power-operated chairs should be asked what sort of switch control is used (joystick, toggle switch, chin control, puff-sip).

c. *Ambulation*—The provider should assess not only whether the patient can walk or whether she falls, but what assistive devices she uses, including walker, crutches, cane, braces, ankle-foot orthosis, knee-ankle-foot orthosis, or prosthesis.

d. *Transportation*—The provider should ask whether she operates a motor vehicle, and if so, the type of controls applied to a car, whether she has any difficulty with motor vehicle operation, and whether she has had any accidents.

2. Activities of daily living

a. *Communication*—This includes an assessment of speech and language abilities as well as questions about difficulties in hearing, seeing, reading, or word finding.

b. *Eating*—This includes an assessment of the patient's ability to prepare food (open containers, cook, serve, and cut food) and to swallow without choking or regurgitating.

c. *Grooming*—This includes an assessment of the patient's ability to brush teeth, comb hair, or apply makeup.

d. *Bathing*—The patient's ability to maintain cleanliness can affect both her physical and emotional well-being. This includes assessing whether she can bathe or shower, what equipment she uses (shower chair, tub bench, long-handled sponge), and whether there are parts of her body that she cannot reach.

e. *Toileting*—Continence of urine and stool is crucial to social adjustment and to prevention of skin breakdown and infection. Questions to ask include how she empties her bladder, any equipment used (catheters, female urinals, pads), how she empties her bowels, whether she has difficulty removing her clothing or cleaning herself after using the toilet, and whether she has difficulty with sanitary napkin or tampon use.

f. *Dressing*—Providers should ask what type of clothing the patient regularly wears and whether she uses adaptive equipment (long-handled shoe horn, elastic laces, button hook, dressing stick, Velcro closures) or requires assistance.

g. *Advanced ADLs*—These include household chores such as cooking, cleaning, yard work, grocery shopping, child care, and any vocational or avocational concerns. Providers should ask about any architectural barriers such as stairs (bedroom on the second floor, laundry in the basement), thresholds, or high shelves. Discussion should include the patient's work place and any difficulties she

may be having in this setting, hobbies she may have, and sports in which she participates. Sports for individuals with disabilities represent an excellent social outlet as well as an opportunity to maintain fitness and improve self-esteem.

THE SOCIAL HISTORY

The social history should include a description of the individual's current living situation; educational status, including specialty training or learning problems; and current and past sexual partners. Drug, alcohol, and cigarette use should be ascertained. The woman should be asked about any incidents of abuse in the past or present. Disabled women may be particularly vulnerable to abuse[4]; in some cases abuse may have caused their handicaps.[5, 6] In particular, conditions that result in cognitive impairment, weakness, and balance or mobility problems increase the risk of assault[7] (see Chapter 70). Chronic pain may be an indication of present or past abuse. Abuse in the developmentally disabled may be particularly difficult to diagnose, as they may be unable to relate the details of the event[8] (see Chapter 74).

THE SEXUAL AND REPRODUCTIVE HISTORY

The sexual history presents an opportunity to gather and to give information. It should include an assurance of confidentiality, an assessment of the patient's level of knowledge of the structure and function of the reproductive system, and an assessment of the patient's sexual orientation and predisability and current sexual functioning. Special difficulties the disability brings to sexual expression, such as limitation of motion, pain, decreased endurance, incontinence, need for and use of contraception, and any negative or traumatic sexual encounters, should be addressed.[7, 9]

Contraception should be discussed with any heterosexually active woman. The choices appropriate for a disabled woman may be somewhat more limited. For example, a woman with a spinal cord injury should not take combination oral contraceptives because of the risk of thromboembolic events with the estrogen component, although they may be appropriate for women with other types of disabilities. Barrier methods may be impossible for a woman to use independently if she has impaired fine motor function, although her partner or an attendant may be willing to assist her. Progestin-only contraceptives in the form of the mini-pill, medroxyprogesterone acetate, or Norplant may be appropriate. The physician should discuss whether the patient can manage the packaging of any method herself or has appropriate assistance available. A reproductive history should include a description of previous pregnancies and deliveries with specific inquiry about urinary tract infections, decubitus ulcers, precipitous labor, and autonomic dysreflexia.

PHYSICAL EXAMINATION

The physical examination of a disabled woman requires patience and creativity. It focuses on a number of different elements: neurologic, respiratory, cardiovascular, orthopedic, rheumatologic, gastrointestinal, and genitourinary evaluation, pelvic examination, and cognitive status and emotional adjustment.

A woman's ability to get onto the examining table may be limited by strength, range of motion, balance, and coordination. It is best to offer assistance rather than assume help is needed as the woman may have devised her own system of transfer from surface to surface. If she does need help, it is important to have adequate staff to provide this assistance to prevent injury. Examination tables are often too high for easy transfer. Ideally, one electrically controlled or height-adjustable table should be available for such a patient in a physician's office.

For a visually impaired woman, orientation to her surroundings is essential to increase her level of comfort and sense of control. Women with disabilities often have clothing adapted to their fine motor impairments. However, they may not have adaptive equipment with them to assist in dressing. If the patient requires assistance to undress owing to fine motor or coordination impairments, it should not be overlooked that she will need assistance putting her clothes back on.

If the woman's hand function is significantly impaired, she should be provided with written instructions in addition to a verbal explanation. For the patient who has visual difficulties, it is preferable to ask the patient whether she uses Braille or tape recorders or has family members or attendants read material to her and then to use her preferred method. For patients with hearing impairments, all information needs to be written out. Exaggerated gesticulations and shouting are not helpful and can be embarrassing. If the physician or office personnel do not know sign language, ask if the patient can read lips. If she can, the communication can continue in a more normal fashion. If not, an interpreter should be made available.

Neurologic Evaluation

Deep tendon reflexes, tone, and the presence of any obligatory reflex patterns or abnormal reflexes should be checked. Motor strength in all muscle groups should be examined and any weakness or paralysis noted. Sensory deficits, including loss of proprioception, should be assessed. This is particularly important because loss of sensation can predispose to decubitus ulcers, accidental burns, and other serious injuries.

Respiratory Evaluation

Patients with chronic obstructive pulmonary disease can become quite debilitated. Their symptoms may include pulmonary orthopnea, dyspnea on exertion, and shortness of breath. Patients with high spinal cord injuries may be using only their diaphragms to breathe as their accessory muscles may no longer be functional. Patients with severe scoliosis or certain types of muscular dystrophy may suffer from restrictive lung disease. Because chest expansion is limited, they are predisposed to pulmonary infections. Inspection, percussion, and auscultation should be performed.

Cardiovascular Evaluation

Patients with cardiac disease can be disabled in the sense that their normal activity may be significantly curtailed. Cardiac disease may be a feature of neuromuscular disorders such as Friedreich's ataxia or Duchenne's muscular dystrophy. Auscultation should be performed to detect signs of cardiac dysfunction. Common entities such as mitral valve prolapse or atrial fibrillation can be detected in this way. The latter can be a significant predisposing factor in thromboembolic events.

Patients who have decreased ambulatory capacity or are wheelchair bound are more at risk for proximal or distal thrombotic events. The clinician should carefully assess any tenderness in the inguinal region or calves. Homans' sign, edema in thighs, calves, or ankles, discoloration, skin breakdown, peripheral pulses, and size discrepancies between lower extremities should also be checked. In the presence of sensory deficits, as in spinal cord injuries, a slight swelling and low-grade fever may be the only signs of an acute deep vein thrombosis.

Orthopedic Evaluation

Many disabling conditions include bony deformities as part of their presentation. The presence of any deformities should be noted, joint range of motion measured, and bone pain assessed. Scoliosis and joint contractures are especially common. Disabled women, especially older women or those who have been immobilized for a long time may develop osteoporotic changes due to lack of weight bearing on extremities and limitations on torque in the spinal column. Occasionally these changes may result in bone pain in the cervical, thoracic, or lumbar regions. More commonly, the first expression of osteoporotic changes is a fracture. Preventive measures against osteoporosis should be provided to all immobilized women, including adequate dietary calcium and vitamin D. Use of estrogens after menopause is also indicated for osteoporosis prevention; unlike oral contraceptives, risk of thrombotic events is not increased, and estrogen is therefore not contraindicated because of immobility.

Rheumatologic Evaluation

Rheumatologic conditions can be especially disabling and may appear at any age but often are exacerbated in the elderly. This can cause significant mobility loss, which affects ambulation and fine motor coordination capabilities. In addition, abnormal gait patterns resulting from spasticity, weakness, or both may cause painful joint instability or osteoarthritis after several years. Physical examination should evaluate joint mobility, ligamentous integrity, the presence of any fluid collections, and any areas of erythema, heat, or fluctuance.

Gastrointestinal Evaluation

Bowel function may be affected by several disabling conditions. Neurogenic bowel is a prominent feature of spinal cord injury. Continence can be maintained by initiating a regular regimen of stool softeners, high-fiber diet, and timed elimination. Even when the bowel remains normal, altered mobility may make elimination difficult, increasing the risk of fecal impaction. Bowel sounds should be auscultated, the abdomen should be palpated, and the integrity of any stomal pouches and surrounding skin should be checked for leaking and ulceration.

Genitourinary Evaluation

The female urinary tract is anatomically more predisposed to infections, especially during sexual activity. The bladder should be palpated, collection devices should be examined, and the patient should be questioned about symptoms of dysuria, urgency, or frequency. Women with spinal cord injuries may not have such symptoms because of sensory deficits; a change in her baseline level of spasticity or a feeling of malaise may be her only symptom. Urinalysis and culture should be done as part of the routine gynecologic examination if the patient has any urinary tract dysfunction. Women who have indwelling catheters should have the integrity and hygiene of the areas surrounding the urethral meatus carefully inspected. Care should be taken to avoid traction on the catheter with the legbag or other suspending apparatus. It is important to distinguish between urinary tract infection and bladder colonization in women with spinal cord injuries. Treating simple colonization with antibiotics will select for progressively more resistant and invasive organisms. Antibiotics should be reserved for when a positive urine culture is accompanied by pyuria, elevated serum white blood cell count, fever, or a change in the baseline level of spasticity. For prophylaxis, acidification with vitamin C and Mandelamine is usually adequate.

Pelvic Examination

The majority of problems in the pelvic examination are due to restrictions in range of motion, especially in the restriction of hip abduction. These difficulties can arise from various conditions including multiple sclerosis, cerebral palsy, traumatic brain injury, arthritic conditions, and spinal cord injury. Creative positioning manipulations may be required. When dealing with spasticity, slow, gentle, sustained stretch is usually more successful than rapid, forceful movement. Examining the upper body first may be helpful by allowing the patient to relax and by enhancing trust.

In women with neurogenic bladders, as in cases of spinal cord injury, traumatic brain injury, and multiple sclerosis, it is important to empty the bladder before bimanual examination and to check that the rectum is empty. Women who have spinal cord injuries with lesions above T6 are subject to autonomic dysreflexia. This condition is a response to noxious sensory input from areas below the level of injury but particularly from the bladder, bowel, and other pelvic organs in which the supraspinal influence over the major parts of the sympathetic outflow has been lost.[10] The symptom complex includes paroxysmal hypertension, fluctuating heart rate, sweating and piloerection above the level of the lesion, severe headache, and blotchy skin. Patients with a history of this condition should have careful attention to body positioning and blood pressure monitoring if they become symptomatic during the examination. Pain medication may be necessary.

Women with muscle atrophy or joint contractures should have legs and buttocks cushioned during the examination. Careful attention to the skin of the perineal area is crucial to detect herpetic, condylomatous, or decubitus lesions.

Cognitive and Emotional Status

In assessing any patient's cognition, it is always useful to have baseline knowledge of the patient. Family may be crucial in supplying this information. There are many standardized tests administered by neuropsychologists to specifically detect and measure psychological disturbances. The clinician's role is to determine when a patient should be evaluated in such a way. It is useful to find out how the patient has been functioning and whether there have been any changes. If there has been a worsening of coping skills, the physician must determine whether this has been of gradual or sudden onset. The patient's physiatrist or a neurologist should be consulted.

If a patient's cognition affects her judgment, it may be warranted to attempt to counsel her specifically around areas of promiscuity and its dangers. This may or may not be successful, but it should be attempted. Often, family dynamics may be altered by cognitive deficits or personality changes. Intervention and assistance by a social worker, psychologist, or psychiatrist may be useful.

EMOTIONAL ADJUSTMENT

Although all women with physical challenges share common stressors in daily life, the interplay between the nature of the disability and the people around her affect her ability to cope. Body image, or an internalized sense of body self,[9] can be distorted for many reasons, including physical impairments.

Three main categories of disability play a role in the formation of a woman's identity, body image, and self-esteem. These include congenital disabilities or those acquired very early in life, those acquired suddenly later in life and remaining static, and those acquired gradually, with progressive effects on function.

A young girl's body image is partially based on comparisons with her peers and surrounding adults. The parents of a congenitally disabled child can enhance her self-esteem in several ways: by imparting information in a positive way, by dealing directly with feelings, by supporting her desire to present an attractive appearance,[11] and by providing her with disabled role models. It is especially important for girls disabled early in life to have a substantial amount of interaction with other similarly impaired girls and women. This reinforces the belief that a physically disabled body is not undesirable, unusual, or unacceptable and gives her the confidence to interact positively with nondisabled children and adults.

For a woman who acquires her disability later in life, body image adjustments can be quite difficult. A newly disabled adult woman may have difficulty emotionally in accepting the fact that her body has changed. Her feelings may result in either acceptance of her condition with motivation to seek support and improve function and adjustment or denial and withdrawal. The latter may be especially pronounced in progressive disabilities, in which a steady state is never reached and the woman is constantly trying to adjust to a new reality. The process of learning to live with losses and the development of coping strategies is a gradual one. The role of the physician in trying to understand the newly disabled woman's perception of losses and how they affect her functioning is crucial in directing appropriate support and intervention.

Self-esteem is another area of emotional adjustment that requires attention.[12] A disabled teen or adult woman may feel so undesirable that she may become vulnerable to exploitation, particularly in sexual relationships. For example, a disabled woman may encounter a man who refuses to use a condom. Whereas before her changed physical status the woman may have refused to participate in unprotected intercourse, she may now feel that if she does not consent, nobody else will approach her. Her insecurities may become paramount, leading her to make dangerous misjudgments.

The constant challenges that disabled women confront may at times seem overwhelming.[13] These are appropriate feelings, and the clinician should not discount or ignore them. Careful attention, however, is mandatory to prevent this frustration from developing into a depression. The health care provider must address individual needs and concerns in a supportive manner. By establishing and maintaining a strong, supportive relationship, the primary care physician can play a crucial role in the positive emotional adjustment of a physically disabled woman. Peer group counseling can help disabled women feel comfortable talking about their disability, promoting improved self-image and improved confidence and coping skills.[14] Others have advocated formal assertiveness training programs for women with disabilities.[15]

THE IMPACT OF DISABILITY ON SEXUAL FUNCTION

As with other emotional adjustment, sexual function and adjustment is affected by the nature of the disability. Disabilities can be broadly classified as disorders of motion, disorders of sensation, disorders of cognition, and invisible disabilities. Some disease entities, such as strokes, spinal cord injuries, and multiple sclerosis, may cross over several of these categories.

Disorders of Motion

Any disorder that can cause weakness, paralysis, spasticity, abnormal movements, or absence of a body part can fit this category. It may limit the individual's ability to embrace a partner, to perform fine finger movements necessary to obtain sexual satisfaction, or to perform various gross movements such as thrusting, arching, and twisting.[16] Disorders resulting in limited joint range of motion may present similar problems. Such disorders include spinal cord injury, cerebral palsy, stroke, arthritis, and amputations.

Multiple sclerosis is a protean disorder, with signs and symptoms referable to the entire central nervous system in multiple combinations. The problems seen in multiple sclerosis include weakness or paralysis, spasticity, pain, and fatigue. Each of these, alone or in combination, can interfere with sexual expression. The best approach may be symptomatic relief, such as spasticity control, emptying urine- and stool-collecting devices before intercourse, and using positions for sexual intercourse that require less energy expenditure, such as side-to-side or on-the-bottom positions. In addition, there is a concern that susceptibility to multiple sclerosis may be inherited[17] and that pregnancy and delivery may bring on an exacerbation. Professional or peer counseling may be helpful in addressing these concerns.[18]

Disorders of Sensation

The most severe sensory problem is a lack of sensation, as in spinal cord injury. Sexual function

after spinal cord injury is the best understood of all disabilities. Classically, individuals with spinal cord injury are insensate below the level of the lesion due to the interruption of afferent sensory impulses on their way to the cortex. These patients sometimes report heightened erotic sensation at their sensory cutoff level.[19–22] Sexual desire remains intact, although sensation and pelvic movement are limited. The vaginal lubrication process is interrupted; artificial lubricants can be used if natural lubrication is not sufficient.[23] Sexual positions in which the disabled partner does not need to move as much may be helpful.[24] The woman should be advised to empty her bladder before intercourse; if she wears an indwelling catheter, it can be taped out of the way. Menstrual periods may cease for several months following an acute spinal cord injury, but fertility is unchanged once the menses return.

The sexual dysfunction present after stroke is believed to be due primarily to sensory impairment, personality changes, and fear of sustaining a second stroke rather than weakness.[25] Sexual function after stroke may be changed due to decreased libido, fear, decreased ability to move, decreased communication skills, and altered sensation. Counseling may be helpful, particularly encouraging communication and advising patients on the effects of antihypertensive drugs and any risks of resuming sexual activity.[7]

Other entities that can interfere with sensation include peripheral neuropathy, diabetes, stroke, chronic pain, and multiple sclerosis. Diabetic women can have difficulty with lubrication and orgasms.[26, 27] The presence of pain, whether acute or chronic, can severely limit enjoyment of sexual activity. Entities in which pain plays a role include all types of arthritis, chronic low back and neck pain, ischemic ulcers, and amputations. Pain management techniques, experimentation with positions that minimize weight bearing, and planning sexual activity for times when pain is less prominent may also help.

Disorders of Cognition

Traumatic brain injury often results in cognitive and personality changes, including impulsivity, memory deficits, concreteness, emotional lability, and impaired judgment. The severity of these impairments depends on the severity of the injury. It is primarily these symptoms over and above any motor or sensory changes that can cause sexual dysfunction.[28] Patients with frontal lobe dysfunction may make overtly sexual and inappropriate remarks, resulting in the erroneous perception that patients with traumatic brain injury are hypersexual.[29] Counseling for these patients and their significant others may ease their adjustment.[30]

Invisible Disabilities

Invisible disabilities are disorders that are not immediately obvious but may affect sexual function. The chronic pain disorders described earlier fall into this category, as do many cardiac and pulmonary disorders. Such disorders can severely limit endurance,[31] and sexual activity may be limited on that basis or owing to fear.[32] Coping strategies include learning to pace oneself and being open regarding one's limitations.

For the woman who becomes disabled later in life, sexual identity adjustments can be extremely difficult. A newly disabled woman often feels that she has not changed and, on an emotional level, may not accept that her body has changed. Loss of innervation to the vaginal area can make it difficult for the woman to obtain adequate lubrication, making intercourse problematic or uncomfortable. Vaginal accommodation may be reduced because of anatomic changes; orgasmic sensation may be delayed, reduced, or absent. The woman may experience some anxiety about her ability to satisfy her partner. Her partner, who may perceive her as fragile, may be afraid to touch her or to find ways to achieve mutual satisfaction.

Often this is a difficult area for couples to broach with the physician. One survey of disabled individuals reported that less than 5% of the respondents ever received sex education or counseling.[33] Therefore, the provider should initiate the discussion. Couples should be encouraged to explore new, nontraditional foci of sensory pleasures. This exploration in itself can be sexually arousing. Some approaches that have been used successfully revolve around residual intact areas. If the couple declines counseling, the clinician may make it clear that the lines of communication are open. Sometimes, couples will return to the office months later and request further information. If the practitioner is uncomfortable or not experienced in counseling the couple on ways to explore their sexual possibilities, referral to a professional able to provide this service is indicated.

CHILDBEARING

When disabled girls are growing up, parents and peers may assume that they will not want or be able to have children. However, many women with disabilities have the desire to become a parent. The decision to become a parent is often filled with some anxiety, because parenting skills do not come naturally but must be learned.[34] Parents with disabilities experience these same doubts and fears. Professional and personal support should focus on sources of stress commonly experienced by pregnant women with physical disabilities. These include accepting the new role of childbearing and the impending stresses of parenthood, accepting extra nurturing and assuming a more dependent role, seeking a less active lifestyle to cope with fatigue, and maintaining strong self-esteem, body image, and confidence about sexuality.[10] The woman should understand how her disability will affect her pregnancy so that she can modify her lifestyle, maximizing safety for both herself and her fetus.

Once a disabled woman becomes pregnant, the pregnancy, labor, and delivery can progress with surprisingly little difficulty as long as common problems are anticipated and preventive measures are taken. Possible problems and solutions are summarized in Table 73–1. Disabled women should receive regular prenatal care. Consultation with a physiatrist may be particularly helpful for the primary care physician.

Problems encountered at delivery vary with the disability and any medical problems associated with it, such as cardiac, pulmonary, and autonomic dysfunction. Delivery of the patient with a spinal cord injury can be relatively straightforward, as the uterus retains its ability to contract despite denervation,[35] but there is the potential for life-threatening complications. The most significant of these is autonomic dysreflexia, caused by the noxious stimulus of uterine contractions, which can be confused with preeclampsia.[36] Differentiating autonomic dysreflexia and preeclampsia is vital, as untreated autonomic dysreflexia can cause hemorrhagic stroke and even death. The use of oxytocin may increase the force of uterine contractions and result in more severe autonomic dysreflexia. In the management of labor in a mother with a spinal cord injury, the best course of action is to maintain a high index of suspicion for autonomic dysreflexia; use a birthing chair, as dysreflexia is more likely to occur in the supine position than in sitting; avoid oxytocin; and use epidural anesthesia if signs of dysreflexia occur.[36] Careful attention should also be paid to positioning to avoid injury from leg spasms or pressure on insensate skin. In vaginal deliveries, forceps can be used if necessary. Indications for cesarean section in disabled women are the same as those in nondisabled women. Outcome studies of pregnancies in women with spinal cord injuries are promising. Miscar-

TABLE 73–1. Common Pregnancy Problems and Solutions

PROBLEM	SOLUTION
Potentially teratogenic medications	Review all medications, discontinue all nonessential or dangerous agents *Note*: antispasmodics may be teratogenic
Urinary tract infections	Acidify urine with vitamin C; increase oral fluid intake
Anemia	Monitor hematocrit; consider iron
Constipation	Increase fluid and fiber intake; use stool softeners, suppositories
Pressure sores	Monitor positioning in seating system; seek advice of physiatrist to modify system
Altered balance (due to expanding uterus)	Use assistive devices or temporary wheelchair ambulation to prevent falls and fractures
Precipitous labor	Consider frequent examination, outpatient fetal monitoring, possible early admission to maternity ward
Autonomic dysreflexia (in spinal cord–injured women with lesions above T6)	Find and control source of noxious stimulus; control pain with epidural anesthesia if this occurs during labor; avoid oxytocin as this may exacerbate dysreflexia

riage rates, birth defects, and birth weights are comparable to those of nondisabled women.[37, 38]

PARENTING

The disabled woman who is pregnant may encounter a significant amount of negative pressure from neighbors and even strangers in public places if they believe that her disability will make it impossible to be a competent mother. She and her partner may need emotional support to combat these prejudices, as well as to address their own anxiety. Education and advice on adaptive equipment can help with practical concerns about caring for her baby. Some possible approaches to feeding, sleeping, and mobility are summarized in Table 73–2. Some adaptive equipment may be available commercially; some may need to be specially designed.[39, 40] It is helpful for a knowledgeable and creative individual to go to the woman's home to

assess the environment and help solve any problems. Advice from disabled peers who have reared children is invaluable.

Disabled mothers may encounter additional difficulties as their children grow older. Prejudicial attitudes may affect the children's social interactions. A disabled mother may feel guilty for having to subject her children to biases that are related to her. It might be helpful to have brief discussions with the children explaining that some people do not understand that "mommy" is different in some ways but in other ways is the same as everyone else and that being different is okay. Preparing children in this way, as well as furnishing them with books or films appropriate to their age, may be helpful. The parent should be encouraged to join other mothers in parent groups, and the health care provider should be available as a sounding board and a referral source should any problems arise.

RESOURCES

The multidisciplinary team approach is most helpful in gathering resources to maximize function, independence, and personal satisfaction for disabled women. The physiatrist, a physician trained in physical medicine and rehabilitation, can help the primary care physician with a knowledge of resources as well as dealing with specific problems such as prescribing adaptive equipment, managing spasticity or autonomic dysreflexia, and assessing functional abilities. The physiatrist works with a team of health care professionals with spe-

TABLE 73–2. Adaptive Strategies for Child Care

PROBLEM	SOLUTION
Feeding	Pillows to support baby and mother for breast-feeding in wheelchair Molded handles to fasten onto baby bottle to adapt for use with weak hand grasp Plastic hoop worn around mother's neck to hold bottle Adjustable-height feeding chair, such as Tripp-Trapp chair
Carrying	Adjustable baby sling such as Sara's Ride Side car or car seat attached to mother's wheelchair
Sleeping	Crib with split cribside for frontal access or that opens from either side and later converts to a youth bed
Changing	Folding baby dresser with storage drawers and foam pads, 33 inches high; this height is convenient for a parent in a wheelchair

cific areas of expertise. These are summarized in Table 73–3.

Choosing the correct adaptive equipment can mean the difference between dependence and independence. Examples of adaptive equipment include mobility aids such as shoe lifts, braces, canes, crutches, wheelchairs, hand controls for cars, and adapted vans. Aids for ADLs include built-up utensils, palm cuffs, static and dynamic splints, button hooks, reachers, long-handled shoe horns, dressing sticks, and sock aids. Sexual aids include lubricants, vibrators, dildos, oils, and contraceptives. Members of the rehabilitation team can help with the task of choosing the most useful pieces of equipment.

The common denominator among disabled women is their need of assistance to conduct some of their ADLs.[4] Without such assistance, individuals with disabilities are unable to work, may prevent a family member from working, and may become susceptible to new health problems.[41] Owing to the lack of a coherent policy for such assistance, care has often fallen to family members or institutions.[42, 43] The independent living movement, begun in the early 1970s by working-age disabled persons, represents a more empowering solution.[44] Under this model, the disabled person recruits, selects, trains, and supervises his or her assistant. It has been used successfully in several states, including Massachusetts, Maine, California, and Pennsylvania.

THE AMERICANS WITH DISABILITIES ACT

The Americans with Disabilities Act (1990) protects disabled individuals from discrimination in employment, transportation, public accommodations, telecommunications, and government. The act defines disability as a physical or mental impairment that substantially limits one or more major life activities.[45] The act requires that places of public accommodation, including hospitals, clinics, physician's offices, shops, and restaurants:

1. Make ''reasonable modifications'' in policies, practices, and procedures to afford services to individuals with disabilities, unless these modifications would ''fundamentally alter'' the nature of the services.

2. Provide ''auxiliary aids and services'' to be sure that disabled individuals are not treated differently, unless the aid would ''fundamentally alter'' the service or cause an ''undue burden.''

3. Remove structural, architectural, and communication barriers if the removal of barriers is ''readily achievable.''

4. Provide services in an alternative way if barrier removal is not readily achievable. Goods and services must be provided in the most ''integrated setting'' available.

5. Make all new facilities accessible.

6. When making alterations to existing facilities, provide accessibility to individuals with disabilities.[46]

To comply with the law, physicians should evaluate their facilities, policies, procedures, and practices, especially for any future structural changes. Physicians may find that they are already in substantial compliance. A physician must treat a disabled individual as he or she would a nondisabled one.[47] The provider may not refuse to see a patient because she has a disability but may refer the

---

TABLE 73–3. **The Rehabilitation Team**

DISCIPLINE	AREAS OF RESPONSIBILITY
Medicine	
Primary care physician	Provide general medical care
Physiatrist	Manage medical problems associated with disabling condition, coordinate provision of adaptive equipment and rehabilitation services
Specialist physicians	Provide consultation services as needed
Nursing	Coordinate patient teaching; reinforce skills stressed in physical and occupational therapy session; often the first team member to learn of problems
Physical Therapy	Gross motor skills training including strengthening, transfers, flexibility, and mobility; in conjunction with physiatrist, recommends adaptive equipment
Occupational Therapy	Fine motor skills training, such as self-care skills, including feeding, hygiene, grooming, dressing; desktop skills, such as writing, typing, computer use; perceptual evaluation; in conjunction with physiatrist, recommends adaptive equipment
Speech Pathology	Assess speech, language, and oromotor skills (including swallowing); works with patients and staff to overcome deficits
Psychology	Provide cognitive assessment and psychotherapy to assist in adjustment to disability; may also provide substance abuse counseling
Social Service	Assist family with adjustment to disability, coordinates financial arrangements and discharge planning, provides liaison wih community agencies

patient to another practitioner more experienced in her care.

The physician should take careful inventory of the physical layout of the office. Physical and architectural barriers should be viewed in terms of how they affect hearing, seeing, moving, communicating, and interpreting. These adaptations may help the nondisabled as well. For example, a parent pushing a stroller will benefit from curb cuts.[48]

Technologies to assist the disabled include clear signs, lower noise levels, visual displays, telephone display devices, signal lighting for incoming calls, and closed captioning to decrease the impact of hearing impairment; nonglare lighting, raised letters, Braille, audio signals, large print, light-emitting diode display telephones, and Braille access to computers for those with a visual impairment; computers with synthetic speech output, speaker phones, built-in printer for those with a speech impairment; and wheelchairs, walkers, pull-out shelves, reachers, environmental control units, pneumatic switches, and wheeled carts for those with a mobility impairment.[48]

Auxiliary aids the physician must provide include written materials, qualified interpreters, large print materials, and audio recordings. Removal of barriers includes structural and communications barriers alike. Strategies for doing this include in-stalling ramps at the office entrance, grab bars and raised toilet seats in restrooms, widening doorways, Braille signs, visual alarms, and telephone display devices. Specifications for these modifications are summarized in Table 73–4.[49]

The costs of these modifications may be shared between the owner and the lessor of the public accommodation. In general, physicians must make changes to their offices and examination rooms, and building owners must modify the entrance and any common areas.[45] The act is enforced via the institution of a lawsuit by an individual who believes that he or she is about to be discriminated against. Those in the rehabilitation community are in a unique position to assist physicians and other health care providers to comply with the law, making their practices more accessible to all.[50]

TABLE 73–4. Dimensions Important for Structural Modifications

STRUCTURAL MODIFICATIONS	DIMENSIONS
Adult wheelchair seat height	19 inches
Eye level	43–51 inches
Chair width (plus hands)	30 inches
Chair length (plus feet)	48 inches
Space required for turns: U-turn between walls	60 inches
Driveway width	32 inches
Aisle (1 wheelchair)	36 inches minimum
Ramps—ratio rise : run	1:12 feet
Elevator width	
Center opening	80 inches minimum
Side opening	68 inches minimum
Control height	54 inches maximum (48 inches maximum Federal Standards)
Drinking fountains	
Spout height	36 inches
Knee clearance	27 inches minimum
Bathrooms	
Floor space	30 × 48 inches minimum
Toilet seat height	17–19 inches
Toilet paper dispenser height	36 inches
Standard stall width	60 inches
Grab bar height	33–36 inches

REFERENCES

1. Deegan MJ. Multiple minority groups: A case study of physically disabled women. J Soc Soc Welfare 1981; 8(2):274.
2. Cole TM. Gathering a sex history from a physically disabled adult. Sex Disabil 1991;9(1):29.
3. Erickson RP, Mc Phee M. Clinical evaluation. In: De Lisa JA, Currie DM, Gans BM, et al. (eds). Rehabilitation Medicine: Principles and Practice. Philadelphia: JB Lippincott, 1988.
4. Thurer S. Women and rehabilitation. Rehabil Lit 1982; 43(7–8):194.
5. Diamond LJ, Jaudes PK. Child abuse in a cerebral palsied population. Dev Med Child Neurol 1983;25:169.
6. Jaudes PK, Diamond LJ. The handicapped child and child abuse. Child Abuse Negl 1985;9:341.
7. Ducharme S, Gill K, Biener-Bergman S, Fertitta L. Sexual functioning: Medical and psychological aspects. In: De Lisa JA, Gans BM, Currie DM, et al. (eds). Rehabilitation Medicine: Principles and Practice. 2nd ed. Philadelphia: JB Lippincott, 1993.
8. Elvik SL, Berkowitz CD, Nicholas E, et al. Sexual abuse in the developmentally disabled: Dilemmas of diagnosis. Child Abuse Negl 1990;14:497.
9. Rieve JE. Sexuality and the physically disabled. Nurs Clin North Am 1989;24(1):265.
10. Carty EM, Conine TA, Hall L. Comprehensive health promotion for the pregnant woman who is disabled: The role of the midwife. J Nurse Midwifery 1990;35(3):133.
11. Strauss D. Biopsychosocial issues in sexuality with the neurologically impaired patient. Sexuality Disabil 1991;9(1):49.
12. Carty EM, Conine TA. Disability and pregnancy: A double dose of disequilibrium. Rehabil Nurs 1988;13(2):85.
13. Peters L. Women's health care: Approaches in delivery to physically disabled women. Nurs Pract 1982;7(1):34.
14. Celotta BK, Kriegsman KH. An evaluation of creative coping: Counseling groups for women with physical disabilities. J Rehabil 1980;47:36.
15. Smith SL, Kirkpatrick M. Changing attitudes of disabled females through assertiveness training. Rehabil Nurs 1985;10(6):19.
16. Zasler N. Sexuality in neurologic disability: An overview. Sex Disabil 1991;9(1):10.
17. Franklin GM, Burkes JS. Diagnosis and medical management of multiple sclerosis. In: Maloney FP, et al. (eds).

Interdisciplinary Rehabilitation of Multiple Sclerosis and Related Disorders. Philadelphia: JB Lippincott, 1985.

18. Barrett M. Sexuality and Multiple Sclerosis. Toronto: M.S. Society of Canada, 1977.

19. Freed MM. Traumatic and congenital lesions of the spinal cord. In: Kottke FJ, Stillwell KG, Lehmann JF (eds). Krusen's Handbook of Physical Medicine and Rehabilitation. Philadelphia: WB Saunders, 1982.

20. Kolodny RC, Masters WH, Johnson VE. Textbook of Sexual Medicine. Boston: Little, Brown & Co, 1979.

21. Duffy Y. All Things Are Possible. Ann Arbor, Mich: AJ Garvin and Associates, 1981.

22. Becker EF. Female Sexuality Following Spinal Cord Injury. Bloomington, Ill: Accent Special Publications, Cheever Publishers, 1978.

23. Griffith ER, Trieschmann RB. Sexual functioning in women with spinal cord injury. Arch Phys Med Rehabil 1975;56:18.

24. Mooney T, Cole TM, Chilgren R. Sexual Options for Paraplegics and Quadriplegics. Boston: Little, Brown & Co, 1975.

25. Sjogren K, Fugl-Meyer A. Adjustment to life after stroke with special reference to sexual intercourse and leisure. J Psychosom Res 1982;26:409.

26. Ellenberg M. Diabetes and female sexuality. Women's Health 1984;9:70.

27. Newman A, Bertelson A. Sexual dysfunction in diabetic women. J Behav Med 1986;9:261.

28. Boller F, Frank E. Sexual Dysfunction in Neurological Disorders. New York: Raven Press, 1982.

29. Ducharme S. Sexuality and disability. In: Caplan B (ed). Rehabilitation Psychology Desk Reference. Rockville, Md: Aspen Publishers, 1987.

30. Valentich M, Gripton J. Facilitating the sexual integration of the head injured person in the community. Sex Disabil 1984;7:28.

31. Keller S, Buchanan DC. Sexuality and disability: An overview. Rehabil Dig 1984;15:3.

32. Friedman JM. Sexual adjustment of the post coronary male. In: Lo Piccolo J, LoPiccolo L (eds). Handbook of Sex Therapy. New York, Plenum Press, 1978.

33. Szasz G. Sex and disability are not mutually exclusive. West J Med 1991;154(5):560.

34. Robmault IP. Sex, Society, and the Disabled. New York: Harper & Row, 1978.

35. Robertson DNS. Pregnancy and labor in the paraplegic. Paraplegia 1972;10:200.

36. Verduyn WH. Spinal cord injured women, pregnancy and delivery. Paraplegia 1986;24:231.

37. Cross LL, Meythaler JM, Tuel SM, et al. Pregnancy following spinal cord injury. West J Med 1991;154:607.

38. Turk R, Turk M, Assejev V. The female paraplegic and mother-child relations. Paraplegia 1983;21:191.

39. Conine TA, Carty EM, Safarik P. Aids and Adaptations for Disabled Parents: An Illustrated Manual for Service Providers and Parents with Physical or Sensory Disabilities. 2nd ed. Vancouver, Canada: School of Rehabilitation Medicine, University of British Columbia, 1988.

40. Hale G. The Source Book for the Disabled. Philadelphia: WB Saunders, 1979.

41. Batavia AI, De Jong G, McKnew LB. Toward a national personal care assistance program: The independent living model of long term care of persons with disabilities. J Health Politics Policy Law 1991;16(3):523.

42. De Jong G. A legal perspective on disability, home care, and relative responsibility. Home Health Services Q 1982;3(3/4):176.

43. De Jong G. Physical disability and public policy. Sci Am 1983;248(6):40.

44. De Jong G. Independent living: From social movement to analytic paradigm. Arch Phys Med Rehabil 1979;60:435.

45. Golden M. Americans with Disabilities Act of 1990— Implications for the medical field. West J Med 1991; 154(5):522.

46. Burke FG. Disabilities discrimination in public accommodations and services—What physicians need to know about the law. Minn Med 1991;74(11):29.

47. Weber SM. The disabilities act. How to comply. Penn Med 1991;94(12):16.

48. De Witt JC. The role of technology in removing barriers. Milbank Q 1991;69(suppl 1–2):313.

49. Rothstein JM, Roy SH, Wolf SL. The Rehabilitation Specialist's Handbook. Philadelphia: FA Davis, 1990.

50. Verville RE. The Americans with disabilities act: An analysis. Arch Phys Med Rehabil 1990;71(12):1010.

The Mentally Retarded Patient

Frances E. Wiltsie

THE MENTALLY RETARDED AS CONSUMERS OF HEALTH CARE

Mentally retarded adults are presenting to general medical providers with increasing frequency. This is the result of improved survival into adulthood, large-scale deinstitutionalization, and visibility of disabled people. There is an accompanying increased sense of entitlement to care among the disabled and their advocates. These changes present a challenge to the general provider with limited familiarity, potential negative bias, and time constraints.

Communication problems usually exist on several levels. The behavior of the mentally retarded patient may not conform to expectations in the office setting. Financial remuneration is poor and paperwork copious. The patient may present complex problems and diagnostic dilemmas. These barriers to care have been well documented.[1, 2] However, there is an important role for primary care in this population and reward in providing it. Primary care has been shown to reduce exacerbations of chronic diseases, hospitalizations, and polypharmacology.[1] Rewards to the provider include the satisfaction of establishing an elusive diagnosis, the sense of meeting a social or moral obligation, the gratitude of caregivers, and a new appreciation of the mentally retarded themselves.

Varying demographic studies find the incidence of mental retardation to be 1 to 3% of the general population.[1] Approximately 85% of mentally retarded people test in the "mild" range (IQ 50–70), and many do not have serious functional liabilities.[1] Most do not have an identified etiology of mental retardation. Down's syndrome, which affects 1 in 1000 live births, is the most common identified cause. Mentally retarded people have a higher incidence of physical disability and chronic disease than the general population. However, the severely physically disabled and those with more

than two other chronic diseases constitute a definite minority among mentally retarded people living in the community.[3, 4]

The majority of mentally retarded patients can be managed by a primary care provider utilizing only occasional specialty consultations.[2, 4, 5] The most frequently indicated specialties are neurology, orthopedics with an emphasis on congenital and developmental problems, psychiatry, and behavioral psychology. The availability of these consultants may determine which individual patients are appropriate for a general medical practice.

Approximately half of the mentally retarded adults living in the community are in structured community residential programs. A small minority live entirely independently. Many live with family, either parents or siblings. The majority of individuals in residential programs have a case manager or staff person who coordinates medical care, may or may not come to office visits, and sometimes coordinates nursing services. It is critical that the physician clarify what level of supervision and assistance is available in the residence. Successful medical care depends on establishing a relationship with the case manager as well as with the patient.

Issues of informed consent may arise, as well as uncertainty about how aggressively to proceed in the presence of client resistance to care. These problems can be referred to the patient's habilitative treatment team, which usually can obtain a competency determination. Limited medical guardianships, often temporary, have become more common than general guardianships. The legal process is slow and should be initiated early in nonemergency situations. In caring for mentally retarded adults, one should not presume family members are empowered to give medical consent. The disabled adult is presumed competent until legally judged otherwise.

Several additional comments may be useful. An

antiphysician bias exists in many parts of the network serving mentally retarded people. This is attributable to the perceived failures of physician-controlled, medically oriented state schools and is quite generalized. This bias should be recognized and not personalized. There is also a very egalitarian style to the typical treatment team in programs for the mentally retarded. This is often disconcerting to the physician who is accustomed to more preferential treatment and authority. Finally, it is helpful to understand that requirements for documentation are often very strict in these programs. This may be burdensome to the physician but is more problematic to program staff who are accountable for its completion.

APPROACH TO HISTORY TAKING

Unless the mentally retarded patient has always lived with family, the past medical history is often incomplete and inconsistent. High staff turnover in residential programs and purging of records contribute to this problem. The case manager can be expected to assemble what is available, including institutional archives. Even with good effort, much of the past history may remain unknown.

In taking the current medical history one should question both the patient and the staff or family members. Begin to assess the patient's language level by asking several simple questions (e.g., "Who came in with you today?", "How did you get here?"). Observe communication between the patient and staff or family, especially the length and complexity of instructions given to the patient and the relative use of nonverbal cues, such as pointing. If the patient is significantly dysarthric, acknowledge your difficulty in understanding her speech and ask staff or family to restate her comments but continue to speak to the patient directly and encourage her direct responses. Many dysarthric people, especially those with cerebral palsy, have cognitive skills much higher than their speech suggests and have valuable information to impart to the physician. Even the moderately mentally retarded person with limited language may be able to answer simple but useful questions.

Form a general impression of the patient by briefly inquiring about the patient's residence, vocational program, and degree of family involvement. Ask if the patient has a guardian. If she appears at least moderately retarded, determine whether she is independent in basic self-help skills, including feeding and toileting. Ask who supervises or administers medications.

The common question "How are you?" usually elicits a stereotypic answer and is fairly useless.

Instead, clearly identify yourself as the doctor (or "like the doctor" for nonphysician providers), and ask the patient why she came to see you today. Clarify the purpose and expectations for the visit with the staff or family, and restate these clearly for the patient. Briefly explain how the encounter will proceed.

In exploring symptoms, keep questions simple, both in content and in sentence length. Beware of relying exclusively on yes or no questions, which may be answered uniformly in the negative (or the affirmative, which is easier to notice). If responses are largely limited to yes or no, structure questioning to validate the responses ("Did your headache go away?" followed by "Do you still have your headache?"). Verify that the patient accurately knows the location of body parts under discussion ("Show me your . . ."). Even very mildly mentally retarded people can have poor vocabulary in this realm. Time concepts may be poor and unreliable. This is difficult to detect. Staff or family's perception of the duration of the problem, frequency of complaints, and timing of symptoms should be elicited in addition to the patient's account. Many mentally retarded patients who can provide good concrete descriptions of symptoms are unable to clarify how these symptoms are changing. They may be influenced by a desire to please with an expected answer. Again, staff or family may be helpful.

Staff or family often present the severely or profoundly mentally retarded patient as simply seeming "different" or having a tantrum. Either of these can be a significant sign of physical illness. Try to differentiate whether the change is in level of alertness, cardiorespiratory status, gastrointestinal function including appetite, or motor activity. Listen carefully to the hypotheses of those who know the patient well. If the patient is having a tantrum, look for sources of pain. Plan to examine carefully any body part being targeted for self-abuse. If she is noncompliant with certain tasks, consider which body parts are involved. If mealtime behavior is suddenly worse, consider dental pain. If behavior problems are intermittent, consider correlation with menstrual cycles. Do not presume behavior problems are entirely psychological or learned until a reasonably thorough medical evaluation has been performed.

Behavior problems are common and should be identified, without the patient present if possible. Begin with a general inquiry. Then ask specifically about assaultive behavior and self-injurious behavior, including head banging, ingestion of inedibles (pica), and hyperactivity. Elicit any known history of psychotropic medications. These have been commonly used, sometimes inappropriately, and do not necessarily indicate major mental illness or dual diagnosis. Unless there are acute behavioral problems or recent major changes, further consideration can usually be deferred to a follow-up visit.

Obtaining a sexual history can be particularly difficult. This is usually best done by separating the patient from the staff or family. Inquire about staff or family's impression of the patient's knowledge base, past history of sexual activity or sexual abuse, current behavior, potential need for contraception, and potential risk of sexually transmitted infections. Then question the patient about whether she has a special friend she "kisses and touches" or with whom she "has sex." The nature of this discussion depends on the cognitive level of the patient. Many mildly mentally retarded adults have received sex education in school or workshops. Pictures, such as those provided in patient education materials, can be used to review vocabulary or clarify some actions ("This is the man's penis. Have you seen your boyfriend's penis? Do you touch it? Does he touch you with his penis? Show me where."). Also try to determine whether she enjoys the activity ("Does it feel good? Do you like it when he does that?"). This gives clues about whether the activity is consensual. Ask the patient about past sexual behavior and whether anyone has, or is, hurting her "here" in the perineum. It is unfortunately difficult to know how to interpret positive responses, but they need to be pursued. Conclude by affirming that it is acceptable to kiss and touch (be sexually active) but that you, the doctor, need to know about it to keep her healthy. Also state that no one has the right to physically hurt her and that she can say "No" if she does not want sex. Patients may have a keen sense that sexual behavior, especially same-sex behavior, is subject to disapproval and may therefore refuse to disclose this. As with any patient, a second attempt at the sexual history may be more successful after a relationship of trust is established. Remember that women who are too severely mentally retarded to give any sexual history may be sexually active or victims of sexual abuse.

Other physical abuse may have occurred and may be ongoing. The patient should be questioned alone. Make vigorous attempts to establish a time context for any alleged abuse. Concrete questions ("Did anyone hit you this week? this month? this year?") are easier to answer and more useful than the commonly used question, "Are you safe today?" Asking if she is afraid and of what is sometimes useful. Question staff and family if possible, but do not allow them to discredit the patient. Cognitively disabled people may misrepresent time or simple events but will rarely be able to construct intricate confabulations. The very mildly retarded person with coexisting mental illness is more capable of this, but never assume her to be unreliable. Health care workers, including physicians, are usually mandated to report abuse of the disabled. Be aware that residential and vocational programs may include assaultive peers. However, these programs should provide for the safety of potential victims. Repeated or severe injury from a peer should not be condoned.

APPROACH TO THE PHYSICAL EXAMINATION

In obtaining the history, the provider has had an opportunity to assess the patient's degree of apprehension and general ability to follow directions. The mentally retarded patient often fails to comprehend the purpose or value of the examination. Some diagnostic procedures, including pelvic examinations, are inherently unpleasant experiences. The patient may not be able to resist the urge to protest vocally, verbally, and physically. Some mentally retarded people are overstimulated and frightened by the unfamiliar office environment. Others dislike being touched (tactile defensiveness). Thus, even a routine physical can be problematic, although this is not usually the case. The presence of a familiar person may be helpful. If able, the patient should be asked to make this decision for herself.

Always explain your intended actions in advance, using brief, concrete sentences. A mildly mentally retarded patient benefits from a simple initial overview. In the anxious, the new, or the severely mentally retarded patient, begin with the most critical portion of the examination, as it may be impossible to complete an entire physical. Demonstrate any equipment immediately before use, either on a third person if one is present or on oneself. The nonverbal patient may indicate familiarity with an instrument by trying to use it, as in grabbing the blood pressure cuff and bringing it to her arm. Nonverbal cues may also show apprehension toward a particular part of the examination, which could then be postponed until the end.

Proceed slowly, praise cooperative behavior, and make frequent eye contact. It is usually better to keep one's hands clearly within the patient's view. One exception is in giving immunizations, which are better tolerated if given from behind while the patient is distracted. This also reduces the chance of the patient grabbing for the needle. The patient should, however, be forewarned. Progress from the less threatening parts of the examination (extremities, heart, lung, abdomen) to the more threatening parts (otoscope and ophthalmoscope, then pelvic and rectal). Stop for the day if cooperation deteriorates, or the patient may be impossible to examine on future visits.

Other strategies may help with specific problems. The patient who is reluctant to undress can return in a loose top and shirt, which allow a partial but meaningful examination without actually disrobing. This is particularly effective in obtaining breast and abdominal examinations. If the patient cannot follow directions to deep breathe, assess the lungs by auscultating while she is encouraged to vocalize. Differences in the quality of the sound can indicate pneumonia, and increased air movement may reveal adventitious sounds. Auscultation of the heart should be done first, as it may be difficult to quiet the patient. Pelvic examinations on apprehensive patients are sometimes successful if performed with a familiar person straddling the examination table behind the patient, and the patient semireclining back against her. In this position the speculum must be inserted with the handle pointing upward.

When the examination is scheduled as a follow-up visit there are opportunities for staff or family to rehearse the examination with the patient and discuss expected behavior. Be specific in describing what will happen on that visit. A doll can be used at home to repeatedly model the examination. This approach is helpful with special procedures. Rewards for cooperative behavior can also be planned. On short notice, even a cup of office coffee can be persuasive.

Medication before the examination is sometimes warranted. Short-acting anxiolytics can be useful in the mildly mentally retarded. Chloral hydrate has a time-honored reputation for use in the moderately to severely mentally retarded, often combined with diazepam. Sedation is not a substitute for time and patience; it often fails, especially if the patient is in a stimulating environment immediately before the examination. The sensation of being medicated may be aversive and frightening, so a low-dose anxiolytic may be more effective than a stronger sedative. Inquire about whether the patient's dentist has found an effective regimen. Also consider drug interactions with existing medications.

Gentle, brief holding may be helpful, but greater physical restraint may predispose the patient to resist future examinations. It may also be surprisingly difficult to accomplish and may elicit attempts to bite the restrainer. Physical restraint of a mentally retarded person lasting more than several minutes is often illegal.

In recording the results of the examination, include whether the patient was cooperative, specific interfering behaviors, and what, if any, medication was given before the examination. Document incomplete examinations thoroughly, as even limited information can be useful. Try to avoid using the general statement that "the patient could not be examined because of behavior."

Over time, many difficult mentally retarded people learn to trust an examiner and give some cooperation. This is accomplished by building on small, limited successes, being patient, and knowing when to stop.

SPECIFIC CONSIDERATIONS

Many chronic medical problems are more frequent in mentally retarded populations. Those most frequently cited include seizures, congenital heart disease, eye disorders, hearing loss, orthopedic deformities, skin problems, and dental disease.[1, 3, 6-11] As previously stated, most mentally retarded persons have only one or two chronic medical problems and are fairly easily managed. Chronic problems cluster in the severely to profoundly mentally retarded. These individuals often have multiple handicaps.

Down's Syndrome

Down's syndrome is associated with an increase in a variety of medical problems.[5, 7, 12, 13] These include thyroid disease, chronic active hepatitis B, and Alzheimer's disease. Table 74–1 summarizes problems commonly encountered.

Seizures

The reported prevalence of seizures in the mentally retarded varies considerably. Two community-based studies[3, 10] found a prevalence of 16%. Other studies of institutionalized or more severely retarded people reported 21 to 34%.[3, 7, 8] Seizures in the mentally retarded are usually generalized, present in early childhood, and controllable with a single medication.[14] Seizures making an initial appearance after adolescence should be investigated for an etiology unrelated to mental retardation.

Often the primary care provider is expected to manage the patient with a seizure history, few or no seizures in recent years, and one or more anticonvulsant medications. If the patient has been seizure-free for 5 years, it is usual practice to try to wean her off anticonvulsants. Electroencephalogram findings are considered irrelevant to this decision. It is imperative to proceed very slowly.

TABLE 74–1.   Medical Problems Frequently Associated with Down's Syndrome

PROBLEM	CLINICAL IMPLICATION
Eye conditions: cataracts, keratoconus, ectropion, chronic blepharitis	Regular ophthalmologic evaluations; topical antibiotics as necessary
Hearing loss, frequent otitis, ceruminosis (complicated by small ear canals)	Regular audiology evaluation; drops for ear wax control; ear, nose, and throat consultation as necessary
Periodontal disease	Aggressive oral hygiene; regular dental care
Thyroid disease (usually hypothyroidism)	Screen every 1–2 yr
Congenital heart disease: atrial septal defect, ventricular septal defect, mitral valve prolapse, aortic regurgitation	Check on initial visit Echocardiogram or cardiology consultation as necessary; subacute bacterial endocarditis prophylaxis as necessary
Respiratory infections	Flu and pneumococcal vaccines; usual management
Cervical spine instability (usually atlantoaxial)	Lateral cervical-spine films (neutral, flexion and extension) at least once; orthopedic referral as necessary
Skin problems: fungal infection, seborrhea, dry skin	Treat aggressively; often chronic
Chronic Hepatitis B	Hepatitis B profile on initial visit; follow-up as necessary
Seizures	Usual management
Alzheimer's disease (presenting after age 35)	Observe for behavioral change, deterioration of language skills, persistent decline in productivity at work; if suspected, maintain structure, familiar setting, and routine

Withdrawal seizures can be worse than the earlier seizures, even if medication compliance was poor. Reduce one drug at a time, by one third or one fourth of the dose every 3 to 4 months. Wait 6 months, then begin to taper the next anticonvulsant according to the same schedule. Seizures recur in about 50% of patients, either during or after the taper.[14]

Occasionally one encounters an unmedicated patient with long-standing sporadic seizures, separated by months or years. This patient does not necessarily require anticonvulsants. Consider the nature and duration of the seizure as well as the safety risk to this individual. Medication should be initiated if seizures become more frequent or more severe. An abnormal electroencephalogram in the absence of clinical seizures does not require treatment.

The stable patient is monitored with a complete blood count, serum chemistries and anticonvulsant levels at least yearly. Side effects of long-term anticonvulsant use are summarized in Table 74–2.

Congenital Heart Disease

Mentally retarded people are more likely to have congenital heart disease. In current community-based adult populations, there is a significant chance that it has been undetected.[3, 6, 10] Sometimes symptoms are minimized or attributed to other disabilities. A previously asymptomatic person may develop problems as she ages or in the presence of a respiratory infection. The need for subacute bacterial endocarditis prophylaxis may be unrecognized. One should consider the possibility of congenital heart disease, especially if a genetic or an early prenatal cause of mental retardation is suspected. One also encounters the patient who has had prior aggressive surgical treatment and finds access to a pediatric cardiologist limited as she ages. The primary care provider may be placed in the role of managing polycythemia or anticoagulants in consultation with the cardiologist.

Orthopedic Problems

Congenital orthopedic deformities are common, as well as acquired deformities associated with cerebral palsy. An increased prevalence of scoliosis has been reported.[5, 9, 11] The adult with orthopedic deformities has "wear and tear" from abnormal use patterns. This presents as joint pain, arthritis, and increasing disability. Orthopedists

TABLE 74–2.   Side Effects of Long-Term Anticonvulsant Use

Phenytoin	Gingival hyperplasia
	Coarsening of facial features
	Hirsutism
	Hypocalcemia
	Osteomalacia and osteoporosis
	Folic acid deficiency
Phenobarbital	Drowsiness
	Hypocalcemia
Carbamazepine	Hyponatremia
	Persistent leukopenia
Valproic acid	Hyperammonemia (asymptomatic)
	Irregular menses

who specialize in managing these patients are unfortunately rare. The primary care physician must often work with the physical therapist in managing symptoms and determining when further intervention is necessary.

Vision and Hearing

Many mentally retarded people living in the community have not been adequately evaluated and treated for sensory deficits.[3, 7, 10] Hearing loss, visual impairment, and other ophthalmologic problems are more prevalent than in the general population. Assessment may be difficult, but specialists exist and can be located through rehabilitative programs. The physician plays an important role by persistently urging evaluation and treatment.

Hepatitis B

Hepatitis B infection was common in state institutions for the mentally retarded.[5, 8, 15] Former residents are at higher risk for chronic active disease. People with Down's syndrome are also at higher risk. Both groups should be screened. Immunization is recommended for anyone living or working with a known carrier. Liver function should be monitored in the patient with active infection.

Dental Care

Numerous studies cite poor dentition and periodontal disease in the mentally retarded.[7-10] These conditions are often painful as well as a potential source of infection. Nutritional status is affected. One large community-based study[7] reported dental care to be the most frequent cause for hospital admission (dental work under anesthesia). Assess the patient's need for dental work and try to locate an appropriate dentist. Some mentally retarded people do well with a family dentist and anxiolytic medication. Dental schools may have a program for moderately to severely mentally retarded patients. Family, staff, and patient may need encouragement to work on improving oral hygiene.

Etiology of the Patient's Mental Retardation

Traditionally, the physician is advised to pursue an etiology for the patient's mental retardation unless one is already established. It is usually unknown. The pursuit is interesting and a worthy cause but seldom useful in the adult. It has much more potential value if the patient's siblings have not already had children. A sibling beginning a family could benefit from genetic counseling. Widespread prenatal screening for Down's syndrome has reduced the importance of identifying people with trisomy 21 translocations. Fragile X syndrome has emerged as the second most common genetic cause of mental retardation.[16] However, this X-linked recessive disorder manifests in males; carrier females are unaffected.

REPRODUCTIVE HEALTH

The gynecologic needs of women with mental retardation vary considerably. Many mildly mentally retarded women are sexually active and in need of health education, contraception, and screening for sexually transmitted infections. Probably more mentally retarded women have never been sexually active and are therefore at low risk for cervical cancer but remain at risk for breast cancer, premenstrual syndrome, endometriosis, and abnormal vaginal bleeding. Most mentally retarded women do not receive routine pelvic examinations.[3, 17-19] Many have never had a pelvic examination. Similarly, many do not receive regular breast examinations or mammograms, and few are capable of breast self-examination. Barriers to adequate care include patient behavior, knowledge deficits of staff and families, and reluctance to perceive these women as adults. Adequate menstrual records are uncommon, and abnormal bleeding may go unrecognized unless it is very profuse or prolonged.

This lack of health care can be readily addressed by the primary care provider, although the pelvic examination may be difficult or impossible. In taking the history, focus on questions that determine the necessity of a pelvic examination. Important symptoms include cyclic behavior problems, pelvic pain, and abnormal bleeding or discharge. The breast examination is almost always possible, although sometimes requires several attempts and sedation. Usually one can get far enough on a pelvic examination to visually inspect and gently palpate the introitus. The presence of an intact hymenal ring often limits further examination. However, one can obtain a "blind" Papanicolaou smear or a sample of vaginal secretions by inserting a small cotton swab. If the vagina admits an examining finger and the patient cooperates, use of a very narrow, short speculum (Smith-Pederson) yields a better specimen, although the cervix probably cannot be located. Inserting the speculum with the handle upward is helpful when the patient is poorly positioned on the examination table. "Blind" Papanicolaou smears are less effective in detecting cervical cancer, but the presence of an intact hymenal ring indicates that this patient is low risk. The bimanual examination is often very limited or impossible to perform. Use the history and whatever findings are possible on the pelvic examination to determine whether further evaluation is necessary. Fortunately, pelvic ultrasound is often well tolerated. Endometrial biopsy is not. Some patients will need referral to a gynecologist for examination under anesthesia.

The sexually active patient needs a thorough pelvic examination, including screening for infection and an adequate Papanicolaou smear. She may be anxious and have limited tolerance for the length of the procedure. Prior patient teaching is helpful. Be certain all materials are set up in advance, including a variety of speculums. If the examination is unsuccessful, try again using anxiolytic medication.

Dysmenorrhea or premenstrual syndrome is suspected when behavior changes are clearly correlated with menstrual cycles. Prostaglandin inhibitors such as ibuprofen, started before menses and continued for 3 to 5 days, can be highly effective for dysmenorrhea. Oral contraceptives may also help but should be preceded by an adequate pelvic examination.

Vulvovaginitis is a frequent clinical problem. This can be evaluated with saline ("wet prep") and potassium hydroxide slides of vaginal secretions, obtained with or without a speculum. A "blind" culture can be used to screen for gonorrhea if the cervix cannot be visualized. Blind swabs are suboptimal for DNA probes intended to detect chlamydial infection. If chlamydial infection is suspected, treat presumptively. Enteric organisms, especially *Escherichia coli,* can cause a rampant vaginitis in women with poor perineal hygiene or incontinence and may require oral antibiotics. Topical treatment of vaginitis often presents practical problems. Yeast infections can be treated with oral antifungal agents if necessary.

Irregular vaginal bleeding is common but often missed without a careful history. Medications, especially phenothiazines, many antidepressants, and some anticonvulsants, can cause irregular menses or amenorrhea by raising prolactin levels.[19] Also consider hypogonadism (associated with Down's syndrome and others) and low body weight (common with cerebral palsy) as etiologies of amenorrhea. Menorrhagia usually requires referral to a gynecologist.

The sexually active mentally retarded woman requires concrete health education. She needs to have a basic vocabulary and an understanding of her body to participate in her health care. She almost always needs contraception as well as an opportunity to discuss why pregnancy is being avoided. Many mildly mentally retarded women enjoy children and may wish they could be mothers. Some can recognize their limitations ("I can learn to take care of myself, but babies are too hard."); others can accept their medical problems as a contraindication ("Seizures are bad if you're pregnant.") or acknowledge social pressure ("My family will be real mad if I get pregnant."). This discussion should be simple and concrete. Finally, one should present the risk of infection and encourage using condoms and limiting the number of sexual partners.

Practical contraceptive options are limited. Mentally retarded people usually do poorly with methods that require implementation at the time of sexual activity. Unfortunately, this includes condoms. It also includes diaphragms, cervical caps, and spermicides. Even individuals who plan well and are motivated may have difficulty with the fine motor tasks required. Oral contraceptives have been the usual method of choice, although they may affect anticonvulsant levels. The patient may require supervision to remember to take the pill daily or help removing it from the package. Long-acting progestational contraceptives are becoming increasingly popular. Irregular vaginal bleeding on these methods may be a hygiene problem for some women, but others may find the lighter flow more manageable. Tubal ligation is a logical but usually very legally complicated alternative for mentally retarded women.

Standard guidelines for mammography should be followed for the mentally retarded patient. Mammography is more successful if the patient is clearly instructed in advance, anticipates some discomfort, and is awaiting some tangible reward for success. Anxiolytic medication may be indicated if a second attempt is required.

PREVENTIVE HEALTH

Obesity and lack of physical exercise are extremely common among the mentally retarded. Their lifestyle is usually very sedentary, and special events usually focus on food. Food is often used as a reward for cooperative behavior. Workshops commonly pay people partially in change and teach use of snack vending machines as a way of demonstrating the value of money. Mentally retarded people living semi-independently usually have limited cooking skills and rely on convenience foods. Family and staff need encouragement to promote more nutritional choices, nonfood alternatives, cooking classes, and general reduction in fatty foods. Patients need simple instruction and lavish praise for weight loss.

Exercise is a challenge because many mentally retarded people lack the basic skills for sports, have impaired mobility, or require close supervision. Walking, dancing, and stationary bicycles are good options for ambulatory people. Movement to exercise videos is appropriate for a wider range of people, even if they copy motions inaccurately. Physical therapists can design programs for the more physically disabled. Swimming may be an alternative but often requires one-to-one supervision.

Tobacco use is uncommon among mentally retarded people but will be encountered. Attempts to change this behavior require the cooperation and motivation of the patient as well as the staff and family. One should make the simple statement that smoking is bad for her health, repeat it at each visit, and express confidence in her ability to quit. It is important to enlist others in supporting her ability to stop smoking, helping her plan a stop date, and finding tangible short-term rewards for not smoking. Use of a nicotine skin patch may also help. Ongoing encouragement to deep trying is important.

REFERENCES

1. Ruben IL, Crocker AC (eds). Developmental Disabilities: Delivery of Medical Care for Children and Adults. Boston: Lea & Febiger, 1989.
2. Garrard S. Health services for mentally retarded people in community residences: Problems and questions. Am J Public Health 1982;72:1226.
3. Minihan PM, Dean DH. Meeting the needs for health services of persons with mental retardation living in the community. Am J Public Health 1990;80:1043.
4. Cole RF. Community based pre-paid medical care for adults with mental retardation: Proposal for a pilot project. Ment Retard 1987;25:233.
5. Rubin IL. Health care needs of adults with mental retardation. Ment Retard 1987;25:201.
6. Ziring PR, Kastner T, Friedmand DL, et al. Provision of health care for persons with developmental disabilities living in the community. JAMA 1988;260:1439.
7. Ziring PR. Outreach programs from tertiary hospitals. In: Rubin IL, Crocker AC (eds). Developmental Disabilities: Delivery of Medical Care for Children and Adults. Boston: Lea & Febiger, 1989, pp 64–71.
8. Nelson RP, Crocker AC. The medical care of mentally retarded persons in public residential facilities. N Engl J Med 1978;299:1039.
9. Larson CP, Lapointe Y. The health status of mild to moderate intellectually handicapped adolescents. J Ment Defic Res 1986;30:121.
10. Beange H, Bauman A. Caring for the developmentally disabled in the community. Aust Fam Physician 1990;19:1555.
11. Howells G. Are the medical needs of mentally handicapped adults being met? J R Coll Gen Pract 1986;36:449.
12. Pueschel SM (ed). New Perspectives on Down Syndrome. Baltimore: PH Brookes Publishing Co, 1987.
13. Crocker AC. The spectrum of medical care for developmental disabilities. In: Ruben IL, Crocker AC (eds). Developmental Disabilities: Delivery of Medical Care for Children and Adults. Boston: Lea & Febiger, 1989, pp 10–22.
14. Alvarez N. Epilepsy. In: Ruben IL, Crocker AC (eds). Developmental Disabilities: Delivery of Medical Care for Children and Adults. Boston: Lea & Febiger, 1989, pp 130–147.
15. Merker EL, Werning DH. Medical care of the deinstitutionalized mentally retarded. Am Fam Physician 1984;29:228.
16. Pueschel SM, Merlick JA (eds). Prevention of Developmental Disabilities. Baltimore: PH Brookes Publishing Co, 1990.
17. Thomas P. Special adults: New challenge to primary care MDs. Med World News 1986;27:68.
18. Kastner T. Who cares for the young adult with mental retardation? J Dev Behav Pediatr 1991;12:196.
19. Jones KP, Douglass J. Gynecologic problems. In: Ruben IL, Crocker AC (eds). Developmental Disabilities: Delivery of Medical Care for Children and Adults. Boston: Lea & Febiger, 1989, pp 276–282.

Occupational and Environmental Health for Women

Elisha H. Atkins, Maxine J. Garbo, and Elise Pechter Morse

Women live and work in an increasingly complex world. Although there is less physical drudgery in homes and factories, women's work is often dull and poorly paid, may conflict with the care of children or aging parents, and may cause exposure to a variety of chemical, biologic, and physical hazards.

Faced with a bewildering amount of information about occupational and environmental problems, women often turn for advice to their primary physicians and nurse practitioners, who in turn may feel unprepared and wary of an area that seems excessively legalistic and time consuming. Our intent in this chapter is to help primary care practitioners develop a practical approach to these problems. We present not an encyclopedic collection of facts but a framework for gathering information, key suggestions concerning the most common problems, and sources for further help or referral.

WHAT IS WOMEN'S WORK

Increasing numbers of women work, doubling their participation over the past 3 decades. By 1990, women accounted for 46% of the total work force and 43% of full-time employees. Most women who work must do so to support themselves or their families: 59% of employed women in 1988 were single, divorced, widowed, separated, or had husbands earning less than $15,000 the previous year. Unlike the early 1960s, the majority of mothers now work outside the home; in 1990, 75% of those with children of school age or

older and 52% of those with children younger than 2 years old also held jobs.

Statistics from 1990 indicate that although women have entered occupations traditionally dominated by men, they remain a minority, accounting for 11% of executive, administrative, or managerial positions; 11% of construction workers; and 14% of those in mining. In contrast, certain occupations have remained overwhelmingly female. Women occupy 80% of administrative support jobs (98% of secretaries) and 75% of hospital workers (94% of registered nurses). Women are still concentrated in low-paying jobs relative to men, with those working full-time in wage and salary jobs receiving median weekly earnings only 72% of men's.[1-3]

HAZARDS THAT WOMEN FACE AT WORK AND AT HOME: SCREENING QUESTIONS

Not all patients need a comprehensive occupational and environmental history. At a routine checkup, a few screening questions will suffice. Occupational physicians have proposed several mnemonics for detecting risk factors at work and at home, much as practitioners routinely ask about risks in diet, substance use, or sexual practice. One such memory aid is WHIP:

What Work do you do?
What Hazards are you exposed to?
What Illnesses do you believe you have experienced from these exposures?
What Protection do you have?

If you or the patient identify a particular hazard, if the patient is having symptoms that might be

The views and statements in this chapter are those of the authors and not necessarily those of the Massachusetts Department of Labor and Industries.

work related, or if the patient has a condition that might require adjustments in her job, you may wish to ask further questions, give the patient sources of further information, or consult with a government agency or a specialist.

ASSESSING EXPOSURE

Exposures of concern for women include toxic chemicals, infectious agents, and physical stresses. For chemicals, the risk depends on the toxicity of the chemical, the amount of absorption that occurs (usually through inhalation but occasionally through skin contact), and any predisposing health problems or sensitivities in the woman exposed. Effects may be immediate or delayed, life threatening or just annoying, or present in all exposed or detectable only in epidemiologic studies as statistically increased rates of common events. Adverse effects from occupational or environmental exposures are of particular concern to pregnant women or those contemplating having a child.

Case Study: Exposure during Pregnancy

A 28-year-old woman comes for her first prenatal visit. She is 7 or 8 weeks' pregnant. She wonders if it is safe to continue using acids and bases in her job as a laboratory technician. She would prefer to delay informing her employer that she is pregnant. What would you advise her to do?

First, ask for more detailed information in the categories listed previously.

Work: Ask her to describe her job tasks. She reports that she does titrations, mounts slides, washes glassware, and does other bench chemistry work in a quality control laboratory in a manufacturing facility with six co-workers.

Hazards: Ask what chemicals she uses, in what quantities, and with what methods. She uses automatic pipettes and eyedroppers to handle dilute hydrochloric and sulfuric acids, saline, and ''546'' on an open bench. No more than 1 liter of any of these is present at one time, and there have been no spills of more than a few milliliters. Ask about exposure to physical stresses, such as repetitive motions, lifting, or prolonged standing. She reports that she does stand about 75% of the day. Also ask whether her partner has been exposed to chemicals. She says he has not.

Illness: Ask about symptoms experienced at work by the patient or co-workers. She denies any, even when there have been small spills, and denies any skin problems from contact.

Protection: Ask about protective measures, such as ventilation, enclosures, respirators, goggles, and gloves. She reports that her work is done on an open bench, not under a hood, even though there are some hoods in the laboratory. There are ceiling vents providing some ventilation. Even though she wears a laboratory coat, gloves are not often worn because they are not readily available.

Exposures: Obtaining More Information

You are concerned about 546. Ask your patient to obtain the chemical name of 546 through a material safety data sheet. Material safety data sheets are fact sheets that describe the ingredients, health effects, and recommended handling and storage of hazardous chemicals. Under federal law, employers must make these available to employees within the work shift and to physicians on written request.[4]

The patient decides to request the material safety data sheet and faxes it to you the next day. You learn that this substance is 100% acetone, which has a threshold limit value and a permissible exposure level of 750 parts per million parts of air (750 ppm). This relatively high level indicates that this substance is considered less toxic than others with a lower threshold limit value or permissible exposure level. The material safety data sheet also indicates that acetone is a skin irritant, but, as is often the case, there is no information about reproductive toxicity. What do you do next?

Reproductive Hazards: Occupational

Occupational and environmental hazards may affect reproduction through interaction with the central nervous system, endocrine system, or gonads of both males and females, leading to altered function, cell death, and mutations. Adverse outcomes can include infertility, changes in libido and menstrual cycle, spontaneous abortion, preterm delivery, low birth weight, congenital anomalies, and childhood cancer. Some agents may be capable of crossing the placenta and affecting a developing fetus. Absolute statements about the risk of a particular chemical to women are difficult: the risk is related to the toxicity of a substance and the dose, duration, and timing of exposure, and nonoccupational risks may play a significant role. Because paternal exposure is also linked to poor outcomes, counseling and reproductive health policies should be aimed at all employees. In the best of circumstances, the outcome of a pregnancy is uncertain. At least 15 to 20% of pregnancies end in spontaneous abortion, and major birth defects are seen in more than 2% of births, usually without an identifiable cause.[5, 6] Women who have been shown to be at increased risk because of their work include some hospital personnel (particularly if exposed to anesthetic gases or antineoplastic agents), laboratory and industrial workers exposed to certain solvents, and those exposed to heavy metals.

You decide to call a local teratogen information service (see Appendix) for further information. The teratogen information service informs you that no specific reproductive health risk has been associated with exposure to acetone. However, as with any other chemical, it is recommended that exposure be kept to a minimum. You recommend that the patient wear gloves and use a hood when working with acetone. You also ask the teratogen information service about prolonged standing, and they report that this may be associated with an increased risk of preterm delivery. You recommend that she use a stool for at least a part of each day.

Preventing Employment Discrimination against Exposed Women

Several weeks later, the patient tells her employer that she is pregnant. He tells her that he wants her ''off the job immediately, for the sake of her unborn child'' on an unpaid leave of absence. What do you advise her?

Tell her that this attempted action on the part of her employer is illegal. The Supreme Court ruled in 1991 (UAW vs. Johnson Controls) that companies may not discriminate against women, forcing them to leave work or accept lower paying jobs, because of their fear of litigation filed by children harmed in utero. Workplace hazards must be reduced or eliminated, not the workers believed to be at risk. You are also concerned that lack of income and loss of medical insurance may be hazardous to her health. You write the following letter:

Dear Employer:
Ms. X is under my care during her pregnancy. She has described her work tasks and provided material safety data sheets for the following chemicals *546—acetone*. Proper use of this substance, including gloves and a hood, is not considered to pose an increased risk, and she may continue her current job without restrictions.

As with any pregnancy, I recommend that workplace provisions be made for more frequent bathroom access, avoidance of prolonged standing, and release time for 3 to 6 appointments.

I would be happy to discuss these recommendations with you. Thank you.
Sincerely,

The patient's employer accepts your advice, and she remains on the job.

A second patient reports exposure to other solvents, such as xylene, toluene, or trichloroethylene. What do you advise her?

You call the teratogen information service and are told that these chemicals are considered reproductive hazards. The company has no air sampling data or biologic monitoring program, so you have little information on the extent of exposure. At this point, you may try to help the patient eliminate exposures, refer her to an occupational physician, or encourage the employer to hire an industrial hygiene consultant.

The employer is willing to consider improved ventilation, training for potentially exposed men or women of reproductive age, or substitution of safer solvents, but these cannot be accomplished for several months. There are no alternative jobs available within the company. Your consultant recommends against the use of respirators, given the discomfort associated with continuous use and uncertain protection in these situations. The employer is willing to place the patient on temporary layoff. Because she is still ''able and available'' for other work, she is able to collect unemployment insurance.

In circumstances in which the employer is less willing to correct dangerous working conditions, you might want to discuss an Occupational Safety and Health Administration (OSHA) investigation with the patient. This agency regulates employees' exposure to physical, biologic, and chemical hazards. Although only 450 out of 60,000 chemicals have specific standards, and these standards were set with scanty information on reproductive risks, OSHA has a general duty to ensure that employers provide a safe and healthful workplace for all employees. Compliance officers may be willing to inspect and cite an employer for clearly unsafe conditions, even if they are not covered by a specific standard. The OSHA also provides a consultative service for employers, and several state governments have separate industrial hygiene programs. The name of the complainant is kept confidential, and reprisals by employers, though feared by many employees, are illegal.

Case Study: Lead

A 30-year-old friend of the laboratory technician also comes to you for care during her pregnancy. She asks whether she should remove the lead paint in their house before the baby's birth. What do you advise her?

Reproductive Hazards: Environmental

Lead remains a common exposure for women and their families both from work and in the home. There are still few women in certain high-risk industries such as battery manufacture, bridge and structural steel work, or automobile radiator repair, but exposures are more commonly seen among women artists who produce stained glass and use lead pottery glaze, cable and wire manufacturing workers, and home painters. Those who attempt their own lead paint removal may cause more problems for themselves and their families than they solve.

At high levels of absorption, lead can cause well-documented problems such as abdominal pain, peripheral and central nervous system dysfunction, joint pain, anemia, and renal dysfunction. A level above 25 μg per dl in adults is considered an indication of undue absorption, and levels higher than 50 μg per dl require employer action to remove and protect exposed workers. However, reproductive problems such as impaired spermatogenesis, an increase in spontaneous abortions and stillbirths, and damage to a fetus' developing nervous system may occur when a mother's or father's lead level is substantially lower.[7]

With this information in mind, you recommend against lead abatement activities during pregnancy unless she can stay away from home from the beginning to the end of the project. You also recommend that the work be done by a licensed lead abatement company and emphasize the need for removal methods that avoid the generation of excess lead dust and the importance of testing the adequacy of the removal by an independent contractor or inspector, following state regulations. She takes your advice and rejects bids from two companies because they included dry scraping and power sanding inside the house and did not include use of a high-efficiency vacuum and an air exhaust system. After finding an acceptable company, she and her husband stay with friends while windows containing lead paint are removed and a caustic paste is used to remove other areas of old paint. Testing after the project reveals successful abatement.

OTHER EXPOSURES

RADON. Radon is an alpha-emitting radioactive gas found in soil and to a lesser degree in well water. It can enter into homes through the foundation, and radon levels are difficult to predict from a home's construction or location. Radon and its decay products are carcinogenic and have been shown to cause a markedly increased risk of lung cancer in occupationally exposed groups such as miners (particularly in those who also smoke cigarettes). By extrapolation, radon is felt to be a serious risk to occupants of homes with markedly elevated levels, although there is debate over the degree of risk of more modest elevations.

Measurement of radon levels is inexpensive and is the only way to determine whether action to reduce exposure is necessary. The Environmental Protection Agency currently considers a level of 4 picocuries per liter as a threshold for further evaluation. Exposure can be lowered by measures including sealing cracks in floors and walls and installing ventilation systems. The cost is reported to range from $500 to $2500.[8]

Advice for patients:

- Measure radon levels in your home or prospective home, using a charcoal device available in hardware stores, measuring for 48 hours in the lowest occupied portion of the house during a time when the windows and doors are shut.
- If the first level is elevated, confirm with a second test.
- If this is high, contact your state radon office (numbers are available through the Environmental Protection Agency) for advice on whether action is needed, and, if so, for help in finding a contractor. Contractors should be willing to guarantee results.

ASBESTOS. Asbestos exposure, through inhalation of small particles, can cause a variety of serious health problems, including pulmonary fibrosis, lung cancer, pleural scarring and effusion, mesothelioma, and cancer of the larynx and gastrointestinal tract. These effects appear after a long latency period. Although a safe level of exposure is not clear, there is a dose-response relationship, and cigarette smoking acts synergistically to increase markedly the risk of lung cancer from asbestos. Occupational exposure to asbestos is decreasing, and trades in which exposure can take place such as construction work or school custodial positions still have relatively few women. Exposures in homes built before the 1970s may occur if there are asbestos products such as pipe and boiler insulation, panels, or tiles, particularly if the softer materials are improperly maintained or removed or if harder materials are disturbed.

Advice for patients:

- All those working with asbestos must have comprehensive training, protective clothing, and appropriate respiratory protection (usually meaning a powered air-purifying respirator). Work practices such as wetting the material, enclosing the work space, and showering before leaving are necessary. Periodic chest radiographs and pulmonary function tests should be performed according to OSHA regulations, and all workers should be counseled not to smoke.

- All occupants of residences built before the 1970s should have their homes checked for asbestos. Often an experienced plumbing contractor can identify the material.
- Removal of the asbestos is not always necessary and should never be done by an inexperienced person. If there is a small area of crumbling material, dust can be cleaned up with a wet mop, the area can be repaired with rewettable fiberglass cloth, and the area can be enclosed with a durable material to prevent further damage. Clean-up should never be done by dusting, sweeping, or using a standard vacuum.
- Asbestos-containing hard material should not be sanded, sawed, or drilled.
- If there are larger areas of asbestos material, if damage is extensive, or if the asbestos is in an area in which it will likely be disturbed during normal activities or renovations, a licensed contractor should be called to remove it following approved procedures. Call the Consumer Product Safety Commission (see Appendix) for advice. Some state governments have asbestos programs.

BLOOD-BORNE PATHOGENS. Exposure to blood-borne pathogens such as hepatitis B and C and human immunodeficiency virus, through percutaneous injuries and splashes to mucous membranes and nonintact skin, is a growing problem. The risk of transmission depends on the type of injury, the particular virus, and the extent of viremia of the source patient. Hepatitis B may be transmissible in up to 30% of significant exposures, human immunodeficiency virus in approximately 0.3%, and hepatitis C carries an intermediate risk.

Employees at risk include health care workers, particularly nurses, midwives, dental workers, physicians, laboratory technicians, emergency medical technicians, housekeepers, and laundry and central supply personnel; waste disposal workers; embalmers; police and security staff; daycare workers; and providers of first aid.

Advice for patients:

- Follow universal precautions, including appropriate disposal of sharps; avoidance of recapping needles; and use of impervious gowns, gloves, and face shields as mandated by OSHA.[9] Training and protective equipment must be provided by the employer.
- Get a hepatitis B vaccination. The series of

three intramuscular injections is safe and effective and must be provided to all potentially exposed employees except those who decline in writing. It is usually given on a 0, 1-, and 6-month schedule and must be given in the deltoid with a 1½-inch needle to ensure intramuscular injection. Up to 10% of those receiving three doses will have an inadequate antibody response; one or more booster doses should be considered for those individuals.

- Encourage and evaluate efforts to reduce potential sharp object injuries by using advances in needleless systems for intravenous infusions; safer syringes for injections, phlebotomy, and venous access; and analytic devices that do not require blood drawing.
- Report all exposures. Promptly clean the exposed area, obtain hepatitis B immune globulin when appropriate, and possibly take zidovudine for higher risk injuries (although its efficacy is uncertain). Receive counseling about sexual practices, blood donations, and reproductive issues to avoid secondary transmission.

VIDEO DISPLAY TERMINALS. The use of video display terminals has increased dramatically in a wide range of occupations, most of them heavily represented by women. Health effects are hotly debated, but prolonged use has been associated with eye strain and repetitive motion disorders of the hands and arms. There is equivocal evidence about adverse pregnancy outcomes, with concern about exposure to electromagnetic radiation.

Advice for patients:

- Avoid exposure to the side or rear of other terminals. This is the location of the fly back transformer, which is the source of nonionizing radiation.
- Limit video display terminal use to less than 20 hours per week or 4 hours per day.
- Have a rest break each hour.
- Use adjustable chairs and adjustable height keyboards.
- Use screens with good contrast, and situate them away from sunlight.

ASSESSING SYMPTOMS

Occupational and environmental exposures can cause a wide range of problems, from peripheral neuropathy to aplastic anemia to pulmonary interstitial fibrosis. Some are common and easy to diagnose; others have yet to be recognized. If you or your patient suspect that her symptoms are related to an exposure at work or at home, further questioning may help establish the association.

Case Study: Respiratory Illness at Work

A 32-year-old cosmetologist comes to you because of persistent cough and chest tightness. She has no prior history of lung problems. She wants to know if her symptoms are due to substances at work. What do you advise her?

First, ask her about the pattern of symptoms over time and among co-workers. An occupational cause is more likely if symptoms lessen on weekends, on vacation, or while assigned to a different task and if co-workers have similar symptoms. She reports that her symptoms began after working at this job for about 6 months. They do get better after several days of vacation. She reports that a co-worker had to quit the job because of similar symptoms. Because these screening questions suggest an occupational cause, you may elect to obtain further information from the patient or refer her for a consultation.

Based on the results of her chest examination, you suspect asthma as the cause of her symptoms and decide to confirm the presence of reversible air flow obstruction. Results of a baseline spirometry are normal, so you give her a hand-held peak flow meter, instruct her in its use, and ask her to record readings and symptoms at 2-hour intervals while awake over a week. This confirms a drop in peak flow early in each work shift, gradually resolving later in the day.

At her next visit, you ask her more questions in the four categories of the occupational history:

Work: She works 7 hours a day doing hair styling in her own shop where she employs two other women.

Hazards: She uses shampoo frequently. She often applies permanent wave solution, uses hair coloring and hair sprays, and mixes bleach, which comes in a powder. She notes her cough is worse after using this product.

Illness: In addition to the chest symptoms mentioned previously, she notes that her hands have become red and chapped.

Protection: There is no ventilation in the shop. She does use latex gloves when applying permanent wave solution but notes that her hands have not improved with the use of these.

Further Evaluation

You can refer the patient now to a specialist in occupational and environmental medicine, such as a member of the Association of Occupational and Environmental Clinics. If none is available, you can get more information through standard textbooks, a MedLine search, or by calling the National Institute for Occupational Safety and Health (see Appendix for a list of resources). Your consultant diagnoses occupational asthma, probably due to persulfates used in bleaches and aggravated by other workplace irritants. She recommends that the patient try a version of bleach that has no persulfates and comes with a ''shaker'' for enclosed mixing. She also refers the patient to a ventilation engineer and suggests she use only nonaerosol hair sprays and consider a no smoking policy. The patient has an exhaust ventilation system installed, with ports at countertop level to draw dusts and fumes away from her and the customers' breathing zone. She follows the other recommendations, and notes a marked decrease in symptoms.

OCCUPATIONAL ASTHMA. Preexisting asthma may be worsened by exposure to irritants or allergens at work. Previously unaffected workers may develop asthma through both allergic and nonallergic mechanisms. Those who develop allergic sensitization begin to have symptoms after weeks or months of work and may present initially with nocturnal cough or with chest tightness and wheezing. Once sensitized, the worker experiences symptoms even with minimal exposure and, unless exposure is markedly reduced or avoided, may develop permanent, nonspecific airway hyperresponsiveness with wheezing after stimuli such as exercise or cold air. Others develop nonallergic asthma after exposure to high levels of a strong irritant. In this case, symptoms caused by bronchial mucosal injury begin rapidly but, as in allergic occupational asthma, nonspecific airway hyperresponsiveness may persist.

Causes. Asthma may be caused by exposure to chemicals used in glues, dyes, plastics, disinfectants, paints, photographic products, insecticides, foams, hair products, and rubber products; metal fumes; vegetable products such as flour, wood dust, gums, enzymes, latex, and molds; or exposure to animals, birds, marine products, and insects. Occupations at risk with a large percentage of women include laboratory workers, hairdressers, textile workers, nurses, animal handlers, bakers, and printers.[10]

Suggestions for evaluation and treatment:

- Ask about prior asthma or allergic symptoms, timing of symptoms, and workplace exposures.
- Consider sputum and peripheral blood eosinophil counts.
- Confirm reversible air flow obstruction by having the patient perform serial peak flow meas-

urements for several weeks during work and for a period away from work.

- If symptoms are severe and association with work seems likely, remove the patient from work or help arrange transfer to a nonexposed area while evaluation and treatment are in progress.

- Consider consultation to help resolve issues of diagnosis, work-relatedness, job modification, and disability. In most cases, continued exposure will be too risky for the patient, but changing jobs may be difficult.

- Encourage the patient to apply for workers' compensation and provide medical documentation as required in your state. Workers' compensation is a system in which employers are required to obtain no-fault insurance coverage for employees who may become injured or ill owing to work. Benefits include payment of lost wages, medical expenses, and rehabilitation. For example, a patient forced to leave a high-paying job owing to occupational asthma may continue to receive medical treatment, payment of a portion of wages lost while unable to work or while working only at lower-paid jobs, and retraining for another occupation. The rules in each state are somewhat different, but patients with occupational illnesses can anticipate that the insurer may contest the claim, requiring the patient to have additional examinations and eventually a hearing before a state-appointed tribunal, which decides contested issues such as work-relatedness, disability, and prognosis. This process can take months and can be extremely trying. Most patients need legal help and continued support from a sympathetic primary physician. Primary physicians themselves are very rarely asked to give depositions or appear at a hearing.

- Report the case, if required, in your state. Many states now require that certain occupational illnesses, such as infectious disease, be reported to the department of public health.

Prevention. Agents known to cause occupational asthma may be controlled by substitution of a less harmful agent, enclosure of a process, or local exhaust ventilation. Personal protection with respirators is generally inadequate by itself.

Other Common Occupational Illnesses

CONTACT DERMATITIS. The cosmetologist in the earlier case has, in addition to occupational asthma, symptoms suggestive of contact dermatitis. This condition is common, is of particular concern in occupations in which nonintact skin may increase the risk of exposure to bloodborne pathogens, and may become so severe as to require a change of occupation. As in the case of occupational asthma, occupational contact dermatitis may be allergic or nonallergic. Most cases are the latter, caused by the direct toxic affect of strong irritants such as solvents and detergents on epidermal cells, an effect aggravated by friction, moisture, and heat. In contrast, allergic contact dermatitis may occur when a chemical, acting as a hapten, binds with epidermal proteins to form a complete antigen, which results in T-lymphocyte sensitization. Rash occurs at least 5 days after the initial exposure but sooner after subsequent exposures. Although it is difficult to distinguish the two on clinical grounds alone, blistering is more common in cases of allergic dermatitis, tending to appear only in more severe cases of irritant dermatitis. Both should be distinguished from contact urticaria, a type I reaction causing hives immediately after contact with, for example, latex.[11] Attempts to treat without identifying the cause may fail, and the gloves and creams used for treatment and prevention may contain unsuspected irritants and allergens that may actually worsen symptoms. In addition, glove material must be carefully chosen to ensure that chemicals and infectious agents cannot penetrate through.

Suggestions for evaluation and treatment:

- Review for prior skin conditions and nonoccupational exposures.

- Mild cases without blistering may be treated with emollients (preferably free of potential sensitizers such as fragrances) and identification and avoidance of irritants.

- More severe cases may require a period away from work, use of compresses for moist lesions, corticosteroid creams (or ointments for thickened, dry rashes), and job modification or transfer.

- If there is exposure to a known sensitizer or blistering, refer to a dermatologist with experience in occupational dermatology and patch testing. Ask the patient to bring to the visit all appropriate material safety data sheets or other information on exposures.

- If there is evidence suggestive of contact urticaria, refer to an allergist.

- Be specific in recommendations concerning job tasks and use of gloves. For all workers, gloves that are low in starch powder (an irritant) and low in accelerators such as thiurams, benzothiazoles, and carbamates (allergens) are preferable. Persons who develop an allergy to these accelerators (usually contact dermatitis) or to latex protein (contact urticaria, angioedema, asthma, anaphylaxis) may select from a variety of alternatives such as vinyl, nitrile, polyethylene, and neoprene gloves, which are appropriate to different exposures and tasks.

SICK BUILDING SYNDROME. Primary practitioners are likely to see women with symptoms they attribute to poor air quality in office buildings. Some building-related illnesses such as asthma, hypersensitivity pneumonitis, and legionellosis are accompanied by abnormalities on physical examination, radiographs, or other objective testing and have identifiable and correctable causes. The sick building syndrome, though, consists of symptoms such as eye, nose, and throat irritation; headache; and fatigue that occur during work in a particular building and are relieved by leaving. The syndrome may affect large numbers in certain buildings, affect productivity and morale, but does not usually have an easily identified cause. Symptoms are more common in new or renovated buildings, particularly those that are air-conditioned or were designed to minimize energy loss.

Although common in all such buildings, the symptoms may be less tolerable for employees who perceive insufficient rewards for or control over their working conditions. Proposed causes, varying from building to building, include inadequate fresh air supply; release of volatile organic compounds and other pollutants from building materials and furnishings, cigarette smoking, photocopy machines, and other interior sources; entry of outside pollutants such as motor vehicle exhaust; and contamination of humidifiers and ductwork or water-damaged materials by microorganisms.[12]

Suggestions for evaluation and treatment:

- If the patient has fever, chills, wheezing, or crackles on chest examination in association with work, she will likely need to be removed from exposure. Further testing or referral may be required and an expedited workplace evaluation requested if a link is confirmed, particularly if others are at risk.
- If the symptoms suggest sick building syndrome, the examination is normal, and similar symptoms are present in co-workers, you might suggest that the patient call the National Institute for Occupational Safety and Health (see Appendix) for guidance in further evaluating and improving the workplace.
- Some patients have symptoms suggesting sick building syndrome but more severe and more generalized. They may experience disabling symptoms, particularly fatigue or confusion, on exposure to a variety of chemical odors both in and outside of work. The cause and treatment

for this syndrome of "multiple chemical sensitivities" is hotly debated. Some practitioners, particularly those in the field of "clinical ecology," suggest unproven methods of diagnosis, detoxification, and rigid avoidance of provocative stimuli. As those recommendations may deepen a patient's isolation and disability, a primary practitioner may want to consult with a psychologist or psychiatrist who stresses gradual deconditioning, functional rehabilitation, and coping mechanisms for dealing with disability and loss of control.

- Prevention: Institute a nonsmoking policy, a ventilation system with an adequate outside air supply, a reduction of materials likely to cause exposure (or their use before occupancy to allow "off gassing" of volatiles), and regular maintenance that includes cleaning of filters and ducts and removal of water-damaged materials.

LOW BACK PAIN. Low back pain is common in adults, usually resolves quickly, but can be a source of prolonged work disability in some. Although about 70% of adults experience low back pain at some time, it is more frequent in persons such as nurses and nurses' aides, whose work requires frequent lifting, especially if the weight is held away from the body and the lifting is accompanied by twisting. In most cases, no specific diagnoses can be determined for the pain, though a minority may have a specific diagnosis such as lumbar disk herniation, compression fracture, or, less likely, spinal metastasis, infection, or visceral disease with referred pain.

Suggestions for evaluation and treatment:

- At the first visit for back pain experienced at work, document the circumstances of the work activity and onset of pain, a description of required job tasks, and a targeted history and physical examination. Findings requiring further urgent work-up include a prior history of cancer, intravenous drug use, unintentional weight loss, fever, urinary retention, or saddle anesthesia. Women who are postmenopausal or who have had an oophorectomy should be considered at risk for compression fracture.
- Leg pain, reproduced by straight-leg raising, suggests lumbar disk herniation. As almost all involve the L5 or S1 level, the screening examination should include ankle and toe dorsiflexor strength (L5), sensation in the medial (L5) and lateral (S1) foot, and ankle deep tendon reflex (S1).[13]
- If there is no evidence of systemic disease or neurologic compromise, advise bed rest or restricted activity for 2 to 3 days; nonsteroidal

anti-inflammatory agents; ice massage, or muscle relaxants, or both. If there is a suggestion of disk herniation, bed rest might be extended several days. Reassure all these patients, including those with sciatica, that chances for recovery are good without the need for surgery. Schedule a follow-up appointment within a week, and inform the patient's supervisor by a note or call.

- At the follow-up visit, review for factors such as work conflict, substance abuse, or depression, which might slow recovery.
- After the initial pain and muscle spasm have improved, active exercise (generally emphasizing back extension) with the guidance of a physical therapist may help those with a slower recovery, and a therapist-taught "back school" is advised for those who must return to lifting at work. All patients should be encouraged to increase aerobic exercise such as walking and be given specific instructions on the type, frequency, and duration of activity.
- If symptoms are improving but not yet resolved, discuss a return to a modified job assignment with the patient and supervisor.
- For those with persistent sciatica, imaging is appropriate. If a disk herniation is documented and there is a corresponding neurologic deficit, surgery has the greatest chance of success.
- Those who have more serious injuries and require prolonged time off work, surgery, or both and who are motivated to return to a previous physically demanding job may benefit from intensive physical conditioning as in a "work hardening" program or a gradual return to modified work responsibilities.
- If pain and perceived disability persist beyond what is expected, consider referral to a chronic pain rehabilitation program.
- If the injury appears to have been due to improper job design, particularly if there are others with similar problems, suggest an ergonomic assessment to the employer. The OSHA consultation program and the employer's workers' compensation insurer can provide advice.
- Prevention: Employees should redesign job layouts to permit lifting in a forward-facing direction. Hydraulic lifts, mechanical hoists, and two-person lifts should be used when possible.

CARPAL TUNNEL SYNDROME. Carpal tunnel syndrome may occur in women whose work requires repetitive flexion and extension of the wrist, particularly if they must use force, a pinch grip, or vibrating tools. Such work may cause increased pressure within the carpal tunnel, leading to diminished blood flow and impaired function of the median nerve as it passes through the wrist.

Some cases may involve damage to distal small nerves, which is less amenable to standard diagnostic and surgical methods.[14] Women at risk include postal workers, supermarket cashiers, keyboard operators, and stitchers. The symptoms include pain and paresthesias in the median nerve distribution of the hand (generally the thenar eminence at the base of the thumb and the first 3½ digits). Symptoms may be worse at night, requiring the patient to shake her hand for relief. Diagnostic criteria are in dispute but include an appropriate "hand diagram" of discomfort, a positive Tinel's sign (reproduction of symptoms by gentle tapping over the median nerve at the wrist), Phalen's sign (symptoms with unforced full flexion of the wrist for 60 seconds), and confirmatory electrodiagnostic studies.

Suggestions for evaluation and treatment:

- Perform a complete occupational and medical history. Ask the patient to demonstrate job tasks and ask about the time course of symptoms. Consider predisposing factors such as pregnancy, rheumatoid arthritis, diabetes, hypothyroidism, and prior wrist fracture, which may aggravate symptoms, or conditions such as cervical radiculopathy, which might mimic the syndrome.
- Symptoms with few findings can often be managed with job modifications such as rest periods, rotation to other tasks, or use of different tools.
- More severe symptoms may require job transfer or time off work. Ice, splinting, nonsteroidal anti-inflammatory agents, and steroid injection may be helpful.
- Surgical referral should generally be reserved for cases in which symptoms persist despite removal from exposure or when atrophy or weakness are present.
- Help the patient with a workers' compensation application, if necessary, and report the case if required to the appropriate state agency.
- Suggest ergonomic evaluation of the workplace if others appear to be at risk.
- Prevention: Use ergonomically designed tools to prevent extreme wrist positions, frequent work breaks and rotation to different job tasks, and early identification of symptomatic workers.

The exposures and effects listed previously are common and often preventable, but are only examples of the multitude of problems women may encounter at work or at home. Primary practitioners can help women identify potential problems, place risks in perspective, and take appropriate action to protect their health.

APPENDIX

Workplace Hazards

Occupational Safety and Health Administration (OSHA):

Office of Information 1-202-219-8148
Office of Occupational Medicine: 1-202-219-5003

National Institute for Occupational Safety and Health (NIOSH):

Information Hotline 1-800-356-4674

Association of Occupational and Environmental Clinics (AOEC): 1-800-347-4976
Centers for Disease Control and Prevention (infectious hazards): 1-404-639-3311
Teratogen Information Services (reproductive hazards):

Arizona	(AZ only) 800-362-0101
California	(CA only) 800-532-3749
Colorado	(CO only) 800-332-2082
Connecticut	(CT only) 800-325-5391
Florida	904-392-3050
Georgia	404-488-4967
Illinois	(IL only) 800-252-4847
Indiana	317-274-1071
Iowa	319-356-3561
	319-356-2674
Kansas	316-688-2362
Massachusetts	(MA only) 800-322-5014

University of Massachusetts Occupational and Environmental Hazards Center
1-508-856-6162

Missouri	314-454-8172
Nebraska	402-559-5071
New Jersey	(NJ only) 800-287-3015
New York	800-724-2454
North Dakota	701-777-4277
Pennsylvania	215-829-3601
South Dakota	800-962-1642
Texas	817-383-3561
Utah	801-583-2229
Vermont	802-658-4310
Washington	206-543-3373
Wisconsin	(WI, MN IA Only) 1-800-362-9567

Environmental Hazards

Environmental Protection Agency (EPA)	1-800-368-5888
Solid waste clearinghouse	1-800-677-9424
Toxic dump sites	1-800-424-9346
Safe drinking water	1-800-426-4791
Pesticides	1-800-858-7378
Chemical Manufacturers' Association Referral Center	1-800-262-8200
Consumer Product Safety Commission Asbestos in homes	1-800-638-2772

Local phone numbers that may be useful:

State Public Health Dept.
City/Town Board of Health
Poison Control Center
Division of Industrial Accidents
Coalition for Occupational Safety & Health
State OSHA office

REFERENCES

1. U.S. Department of Labor, Bureau of Labor Statistics. Working Women: A Chartbook. Bulletin 2385, Washington, DC: US Government Printing Office, August 1991.
2. U.S. Department of Labor, Women's Bureau. 20 Facts on Women Workers, No. 90-2, September 1990.
3. US Department of Labor, Bureau of Labor Statistics. Employment and earnings. Washington, DC. US Government Printing Office, January 1994.
4. Occupational Safety and Health Administration, Hazard Communication Standard (29 CFR 1910, 1200) Washington, DC: US Government Printing Office, 1990.
5. Bloom AD. Guidelines for Studies of Human Populations Exposed to Mutagenic and Reproductive Hazards. White Plains, NY: March of Dimes Birth Defects Foundation, 1981.
6. Paul M. Occupational and Environmental Reproductive Hazards: A Guide for Clinicians. Baltimore: Williams & Wilkins, 1992.
7. Rempel D. The lead-exposed worker. JAMA 1989; 262(4):532.
8. Environmental Protection Agency. A Citizen's Guide to Radon. 2nd ed. Washington, DC: US Government Printing Office, 1992.
9. Occupational Safety and Health Administration. Occupational exposure to bloodborne pathogens (29 CFR 1910, 1030) Washington, DC: US Government Printing Office, 1991.
10. Chan-Yeung M, Lam S. Occupational asthma. Am Rev Resp Dis 1986;133:686.
11. Gonzalez E. Latex hypersensitivity, a new and unexpected problem. Hosp Pract 1992; 27(2):137.
12. The Sick Building Syndrome: Where is the Epidemiologic Basis? (editorial). Am J Public Health 1990;80(10):1172.
13. Deyo RA, Rainville J, Kent DL. What can the history and physical tell us about low back pain? JAMA 1992;286(6):760.
14. Cullen M, Rosenstock L. Occupational medicine. N Engl J Med 1990;322(10):677.

Sports Medicine

Michael L. Corbett and Coleman D. Fowble

Although "a strong mind in a strong body" has been the ideal since antiquity, it is only in the last few years that women have been afforded full participation in athletic activity. The history of organized athletics dates back to 776 B.C. with the Olympic Games. Before this, athletic competition undoubtedly took place but not in an organized fashion. Women not only were excluded from participating in these Olympic Games, but also were forbidden to view them. However, there were athletic competitions for women, the Herean Games, which took place every 4 years. During the time of the Roman Empire, women were allowed to compete in certain activities. Most of the women's athletic activities, such as dancing, were derived from religious, agricultural, or fertility rituals. Systems of physical training that subsequently developed in Europe were designed primarily to prepare men for their role as warriors in battle, in which speed, strength, and power were the most effective weapons. Because there was no military role for women, they did not participate in these activities.

In 1900, women began to compete in sports such as golf and tennis. It was not until 1920 that women competed in the modern Olympics. For the next 40 years, debate concerning the proper role of women in sports continued. Most issues revolved around questions of safety, ability to compete, social norms, and political control of women's sports. A more feminist interpretation of this period is that it represented an ongoing process of denying women their equal right to the physical, psychological, and social benefits of sports. Finally, the Civil Rights Act of 1964, the rise of the women's movement, and, most important, Title IX of the Education Act of 1972 ensured women the opportunity for full athletic participation.

PHYSIOLOGIC CONSIDERATIONS

When the athletic performance of women is studied, it is difficult to distinguish the residuum of low sports participation, less intense coaching, and poor training techniques from true physiologic parameters that affect athletic performance. For example, an untrained teenaged boy can usually throw a softball farther than an untrained teenaged girl. Does this represent a difference in strength and coordination, or does it reflect a difference in training and throwing experience? Among the first to attempt to answer this question were the United States military academies, who admitted their first female cadets in 1976. At this time, no standards of physical performance had been outlined for women. Hence, the institutions developed their own guidelines.

The major physiologic differences between men and women that affect athletic performance relate to body composition and certain parameters of cardiovascular function. Body composition can be determined either directly or indirectly. Accepted methods divide the body into different components, such as fat, bone, and muscle. The most useful for the sports physiologist subdivides the body into two components: fat and lean body mass. In the clinical setting, indirect assessment is used to determine body fat percentage. From this measurement and total body weight, lean body mass can be calculated. However, it should be recognized that indirect measurements of body fat percentage, such as skin fold thickness or abdominal girth, tend to be inaccurate.

Several studies have established the statistical average (reference) standard for male and female body composition. For males, the reference body fat standard is 15%. For females, the body fat standard is 27%. The lowest standard body fat for an otherwise healthy male is 3%, and the minimal standard for a female is 12%. The approximately 10% difference is maintained across specific sports. For instance, a male elite-level distance runner may have a 5% total body fat composition; an elite female distance runner may have 15% total body fat. Both a male and a female shot putter would have higher body fat percentages, but the 10% difference between the sexes would be maintained.

A similar pattern is seen in height and weight. A reference male is 10 cm taller and 16 kg heavier than a reference female. Like body fat percentage, the actual height and weight are somewhat sport specific, but the percentage difference is maintained. A female basketball player is taller than an average woman but shorter than a male basketball player.

There are certain anatomic differences between males and females that contribute to the distinct performance capabilities of each sex. Because the female pelvis is wider than the male's, the femoral tibial angle is increased. In addition, women tend to have more femoral neck anteversion and foot pronation. These factors along with an increased Q angle (quadriceps to patella-tibial tubercle line) (Fig. 76–1) in females have been implicated in patellofemoral disorders.

Cardiovascular function is different in women. A woman has a statistically lower stroke volume and serum hemoglobin. Therefore, cardiac output as well as maximum tissue oxygenation are reduced. Other factors affecting cardiovascular function are addressed later in the endurance training section of this chapter.

There is no evidence of any difference in either the ratio of fast (white) to slow (red) twitch muscle fibers or alternate metabolic pathways between men and women.

PHYSICAL FITNESS AND ATHLETIC TRAINING

Physical fitness is an easily understood but hard to define term. It implies the presence of sufficient

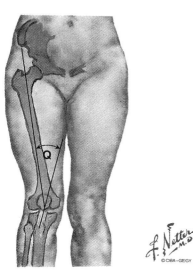

Figure 76–1. The Q angle.

neuromuscular skeletal function to easily perform work and recreational activities. Fitness is defined differently for each individual, as a physically fit steelworker has different physical characteristics than a physically fit pianist. Components of fitness include strength, endurance or aerobic function, and flexibility.

Strength is the ability to perform work. It is defined by the maximum tension developed in a contracting muscle. Power is strength measured as a function of time. Both strength and power correlate directly with lean body mass. A male, possessing a larger total body weight and a higher percentage of lean body mass, has greater strength than a female athlete. In fact, world records in sports requiring strength and power usually demonstrate a 10% difference reflecting the reported 10% difference in lean body mass between male and female athletes. However, the difference in strength is somewhat dependent on which muscle group is studied. If the upper body is studied, the male-female strength difference is 40 to 60%. In the lower body the disparity drops to 25%. The explanation of this finding is not obvious. It may relate to the virtual lack of upper body strength training undertaken by female athletes. The experience of the United States military academies appears to support this hypothesis. Initially, many female recruits could do less than one pull-up. Therefore, hanging flexed-arm time was used as the measure of upper body strength. With the introduction of upper body training into the overall training regimen, this method has been discontinued and conventional pull-ups are now the standard. In sports relying on upper body strength such as the shot put, European athletes, who do employ upper body training, have long dominated these sports. Data from wheelchair athletes also reveal that smaller cross-sectional muscle area requires more metabolic energy to produce the same amount of work as a muscle of greater cross-sectional area. This may also be a factor in the upper-lower body strength differences between males and females.

What if the strength is measured on the basis of lean body mass? If a male and female athlete of identical percentage of lean body mass are compared, the male still tests slightly stronger. The reason for this is not clear. The theory is that the measured difference is purely quantitative, and it is a function of body composition. Baeche, in an excellent review of strength training in women, discussed several important points. He agrees the strength difference is a function of body composition and that it is a quantitative, not qualitative, difference. He also reports a 12 to 38% increase in strength following a resistive training program.

This type of program gives the greatest increase in the strength of the female athlete, yet it does not lead to excessive hypertrophy. The increase in muscle bulk itself is somewhat offset by the diminution of intramuscular adipose tissue. The overall result is a minute increase in limb girth and no change in body weight. The bulky changes seen in male weight lifters are secondary to higher serum levels of testosterone. In the absence of exogenous steroids, these changes do not occur in women. The female athlete who incorporates resistive training suffers no loss of flexibility and can actually anticipate an increase in her speed.

The second component of physical fitness is endurance or aerobic function. Any activity that lasts more than a few minutes needs an aerobic pathway to provide energy. Aerobic metabolism requires oxygen to be taken in by the lungs, distributed by the cardiovascular system, and utilized by the muscles. The best measure of aerobic function is VO_{2max} (Vmax). This is the maximum amount of oxygen that can actually be utilized for energy at the cellular level. VO_{2max} is defined as the point at which increasing work intensity does not further oxygen consumption. Any additional energy requirements must be met anaerobically. It is expressed as liters per minute or better as ml per kg per minute. For an athlete, the higher the Vmax, the greater the aerobic capacity. In the absence of pulmonary or vascular disease, as is the case of most competitive athletes, the rate-limiting step in this system is cardiac output.

Cardiac output is the product of stroke volume and heart rate. Females generally have a smaller heart volume and hence a lower stroke volume. In addition, women tend to have lower serum hemoglobin values, which decrease their ability to deliver oxygen to the tissues. Based on these concepts, it is not surprising that Vmax is 15 to 20% lower in females than in males. An untrained female has a Vmax in the range of 30 to 35 ml per kg per minute compared with an untrained male, whose Vmax is 36 to 40 ml per kg per minute. Despite the physiologic differences, the woman athlete can dramatically improve her Vmax and aerobic capacity with an intensive training program. A typical training schedule designed to enhance aerobic function can be as simple as exercising three times a week at a heart rate of 60 to 80% of the maximum recommended heart rate. A more complicated program, usually involving running, would vary the frequency, intensity, and duration of each training activity. Elite level female distance runners often have a Vmax of 60 to 65 ml per kg per minute.

Although physiologic conditions affect performance significantly, races are not won and lost in a research laboratory. Many times, the winner is not the competitor with the highest Vmax but the one who performs most efficiently. In other words, successful endurance athletes can perform more work for a sustained period of time with less effort. At the same time, the requirements of their bodies for oxygen, lactic acid removal, and the like are met more efficiently than are those of unsuccessful athletes. This may be a function of lactic acid metabolism and is probably not a trainable characteristic. There is no conclusive evidence that women possess any unusual metabolic pathways that allow them to utilize increased body fat as an energy substrate.

Flexibility is another component of physical fitness that affects both performance and the ability to protect the body from injury. Flexibility is defined as the ability to move a joint or joints through a full range of motion. If a full range of motion is not maintained, capsular and ligamentous contraction can occur. The occurrence of this in an athlete can hinder her performance and increase the incidence of injury. Unlike strength and endurance, there is a limit to the amount of desired flexibility that can be achieved. A certain amount of ligamentous structure is needed to provide stability to the joints. Particularly in teenaged female athletes, excess joint laxity is associated with orthopedic pathology, especially in the knee and shoulder. Also, excess laxity is seen in many primary connective tissue disorders. Flexibility can best be maintained by slow stretching and maintaining the stretch for 15 to 20 seconds. Evidence suggests that stretching after exercise is particularly efficacious.

COMPLICATIONS OF ATHLETIC ACTION

Athletic Amenorrhea

Of prime concern to the physician who treats female athletes is the occurrence of amenorrhea, decreased bone mass, and stress fractures. Athletic amenorrhea or menstrual changes can affect up to 40% of elite endurance female athletes. Despite exhaustive research efforts, the precise etiology and optimal treatment are unknown. Most researchers agree that some combination of low body weight, an overly zealous training program, reproductive immaturity, and psychic or physical stress is usually present.

For a physician, a review of the literature to provide guidance in diagnosing and treating these patients is neither comforting nor reassuring. The terms amenorrhea, trained athlete, normal body composition, and others are defined differently by various investigators. To look for a hormonal cause of athletic amenorrhea is not definitive because the methodology of hormone measurement is difficult. Exercise itself in a healthy individual causes an increase in prolactin, cortisol, testosterone, estradiol, progesterone, and growth hormone. As changes in menstrual function are linked to hormonal fluctuations, the accurate measurement of all these hormones, many of which are released in a pulsatile manner, would have to be monitored continually. At the present time, this is not technically feasible.

The precise anatomic and secondary hormonal defects in athletic amenorrhea are unknown. A simplified schematic of normal endocrine function in the menstrual cycle based on available data suggests the pathway through the hypothalamus and the pituitary to the ovary is disrupted, possibly by the failure of the hypothalamus to secrete gonadotropin-releasing hormone (Gn-RH). At the present time, this should be considered the best theory, although it is unproven. The actual gynecologic changes of athletic amenorrhea begin with a shortening of the luteal phase. This is not a clinical manifestation and would be detected only as part of an infertility evaluation. Anovulatory cycles follow the shortening of the luteal phase, and eventually estrogen levels decrease. Most reports state that 3 months without a menstrual cycle is an indication for evaluation of amenorrhea. Pregnancy, pituitary neoplasia, and primary ovarian failure are conditions that must be excluded (see Chapter 19).

Several factors have been implicated in contributing to athletic amenorrhea. The most common is low body weight. Virtually every published series on this condition reports the amenorrheic athletes to be significantly lighter than eumenorrheic women. Because adipose tissue is a site of estrogen production, it is tempting to postulate that lower estrogen is secondary to less adipose tissue in these athletes. However, many athletes with low body fat have normal menstrual cycles, and athletes with higher body fat may be amenorrheic. Furthermore, reports show that cessation of training leads to the recurrence of menses without concomitant weight gain. Therefore, low body weight alone does not explain this syndrome.

Training regimens can cause alterations in the menstrual cycle. Most reports correlate the incidence of amenorrhea to the intensity of training. The many technical differences in these studies make it difficult to compare and quantify the different training programs. For example, a 10-kilometer race for one athlete may represent a major effort, but for another it may be closer to daily training exercises. Analogous to the body fat and menstrual cycle findings, studies have shown that many highly trained athletes on tremendously demanding training schedules are eumenorrheic, whereas some less highly trained women are amenorrheic. The specific role of training in this syndrome remains obscure. The effect of training regimens on male athletes has also been studied. The hypothalamic function in these high-level male athletes is quite similar to the proposed pathway that leads to secondary amenorrhea in women.

Stress is another factor that may contribute to the development of athletic amenorrhea. Many researchers refer to stress as a contributing factor; however, they all find it difficult to accurately and objectively measure stress levels. A certain amount of stress is intrinsically involved in the demands of intense training and actual competition. Psychological testing has been performed on many of these athletes with no evidence of unusual psychological profiles.

Reproductive maturity may also affect the risk of developing athletic amenorrhea. A woman who has a history of normal menses or, more important, has been pregnant is at low risk for developing athletic amenorrhea. Many affected individuals who develop athletic amenorrhea have never experienced normal menstrual cycles. In addition, there may be an element of self-selection involved. A woman with early onset of menses is statistically heavier and shorter, and has a higher body fat percentage. Many of these qualities may be detrimental to athletic performance. A late-maturing female will be taller, leaner, and stronger, thus making her more likely to participate in endurance sports. The risk of developing athletic amenorrhea is higher for the latter group.

Another factor that may play a role in athletic amenorrhea is diet. Of the components mentioned earlier, diet is the least implicated. It is difficult to separate the isolated effects of diet from the effects of low body weight. Studies have shown that female endurance athletes have a lower total caloric and decreased amino acid intake compared with that of controls. Irregularities in calcium metabolism have also been described but have not been substantiated.

Originally, it was felt that excessive training caused athletic amenorrhea and that it would resolve spontaneously when training ceased. So far, the etiology is unknown and is likely multifactorial. Successful treatment of athletic amenorrhea should be possible without eliminating female athletic participation. Athletic amenorrhea, whether it is a reaction phenomenon or a primary disease, causes low estrogen levels, which must be evaluated and treated with appropriate hormone therapy. It is somewhat perplexing that a vigorous exercise program often prescribed for older women to prevent osteopenia may actually cause the same problem in a young active athlete. Initial treatment includes weight gain if body weight is low. Next, the training schedule is altered by substituting strength training activities for endurance training. If menstruation does not resume, a complete endocrinologic evaluation is indicated.

Athletic Injuries

In addition to the physiologic aspects that influence an athlete's performance, training practices have a tremendous impact on the athlete's endurance, power, and risk of injury. A combination of these three facets of physical training (cross training) is now thought to be the most effective method of enhancing performance. In addition, varying training schedules helps prevent many stress or overuse injuries. Many injuries in athletes occur because of asymmetric development of strength, flexibility, or both. In a study of 138 female collegiate athletes, Knapik and colleagues found that athletes with a greater than 15% discrepancy in lower extremity strength were 2.6 times more likely to suffer a strain or sprain injury to the weaker extremity compared with athletes without this discrepancy. Similar findings were noted when a 15% difference in flexibility was present between the lower extremities. All of the injuries that occurred forced these athletes to miss some practice or competition.

With the increase in the number of women involved in athletic competition, the frequency of injuries is also on the rise. Many of these injuries are the same as those that male athletes suffer. It was once thought that women were more susceptible to ligamentous injury because of greater ligamentous laxity. However, it has been shown that most ligament injuries are not due to excess laxity but to lack of supporting muscular strength around the joint and inadequate conditioning. Because the female athlete does not generate the speed or power of the male (as discussed previously), female athletic injuries are usually low-velocity injuries. In a low-velocity injury, less energy is involved, and the body is given more time to compensate protectively before a bone, ligament, or tendon fails. Before the Title IX legislation, little data were available comparing injury rates of male and female athletes participating in the same sports. The early data from this period were reported by the military academies, which described an increased rate of injury, especially overuse syndromes and stress fractures, in female cadets. This undoubtedly represents poor previous training and

conditioning. Later studies show that the types and frequencies of injuries between male and female athletes is similar. It would appear that the injuries are more sport specific than sex specific.

The two major causes of athletic injuries are a traumatic event or, more commonly, an overuse syndrome. Overuse or stress injuries generally occur in the lower extremities because of the increased force of weight-bearing loads. The sequence of events leading to a stress injury is multifactorial. Conditions such as training errors, biomechanical problems, and accumulation of microtrauma play a role in injuries of overuse. Injuries associated with overuse syndromes include stress fractures, muscle strains, tendonitis, and tendon ruptures. It is unclear why some athletes experience stress injuries, whereas others on the same training schedule do not.

Stress Fractures

Stress fractures appear to be a common occurrence in female athletes. As bone is mechanically loaded by muscle forces acting on it, hypertrophy of the cortex occurs. A stress fracture appears when the rate of bone destruction from increased mechanical demands exceeds the rate of bone formation. In women, tibial stress fractures are the most common (Fig. 76–2); however, the fibula and metatarsals also can be affected. Numerous investigators describe significant osteopenia associated with athletic amenorrhea. Presumably, this would lead to a higher incidence of stress fractures reported in these women. More recent studies have confirmed that stress fractures occur in regions of osteopenia. Barrow and Saha retrospectively studied collegiate female distance runners. They found a 49% rate of stress fractures in subjects with irregular menses as opposed to a 29% rate in those with a normal menstrual cycle. Myburgh and as-

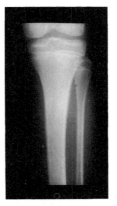

Figure 76–2. Stress fracture of the tibia.

sociates studied low bone density as an etiologic factor in stress fractures in some athletes. The group of injured athletes had a higher incidence of menstrual irregularity, and this was associated with low trabecular bone density in the spine. They also noted that the bone loss from estrogen deprivation was reversed with the restoration of menses. Of interest in both of these studies is that the athletes with fractures had either a decreased dietary intake of calcium or an increased incidence of eating disorders. In addition, the use of oral contraceptives seemed to protect against the development of stress fractures.

Although the relationship among endurance training, secondary amenorrhea, osteopenia, and stress fractures has been firmly established, the exact etiology and precise mechanism of stress fractures remain controversial. Any woman athlete who presents with a stress fracture should be questioned regarding her menstrual history. An athlete with amenorrhea should be referred for further evaluation. A woman with multiple stress fractures should have bone densitometry studies performed.

A patient with a stress fracture usually presents with pain over a specific area. The pain is usually not present at rest but becomes worse with activity. Patients are usually able to ambulate without pain. Radiographs may or may not be helpful. Because a stress fracture is really a series of microfractures, radiographs may only show a fracture line in fractures that are several weeks old. The presence of sufficient healing callus will be evident on plain radiographs. A bone scan is the most effective study for diagnosing an early stress fracture. These studies can detect osteoblastic activity as soon as the fracture occurs.

Treating a stress fracture is based on one premise: removal of the stress from the affected bone. Usually casting is not required to accomplish this. The athlete should use aids for ambulation until she is able to walk without pain. Once walking long distances causes no symptoms, other activities can be introduced. All of these fractures heal at different rates. The level of pain should be the primary factor in establishing progress.

Running Injuries

Running injuries are probably the most common injuries encountered by athletes at all levels. There are approximately 25 million joggers in the United States. Of these runners, there is a 60 to 70% incidence of injury each year. The accumulated impact of 800 to 2000 heel strikes per mile with three to five times body weight places tremendous force on the lower extremities. Forty percent of the running injuries involve the knee. The injuries are related to poor training techniques, biomechanical factors such as alignment, or abnormal gait patterns. Other injuries associated with running include shin splints, stress fractures, tendonitis, and muscle strains.

Patellofemoral Stress Syndrome

Patellar pain is the most frequent type of knee pain in runners (AAOS Course lectures). Anterior knee pain, "runners knee," accounts for 25% of these knee complaints and probably represents an inflammatory syndrome of the parapatellar tissue or irritation of the patellar cartilage. Women have a greater valgus angle at the knee joint, and, in addition, females frequently have femoral neck anteversion and pronation of the foot, which creates an increased Q angle (>20 degrees) at the knee (see Fig. 76–1). This makes women more likely to have a laterally tracking patella, especially in flexion, which predisposes them to retropatellar pain. This retropatellar pain was once referred to as chondromalacia, but it has been replaced by the term patellofemoral stress syndrome.

Because women are more anatomically susceptible to patellofemoral stress syndrome training regimens should emphasize quadriceps exercises to stabilize the patella. Preventing patellofemoral stress syndrome is easier than treating it. Quadriceps exercises should not include full range of motion with maximal weights but short arch activities with lighter weights and increased repetitions. Activities such as squats or stair climbing may increase the risk of patellofemoral stress syndrome in the female athlete. Treating patellofemoral stress syndrome starts with an attenuation of activity. Exercises that emphasize development of the quadriceps, particularly the vastus medialus obliquus, are encouraged to alter the distribution of force on the patella. Patellar braces have been used to hold the patella in a more medial position or to decrease the load from the quadriceps. Also, orthotics have been used to decrease the amount of foot pronation in some athletes. By reducing pronation, the valgus angle at the knee is decreased. Finally, the athlete should be reassured that this condition is generally temporary and does not cause any permanent joint damage. Participation should be allowed within the athlete's pain tolerance.

Iliotibial Band Friction Syndrome

Another injury around the knee is iliotibial band friction syndrome. Patients generally present with point tenderness where the iliotibial band crosses over the lateral femur. The main component is an inflammatory response to the friction created by the lateral structure's rubbing the lateral femoral excrescence. These conditions are often seen in runners who have a crossover or narrow-based gait pattern. When running, women tend to narrow their base more than men. Iliotibial band problems occur as a result of anatomic and biomechanical causes. A cavus foot tends to maintain its varus alignment. The effect on the tibia from the foot prevents internal rotation during flexion of the knee, so the knee remains in varus, thus tightening the lateral structures.

A set of iliotibial stretching exercises is the initial treatment for this syndrome. Patients are encouraged to change their training pattern, change the running surface, and use ice and nonsteroidal inflammatory drugs. Orthotics have not been shown to work effectively. If pain persists, steroids injected under the ligament into the bursa have been successful in some cases. In patients whose symptoms have persisted for 1 year or more, surgical release of the superior portion of the iliotibial band allows increased laxity. Some reports recommend complete division of the ligament. Patients with iliotibial band syndrome should be instructed to wait approximately 3 months before returning to their running routine.

Medial Tibial Stress Syndrome

Another overuse injury of the lower extremity is referred to as ''shin splints'' or medial tibial stress syndrome. This term is used to describe pain between the knee and ankle that is not a compartment syndrome or a stress fracture—more specifically, pain along the origin of the posterior tibial muscle, which courses along the anteromedial aspect of the tibia. Causes of shin splints are linked to running on hard surfaces, improper footwear, improper training techniques, or a combination of these. Diagnosis is usually made by history and physical examination. Shin splints must be differentiated from a stress fracture of the tibia. In shin splints, the pain increases with the initiation of activity, improves as participation continues, and returns after completion of activity. A stress fracture of the tibia has increased pain with activity that diminishes with rest. Also, the pain is discretely identifiable on the tibia.

Like treating other overuse syndromes, initial conservative therapy should include rest, ice, nonsteroidal anti-inflammatory drugs, and physical therapy. Changing activity until symptoms resolve may allow an athlete to continue training while waiting to return to a specific activity. Stretching and strengthening exercises for the posterior tibial muscle are also beneficial. Arch supports and tap-

ing may alleviate the symptoms during athletic participation. In athletes with chronic pain, participation may continue with the persistence of mild pain if a stress fracture has been ruled out. Proper warm-up and stretching are essential before starting activity.

Ankle-Foot Injuries

Achilles tendonitis is an injury that can be caused by overuse in sports requiring repeated flexion and extension of the ankle or direct trauma from boots in hockey and skiing. The pathology can involve either the fibers of the tendon itself or the damage to the tendon sheath. Acutely, Achilles tendonitis is painful along the distal portion of the tendon or its insertion point on the calcaneus. The pain is more severe with active plantar flexion or when resisting passive dorsiflexion. Athletes with chronic tendonitis generally experience more pain at the beginning of an activity that diminishes as their participation progresses. Physical examination may reveal some crepitation with plantar and dorsiflexion, and there may be mild swelling around the posterior aspect of the ankle.

Resting the tendon is the most effective method of treatment. Heel lifts or casts may be applied to relax the tendon. In acute situations, ice, nonsteroidal anti-inflammatory drugs, and changing activity can decrease the inflammation. Steroid injections should not be used indiscriminately because of the risk of further compromising the tendon by injecting it instead of the sheath. Stretching can retard healing of acute tendonitis. However, once the acute inflammation has subsided, exercises to stretch and strengthen the Achilles tendon should be initiated. Once the pain has resolved, the athlete may gradually begin training again. Ice should be used after training for several weeks. Pre-exercise warm-up and stretching are essential. Rarely, an athlete requires surgical resection of the tendon sheath.

Ankle sprains result from a traumatic event usually involving inversion of the foot. All running sports (e.g., soccer, field hockey, lacrosse) or jumping sports (basketball and volleyball) have a high incidence of ankle sprains. There are several systems for classifying ankle sprains. For example, one type deals with grading individual ligaments (e.g., grade II talofibular ligament sprain). The most common system describes a grade I as a minor injury, grade II as ligament injury with instability, and grade III as a complete ligamentous rupture.

The method of treatment is somewhat guided by the severity of the injury. A radiograph should be obtained if any bony tenderness to palpation is present. Initially, all sprains are iced and elevated. The eponym for this is RICE, *r*est, *i*ce, *c*ompression, and *e*levation. Nonsteroidal anti-inflammatory drugs may be given for pain and inflammation. After the acuteness of the injury has subsided, patients with less severe sprains can begin immediate rehabilitation. Patients with more severe sprains may need cast immobilization for a short period (1 to 2 weeks) and more rarely surgery. Generally, they receive the same rehabilitation as less severe injuries at a later time. The most important goal of the ankle rehabilitation process is to restore the proprioceptive function of the affected foot. This not only stabilizes the joint, it provides a protective function for the ankle to prevent further injury. The tilt board is used to regain proprioception after an ankle sprain. Ankle strength can be increased using exercises with heavy rubber bands. Taping or pneumatic ankle splints may give the athlete added support while training or competing. However, no athlete should be allowed to return to competition until she has demonstrated the ability to protect the ankle on the tilt board.

Common injuries in the foot include not only stress fractures, but also pathology of the first metatarsophalangeal joint (bunions). Women in general have a higher incidence of bunions than males owing in part to differences in shoes and heels. As a result, female athletes have more frequent problems with them than male athletes. Bunions are caused by inflammation and bursitis around the medial flare of the first metatarsal head. Metatarsus primus varus may predispose one to bunion formation. However, many women without this condition develop bunions.

Usually this condition can be managed with pads in the shoe or change in the type of shoes worn by the athlete. When degenerative changes (hallux rigidus) in the joint have occurred because of this condition, treatment is a little more difficult. Steroid injection and orthotics may be helpful in this situation. If the pain becomes unbearable, a bunionectomy may be performed. Surgery should be a last resort because of the possibility of changing the anatomic and biomechanical function of the foot.

Upper Body Injury

As noted earlier in this chapter, upper body strength in females is significantly lower than in males. Some researchers blame this lack of upper body strength on the injuries frequently seen in female athletes. The most common upper extremity injuries are impingement syndromes. Women who participate in swimming, throwing sports, and racquet sports are most susceptible to these injuries.

Shoulder impingement is a common condition seen in female athletes. No matter what the cause, weakened rotator cuff muscles (supraspinatus, infraspinatus, subscapularis, and teres minor) initiate a cycle of inflammation, pain, and swelling. In shoulder impingement the humeral head actually rides up in the glenoid and traumatizes the subacromial bursa. The pain of impingement can be reproduced by holding down the acromion, while elevating the arm in abduction or forward flexion. Impingement syndrome should be differentiated from recurrent subluxation of the shoulder, which is tested by externally rotating and abducting the arm. If the patient feels the shoulder is "popping out," then there is some instability present.

Treating impingement syndrome in the shoulder is a slow process. First, the athlete's training practices should be assessed. Is there a proper warm-up? Are the weight training exercises strengthening the rotator cuff muscles? Are the mechanics of the activity correct? Too much internal rotation of the shoulder facilitates impingement on the acromion. Alterations in activity may help alleviate some symptoms. Physical therapy and nonsteroidal anti-inflammatory drugs may also be beneficial. If these measures fail to eliminate the symptoms, steroid injections may be used with caution. Finally, surgical resection of the acromion, either open or arthroscopically, is used for patients with impingement symptoms that are affecting the activities of daily living or are preventing an athlete from competing at the level she desires.

SUMMARY

Even though differences in body composition and physiologic, anatomic, endocrine, and mechanical function exist between men and women, injuries in female athletes appear to be more sport specific than sex specific. Injuries in endurance athletes are not the same as those in power athletes. However, because of these differences, the incidence of certain injuries will always be different between the sexes. As female participation in athletics has increased, improvements in training techniques have actually lowered the frequency of injuries. The most important aspect of sports medicine is managing training principles to prevent and minimize athletic injuries. The injuries that do occur are caused by acute trauma or overuse syndromes. Thorough and accurate evaluation of these injuries is necessary to initiate successful treatment and safely return the athlete to a preinjury activity level.

REFERENCES

Barrow GW, Saha S. Menstrual irregularity and stress fractures in collegiate female distance runners. Am J Sports Med 1988;16(3):209.

Bodnar LM. Historical role of women in sports. Am J Sports Med 1980;8(1):54.

Cann CE, Martin MC, Genant HK, et al. Decreased spinal mineral content in amenorrheic women. JAMA 1984; 251(5):626.

Chang FE, Dodds WG, Sullivan M, et al. The acute effects of exercise on prolactin and growth hormone secretion: Comparison between sedentary women and women runners with normal and abnormal menstrual cycles. J Clin Endocrinol Metabol 1986;62(3):551.

Clarke DH. Sex differences in strength and fatigability. Res Q Exerc Sport 1986;57(2):144.

Dale E, Gerlach DH, Wilhite AL. Menstrual dysfunction in distance runners. Obstet Gynecol 1979;54(1):47.

Drinkwater BL, Nilson K, Chesnut CH, et al. Bone mineral content of amenorrheic and eumenorrheic athletes. N Engl J Med 1984;311(5):277.

Drinkwater BL, Nilson K, Ott S, et al. Bone mineral density after resumption of menses in amenorrheic athletes. JAMA 1986;256(3):380.

Hunter LY. Women's athletics: The orthopedic surgeon's viewpoint. Clin Sports Med 1984;3(4):809.

Hunter-Griffin LY. Orthopedic concerns. In: Shangold M, Mirkin G (eds). Women and Exercise, Physiology and Sports Medicine. Philadelphia: FA Davis Company, 1988, p 195.

Knapik JJ, Bauman CL, Junes B, et al. Preseason strength and flexibility imbalances associated with athletic injuries in female collegiate athletes. Am J Sports Med 1991;19(1):76.

Loucks AB, Horvath SM. Athletic amenorrhea: A review. Med Sci Sports Exerc 1985;17(1):57.

Lanese RR, Strauss RH, Leizman DJ, et al. Injury and disability in matched men's and women's intercollegiate sports. Am J Public Health 1990;80(12):1459.

Litt IF. Amenorrhea in the adolescent athlete: Exploration of a growing phenomenon. Postgrad Med 1986;80(5):245.

Monahan T. Treating athletic amenorrhea: A matter of instinct? Physician Sports Med 1987;15(7):184.

Myburgh KH, Hutchins J, Fataar AB, et al. Low bone density is an etiologic factor for stress fractures in athletes. Ann Intern Med 1990;113:754.

Nelson ME, Fisher EC, Catsos PD, et al. Diet and bone status in amenorrheic runners. Am J Clin Nutr 1986;43:910.

Nelson RC, Brooks CM, Pike NL. Biomechanical comparison of male and female distance runners. Ann NY Acad Sci 1977;301:793.

Protzman RR. Physiologic performance of women compared to men. Am J Sports Med 1979;7(3):191.

Protzman RR. Women athletes: Historical evolution of their participation. Am J Sports Med 1980;8(1):53.

Protzman RR. Stress fractures in men and women undergoing military training. J Bone Joint Surg 1977;59A(6):825.

Thomas JC. Women's sports and fitness programs at the US Air Force Academy. Physician Sports Med 1979;7(4):59.

Medical Care of Lesbian Patients

Jocelyn White

Lesbians are a diverse group of women with unique medical and psychosocial needs. Although 2 to 10% of women are lesbians, they often go unrecognized and may not be cared for adequately by their physicians. Unfortunately, physicians seldom receive specific training to care for these patients. This chapter provides physicians with the knowledge and skills necessary to identify the sexual orientation of patients, address lesbian and bisexual issues, screen appropriately for medical and psychosocial conditions, and educate patients in ways specific to their identity and behaviors.

SEXUAL ORIENTATION

The latest research suggests that sexual orientation—heterosexual, homosexual, and bisexual—is probably determined by a combination of biologic and environmental factors. The dictionary defines a lesbian as ''a female homosexual,'' meaning a woman who is sexually attracted to other women. Practically speaking, however, lesbianism is not only a sexual orientation but also an identity based on emotions and psychological responses, societal expectations, and the individual's own choices and identity formation. Therefore, some women call themselves lesbians but are not sexually active with women. Others are sexually active with women but do not identify themselves as lesbians.

Lesbians are a diverse group from all racial, economic, geographic, religious, cultural, and age populations. Amid this diversity, lesbians have created a culture of their own filled with music, art, literature, history, spiritual beliefs, ethics, and politics. Not all women have access to or feel themselves a part of such a community; in fact, many older women may feel less connected to this culture. These older women may be more reluctant

to reveal their identity even to peers because of experience with or fears of discrimination. In addition, many women believe that a common thread held by members of the community is a belief in feminist ideals. Many adolescent women forming their lesbian identity may not share these ideals and may feel less a part of a well-formed community. Nonetheless, a lesbian community is an important source of support to many women and can provide an alternative family or kin group to its members. Community resources may also be useful to health care providers looking for lesbian-sensitive referrals for social services, counseling, or peer support.

Sexual orientation is not only an important determinant of sexual behavior but also an influence on the structure of a woman's immediate family and her social support system. Therefore, specific lesbian health care needs include any medical condition in which family dynamics and social support play a role as well as those usually considered, such as sexually transmitted diseases and cancer screening.

THE DOCTOR-PATIENT INTERACTION

Many lesbians are reluctant to reveal their sexual orientation to physicians for fear of provoking a negative response. Some lesbians do not share this information even when asked. Negative experiences with health care professionals make lesbians more likely to avoid health care and routine screening. Physicians need to ensure that lesbians and bisexual women have access to sensitive, competent care. Many physicians, however, are not sure what language to use to elicit information respectfully from lesbian patients. Discomfort on the part of both patient and doctor means important information is often not shared.

Gathering information about the lesbian lifestyle and sexual practices is the first stumbling block encountered by health care providers. The most commonly used questions often lead to inaccurate or incomplete information. They set up barriers between the physician and the lesbian patient because they assume she is heterosexual: "What form of birth control do you use?"; "Are you married or single?"; and "When was the last time you had intercourse?" are common examples. All of these questions are difficult for lesbians.

Appropriate questions make no assumption about sexual orientation. Physicians may feel most comfortable beginning with questions related to the social history such as "Are you single, partnered, married, widowed, or divorced?"; "Whom do you include in your immediate family?"; "Are you in a relationship? With a man or a woman?" Physicians should ask questions like these of all women irrespective of age.

Relevant questions in the sexual history include "Have you been sexually active with men, women, or both?" and "Do you have a need for birth control?" For some women it may be important for physicians to explain that they need information on sexual practices to make an accurate diagnosis and to counsel patients on prevention or transmission of disease.

Physicians who demonstrate a nonjudgmental attitude will win the trust of lesbian patients. Physicians can also build rapport with lesbians by offering to include a partner in discussions and by ensuring that a lesbian's partner is treated as any other spouse. Partners should be included in discussions of next-of-kin policies and advance directives. Physicians may also demonstrate their acceptance by using office and hospital forms with words that do not assume a heterosexual family structure. Terms such as "living with a partner" or "living as a couple" in addition to the usual "spouse" can be helpful.

Once information gathering is completed and rapport is established, the physician faces the task of providing education for lesbian patients that is specific to their needs. This includes both verbal and written instructions. Instruction in preventing the transmission of sexually transmitted diseases including the human immunodeficiency virus (HIV) should be clear and specific to lesbian sexual practices. Explanations of a lesbian's risk for cervical cancer should be based on her sexual history. Counseling on topics such as parenting, domestic violence, and substance abuse should be specific to the lesbian's support system and family structure. Written materials that avoid the assump-

tion of heterosexual orientation are provided. Physicians should be able to refer patients to other providers and community resources that are sensitive to the needs of lesbians. Hotlines, bookstores, lesbian and gay youth groups, senior groups, 12-step programs, community centers, and religious organizations may also be of help.

In the initial visit with a patient, it is also important to discuss explicitly the documentation of sexual orientation in the chart. When a lesbian does not want her sexual orientation documented, physicians should use a coded entry and inform the patient that this is being done. Using a code will remind physicians of the patient's sexual orientation for medical purposes but will prevent inadvertent breaches of confidentiality through use of the chart.

SEXUALLY TRANSMITTED DISEASES

CASE. *A 26-year-old African American architect presents to your office for the first time with a vaginal discharge. Which tests should you perform and how will you counsel her?*

Lesbians are a diverse group in terms of sexual practices. They may be celibate or sexually active with women or men or both. Although 77% of lesbians have had a heterosexual partner (at some point), most women who identify as lesbian are either currently sexually active with women only or are celibate. It is important to remember that the specific sexual practices of an individual woman determine her risk for a particular condition. Physicians should base medical recommendations on the history of the individual patient.

Sexually transmitted diseases are less common in lesbians than in heterosexual women or gay men. Lesbian sexual practices include kissing, breast stimulation, manual and oral stimulation of the genitals and anus, friction of the clitoris against the partner's body, and penetration of the vagina and anus with fingers and devices. There are no gynecologic problems unique to lesbians and none that occurs more often in lesbians than in bisexual or heterosexual women. This may be due in part to the lack of penile vaginal intercourse among lesbians and the relative epidemiologic isolation of this population from men.

Based on uncontrolled clinical and survey data, lesbians appear to have a lower incidence of syphilis and gonorrhea than any other population except those who have never been sexually active at all. Therefore, routine screening for these diseases in lesbians does not appear to be cost-effective. Testing is appropriate only in the setting of other risk factors, particularly recent heterosexual exposure.

Other sexually transmitted diseases common among heterosexual women are uncommon or rare in the lesbian population. *Chlamydia* and herpes are rarely cultured from lesbians who have been sexually active exclusively with women. Herpes can be transmitted between women, but the prevalence in the lesbian population seems to be low. Pelvic inflammatory disease also appears to be rare among lesbians. Venereal warts caused by human papilloma virus are uncommon unless the patient has had heterosexual contact. However, because a woman with venereal warts may theoretically transmit them to her female partner, the partner should also be evaluated. Enteric infections due to hepatitis A, *Amoeba*, *Shigella*, and helminths have a low prevalence in lesbians, in contrast to their prevalence in the gay male population. Hepatitis B does not occur unless other risk factors are present.

Unlike sexually transmitted diseases, vaginitis and bacterial vaginosis occur with similar frequency among lesbians. Physicians should inquire about a vaginal discharge and evaluate partners of infected lesbians who have symptoms. Bisexual women report vaginal candidiasis more often than lesbians but not as often as heterosexual women. This may be related to heterosexual contact, but it is believed that transmission of *Candida* is possible between women. Partners of lesbians with vaginal candidiasis may be treated if they have symptoms or evaluated if they have been exposed and lack symptoms.

Trichomonas vaginalis has been found in women who are sexually active exclusively with women, women with no sexual contact at all, and lesbians with a bisexual woman as contact. *Trichomonas* may be transmitted by fomites such as damp towels and underwear or possibly by hand-genital contact. Based on this information, clinicians should include trichomonal infection in the differential diagnosis of vaginal discharge in lesbians. Sexual partners of lesbians diagnosed with trichomonal infection should also be treated.

MANAGEMENT. *In taking a history you learn that this patient has a long-standing relationship with another woman. They are monogamous, and the partner is asymptomatic. Your patient is very unlikely to have syphilis and gonorrhea. Chlamydial infection is also unlikely. You should examine her and test for bacterial vaginosis, yeast infection, and trichomonal infection. You diagnose bacterial vaginosis and treat accordingly. You counsel her to ask her partner again about symptoms. If she is symptomatic or if they choose to be cautious about transmissibility, her partner should seek care. Until any infection is resolved, they should* avoid transfer of vaginal fluid. Oral-genital contact is probably not contraindicated, but this is not yet clear.

HUMAN IMMUNODEFICIENCY VIRUS AND ACQUIRED IMMUNODEFICIENCY SYNDROME

CASE. *During a preventive medicine visit, a lesbian musician asks you if she should have an HIV test. What are her chances of being infected? Should you offer the test? How would you advise her about safer sex practices?*

Intravenous drug use accounts for 93% of AIDS cases in lesbians. Yet transmission of HIV between women as a result of sexual contact may have occurred in up to nine cases (SY Chu, personal communication, April 1993). Exposure to menstrual and traumatic bleeding was probably the source of transmission. However, because HIV is present in cervical tissue and vaginal secretions, it may be transmitted by infected women who are not bleeding. Nonetheless, the rate of this transmission between women is probably low.

Although HIV infection is rare in lesbians without risk factors, physicians should counsel lesbians to avoid contact with cervical and vaginal secretions, menstrual blood, and blood from vaginal and rectal trauma in partners who have not tested negative for the virus. Methods believed to protect against HIV transmission for oral-genital contact include latex squares, known as dental dams, and latex condoms or gloves or gloves cut open and laid flat; nonmicrowavable plastic wrap may also be an effective barrier. For vaginal penetration, latex gloves used on hands and condoms on sexual toys are appropriate.

Artificial insemination also places lesbians at risk for HIV infection. Sperm banks routinely test donors for HIV infection at the time of donation and 6 months later before releasing the sample for use. Rarely, due to delays in seroconversion of the donor, a lesbian may be exposed to HIV from a tested frozen sperm sample. Fresh semen, however, can be much riskier, especially if the HIV status of the donor is unknown or uncertain. Physicians should recommend screening of all sperm donors and HIV testing of the donor at least 6 months after the last possible exposure to HIV.

MANAGEMENT. *Your patient informs you that her new partner had been sexually active with a woman who was using intravenous drugs. You explain that lesbians who have had unprotected sexual contact with intravenous drug users are at risk for HIV. Because it is possible for HIV to be transmitted between women, your patient and her* *partner should both be serially tested. You counsel her to use safer sex practices with her new partner until all tests are negative. You explain about dental dams, plastic wrap, condoms on toys, and gloves on hands. You tell her to avoid passing vaginal secretions from genitals to other genital membranes, hands, or mouth. Finally, you refer her and her partner to a safer sex workshop you know of at your local women's bookstore.*

CANCER

CASE. *A 44-year-old European American computer programmer is in your office for her preventive medicine visit. She is a lesbian in a 15-year relationship with a woman. She has never been sexually active with a man. Her last Papanicolaou test and physical examination were 7 years ago. She has never had a mammogram. She asks if she really needs to have them now. What is your advice?*

Very little is known about the risks of cancer in lesbians, women sexually active with women, or single women. Most population-based studies of cancer in women have not distinguished between women sexually active with women and the rest of the population. Until more information is available, physicians should screen lesbians for cancer based on current screening guidelines for all women. However, based on individual reproductive histories, sexual practices, or other covariants of the lesbian lifestyle, certain cancers may be more or less common in lesbians.

Women who are sexually active exclusively with women have fewer abnormal Papanicolaou smear results than either bisexual or heterosexual women. This may be because women who are sexually active only with women have fewer risk factors for cervical cancer such as total number of male sexual partners, early age of first intercourse with a man, and infection with human papilloma virus. These data suggest that lesbians may have a lower incidence of cervical cancer than other women.

None of the current preventive health guidelines for cervical cancer screening addresses women who are celibate or women who are sexually active exclusively with women. Women who have a significant history of sexual contact with men or who have other known risk factors should be screened according to published guidelines. Women with no known risk factors for cervical cancer should be screened according to general guidelines (see Chapter 11).

There is no specific information on breast cancer, endometrial cancer, or ovarian cancer in les-

bians. Studies suggest that women who have never given birth, women who are older with their first birth, or women who have never breast-fed may be at increased risk of breast cancer. Single women are less likely to have heard of mammography and to have a yearly breast examination than married women. Many lesbians fall into these categories, and their physicians should adhere to current guidelines for breast examination and mammography (see Chapter 17).

Ovarian cancer may occur more frequently in women who have not used oral contraception or who have not given birth. Endometrial cancer is also more common in nulliparous women. Therefore, some lesbians may be at a higher risk for these cancers. However, there are no specific guidelines on screening for these cancers in the population at large or among lesbian patients.

Lesbians older than 45 report smoking and drinking alcohol more often than their heterosexual counterparts. There are no data on lung or head and neck cancers in lesbians. Physicians should emphasize the health risks of smoking and alcohol use in the lesbian population and strongly encourage smoking cessation.

MANAGEMENT. *In exploring why she has not had regular checkups, you discover that she had a difficult experience with a physician years ago who appeared uncomfortable with her lesbian lifestyle. She has avoided doctors since. Your rapport with her is good, and, after explaining current theories on cervical cancer and your belief that she is probably at a lower risk of cervical cancer than most heterosexual women, you recommend three yearly Papanicolaou tests and if all are normal every 3 years thereafter. You emphasize, however, a need for yearly physician breast examinations, mammography every 1 to 2 years, and monthly breast self-examination.*

PARENTING AND REPRODUCTIVE ISSUES

CASE. *A 34-year-old Mexican American teacher has come in to discuss parenting options with you. She and her partner are considering insemination and want your advice. What are their options? Where can they obtain insemination services? How can you help your patient and her partner during the pregnancy?*

Many lesbians are or want to become parents. They may have children from previous heterosexual relationships or by adoption, artificial insemination, or foster parenting. Although some members of society may oppose motherhood for lesbians owing to concerns about the sexual development and orientation of the children, no studies have demonstrated any differences between children raised by lesbians and those raised by heterosexuals. Some lesbians have concerns about how to address the issues of their lesbian lifestyle with their children. It appears that open communication with children about the lesbian lifestyle is an important factor in maintaining family function.

Lesbians often ask their physicians for advice on the best methods of conception. Most lesbians find artificial insemination, also called alternative insemination or alternative fertilization, the preferred method. Many women perform the insemination at home with the help of a partner or friends. Others ask their primary physician to perform insemination with samples from a known donor or samples from a sperm bank.

Some physicians feel uncomfortable performing insemination for lesbians either because of legal statutes, social pressures, or misconceptions about lesbians' ability to be mothers. Legal statutes on artificial insemination vary from state to state, but most address only married women and assume that a physician will perform the procedure. Often the law is not clear regarding the physician's responsibility or liability toward a lesbian who has been inseminated. It is ethically justifiable and medically reasonable for physicians to inseminate lesbians; however, physicians cannot be mandated to participate in a procedure that they personally believe to be immoral. A physician who feels unable to provide insemination services to a lesbian should refer the patient to another provider.

Lesbians may also ask their physicians to help ensure that the birthing team and the hospital or delivery staff will be accepting of a lesbian and her partner through the pregnancy and the delivery. Physicians can support the pregnant lesbian by demonstrating nonjudgmental attitudes, encouraging acceptance of lesbian motherhood at hospitals, birthing centers, and childbearing classes, and by including partners in the process of conception, prenatal care, and delivery.

MANAGEMENT. *You and your patient discuss fresh versus frozen semen and decide on frozen for its relative safety. In your small city it is well known that none of the clinics or specialists will provide insemination services to lesbians. Your patient is unwilling to lie to them about her relationship because she wants her partner involved in the process. You refer her to a sperm bank out of state that will express samples when needed with physician preapproval. You recommend a prepregnancy checkup and encourage her to bring her partner in to meet you. You also offer to help ensure that they are treated respectfully as* *a couple by the birthing team and ancillary personnel.*

PSYCHOSOCIAL AND PSYCHOLOGICAL ISSUES

CASE. *A 15-year-old high school student is brought in by her mother for complaints of fatigue. She appears anxious. You see her alone and she simply states she's "tired all the time." What psychosocial issues should you explore?*

The American Psychiatric Association removed homosexuality from its list of mental illnesses in 1973. Although homosexuality itself is not an illness, lesbians experience unique psychosocial stressors. These stressors often affect their physical and emotional well-being. Physicians are in a unique position to screen for these stressors in their lesbian patients and to help them find resources for coping more effectively with them. The psychosocial issues most relevant for primary care providers include homophobia, "coming out," alcohol use, suicide, lesbian battery, and hate crimes.

Society's negative attitude toward or fear of lesbians and gay men is known as homophobia. Although, overall, lesbians' self-esteem is similar to that of heterosexual women, some individuals internalize society's homophobia. These internalized negative thoughts and fears can create a stressful conflict in lesbians between what they believe their sexual orientation to be and how they express themselves to the outside world. As a result, many lesbians have not only the stresses of dealing with societal attitudes but the stress of an inner conflict as well.

A lesbian patient's support network may be different from that of heterosexual women. Many families have difficulty accepting a lesbian's sexual orientation. Lesbians surveyed most often report receiving support from partners, friends, and lesbian and gay community organizations. Because of potential isolation from other family members, the quality of the relationship with a partner can be particularly important to a lesbian's psychological well-being. As a result, discord in this relationship can be even more stressful than that in a typical heterosexual couple. Assessment of a lesbian's support network should be a routine part of the social history.

The process of discovering one's sexual orientation and revealing it to others is known as "coming out" and may begin at any age. Indeed, it may be a lifelong process. Coming out involves a shift in core identity that takes place in four stages: (1) awareness of homosexual feelings, (2) testing and exploration, (3) identity acceptance, and (4) identity integration and disclosure to others. Prevailing social and family attitudes strongly influence the experience of coming out and can cause significant emotional distress in a lesbian. Societal and internalized homophobia cause the lesbian to perform a sophisticated and fatiguing ''cost-benefit'' analysis for every situation in which she considers coming out. When the costs of coming out are perpetually high, a lesbian may become socially isolated or attempt to deny her sexual orientation.

Lesbian adolescents are particularly vulnerable during this process, and any distress incurred in coming out can confound other developmental tasks. Parental, especially maternal, acceptance during the coming out process may be the primary determinant of the development of healthy self-esteem in adolescent lesbians. Sexual orientation confusion may appear to the physician to be depression, diminished school performance, alcohol and substance use, acting out, and suicidal ideation. In fact, lesbian and gay youth are two to three times more likely to attempt suicide than other adolescents and may account for 30% of completed youth suicides. For these reasons, it is extremely important for the primary care provider to identify the sexual orientation of adolescents, to screen for these signs of sexual orientation confusion, and to consider this confusion in the differential diagnosis of depression and substance abuse.

As part of a comprehensive clinical evaluation, primary care providers should screen all women, including their lesbian patients, for alcohol abuse, depression, and violence. Older studies report that alcohol use may be higher among lesbians than among heterosexual women, but rigorous epidemiologic studies are still lacking. In fact, some research suggests that lesbians are more sensitive to the issues of alcohol abuse than the heterosexual population. Until appropriate data are available, we have no reason to believe that alcoholism is more common in lesbians than in heterosexual women. Physicians should screen all women for alcohol use.

Domestic violence is an issue in lesbian relationships as well as in heterosexual ones. One small study reported that more than one third of lesbians have experienced battery by a partner and a majority of these involved alcohol or drug use. The primary care provider should screen all women, including lesbians, for domestic violence. Once violence has been identified in a relationship, the provider should have on hand resources available to the patient. Many shelters and agencies do not deal well with lesbian battery, and lesbians report having difficulty in many battered women's shelters. Care should be taken to refer lesbian patients to shelters that are skilled in dealing with the needs of these women.

According to the U.S. Department of Justice, lesbians and gay men may be the most victimized group in the nation. Hate crimes, or bias crimes, against lesbians including verbal abuse, threats of violence, property damage, physical violence, and murder are increasing each year. In addition, lesbians at universities report being victims of sexual assault twice as often as heterosexual women. Perpetrators of hate crimes often include family members and community authorities. Many lesbian and gay teenagers may leave home because of abuse related to their sexual orientation. Primary care providers should consider hate crime violence in the differential diagnosis of a lesbian who presents with symptoms of depression or anxiety.

MANAGEMENT. *A history and physical examination reveal no obvious causes for this girl's fatigue. You plan to do basic testing, but you also explore psychosocial issues. You ask about school performance, friends, mood, suicidal thoughts, substance use, sexual activity and sexual orientation, physical and sexual abuse, and date rape. You discover that she is dating boys and is sexually active with them. She has been disturbed, however, by an attraction to a girlfriend. They have kissed and ''messed around'' once. She hasn't told anyone else but you. She is afraid of her parents' reaction. You reassure her that there is nothing wrong with her. You encourage her to talk with her parents and the school counselor. You offer to talk to her parents as well if she wishes. You recommend books to read. You explain that her worry may be the cause of her fatigue but that you will proceed with the tests. Finally, you schedule a follow-up appointment and make it clear that you will continue to support her.*

SUMMARY

Many primary care providers are presently caring for lesbian patients without recognizing their sexual orientation or their unique medical and psychosocial needs. The first step in providing sensitive competent care for all women is the routine use of appropriate questions regarding primary relationships. Physicians who use nonjudgmental language in taking a history and in educating patients allow lesbians to express the medical needs and psychosocial issues that affect their health and well-being. Improvement in communication skills and knowledge about lesbian health care issues allow practitioners to provide optimal care for their patients. Clearly, much more research on lesbian health issues is needed to provide appropriate guidelines for clinicians.

REFERENCES

1. White J, Levinson W. Primary care of lesbian patients. J Gen Intern Med 1993; 8:41.
2. Stevens PE. Lesbian health care research: A review of the literature from 1970 to 1990. Health Care Women Int 1992; 13:91.
3. Diamond M. Homosexuality and bisexuality in different populations. Arch Sex Behav 1993; 22(4):291.
4. Byne W, Parsons B. Human sexual orientation: The biologic theories reappraised. Arch Gen Psychiatry 1993; 50:228.
5. Bradford J, Ryan C. The National Lesbian Health Care Survey: Final report. National Lesbian and Gay Health Foundation, 1992.
6. The Michigan Lesbian Health Survey. Michigan Organization for Human Rights (Special Report) August 1991.
7. Warshafsky L. Lesbian Health Needs Assessment: Prepared for the Los Angeles Gay and Lesbian Community Services Center, April 1992.
8. Trippet SE, Bain J. Physical health problems and concerns of lesbians. Women Health 1993; 20(2):59.
9. Chu SY, Hammett TA, Buehler JW. Update: Epidemiology of reported cases of AIDS in women who report sex only with other women, United States, 1980–1991. AIDS 1992; 6(5):518.
10. Patterson CJ. Children of lesbian and gay parents. Child Dev 1992; 63:1025.
11. Smith S, McClaugherty LO. Adolescent homosexuality: A primary care perspective. Med Society 1993; 48(1):33.
12. Alcohol, Drug Abuse, and Mental Health Administration. Report of the Secretary's Task Force on Youth Suicide. Volume 3: Prevention and Interventions in Youth Suicide. DHHS Pub. No. (ADM) 89-1623. Washington, DC: US Government Printing Office, 1989.
13. Quam JK, Whitford G. Adaptation and age-related expectations of older gay and lesbian adults. Gerontologist 1992; 32(3):367.

Health Care for Homeless Women

Roseanna H. Means

OVERVIEW

Almost one third of all homeless adults are women. Homelessness produces profound personal loss and destruction of social context. Homeless women live at risk for serious infections, chronic diseases, and physical harm. They constitute a growing portion of individuals infected with the human immunodeficiency virus (HIV) and victims of physical battery. They live as outsiders in our society, often with no access to primary care. These are all conditions that bring them into our hospitals and emergency departments.

At a time when women's health issues are being addressed in a scientific and systematic way, it is important that the perspective of homeless women not be overlooked. Yet scientific studies on the health problems of the homeless are poorly represented in the traditional medical literature. Much of what is written is based on small selected samples. The most difficult patients to reach are not included because they are physically, emotionally, or culturally isolated.

Nonetheless, what emerges from the literature and working experience is the following:

- The causes of homelessness are numerous.
- The number of homeless persons in the United States is rising every year, and women constitute the fastest growing portion.
- The stereotyped images of homeless women as bag ladies, prostitutes, and drug addicts are often inaccurate and only serve to distance, and depersonalize these individuals.
- Men and women become homeless in different ways and have different concerns.
- There are different kinds of shelters for women, with varying degrees of safety.
- Homeless mothers of minor children live in family shelters and take some or all of their children with them; or they give up custody of

their children and live alone in single adult shelters or on the streets.
- A background history of childhood or adult emotional, sexual, or physical abuse is common to many homeless women and has serious ramifications for how they cope, survive, trust, and form relationships.

Homeless persons are being identified in clinics and emergency departments more frequently. However, physicians who are not used to caring for homeless patients often feel overwhelmed by the many daunting medical, social, emotional, and mental health challenges that accompany these patients. Providers may want to help but lack the training or tools to do so. Taking care of homeless persons is time consuming and difficult. The physician must work with a multidisciplinary team of professionals and paraprofessionals without always being in control and must be more of a "facilitator" than a "gatekeeper." The outcomes are improved service to an underserved population, prevention of serious disease, and a decrease in acute care emergency department costs and inpatient hospital stays.

The purpose of this chapter is to define the problems that are unique to homeless women and to offer strategies to overcome those problems.

DEFINITION OF HOMELESS

Being homeless is defined as having no permanent residence. This can mean living on the streets or in a shelter or being "precariously housed," that is, living below the poverty level, doubled up temporarily with friends or relatives, or living in single-room-occupancy hotels. Often the resources (physical, social, or psychological) to get housing and community support are lacking. Being homeless does not necessarily mean being unemployed.

DEMOGRAPHICS

Demographics on the homeless are only estimates. Discrepancies in the numbers are due to variations in the definitions of homelessness, difficulties in studying a transient population, methodologies of the populations studied, and exclusionary criteria. Women are counted least consistently. For instance, women living in battered women's shelters are not always counted among the homeless. Many adult women choose to avoid the shelters out of fear for their safety; they will be omitted if a study is counting only shelter clients. Patients who distrust the interviewers may also be excluded.

Several million persons are counted as homeless by the National Coalition for the Homeless, of which 45% are ''unaccompanied'' men, 14% are ''unaccompanied'' women, and the remainder are families that are mostly headed by single mothers. ''Unaccompanied'' in the literature refers to adults who are alone, not living with a mate or children. It is estimated that 100,000 children are homeless on any given night. Fifty percent of homeless children are under the age of 5 years.[1]

A separate report, ''The Health Care for the Homeless Program Report to the Congress for Calendar year 1992,'' documented 400,468 clients served by their clinic system. Of these, 25% were adult women and 51% were adult men. The women were not identified as alone or as accompanied by children. The rest of this population was younger than 20 years. By race, 42% of the entire population were African American, 34% white, 15% Hispanic, 2% Native American, and 2% Asian or Pacific Islander. Of the women served, 23% were African American, 24% white, and 23% Hispanic.

ETIOLOGY: RISK FACTORS AND GENDER DIFFERENCES

Women have borne the brunt of events that have adversely affected the poor: rising numbers of poor Americans, high levels of unemployment, and lack of affordable housing, paralleled with a rise in existing rental costs, lack of federally funded daycare, and reductions in federal and state housing and assistance programs.[1-3] The number of families headed by single women because of divorce, teenage pregnancies, and cultural lifestyles has increased considerably. In 1988, one in five families with dependent children was headed by a single parent.[4] Many of these working women are in low-paying service jobs that offer few or no benefits. At the same time, the amount of benefits

offered by Aid to Families of Dependent Children has been decreased so that families living at the economic margins have been forced to pay more than 50% of their income for rent, even though the government standard is for less than 30% of household income to be spent on rent.[3] Women whose husbands have left them have few legal guarantees for child support payments. Deinstitutionalization of the chronically mentally ill[5] followed by inadequate follow-through by government and community agencies forced thousands of individuals with inadequate coping skills into the streets.

The role of domestic violence as a single cause of homelessness is unclear. Estimates vary in the literature but range from 40 to 70% of homeless women who report being battered.[6, 7] Battered women who leave their homes are not perceived by statisticians as permanently homeless. Further complicating the estimates, all battered women do not go to battered women's shelters. Some are in hiding with friends or in family shelters. They may not identify themselves as battered to protect their anonymity. Many battered women's shelters set limits on the length of stay. If the woman does not have a support system in place, she and her children may be forced to live in the street or in a family shelter or return to the batterer. Thus, battered women can be a transient population. Homeless advocates consider battered women to be ''precariously housed.''

Risk Factors

Risk factors identified as strongly associated with adult homelessness are profound childhood traumas: physical or sexual abuse,[8, 9] foster care placement,[8-10] and impaired parenting caused by substance abuse or mental illness.[8]

Any of these disruptions occurring individually or collectively at vulnerable periods in a child's development can cause psychopathology, including low self-esteem, major depression, poor ability to trust, poor coping skills, poor relationship skills, poor impulse control, a sense of hopelessness, anxiety and panic disorders, personality disorders, trouble with authority figures, or poor parenting skills. If homelessness occurs, the person is more vulnerable to alcohol or substance abuse, which only exacerbate the problems. Padgett and Struening found that the majority of homeless women alcoholics reported a prior history of having been physically or sexually assaulted.[11]

Gender Differences

Alcoholism is more prevalent among homeless men than women, 45% versus 15%, respectively.[12]

More men than women have criminal records and cite physical injury or illness or job loss as precipitating their homelessness. "Job loss" may mask alcohol or drug abuse. Homeless women veterans, although small in number, are younger than male veterans, are less likely to be employed, are homeless for a shorter period of time, are less likely to have a dual diagnosis (coexisting substance abuse and mental illness), but are more likely to carry a major psychiatric diagnosis.[13] Men who are alone tend to be homeless longer than women with families, and the longer single women are homeless, the greater the risk of alcoholism, mental illness, or both.[14]

More homeless women than homeless men have been married.[15] Women report more instances of physical and sexual abuse. Women more often cite family conflict or extreme poverty as reasons for becoming homeless. Fewer women are employed before becoming homeless, or if they are employed, they are in very low paying jobs and usually for only a short time. The day labor pool has a higher preponderance of jobs for men. More women than men stay connected to their children.[16] Single male parents are rare. Women who have dependent children but are unable to care for them are forced to forfeit custody of their children to the state. Sometimes the children are placed within the extended family; otherwise they are placed in foster care. Homeless men who have had children and left them or have been separated from them tend to lose track of their children more frequently than women. Maurin and colleagues commented that homeless women who had given up their children were more likely to voice the expectation that they would regain their children.[17] Mothers who have given up custody of their children often remain in contact with them and voice more psychological distress over the loss and separation than do the fathers.

Studies comparing causes and risk factors in different subpopulations of homeless women are limited. Women who keep their dependent children with them stay at a family shelter or state-subsidized motel for homeless families. In a small study comparing unaccompanied homeless adult women with single homeless mothers with children in St. Louis in 1989, the single homeless mothers were younger, nonwhite, less likely to abuse alcohol, and less likely to have had an inpatient admission for psychiatric reasons.[14]

SHELTERS FOR WOMEN

Shelter space for women has historically been an afterthought. Although fewer in number, there have always been homeless women. In the 1970s, Kip Tiernan, a lay minister in Boston, noticed women dressing up as men to gain admission to the then all-male Pine Street Inn, the largest shelter. She had been told there were no homeless women in Boston. Tiernan founded Rosie's Place, the first emergency shelter for women in the United States.[18] Shelter choices now include churches, single adult shelters, battered women's shelters, family shelters, or motels when the family shelters are full. Historically, the "homeless" were skid row men. Now with more homeless families, there are more family shelters and overall fewer beds for women who are alone. Women who are pregnant or accompanied by their children go to the family shelters, which are smaller and somewhat safer than the large single adult shelters, some of which are converted armories. Women in family shelters in general are homeless for shorter periods of time than women who are alone (months vs. years). Many homeless women who are forced to raise their children in family shelters ultimately move on to transitional or permanent housing. Women who have poor parenting skills because of a family history of the same or because of the negative influence of drugs, mental illness, or poor physical health run the risk of losing their children to state custody and ending up on the streets alone.

Except for the family shelters, shelters must be vacated each morning, so the homeless spend the majority of their time on their feet. To get back into the shelters and to avail oneself of the services often requires lining up by a certain hour. Homeless persons who miss the line for the main meal or a bed for the night have no recourse. Physicians, nurses, or social workers can help by calling the shelters and explaining the situation. Family shelters are often in unfamiliar areas, so that the families are cut off from friends, neighborhoods, access to medical care, and their children's schools. Families are frequently quite transient and are sometimes moved from one shelter to another or from a motel to subsidized housing and then back into a family shelter. Transportation for prenatal care, immunizations, or follow-up appointments is time-consuming and expensive. Usually no child care is available. Homeless persons who are put on medications generally carry them on their person. Some clinics in the shelters will keep the medications and dispense them, but patients must be able to get to the clinic for the medications. Many homeless persons lack a watch or a calendar to comply with appointments and medication schedules. Complicated medication regimens have a low compliance rate. Access to necessities such as water with which to take medications can also be problematic.

COMMON MEDICAL PROBLEMS EXACERBATED BY BEING HOMELESS

Medical problems of homeless women include acute and chronic ones that are exacerbated by being homeless and those that are more directly caused by being homeless. Conditions of homelessness that contribute to illness are exposure to the elements, poor hygiene, inadequate nutrition, overcrowding in shelters, prolonged standing and walking, and a high prevalence of mental illness, alcoholism, drug abuse, and physical and sexual trauma.[19–22]

Homeless persons are chronically poorly nourished. Single adults who use the shelters and soup kitchens rely on one or two meals a day. Homeless adults who live solely in the streets scrounge in the trash for food and clothing. Some family shelters have kitchen facilities, but food choices are poor and limited, and there is little refrigeration or storage space. Even in the "best" shelter systems, serious vitamin deficiencies have been documented.[23, 24]

Common medical problems seen with more frequency in the homeless are sexually transmitted diseases (STDs) including HIV,[25] chronic diseases,[21] gastrointestinal disorders, urinary tract infections, trauma, peripheral vascular disease, injections, tuberculosis, skin disorders, and dental disease.[26] Complications of substance abuse, such as peripheral neuropathy and lack of attention to personal hygiene, play an important part in affecting the pathology of the other disorders. Women frequently have unattended gynecologic problems and receive inadequate prenatal care.[27] Chronic illnesses are ignored until an emergency intervenes. Preventive health is overlooked in favor of more acute needs.[28]

Sexually Transmitted Diseases

Sexually transmitted diseases are often neglected in the homeless, particularly if they are asymptomatic.[29] Many women are exposed to STDs through their sexual partners and rape. Many rapes are unreported. Women who have been sexually assaulted are not always willing to have gynecologic examinations performed, particularly by male physicians. Nevertheless, every effort must be made to examine and culture homeless women for *Chlamydia*, gonorrhea,

Trichomonas, yeast, and bacterial pathogens. Papanicolaou smears must be taken whenever possible because of the association of abnormal results on Papanicolaou smears with STDs. Blood tests for syphilis are encouraged. All women with STDs must be counseled and HIV testing is recommended.

Birth control counseling is important when discussing STDs. Condoms are the usual method of contraception in this population because they are given out free at the shelters. Nevertheless, the pregnancy rate is high among homeless women. Poor access to prenatal care, malnutrition, and smoking contribute to poor birth outcomes for homeless women.[27] Concomitant drug or alcohol abuse further compromises the mother and the unborn child.[30] Cocaine and heroin abuse during pregnancy are associated with earlier gestational age at delivery, lower birth weights, stillbirths, and neurologically impaired newborns.[31, 32] Even though the majority of homeless pregnant women do not abuse drugs, all homeless pregnant women need access to early intervention. Prenatal counseling, including prenatal vitamins, should be initiated along with referral for early obstetric evaluation and management (see Chapter 30). Some pregnant addicts will not go to prenatal clinics because they are afraid that their babies will be taken from them at birth. Positive results on urine screens in the third trimester are reportable to the state. However, they are not reportable in the first trimester, so that information acquired at this time can be used to motivate the patient to seek treatment early on for substance abuse.[27]

All homeless women should be counseled about HIV status. The prevalence of HIV seropositivity in homeless women is unknown. O'Connell and Lebow retrospectively reviewed clinical records of Boston Health Care for the Homeless from July 1985 through March 1990. Out of 40 homeless individuals with acquired immunodeficiency syndrome (AIDS), 18% were women.[33] Routine testing of asymptomatic individuals remains a controversial issue, particularly if the patient is unlikely to change her lifestyle and habits, and the patient's access to the full complement of medical, social, addiction, and psychological counseling services is limited. Patients who are HIV positive, however, qualify for free medications through government programs and in some cities get priority housing. Despite the obstacles, a multidisciplinary team approach can successfully manage and support motivated homeless AIDS patients.[25] Some patients when told they have AIDS are motivated to stay healthy and resolve some long-standing personal issues, but others decompensate. This is true for both the homeless and the nonhomeless. Education about AIDS and the risks of AIDS through sexual transmission, blood contact, and needle sharing should be done at every opportunity.

Chronic Illnesses

Chronic illnesses present a special problem because interventional medical care usually comes when the illness reaches a crisis. Common chronic illnesses that are seen frequently in the homeless are chronic obstructive pulmonary disease, hypertension, congestive heart failure, arthritis, coronary heart disease, diabetes, alcoholic liver disease, cancer, and seizure disorders.[21] All homeless patients with chronic conditions are candidates for the annual flu vaccine and at least one pneumococcal vaccine.[28] Medication regimens must be kept simple. Diabetics may not have access to refrigeration for insulin, and insulin syringes are often stolen because of their high street value. Food sources are not predictable. Health care sources are not readily available for extremes of hypo- or hyperglycemia. Consequently, diabetics do better when kept under moderately good control on oral agents or at most a simple once or twice a day dosing schedule of long-acting insulin.

Chronic illnesses are difficult to treat in elderly homeless women.[34] Although few in number, there are elderly homeless women. Some of these women are mentally ill patients who were deinstitutionalized in the last 20 years; others are women who lived normal lives until the death of a spouse or other events of economic difficulty. Some women, although chronologically younger, are impaired by virtue of their health and functional disabilities.[35] Mental illness and profound social isolation in this population affect their ability to seek or accept help. Despite multiple medical problems, these patients often seek help only when a medical crisis intervenes such as congestive heart failure, myocardial infarction, or pneumonia. At that point, intensive efforts must be made to provide multidisciplinary support and explore housing options in addition to treating the medical illnesses.

Homeless patients with cancer present a special challenge, particularly if they have other psychological or substance abuse issues that impair their insight and judgment. In the most seriously impaired, legal and competency issues must be addressed, but for patients with personality disorders, the physician must utilize patience and interpersonal skills.

Case 1

A 47-year-old woman with a palpable breast mass and a suspicious result on mammography was referred for surgery. Excision was proposed, and the patient agreed. Her surgery was scheduled, but she missed appropriate preoperative tests and failed to appear on the day of admission. Over the next 4 months, her surgery was scheduled and cancelled on two further occasions. Admitting office staff, the surgeon, nurses, and secretaries were on the verge of refusing to help the patient. The homeless team doctor met with the patient many times to alleviate the patient's fears and anxieties and to educate the patient that her behavior was interfering with her health. The patient ultimately went through with the surgery, and the cancer was completely excised. Two years later, the patient remains disease free and housed. Her relationship with the homeless team doctor is the longest one she has ever had with a doctor.

Substance Abuse

Alcohol and drug abuse are enormous problems in the homeless population. Many patients deny substance abuse even in the face of overt inebriation or documented positive results on urine screens. Actual numbers on the prevalence of substance abusers vary. In a small sample of 203 homeless men and women in Baltimore in 1989, Breakey and associates found that 69% of the men and 38% of the women were identified as probable alcoholics by the Michigan Alcoholism Screening Test.[19] More detailed examinations on these same persons by psychiatrists identified alcohol dependence syndrome in 56% of the men and 17% of the women. Other surveys have identified at least 50% of the entire homeless population as active alcohol or drug users.[12, 36]

Hard data on the existence of alcohol and drug use among subpopulations of women are lacking. Claims are made that as much as a 30 to 40% alcohol and drug abuse rate exists among parents in homeless families,[37] but alcoholism is also described as occurring just as frequently (38%) among populations of single unaccompanied women.[13, 19]

The medical complications of alcohol and drug abuse are legion.[30, 38–40] Women who are alcoholics suffer a higher rate of alcoholic liver disease than men due to decreased gastric alcohol dehydrogenase activity and first-pass metabolism.[41] Homeless women who are abusing drugs or alcohol or both require hospitalization repeatedly. Because of the high morbidity and mortality associated with these conditions, detoxification and treatment should be offered at every opportunity. Signs of withdrawal should be attended to in every admission, regardless of the admitting diagnosis.

Patients with personality disorders can be disruptive to nursing and house staff and often manipulate and split the health care team. The use of a written contract of limits and expectations for both parties to agree on and sign is often valuable. It is vital that the health care team follow through on any promises made, because trust and control are important issues for the psychologically impaired. Despite the high recidivism rate in this population, it is important to maintain a professional and nonjudgmental approach. Many of these patients will leave care against medical advice. It is important to remain objective and to assure the patient that she is still welcome to return. This aids in continuity of care and ultimately decreases the cost of care if she does not seek repetitive care at another institution.

Homeless mothers with minor children who require drug or alcohol detoxification or an inpatient psychiatric admission require care of their children for that period of time. If no one is available to provide care, the children go into temporary custody with the state. This decision for the mother is extremely difficult and requires support and counseling.

Preventive Care

Few homeless women have the time, money, or resources for preventive health care. Providers who see homeless women for acute illness are urged to take the time for preventive care. As mentioned previously, women need Papanicolaou smears and gynecologic examinations whenever possible. Breast examinations and mammography, when indicated, are important, particularly because of the suggestion in the literature that alcohol abuse may be linked to breast cancer.[42, 43] Immunizations against tetanus and pneumococcal species can be given at any time of year. Flu vaccines should be given yearly. Intravenous drug users and contacts should be screened for hepatitis B and offered the vaccination series. Public health nurses can often obtain the medications and dispense them in the shelter. Multivitamins are often available at no cost in the shelters, but patients are not always aware of it.

MEDICAL PROBLEMS CAUSED BY BEING HOMELESS

Medical problems that are more directly caused by being homeless include the infectious complications of overcrowding, particularly tuberculosis,

skin diseases and infestations, other respiratory illnesses, vascular dysfunction, diarrhea, measles, rubella, and herpes zoster.[29] Outbreaks of infectious disease in shelters have been documented.[44–47] During the infectious stage of these illnesses, the patients require hospitalization as a public health mandate, and the shelter needs to be notified.

Every homeless patient needs tuberculosis screening. If the patient does not remember if she was positive in the past, the state department of public health may have a record if she has ever been positive. Because the homeless represent a high-risk population, a response of 5 mm or more of induration is considered positive. High-risk patients who require tuberculosis prophylaxis (HIV-positive, HIV-positive who are anergic, active tuberculosis contacts, converters, patients with a history of inadequately treated tuberculosis, patients with an abnormal result on chest radiography, or those with any risk factor for reactivation such as diabetes, malnutrition, uremia, cancer, gastrectomy, or silicosis) should be reported to the department of public health and enrolled in a preventive therapy program. If a patient states that she was "already treated" at another time and place, it is very important that documentation of the regimen and length of time it was given be obtained. Because of the epidemic of tuberculosis in the United States in parallel with the HIV epidemic, aggressive control of tuberculosis is mandated by departments of public health. Many public health departments have implemented programs of directly observed therapy according to the Centers for Disease Control and Prevention guidelines to reduce the number of treatment failures.[44] Multiply drug-resistant tuberculosis is increasingly being seen, particularly in the HIV-positive population, among intravenous drug abusers, and in those who did not complete tuberculosis treatment regimens in the past.[48, 49] Patients in methadone programs who are treated with rifampin require an increase in their methadone dose because of accelerated metabolism. Patients with active tuberculosis who refuse hospitalization can legally be held involuntarily.

Other respiratory illnesses, particularly upper respiratory infections, bronchitis, asthma, pneumonia, and chronic obstructive pulmonary disease, are common and clearly influenced by the large number of smokers in this population. Respiratory deaths accounted for 36 (20%) of 184 deaths in Boston's homeless population between 1986 and 1988.[50] Cultures are not always possible or useful if the patient cannot or will not follow up. Simple regimens of empiric antibiotics are frequently successful. Metered-dose inhalers have a higher compliance rate than oral bronchodilators.

Skin conditions seen frequently include cellulitis, infestations (scabies and lice), frostbite, gangrene, impetigo, abscesses from intravenous drug use, eczema and fungal dermatoses, wounds, and abrasions.[51] Smoking cocaine can singe eyebrows and eyelashes. Needle marks, skin popping scars, tattoos in odd places to cover scars, phlebitis, and vasculitis can be seen in intravenous drug users. Atypical bruises, marks, and burns can be clues to physical abuse.[52]

Immunologic compromise allows scabies to advance to a variant called crusted (Norwegian) scabies, which is highly contagious and is characterized by generalized hyperkeratotic scaly plaques or papules. This form of scabies can be the first sign of HIV infection.[53] Treatment of scabies and lice requires access to a shower. One percent lindane cream (Kwell), a standard treatment, carries a risk of neurotoxicity, especially if used improperly. Often these treatments are also used on children. Five percent permethrin cream (Nix) is a good scabicide and has less toxicity.[54] Both agents are considered unsafe for pregnant women.

Lower extremity vascular disease is very common, owing to chronic dependence, and often leads to venous stasis and ulcers.[55] Other common lower extremity disorders are immersion foot, tinea pedis, edema and other manifestations of peripheral vascular disease, corns, calluses, and blisters. The many foot and lower extremity problems in the homeless come from prolonged standing and walking, exposure, and poor footwear exacerbated by the influences of drug or alcohol abuse or mental illness, or a combination of these.[56, 57] Sometimes creative solutions must be devised to treat cellulitis and leg ulcers in this population.

Case 2

A 53-year-old massively obese woman with chronic venous insufficiency, stasis dermatitis, and edema developed bilateral cellulitis and multiple draining leg ulcers. Despite the entreaties of multiple caregivers in the shelter clinics, she adamantly refused to go to the emergency department for treatment. She was terrified of hospitals and doctors and of losing the little control she had in her life. Careful explanations of the dire consequences of not attending to these problems did not persuade her. Finally, she consented to a regimen of daily dressing changes and parenteral shots of antibiotics carefully orchestrated between two shelter clinics and a drop-in center. After 3 weeks, the ulcers began to heal, and she was started on an oral antibiotic regimen. At the end of 6 weeks her legs had healed.

Medical problems from exposure include the skin conditions mentioned earlier, hypo- and hyperthermia, and frostbite.[58] The San Francisco Department of Public Health documented that 35% of all deaths of homeless persons between 1985 and 1990 occurred outdoors.[59] In 78% of the deaths, drugs or alcohol were detected. Many orthopedic problems ensue from exposure, overuse, and trauma, principally arthritis, arthralgias, fractures, sprains, and osteomyelitis.

Trauma is highly prevalent in this population and is the leading cause of emergency department visits by the homeless.[20] Homeless men have more trauma-related diagnoses than women, but homeless women are also subject to assault, rape, fracture, head injury, gunshot wounds, lacerations, and burns. Women brought into the emergency department for trauma should be asked carefully about where they will go to recuperate. Unless asked, many women do not volunteer that they are homeless. Complications of healing can occur if the patient is discharged to the street. Social Service should be contacted to facilitate finding a bed for the night.

MENTAL HEALTH PROBLEMS OF HOMELESS WOMEN

Often it is impossible to determine if homelessness preceded or postdated any mental illness, substance abuse, physical problems, or emotional or sexual abuse. Many of the women have or had parents or loved ones who hurt them and abandoned them or partners who abused them. Many had children whom they are struggling to raise or were forced to give up. Some are struggling with a major psychiatric diagnosis. Some have developed difficult personality disorders or have turned to drugs or alcohol.

The many psychodynamic paths the patient has traveled before she presents for medical attention are not going to be fixed by a pill, traditional psychotherapy, or therapeutic strategies that separate the overlapping needs and concerns of this population. Physicians who wish to care for homeless persons must integrate the disciplines of medicine, psychiatry, nursing, social work, and outreach. Outreach means professionals who go where the homeless are and treat them on their own turf. That turf can be in a shelter, standing in a food line, on the street, or in a doorway. The outreach worker links the traditional with the nontraditional delivery of care.

Many patients report distrust and disillusionment with the mental health system. This is due in part to the fact that few training programs in psychiatry or even addiction have any exposure to homeless clinics or shelters. Patients often ask that their primary care physician write for their medications or counsel them. Doctors who work with the homeless are then faced with the dilemma of knowing about the realities of the life of their patient but having inadequate formal training in psychiatry. It helps the patient in the long run to broaden her base of support among several caregivers, but until the patient finds a suitable mental health provider, the consistent support of the primary provider can be invaluable.

Case 3

A 42-year-old woman came to the homeless clinic with multiple somatic symptoms. She had diffuse pains in her head and throughout her body. She had marked memory losses for events of her life and suffered from nightmares and anxiety. She did not abuse alcohol or drugs. A complete neurologic evaluation was negative. She met with the physician weekly for several weeks, which revealed more background information. She had been born poor. As a child she had been raped by her father. She had her first of 10 babies, only five of whom had lived, when she was 16. Her husband and one of her sons raped and beat her. She began to hear voices and became increasingly depressed, attempting suicide several times. She was hospitalized in a psychiatric facility twice but was never able to follow through with the outpatient medication regimen. She found herself in strange cities she did not recall traveling to. In Boston she went to a shelter where she was referred to the homeless clinic. Over three or four visits in which she was allowed the chance to talk, she began to relax and be more comfortable. She agreed to be seen by a psychiatrist and entered into a therapeutic relationship. The physician and psychiatrist kept in close contact during the next year while the patient worked through the traumas she had suffered and accepted psychopharmacologic intervention. Two years later, the patient was housed and stable on medications.

PREVALENCE OF MENTAL ILLNESS

The prevalence of mental illness among the homeless is unknown. Estimates vary widely, but the majority hover around 30%.[60] By gender, prevalence rates for men range between 20 and 40% and for women between 50 and 60%. These numbers are very hard to interpret. The problems are inadequate sampling and varying criteria and definitions of what constitutes mental illness. Some studies only look at axis I disorders such as major depression and schizophrenia, whereas others include personality disorders and substance abuse. Another method used to estimate prevalence is measurement of documented inpatient psychiatric hospitalization, but that often excludes patients with personality disorders and substance abuse. Prevalence studies also do not always explain causality. Personality disorders can be manifestations of chronic drug abuse. It is not always clear which came first; the personality disorder or the addiction. Addiction in women is often the result of attempts to escape from posttraumatic symptoms. Patients who appear hypervigilant and paranoid may have a thought disorder, or they may be reflecting the reality of life on the streets. This point illustrates the main difficulties in understanding mental illness in the homeless: not knowing the exact roles of each comorbid disability and not knowing the exact precipitant that caused the patient to go from mental wellness to mental illness. It is important to document or attempt to establish a time line of psychological and physical insults. For example, evidence of major depression by clinical symptomatology before substance abuse is more likely to implicate a primary affective disorder than solely an affective response to substance abuse. This is helpful therapeutically and interventionally.

Homeless advocates know from experience that not all homeless people are mentally ill, but few studies have directly investigated the proportions without mental disorders. In Winkleby and White's survey of single adult men and women in shelters in California, 46% of the population reported no physical or addictive disorders or psychiatric hospitalizations before their first episode of homelessness.[9] The number of women was small, only 169, and women from family shelters were excluded. More of those persons who lacked a mental disorder when they became homeless were from an ethnic minority group, were younger, were married, and had lower educational attainment and a lower frequency of childhood abuse and foster care. However, patients in this group had also been homeless a shorter period of time and were more frequently immigrants. In the group that had established problems before becoming homeless, the most prevalent conditions were alcohol abuse and physical injury. Among all groups, the longer the period of homelessness, the greater the risk of mental or physical illness, substance abuse, or a combination of these.

MAJOR PSYCHIATRIC DIAGNOSES

Few psychiatric disorders occur in isolation in the homeless. Comorbidity is high. For example, in Breakey and colleagues' study of 203 homeless in Baltimore, 91% of the men and 80% of the women had axis I disorders (major mental illness, substance abuse, or anxiety or phobias).[19] Forty-seven percent of the men and 45% of the women had axis II (personality) disorders. The major axis I diagnoses were schizophrenia (12% of men, 17% of women) and depression (19% of men and 24% of women). Of the patients with dual diagnosis (major mental illness plus substance abuse), 31% were men and 32% were women.

The recognition of dual diagnosis and posttraumatic stress disorder in homeless women is helpful for treatment and intervention. Smith interviewed 300 women in shelters in St. Louis. The lifetime incidence of major depression (25% vs. 12%), antisocial personality (10% vs. 4%), alcohol abuse (17% vs. 10%), drug abuse (23% vs. 5%), and posttraumatic stress disorder (34 percent vs. 3%) was significantly higher in the homeless group than in women in low-income housing in the same area. Substance abuse was approximately twice as frequent in those with another axis I diagnosis. Antisocial personality disorder was associated with more than doubled rates of substance abuse for both alcohol and drugs.[61] Interestingly, the diagnosis of schizophrenia was similar in the homeless group and the low-income housed group (4% vs. 3%). Although 40% of the homeless had received mental health treatment at some point in their lives, the mental health issues were not resolved. Treatment of patients with dual diagnosis is difficult and challenging even when patients have homes and social supports. In the homeless population, resolution of complex and long-standing psychiatric dysfunction has to be continuous and long-term with ongoing support in the areas of most immediate concern to the patient: housing, food, and clothing.

Posttraumatic stress disorder has been described in homeless women who have suffered devastatingly traumatic events.[7] Patients describe frequent nightmares and flashbacks of the traumatic event that are so intrusive as to preclude normal function. Posttraumatic stress disorder also manifests as maladaptive behavior, sleep disorders, somatization, dissociative states, and chronic anxiety. Unlike the posttraumatic stress disorder experienced by combat veterans, that suffered by women in the homeless population cannot be explained by events that occurred under unusual circumstances of wartime conditions. The risk of a similarly traumatic event is always present, and they rarely feel completely safe.

North and Smith examined posttraumatic stress disorder separately in the women in St. Louis.[62] Seventy-four percent of the women with a clinical diagnosis of posttraumatic stress disorder developed symptoms before they became homeless. Earlier onset of posttraumatic stress disorder in women was associated with childhood sexual abuse. Symptoms of posttraumatic stress disorder can be masked by more obvious comorbid conditions such as behavioral or physical manifestations of substance abuse.

In the absence of a formal axis I or II diagnosis, the psychological stress itself of being homeless takes an enormous toll. Even for the woman who is not compromised by physical, mental, or substance abuse issues when she becomes homeless, other problems are devastating: the many losses—of one's home, one's self-image, one's self-confidence, the routine of a familiar neighborhood, one's children, parents, siblings, and society—are all appropriate reasons for unresolved grief. When these are burdened with complexities of welfare and social services, a gradual decline in health, exposure, poor sleep, lack of privacy, social isolation, crime, violence and the constant fear for one's safety, or demands of children who have their own coping issues and their own illnesses, some women develop maladaptive responses and emotional numbing.

The longer one is homeless, the greater the risk of psychological stress and breakdown. Women with families tend to get housed within months, whereas women alone can spend years on the streets. It is important to ask homeless women if they have children and, if so, where the children are. The woman who had her children with her when she became homeless and later lost them to the department of social services is different from the woman who lost her children to state custody as she became homeless and can often reacquire her children and housing.

MEDICAL CARE FOR THE HOMELESS

Homeless persons use hospital emergency departments, free clinics, and neighborhood health centers for health care and often only when a crisis intervenes. It is common for homeless persons to go to the first available place. Consequently, they have spotty records at dozens of institutions. Homeless persons requiring acute medical or psychiatric hospitalization are discharged back to the street and require hospitalization 15 to 20% longer than nonhomeless persons. Use of services in this manner is costly and preventable.

Homeless persons who are referred to the clinic or hospital are not always able to get adequate care. Physical barriers such as distance and lack of money for transportation often prevent initial care or follow-up. Clinics often have long waiting times or do not allow walk-ins. Appointments made months in advance are difficult to remember. Prescriptions made out for medicines that are either not covered by Medicaid or not affordable for the patient will not be filled. Outpatient mental health programs that have strict attendance criteria are a set-up for failure.

The medical evaluation of a homeless woman requires not only a diagnosis and treatment but also consideration of other issues (Table 78–1): what factors in her life contribute to this diagnosis? What does she need to get better? How did she make it here, and how is she going to get back? Can she pay for a prescription, and is the therapy prescribed in such a way as to maximize compliance? Does she need leg elevation or other intervention that requires staying inside for a few days? Does she have a bed and a meal for the day, or can you call and find her one? Is she wearing appropriate clothing, particularly shoes? Can she get to a shower if you give her Kwell? Is she immunized properly? Has she had a recent pelvic or breast examination? Does she have children who might be sick? What benefits does she have and what other supports? Is she alone, or does she have custody of her children? If she lost her children, why, and is she able to maintain contact?

NEW MODELS

In the last decade there has been a move to improve health care for homeless patients, by establishing links among the shelters, the homeless population, and the traditional clinics and hospitals. These links include physician, nurse practitioner, and physician assistant outreach teams that work in the shelter clinics, on the streets, or in mobile vans; case managers that coordinate the benefits and medical and social services; and hospital-based homeless clinics specifically designed to meet the needs of homeless persons. These programs vary in scope from city to city and are usually funded by grants. Some are more comprehensive than others. Although the concept has improved access to medical care for many homeless persons, it remains an emergency response to a dire social problem.

The Health Care for the Homeless program is an example of a successful effort. It began as nineteen demonstration programs funded by the Robert Wood Johnson Foundation and the Pew Memorial Trust, which have expanded through additional funding to 119 Health Care for the Homeless Programs in the country. Each is a nonprofit program funded by federal McKinney Act funds, public grants, and private donations.[63, 64] The goal of this model is to improve access to medical care for homeless persons by integrating the service delivery systems for homeless persons into existing traditional health care systems.

In some cities, shelters offer clinic services run by nurses. The nurses screen and assess the clients; review their medications; refer them to a hospital, clinic, or detoxification facility when necessary; and perform routine nursing care. Shelter clinics require medical backup for serious cases and therefore rely on hospital emergency departments. In addition, in some cities, teams of doctors, nurse practitioners, and physician assistants also work as outreach staff in shelter clinics and in the hospital clinics (private and public) of their parent institutions, thus allowing patients seen in the shelters to be referred to an existing hospital network. Similar teams also visit the family shelters and motels to provide physician, nursing, case manager, mental health, and nutritional services.

The Boston Health Care for the Homeless Program was one of the first 19 demonstration projects funded by the Robert Wood Johnson Foundation and the Pew Memorial Trust in 1985. The program has hospital-based teams in primary care and HIV, outreach teams, case managers who speak English and Spanish, social workers, family health teams, a nutritionist, substance abuse counselors, a prenatal and perinatal nurse practitioner, and a mental health team. Patients are seen in clinics on a scheduled and walk-in basis, thus allowing flexibility for patients who cannot always comply with schedules but who require urgent care. Sometimes patients are booked for weekly returns, which introduces structure into the relationship. It also allows the physician to maintain contact, provide support, counseling, and build trust, as well as to help with entitlements and housing. In this they are assisted by social workers who know the government programs and the shelter system. Boston Health Care for the Homeless staff assist their patients with detoxification unit referrals, educate house staff about substance abuse issues, and keep abreast of the available hospital-based and community-based substance abuse and mental health services. The hospital team makes rounds on all homeless inpatients on all services, providing a link to the shelter network and advice and education to hospital staff. The Boston Health Care for the Homeless Program also owns and runs a 50-bed respite facility where male and female homeless persons who require recuperation or short-term intense nursing care can remain at less cost than at a traditional hospital.

TABLE 78–1. Health Care Provider Contact Checklist for Homeless Women: A Tool for Primary Care

1. Name
2. Social Security Number
3. Where staying
4. Date of birth
5. Contact person at shelter (e.g., nurse, counselor)
6. Benefits (General Relief/Emergency Aid; SSI; SSDI; AFDC; WIC; Medicare; hospital free care; food stamps; public transportation pass; VA; other; none)
   A. Card numbers
7. Social history:
   (Why?)/Separated (Why?)/Single/Gay/Straight/Bisexual
   A. Married/divorced
   B. Parents/siblings/any contact?
8. Veteran?
   A. Branch of service/years served/combat?
   B. Honorable/general/dishonorable discharge?
   C. Any service-connected disabilities?
9. If immigrant, do you have a green card?
10. How did you become homeless?
    A. How long homeless?
11. Last Papanicolaou test? Ever abnormal? Menstrual history:
    How many pregnancies/live births:
    Where are your children?
    Ever had a mammogram? Why? Results:
    Birth control:
12. Have you ever had a sexually transmitted disease? Do you practice safe sex?
13. Last PPD/History of tuberculosis?
    Where?   When?
    Result: Controls?
    A. Last chest radiograph/result:
    B. Prior treatment for tuberculosis?
14. Alcohol history
    A. At what age did you start?
       Why?
    B. Complications? (seizure, pancreatitis, gastrointestinal bleed, blackouts, delirium tremens, trauma, job loss, relationship loss, etc)
    C. Ever been in detox? How many? How long? (e.g., 5, 7, 28 days, 6 wk). Halfway house? Names of detoxes:
    D. Longest sobriety? How did it feel? Reason for relapse?
15. Drug history
    A. At what age did you start?
       Why?
    B. Which drugs? (pot, cocaine, heroin, amphetamines, narcotic analgesics, anxiolytics, other)
       Route? (e.g., orally/snort/IV/smoke)
    C. Complications? (e.g., OD, skin infections, endocarditis, hepatitis A/B/or C, cardiac, muscle, nasal, HIV/AIDS)
    D. Ever been in detox?   Names:
    E. Ever been in a methadone program?
    F. Ever been HIV tested?   Where?
       When?   Result:
16. Psychological history:
    A. Ever been treated for depression, nervous breakdown, anxiety, voices (AH), wanting to kill yourself (SI) or someone else (HI)? Any symptoms (describe) before you became homeless?
    B. Names/dates of psychiatric hospitalizations, counselors/therapists
    C. Is there anyone you can count on for emotional support?
    D. Have you ever been physically or sexually hurt? By someone you loved? Where you able to get any help? Do you worry about it happening again? Do you have dreams and thoughts about it? Do you know how to get help if it happens again?
17. What do you want most from me?

SSI, Supplementary Security Income; SSDI, Social Security Disability Insurance; AFDC, Aid to Families with Dependent Children; WIC, Women, Infants, and Children; PPD, purified protein derivative; IV, intravenous; OD, overdose; HIV, human immunodeficiency virus; AIDS, acquired immunodeficiency syndrome; AH, auditory hallucinations; SI, suicidal ideation; HI, homicidal ideation.

SUMMARY

Homelessness in America is a huge problem. A growing number of women have fallen through the social safety net. Efforts to understand the issues that affect homeless women and to find creative solutions to their medical problems are necessary. Unlike other disciplines of medicine, health care for homeless persons cannot be done alone. Physicians who care for homeless persons must work with the network of professionals who exist in the homeless person's world. There is no single "homeless expert" but rather a multidisciplinary team that together provides comprehensive care for homeless patients.

REFERENCES

1. National Coalition for the Homeless Fact Sheets. The Problem of Homelessness, Causes and Trends; Women and Homelessness; How Many People Are Homeless in the US-And Recent Increases in Homelessness. Homeless Information Exchange (HIE), a project of the National Coalition for the Homeless. Washington, DC, 1993.
2. Tull J. Homelessness: An overview. N Engl J Public Policy 1992; 8(1):25.
3. Bassuk EL. Social and economic hardships of homeless and other poor women. Am J Orthopsychiatry 1993; 63(3):340.
4. Mulroy A. The housing affordability slide in action. How mothers slip into homelessness. N Engl J Public Policy 1992; 8(1):203.
5. Surber RW, Dwyer E, Ryan KJ, et al. Medical and psychiatric needs of the homeless—A preliminary response. Social Work 1988; 33(2):116.
6. Fleischman S. Trauma and victimization. In: Wood D (ed). Delivering Health Care to Homeless Persons. New York: Springer, 1992, pp 133–140.
7. Browne A. Family violence and homelessness: The relevance of trauma histories in the lives of homeless women. Am J Orthopsychiatry 1993; 63(3):370.
8. Blankertz LE, Cnaan RA, Freedman E. Childhood risk factors in dually diagnosed homeless adults. Social Work 1993; 38(5):587.
9. Winkleby MA, White R. Homeless adults without apparent medical and psychiatric impairment: Onset of morbidity over time. Hosp Community Psychiatry 1992; 43(10): 1017.
10. Susser ES, Lin SP, Conover SA, Struening EL. Childhood antecedents of homelessness in psychiatric patients. Am J Psychiatry 1991; 148(8):1026.
11. Padgett DK, Struening EL. Victimization and traumatic injuries among the homeless: Associations with alcohol, drug, and mental problems. Am J Orthopsychiatry 1992; 62(4):525.
12. Wright JD, Knight JW, Weber-Burdin E, Lam J. Ailments and alcohol. Health status among drinking homeless. Alcohol Health Res World 1987; 11(3):22.
13. Leda C, Rosenheck R, Gallup P. Mental illness among female veterans. Hosp. Community Psychiatry 1992; 43(10):1026.
14. Johnson AK, Kreuger LW. Toward a better understanding of homeless women. Social Work 1989; 34:537.
15. Hodnicki D, Horner SD, Boyle S. Women's perspectives on homelessness. Public Health Nurs 1992; 9(4):257.
16. Calsyn RJ, Morse G. Homeless men and women: Commonalities and a service gender gap. Am J Community Psychiatry 1990; 18(4):597.
17. Maurin JT, Russell L, Memmott RJ. An exploration of gender differences among the homeless. Res Nurs Health 1989; 12:315.
18. Tiernan K. Homelessness. The politics of accommodation. N Engl J Public Policy 1992; 8(1):647.
19. Breakey WR, Fischer PJ, Kramer M, et al. Health and mental health problems of homeless men and women in Baltimore. JAMA 1989; 262(10):1352.
20. Brickner PW, et al. Homeless persons and health care. Ann Intern Med 1986; 104(3):405.
21. Gelberg L, Linn LS, Usatine RP, Smith MH. Health, homelessness, and poverty. A study of clinic users. Arch Intern Med 1990; 150:2325.
22. Vredevoe DL, Brecht M-L, Shuler P, Woo M. Risk factors for disease in a homeless population. Public Health Nurs 1992; 9(4):263.
23. Wiecha JL, Dwyer JT, Jacques PF, Rand WM. Nutritional and economic advantages for homeless families in shelters providing kitchen facilities and food. J Am Diet Assoc 1993; 93(7):777.
24. Bunston T, Breton M. The eating patterns and problems of homeless women. Women Health 1990; 16(1):43.
25. Avery R, O'Connell JJ. Human immunodeficiency virus and homeless persons. In: Wood D (ed). Delivering Health Care to Homeless Persons. New York: Springer Publishing, 1992, pp 114–132.
26. Gelberg L, Linn LS, Rosenberg DJ. Dental health of homeless adults. Spec Care Dentist 1988, 8(4):167.
27. McNally E, Wood J. Obstetrical care and family planning for homeless women. In: Wood D (ed). Delivering Health Care to Homeless Persons. New York: Springer Publishing, 1992, pp 181–195.
28. Weinreb L. Preventive medical care for homeless men and women. In: Wood D (ed). Delivering Health Care to Homeless Persons. New York: Springer Publishing, 1992, pp 61–75.
29. O'Connell JJ, Groth J (eds). The Manual of Common Communicable Diseases in Shelters. Boston: Boston Health Care for the Homeless Program, 1991.
30. Morgan R, Geffner EI, Kiernan E, Cowles S. Alcoholism and the homeless. In: Bricker PW, Brickner PW, Scharer LK, Conanan B, et al (eds): Health Care of Homeless People. New York: Springer Publishing, 1985, pp 131–150.
31. Lindenberg CS, Alexander EM, Gendrop SC, et al. A review of the literature on cocaine abuse in pregnancy. Nurs Res 1991; 40(2):69.
32. Zuckerman B, Frank DA, Hingson R, et al. Effects of maternal marijuana and cocaine use on fetal growth. N Engl J Med 1989; 320(12):762.
33. O'Connell JJ, Lebow J. AIDS and the homeless of Boston. N Engl J Public Policy 1992; 8(1):541.
34. Kutza EA, Keigher SM. The elderly "new homeless": An emerging population at risk. Soc Work 1991; 36(4):288.
35. Gelberg L, Linn LS, Mayer-Oakes SA. Differences in health status between older and younger homeless adults. J Am Geriatr Soc 1990; 38:1220.
36. Koegel P, Burnam MA. Traditional and nontraditional homeless alcoholics. Alcohol Health Res World 1987; 11(3):28.
37. Hausman B, Hammen C. Parenting in homeless families: The double crisis. Am J Orthopsychiatry 1993; 63(3):358.
38. Lockyer JR. Management of substance abuse in primary care setting. In: Wood D (ed): Delivering Health Care to Homeless Persons. New York: Springer Publishing, 1992, pp 92–113.

39. Warner EA. Cocaine abuse. Ann Intern Med 1993; 119(3):226.

40. Cherubin CE, Sapira JD. The medical complications of drug addiction and the medical assessment of the intravenous drug user: 25 years later. Ann Intern Med 1993; 119(10):1017.

41. Frezza M, di Padova C, Pozzato G, et al. High blood alcohol levels in women. The role of decreased gastric alcohol dehydrogenase activity and first-pass metabolism. N Engl J Med 1990; 322(2):95.

42. Harris M, Bachrach LL. Perspectives on homeless mentally ill women. Hosp Community Psychiatry 1990; 41(23):253.

43. Longnecker MP, Berlin JA, Orza MJ, Chalmers TC. A meta-analysis of alcohol consumption in relation to risk of breast cancer. JAMA 1988; 260(5):652.

44. Centers for Disease Control. Tuberculosis among homeless shelter residents. MMWR 1991; 40:869.

45. DeMaria A, Browne K, Berk SL, et al. An outbreak of type 1 pneumococcal pneumonia in a men's shelter. JAMA 1980; 244(13):1446.

46. Felice GA, Englander SJ, Jacobson JA, et al. Group A meningococcal disease in skid rows: Epidemiology and implications for control. Am J Public Health 1984; 74(3):253.

47. Gross TP, Rosenberg ML. Shelters for battered women and their children: An under-recognized source of communicable disease transmission. Am J Public Health 1987; 77(9):1198.

48. Frieden TR, Sterling T, Pablos-Mendez A, et al. The emergence of drug-resistant tuberculosis in New York City. N Engl J Med 1993; 328(8):521.

49. Small PM, Shafer RW, Hopewell PC, et al. Exogenous reinfection with multidrug-resistant *Mycobacterium* tuberculosis in patients with advanced HIV infection. N Engl J Med 1993; 328(16):1137.

50. O'Connell JJ. Nontuberculous respiratory infections among the homeless. Semin Respir Infect 1991; 6(4):247.

51. Usatine R. Skin diseases of the homeless. In: Wood D (ed). Delivering Health Care to Homeless Persons. New York: Springer Publishing, 1992, pp 141–159.

52. Moy JA, Sanchez MR. The cutaneous manifestations of violence and poverty. Arch Dermatol 1992; 128(6):829.

53. Jessurun J, Romo-Garcia J, Lopez-Denis O, Olvera-Rabiela JE. Crusted scabies in a patient with the acquired immunodeficiency syndrome. Virchows Arch A Pathol Anat Histopathol 1990; 416(5):461.

54. Schultz MW, Gomez M, Hansen RC, et al. Comparative study of 5% of permethrin cream and 1% lindane lotion for the treatment of scabies. Arch Dermatol 1990; 126:167.

55. McBride K, Mulcare RJ. Peripheral vascular disease in the homeless. In: Brickner PW, Scharer LK, Conanan B et al. (eds). Health Care of Homeless People. New York: Springer Publishing, 1985, pp 121–129.

56. Wrenn K. Foot problems in homeless persons. Ann Intern Med 1990; 113(8):567.

57. Wrenn K. Immersion foot. A problem of the homeless in the 1990s. Arch Intern Med 1991; 151:785.

58. Lockyer R. Hypothermia and exposure among homeless persons. In: Wood D (ed). Delivering Health Care to Homeless Persons. New York: Springer Publishing, 1992, pp 160–167.

59. Centers for Disease Control. Deaths among homeless persons—San Francisco, 1985–1990. MMWR 1991; 40:877.

60. Koegel P, Sherman D. Assessment and treatment of homeless mentally ill adults. In: Wood D (ed). Delivering Health Care to Homeless Persons. New York: Springer Publishing, 1992, pp 231–254.

61. Smith EM, North CS, Spitznagel EL. Alcohol, drugs, and psychiatric comorbidity among homeless women: An epidemiologic study. J Clin Psychiatry 1993; 54(3):82.

62. North CS, Smith EM. Posttraumatic stress disorder among homeless men and women. Hosp Community Psychiatry 1992; 43(10):1010.

63. Doblin BH, Gelberg L, Freeman HE. Patient care and professional staffing patterns in McKinney Act clinics providing primary care to the homeless. JAMA 1992; 267(5):698.

64. Jahiel I. Health and Health care of homeless people. In: Robertson MJ, Greenblatt M (eds). Homelessness—A National Perspective. New York: Plenum Press, 1992; pp 133–163.

BIBLIOGRAPHY

Bachrach LL. Chronic mentally ill women: Emergence and legitimation of program issues. Hosp Community Psychiatry 1985; 36(10):1063.

Bachrach L. Homeless women: A context for health planning. Milbank Q 1987; 65(3):371.

Brickner PW, Scharer LK, Conanan B, et al. (eds). Under the Safety Net. The Health and Social Welfare of the Homeless in the United States. New York: WW Norton, 1990.

Buckner JC, Bassuk EL, Zima BT. Mental health issues affecting homeless women: Implications for intervention. Am J Orthopsychiatry 1993; 63(3):385.

Chavkin W, Kristal A, Seabron C, Guigli PE. The reproductive experience of women living in hotels for the homeless in New York City. NY State J Med 1987; 87:10.

Christiano A, Susser I. Knowledge and perceptions of HIV infection among homeless pregnant women. J Nurse-Midwife 1989; 34(6):318.

Cousins A. Profile of homeless men and women using an urban shelter. J Emerg Nurs 1983; 9(3):133.

Fischer PJ. Victimization and homelessness—Cause and effect. N Engl J Public Policy; 8(1):229.

Fleischman S, Farnham T. Chronic disease in the homeless. In: Wood D (ed). Delivering Health Care to Homeless Persons. New York: Springer Publishing, 1992, pp 79–91.

Flynn K. The toll of deinstitutionalization. In: Brickner PW, Scharer LK, Conanan B et al. (eds). Health Care of Homeless People. New York: Springer Publishing, 1985; pp 189–203.

Harris RE, Wynder EL. Breast cancer and alcohol consumption. A study in weak associations. JAMA 1988; 259(19):2867.

Health Care for the Homeless Report to the Congress on the Utilization and Costs of Health Care Services Provided Under Section 340 of the Public Health Service Act—Calendar Year 1992.

Herman JL. Trauma and Recovery. New York: Basic Books, 1992.

Iseman MD. Treatment of multidrug-resistant tuberculosis. N Engl J Med 1993; 329(11):784.

Iseman M. Tuberculosis: An overview. In: Brickner PW, Scharer LK, Conanan B et al. (eds). Health Care of Homeless People. New York: Springer Publishing, 1985; pp 151–154.

Iseman MD, Cohn DL, Sbarbaro JA. Directly observed treatment of tuberculosis—We can't afford not to try it. N Engl J Med 1993; 328(8):576.

Kellermann SL, Halper RS, Hopkins M, Nayowith GB. Psychiatry and homelessness: Problems and programs. In: Brickner PW, Scharer LK, Conanan B, et al. (eds). Health Care of Homeless People. New York: Springer Publishing, 1985; pp 179–188.

Kline EN, Saperstein AB. Homeless women. The context of an urban shelter. Nurs Clin North Am 1992; 27(4):885.

Martin M. The homeless mentally ill and community-based care: Changing a mindset. Community Mental Health J 1990; 26(5):435.

Merves ES. Homeless women. Beyond the bag lady myth. In: Greenblatt M, Robertson MJ (eds). Homelessness. A National Perspective. New York: Plenum Press, 1992, pp 229–244.

Morse GA, Calsyn RJ. Mental health and other human service needs of homeless people. In: Greenblatt M, Robertson MJ (eds). Homelessness. A National perspective. New York: Plenum Press, 1992, pp 117–130.

Nyamathi A, Shuler P. Factors affecting prescribed medication compliance of the urban homeless adult. Nurse Pract 1989; 14(8):47.

Osher FC, Kofoed LL. Treatment of patients with psychiatric and psychoactive substance abuse disorders. Hosp Community Psychiatry 1989; 40(10):1025.

Padgett DK, Struening EL. Influence of substance abuse and mental disorders on emergency room use by homeless adults. Hosp Community Psychiatry 1991; 42(8):834.

Padgett D, Struening EL, Andrews H. Factors affecting the use of medical, mental health, alcohol, and drug treatment services by homeless adults. Med Care 1990; 28(9):805.

Panosian CB. Tuberculosis in the homeless. In: Wood D (ed). Delivering Health Care to Homeless Persons. New York: Springer Publishing, 1992; pp 168–178.

Prevention and control of tuberculosis among homeless persons. Recommendations of the Advisory Council for the Elimination of Tuberculosis. MMWR 1992; 41(RR-5):13.

Roob N, McCambridge R. Private-sector funders: Their role in homelessness projects. N Engl J Public Policy 1992; 8(1):623.

Schutt RK, Garrett GR. Homeless people with alcohol problems. In: Schutt RK, Garrett GR (eds). Responding to the Homeless. Policy and Practice. New York: Plenum Press, 1992; pp 97–138.

Schutt RK, Garrett GR. Homeless people with drug problems. In: Schutt RK, Garrett GR (eds). Responding to the Homeless. Policy and Practice. New York: Plenum Press, 1992; pp 139–162.

Schutt RK, Garrett GR. The homeless alcoholic. Past and present. In: Robertson MJ, Greenblatt M (eds). Homelessness. A National Perspective. New York: Plenum Press, 1992; pp 177–186.

Segal SP, Hines AM, Florian V. Early life experiences and residential stability: A ten-year perspective on sheltered care. Am J Orthopsychiatry 1992; 62(4):535.

Somers A. Domestic violence survivors. In: Robertson MJ, Greenblatt M (eds). Homelessness. A National Perspective. New York: Plenum Press, 1992; pp 265–272.

Tynes LL, Sautter FJ, McDermott BE, Winstead DK. Risk of HIV infection in the homeless and chronically mentally ill. South Med J 1993; 86(3):276.

Usatine RP, Gelberg L. Health care for the homeless: A family medicine perspective. Am Fam Physician 1994; 49(1):139–146.

Weinreb L, Buckner JC. Homeless families: Program responses and public policies. Am J Orthopsychiatry 1993; 63(3):400.

Index

Note: Page numbers in *italics* refer to illustrations; page numbers followed by t refer to tables.